European Manual of Medicine

Series Editors

W. Arnold
München, Germany

U. Ganzer
Düsseldorf, Germany

Presenting state-of-the-art procedures in all clinical medicine disciplines, the European Manual of Medicine book series aims to educate postgraduate students and residents in accordance with the U.E.M.S. charter on training medical specialists in the European Union. Each volume is a comprehensive reference devoted to a specific discipline, and the editors are internationally renowned specialists from different European Countries. The contents cover both diagnostic and therapeutic methods which are subdivided into essential procedures (those that are commonly employed in all European countries) and helpful procedures (which might be of further interest as well). The reader-friendly layout allows quick retrieval of information, and concise checklists and algorithms throughout each volume clearly present the pathway from patient complaint to diagnosis. This text book series is ideal for any practitioner in the European Union looking to gain a thorough understanding of the latest procedures in their field of interest. The European Union of Medical Specialists (U.E.M.S.) represents national associations of medical specialists in the European Union and its associated countries. Active at the European level since 1958, the UEMS promotes the free movement of European medical specialists while ensuring the highest quality of medical care for European citizens. More information can be found online at: http://www.uems.net

More information about this series at http://www.springer.com/series/4640

Antoinette am Zehnhoff-Dinnesen
Bożena Wiskirska-Woźnica
Katrin Neumann · Tadeus Nawka
Editors

Phoniatrics I

Fundamentals – Voice Disorders – Disorders of Language and Hearing Development

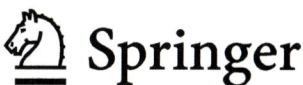
Springer

Editors
Antoinette am Zehnhoff-Dinnesen
Clinic of Phoniatrics
University Hospital Münster
Münster
Germany

Katrin Neumann
St. Elisabeth-Hospital, Abt. für
Phoniatrie und Pädaudiologie
Ruhr University Bochum
HNO-Universitätsklinik
Bochum
Germany

Bożena Wiskirska-Woźnica
Department of Phoniatrics and Audiology
University of Medical Sciences
Poznan
Poland

Tadeus Nawka
Klinik für Audiologie und Phoniatrie
Charité - Universitätsmedizin Berlin
Campus Charité Mitte
Berlin
Germany

ISSN 2626-7845   ISSN 2626-7853   (electronic)
European Manual of Medicine
ISBN 978-3-662-46779-4   ISBN 978-3-662-46780-0   (eBook)
https://doi.org/10.1007/978-3-662-46780-0

Foreword of the Series Editors

The European Manual of Medicine (EMM) offers medical graduates and clinicians the current state-of-the-art knowledge based on the training book and logbook of clinical disciplines accepted by the European Union of Medical Specialists (UEMS) in Brussels.

This Volume *Phoniatrics I* of the EMM series provides phoniatric and ENT trainees, as well as members of related disciplines, with a comprehensive textbook. To ensure the best quality of patient care, the book is supported by electronic material as a necessary basis for training standards in Phoniatrics. Volume I includes the parts "Voice Disorders" and "Disorders of Language and Hearing Development", following the training programme and logbook "Medical Speech, Voice and Language Pathology, and Hearing and Swallowing Disorders" of the UEMS Section Oto-Rhino-Laryngology. According to the phoniatric logbook, fundamentals concerning all mentioned communication disorders are presented in this volume.

"Speech and Speech Fluency Disorders", "Literacy Development Disorders", "Acquired Motor Speech and Language Disorders" and "Dysphagia" are parts of Volume II. Since Phoniatrics is an interdisciplinary specialty, both volumes may be of interest to members of related clinical disciplines, e.g. neurology and paediatrics.

In accordance with the principles of EMM, a standardised structure is used in addressing basics, special kinds of disorders, diagnosis/differential diagnosis, prevention and rehabilitation/prognosis. Case studies, colour photos, tables and supplementary audio and video samples, as well as detailed reference lists, provide a substantial amount of useful information to the reader.

Prof. Antoinette am Zehnhoff-Dinnesen, as editor-in-chief (Münster, Germany), and the editors Prof. Bożena Wiskirska-Woźnica (Poznan, Poland) and Prof. Katrin Neumann (Bochum, Germany) have recruited interdisciplinary experts from different European countries and other continents to fulfil the demands of the book series. Supplementary electronic material, including audio and video samples, was collected and provided by the editor Prof. Tadeus Nawka (Berlin, Germany).

Special thanks go to Springer, especially to Sandra Lesny and Claus-Dieter Bachem, for their valuable help and assistance.

The Series Editors are extremely grateful for the work of the editors and the immense effort the editor-in-chief, Prof. Antoinette am Zehnhoff-Dinnesen, has shown in creating this comprehensive textbook, which is both timely and of extraordinary quality.

München, Germany   Wolfgang Arnold
Düsseldorf, Germany   Uwe Ganzer
Summer 2018

Preface of the Editors

Volume I of the textbook *Phoniatrics* in the European Manual of Medicine series provides a basis of standards and good quality in patient care for improving training and education in Phoniatrics. It gives orientation in the current situation where the extent and intensity of phoniatric training vary in different countries. In addition to the complete textbook, separate e-chapters and e-books are offered to the reader. The book is written for phoniatric trainees, ENT trainees and specialised clinicians, but—because of the interdisciplinarity of Phoniatrics—it may also be interesting for medical students, other physicians with a special interest in Phoniatrics and members of related disciplines.

In order to improve the understanding of the field, *Phoniatrics I* offers a large number of colour photos, figures, tables and case studies, supplemented by more than 150 audio and video samples. To follow the consensual aims of the book series, most of the articles are written by more than one author, coming from different countries. A total of 162 authors and co-authors provided contributions for this volume, representing 23 countries from five continents and 36 disciplines. In addition, singers and musicians participated in preparing *Phoniatrics I*, which comprises 181 contributions. All topics concerning Fundamentals, Voice Disorders and Disorders of Language and Hearing Development have been prepared following the training programme and logbook "Medical Speech, Voice and Language Pathology, and Hearing and Swallowing Disorders" within the Section Oto-Rhino-Laryngology of the European Union of Medical Specialists (UEMS). The latter were elaborated by members of the Union of the European Phoniatricians (UEP) and provide a basis of the Courses organised by the European Academy of Phoniatrics (EAP).

We thank all authors and co-authors who invested their time and effort, precious contributions and support in this project.

We thank the following trainees and colleagues, who helped us as test readers, for their valuable hints: Katarina Smatanova, Czech Republic; Mohamed Gad-el-Hak, Egypt; Miia Ruuskanen, Finland; Docent Dirk Deuster, Dr. Seo-Rin Ko, Dr. Sabrina Regele, Dr. Ken Roßlau and Dr. Amélie Tillmanns, Germany; Rosa Mora, Spain; and Docent Erhan Demirhan and Muhittin Demir, Turkey.

Special thanks go to the external lectors who, in addition to the editors, provided in-depth research and analysis that significantly helped to achieve a high standard of knowledge transfer by their particular competence, proficiency and expertise: Prof. Philippe Dejonckere, Belgium; the late Prof. Manfred Gross, Germany, Prof. Jürgen Wendler, Germany; Dr. Jochen Rosenfeld, Switzerland; and Ross Parfitt and John Rubin, the United Kingdom.

The editors are much obliged and deeply grateful to the editors of the manual series, Prof. Wolfgang Arnold, Munich, and Prof. Uwe Ganzer, Düsseldorf, who initiated and decisively supported this important project.

Our special thanks go to Springer Company, especially Mrs. Sandra Lesny, Mr. Claus-Dieter Bachem, Wilma McHugh, Daniela Heller and Ms. Shanjini Rajasekaran for their substantial assistance and valuable advice.

The editors are deeply indebted to Dr. Trevor Cooper, lector for English language, for his excellent work and continued invaluable support as experienced scientist.

We also thank Nicole Neptun for her untiring contributions, especially to the layout and the reference lists; Ross Parfitt for his diligent work, especially on the refinement of the figures and tables in this book; and Peter Matulat for his valuable support and advice in technical and IT matters.

We hope that the book, as well as its e-version and the supplementary electronic material, will provide a comprehensive training tool for everybody who is interested in the field of communication disorders.

Münster, Germany	Antoinette am Zehnhoff-Dinnesen
Poznan, Poland	Bożena Wiskirska-Woźnica
Bochum, Germany	Katrin Neumann
Berlin, Germany	Tadeus Nawka
Summer 2018	

Contents

3   Basics of Related Medical Disciplines   155
Hanno J. Bolz, Tiemo Grimm, Gereon Heuft,
Christian Postert, Georg Romer, Eva Seemanova,
Esther Strittmatter, Dagmar Weise, and Klaus Zerres

Part II   Voice Disorders Including Rehabilitation of Tumour Patients

Sevtap Akbulut, Antoinette am Zehnhoff-Dinnesen,
Felix de Jong, Matthias Echternach, Ulrich Eysholdt,
Michael Fuchs, Tamás Hacki, Krzysztof Izdebski,
Annerose Keilmann, Peter Kummer, Sanila Mahmood,
Willy Mattheus, Dirk Mürbe, Tadeus Nawka, Haldun Oguz,
Ekaterina Osipenko, Friedemann Pabst, Mette Pedersen,
Rainer Schönweiler, Amélie Elisabeth Tillmanns,
and Erkki Vilkman

5 **Special Kinds and Clinical Manifestation of Voice Disorders**

Antoinette am Zehnhoff-Dinnesen, Sevtap Akbulut,
Eugenia Chávez Calderón, Muhittin Demir, Dirk Deuster,
Michael Fuchs, Ahmed Geneid, Thomas Murry,
Tadeus Nawka, Christiane Neuschaefer-Rube,
Ewa Niebudek-Bogusz, Andrzej Obrębowski, Haldun Oguz,
Arno Olthoff, Anders Overgård Jønsson, Mette Pedersen,
Bernhard Richter, John Rubin, Berit Schneider-Stickler,
Kevin Shields, Mariola Śliwińska-Kowalska,
Bożena Wiskirska-Woźnica, Virginie Woisard,
and Waldemar Wojnowski

6 Diagnosis and Differential Diagnosis of Voice Disorders...... 349

Wolfgang Angerstein, Giovanna Baracca, Philippe
Dejonckere, Matthias Echternach, Ulrich Eysholdt,
Franco Fussi, Ahmed Geneid, Tamás Hacki,
Katarzyna Karmelita-Katulska, Renate Haubrich,
František Šram, Jan G. Švec, Jitka Vydrová,
and Bożena Wiskirska-Woźnica

Part III   Developmental Disorders of Speech and Language

Antoinette am Zehnhoff-Dinnesen,
Doris-Maria Denk-Linnert, Mona Hegazi,
Annerose Keilmann, Christiane Kiese-Himmel,
Katrin Neumann, Sabrina Regele, Rainer Schönweiler,
and Eva Seemanova

Part IV   Disorders of Hearing Development

14 Basics of Disorders of Hearing Development 751

Antoinette am Zehnhoff-Dinnesen, Wendy Albuquerque,
Hanno J. Bolz, Steffi Johanna Brockmeier, Thorsten Langer,
Radha Narayan, Ross Parfitt, Simona Poisson-Markova,
Ewa Raglan, Sabrina Regele, Rainer Schönweiler,
Pavel Seeman, Eva Seemanova, Amélie Tillmanns,
and Oliver Zolk

16 Diagnosis and Differential Diagnosis of Disorders of Hearing Development

Ahmet Atas, Songul Aksoy, Antoinette am Zehnhoff-Dinnesen,
Doris-Eva Bamiou, Sylva Bartel-Friedrich, Claire Benton,
Hanno J. Bolz, Nicole G. Campbell, Frans Coninx,
Martine de Smit, Jakub Dršata, Mona Hegazi,
Armagan Incesulu, Kristin Kerkhofs, Arne Knief,
Sabrina Kösling, Jill Massey, Peter Matulat, David R. Moore,
Dirk Mürbe, Katrin Neumann, Haldun Oguz,
Levent N. Ozluoglu, Waheeda Pagarkar, Ross Parfitt,
Simona Poisson-Markova, Ewa Raglan, Charlotte Rogers,
Mustafa Asim Safak, Pavel Seeman, Eva Seemanova,
Tony Sirimanna, Piotr Swidzinski, Monika Tigges,
and Thomas Wiesner

18 Rehabilitation and Prognosis of Disorders of Hearing Development

Songul Aksoy, Antoinette am Zehnhoff-Dinnesen,
Ahmet Atas, Doris-Eva Bamiou, Sylva Bartel-Friedrich,
Claire Benton, Steffi Johanna Brockmeier,
Nicole G. Campbell, Gwen Carr, Marco Caversaccio,
Hatice Celik, Jakub Dršata, Kate Hanvey, Mona Hegazi,
Reinhild Hofmann (born Glanemann), Malte Kob,
Martin Kompis, Peter Matulat, Wendy McCracken,
David R. Moore, Dirk Mürbe, Haldun Oguz,
Levent N. Ozluoglu, Kayhan Öztürk, Ross Parfitt,
Stefan Plontke, Ute Pröschel, Karen Reichmuth,
Debbie Rix, Charlotte Rogers, Mustafa Asim Safak,
Tony Sirimanna, Konstance Tzifa, Christoph von Ilberg,
Thomas Wiesner, and Katherine Wilson

Contributors

Tahany AbdelKarim Elsayed Speech-Language Pathology and Psychology, Salmiya, Kuwait

Sevtap Akbulut Department of Otolaryngology, Yeditepe University, Istanbul, Turkey

Songul Aksoy Department of Audiology, Hacettepe University, Sıhhiye-Ankara, Turkey

Wendy Albuquerque Department of ENT and Audiovestibular Medicine, St Georges Healthcare NHS Trust, London, UK

Antoinette am Zehnhoff-Dinnesen Clinic of Phoniatrics and Pedaudiology, University Hospital Münster, Münster, Germany

Wolfgang Angerstein Phoniatrie und Pädaudiologie, Univ.-Klinikum Düsseldorf, Düsseldorf, Germany

Ojan Assadian Landesklinikum Neunkirchen, Neunkirchen, Austria

Ahmet Atas Department of Audiology, Faculty of Health Science, Istanbul University Cerrahpasa, İstanbul, Turkey
Department of ENT—Audiology and Speech Pathology, Faculty of Medicine, Istanbul University Cerrahpasa, İstanbul, Turkey

Doris-Eva Bamiou National Hospital for Neurology and Neurosurgery, London, UK

Giovanna Baracca ENT Department, AO Niguarda Cà Granda, Milan, Italy

Sylva Bartel-Friedrich Department of Otorhinolaryngology—Head and Neck Surgery, University Hospital Martin Luther University Halle-Wittenberg, Halle (Saale), Germany

Lisa Bartha-Doering Department of Pediatrics and Adolescent Medicine, Medical University of Vienna, Vienna, Austria

Ulrike Becker-Redding Praxis für Logopädie, Bochum, Germany

Claire Benton Nottingham Audiology Services, Ropewalk House, Nottingham, UK

Jan Betka Department of Otorhinolaryngology, Head and Neck Surgery, Charles University in Prague and University Hospital Motol, Prague, Czech Republic

Maria Bielsa Corrochano Clinica Foniatria Y. Logopedia Bielsa, Talavera de la Reina, Spain

Peter Birkholz Institute of Acoustics and Speech Communication, Technische Universität Dresden (TU Dresden), Dresden, Germany

Hanno J. Bolz Senckenberg Centre for Human Genetics, Frankfurt am Main, Germany

Steffi Johanna Brockmeier ENT Clinic, Audiology, Phoniatrics, Neuro-Otology, Kantonsspital Aarau AG, Aarau, Switzerland

Nicole G. Campbell Auditory Implant Service, University of Southampton, Southampton, UK

Gwen Carr UCL Ear Institute, University College London, London, UK

Cori Casanova Voice and Communication, Universitat Ramon Llull, Barcelona, Spain

Marco Caversaccio Universitätsklinik für Hals-, Nasen- und Ohrenkrankheiten (HNO), Kopf- und Halschirurgie, Inselspital, Bern, Switzerland

Hatice Celik Department of Otorhinolaryngology, Ankara Training and Research Hospital, Ankara, Turkey

Eugenia Chávez Calderón Centro de Foniatría y Audiología, Mexico City, Mexico

Viktor Chrobok Department of Otorhinolaryngology and Head and Neck Surgery, University Hospital Hradec Kralove, Hradec Kralove, Czech Republic

Frans Coninx Institut für Audiopädagogik, University of Cologne, Solingen-Ohligs, Germany

Hanna Czerniejewska-Wolska Department of Phoniatrics and Audiology, Poznan University of the Medical Sciences Poland, Poznan, Poland

Karina Dancza Singapore Institute of Technology, Health and Social Sciences Cluster, Singapore, Singapore

Felix de Jong Research Group ExpORL, University Hospitals KU Leuven, Leuven, Belgium

Martine de Smit Artevelde University College, Ghent, Belgium

Wivine Decoster Research Group ExpORL, KU Leuven, Leuven, Belgium

Philippe Dejonckere Federal Agency for Occupational Risks, Brussels, Belgium

Muhittin Demir Section of Phoniatrics and Audiology, ENT Clinic, University Hospital Essen, Essen, Germany

Ilter Denizoglu Medical Park Hospital Imbatli Mahallesi, Izmir, Turkey
Otolaryngology Department, Faculty of Medicine, Izmir University, Izmir, Turkey

Doris-Maria Denk-Linnert Division of Phoniatrics-Logopedics, Department of Otorhinolaryngology, Medical University of Vienna, Wien, Austria

Dirk Deuster Clinic of Phoniatrics and Pedaudiology, University Hospital Münster, Münster, Germany

Rolf Dierichs Former Institute of Anatomy, University Clinic of Münster, Münster, Germany

Christian Dobel Medical Faculty, Department of Otorhinolaryngology, Friedrich-Schiller-University, Jena, Germany

Jakub Dršata Department of Otorhinolaryngology and Head and Neck Surgery, University Hospital Hradec Kralove, Hradec Kralove, Czech Republic

Matthias Echternach Department of Otorhinolaryngology, Division of Phoniatrics and Pediatric Audiology, Munich University Hospital (LMU), Campus Großhadern, Munich, Germany

Andrea Joe Embacher Clinic of Phoniatrics and Pedaudiology, University Hospital Münster, Münster, Germany

Ulrich Eysholdt Department of Medical Physics and Acoustics/Medical Physics and Cluster of Excellence Hearing4all, Carl von Ossietzky-Universität Oldenburg, Oldenburg, Germany

Michael Fuchs Section of Phoniatrics and Audiology, University of Leipzig, Leipzig, Germany

Franco Fussi AudioPhoniatric Centre, Azienda USL Romagna, Ravenna, Italy

Ahmed Geneid Department of Otolaryngology and Phoniatrics – Head and Neck Surgery, Helsinki University Central Hospital, Helsinki, Finland

Tiemo Grimm Department of Human Genetics, Biocenter, University of Würzburg, Würzburg, Germany

Manfred Gross Department of Audiology and Phoniatrics, Campus Virchow-Klinikum, Berlin, Germany

Tamás Hacki Department of Otorhinolaryngology, Head and Neck Surgery, Semmelweis University Budapest, Budapest, Hungary

Uta Hanning Department of Neuroradiological Diagnostics and Intervention, University Hospital Hamburg, Hamburg, Germany

Kate Hanvey Aston University Day Hospital, Birmingham Children's Hospital, The Midlands Hearing Implant Programme, Birmingham, UK

Renate Haubrich Evangelisches Klinikum Niederrhein Duisburg-Nord, Zentrale Abteilung für Diagnostische und Interventionelle Radiologie, Duisburg, Germany

Mona Hegazi ENT Department, Ain Shams University, Cairo, Egypt

Gereon Heuft Department of Psychosomatics and Psychotherapy, University Clinic Münster, Münster, Germany

Reinhild Hofmann (born Glanemann) ICBF Germany International Talent Centre, Westphalian Wilhelms-University Münster, Münster, Germany

Armagan Incesulu Faculty of Medicine, Department of Otolaryngology-Head and Neck Surgery, Eskisehir Osmangazi University, Eskişehir, Turkey

Krzysztof Izdebski Department of Otolaryngology, Head and Neck Surgery, David Geffen School of Medicine, UCLA, Los Angeles, CA, USA

Katarzyna Karmelita-Katulska Department of Neuroradiology, University of Medical Sciences in Poznan, Poznan, Poland

Michèle Kaufmann-Meyer Tüscherz-Alfermée, Switzerland

Annerose Keilmann Voice Care Center Bad Rappenau, Bad Rappenau, Germany

Kristin Kerkhofs Rehabilitationcentre De Poolster, Brussels, Belgium

Christiane Kiese-Himmel Phoniatrics/Pediatric Audiological Psychology, University Medical Center Göttingen, Göttingen, Germany

Mehmet Akif Kilic Department of Otolaryngology, Faculty of Medicine, Medeniyet University, Istanbul, Turkey

Arne Knief Clinic of Phoniatrics and Pedaudiology, University Hospital Münster, Münster, Germany

Malte Kob Detmold University of Music, Erich Thienhaus Institute, Music Acoustics and Theory of Music Transmission, Detmold, Germany

Claudia Koch-Günnewig Physiotherapy Practice for Children, Münster, Germany

Martin Kompis Universitätsklinik für Hals-, Nasen- und Ohrenkrankheiten, Inselspital, Bern, Switzerland

Sabrina Kösling Department of Diagnostic Radiology, Martin-Luther University Halle-Wittenberg, Halle (Saale), Germany

Nasser Kotby Otolaryngology and Phoniatrics, Ain Shams University Cairo, Cairo, Egypt

Peter Kummer Phoniatrics and Pediatric Audiology, University Hospital Regensburg, Regensburg, Germany

Thorsten Langer Department of Pediatric Oncology and Hematology, University Hospital Schleswig-Holstein, Campus Lübeck, Lübeck, Germany

Anders Löfqvist Department of Logopedics, Phoniatrics and Audiology, University Hospital Lund, Lund, Sweden

Ben A.M. Maassen Center for Language and Cognition Groningen and Department of Neurosciences/BCN, University Medical Center Groningen, University of Groningen, Groningen, The Netherlands

Barbara Maciejewska Department of Phoniatrics and Audiology, Poznan University of Medical Sciences, Poznan, Poland

Sanila Mahmood Voice Unit, The Medical Center, Copenhagen, Denmark

Jean-Paul Marie Otolaryngology, Head and Neck Surgery Department, Centre Hospitalier Universitaire, Rouen, France

Sławomir Marszałek Department of Head and Neck Surgery, Poznan University of Medical Sciences, Poznan, Poland

Ana Martínez Arellano Clinica Foniatria Y Logopedia, Pamplona, Spain

Jill Massey Evelina London Children's Hospital, Guys and St Thomas' NHS Foundation Trust, London, UK

Willy Mattheus Division of Phoniatrics and Audiology and Saxonian Cochlear Implant Center, University Hospital Carl Gustav Carus, Technische Universität Dresden, Dresden, Germany

Peter Matulat Clinic of Phoniatrics and Pedaudiology, University Hospital Münster, Münster, Germany

Wendy McCracken School of Psychological Sciences, University of Manchester, Manchester, UK

David R. Moore Communication Sciences Research Center, Cincinnati Children's Hospital, Cincinnati, OH, USA

Andreas Müller Department Otorhinolaryngology/Plastic Surgery, SRH Wald-Klinikum Gera gGmbH, Teaching Hospital of the Friedrich-Schiller-University Jena, Gera, Germany

Dirk Mürbe Department of Audiology and Phoniatrics, Charité—University Medicine Berlin, Berlin, Germany

Thomas Murry Department of Otolaryngology-Head and Neck Surgery, Loma Linda Voice and Swallowing Center, Loma Linda Medical University, Loma Linda, CA, USA

Radha Narayan The Whittington Hospital, London, UK

Tadeus Nawka Department of Audiology and Phoniatrics, Charité—University Medicine Berlin, Berlin, Germany

Katrin Neumann Department of Phoniatrics and Pediatric Audiology, ENT Clinic, St. Elisabeth Hospital, University of Bochum, Bochum, Germany

Christiane Neuschaefer-Rube Clinic of Phoniatrics, Pedaudiology and Communication Disorders, School of Medicine of the RWTH Aachen University, University Hospital Aachen, Aachen, Germany

Ewa Niebudek-Bogusz Department of Audiology and Phoniatrics, Nofer Institute of Occupational Medicine, Łódź, Poland

Thomas Niederstadt Department of Clinical Radiology, University Hospital Münster, Münster, Germany

Andrzej Obrębowski Clinic of Phoniatrics and Audiology, Poznan University of Medical Sciences, Poznan, Poland

Haldun Oguz Fonomer, Ankara, Turkey

Arno Olthoff Department of Otorhinolaryngology, Phoniatrics and Pedaudiology, University Medical Center Göttingen, Göttingen, Germany

Ekaterina Osipenko Phoniatrics Department, Federal Research Clinical Centre of Otorhinolaryngology, Moscow, Russia

Anders Overgård Jønsson University of Copenhagen, Copenhagen, Denmark

Levent N. Ozluoglu Department of Otolaryngology, Baskent University, Etimesgut/Ankara, Turkey

Kayhan Öztürk Department of Otolaryngology, Selcuk University, School of Medicine, Yeni Istanbul, Caddesi, Konya, Turkey

Friedemann Pabst ENT Department, Municipal Hospital Dresden, Dresden, Germany

Waheeda Pagarkar Royal National Throat, Nose & Ear Hospital, Nuffield Hearing and Speech Centre, London, UK

Christo Pantev Institute for Biomagnetismus and Biosignalanalysis, University of Münster, University Hospital Münster, Münster, Germany

Ross Parfitt Clinic of Phoniatrics and Pedaudiology, University Hospital Münster, Münster, Germany

Mette Pedersen Voice Unit, The Medical Center, Copenhagen, Denmark

Stefan Plontke Department of Otorhinolaryngology—Head and Neck Surgery, University Hospital Martin Luther University Halle-Wittenberg, Halle (Saale), Germany

Simona Poisson-Markova Department of Child Neurology, 2nd Medical School of Charles University Prague, Prague, Czech Republic

Christian Postert Department of Applied Health Sciences, University of Applied Health Science, Bochum, Germany

Ute Pröschel Institut für Phoniatrie und Pädaudiologie, Vestische Kinder- und Jugendklinik Datteln, Datteln, Germany

Antoni Pruszewicz Department of Phoniatrics and Audiology, Poznań University of the Medical Sciences, Poznan, Poland

Ewa Raglan Department of Audiology and Audiovestibular Medicine, Great Ormond Street Hospital for Children NHS Foundation Trust, London, UK

Sabrina Regele Clinic of Phoniatrics and Pedaudiology, University Hospital Münster, Münster, Germany

Karen Reichmuth Clinic of Phoniatrics and Pedaudiology, University Hospital Münster, Münster, Germany

Barbora Řepova Department of Otorhinolaryngology, Head and Neck Surgery, Charles University in Prague and University Hospital Motol, Prague, Czech Republic

Bernhard Richter Freiburger Institut für Musikermedizin, Hochschule für Musik und Universitätsklinikum Freiburg, Freiburg, Germany

Debbie Rix Wandsworth Hearing Support Service, Linden Lodge School, London, UK

Ken Roßlau Praxis, Hannover, Germany

Charlotte Rogers Leicester School of Allied Health Sciences, De Montfort University, Hawthorn Building, Leicester, UK

Georg Romer Klinik für Kinder- und Jugendpsychiatrie, -psychosomatik und –psychotherapie, Univeritätsklinikum Münster, Münster, Germany

Jan Romportl Department of Man-Machine Interaction, New Technologies Research Centre, University of West Bohemia, Pilsen, Czech Republic

Jochen Rosenfeld Abteilung Gehör-, Sprach- u. Stimmheilkunde, Kantonsspital St.Gallen, St. Gallen, Switzerland

John Rubin University College London, London, UK

Mustafa Asim Safak Department of Otolaryngology, Near East University, Lefkosa, Turkey

Antonio Schindler Department of Surgical Sciences, University of Turin, Turin, Italy

Oskar Schindler Department of Surgical Sciences, University of Turin, Turin, Italy

Josef Schlömicher-Thier International Voice Center Austria (IVCA), Neumarkt am Wallersee, Austria

Claus-Michael Schmidt Gemeinschaftspraxis im Vitalcenter, Münster, Germany

Berit Schneider-Stickler Division of Phoniatrics-Logopedics, Department of Otorhinolaryngology, Medical University Vienna, Wien, Austria

Rainer Schönweiler Department of Phoniatrics and Pediatric Audiology, University Clinic of Schleswig-Holstein, Campus Lübeck, Lübeck, Germany

Harm K. Schutte Voice Research Lab. Groningen, Groningen, The Netherlands

Pavel Seeman Department of Child Neurology, 2nd Medical School of Charles University Prague, Prague, Czech Republic

Eva Seemanova Department of Child Neurology, 2nd Medical School of Charles University Prague, Prague, Czech Republic

Wolfram Seidner Former Department for Phoniatrics and Pediatric Audiology, University ENT Clinic Charité (Campus Mitte), Berlin, Germany

Kevin Shields National Hospital for Neurology and Neurosurgery, London, UK

Tony Sirimanna Audiological Medicine and Cochlear Implant Department, Great Ormond Street Hospital, London, UK

Mariola Śliwińska-Kowalska Department of Audiology and Phoniatrics, Nofer Institute of Occupational Medicine, Łódź, Poland

Ad Snik Audiologisch Centrum, KNO Klinik, Radboud University Medical Center, Nijmegen, The Netherlands

Claudia Spahn Freiburger Institut für Musikermedizin, Hochschule für Musik und Universitätsklinikum Freiburg, Freiburg, Germany

František Šram Voice and Hearing Centre Prague, Prague 2, Czech Republic

Kurt Stephan Department for Hearing, Speech and Voice Disorders, Medical University of Innsbruck, Insbruck, Austria

Esther Strittmatter Health Care Centre Walstedde Day Hospital, Drensteinfurt, Germany

Jan G. Švec Department of Biophysics, Palacky University, Olomouc, Czech Republic

Piotr Swidzinski Department of Phoniatrics and Audiology, Poznan University of Medical Sciences, Poznan, Poland

Monika Tigges Städt. Klinikum Karlsruhe GmbH, ENT Clinic, Phoniatrics and Pedaudiology, Karlsruhe, Germany

Amélie Elisabeth Tillmanns Clinic of Phoniatrics and Pedaudiology, University Hospital Münster, Münster, Germany

Sharon Tuppeny Royal College of Occupational Therapists, London, UK

Konstance Tzifa Birmingham Children's Hospital, Birmingham, UK

Melanie Vauth Clinic of Phoniatrics and Pedaudiology, University Hospital Münster, Münster, Germany

Dorothe Veraguth Clinic of ENT, Head- and Neck-Surgery, University Hospital Zurich, Zurich, Switzerland

Erkki Vilkman Department of Otolaryngology and Phoniatrics – Head and Neck Surgery, Helsinki University Hospital, Helsinki, Finland

Adam P. Vogel Centre for Neuroscience of Speech, The University of Melbourne, Parkville, VIC, Australia

Christoph von Ilberg Meniere-Center-Frankfurt, Frankfurt am Main, Germany

Jitka Vydrová Voice and Hearing Centre Prague, Prague 2, Czech Republic

Matthias Weikert Clinic St. Hedwig, Barmherzige Brüder, Regensburg, Germany

Dagmar Weise Abteilung Neuropädiatrie, Universitätsmedizin Göttingen, Göttingen, Germany

Jürgen Wendler Berlin, Germany

Thomas Wiesner Department of Phoniatrics and Pediatric Audiology, Werner Otto Institut gGmbH, Hamburg, Germany

Katherine Wilson St Thomas' Hearing Implant Centre, St Thomas' Hospital, London, UK

Bożena Wiskirska-Woźnica Department of Phoniatrics and Audiology, Poznan University of Medical Sciences, Poznan, Poland

Virginie Woisard Voice and Deglutition Unit, ENT Department, Toulouse University Hospital, Toulouse, France

Waldemar Wojnowski Department of Phoniatrics and Audiology, Poznan University of Medical Sciences, Poznan, Poland

Klaus Zerres Institute of Human Genetics, University Clinic RWTH Aachen, Aachen, Germany

Oliver Zolk Institute of Pharmacology of Natural Products and Clinical Pharmacology, University Hospital Ulm, Ulm, Germany

Abbreviations

A(section)E	Auditory speech sounds evaluation
AAA	American Academy of Audiology
AABR	Automated auditory brainstem response
AAC	Augmentative and alternative communication
AAST	Adaptive auditory speech test
ABI	Auditory brainstem implant
ABR	Auditory brainstem response
AC	Alternating current
ACALOS	Adaptive categorical loudness scaling
ACCP	American College of Chest Physicians
ACE	Advanced combination encoder
aCGH	array comparative genomic hybridisation
ACIP	Advisory committee on immunization practices
AD	Auditory dyssynchrony
AD	Autosomal dominant
ADHD	Attention-deficit/hyperactivity disorder
ADI-R	Autism diagnostic interview-revised
ADL	Activities of daily living
ADNSHL	Autosomal dominant non-syndromic hearing loss
ADOS	Autism diagnostic observation schedule
ADOS	Autosomal dominant Opitz syndrome
ADR	Adverse drug reactions
AE	Aryepiglottic
AEP	Acoustic-evoked potentials
AEP	Auditory evoked potentials
AI	Articulation index
AIDS	Acquired immunodeficiency syndrome
ALS	Amyotrophic lateral sclerosis
AM	Accent method
AMC	Academisch Medisch Centrum
AMCD	Association for Multicultural Counseling and Development
aMEI	active middle ear implant
AMFR	Amplitude modulated frequency response
AN	Auditory neuropathy
ANCA	Anti-neutrophil cytoplasmic autoantibody
ANDD	Auditory neuropathy dyssynchrony disorders
ANSD	Auditory neuropathy spectrum disorder

APA	American Psychiatric Association
APA	Auditory perceptual assessment
APD	Auditory processing disorder
APM	Ambulatory phonation monitor
APPD	Auditory processing and perception disorder
AR	Autosomal recessive
ARNSHL	Autosomal recessive non-syndromic hearing loss
ART	Acoustic reflex threshold
AS	Angelman syndrome
AS	Auditory synaptopathy
ASB	Arylsulfatase B
ASD	Autism spectrum disorder
ASHA	American Speech-Language-Hearing Association
ASQ	Ages and stages questionnaires
ASR	Automatic speech recognition
ASSR	Auditory steady state response
AT-MSC	Adipose tissue-derived mesenchymal stem cells
ATNR	Asymmetrical tonic neck reflex
AVQI	Acoustic voice quality index
AVT	Auditory verbal therapy
AVWS	Auditive Verarbeitungs- und Wahrnehmungsstörung
BA	Brodmann's area
BAHA	Bone-anchored hearing aid
BBS	Bardet-Biedl syndrome
BC	Bone conduction
BCNC	Bony cochlear nerve canal
BERA	Brain-evoked response audiometry
bFGF	basic fibroblast growth factor
BFLA	Bilingual first language acquisition
BIAP	Bureau International d'Audiophonologie
BIT	Beginner's intelligibility test
BM-MSC	Bone marrow-derived mesenchymal stem cells
BNL	Background noise level
BOA	Behavioural observation audiometry
BOR	Branchio-otorenal syndrome
BPPV	Benign paroxysmal positional vertigo
BPS	Bilateral Perisylvian syndrome
BRAT	Behaviour readjustment therapy
BSA	British Society of Audiology
BSL RST	British sign language development: receptive skills test
BSL	British sign language
BTD	Biotinidase
BTE	Behind the ear
bVFP	Bilateral vocal fold palsy
cABR	ABR with complex sounds
CAG	Cytosine-adenine-guanine
CAMHS	Child and adolescent mental health service
C-ANCA	Cytoplasmic ANCA

CANS	Central auditory nervous system
CAP	Compound action potentials
CAPD	Central APD
CAPD	Central auditory processing disorders
CAPE-V	Consensus auditory-perceptual evaluation of voice
CAS	Childhood apraxia of speech
CASL	Comprehensive assessment of spoken language
CBCL	Child behavioural checklist
CB-CT	Cone-beam CT
CBGD	Corticobasal degeneration
cCMV	congenital CMV
CDD	Coupler-to-dial difference
CDG	Congenital disorder of glycosylation
CDI	Communicative development inventory
CELF	Clinical evaluation of language fundamentals
CELF-FS	CELF formulated sentences
CELF-WS	CELF word structure
CERA	Cerebral-evoked response audiometry
CERA	Cortical ERA
CHARGE	Coloboma, Heart defect, Atresia choanae, Retarded growth and development, Genital hypoplasia, and Ear anomalies/deafness
CHEP	Cricohyoidoepiglottopexy
CHILDES	Child language data exchange system
CHIP	Colorado home intervention program
CHL	Conductive hearing loss
CHP	Cricohyoidopexy
CHSWG	Children's Hearing Services Working Group
CI	Cochlear Implant
CIS	Common intelligibility scale
CIS	Continuous interleaved sampling
CLAN	Computerized language analysis-program
CM	Cochlear microphonics
CM	Congenital malformation
CMV	Cytomegalovirus
CN	Cochlear nerve
CND	Cochlear nerve deficiency
CNRep	Children's test of nonword repetition
COR	Conditioned orientation reflex audiometry
COT	College of Occupational Therapists
CP	Cerebral palsy
CP	Cricopharyngeal
CPA	Cerebellopontine angle
CPA	Conditioned play audiometry
CPCI-S	Conference proceedings citation index-science
CPM	Coloured progressive matrices
CPT	Continuous performance test
CQ	Contact quotient

CRIDE	Consortium for research into deaf education
CROS	Contralateral routing of signal
CRS	Congenital Rubella syndrome
CSDB	Colorado School for the Deaf and the Blind
CSF	Cerebral spinal fluid
CSF	Cerebrospinal fluid
CSID	Cepstral spectral index of dysphonia
CSVHI	Classical singing voice handicap index
CT	Computed tomography
CT	Cricothyroid
CTAF	Conotruncal anomaly face syndrome
CTCAE	Common terminology criteria for adverse events
CTOPP	Comprehensive test of phonological processing
CVC	Consonant-vowel-consonant
cVEMP	cervical VEMP
CW	Continuous wave
CWMT	Cogmed working memory training
DAD	Developmental articulatory dyspraxia
DAS	Developmental apraxia of speech
dB HL	decibel hearing level
dB SPL	decibel sound pressure level
DC	Direct current
DDK	Diadochokinetic
DDON	Deafness-dystonia-optic neuronopathy
DDSL	Developmental disorders of speech and language
DDSLC	DDSL associated with language-relevant Comorbidities
DDST	Denver developmental screening test
DEAP	Diagnostic evaluation of articulation and phonology
DEF-TK	Diagnostischer Elternfragebogen zur taktil-kinästhetischen Responsivität im frühen Kindesalter
DFNB1	Deafness type B1
DGfMM	German Association for Music Physiology and Musicians' Medicine
DGPP	German Society of Phoniatrics and Pedaudiology
DGS	German sign language
DIMAH	Diversity in medicine and health
DKG	Digital kymography
DPOAE	Distortion product OAE
DR	Dynamic range
DSD	Disorders of sexual development
DSI	Dysphonia severity index
DSL	Desired sensation level
DSM	Diagnostic and statistical manual of mental disorders
DTI	Diffusion tensor imaging
DVD	Developmental verbal dyspraxia
DVT	DoctorVox voice therapy
DWI	Diffusion-weighted imaging
EA	Estimated audiogram

EAC	External auditory canal
EACEA	Education, Audiovisual and Culture Executive Agency
EARS	Evaluation of auditory responses to speech
EAS	Electric-acoustic stimulation
EBD	Emotional or behavioural disorder
EBM	Evidence-based medicine
ECG	Electrocardiography
ECMO	Extra-corporal membrane oxygenation
ECochG	Electrocochleography
EE	Endoscopic-positive esophagitis
EECV	Equivalent ear canal volume
EEG	Electroencephalography
EGG	Electroglottography
EHDI	Early hearing detection and intervention
EHF	Extended high-frequency
EIA	Enzyme immunoassays
ELA	Environmental language abnormality
ELISA	Enzyme-linked immunosorbent assay
ELS	European Laryngological Society
EMA	Electromagnetic articulography
EMG	Electromyography
ENT	Ear nose and throat
EPG	Electropalatography
ERA	Evoked response audiometry
ERG	Electroretinography
ERP	Event-related responses
ESP	Estimated subglottal pressure
ET	Eustachian tube
ETPG	European Test Publisher Group
EVA	Enlarged vestibular aqueduct
EVT	Expressive vocabulary test
F0	Fundamental frequency
F1	First formant
FAS	Foetal alcohol syndrome
FASD	Foetal alcohol spectrum disorder
FDA	Food and Drug Administration
FDG	Fludeoxyglucose
FEES	Fibre-optic endoscopic examination of swallowing
FEIA	Fluorescence-enzyme-immunoassays
FEM	Finite element method
FFR	Frequency-following responses
FFT	Fast Fourier transform
FFW	Fast ForWord®
FHP	Forward head posture
FIM	Freiburg Institute for Musicians' Medicine
FLIP	Familienzentriertes Linzer Interventions Programm
FLOG	Flow glottography
FM	Female-to-male

FM	Frequency modulation
FMAER	Frequency-modulated auditory evoked responses
FMR1	Fragile X mental retardation 1
fMRI	functional MRI
FN	Facial nerve
FSHD	Facioscapulohumeral muscular dystrophy
FSP	Fine structure processing
FSP4	Fine structure processing on 4 channels
fT3	free tri-iodothyronine
fT4	free thyroxine
GABA	Gamma aminobutyric acid
GER	Gastroesophageal reflux
GERD	Gastroesophageal reflux disease
GFR	Glottal flow rate
GH	Geniohyoid
GH	Growth hormone
GJB2	Gap Junction Beta 2 protein, encoding connexin 26
GJB6	Gap Junction Beta 6 protein, encoding connexin 30
GNE	Glottal-to-noise excitation
HA	Hearing aid
HAAT	Highly-active antiretroviral therapy
HDR	Homology-directed repair
HDR	Hypoparathyroidism, sensorineural deafness and renal dysplasia
HEPA	High-efficiency particulate air
HGF	Hepatocyte growth factor
HHV	Human herpes virus
HI	Hearing impairment
HiRes120	High-Resolution fidelity—120 virtual channels
HIV	Human immune deficiency virus
HL	Hearing loss
HLA	Human leukocyte antigen
H-LAD	Heidelberger Lautdifferenzierungstest
HM	Hyomandibular
HME	Heat and moisture exchanger
HMM	Hidden Markov model
HNR	Harmonics-to-noise ratio
HOT	Hyperbaric oxygen treatment
HP	Hearing preservation
HPV	Human papilloma virus
HRQOL	Health-related quality of life
HRTF	Head-related transfer function
HSN	Hereditary sensory neuropathy
HSV	Herpes simplex virus
HSV	High-speed video
HT	Hyothyroid
IAC	Internal auditory canal
IAM	Internal auditory meatus

IASSID	International Association of Scientific Studies on Intellectual Disability
ICA	Internal carotid artery
ICD	International statistical classification of diseases and related health problems
ICF	International classification of functioning, disability and health
ICF-CY	Children and youth version of the ICF
ICF-CY	International classification on functioning, disability and health—child and youth version
ICS	Intelligibility in context scale
ICSOM	International Conference of Symphony and Opera Musicians
ICU	Intensive care unit
IEA	International Ergonomics Association
IFFM	International female fluctuating masker
IFOS	International Federation of Otorhinolaryngological Societies
IGV	Integrative genomics viewer
IHC	Inner hair cell
ILD	Inter-aural level difference
ILO	Inducible laryngeal obstruction
IPA	International Phonetic Association
IQ	Intelligence quotient
ISAAC	International Society for Augmentative and Alternative Communication
ITC	In the ear canal
ITD	Inter-aural time difference
ITE	In the ear
ITG	Inferior temporal gyrus
ITS	Intratympanic steroids
JC	John Cunningham viruses
JCIH	Joint Committee on Infant Hearing
JLNS	Jervell and Lange-Nielsen syndrome
K-ABC	Kaufman-assessment battery for children
KiSS	German Kindersprachscreening
KSS	Kearns-Sayre syndrome
LAEP	Late auditory evoked potential
LAR	Laryngeal adductor reflex
LCA	Linear component analysis
LDL	Loudness discomfort level
LDS	Language development survey
LED	Light-emitting diode
LEDS	Large endolymphatic duct and sac syndrome
LFS	Laryngeal framework surgery
LGOB	Loudness growth in 1/2-octave bands
LI	Language impairment
LIFG	Left inferior frontal gyrus

LKS	Landau-Kleffner syndrome
L_{min}	Phonation threshold
LNT	Lexical neighborhood test
LP	Lamina propria
LP	Laryngopharyngeal
LPL	Laryngoplasty
LPR	Laryngopharyngeal reflux
LSTG	Left superior temporal gyrus
LTAS	Long-time average spectra
LTASS	Long-term average speech spectrum
LVAS	Large vestibular aqueduct syndrome
LVPM	Levator veli palatini muscle
MAGIC®	Multiple-choice auditory graphic interactive check
MAIS	Meaningful auditory integration scale
MAOI	Monoamine oxidase inhibitor
MAP	Muscle action potential
MAPL	Minimal associated pathological lesion
MC	Most comfortable
MCDI	MacArthur communicative development inventories
M-CHAT-R	Modified checklist for autism in toddlers, revised
MCL	Maximum comfortable level
MD	Menière's disease
MDCT	Multi-detector CT
MDI	Mental development index
MDVP	Multi-dimensional voice program
ME	Middle ear
MEG	Magneto-encephalography
MELAS	Mitochondrial encephalopathy, lactic acidosis and stroke-like episodes
MERRF	Myoclonus epilepsy associated with ragged-red fibres
MF	Male-to-female
MFDR	Maximum flow declination rate
MIDD	Maternally-inherited diabetes and deafness
MLNT	Multisyllabic lexical neighborhood test
MLPA	Multiple ligation-dependent probe amplification
MLR	Middle latency response
MLST-C	Multimodal lexical sentence test for children
MLU	Mean length of utterances
MML	Minimum masking level
MND	Motor neuron disorders
MPO	Maximum power output
MPP	Muenster parental programme
MPPA	Medical problems of performing artists
MPS	Massively parallel sequencing
MPS1 H	Mucopolysaccharidosis Hurler disease
MPS1H	Mucopolysaccharidosis type 1H
MPS1S	Mucopolysaccharidosis type 1S
MPSII, MPS2	Mucopolysaccharidosis type II

MPSIII, MPS3	Mucopolysaccharidosis type III
MPSIV, MPS4	Mucopolysaccharidosis type IV
MPSVI, MPS6	Mucopolysaccharidosis type VI
MPT	Maximum phonation time
MRI	Magnetic resonance imaging
MRL	Minimal response level
MRR	Maximum repetition rate
MSA	Multiple systems atrophy
MSB	My Sentence Builder ©
MSVHI	Modern singing voice handicap index
MTG	Middle temporal gyrus
MTS	Monosyllable-trochee-spondee
MUSS	Meaningful use of speech scale
MVPT	Motor-free visual perception test
NAL	National Acoustics Laboratories
NC	Noise criteria
NCI	National Cancer Institute
NCV	Nerve conduction velocity
NeAR	Newcastle audio ranking
NELP	National Early Literacy Panel
NF2	Neurofibromatosis type 2
NGS	Next-generation sequencing
NH	Normal-hearing
NHS	Newborn hearing screening
NHSP	Neonatal hearing screening programme
NHSP	Newborn hearing screening programme
NICU	Neonatal intensive-care unit
NIDCD	National Institute on Deafness and Other Communication Disorders
NIH	National Institutes of Health
NIHL	Noise-induced hearing loss
NIT	Noise-induced tinnitus
NMEPS	Neuromuscular electro-phonatory stimulation
NMES	Neuromuscular electro-stimulation
NNE	Normalised noise energy
NOHL	Non-organic hearing loss
NRT	Neural response telemetry
NSAID	Non-steroidal anti-inflammatory drug
NSHL	Non-syndromic hearing loss
NU-CHIPS	Northwestern University Children's Perception of Speech
OAE	Oto-acoustic emission
OAV	Oculoauriculovertebral
OAVS	Oculoauriculovertebral syndrome
OBT	Open bedside tracheostomy
ODD	Oculodentodigital
ODDD	Oculodentodigital dysplasia
ODOD	Oculodentoosseous dysplasia
OHC	Outer hair cell

OM	Otitis media
OME	Otitis media with effusion
OMIM	Online Mendelian inheritance in man
OPD I	Otopalatodigital syndrome type I
OSEP	Office of Special Education Programs
OSH	Occupational safety and health
oVEMP	ocular VEMP
PAR	Pseudo-allergic reactions
PARAFAC	Parallel factor analysis
PBD	Peroxisome biogenesis disorders
PCA	Posterior cricoarytenoid
PCA	Principal component analysis
PCD	Permanent childhood deafness
PCHI	Permanent childhood hearing impairment
PCR	Polymerase chain reaction
PDD-NOS	Pervasive developmental disorders not otherwise specified
PDMS	Peabody developmental motor scales
PDS	Pendred syndrome
PDT	Percutaneous dilational tracheostomy
PE	Pharyngo-esophageal
PECS	Picture exchange communication system
PEDS	Parents' evaluation of developmental status
PEG	Percutaneous endoscopic gastrostomy
PET	Positron emission tomography
PIAT	Peabody individual achievement test
PKU	Phenylketonuria
PL	Preferential looking
PLAKKS-II	Psycholinguistische Analyse kindlicher Aussprachestörungen-II
PLS	Preschool language scale
PM	Particulate matter
PM	Pre-motor
PPI	Proton pump inhibitor
PPVT	Peabody picture vocabulary test
PQ	Phonation quotient
PSP	Progressive supranuclear palsy
PTA	Pure tone audiometry
PTP	Phonation threshold pressure
PUP	Prosodic utterance production
PVFM	Paradoxical vocal fold motion
PVG	Phonovibrogram
pVHI	pediatric voice handicap index
PVSQ	Pediatric voice symptom questionnaire
PW	Pulsed wave
PWS	Prader-Willi syndrome
RA	Rheumatoid arthritis
RAST	Radioallergosorbent test
RASTI	Room acoustics speech transmission index

RAVI	Rastreamento de Alteracoes Vocais em Idosos
R_{AW}	Airway resistance
RBH	Roughness-breathiness-hoarseness
RCT	Randomised controlled trial
RDLS	Reynell developmental language scales
RECD	Real ear-to-coupler difference
RF	Radio frequency
RFS	Reflux finding score
RLN	Recurrent laryngeal nerve
RP	Retinitis pigmentosa
RSI	Reflux symptom index
rTMS	repetitive transcranial magnetic stimulation
RVT	Resonant voice therapy
SAEVD-R	Stark assessment of early vocal development-revised
SALT	Systematic analysis of language transcripts
SAT-HI	Stanford achievement test for hearing-impaired students
SCA7	Spinocerebellar ataxia type 7
SCC	Semicircular canal
SCIT	Subcutaneous immunotherapy
SD	Spasmodic dysphonia
SD	Standard deviation
SDDSL	Specific developmental disorder of speech and language
SEA	State Education Agency
SGD	Speech-generating devices
SGS	Schinzel-Giedion syndrome
SH	Sternohyoid
SI	Primary somatosensory cortex
SIL	Speech intelligibility index
SIOP	International Society of Paediatric Oncology
SIPT	Sensory integration and praxis tests
SIR	Speech intelligibility rating test
SIVD	Screening index for voice disorders
SLI	Specific language impairment
SLIT	Sublingual immunotherapy
SLN	Superior laryngeal nerve
SLO	Smith-Lemli-Opitz
SLP	Speech and language therapist
SM	Selective mutism
SM	Stapedius muscle
SMG	Supra-marginal gyrus
SNHL	Sensorineural hearing loss
snoRNA	small nucleolar RNA
SNR	Signal-to-noise ratio
SOAE	Spontaneous OAE
SOC	Sense of coherence
SOC	Superior olivary complex
SOP	Standard operating procedure
SOT	Sensory organisation test

SOVT	Semi-obstructive vocal tract
SP	Summation potentials
SP	Sustained potential
Speak	Spectral peak
SPL	Sound pressure level
SPM	Standard progressive matrices
SPT	Skin-prick test
SPT	Sylvian parietal temporal
SRT	Speech recognition threshold
SSD	Speech sound disorder
SSEP	Somatosensory evoked potentials
SSEP	Steady state evoked potential
SSRI	Selective serotonin reuptake inhibitors
SST	Stop signal task
ST	Spontaneous tinnitus
ST	Sternothyroid
ST	Surgical tracheostomy
STG	Superior temporal gyrus
STI	Speech transmission index
STI-PA	Sound transmission index (for public address systems)
STNR	Symmetrical tonic neck reflex
STORCH	Syphilis toxoplasmosis others rubella *cytomegalovirus* herpes
STS	Superior temporal sulcus
SVAS	Supravalvular aortic stenosis
SVH	Subjective visual horizontal
SVHI	Singing voice handicap index
SVKG	Strobo-videokymography
SVV	Subjective visual vertical
SWOT	Strengths, weaknesses, opportunities and threats
TA	Thyroarytenoid
TAKIWA	Göttingen developmental test of tactile-kinaesthetic perception
TBE	Tick-borne encephalitis
TBEV	Tick-borne encephalitis virus
tDCS	Transcranial direct current stimulation
TEACCH	Treatment and education of autistic and related communication handicapped children
TEN	Threshold-equalising noise
TENS	Transcutaneous electrical nerve stimulation
TEOAE	Transient evoked OAE
TEOAE	Transitory evoked OAE
TERA-D/HH	Test of early reading ability: deaf hard of hearing
TF	Transfer factor
TFI	Tinnitus functional index
THI	Tinnitus handicap inventory
THR	Threshold level
THS	Tinnitus and hearing survey

TIE	Touch inventory for elementary-school-aged children
TLR	Tonic labyrinthine reflex
TM	Time motion
TM	Tympanic membrane
TMS	Transcranial magnetic stimulation
TNM	Tumour, node and metastasis
TOAE	Transient OAE
ToCS	Test of child speechreading
ToD	Teacher of the deaf
TOLD-I	Test of language development: intermediate
TORC	Test of reading comprehension
TORCH	Toxoplasmosis others rubella *cytomegalovirus* herpes
TP	Thyropharyngeal
TPT	Toddler phonology tests
TROCA	Tangible reinforced operant conditioning audiometry
TRT	Tinnitus retraining therapy
TS	Turner syndrome
TSH	Thyroid-stimulating hormone
TTM	Trans-theoretical model
TTS	Temporary hearing-threshold shift
TTS	Text-to-speech
TVL	Teacher's voice level
TVPM	Tensor veli palatini muscle
TVPS	Test of visual-perceptual skills
UEMS	European Union of Medical Specialists
UEP	Union of European Phoniatricians
UHL	Unilateral hearing loss
ULL	Uncomfortable loudness level
UNHS	Universal newborn hearing screening
URT	Upper respiratory tract
URTI	URT infection
VA	Vestibular aqueduct
vAm	Peak Amplitude variation
VAP	Voice assessment protocol
VAS	Visual analogue scale
VC	Vital capacity
VCFS	Velocardiofacial syndrome
VCV	Vowel-consonant-vowel
VDCQ	Voice disability coping questionnaire
VEMP	Vestibular evoked myogenic potential
VEP	Visual evoked potential
VEP	Visually evoked potential
vF0	Fundamental frequency variation
VFD	Vocal fold dysfunction
VFR	Vertical focus of resonance
VHF	Viral haemorrhagic fever
VHI	Voice handicap index
vHIT	video head impulse test

VKG	Videokymography
VN	Vestibular nerve
VOCA	Voice output communication aids
VoiSS	Voice symptom scale
VOR	Vestibulo-ocular reflex
VOS	Voice outcome survey
VOT	Voice onset time
VPQ	Vocal performance questionnaire
VR	Vestibular rehabilitation
VR	Volume rendering
VRA	Visual reinforcement audiometry
VRP	Voice range profile
VRQOL	Voice-related quality of life
VSCM	Vestibular and semicircular canal
VSR	Vestibulo-spinal reflex
VTDS	Vocal tract discomfort scale
WADT	Wepman auditory discrimination test
WES	Whole exome sequencing
WHO	World Health Organization
WiLD	Wireless listening devices
WISC	Wechsler intelligence scale for children
WPPSI	Wechsler preschool and primary scale of intelligence
WRMT	Woodcock reading mastery test
WS	Waardenburg syndrome
WS	Williams syndrome
WVA	Widened vestibular aqueduct
X-ALD	X-linked adrenoleukodystrophy
XLA	X-linked agammaglobulinaemia
XNSHL	X-linked non-syndromic hearing loss

Part I

Fundamentals

Editor: Antoinette am Zehnhoff-Dinnesen

Lector: Philippe Dejonckere

Basics of Phoniatrics

1

Lisa Bartha-Doering, Peter Birkholz,
Cori Casanova, Felix de Jong, Wivine Decoster,
Ilter Denizoglu, Rolf Dierichs, Christian Dobel,
Michèle Kaufmann-Meyer, Malte Kob,
Anders Löfqvist, Dirk Mürbe,
Christiane Neuschaefer-Rube, Christo Pantev,
Bernhard Richter, Ken Roßlau, Oskar Schindler,
Harm K. Schutte, Ad Snik, Claudia Spahn,
Kurt Stephan, and Jürgen Wendler

Electronic Supplementary Material The online version
of this chapter (https://doi.org/10.1007/978-3-662-46780-
0_1) contains supplementary material, which is available
to authorized users.

L. Bartha-Doering
Department of Pediatrics and Adolescent Medicine,
Medical University of Vienna, Vienna, Austria
e-mail: elisabeth.bartha-doering@meduniwien.ac.at

P. Birkholz
Institute of Acoustics and Speech Communication,
Technische Universität Dresden (TU Dresden),
Dresden, Germany
e-mail: peter.birkholz@tu-dresden.de

C. Casanova
Voice and Communication, Universitat Ramon Llull,
Barcelona, Spain
e-mail: 29646mcb@comb.cat

F. de Jong
Research Group ExpORL, University Hospitals KU
Leuven, Leuven, Belgium
e-mail: Felix.DeJong@med.kuleuven.be

W. Decoster
Research Group ExpORL, KU Leuven, Leuven,
Belgium
e-mail: wivine.decoster@med.kuleuven.be

I. Denizoglu
Medical Park Hospital Imbatli Mahallesi, Izmir,
Turkey

R. Dierichs
Former Institute of Anatomy, University Clinic of
Münster, Münster, Germany
e-mail: kontakt@rolf-dierichs.de

C. Dobel
Medical Faculty, Department of Otorhinolaryngology,
Friedrich-Schiller-University, Jena, Germany
e-mail: christian.dobel@med.uni-jena.de

M. Kaufmann-Meyer
Tüscherz-Alfermée, Switzerland
e-mail: michele.kaufmann@arld.ch

M. Kob
Detmold University of Music, Erich Thienhaus
Institute, Music Acoustics and Theory of
Music Transmission, Detmold, Germany
e-mail: kob@hfm-detmold.de

A. Löfqvist
Department of Logopedics, Phoniatrics and
Audiology, University Hospital Lund, Lund, Sweden
e-mail: Anders.Lofqvist@med.lu.se

D. Mürbe
Department of Audiology and Phoniatrics, Charité–
University Medicine Berlin, Berlin, Germany
e-mail: dirk.muerbe@charite.de

C. Neuschaefer-Rube
Clinic of Phoniatrics, Pedaudiology and
Communication Disorders, School of Medicine of the
RWTH Aachen University, University Hospital
Aachen, Aachen, Germany

© Springer-Verlag GmbH Germany, part of Springer Nature 2020
A. am Zehnhoff-Dinnesen et al. (eds.), *Phoniatrics I*, European Manual of Medicine,
https://doi.org/10.1007/978-3-662-46780-0_1

e-mail: cneuschaefer@ukaachen.de

C. Pantev
Institute for Biomagnetismus and Biosignalanalysis,
University of Münster, University Hospital Münster,
Münster, Germany
e-mail: pantev@uni-muenster.de

B. Richter
Freiburger Institut für Musikermedizin, Hochschule
für Musik und Universitätsklinikum Freiburg,
Freiburg, Germany
e-mail: Bernhard.Richter@uniklinik-freiburg.de

K. Roßlau
Praxis, Hannover, Germany
e-mail: ken.rosslau@uni-muenster.de

O. Schindler
Department of Surgical Sciences, University of Turin,
Turin, Italy
e-mail: antonio.schindler@unimi.it

H. K. Schutte
Voice Research Lab. Groningen,
Groningen, The Netherlands

A. Snik
Audiologisch Centrum, KNO Klinik, Radboud
University Medical Center,
Nijmegen, The Netherlands
e-mail: A.Snik@kno.umcn.nl

C. Spahn
Freiburger Institut für Musikermedizin, Hochschule
für Musik und Universitätsklinikum Freiburg,
Freiburg, Germany
e-mail: claudia.spahn@uniklinik-freiburg.de

K. Stephan
Department for Hearing, Speech and Voice Disorders,
Medical University of Innsbruck, Insbruck, Austria
e-mail: Kurt.stephan@i-med.ac.at

J. Wendler
Berlin, Germany
e-mail: juergen.wendler@alumni.charite.de

1.1 History of the Discipline

Jürgen Wendler

Phoniatrics is, as of the current definition from the Union of the European Phoniatricians (UEP) and the European Union of Medical Specialists (UEMS), the medical field for communication disorders, concerned with functions and diseases of voice, speech, language, hearing (especially in so far as hearing impairment has its effects on any of the areas previously mentioned) and swallowing. In practice, phoniatrics is a multidisciplinary speciality combining information from medical and non-medical sciences. In addition to general medical investigations and treatment procedures, phoniatrics encloses complex areas of competence in the fields of cognition, learning abilities, psychological behaviour and rehabilitation procedures. The more important medical fields for clinical practice are otorhinolaryngology (ENT), neurology, neuropaediatrics, (child) psychiatry, paediatrics, radiology, genetics, endocrinology, dentistry, gerontology and musicians' medicine. On the other hand, the fundamentals of many non-medical disciplines, for instance, linguistics, phonetics, (neuro-) psychology, pedagogy, acoustics, information and communication sciences, also need to be included in phoniatric training programmes (Vilkman et al. 2010).

The following overview of the history of this discipline is based on these integrative interrelations. At the same time, it has to be stressed that the profile of phoniatrics as a medical speciality has always to be determined with reference to the aspects of disease and health in terms of specific approaches to clinical understanding, diagnostics and therapy of communication disorders.

1.1.1 Scientific Background

1.1.1.1 Antiquity

In antiquity, language and also speech often appeared as a type of divine mystery, a phenomenon, obvious when Pythia was announcing the Delphi oracles. This irrational approach to language can be followed in many parts of the world up to the present time, and we have come a long way to a more rational approach to speech and language, a road that can be marked here by only a very few towering giants as mentioned by Hans von Leden (1981, 1997a).

In contrast to his distinguished predecessors, such as Hippocrates and Aristotle, who thought of themselves as philosophers and based their wisdom largely on thoughtful speculation, Claudius Galenus (circa 131–216) was the first to derive his knowledge of anatomy and physiology from the dissection of animals (mainly pigs and dogs) and to base his judgement on these personal observations. In his book *De usu partium corporis humani*, he described the most important cartilages and muscles of the vocal system as well as its innervation and compared the production of the voice to the sound from a flute. He correctly identified the larynx as the instrument of voice or *principalissimum organum vocis*. He separated speech from voice, and he ascribed different types of hoarseness to various diseases and disorders of the vocal system. This medical colossus reigned like a dictator over the world of medical science; and his dominance extended throughout Europe and far into the sixteenth century.

1.1.1.2 Renaissance

The Renaissance began its work of enlightenment in the field of art, and some of the bolder artists did not hesitate to exchange brush for scalpel in order to explore the human body. Among them was Leonardo da Vinci (1452–1519), the versatile genius who contributed remarkable discoveries to the anatomy of the larynx and the physiology and pathology of the voice. His major anatomical study *Quaderni d'anatomia* that was completed about the year 1500 includes several rather lifelike drawings of the larynx. He also described the parts played by the structures of the mouth, lips and teeth for articulation and assigned phonetic terms to the acoustic signals.

The new spirit of freedom for scientific exploration found its zenith in the Italian universities. In Padua, the Fleming Andreas Vesalius's (1514–1564) great work *De humani corporis fabrica* reformed the knowledge of anatomy including detailed depictions of the larynx; some of the magnificent woodcuts in this volume have been attributed to Titian. One of the successors of Vesalius as professor of anatomy at Padua was Hieronymus Fabricius of Aquapendente (1537–1619). A diligent student of comparative anatomy, Fabricius, published a textbook on the organs of vision, voice and hearing: *De Visione, Voce et Auditu*. This book and two others present anatomically correct pictures of the vocal organ, and the author states categorically that 'the vocal cords and the gap between them cause the voice'. Giovanni Battista Morgagni (1682–1771) was the last and the greatest of the celebrated professors who made Padua the leading medical school of Europe. He stressed the organic pathological state of the organism and followed a topographic classification system (*The Seat and Causes of Diseases*, 1769). He assumed, for instance, that hyoid bone deviations were the cause of the majority of cases of stuttering, and he described various cases of speechlessness associated with apoplexy, head injury and cerebral disease. His painstaking observations called attention to the larynx as the primary site of diseases and formed the basis of laryngeal pathology, far beyond the description of the ventricles erroneously named after him. (Morgagni himself had stressed that these structures had been clearly identified before him by Galenus and Fabricius.) Also in Padua, Hieronymus Mercurialis (1530–1696) held the Chair of Practical Medicine. As early as 1583, he made an attempt that can be considered most striking even today. In an excellent review on stuttering in the view of mediaeval physiology, the classical theories of Galen, Aristotle, Hippocrates and others are discussed in terms of aetiology and therapy in order to explain conflicting points of view (Rieber and Fröschels 1966).

1.1.1.3 From the Seventeenth to Nineteenth Centuries

With the formation of the Royal Society in England during the second half of the seventeenth century, an important scientific forum came into being, where, among many other topics, questions of phonetics were discussed, as well as teaching of speech for the deaf.

The Swiss physician Johann Conrad Amman (1669–1724), often considered the father of logopaedics, published in Amsterdam in 1700 his *Dissertatio de Loquela* (based on his dissertation *Surdus Loquens* (the speaking deaf) 1692), dealing profoundly with general basics of human language and speech.

Francisco Boissier de Sauvages (1706–1767), Montpellier and Paris, botanist and physician, presented (probably stimulated by the systema-tology of Carl von Linné) the first overall system-atic classification of diseases based on clinical similarities of aetiology, anatomy and therapy in 1768: 'Nosologia methodica sistens morborum classes'. Regarding our field of interest, he grouped the following clinical entities under 'Dyskinesia': Mutitas (today analogous to com-plete loss of voice and speech), aphonia (loss of voice), psellismus (disorders of rate and rhythm such as stuttering and cluttering) and paraphonia (defects of vocal quality).

The fundamental change to a medicine gener-ally based on natural science finally occurred in the nineteenth century. Johannes-Müller (1801–1858) in Berlin (Müller 1839), for instance, per-formed precise experiments on the excised larynx (1839), confirming earlier results achieved by the French anatomist Antoine Ferrein (1693–1769), the first scholar to conduct acoustic experiments on the isolated cadaver larynx (1741). With his exact measurements of vocal folds tension and subglottal pressure in relation to pitch and loud-ness, Müller created a solid basis for the aerodynamic-myoelastic theory of voice produc-tion still valid today.

Hermann von Helmholtz (1821–1894), an outstanding physiologist and physicist in Berlin, explored the acoustic structure of vowels through sophisticated subjective analyses and syntheses using rather simple resonators (1859) (von Helmholtz 1859). He described exactly the two spectral areas that characterise each individual vowel, which Ludimar Hermann (1838–1914), physiologist in Königsberg, named 'formants' later on (1894), identified by objective phono-photographic recordings and mathematical pro-cessing of the data. Helmholtz also based his theory of hearing on the principles of resonance still reflected in current frequency distribution on the basilar membrane.

1.1.1.4 From the Twentieth Century to Present Times

The recent century has been characterised by rap-idly growing knowledge and technological prog-ress in every respect:

The theoretical-linguistic construct of a 'lan-guage acquisition device' (Chomsky 1965), an instinctive mental capacity that enables an infant to acquire and produce language, an instinct or 'innate facility' for acquiring language (Chomsky 1965), was encouragingly supported or even con-firmed by the discovery of the *FOXP2*-gene by Cecilia S. Lai et al. in 2001, a gene on chromo-some No. 7 that obviously plays a major role in this connection (Lai et al. 2001), a milestone on 'a long and winding road' (Felsenfeld 2002). Practical consequences regarding specific devel-opmental disorders of speech and language may be expected in the near future.

Independent of numerous theoretical concepts in the frame of Aphasiology, therapeutic concepts for the treatment of aphasia have changed funda-mentally during the recent century (Schindler et al. 2014; Wendler et al. 2005). Starting out from a symptomatic-linguistic approach (language-orientated, restitution of verbal capac-ities as the definite goal and termination of ther-apy if this is not possible), followed by a communicative model (information-orientated, use of all means, linguistic or nonlinguistic, natu-ral, supporting or artificial, to make possible any exchange of information; the restitution of lin-guistic capacities is not primarily crucial any more), the development finally arrived at an eco-logical concept (action-orientated, show and imi-tate, transfer of action to make possible basic daily activities such as personal hygiene, dress-ing oneself, ingestion of food; the restitution of communicative capacities is not primarily crucial any more). These changes stand for a consider-able extension of rehabilitative perspectives to the benefit of the aphasic patients themselves as well as for their personal environment.

On the other hand, stuttering still continues to be an issue of intense investigations without a real breakthrough in terms of an evidence-based causal therapy. However, there is good reason to hope for relevant results from molecular genetic research.

With the discovery of otoacoustic emissions by David T. Kemp 1976 (Kemp 2007) and the introduction of the measurements of these signals for newborn hearing screening, the door was opened for the early detection of relevant hearing losses and effective treatment decisions including the application of cochlear implant systems (by

Clark et al. 1979), the most successful electronic prosthesis for the time being (Clark 2003). In recent years there has been a dramatic upsurge in professional and public awareness of Auditory Processing Disorders (APD), also referred to as Central Auditory Processing Disorders (CAPD) (Bellis 1997; Schönweiler et al. 2012).

In the middle of the last century, Raoul Husson (1901–1967), a French physicist and singer, perplexed the scientific world by a ground-breaking, unbelievable idea about the production of the voice. He claimed that the vocal folds are brought to vibratory motion by rapid contractions of the vocalis muscles themselves, following 'coup par coup', nervous excitations from the recurrent nerve, instead of being passively set in vibration by air blowing from below (Husson 1950). This meant that the laryngeal sound was produced by active movements of the glottis. After a short while of paralysis-like silence, scientists all over the world started a great variety of research programmes to check this new philosophy, most of them deeply convinced that this could be nothing but a fundamental error. One of them was Janwillem van den Berg (1920–1985) who essentially contributed a convincing confirmation of the aerodynamic-myoelastic theory of voice production (van den Berg 1958). Among many other profound studies, he repeated the Johannes-Müller experiments according to his current technical possibilities and produced, together with the American singer William Vennard, a fascinating instructional film on the vibrating larynx (1969) clearly demonstrating the aerodynamic-myoelastic principle.

Aatto Sonninen's (1922–2009) comment on Husson at a symposium in Wendler (2010):

His work was by no means in vain. On the contrary, without his work our knowledge of vocal physiology would certainly be much more fragmentary. Hardly anyone but Husson has had such a stimulating effect on the research of vocal fold anatomy and the role of the central nervous system in phonation. In my opinion, the life work of Husson deserves the deference and commendation of succeeding generations. The lesson that can be learned from the scientific "war" described above is on one hand the fact that the bold and unprejudiced framing of questions - possibly leading to erroneous conclusions - is not dangerous, something to be feared. On the contrary, it may help in

opening quite new perspectives. On the other hand, however, a scientist must always aim at confirming in all respects the validity and reliability of his observations.

Van den Berg's research has been successfully carried on by Harm K. Schutte (1992).

Of course, the aerodynamic-myoelastic aspects of voice production reveal a rather mechanical view on this process, often belittled as mechanistic by scientists concentrating on psychological conditions and considered to be of, at the most, peripheral importance. Thus, they looked quite sceptically at surgical attempts to correct morphological changes of laryngeal structures, but these interventions proved to be very successful. Hans von Leden and Godfrey Arnold (1914–1989) coined the term *phonosurgery* in 1963 for surgical procedures to improve or to restore vocal function (von Leden 1997b). Afterwards, Hirano (1975) and Isshiki (1989) presented extended histo-anatomical and acoustic studies as a basis for specific microsurgical procedures that were soon in common use worldwide, and since the 1970s, biomechanics has increasingly attracted attention as a powerful tool in many medical fields. This does not mean that psychological and behavioural dimensions of voice production should be neglected. Another milestone in voice therapy, competing with psychological approaches, was the courageous introduction of botulinum neurotoxin, one of the strongest poisons, by Blitzer et al. (1986) for the successful symptomatic treatment of muscular dystonias such as spasmodic dysphonias (Blitzer et al. 1986). In 2000, the International Association of Phonosurgeons extended the definition of phonosurgery from voice to speech, taking in account the essential contributions of phoniatrics to the rehabilitation of cleft palate patients (Hirschberg 1997).

1.1.2 Medical Specialisation Towards Voice, Speech, Language and Hearing

From both Paris and London, the itinerant Spanish teacher of song, Manuel García (1805–1906) (García 1854), promoted enthusiastically the use of a mirror to observe the acting larynx deep in the throat and thus opened the door to the development of laryngology, pioneered by Ludwig Türck (1810–1868) (Türck 1860) in Vienna and Johann Nepomuk Czermak (1829–1873) (Czermak 1863) in Pest, Hungary.

Only a few years later, the leading surgeon in Tubingen, Germany, Victor von Bruns (1812–1883), succeeded via laryngeal mirror (without today's anaesthesia, not available then) in removing a polyp from the vocal folds (von Bruns 1862). He designed special instruments, quite similar to those still in use today, and he left a collection of excellent pictures (von Bruns 1873). Von Bruns contributed significantly towards establishing medical competence in voice disorders.

In contrast, 20 years previously in Berlin, the well-acknowledged surgeon of outstanding merit, Johann Friedrich Dieffenbach (1792–1847), had attempted to treat stuttering with horrible wedge excisions of the tongue and brought approximately equal damage to the developing reputation of medical speech therapy.

In Paris, the surgeon (and anthropologist) Pierre Paul Broca (1824–1880) localised the origin of expressive, motor language problems in the frontal lobe of the brain of 'Mr. Tan' (1861), a patient of his who was able only to produce repeatedly the stereotypic utterance 'tan, tan' (Broca 1861).

The German neurologist Carl Wernicke (1848–1905) from Breslau supplemented these findings in describing lesions of the temporal lobe associated with impressive or sensory language impairments (Wernicke 1874). Broca and Wernicke together represent a turning point, when largely speculative ideas on the phenomenon of aphasia were replaced with evidence from anatomy and physiology as the cornerstones of diagnosis and therapy.

Now the time was ripe for a comprehensive medical treatise on disorders of speech and language. It came from Adolph Kussmaul (1822–1902) (Fig. 1.1), internist in Strasbourg, Alsace. His book, *The Disorders of Speech* (*Die Störungen der Sprache*, 1877), became the standard work for more than a generation (Kußmaul 1877). A fourth edition was published 8 years after his death.

The new medical field was at first denominated as *voice and speech pathology* (*Stimm- und Sprachheilkunde*). The closest approximation,

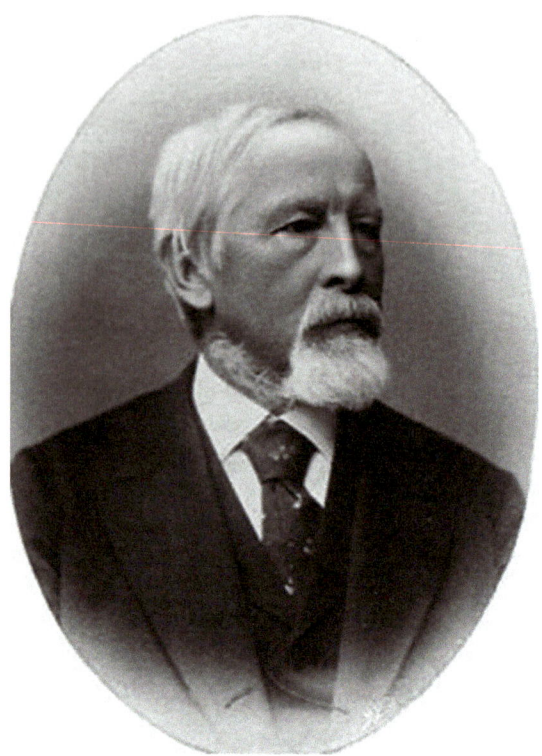

Fig. 1.1 Adolph Kussmaul

however, to the present term 'phoniatrics' was found in the term 'phoniatros' (1886), the telegram address of the London laryngologist Morell Mackenzie (1837–1892).

Voice and speech pathology was initially developed from two centres: Berlin and Vienna. Albert Gutzmann (1839–1910), a highly motivated teacher of the deaf in Berlin, also worked with speech/language impairment, particularly stuttering. He organised courses and edited a journal of medicine and pedagogy (*Medizinisch-pädagogische Monatsschrift*) as of 1891 together with his son Hermann, then a medical student.

In 1905, Hermann Gutzmann (1865–1922) (Fig. 1.2) completed his Ph.D. thesis on 'Respiratory Movements in their Relation to Speech/Language Disorders' and gave the probative lecture at the Medical Faculty of the Berlin Kaiser-Wilhelm-University on 'Speech/Language Disorders as a Topic of Clinical Education'. With his pioneering inauguration, he established medical Voice and Speech Pathology as an academic discipline and made the Berlin Charité Hospital the cradle of phoniatrics.

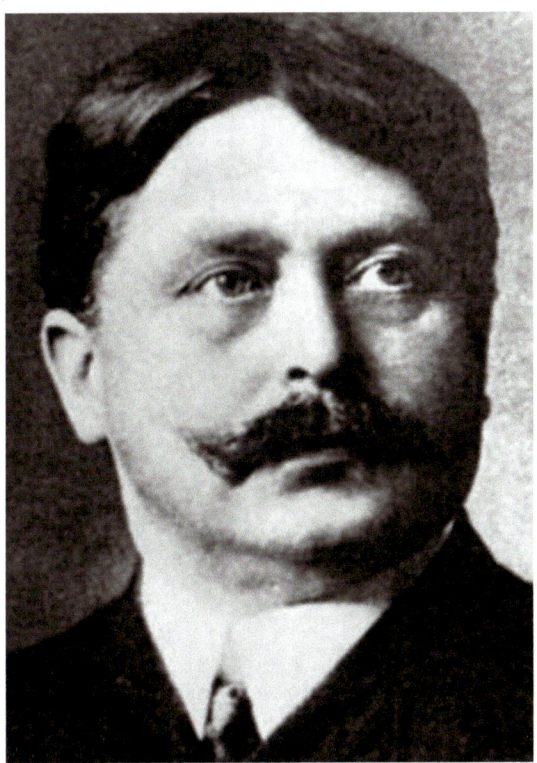

Fig. 1.2 Hermann Gutzmann Sr.

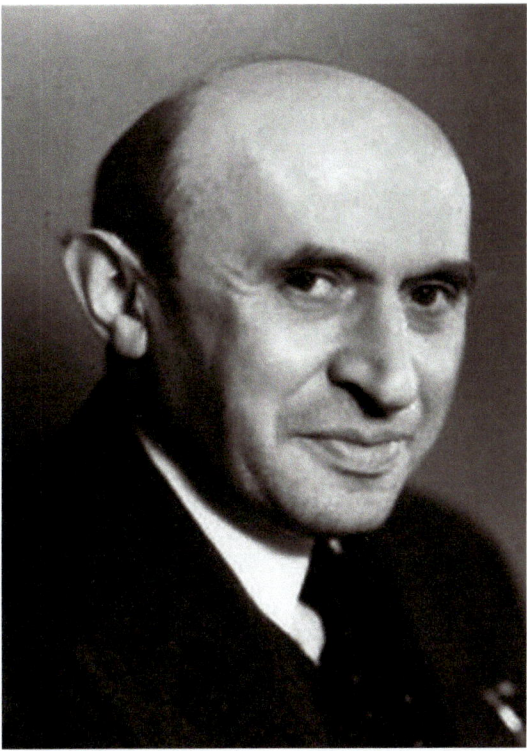

Fig. 1.3 Emil Fröschels. With kind permission from Josephinum, Ethics, Collections and History of Medicine, MedUni Vienna

International students worldwide flocked to Berlin to study under Hermann Gutzmann. Thirteen books and more than 300 articles offer evidence of his scientific achievement (complete bibliography in Wendler 1980). His main work, 'Sprachheilkunde' (Gutzmann 1912), was standard reference of the discipline for many years. The Berlin school of phoniatrics was based on natural sciences, physiology and phonetics; its students were known as the 'organists'.

In contrast, the Vienna school led by Gutzmann's student Emil Fröschels (1884–1972) (Fig. 1.3), as of 1909, emphasised the psychological basis, and its students were tipped as the 'psychologists' (Fröschels 1913). Being a Jewish scientist, Fröschels was expelled from his academic position. He emigrated from Austria to the United States in 1939 where he continued his work in St. Louis and in New York for many more years and, very successfully, held in high esteem all over the world owing to his outstanding achievements.

The internist Kussmaul had demonstrated multiple close relations between speech and language disorders with neurology and psychiatry and detailed the cerebral origins of language and speech. Both Gutzmann and Fröschels attached their departments to otolaryngology with the more peripheral structures and functions in focus, covering the fields of voice, speech/language and hearing, without ignoring the central functions. This latter tradition is still alive in several areas and corresponds to a communicative approach.

1.1.3 After the Second World War

After the Second World War, with large areas of Europe in ruins, Prague assumed the leadership in phoniatrics. Miloslav Seeman (1892–1975) (Fig. 1.4), a student of Gutzmann, succeeded here in 1967 in establishing the first University-Clinic for Phoniatrics, and young students from across the world met there for advanced studies in the field. These students included many Germans of the post-war generation who rediscovered their

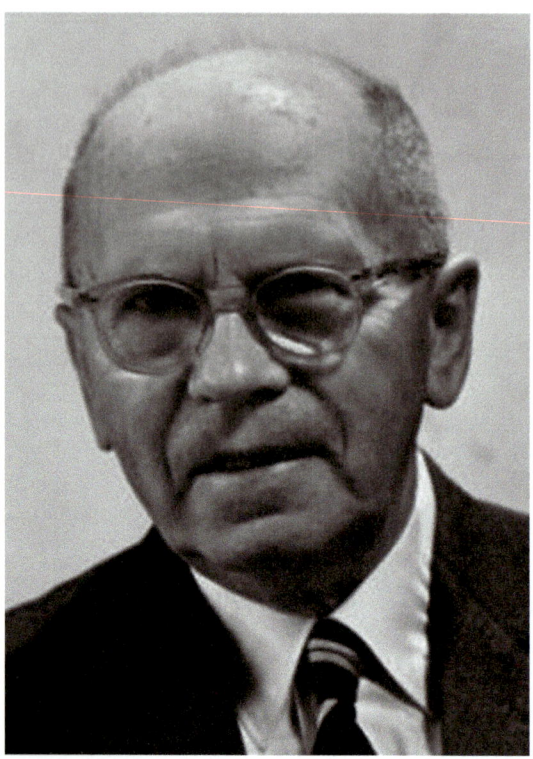

Fig. 1.4 Miloslav Seeman (from Sedláček E, Sedláček K (1973) Zum 80. Geburtstag von Prof. Dr. Miloslav Seeman. Folia Phoniatr Logop 25:1–8 with permission from S. Karger AG, Basel)

nation's contributions to the field and were able to re-establish phoniatric competence in Germany: good reason for them to be very grateful for this guidance and friendship offered by the colleagues of the Prague school under Miloslav Seeman and Eva Sedláčková (1913–1976). In 1958, phoniatrics was established as an official subspeciality to ENT in Czechoslovakia, a model later on for the further development in Europe. Seeman's textbook *Poruchy détski reči* (*Language Disorders in Children*), 1955, seven editions, translated into German, French and Russian, contributed essentially to shaping the phoniatric profile in post-war Europe (Seeman 1955). The same is true for Richard Luchsinger (1900–1993) and Gottfried (Godfrey) Arnold (1914–1989) with their textbook from 1948 and 1959 that in 1970 was extended to two volumes as *Handbuch der Stimm- und Sprachheilkunde* (Luchsinger and Arnold 1970) and also appeared in English. All of them were students of Hermann Gutzmann, and they followed his ideas in the same way that Karl Wilhelm

Weinberg (1862–1935) did in Sweden, where phoniatrics achieved the acknowledgement of a medical speciality of its own standing as early as in 1931 owing to the activities of Bertil Borg (1894–1931) and Bertil Kågen (1905–1978) and supported by the holder of the first professorial chair in ORL in Sweden, Gunnar Holmgren (1875–1954). In Finland (phoniatrics became an independent speciality in 1948), it was Rauha Hammar (1878–1964) together with Lennart Sjöström, in Switzerland, Max Nadoleczny (1874–1940) and in Poland Wladyslaw Ołtuszewski (1855–1922) (Wendler 1980). Besides this so-called German-speaking group, there was a very active 'francophone group' led by Jean Tarneaud (1888–1972), France, and completed by Bernard Vallancien (1907–1980), France; Jean-Claude Lafon (1922–1998), France; Jordi Perelló (1918–1999), Spain; Lucio Croatto (1920–2001), Italy; and André Muller (1918–2015), Switzerland (Perelló 1977). Regrettably, there was little if any contact between the two groups, even after the edition of *Folia phoniatrica*, the pioneering international journal of phoniatrics, by Luchsinger, Seeman and Tarneaud in 1947, with contributions in English, French and German. Meantime, quite a number of phoniatric textbooks have appeared in several European languages; only a few of them can be quoted here (Böhme 2001, 2003; Friedrich et al. 2013; Hirschberg et al. 2013; Obrębowski and Tarkowski 2003; Pruszewicz 1992; Schindler and Schindler 2001; De Vincentiis 2001; Vasilenko 2002; Wendler et al. 2005). With his 'Lexicón de Comunicologia' (Perelló 1977), Perelló provided a multilingual dictionary comprising relevant terms of the discipline in Spanish, French, English, German, Catalan, Italian and Latin as well as biographical essentials of outstanding historical personalities.

In post-war Germany, it was Peter Biesalski (1915–2001) who in 1969 opened in Mainz the first German University-Clinic for Communication Disorders. His domain was pedaudiology. Together with Gerhard Kittel (1925–2011) (Erlangen), Oskar Schindler (Torino) and Dušan Cvejić (1923–1998) (Belgrade), he founded in 1971 the *Union of the European Phoniatricians, UEP* (Fig. 1.5).

This became, mainly owing to the untiring efforts of Biesalski and Kittel, an extremely effective organisation, bringing together not only the two groups mentioned above but offering a channel for permanent contacts among people, even from the two sides of Europe divided by the iron curtain and the cold war. Annual congresses were organised, the venues of which alternated regularly between Western and Eastern Europe with a special highlight: the Gutzmann Anniversary in East Berlin in 1980 under the heading '75 Years of Phoniatrics'. In a Festschrift, the history and the present state of phoniatrics from 21 countries

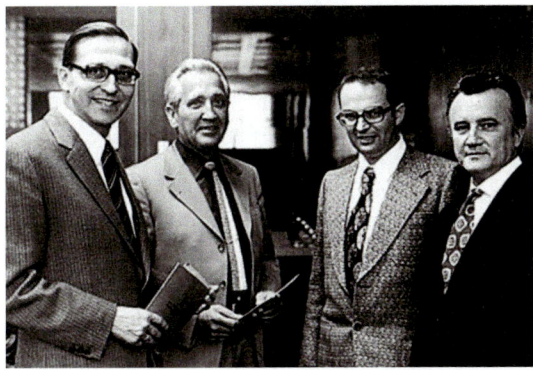

Fig. 1.5 The initiators of the UEP. Left to right: Gerhard Kittel, Peter Biesalski, Oskar Schindler, Dušan Cvejić

could be presented (Wendler 1980), and a Gutzmann-Medal was awarded to internationally leading personalities for the first time (Fig. 1.6).

The structure and content of the field of phoniatrics were defined and determined through close cooperation among several partners, of especial importance are the *European Union of the Medical Specialists* (*UEMS*) with Willy Wellens representing the UEP in the beginning and the *International Federation of Oto-Rhino-Laryngological Societies, IFOS.*

The UEP has launched numerous programmes to shape and define phoniatrics further as the medical speciality for communication disorders and to develop programmes to train and educate competent phoniatricians. A first draft was published by Wendler and Wellens in 1983 (Wendler and Wellens 1983). Within the EU, the harmonisation of such programmes is continuously advancing, after Christiane Neuschaefer-Rube (Germany) currently with Tamer Abou-Elsaad (Egypt) and Tadeus Nawka (Germany) representing phoniatrics within the framework of UEMS with a well-elaborated training programme and logbook (Vilkman et al. 2010, updated 2018),

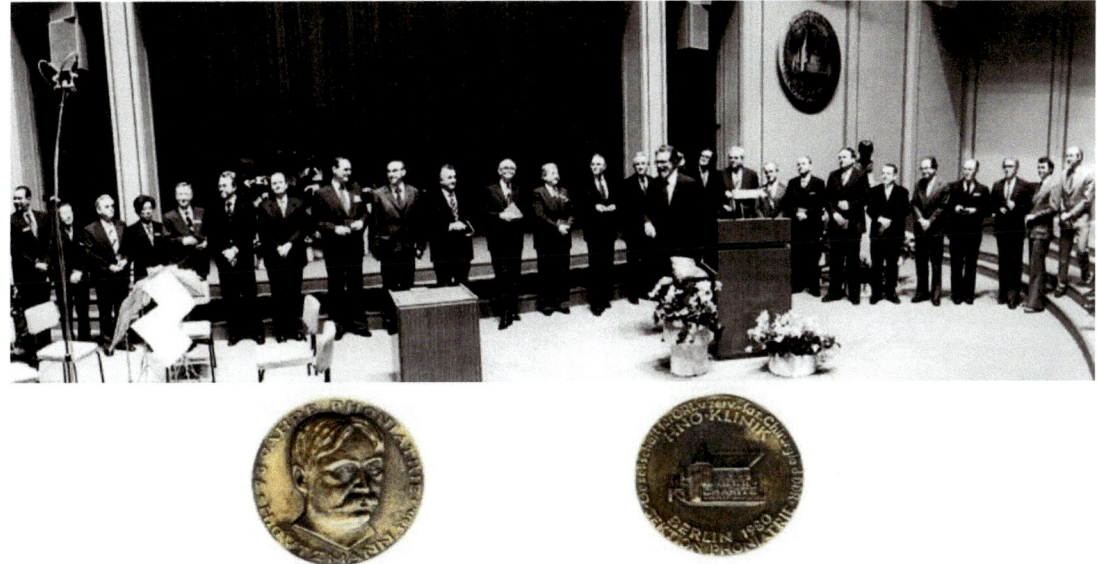

Fig. 1.6 Awarding the Gutzmann-Medal, Berlin 1980, the laureates. Left to right: N.M. Kotby (Egypt), N. Isshiki (Japan), J. Hirschberg (Hungary), M. Hirano (Japan), L. Handzel (Poland), B. Fritzell (Sweden), T. Frint (Hungary), F. Frank (Austria), L. Dmitriev (Soviet Union), D. Cvejić (Yugoslavia), O. Caprez (Switzerland), L. Croatto (Italy), O. von Arentsschild (Western Germany), P. Biesaslski (Western Germany), C.I.E. Jansen (the Netherlands, hidden by J. Wendler, at the desk, laudator), G. Kittel (Western Germany), I. Maximov (Bulgaria), J. Perelló (Spain), E. Loebell (Western Germany), A. Pruszewicz (Poland), K. Sedláček (Czechoslovakia), C. Siegert (Eastern German), A. Sonninen (Finland), F. Šram (Czechoslovakia), R. Tostmann (Eastern Germany), H. Lindholm (Sweden). Not in the picture: H. von Leden (USA), W. Pfau (Eastern Germany)

and the European concept of phoniatrics attracts increasing attention worldwide.

Under the *Standing IFOS Committee on Phoniatrics and Voice Care* (Chair J. Wendler), the special profile of phoniatrics has been generally acknowledged (International Federation of Oto-Rhino-Laryngological Societies 1986). This Committee can be traced back to the *Committee on the Care of Voice* established in 1969 by the pioneer of phonosurgery, Hans von Leden. In 1993, IFOS recommended that selected phoniatric topics be included in postgraduate ENT training programmes as a basic requirement for their completion (International Federation of Oto-Rhino-Laryngological Societies 1993).

An interdisciplinary organisation, the *International Association of Logopedics and Phoniatrics*, had been founded in Vienna on the initiative of Emil Fröschels as early as in 1924 (Perelló 1982). He originally named the medical field of speech/language pathology 'Logopedics'. Hugo Stern and Miloslav Seeman later introduced the term *Phoniatrics*, which is in common use today to describe communication medicine, whereas the term *Logopedics* denotes the corresponding non-medical speciality.

1.1.4 Present and Future

Since the 1960s, phoniatrics has extended its scope from the above-outlined concept of physiological and psychological aspects of voice, speech/language and hearing to an all-encompassing perspective of communication including all input, central and output functions as well as sociocultural and ecological dimensions. As the primary function of the articulatory system, swallowing has also been included in the competence of the field. Regarding aetiological studies, molecular genetics has already contributed essential insights, particularly in the field of hearing and developmental language disorders, and as far as stuttering is concerned, genetic factors are being explored with encouraging perspectives. Neurosciences, especially in terms of neurolinguistics, are opening up new ways to the understanding and management of central language

processing by means of functional imaging technologies. As the medical speciality for communication disorders, phoniatrics is a worldwide issue today, although with significant geographical differences. The status of phoniatrics varies, in a global view, from an independent speciality on its own to a rather unknown peculiarity, whereas in continental Europe, the cradle of phoniatrics, the speciality is generally well established.

According to an international inquiry in 2012 (Wendler 2012), there were some 1200 specialists in the field: 300 in Italy, 290 in Germany, 210 in Poland, 96 in Czechoslovakia and altogether some 100 university departments. According to a survey from 2016 (Antoinette am Zehnhoff-Dinnesen et al. 2016) we got data about colleagues active in phoniatrics concerning the following countries: 40 in Austria, 10 in Belarus, a couple of dozen in Belgium, 120 in the Czech Republic, many hundreds in Egypt, 23 in Finland, 319 in Germany, 23 in Hungary, 150 in Mexico, more than 200 in Poland, 150 in Russia, 13 in Saudi Arabia, about 100 in Spain, 32 in Switzerland, about 20 in the Netherlands, 15 in Turkey and 135 in Venezuela, in total more than 1650.

According to that survey phoniatrics is an independent specialty in Finland, Germany, Italy, Poland, Egypt, Mexico and Venezuela. It is an officially recognised subspeciality to ENT in many other countries. In several countries, hearing-impaired children are cared for through pedaudiology as an integrated part of phoniatrics. In others, this is a special area of audiology. Considerations to bring phoniatrics and audiology together in terms of a speciality 'communication medicine' are being discussed.

For the near future, when rules and regulations for medical specialisation regarding professional profiles and official recognition can be expected to be continuously under discussion, successful cooperation is of greatest importance between UEP with their untiring past president Antoinette am Zehnhoff-Dinnesen (Germany), because of her outstanding merits in rebuilding and further developing the UEP appointed honorary president in 2018, with her inspiring successor Ahmed Geneid (Finland), and with the phoniatric representatives within UEMS. An eminent milestone on the way towards a high level standard of the discipline in all of Europe was the foundation of the European Academy of Phoniatrics in 2013, initiated and finally well established after sustained multiple efforts by Antoinette am Zehnhoff-Dinnesen as the founding director. Christiane Neuschaefer- Rube was elected first president of the academy, mean-time followed by Tadeus Nawka (Germany).

In spite of differing concepts of formal professional formats and independently from systematic orders, the medical challenges of the information age require the general adoption of a recognised special medical field with encompassing compe tence for communication disorders, and that is phoniatrics.

1.2 Developmental and Anatomical Background of Communication and Swallowing Disorders

Rolf Dierichs

1.2.1 Embryology

1.2.1.1 Cranium and Face
Normal Craniofacial Development (Figs. 1.7, 1.8, 1.9 **and** 1.10) (Kliegman and Nelson 2007) The human skull comprises three components of different origin: the chondrocranium, which forms from three parasagittal cartilages and three sensory capsules via endochondral ossification; the membrane (dermal) bones, ossifying directly from mesenchyme of the skin; and the branchial skeleton of the pharyngeal arches, forming via endochondral ossification. The parasagittal cartilages form the base and median elements of the skull, and the primitive sensory capsules are the origins for elements of the nose, orbit and temporal bone.

The membrane bones of the human skull include the cranial vault (calvaria) and the bones of the face. The bones of the calvaria are separate at birth but will fuse to form sutures, and the fontanelles between these bones will join later after the brain has finished growing.

From week 4 to week 10, the face develops from five facial swellings: paired maxillary swellings, paired mandibular swellings and an unpaired medial frontonasal process. The maxillary swellings enlarge in the fifth week; they lengthen medially and form the primordia of the cheeks and the lateral portions of the upper lip. The lateral portions of the maxillary and mandibular swellings fuse to produce the final shape of the mouth. The mandibular swellings enlarge to form the primordia of the lower lip and jaw in the fourth and fifth weeks. The buccopharyngeal membrane, which separates the ectodermal stomodeum from the endodermal foregut, breaks down on day 24.

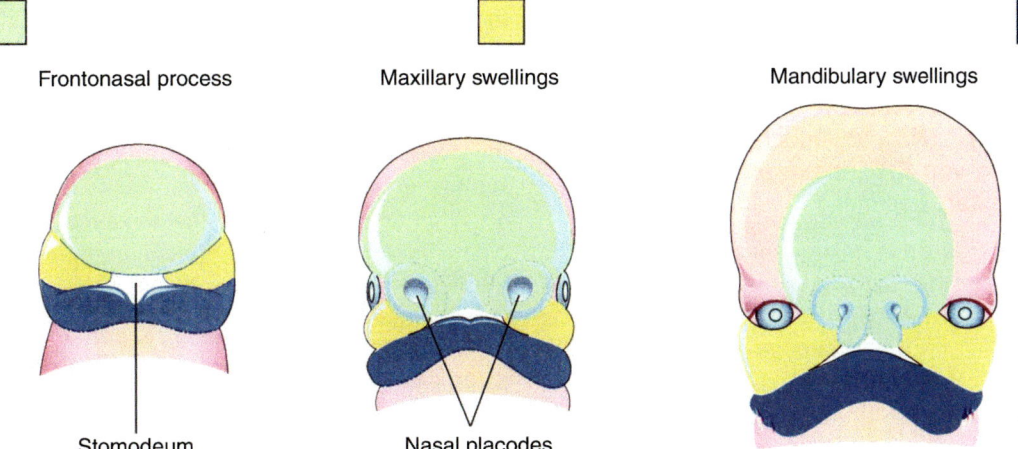

Fig. 1.7 Facial development, day 24, day 33, day 48 (from Moore and Persaud 2003, courtesy of Elsevier)

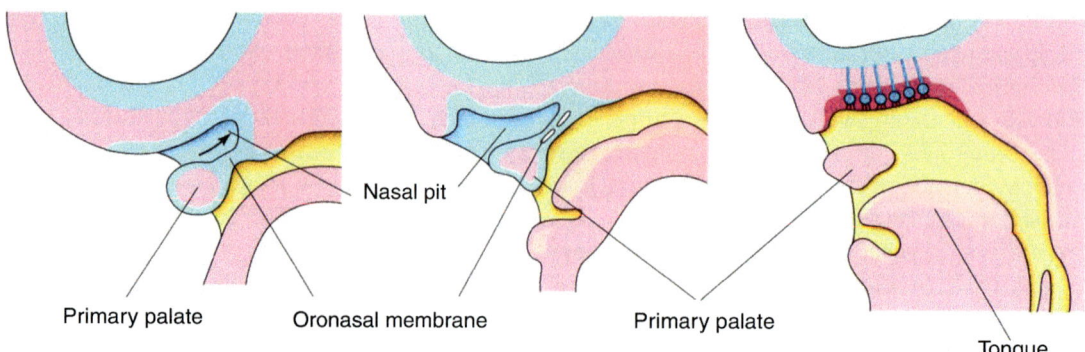

Fig. 1.8 Sagittal section through the head; the nasal septum has been removed. Week 5, week 6, week 7 (from Moore and Persaud 2003, courtesy of Elsevier)

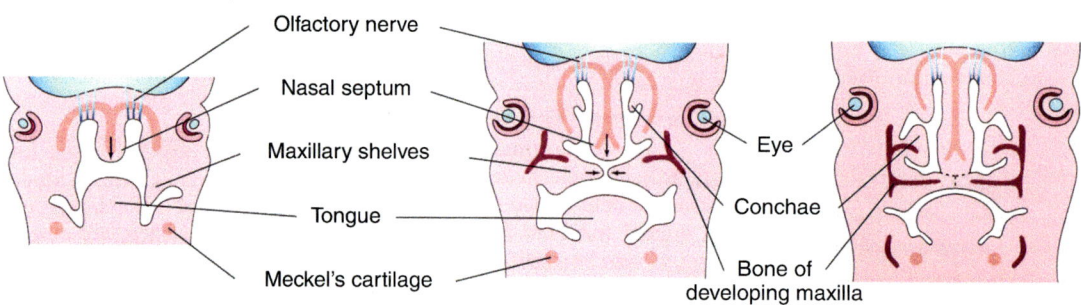

Fig. 1.9 Frontal section through the head, weeks 6–12, fusing of the maxillary shelves with the nasal septum (from Moore and Persaud 2003, courtesy of Elsevier)

In the fifth week, ectodermal thickenings, called nasal placodes, appear on the frontonasal process, which will give rise to the nose and philtrum. Each placode develops a nasal pit in its centre. In the sixth week, its lateral edge, the lateral nasal process, will form the sides of the nose; its medial rim, the medial nasal process, will fuse with its contralateral partner to form the bridge of the nose. During the seventh week, the inferior portion of the fused material forms the intermaxillary process that will join the maxillary swellings to form the philtrum of the upper lip.

The nasal pits enlarge and fuse to form the nasal sac, with the nasal fin developing from its floor to separate the nasal and oral cavities. The nasal fin thins to form the oronasal membrane. It finally ruptures, forming an opening into the oral cavity, called the primitive choana. The primary palate grows posteriorly from the intermaxillary process as a ridge to form the floor of the primitive nasal cavity.

In the eighth week, a pair of palatine shelves initially grows inferiorly from the maxillary swellings into the oral cavity, on either side of the tongue. The shelves rotate horizontally in the ninth week and fuse medially to form the secondary palate. The anterior portion of the secondary palate ossifies to form the hard palate, while muscles of the soft palate develop in its posterior portion. Meanwhile, the nasal septum grows inferiorly from the roof of the nasal cavity, fusing with the top of the hard palate to form two nasal passages that communicate with the pharynx through the definitive choanae.

Malformations of Lips and Palate (Figs. 1.11, 1.12 and 1.13) Cleft lips occur about once in 100 births. Males dominate by 60–80%. The

Fig. 1.10 Roof of the oral cavity, weeks 6–12, demonstrating the developing palate (from Moore and Persaud 2003, courtesy of Elsevier)

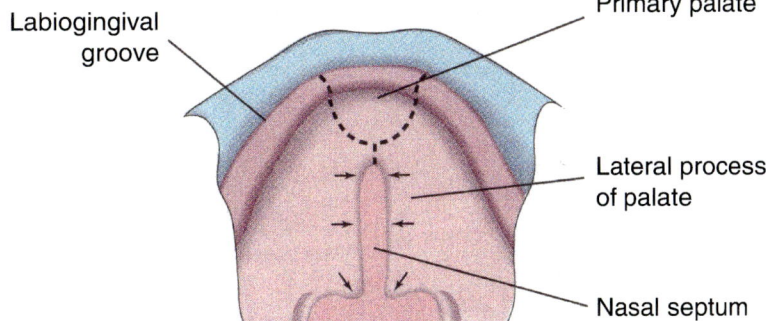

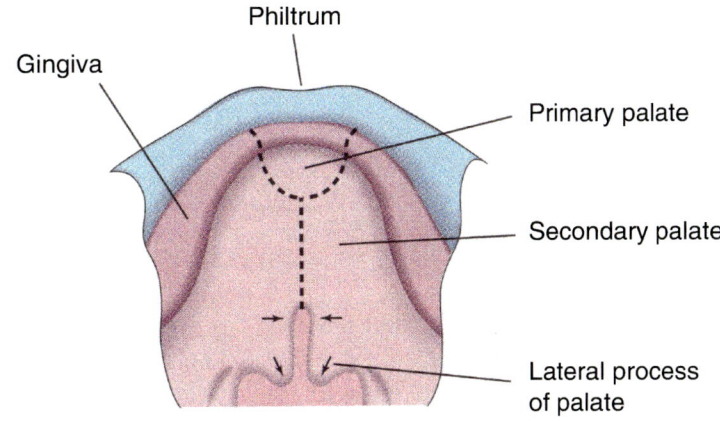

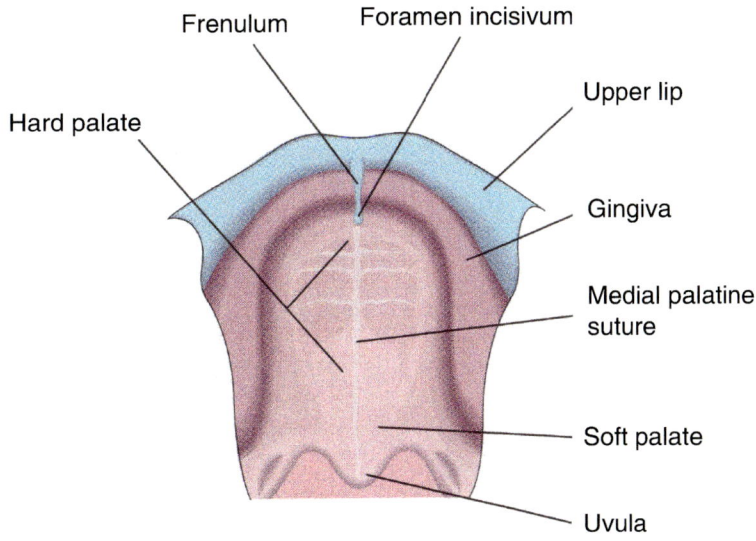

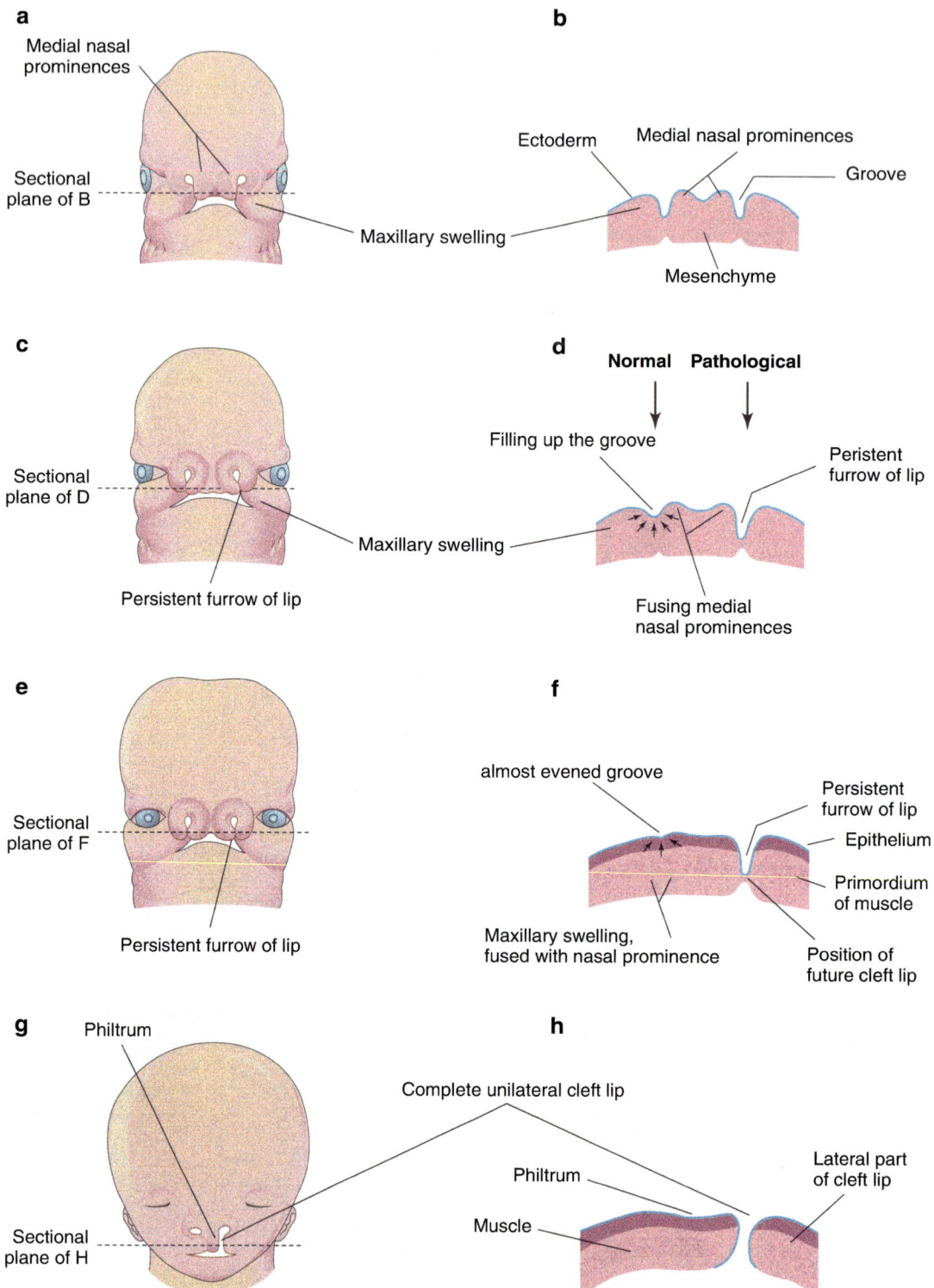

Fig. 1.11 Development of a cleft lip: (**a**, **c**, **e**, **g**): week 5, week 6, week 7, week 10, foetus with a complete unilateral cleft lip. (**b**, **d**, **f**, **h**): Horizontal section through the upper lip (from Moore and Persaud 2003, courtesy of Elsevier)

Fig. 1.12 Various forms of split palate: (**a**) Normal development. (**b**) Split uvula. (**c**) Unilateral cleft of the secondary palate (posterior cleft palate). (**d**) Bilateral cleft palate. (**e**) Complete unilateral cleft of the lip, the maxillary process and cleft between the primary and secondary palate. (**f**) Complete bilateral cleft of lip and maxillary process with continuation between the primary and secondary palate. (**g**) Complete bilateral cleft lip, cleft between primary and secondary palate and unilateral cleft of the secondary palate. (**h**) Complete bilateral cleft lip, cleft between primary and secondary palate and bilateral cleft of posterior palate (from Moore and Persaud 2003, courtesy of Elsevier)

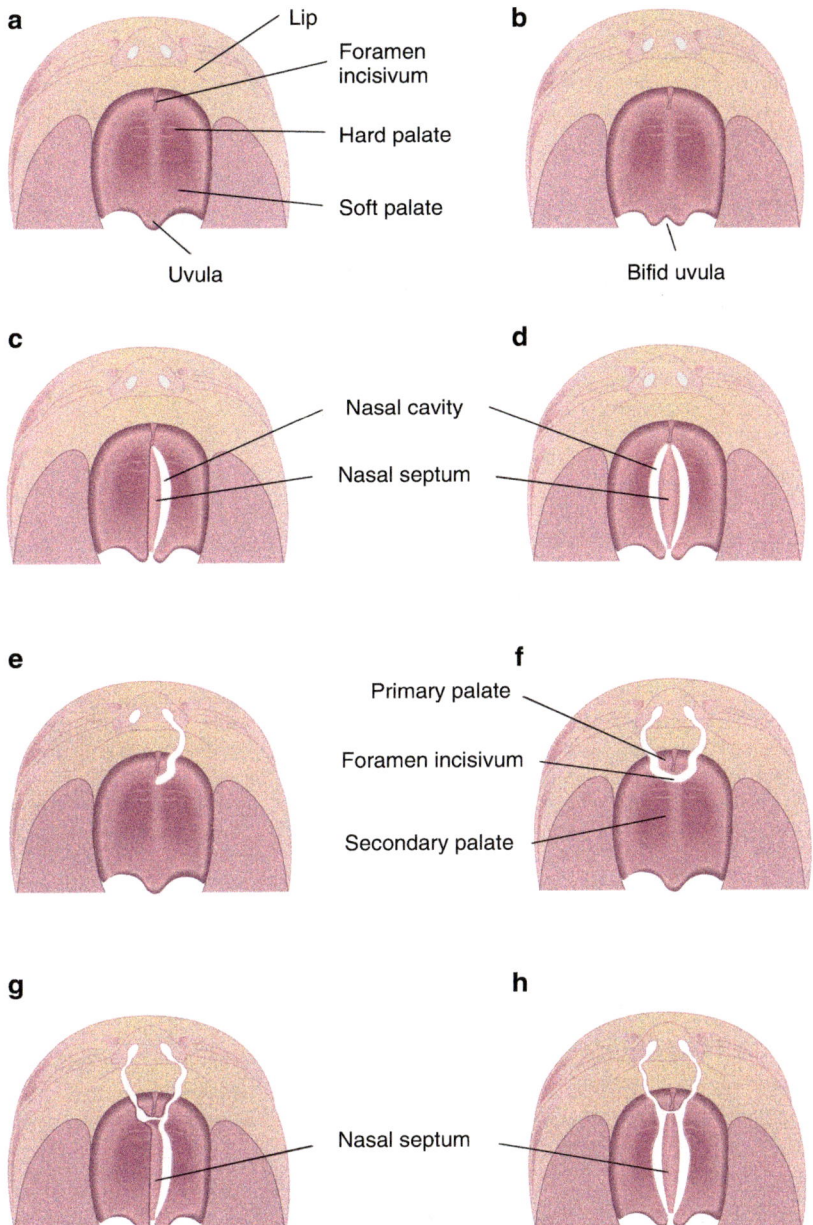

clefts vary from small notches in the red of the lip to larger gaps, including the floor of the nose and the alveolar process of the maxilla. They may appear uni- or bilaterally and are caused by a failure of the maxillary swelling and the nasal prominence to merge. The median cleft lip (Figs. 1.7, 1.8, 1.9, 1.10, 1.11, 1.12 and 1.13a) is an extremely rare malformation, probably induced by a deficiency of mesenchyme and an incomplete fusion of the medial nasal processes.

A split palate may occur solely or combined with a cleft lip. The cleft may be limited to the uvula but may extend across the soft and hard palate. The reason lies in an insufficient generation of mesenchyme, resulting in a dis-

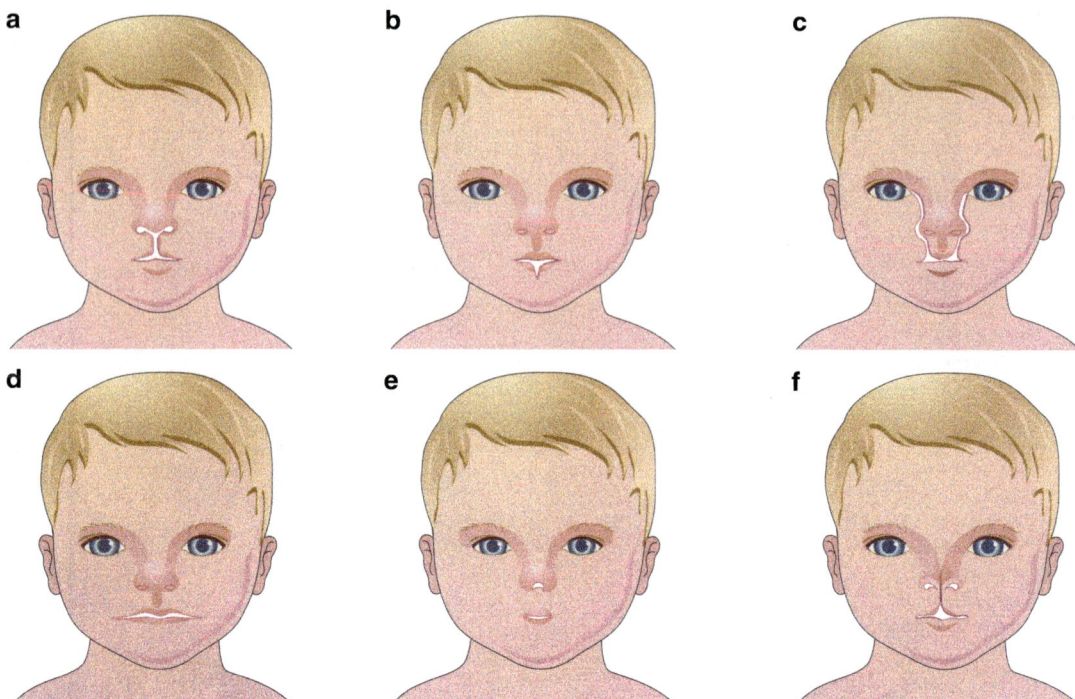

Fig. 1.13 Rare congenital anomalies of the face: (**a**) Median cleft of the upper lip. (**b**) Median cleft of the lower lip. (**c**) Bilateral oblique facial clefts and complete bilateral cleft lip. (**d**) Macrostomia. (**e**) Microstomia and singular nostril. (**f**) Split nose and incomplete cleft lip (from Moore and Persaud 2003, courtesy of Elsevier)

turbed fusion of the lateral maxillary shelves with the nasal septum and the posterior edge of the primary palate.

1.2.1.2 Pharyngeal Arches, Clefts and Pouches

During early development, five pharyngeal (branchial) arches are generated, which appear as bar-like ridges on the ventrolateral surface of the head and neck region. They are covered by ectoderm and are separated from each other by invaginations called pharyngeal clefts. The pharyngeal clefts have counterparts on the interior in the form of endoderm-lined pharyngeal pouches. Ectoderm and endoderm are isolated by a mesodermal core. Pharyngeal membranes separate the clefts from the pouches (Graham 2001).

The pharyngeal arches are numbered 1, 2, 3, 4 and 6; they develop in cranio-caudal sequence with the first pair appearing on day 22, the second and third pairs on day 24 and the fourth and sixth pairs on day 29. Each pharyngeal arch contains an arch cartilage, an arch artery, a mesodermal component as precursor for muscles and a specific cranial nerve.

The first branchial arch is divided into a maxillary and a mandibular process; the former develops to the palatopterygoquadrate bar cartilage, which will become the greater wing of the sphenoid and the incus; the latter contains Meckel's cartilage, a precursor of the malleus and the fibrous core of the mandible. The jaws mainly consist of membrane bones formed by direct ossification; the maxillary process gives rise to the upper jaw, the maxilla, the zygomatic and the temporal squama, and the mandibular process generates the lower jaw.

The second arch cartilage, Reichert's cartilage, forms the stapes, styloid process, stylohyoid ligament and parts of the hyoid. The third arch cartilage also contributes to the hyoid; the fourth and sixth arch cartilages form the larynx; and the

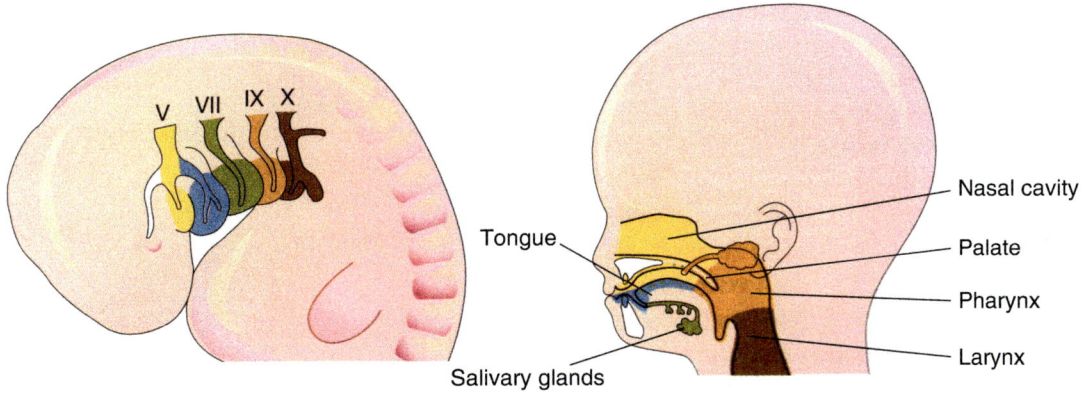

Derivates of branchial cartilages

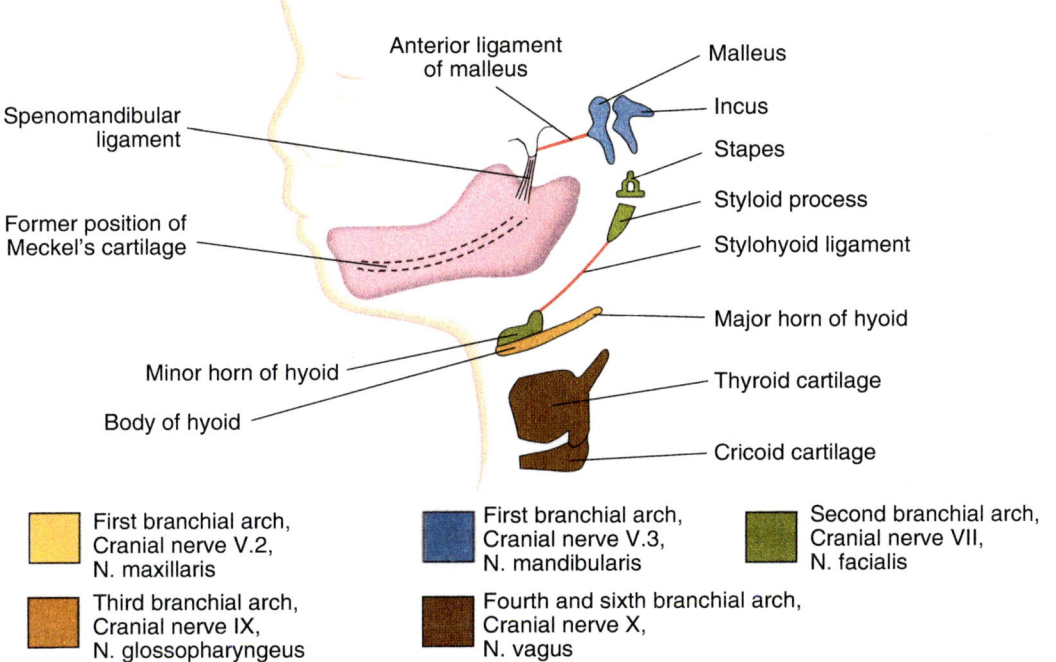

First branchial arch,
Cranial nerve V.2,
N. maxillaris

First branchial arch,
Cranial nerve V.3,
N. mandibularis

Second branchial arch,
Cranial nerve VII,
N. facialis

Third branchial arch,
Cranial nerve IX,
N. glossopharyngeus

Fourth and sixth branchial arch,
Cranial nerve X,
N. vagus

Fig. 1.14 Branchial arches, their innervation by cranial nerves and the definitive structures to which they develop (from Moore and Persaud 2003, courtesy of Elsevier)

epiglottis arises in the location of the fourth arch (Fig. 1.14).

The first arch is innervated by the trigeminal nerve, the maxillary swelling by V2 and the mandibular swelling by V3. The second arch is innervated by the facial nerve (VII), the third arch is innervated by the glossopharyngeal nerve (IX), the fourth arch is innervated by the superior branch and the sixth arch is innervated

by the recurrent laryngeal branch of the vagus nerve (X).

The following Table 1.1 summarises the derivatives of the five pharyngeal arches:

1.2.1.3 Development of the Larynx
Normal Development (Fig. 1.15) The respiratory system is an outgrowth of the primitive pharynx. Between the 20th and the 26th days

Table 1.1 Branchial arches and their derivatives

Arch/ nerve	Skeletal	Muscles	Ligaments	Pouch
First/V	Malleus Incus	Muscles of mastication Tensor tympani Tensor v. palatini Mylohyoid Ant. belly of digastric	Ant. Ligament of the malleus Sphenomandibular ligament	Auditory tube Tympanic cavity
Second/ VII	Stapes Styloid process Hyoid bone, minor horn, upper part of body	Mimic muscle system Stapedius Styloid Post. belly of digastric	Styloid ligament	Lining (crypts) of the palatine tonsils (lymphatic follicles have mesodermal origin)
Third/IX	Hyoid, major horn, lower part of the body	Stylopharyngeus	–	Thymus Lower parathyroid Gland
Fourth/X (sup.)	Cartilages of the larynx	Cricothyroid All muscles of the pharynx (except the stylopharyngeus) All muscles of the soft palate (except the tensor v. palatini)	–	Upper parathyroid gland Telopharyngeal body C cells of thyroid
Sixth/X (rec.)	Cartilages of the larynx	All intrinsic muscles of the larynx except the cricothyroid	–	–

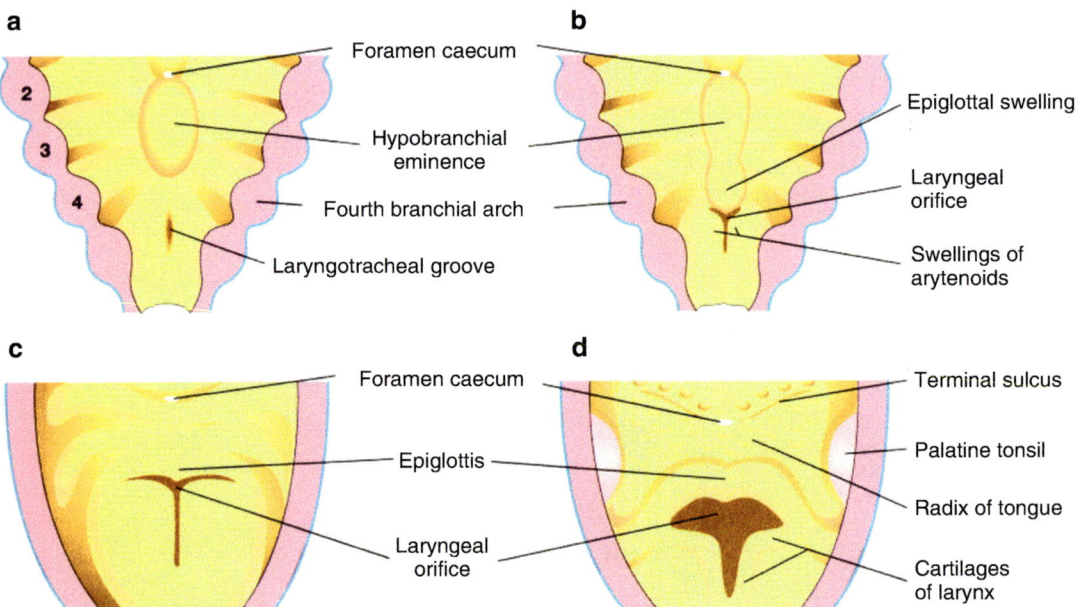

Fig. 1.15 Stages of laryngeal development. (**a**) Week 4. (**b**) Week 5. (**c**) Week 6. (**d**) Week 10 (from Moore and Persaud 2003, courtesy of Elsevier)

of gestation, a ventral laryngotracheal groove in the primitive foregut differentiates into the laryngeal sulcus and the respiratory primordium. The tracheo-oesophageal folds between these tubular hollows later fuse to form the tracheoesophageal septum, separating the laryngotracheal groove from the foregut. From now on the foregut is divided into the ventral laryngotracheal tube and the dorsal oesophagus.

The larynx develops from the fourth and sixth branchial arches. The laryngotracheal opening lies between these two arches. The internal lining of the larynx originates from endoderm, whereas cartilages and muscles emanate from mesenchyme. The mesenchyme proliferates rapidly, and the sagittal slit of the laryngeal orifice changes into a T-shaped opening by the growth of three tissue masses: one is the hypobranchial eminence, which later becomes the epiglottis. The second and third growths are two arytenoid precursors. They grow between the fifth and seventh week, resulting in a temporary occlusion of the lumen. Recanalisation occurs by the tenth week and produces a pair of lateral recesses, the laryngeal ventricles that are bounded by folds of tissue that differentiate into the false and true vocal cords. Failure to recanalise may result in atresia, stenosis or web formation in the larynx.

The development of the larynx begins with the appearance of the mesenchymal-arytenoid swellings from the sixth branchial arches on the 32nd day of gestation on both sides of the opening of the laryngotracheal tube. These swellings approach each other in the midline and converge at the caudal end of the hypobranchial eminence to convert the vertical laryngotracheal opening into a T-shaped aditus. Midline compression of the tube by these swellings results in the fusion of the epithelial lamina, thereby closing the tube from the pharynx. If the closing does not occur, a posterior laryngeal cleft can result leading to severe aspiration in the newborn. The arytenoid swellings differentiate into the arytenoid and corniculate cartilages and the primitive aryepiglottal folds.

The epiglottal and cuneiform cartilages are formed by the hypobranchial eminence. Chondrification of both fourth branchial arches gives rise to the thyroid cartilage, whereas the cricoid cartilage derives from the chondral tissue of the sixth branchial arch. The laryngeal lumen obliterates to give rise to the epithelial lamina. The larynx recanalises by the tenth week of gestation.

The intrinsic muscles have gained their shapes and positions by the 40th day of gestation, and by the end of the eighth week, all components of the larynx are present including innervation and blood supply.

During the foetal period, the vocal processes develop from the arytenoids, and the thyroid cartilage laminae fuse in the midline. The epiglottal cartilage matures between the fifth and seventh months. During this period, the corniculate and cuneiform cartilages become evident. The foetal period ends with the cricoid cartilage changing from interstitial to perichondrial growth.

Malformations of the Larynx (Figs. 1.16, 1.17 and 1.18) From the location of laryngeal malformations (Sidrah et al. 2007), one discriminates between supraglottal, glottal and subglottal anomalies.

The most abundant congenital anomaly of the larynx is the laryngomalacia, accounting for more than a half of all cases (Ahmad and Soliman 2007). The ratio between males and

Fig. 1.16
Laryngomalacia:
(**a**) anterior prolapse.
(**b**) Posterior prolapse
(from Rutter and Dickson 2014, courtesy of Elsevier)

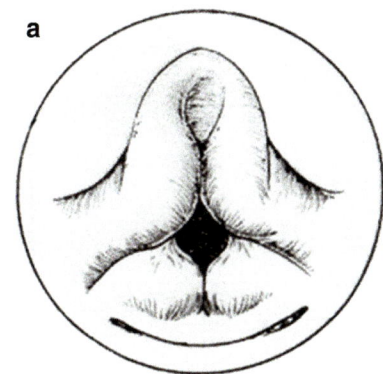
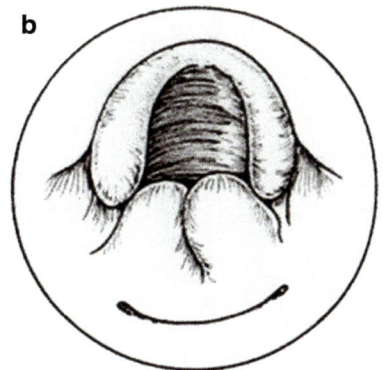

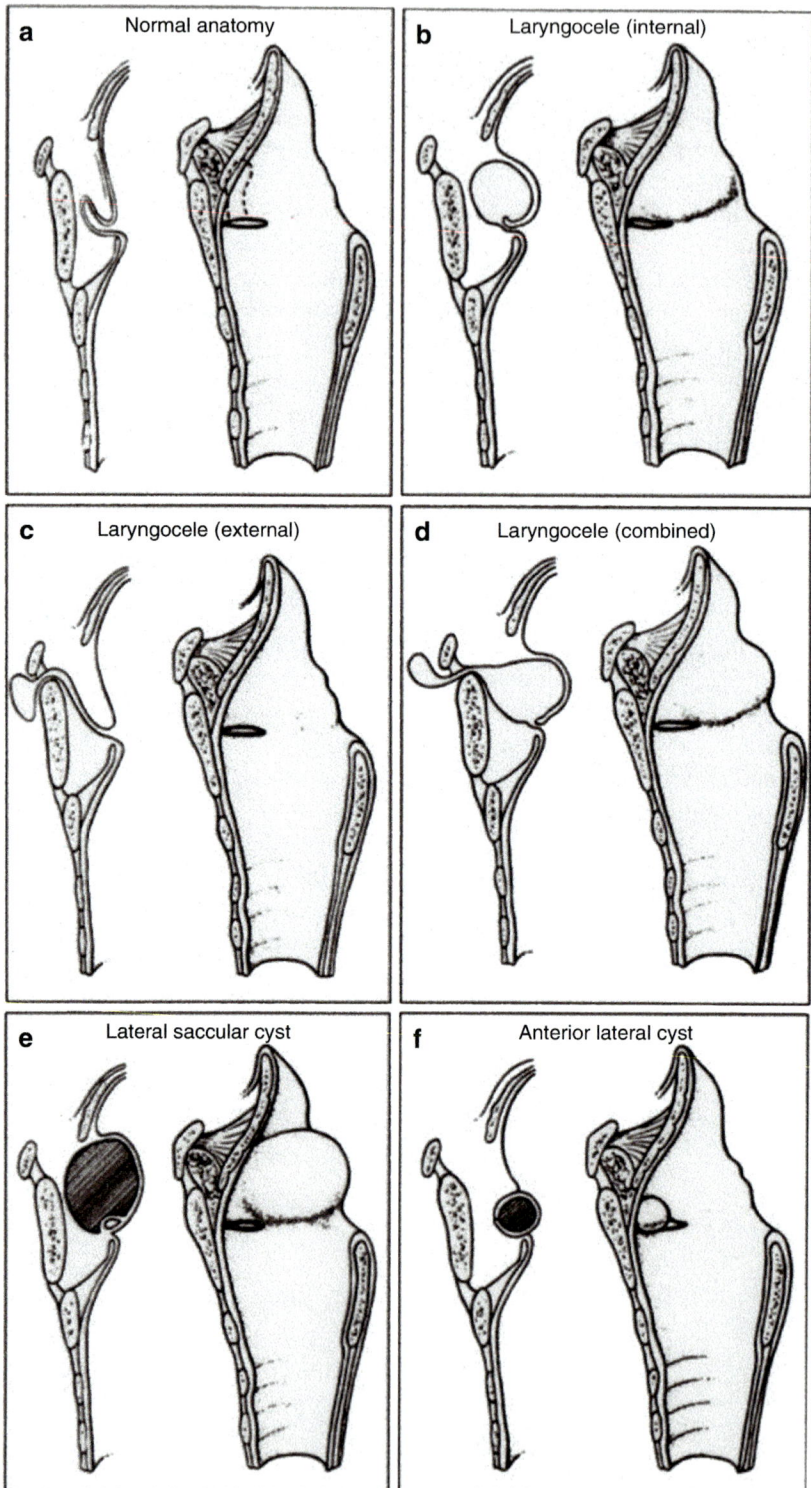

Fig. 1.17 (**a**) Differences between laryngoceles (**b–d**) and saccular cysts (**e, f**) (from Rutter and Dickson 2014, courtesy of Elsevier)

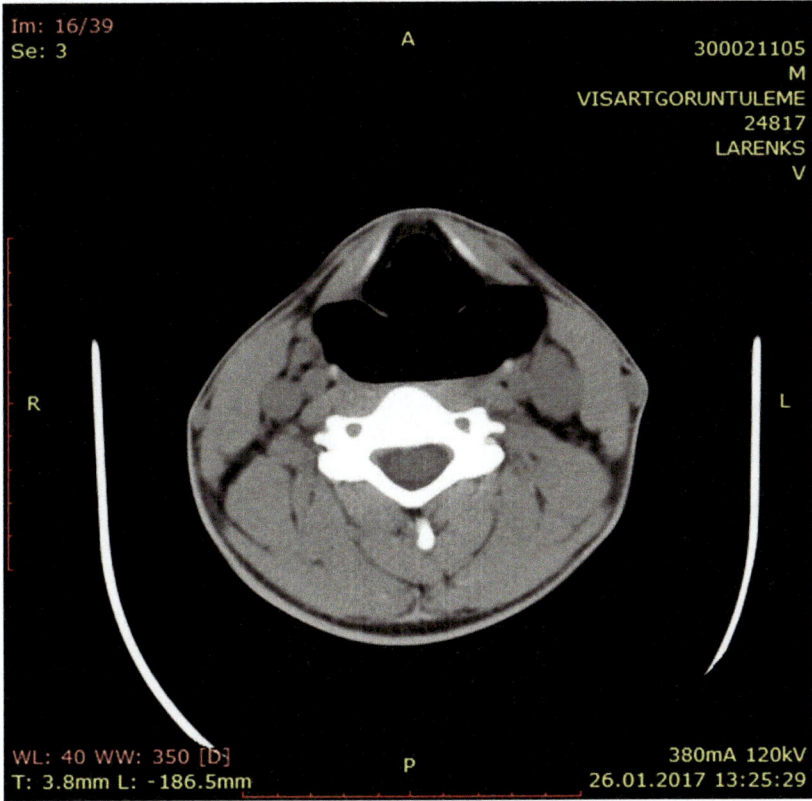

Fig. 1.17 (**b**) Computerised tomographic view of a patient with combined laryngocele. Prof. Dr. Haldun Oguz, personal archive photo, with permission

Fig. 1.18 Four types of laryngeal cleft: supraglottal interarytenoid cleft, partial cricoid cleft, total cricoid cleft and laryngo-oesophageal cleft (from left to right) (from Rutter and Dickson 2014, courtesy of Elsevier)

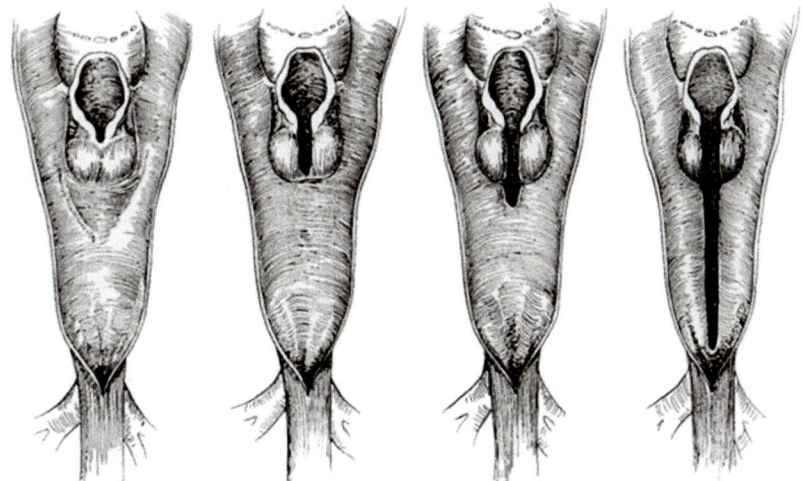

females is about 2:1. It is classified as Type 1, Type 2 or Type 3 on the basis of patterns of supraglottal collapse. In Type 1 laryngomalacia, redundant supraglottal mucosa prolapses; Type 2 is characterised by shortened aryepiglottic folds; and Type 3 displays posterior displacement of the epiglottis coincident with a deformation, due to an imbalance in its development. The epiglottis develops from the cartilages of the third and fourth branchial arches, and an overgrowth of the third arch portion results in an omega-shaped organ. In addition, an arytenoid prolapse may result from immature neuromuscular control.

The second-most common congenital laryngeal disorder, in about 15–20% of all congenital anomalies, affects vocal fold movement. It may occur unilaterally or, less frequently, bilaterally. Unilateral paralysis is usually idiopathic but may be secondary to peripheral nerve pathology. Strain injuries to the recurrent laryngeal nerve during birth may be one of the causes.

The glottal sulcus (or sulcus vocalis) is characterised by dysphonia due to hampered movement of the mucous membrane, absence of Reinke's space and adhesion of the epithelium to the vocal ligament or the vocal muscle itself.

The congenital subglottal stenosis takes third place in laryngeal anomalies with approximately 15% of the cases, twice as often in boys than in girls. It may be subdivided into two types, the more abundant is membranous congenital subglottal stenosis, due to submucosal hypertrophy. The second, cartilaginous congenital subglottal stenosis, results from an abnormal growth of the cricoid cartilage.

Subglottal haemangioma accounts for 1.5% of congenital anomalies of the larynx, in girls twice as often than in boys. It results from a malformation of the mesenchymal vascular precursors.

Laryngoceles are rare congenital anomalies of the supraglottal larynx. They form as a result of air- or fluid-filled dilations of the laryngeal ventricle communicating with the laryngeal lumen. They may occur internally or externally or both.

About 25% of all laryngeal cysts are saccular cysts. In contrast to the laryngoceles, they do not communicate with the laryngeal lumen.

Laryngeal webs are rare congenital anomalies. They are due to an incomplete recanalisation of the laryngotracheal tube, which occurs in the third month of gestation. They appear mostly at the anterior level of the vocal folds.

Laryngeal or laryngotracheo-oesophageal clefts are posterior fusion defects between the airway and oesophagus during embryogenesis.

These clefts may be minor and short or may even extend beyond the carina. They are classified according to their anatomical extent.

Laryngeal atresia is considered to be the rarest of the congenital anomalies of the larynx. It occurs when the recanalisation of the laryngotracheal tube during the third month of gestation fails.

1.2.1.4 Tongue Development

Normal Development (Figs. 1.19, 1.20 and 1.21) Tongue development starts with a triangular elevation in the floor of the first pharyngeal arch during the end of the fourth week of gestation, which is called the median tongue bud (tuberculum impar). A pair of mesenchymal swellings in the ventromedial areas of the first pharyngeal arch forms the distal tongue buds (lateral lingual swellings) on either side of the tongue. They are covered by epithelium of ectodermal origin, overgrow the median tongue bud and fuse medially to form the midline sulcus. Sensory innervation of this part is by the lingual branch of the mandibular division of the trigeminal nerve, the nerve of the first pharyngeal arch.

Behind the foramen cecum, the second pharyngeal arch develops the copula in the midline. A second elevation, arising from the third and partly the fourth pharyngeal arch, forms the hypobranchial eminence, which will become the pharyngeal part of the tongue.

The copula is overgrown by the hypobranchial eminence in the fifth and sixth week. It will fuse anteriorly with the distal tongue buds, thereby creating the terminal sulcus.

The median and pharyngeal sections of the organ then become joined at the terminal sulcus. This posterior compartment of the tongue is innervated by the glossopharyngeal nerve, the nerve of the third pharyngeal arch, whereas the chorda tympani from the cranial nerve VII supplies the taste buds on the anterior two thirds. The growing tongue extends out into the oral cavity; its anterior part is covered by a layer of ectodermal epithelium. In contrast, the root of the tongue is covered with endodermal epithelium.

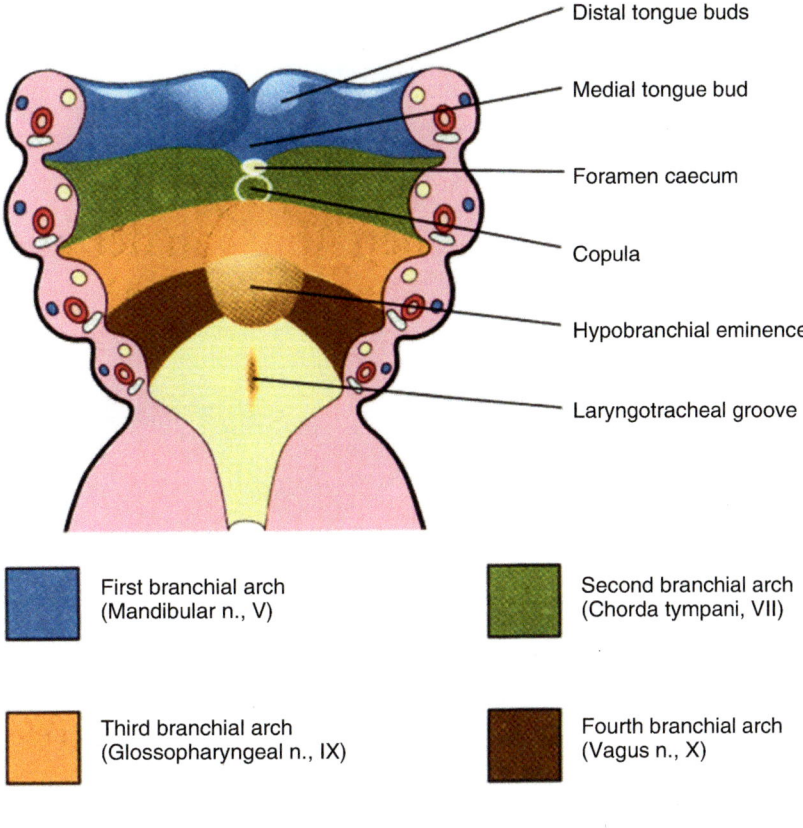

Fig. 1.19 Tongue development, early phase from the fourth week on (from Moore and Persaud 2003, courtesy of Elsevier)

Distal tongue buds

Medial tongue bud

Foramen caecum

Copula

Hypobranchial eminence

Laryngotracheal groove

First branchial arch (Mandibular n., V)

Second branchial arch (Chorda tympani, VII)

Third branchial arch (Glossopharyngeal n., IX)

Fourth branchial arch (Vagus n., X)

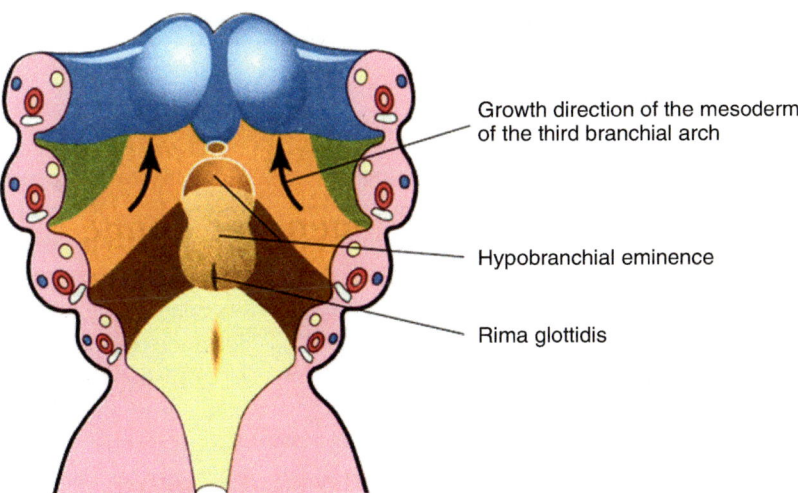

Fig. 1.20 Tongue development, later stage, fourth to fifth month (from Moore and Persaud 2003, courtesy of Elsevier)

Growth direction of the mesoderm of the third branchial arch

Hypobranchial eminence

Rima glottidis

So far, only the epithelial and mucosal tissues of the tongue have been considered, which develop from the four pharyngeal swellings as described above. The muscular compartment of the tongue descends from myoblasts that differentiate after migrating from the myotomes of the occipital cervical somites. Following these myoblasts is the hypoglossal nerve, which generates the nerve supply for the tongue musculature.

Tongue Abnormalities The tongue may vary in its size from microglossia, an abnormal

Fig. 1.21 Adult tongue, indicating the derivatives of the branchial arches (from Moore and Persaud 2003, courtesy of Elsevier)

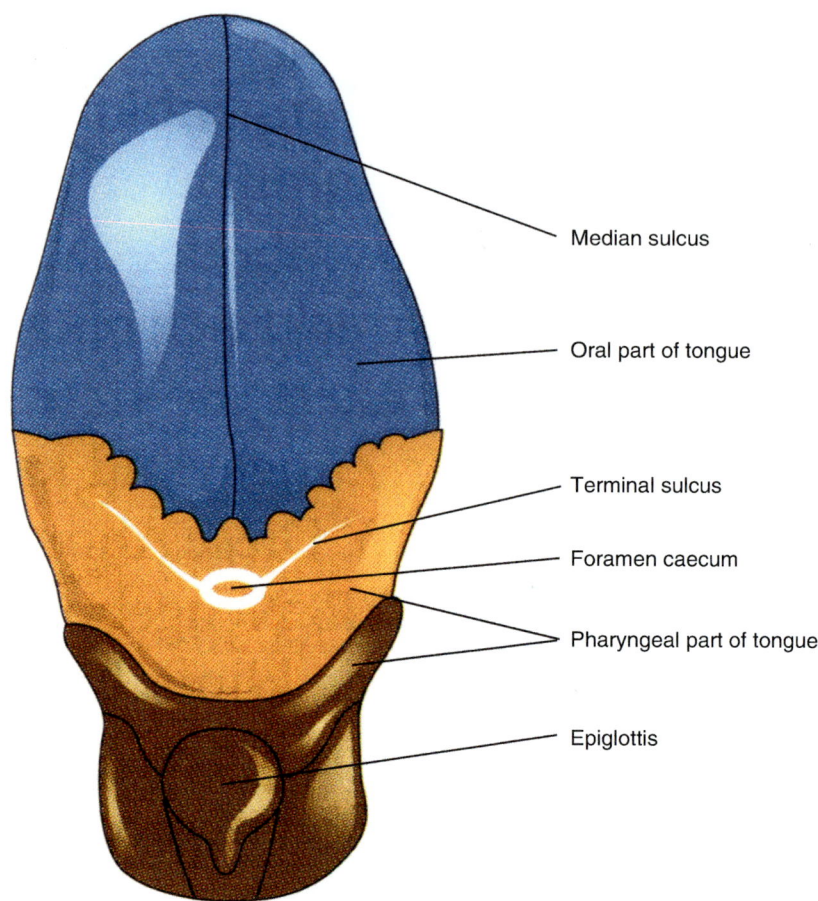

Median sulcus

Oral part of tongue

Terminal sulcus

Foramen caecum

Pharyngeal part of tongue

Epiglottis

smallness of the tongue, which occurs very rarely, to macroglossia, a more abundant phenomenon, which means that the tongue is extraordinarily large.

Ankyloglossia affects the frenulum of the tongue; it develops short and thick and fixes the tongue to the floor of the mouth (tongue-tied) or at least restricts the movement of the tongue.

A cleft or bifid tongue has a cleft running vertically right across it. Complete clefting is extremely rare and occurs as a result of lack of developmental forces that push both halves of the tongue towards each other. Partial clefting presents as a deep groove in the middle of the tongue.

When the two lateral parts of the tongue fail to overgrowth the tuberculum impar, a bald patch will appear in the centre of the tongue, known as medial rhomboid glossitis.

1.2.1.5 Development of the Ear

Inner Ear, Normal Development (Figs. 1.22 and 1.23) In the third week of embryonic development, the ectoderm on both sides of the rhombencephalon (hindbrain) begins to thicken and form the otic placodes. They shift caudally to the level of the second pharyngeal arch and invaginate during the fourth week to form the otic pits. The pits separate from the surface to form the otic vesicles, which are the precursors of the membranous labyrinth.

Each otic vesicle differentiates into three parts: a dorsomedial, elongated endolymphatic extension, origin of the endolymphatic duct and, at its distal end, the endolymphatic sac; a central partition, which will expand to form the utricle and the three semicircular ducts, arising from utricular diverticula; and a ventral, conical sac-

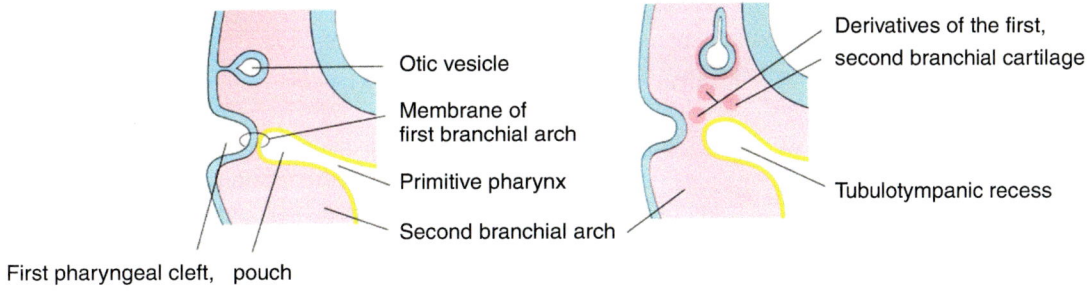

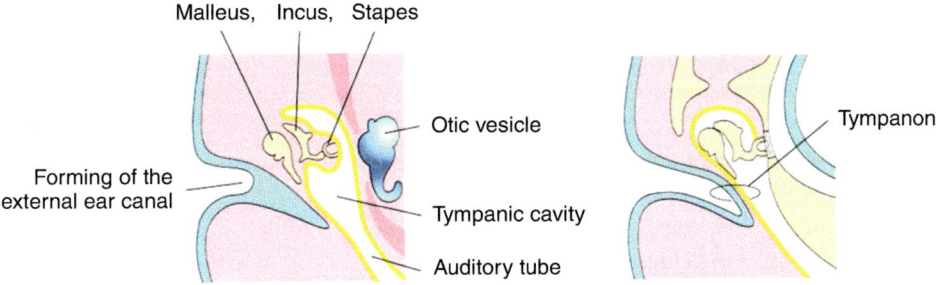

Fig. 1.22 Development of the ear: week 4, 5 (top left, right) and two later stages (bottom left, right) (from Moore and Persaud 2003, courtesy of Elsevier)

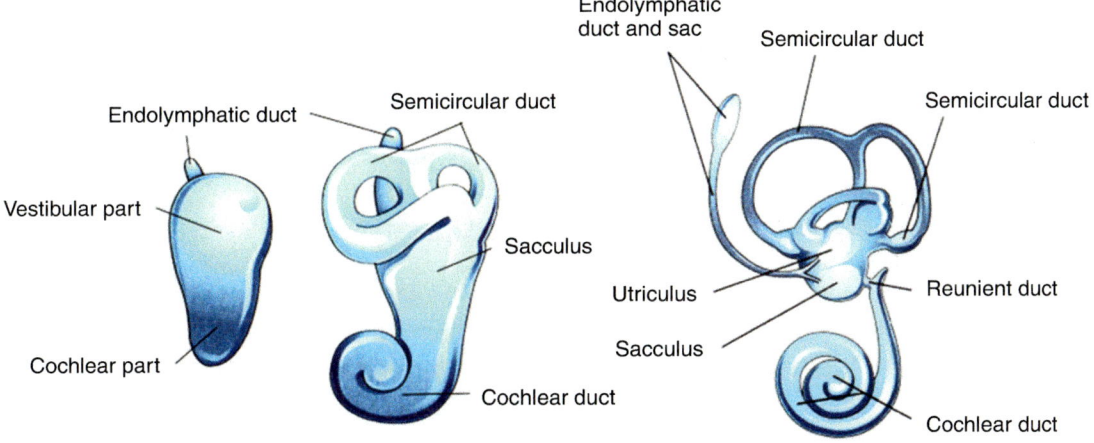

Fig. 1.23 Development of the otic vesicle, weeks 5–8 (from Moore and Persaud 2003, courtesy of Elsevier)

cular region, which forms the saccule and the cochlear duct, as well as the ductus reuniens joining the saccule and cochlear duct. The duct elongates in the fifth week and starts to coil, with the spiral organ of Corti differentiating in the seventh week. By this time, the organ of Corti is inner-vated by the cochlear ganglion, which will elongate and wind up together with the organ of Corti.

At the end of the ninth month, the auricular pathway is completed; myelinisation, however, has not taken place, and axo-dendritic synapses are not yet established.

Malformations of the Inner Ear Malformations in otic vesicle development result in anomalies of the membranous labyrinth and its bony envelope as well. In descending order of intensity and time course of appearance during development, they are complete labyrinthine aplasia; cochlear aplasia; common cavity (single cystic cavity of coalesced cochlea and vestibulum); cochlear hypoplasia; incomplete partition Type I, II or III; and enlargement of the vestibular or cochlear aqueduct.

Tympanic Cavity, Normal Development The first pharyngeal pouch elongates to form the tubotympanic recess, which will give rise to the tympanic cavity and the auditory tube. By the seventh week, the auditory ossicles begin to condense within the mesenchyme of the first and second pharyngeal arches, whereas the muscles of the middle ear begin to form in the ninth week. The cartilage of malleus and incus develop within the first pharyngeal arch, and its mesoderm gives rise to the tensor tympani muscle, which will be innervated by the nerve of the first pharyngeal arch, the mandibular nerve (CN V/3). The cartilage of the stapes is formed within the second pharyngeal arch, as well as the stapedius muscle. It is therefore innervated by the facial nerve (CN VII), which is the nerve of the second pharyngeal arch.

The first pharyngeal cleft develops to the external acoustic meatus, and the membrane, separating the first pharyngeal cleft from the first pharyngeal pouch, becomes the tympanic membrane, which consists of three layers: an outer covering of ectoderm, a mesodermal layer (the fibrous stratum) and an inner lining of endoderm.

In the ninth month, the ossicles assume their functional relationships, with the malleus attaching to the eardrum and the stapes attaching to the oval window. Sound vibrations can now be transmitted from the eardrum to the cochlea via the ossicles and oval window and then transduced into neural impulses via the organ of Corti.

Malformations of the Middle Ear The close relationship of the external ear canal and the tympanic cavity gave rise to the classification of a common malformation termed atresia auris congenita:

- First-degree malformations are characterised by moderate deformations of the external ear canal, a normal or slightly hypoplastic tympanic cavity, deformed ossicles and normal pneumatisation of the mastoid.
- The second-degree malformation exhibits intermediate deformities including an absence of the external ear canal or its blind ending, a narrow tympanic cavity, deformations and fixations of the ossicles and reduced mastoid pneumatisation.
- Third-degree malformations include the absence of an external ear canal, hypoplastic tympanic cavity, severely deformed ossicles and a failure in mastoid pneumatisation.

External Ear, Normal Development (Fig. 1.24) Each of the adjacent ectodermal parts of the first and second pharyngeal arches differentiates into three auricular hillocks. They arise in the fifth week. In the seventh week, the auricular hillocks begin to enlarge, differentiate and fuse, producing the final shape of the ear, which is gradually translocated from the side of the neck to a more cranial and lateral site. The first pharyngeal arch gives rise to the tragus, the helix and the cymba conchae; the second pharyngeal arch forms the antitragus, the antihelix and the concha.

Anomalies of the External Ear Malformations of the external ear have their causes in an inaccurate development of a single or a combination of several auricular hillocks. They result in deformities of three grades of severity: dysplasia grade I represents only a slight deformation, most elements of a normal pinna are present. Moderate deformations are summarised in dysplasia grade II. Only some structures of a normal ear are identifiable. Dysplasia grade III is characterised by severe deformations. Nothing of a normal pinna is recognisable.

Fig. 1.24 Development of the external ear (from Paulsen et al. 2010, courtesy of Elsevier)

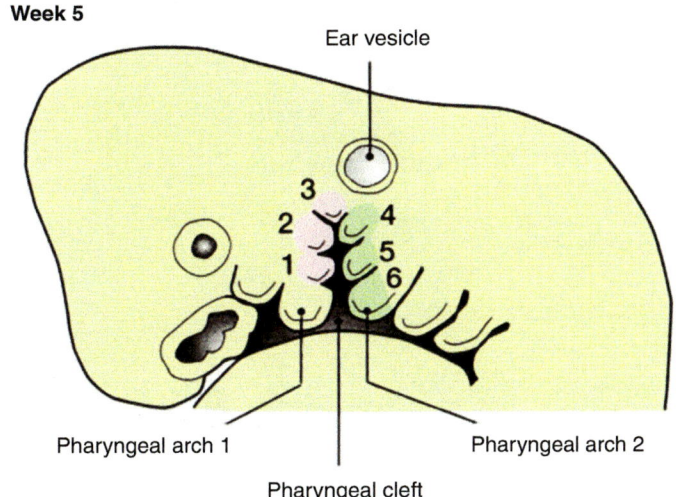

Week 5

Ear vesicle

Pharyngeal arch 1

Pharyngeal cleft

Pharyngeal arch 2

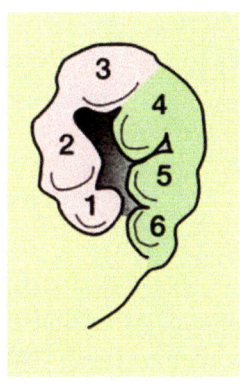

Week 7

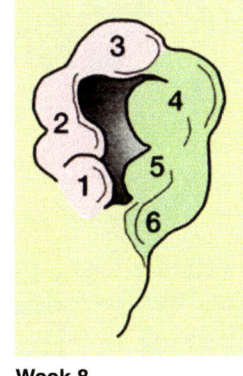

Week 8

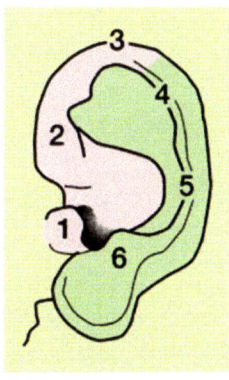

Birth

Malformations may be further classified according to the size of the auricle (macrotia, microtia, anotia), the shape of the ear (cup-shaped, lop ear, ear dysplasia, elfin (pointed) ear, lobe malformations), the position of the ears (melotia, low set ears, synotia) and other malformations such as auricular fistulas or appendages.

1.2.2 Anatomy

1.2.2.1 The Palate

The hard palate is generated by two types of bone, which are covered by a mucous membrane: the palatine processes of the maxillae and the horizontal parts of the palatine bones (Fig. 1.25).

These bones continue into the soft palate, which contains a membranous aponeurosis. The soft palate, also called velum palatinum, is a movable, fibromuscular fold that is attached to the posterior edge of the hard palate. It separates the superior nasopharynx from the inferior oropharynx. Laterally, the soft palate is continuous with the wall of the pharynx and is joined to the tongue and pharynx by the palatoglossal and palatopharyngeal folds.

The components are as follows:

The levator veli palatini, extending from the cartilage of the auditory tube and petrous part of temporal bone to the palatine aponeurosis. It elevates the soft palate, drawing it superiorly and posteriorly and also opens the auditory tube to

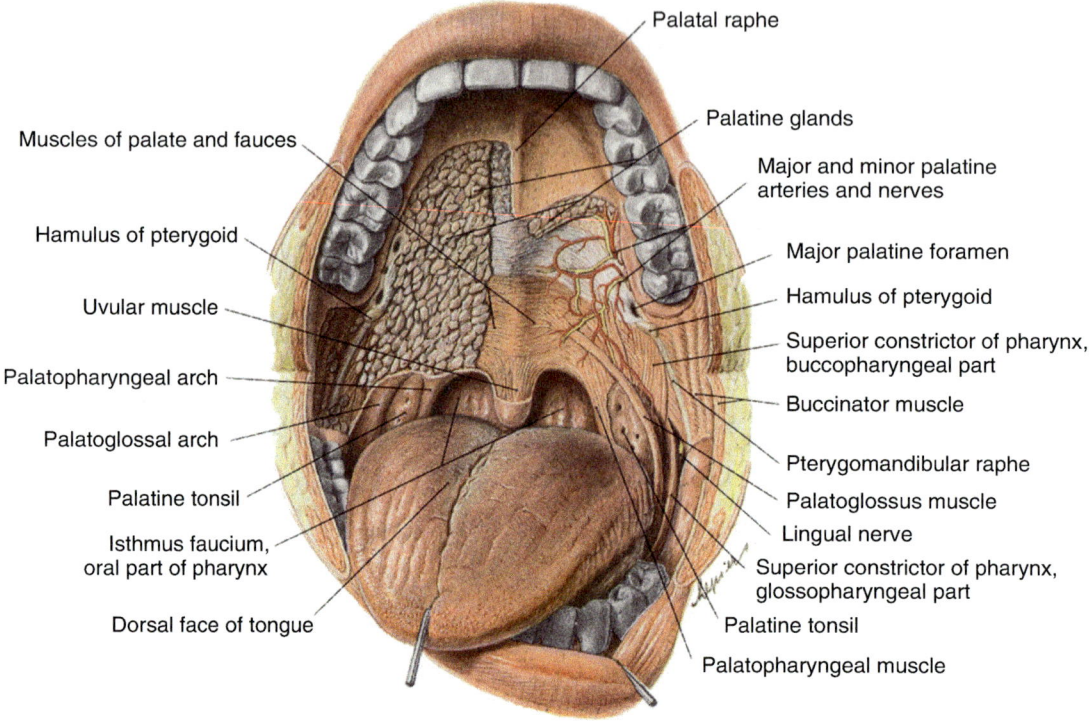

Palatal raphe

Muscles of palate and fauces

Hamulus of pterygoid

Uvular muscle

Palatopharyngeal arch

Palatoglossal arch

Palatine tonsil

Isthmus faucium,
oral part of pharynx

Dorsal face of tongue

Palatine glands

Major and minor palatine
arteries and nerves

Major palatine foramen

Hamulus of pterygoid

Superior constrictor of pharynx,
buccopharyngeal part

Buccinator muscle

Pterygomandibular raphe

Palatoglossus muscle

Lingual nerve

Superior constrictor of pharynx,
glossopharyngeal part

Palatine tonsil

Palatopharyngeal muscle

Fig. 1.25 Aspect of the mouth and palate (from Paulsen et al. 2010, courtesy of Elsevier)

regulate air pressure in the middle ear. It is innervated by a pharyngeal branch of the vagus via the pharyngeal plexus.

The tensor veli palatini arises from the scaphoid fossa of the medial pterygoid plate, spine of sphenoid bone and cartilage of auditory tube to the palatine aponeurosis. It tenses the soft palate by using the hamulus as a pulley. It also acts on the membranous portion of the auditory tube in the same sense as the levator muscle. Innervation is through the medial pterygoid nerve (a branch of the mandibular nerve).

The musculus uvulae, which emanates at the posterior nasal spine and palatine aponeurosis and inserts into the mucosa of uvula. When the muscle contracts, it shortens the uvula and pulls it upwards. The pharyngeal branch of vagus innervates the muscle via the pharyngeal plexus.

The palatoglossus muscle between the palatine aponeurosis and the side of tongue. The mucous membrane covering the muscle forms the palatoglossal arch. The muscle elevates the posterior part of the tongue and draws the soft palate downwards onto the tongue.

The palatopharyngeus muscle, extending from the hard palate and palatine aponeurosis to the lateral wall of pharynx. Its mucous membrane forms the palatopharyngeal arch. The muscle tenses the soft palate and pulls the walls of the pharynx upwards, forwards and medially during swallowing. Both muscles are supplied by the cranial part of accessory nerve (CN XI) joining with the pharyngeal branch of vagus via the pharyngeal plexus.

The sensory nerves of the palate, which are branches of the pterygopalatine ganglion, are the greater (major) and lesser (minor) palatine nerves (Fig. 1.26). They accompany the arteries through the greater and lesser palatine foramina, respectively.

The palate has an abundant blood supply from branches of the maxillary artery.

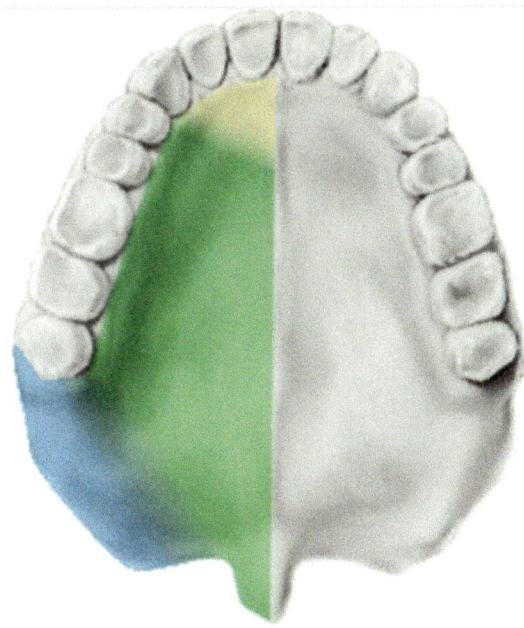

Sensory innervation of soft palate

☐ Nasopalatine nerve

▇ Major palatine nerve

▇ Minor palatine nerves

Fig. 1.26 Sensory innervation of the soft palate

1.2.2.2 The Pharynx

The pharynx is a fibromuscular tube that spans vertically from the base of the skull to the oesophagus. Being situated posterior to the nasal and oral cavities and posterior to the larynx, it is therefore divisible into the nasopharynx, oropharynx and laryngopharynx, which ends at the inferior border of the cricoid cartilage, where it becomes continuous with the oesophagus.

The anterior part of the nasopharynx communicates through the choanae with the nasal cavities. Its lateral walls contain the pharyngeal ostia of the auditory tube, bounded behind by the torus tubarius, a prominence of the mucous membrane caused by the medial end of the cartilage of the tube. On the posterior wall of the nasopharynx, an assembly of lymphatic tissue is located, known as the pharyngeal tonsil.

The oropharynx, or mesopharynx, lies behind the oral cavity, extending from the uvula to the level of the hyoid bone. It opens anteriorly, through the isthmus faucium, into the mouth. The anterior wall consists of the base of the tongue; the superior wall consists of the inferior surface of the soft palate and the uvula. Its entrance, the isthmus faucium, is formed by the palatoglossal and palatopharyngeal arches of each side of the oral cavity, between them the palatine tonsil is positioned.

The laryngopharynx extends from the superior border of the epiglottis to the inferior border of the cricoid cartilage, where it becomes continuous with the oesophagus. Its anterior wall is the rear of the epiglottis and the posterior aspects of the arytenoid and cricoid cartilages. The piriform recess is part of the cavity of the laryngopharynx, situated on each side of the inlet of the larynx.

The lateral and posterior walls (Fig. 1.27) of the three parts of the pharynx are formed by various muscles: two of them, the palatopharyngeal muscle with its origin in the soft palate and the salpingopharyngeal muscle, originating at the auditory tube, are longitudinally orientated and form the innermost muscular layer. They are covered by the three constrictors, the upper (superior), middle and lower (inferior) constrictor muscle.

These three pharyngeal constrictors originate from antero-laterally placed structures:

- The superior constrictor emanates from the pterygomandibular raphe, the pterygoid hamulus and the buccinator ridge of the mandible. The right and left muscles run posteriorly and superiorly. Their superior attachment is to the pharyngeal tubercle on the base of the skull, and the largest part of the muscle meets its companion muscle from the opposite side to form a midline pharyngeal raphe.

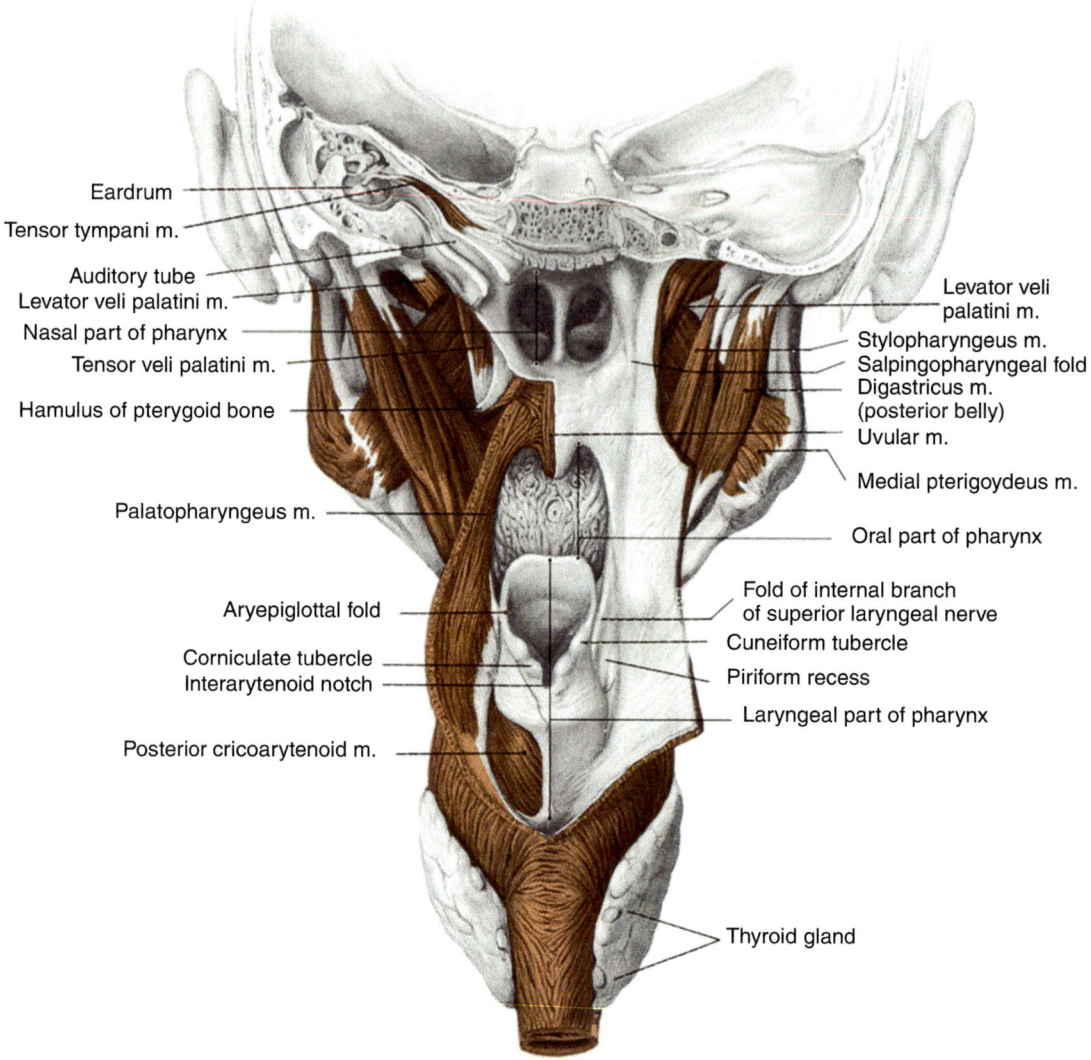

Fig. 1.27 Dorsal aspect of the pharynx (from Benninghoff and Drenckhahn 2003, courtesy of Elsevier)

- The middle constrictor originates from the hyoid bone and the stylohyoid ligament and meets its partner at the pharyngeal raphe.
- The inferior constrictor originates from the oblique line on the cricoid and thyroid cartilages. It meets its partner to contribute to the midline posterior raphe.

Finally, the stylopharyngeus muscle, beginning at the styloid process, runs into a gap between the upper and the middle constrictor and ends at the thyroid cartilage. All of these muscles are of the striated type.

Altogether, the tubulo-muscular wall of the pharynx consists of four layers: a mucous membrane, the pharyngeal aponeurosis, the muscle layer and the buccopharyngeal fascia.

The motor nervous and most of the sensory nervous supply to the pharynx is by way of the pharyngeal plexus, which, situated mainly on the middle constrictor, is formed by the pharyngeal branches of the vagus and glossopharyngeal nerves and also by sympathetic nerve fibres.

Blood supply of the pharynx is ensured by pharyngeal branches of the ascending pharyngeal artery, ascending palatine artery, descending palatine artery and pharyngeal branches of inferior thyroid artery. Veins collect the blood into the pharyngeal plexus.

1.2.2.3 The Larynx

The larynx is located in the anterior neck, ventrally of the cervical vertebrae 3–6. It connects the pharynx with the trachea and regulates the flow of air to and from the lungs for respiration and vocalisation and guards the air passages against food and liquids entering it. Its ventral prominence is called Adam's apple. The larynx extends from the tip of the epiglottis to the inferior border of the cricoid cartilage. Its interior can be divided into three parts, the supraglottis, the transglottis and the subglottis (see below).

The skeleton of the larynx is composed of nine cartilages, three single and three paired (Fig. 1.28):

First is the thyroid cartilage, of hyaline nature. Its superior margin and its superior horn are attached to the hyoid bone by the thyrohyoid membrane, centrally and laterally enhanced as the medial or lateral thyrohyoid ligament. Its inferior horn connects to the cricoid cartilage and takes part in the cricothyroid articulation.

The hyaline cricoid cartilage is situated below the thyroid cartilage. It is the only one that encircles the entire larynx. It is attached to the thyroid cartilage via the median cricothyroid ligament and to the first ring of the trachea via the cricotracheal ligament.

Two mostly hyaline arytenoid cartilages of pyramidal shape are positioned dorsally on the superior margin of the cricoid cartilage. They are connected to the vocal ligaments by their vocal process, and their muscular process serves for muscular attachment. Each of them has an elastic corniculate cartilage on its top. The latter connect to the cricoid cartilage via the posterior cricoarytenoid ligament.

Behind the thyroid cartilage protrudes the epiglottis, a spoon-shaped elastic cartilage, which is connected to the thyroid cartilage by the thyroepiglottic ligament. It contacts the arytenoid cartilages via the quadrangular membrane, into which two elastic cuneiform cartilages are embedded.

The most prominent and most important ligaments of the larynx are the vocal ligaments, converging from the vocal processes of the arytenoids to the posterior surface of the thyroid. They serve as a margin for the conus elasticus, extending downwards to the cricoid cartilage.

Two pairs of joints affect the vocal ligaments: the cricothyroid joints allow tilting, and to a small extent gliding between the thyroid and cricoid cartilage, they thereby stretch or loosen the vocal ligaments. The cartilages move by action of the straight and oblique parts of the external cricothyroid muscle (Fig. 1.29). The muscle is innervated by the superior laryngeal nerve, which branches from the main trunk of the vagus nerve.

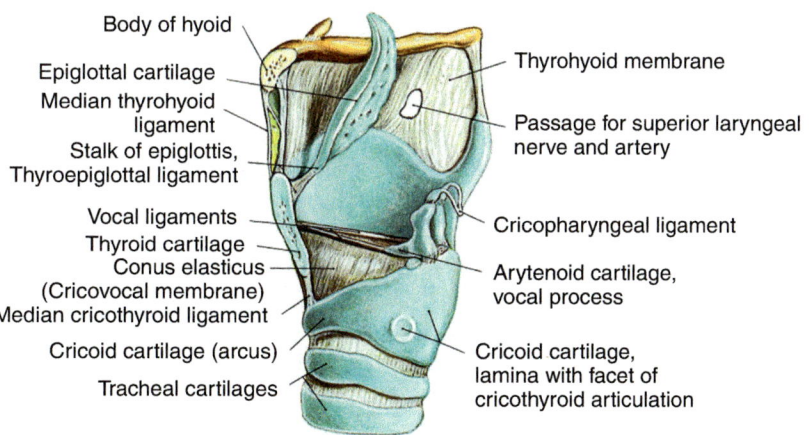

Fig. 1.28 Skeleton of the larynx, the thyroid cartilage has been dissected (from Paulsen et al. 2010, courtesy of Elsevier)

Body of hyoid

Epiglottal cartilage
Median thyrohyoid ligament
Stalk of epiglottis, Thyroepiglottal ligament

Vocal ligaments
Thyroid cartilage
Conus elasticus (Cricovocal membrane)
Median cricothyroid ligament

Cricoid cartilage (arcus)

Tracheal cartilages

Thyrohyoid membrane

Passage for superior laryngeal nerve and artery

Cricopharyngeal ligament

Arytenoid cartilage, vocal process

Cricoid cartilage, lamina with facet of cricothyroid articulation

34

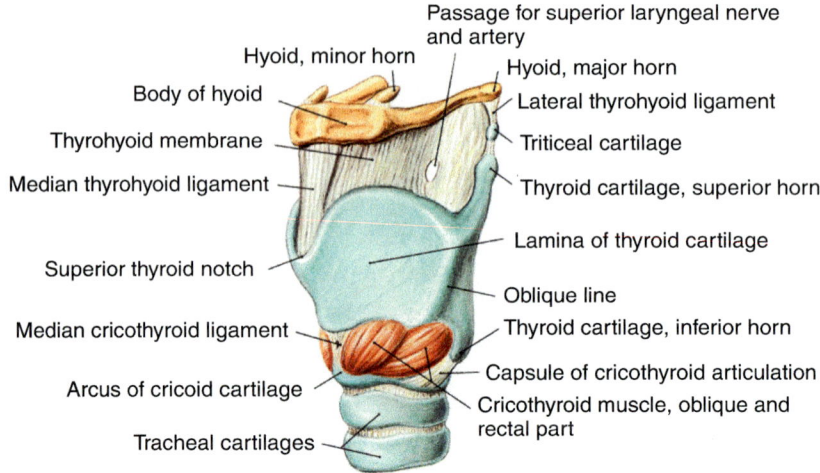

Fig. 1.29 Outer muscles of the larynx (from Paulsen et al. 2010, courtesy of Elsevier)

Hyoid, minor horn

Body of hyoid

Thyrohyoid membrane

Median thyrohyoid ligament

Superior thyroid notch

Median cricothyroid ligament

Arcus of cricoid cartilage

Tracheal cartilages

Passage for superior laryngeal nerve and artery

Hyoid, major horn

Lateral thyrohyoid ligament

Triticeal cartilage

Thyroid cartilage, superior horn

Lamina of thyroid cartilage

Oblique line

Thyroid cartilage, inferior horn

Capsule of cricothyroid articulation

Cricothyroid muscle, oblique and rectal part

The cricoarytenoid joints permit gliding and rotation of the arytenoid cartilages, thus changing the positions of the vocal ligaments. Adductors of the vocal ligaments are the lateral cricoarytenoid muscle, the oblique and transverse arytenoid muscles and the vocalis muscle (by increasing its diameter in isometric contraction). The posterior cricoarytenoid muscle acts as an abductor of the vocal ligaments, whereas the aryepiglottic, thyroarytenoid and vocalis muscles are effective in reducing the tension of the vocal ligaments (Fig. 1.30). All of these muscles are innervated by the recurrent laryngeal nerve, a branch of the vagus nerve.

The internal cavity of the larynx (Fig. 1.31) is divided into three parts. It starts with the vestibule of larynx (supraglottis), the laryngeal inlet, which extends from the upper border of the epiglottis down to the ventricular folds. These are mucus membrane folds forming the lower free edge of the quadrangular membrane, they run from the thyroid cartilage above the vocal ligament to the arytenoid cartilages. They contain large sero-mucous glands, which serve to moisten the vocal folds. The vestibule continues into the ventricle of the larynx (transglottis), which extends between the vestibular and vocal folds.

The vocal folds extend from the angle of thyroid to the vocal processes of arytenoid cartilages. They are important for phonation by controlling the stream of air through the rima

glottidis, the variable cleavage between them. They alter the shape and size of the wedge-shaped rima glottidis by movement of the arytenoids to ensure respiration or phonation.

Below the vocal folds, the subglottal space extends to the lower border of the cricoid cartilage.

On both sides of the laryngeal inlet, the piriform recesses ensure continuity between the pharynx and the beginning of the oesophagus, where they meet. They are bordered medially by the aryepiglottic fold, laterally by the thyroid cartilage and the thyrohyoid membrane (Fig. 1.32).

The epithelium of the vocal fold (Fig. 1.33) is of the non-keratinised stratified squamous type. It changes to a ciliated pseudostratified epithelium on the posterior glottis, ventricular folds and trachea. The lamina propria may be divided into three layers according to its histological composition: a superficial layer, pliable and flexible, also called Reinke' space, of loose connective tissue. It is densely interwoven with the epithelium by digital projections containing small vessels. It continues into an intermediate and a deep layer. There is an increase in the presence of fibrous and interstitial proteins in the intermediate and, to a greater extent, in the deep layer of the lamina propria, both making up the vocal ligament. The intermediate layer is marked with a distinct elevation in the relative amount of elastin and collagen, and this increases even more within the

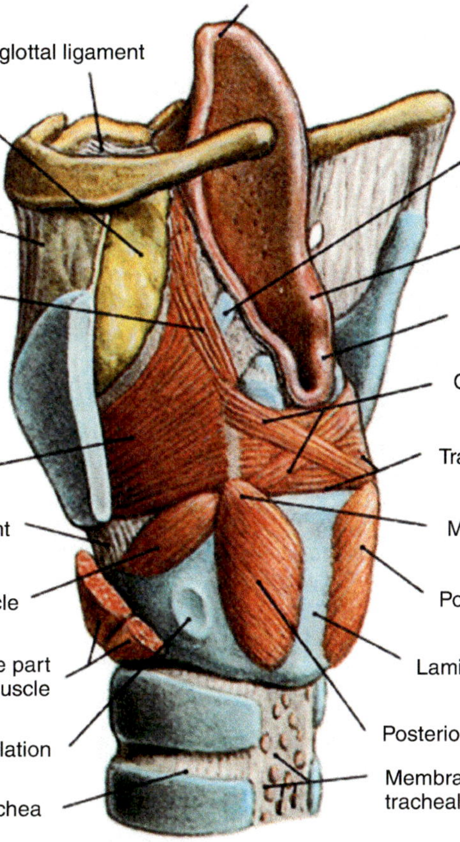

Epiglottis

Hypoepiglottal ligament

Laryngeal fat body

Cuneiform cartilage

Thyrohyoid membrane

Cuneiform tubercle

Aryepiglottal muscle

Corniculate tubercle

Oblique arytenoid muscles

Thyroarytenoid muscle

Transverse arytenoid muscle

Median cricothyroid ligament

Muscular process of arytenoid cartilage

Lateral cricoarytenoid muscle

Posterior cricoarytenoid muscle

Rectal and oblique part
of cricothyroid muscle

Lamina of cricoid cartilage

Facet of cricothyroid articulation

Posterior cricoarytenoid muscle

Annular ligament of trachea

Membranceal part of trachea with
tracheal glandules

Fig. 1.30 Inner muscles of the larynx (from Paulsen et al. 2010, courtesy of Elsevier)

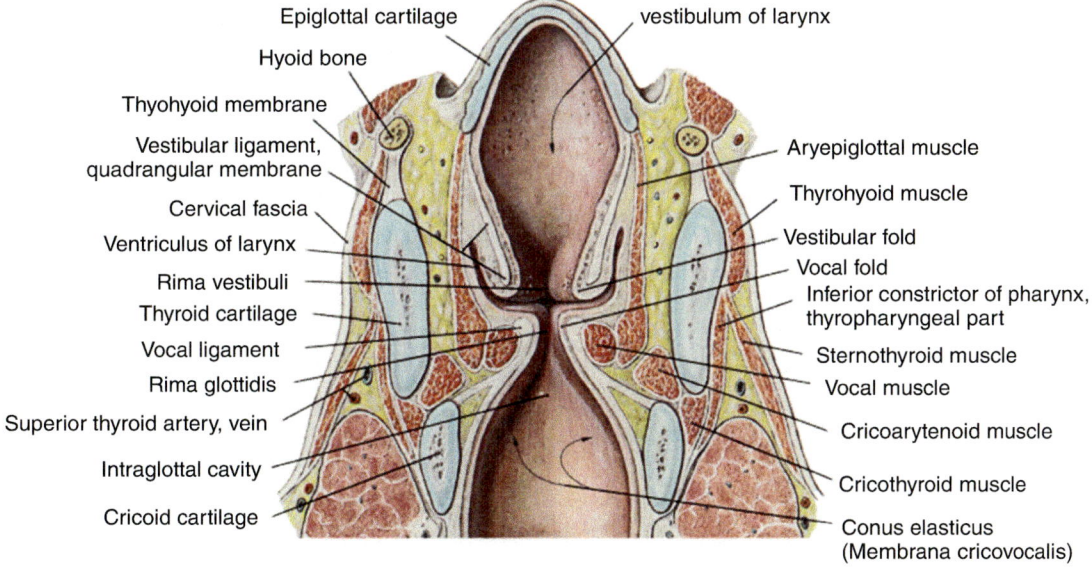

Epiglottal cartilage

vestibulum of larynx

Hyoid bone

Thyohyoid membrane

Vestibular ligament,
quadrangular membrane

Aryepiglottal muscle

Thyrohyoid muscle

Cervical fascia

Ventriculus of larynx

Vestibular fold

Rima vestibuli

Vocal fold

Thyroid cartilage

Inferior constrictor of pharynx,
thyropharyngeal part

Vocal ligament

Sternothyroid muscle

Rima glottidis

Vocal muscle

Superior thyroid artery, vein

Cricoarytenoid muscle

Intraglottal cavity

Cricothyroid muscle

Cricoid cartilage

Conus elasticus
(Membrana cricovocalis)

Fig. 1.31 Interior of the larynx seen from the dorsal aspect (from Paulsen et al. 2010, courtesy of Elsevier)

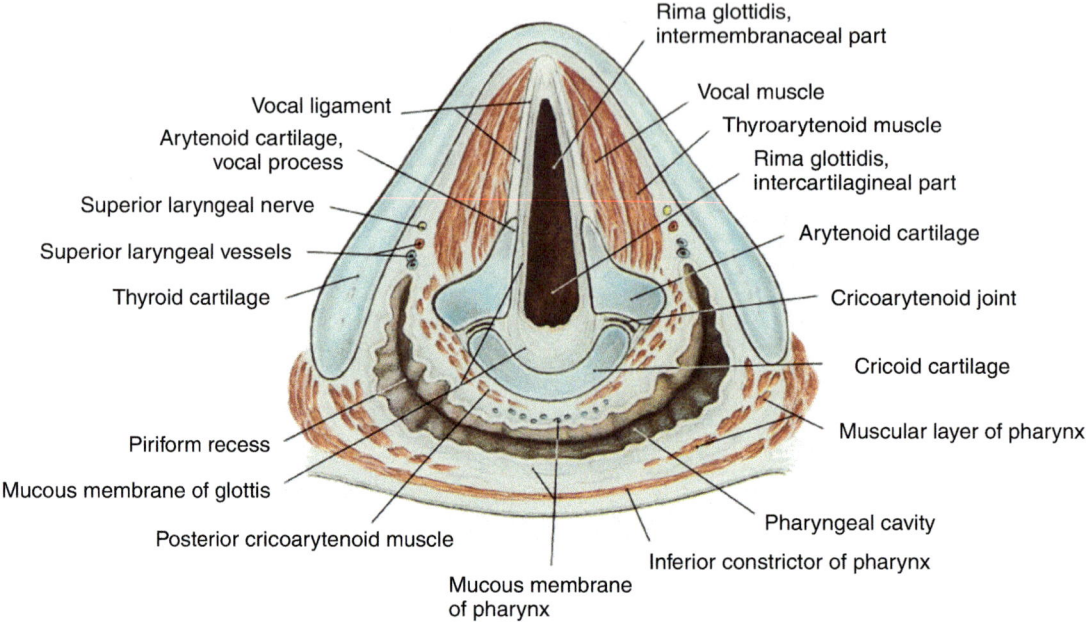

Rima glottidis, intermembranaceal part

Vocal ligament

Arytenoid cartilage, vocal process

Superior laryngeal nerve

Superior laryngeal vessels

Thyroid cartilage

Vocal muscle

Thyroarytenoid muscle

Rima glottidis, intercartilagineal part

Arytenoid cartilage

Cricoarytenoid joint

Cricoid cartilage

Muscular layer of pharynx

Piriform recess

Mucous membrane of glottis

Posterior cricoarytenoid muscle

Mucous membrane of pharynx

Pharyngeal cavity

Inferior constrictor of pharynx

Fig. 1.32 Horizontal section of the larynx above the vocal ligaments (from Paulsen et al. 2010, courtesy of Elsevier)

Fig. 1.33 Histology of the vocal fold (from Klinger and Schramm 2001, courtesy of Prof. Klinger)

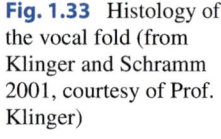

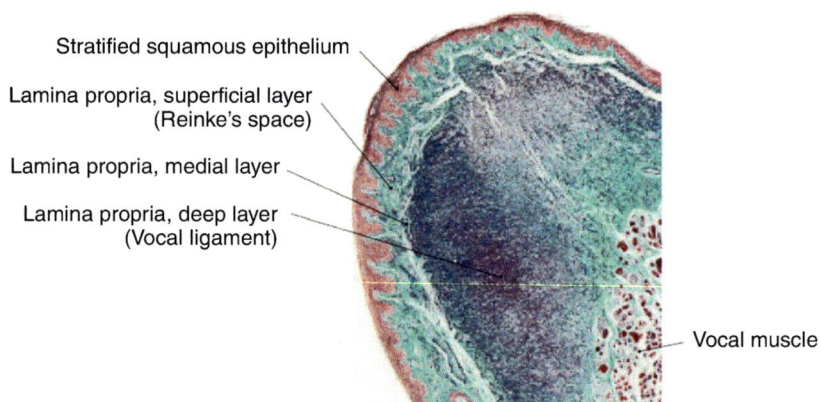

Stratified squamous epithelium

Lamina propria, superficial layer (Reinke's space)

Lamina propria, medial layer

Lamina propria, deep layer (Vocal ligament)

Vocal muscle

deep layer (Jette and Thibeault 2011). The deep layer is adjacent to the vocal muscle, which may be considered as a medial part of the thyroarytenoid muscle.

The larynx as a whole is embedded into the vertically running muscle cords of the anterior neck (Fig. 1.34). Two longer muscles, the sternohyoid and the omohyoid, cover a group of shorter muscles ventrally, inserting directly at the thyroid. These extrinsic muscles may be divided into two groups: to the elevators (mainly suprahyoid muscles) of the larynx belong muscles that pull

the hyoid upwards (the digastric muscle, the mylohyoid, the genioglossus, the stylohyoid and the stylopharyngeus) and, acting directly on the thyroid, the thyrohyoid muscle; depressors of the larynx are the sternothyroid, the omohyoid and the sternohyoid muscle, the latter two by pulling the hyoid downwards.

The entire larynx is innervated by the vagus nerve: the nerve separates a superior branch that leaves the main trunk high in the neck. Approximately at the level of the hyoid bone, this superior laryngeal nerve divides into an external

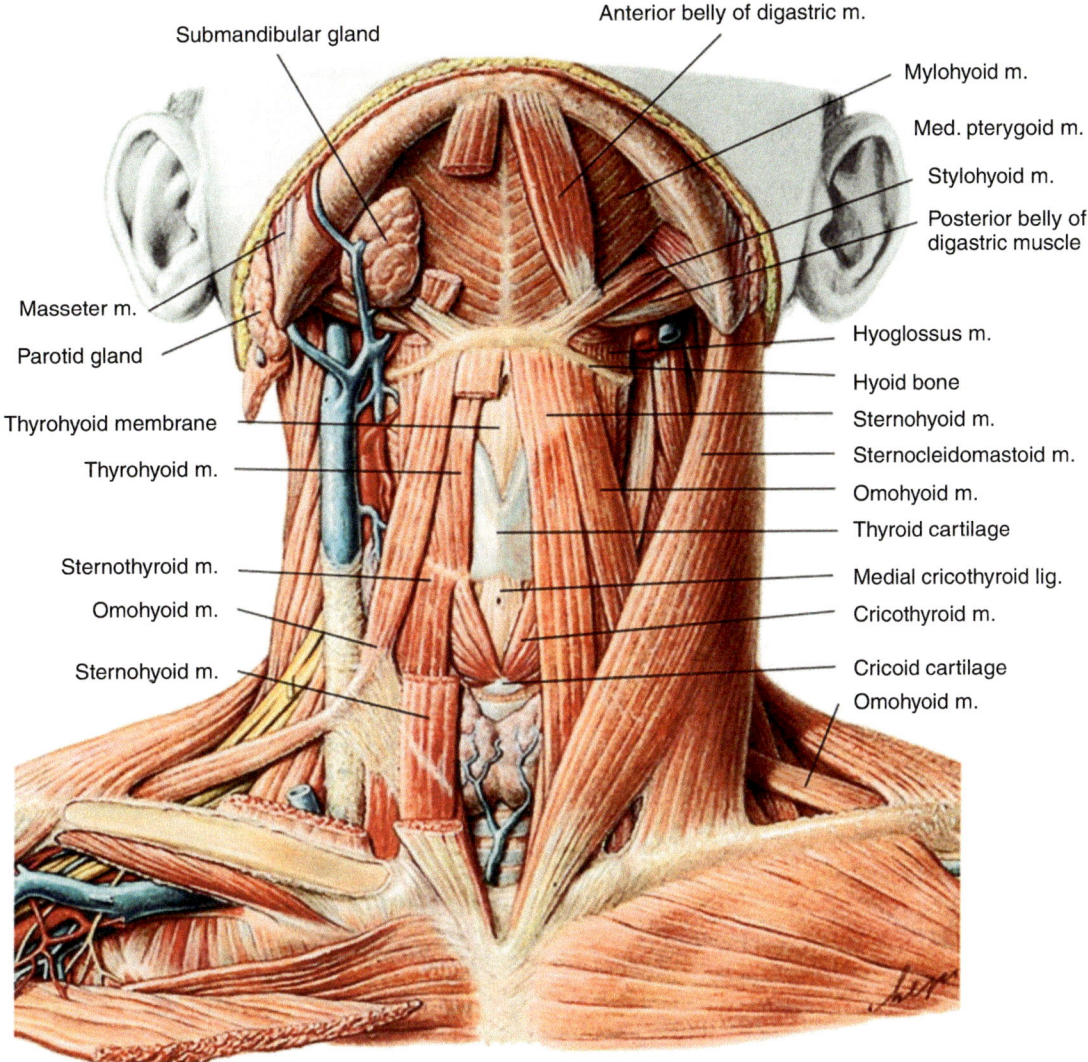

Fig. 1.34 Muscles of the anterior neck (from Paulsen et al. 2010, courtesy of Elsevier)

and an internal branch. The only function of the external branch is the motoric innervation of the cricothyroid muscle.

The internal branch passes through a foramen in the thyrohyoid membrane together with the superior laryngeal artery and vein. It provides general sensation, including pain, touch and temperature for the tissue superior to the vocal folds.

The lower part of the larynx is supplied by the recurrent laryngeal nerve. It contains motor fibres to innervate all the intrinsic muscles of the larynx—except for the cricothyroid muscle—as well as both sensory and secretory fibres to the glottis, subglottis and trachea. The right recurrent laryngeal nerve leaves the vagus nerve, which parallels the internal jugular vein, near the point where the brachiocephalic trunk divides. The left recurrent laryngeal nerve emanates from the vagus nerve near the aortic arch. Both branches cross dorsally below the adjacent vessel and ascend laterally next to the trachea. They often terminate in forming an anastomosis with the ipsilateral internal branch of the superior laryngeal nerve.

The larynx has its arterial supply from the superior laryngeal artery, a branch of the superior thyroid artery, which accompanies the internal laryngeal nerve, and by the inferior laryngeal artery from the inferior thyroid artery, which runs parallel to the recurrent laryngeal nerve.

1.2.2.4 The Tongue

The relaxed tongue takes up most of the space inside the oral cavity. It basically comprises muscles surrounded by a mucous membrane. The posterior one third of the tongue, the root, is attached to the floor of the oral cavity. The mobile anterior two thirds of the tongue is called the body, and the tip is the apex.

The surface, or dorsum, contains numerous projections of the mucous membrane called papillae. They contain taste buds, which can sense five types of sensations: sweet, salty, sour, bitter and umami, which is a savoury meaty flavour. In addition, serous glands of the mucosa secrete some of the fluid of the saliva.

The inferior surface of the tongue is covered by a thin transparent membrane. A large fold of mucosa, called the frenulum, runs down the midline. The ducts of the submandibular salivary glands open at the base of the frenulum.

The muscles of the tongue are divided by the lingual septum. Four pairs are intrinsic, and four pairs are extrinsic (Table 1.2, Fig. 1.35).

All muscles of the tongue, except for the palatoglossus, are innervated by the hypoglossal nerve (CN XII). The palatoglossus is innervated by the pharyngeal plexus (CN X).

The somatosensory innervation of the anterior two thirds of the tongue comes with the mandibular nerve via the lingual nerve; the visceral sensory innervation is by the facial nerve via the chorda tympani. The posterior 1/3 part of the tongue has somatosensory and visceral innervation from the glossopharyngeal nerve. The somatosensory innervation of the root is by the vagus nerve (Fig. 1.36).

The tongue gains its blood by the lingual artery, a branch of the external carotid artery. It is drained by lingual veins, which continue into internal jugular vein.

1.2.2.5 Swallowing

Swallowing is a complex series of sequential neuromuscular events that are integrated into a smooth and continuous process, which is divided into three stages: oral, pharyngeal and oesophageal.

Table 1.2 Internal and external muscles of the tongue

Muscles	Origin	Insertion	Function
Internals			
Superior longitudinal muscle	Submucosal fibrous layer and septum	Margins of the tongue and mucous membrane	Curls the tongue upwards and shortens it
Inferior longitudinal muscle	Root of the tongue and hyoid bone	Apex	Curls the tongue downwards and shortens it
Transverse muscle	Septum of the tongue	Lateral margins of the tongue	Narrows and protrudes the tongue
Vertical muscle	Submucosal fibrous layer of the dorsum of the tongue	Inferior surfaces of the borders of the tongue	Flattens and broadens the tongue
Externals			
Genioglossus muscle	Mandible	Entire dorsum of the tongue and hyoid bone	Protrudes the tongue and assists with other movement
Hyoglossus muscle	Hyoid bone	Inferior and lateral parts of the tongue	Depresses and shortens the tongue
Styloglossus muscle	Styloid process of temporal bone	Posterior parts of the tongue	Retracts the tongue and curls its sideways
Palatoglossus muscle	Palatine aponeurosis	Posterolateral parts of the tongue	Elevates the posterior part of the tongue and depresses the soft palate

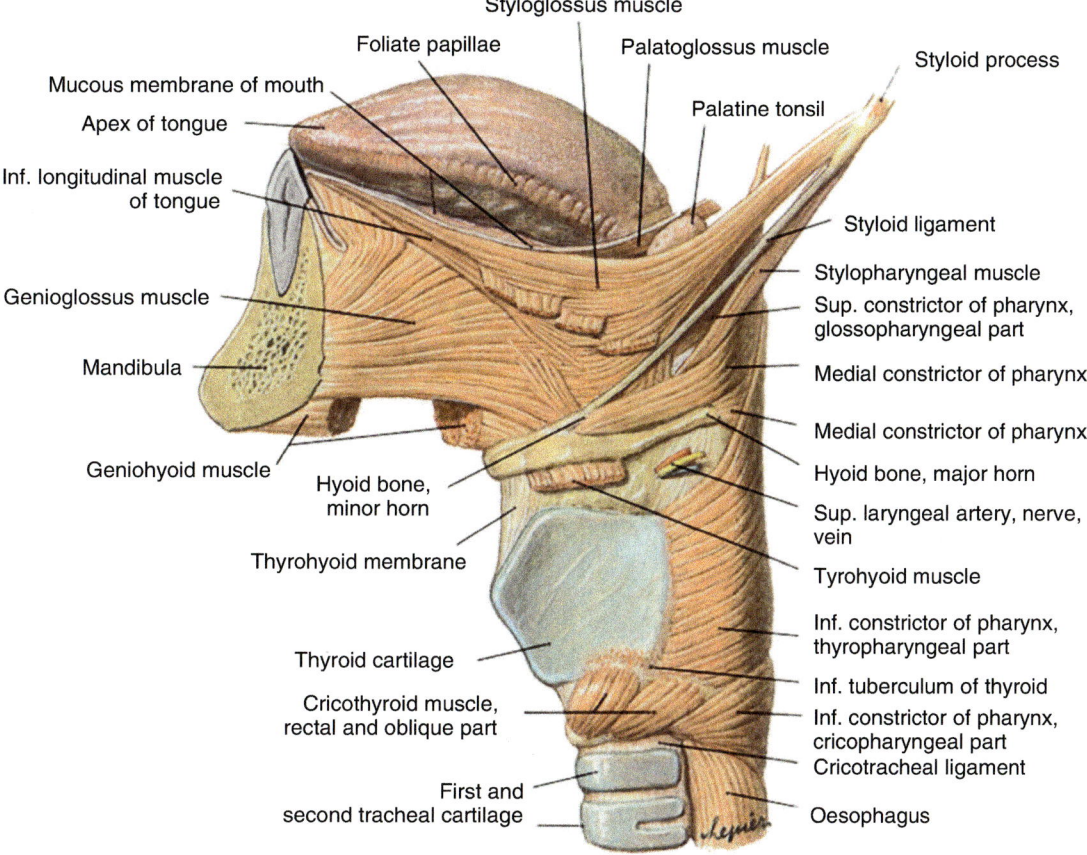

Fig. 1.35 External muscles of the tongue (from Paulsen et al. 2010, courtesy of Elsevier)

The oral phase of swallowing can be further subdivided into the oral preparatory and the oral transport phase. In the oral preparatory phase, the lips, tongue, mandible, palate and cheeks act in common with salivary flow to form food into a consistency and position appropriate for the subsequent phases of swallowing. Once the food bolus is prepared, the oral transport phase occurs, as the musculature of the lips and cheeks contract, followed by tongue contraction against the hard palate. The soft palate elevates as a consequence of contraction of the tensor veli palatini, levator veli palatini and palatopharyngeus muscles. Thereby a reflux of food into the nasal cavity is prevented.

The anterior two thirds of the tongue are critical in the oral phase of deglutition. The posterior one third of the tongue, the tongue base, plays an important role in propelling a food bolus posteriorly towards the pharynx.

The nerves involved so far are the trigeminal nerve (CN V) to control general sensation to the face and motor supply to the muscles of mastication, the facial nerve (CN VII) to supply taste to the anterior two thirds of the tongue and motor function to the lips, the glossopharyngeal nerve (CN IX) to provide general sensation to the posterior third of the tongue and the hypoglossal nerve (CN XII) to enable movements of the tongue.

Once the food bolus touches the palatoglossal folds, the pharyngeal phase of swallowing reflexively begins.

When the swallowing reflex is initiated, the following reactions take place: velopharyngeal closure to prevent reflux of material into the

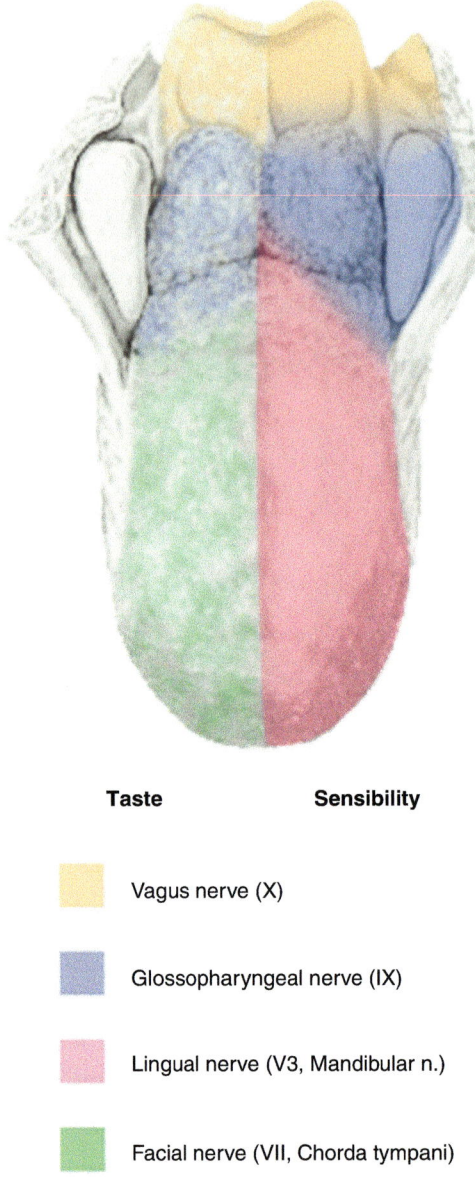

Taste   **Sensibility**

Vagus nerve (X)

Glossopharyngeal nerve (IX)

Lingual nerve (V3, Mandibular n.)

Facial nerve (VII, Chorda tympani)

Fig. 1.36 Sensory innervation of the tongue

posterior choana. This is affected by contraction of the levator veli palatini muscles, which elevate the soft palate against the posterior nasopharyngeal wall. Medial contraction of the lateral pharyngeal wall musculature and a slight anterior movement of the posterior pharyngeal wall create Passavant's ridge, against which the velum is approximated during the initiation of the pharyngeal phase of swallowing. The pharyngeal con-

strictor muscles contract in a superior-to-inferior direction. The epiglottis inverts to cover the larynx and prevent aspiration of contents into the airway. This retroversion of the epiglottis directs the food bolus laterally towards the pyriform sinuses. The vocal folds adduct to prevent aspiration.

With contraction of the superior pharyngeal constrictor muscle, laryngeal elevation occurs. The larynx elevates following the anterior movement of the hyoid bone and tongue base owing to contraction of the mylohyoid, geniohyoid, stylohyoid and anterior digastric muscles. This anterior movement of the larynx combined with the contraction of the middle and inferior constrictor muscles forces the food bolus inferiorly, initiating the final portion of the pharyngeal phase, which is the entry of the food bolus into the cervical oesophagus.

The mylohyoid nerve, branch of CN V3, supplies the mylohyoid and the anterior digastric muscles. The stylohyoid muscle is innervated by branches of the facial nerve (CN VII), and the geniohyoid muscle receives fibres from the first cervical nerve, which joins the hypoglossal nerve. The pharyngeal constrictors have their nervous supply through the glossopharyngeal (CN IX) and the vagus (CN X) nerves.

1.2.2.6 The Ear

Outer Ear

The pinna or auricle (Fig. 1.37) is a prominent skin-covered flap located on the side of the head and is the external visible part of the ear. It is shaped and supported by cartilage except for the earlobe. The outer verge of the ear is called the helix, and the inner elevated rim is the antihelix, which originates from the fusion of two crura, between which is a triangular depression, the fossa triangularis. The deepest depression, which leads to the ear canal, is known as the concha. It is overlapped by the tragus, a small cartilaginous flap that can be pushed down to block the opening to the ear canal.

The pinna collects sound waves and directs them to the external ear canal. Its shape also

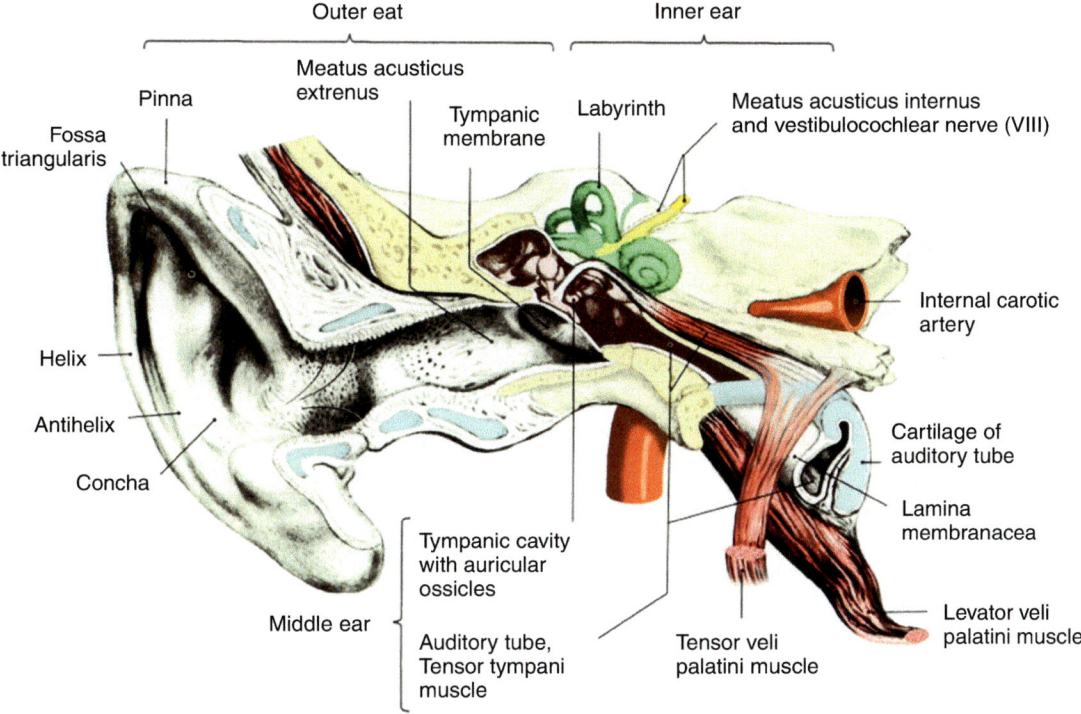

Fig. 1.37 The ear, overview (from Benninghoff and Drenckhahn 2003, courtesy of Elsevier)

partially shields sound waves that approach the ear from the rear, therefore enabling a person to tell whether a sound is coming directly from the front or the back.

The external auditory canal (meatus acusticus externus) begins at the bottom of the concha and ends at the tympanic membrane. It is approximately 2.5–3 cm long and slightly S-curved. It is supported by cartilage at its first third and by the bone for the rest of its length. It exhibits two narrowings, one near the inner end of the cartilaginous portion and another, the isthmus, within the osseous part. The whole tube is lined by the skin and contains glands that produce secretions that mix with dead skin cells to produce cerumen (earwax).

Middle Ear

The outer ear ends, and the middle ear (Fig. 1.38) begins, at the tympanic membrane, commonly known as the eardrum. It lies in the tympanic cavity within the temporal bone. The cavity connects to the nasal part of the pharynx via the auditory

tube. It is therefore filled with air, normally of the same atmospheric pressure as the outer ear. This ensures that the tympanic membrane can swing freely between both ear parts. Within the tympanic cavity, the vibrations of the tympanic membrane are transmitted to the oval window, the beginning of the inner ear, by a chain of ossicles: the malleus, which has a handle that attaches to the inner surface of the eardrum and a head that is suspended from the wall of the tympanic cavity; the incus, which is connected by its body to the head of the malleus and by its long arm to the stapes. Both its body and its short arm are fixed to the wall of the tympanic cavity by ligaments. The third ossicle, the stapes, has an arch and a footplate. The arch connects to the incus, whereas the footplate is held by a ring-like piece of tissue in the oval window, which is the entrance into the inner ear.

Two muscles exert influence on the movements of the middle ear bones: the tensor tympani (innervated via a branch of the mandibular nerve), whose tendon inserts on the medial part

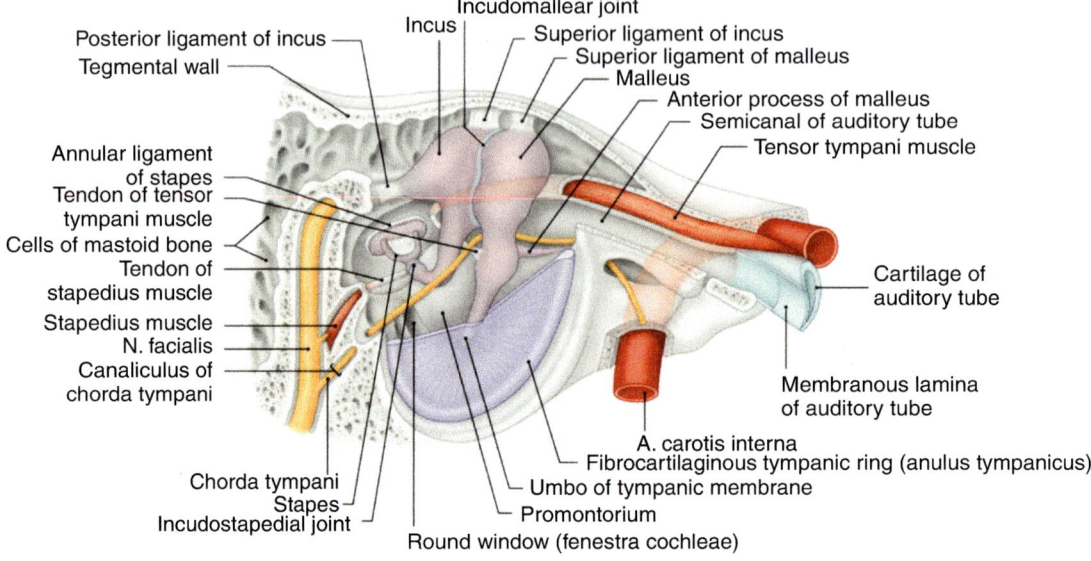

Fig. 1.38 The middle ear (from Zilles and Tillmann 2010, courtesy of Springer)

Fig. 1.39 The labyrinth of the inner ear (from Paulsen et al. 2010, courtesy of Elsevier)

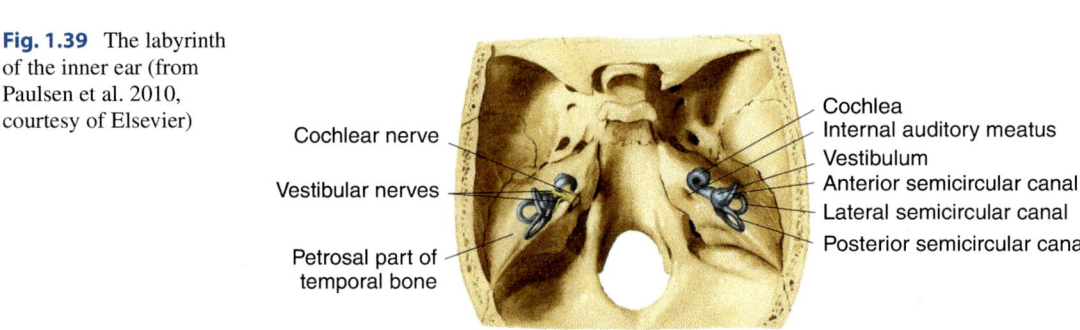

of the malleus, pulls the malleus medially, tensing the tympanic membrane, damping its vibration and thereby reducing the amplitude of sounds. The other one, the stapedius muscle (innervated by a branch of the facial nerve), inserts into the posterior neck of the stapes and reflexively lessens its vibrations by pulling its head backwards.

Inner Ear

The oval window, where the footplate of the stapes is fixed, is the beginning of the inner ear, a system of osseous cavities within the petrosal part of the temporal bone, called the labyrinth (Fig. 1.39). It consists of three components, the vestibule (vestibulum), the three semicircular canals and the cochlea.

The Organs of Equilibrium: Vestibulum and Semicircular Canals The organ of equilibrium (Fig. 1.40) consists of five compartments, two saccular organs, the utriculus and the sacculus, and three semicircular canals, orientated at right angles to each other, corresponding to the three dimensions of space (Speckmann et al. 2013). The inner membranous compartments of these cavities contain endolymph and do not directly contact their osseous walls but are separated by a small space filled with perilymph. Via the ductus endolymphaticus, the five membranous compartments are continuous to the endolymphatic sac, which in turn has contacts to the dura mater. Both of them have absorptive and secretory functions and regulate the volume and composition of the endolymph. This endolymph is not identical with

Fig. 1.40 Components of the organ of equilibrium (green) and their sensory areas (from Speckmann et al. 2013, courtesy of Elsevier)

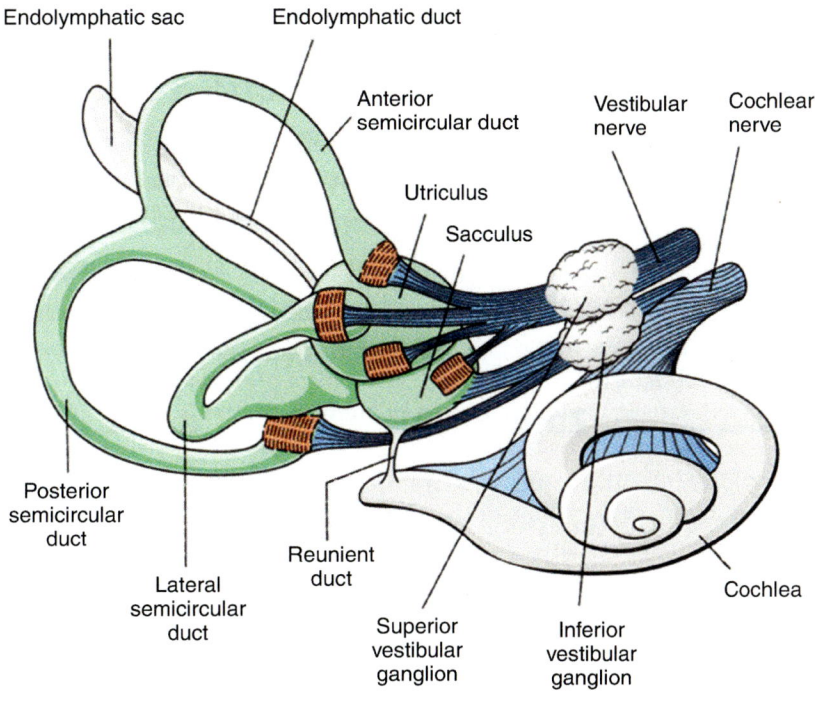

Endolymphatic sac   Endolymphatic duct

Anterior semicircular duct

Utriculus

Sacculus

Vestibular nerve   Cochlear nerve

Posterior semicircular duct

Lateral semicircular duct

Reunient duct

Superior vestibular ganglion

Inferior vestibular ganglion

Cochlea

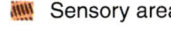 Sensory area

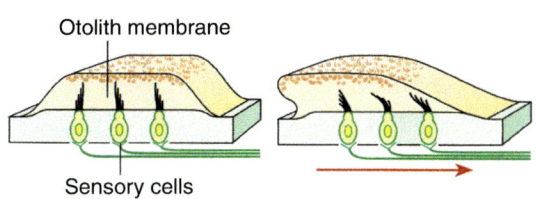

Otolith membrane

Sensory cells

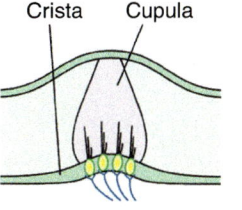

Crista   Cupula

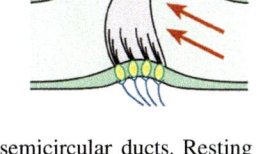

Turning of head

Fig. 1.41 The macula organ. Resting position (left), macula in action (right) (from Speckmann et al. 2013, courtesy of Elsevier)

Fig. 1.42 The organ of the semicircular ducts. Resting position (left), activation by turning of the head (right) (from Speckmann et al. 2013, courtesy of Elsevier)

the endolymph of the cochlear duct (see below) but differs in its ion content.

The sensory element of the sacculus, as well as of the utriculus, is named the macula (Fig. 1.41). It is a plain area containing roughly 16,000 or 30,000 hair cells. They are covered by a gelatinous layer, in which otoliths, small crystals of calcium carbonate, are embedded. This layer has a higher density than the endolymph, and when the otolith membrane is moved, induced either by bending the head or by linear acceleration or deceleration, the ciliary hairs of the sensory cells are declined and evoke

depolarisations or hyperpolarisations that trigger the spontaneous activity of the vestibular nerve fibres. The macula utriculi is nearly horizontally orientated and reacts mainly to changes of horizontal movements (e.g. to increasing or reducing speeds of a car); the macula sacculi, on the other hand, is in an approximately vertical position and therefore registers vertical accelerations (e.g. to movements of a lift).

The semicircular ducts (Fig. 1.42), the membranous components of the semicircular canals, start and end within the recessus ellipticus of the vestibulum. The end of one haunch of each of them is enlarged to an ampulla and is the domicile of the sensory organ. Each ampulla contains a so-called crista ampullaris, a specialised connective tissue with approximately 7000 hair cells. They are covered by a dome of jelly-like material (cupula ampullaris), which does not touch the cells directly: only the sensory hairs of the cells contact the cupola through a small gap. The cupola has nearly the same density as the endolymph, so it exerts no direct pressure on the sensory cells. Inertness of the endolymph together with the cupola evokes an opposite movement within the semicircular ducts, contrary to turning movements of the head, and induces a shear force on the hairs of the sensory cells, which causes depolarisation or hyperpolarisation, depending on the direction of turning.

The Cochlea (Fig. 1.43) The vestibulum continues into the cochlea, which winds by 2½ turns around a section of spongy bone called the modiolus. The modiolus is shaped like a screw whose threads, the lamina spiralis ossea, form a spiral platform that supports the membranous parts of the cochlea. The cochlea measures about 35 mm in length. It contains three fluid-filled chambers separated by membranes. The upper chamber, scala vestibuli, and the bottom chamber, scala tympani, are filled with perilymph. They communicate with each other at the top of the modiolus, the helicotrema and the scala tympani ends at the round window, which again continues into the middle ear but is closed by the secondary tympanic membrane. Between these two

perilymphatic ducts, the triangular scala media or ductus cochlearis is expanded. Its basilar membrane extends laterally from the osseous spiral lamina to the outer wall of the cochlea. It separates the scala media from the scala tympani and carries the organ of Corti. Its inclining roof, a more subtle membrane, is called Reissner's membrane and serves as boundary against the scala vestibuli. The lateral wall of the scala media consists of a specialised epithelium, the stria vascularis (as it contains blood vessels); it generates the endolymph, with which the scala media is filled.

The basilar membrane and its medial continuation, the osseous spiral lamina, carry the organ of Corti, which changes pressure waves into nervous impulses.

The organ of Corti (Fig. 1.44) is composed of a series of epithelial structures. As a central part, the inner and outer rods or pillars of Corti flank a triangular tunnel, the tunnel of Corti. On both sides of the tunnel, the inner and outer hair cells are located. These are short columnar cells; their free ends are level with the heads of Corti's rods. The approximately 3500 inner hair cells are arranged in a single row on the medial side of the inner rods. They do not reach the basilar membrane but are positioned within supporting phalangeal cells. This facilitates abundant contacts of nerve endings with the cell bodies. The name 'hair cells' originates from ciliary structures on their tips, which contact the tectorial membrane. The outer hair cells (approx. 12,000) are nearly twice as long as the inner ones. They are

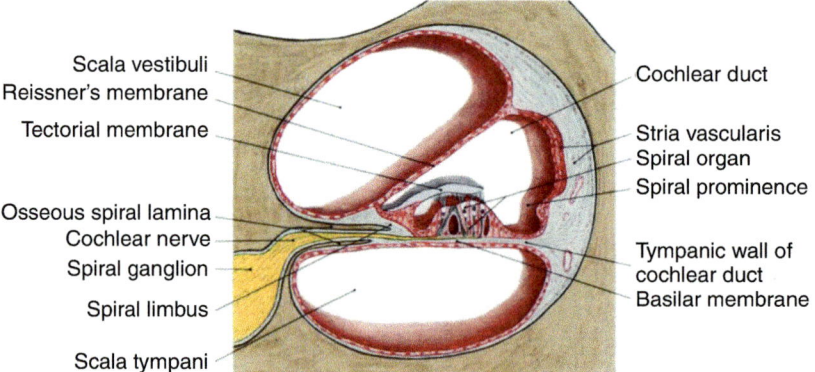

Fig. 1.43 Cross-section of cochlear spiral canal (from Paulsen et al. 2010, courtesy of Elsevier)

Scala vestibuli
Reissner's membrane
Tectorial membrane
Osseous spiral lamina
Cochlear nerve
Spiral ganglion
Spiral limbus
Scala tympani

Cochlear duct
Stria vascularis
Spiral organ
Spiral prominence
Tympanic wall of cochlear duct
Basilar membrane

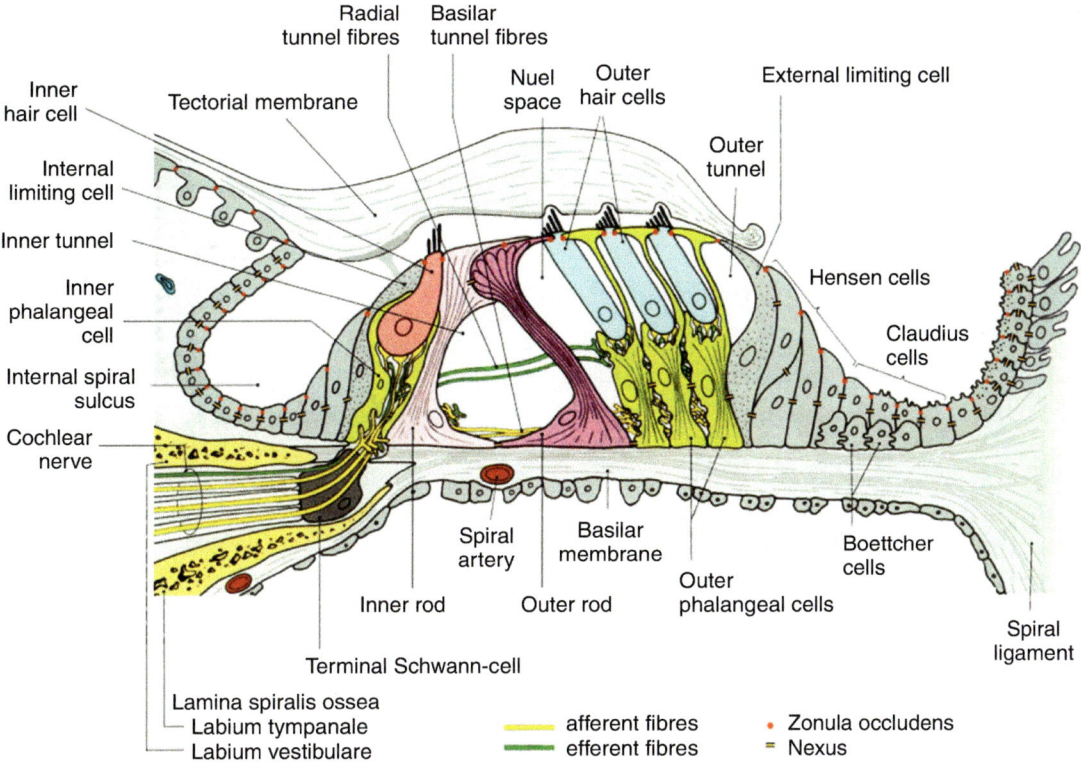

Fig. 1.44 The organ of Corti (from Benninghoff and Drenckhahn 2004, courtesy of Elsevier)

supported by outer phalangeal cells, the cells of Deiters. A space exists between the outer rods of Corti and the adjacent hair cells; this is called the space of Nuel. The Deiters' cells are neighboured by five or six rows of columnar cells, the supporting cells of Hensen, followed by another group of columnar cells, the cells of Claudius. Covering the sulcus spiralis internus and the spiral organ of Corti is the tectorial membrane, which is attached to the limbus laminae spiralis close to the inner edge of the vestibular membrane. It has contact with the cilia of the inner as well as of the outer hair cells.

The so-called cochlear transduction process of sound, from air waves to nervous impulses, is the result of several steps.

Vibrations of the eardrum are transmitted through the three ossicles of the middle ear, which induce pressure waves within the scala vestibuli. These pressure waves generate a travelling wave on the basilar membrane of the scala media. The basilar membrane vibrations cause shear movements between the tectorial membrane and the stereocilia of both types of hair cells, resulting in deflection of the stereocilia and activation of ion channels. Thereby the mechanical stimulus is transduced, and receptor potentials are generated. In inner hair cells, these receptor potentials induce neurotransmitter release and action potential generation in the synapses of auditory nerve fibres.

The receptor potentials of the outer hair cells, however, initiate a contraction in the longitudinal axis of the cells, which influences the basilar membrane's motions (Fettiplace and Hackney 2006; Ashmore 2008). The cells act in a sense of a 'cochlear amplifier', a mechanism that increases both the amplitude and frequency selectivity of basilar membrane vibration for low-level sounds. These activities of the outer hair cells can be measured as otoacoustic emission (OAE). Efferent nerve fibres contact the outer hair cells by crossing the tunnel of Corti medially as radial fibres. They are thought to adjust the resting membrane potential of these cells, thereby regulating the amount of feedback provided to the basilar membrane.

1.2.2.7 Auditory Pathway and Vestibular Tracts

Auditory Pathway

About 90% of the afferent nerve fibres that leave the organ of Corti come from the inner hair cells. They are Type I nerve fibres, i.e. thick, myelinated and fast conducting. The remaining 10% are afferent fibres from the outer hair cells; they are slow-conducting Type II fibres and cross the tunnel of Corti as basilar tunnel fibres. The cell bodies of all of these fibres form the spiral (or cochlear) ganglion, embedded within the central part of the modiolus. Their axons continue as the acoustic nerve (pars cochlearis of the vestibulocochlear nerve, cranial nerve VIII) and enter the brainstem (Fig. 1.45) (ten Donkelaar 2011).

Each of the nerve fibres diverges, one branch projects rostrally to the dorsal cochlear nucleus,

the other projects caudally to the ventral cochlear nucleus. The cochlear nuclei contain second-order neurons, which generally project to higher centres by an ipsilateral or, after decussating, by a contralateral pathway.

The ventral cochlear nucleus projects to the superior olivary complex, whereas fibres of the dorsal cochlear nucleus bypass the superior olivary complex and directly enter the lateral lemniscus to reach the inferior colliculus.

The superior olivary complex consists of the medial nucleus of the superior olive, the lateral nucleus of the superior olive and the medial nucleus of the trapezoid body. Both nuclei of the superior olive receive fibres from the ipsilateral and contralateral ventral cochlear nucleus. The medial nucleus analyses time differences of neuronal signals; the lateral nucleus evaluates differences in intensities. On their way to the nuclei of the superior olive, the contralateral fibres pass through the trapezoid body as a passive relay. In mammals as well as in man, its nuclei, however, are thought to play a role in distinguishing interaural intensity differences.

The superior olivary complex sends outputs to the cranial nerves V and VII for reflex contractions

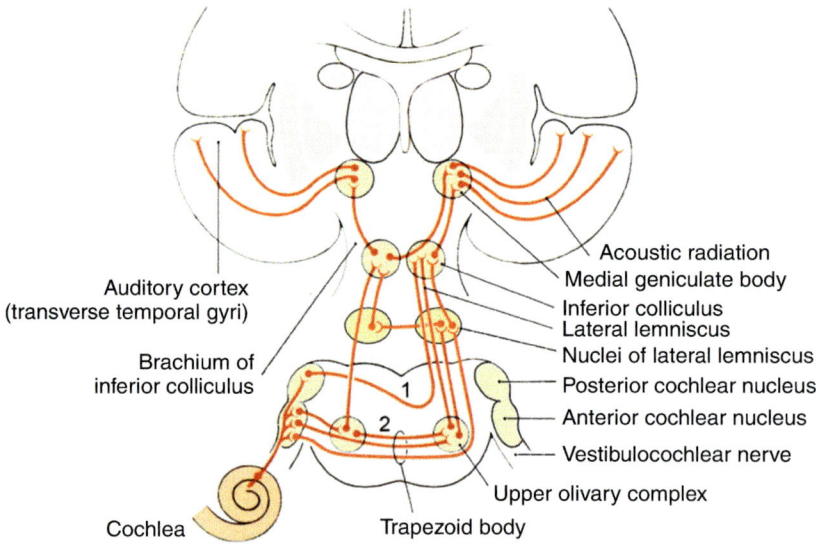

Fig. 1.45 The auditory pathway (from Benninghoff and Drenckhahn 2004, courtesy of Elsevier)

Auditory cortex (transverse temporal gyri)

Brachium of inferior colliculus

Cochlea

Trapezoid body

Acoustic radiation
Medial geniculate body
Inferior colliculus
Lateral lemniscus
Nuclei of lateral lemniscus
Posterior cochlear nucleus
Anterior cochlear nucleus
Vestibulocochlear nerve
Upper olivary complex

1 direct auditory pathway
2 indirect auditory pathway

of the tensor tympani and stapedius muscles to dampen loud sounds.

The fibres connecting the olivary complex with the inferior colliculus form a lateral tract in the brainstem, called the lateral lemniscus. Within this tract a mass of grey matter is embedded, called the nuclei lemnisci lateralis dorsalis and ventralis. They serve as synaptic relay stations for some of the fibres of the lateral lemniscus.

The end point of the lateral lemniscus is the inferior colliculus. It serves as an auditory relay and reflex centre, where information derived directly from the dorsal cochlear nucleus and from the olivary complex may be compared. Moreover, it receives inputs from the somatosensory system. The inferior colliculi of both sides contact each other by commissural fibres.

The inferior colliculus projects to the medial geniculate nucleus or medial geniculate body. This nucleus is part of the thalamus and serves as a thalamic relay on the way to the auditory cortex. From their neuronal morphology, a number of subdivisions can be distinguished. They have different afferent and efferent connections, and they are thought to be involved together in the direction and maintenance of attention. The fibres leaving the medial geniculate body join the internal capsule as the radiatio acustica and terminate in the primary auditory cortex, the Brodmann's areas 41 and 42 within the superior temporal gyrus.

Nervous activation of individual parts of the auditory pathway may be recorded as the auditory brainstem response (ABR) upon a stimulus that evokes a response of the cochlea. The first two waves correspond to true action potentials of the cochlear nerve. Later waves may reflect postsynaptic activities (afferent and efferent) in brainstem auditory centres:

- Wave I is a response of the auditory nerve action potential in the distal portion of the cochlear nerve (cranial nerve VIII).
- Wave II is generated by the proximal part of the cochlear nerve as it enters the brainstem.
- Wave III arises from second-order neuron activities in or near the cochlear nucleus.

- Wave IV is said to arise from the superior olivary complex, but additional contributions may come from the cochlear nucleus and nucleus of lateral lemniscus.
- Wave V is believed to originate from the vicinity of the inferior colliculus.
- Waves VI and VII are suggested to have their origins in the medial geniculate body of the thalamus.

Beginning in the auditory cortex, several descending pathways exist. The centrifugal fibres run close to, but usually not within, the tracts containing the auditory afferent pathways. They project to the medial geniculate bodies, the inferior colliculi and other midbrain nuclei; from the inferior colliculi, they descend to the superior olivary complex. From here the olivo-cochlear bundles travel down to the inner and outer hair cells of the cochlea. They carry information from the superior olivary complex, the nuclei of the lateral lemniscus, the reticular formation and the inferior colliculus. These bundles have two compartments: a lateral one, containing unmyelinated fibres, which end on the afferent fibres of the inner hair cells, and a medial one with myelinated fibres, which medially crosses the tunnel of Corti and terminates directly on the bodies of the outer hair cells.

The pathway of the acoustic startle reflex is part of the auditory pathway from the ear up to the nucleus of the inferior colliculus. Mainly from there but also from the dorsal nucleus of the lateral lemniscus and from parts of the superior olivary complex, it follows connections to nuclei of cranial nerves and motor centres in the reticular formation. The motoneurons of the ventral root are activated, and moving of the body is initiated, by the reticulospinal tract in the anterolateral part of the spinal cord. The inferior colliculi also project to the superior colliculi, important relay stations in the visual pathway, coordinating optical reflexes.

Learned reflexes (e.g. turning upon hearing one's name) are conditioned reflexes. They include the auditory pathway and other complex parts of the central nervous system.

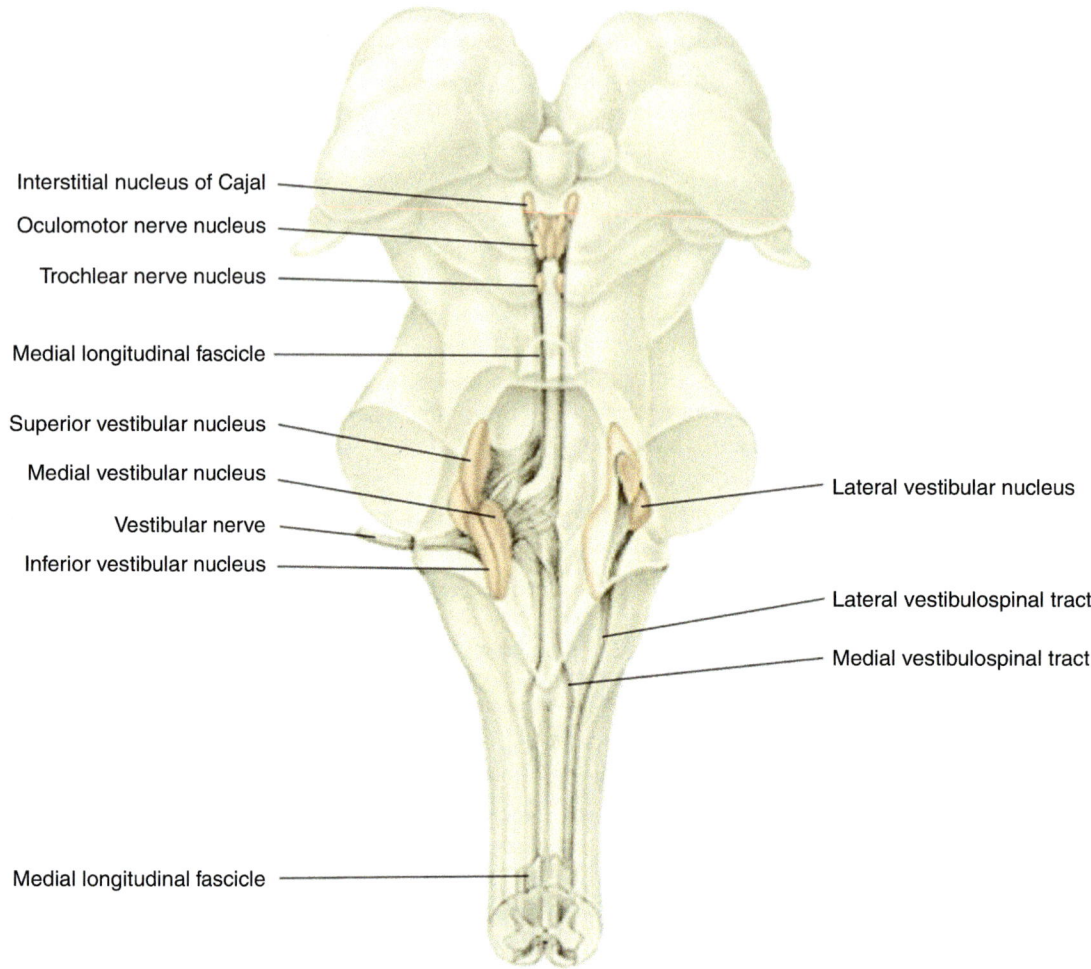

Interstitial nucleus of Cajal

Oculomotor nerve nucleus

Trochlear nerve nucleus

Medial longitudinal fascicle

Superior vestibular nucleus

Medial vestibular nucleus

Vestibular nerve

Inferior vestibular nucleus

Lateral vestibular nucleus

Lateral vestibulospinal tract

Medial vestibulospinal tract

Medial longitudinal fascicle

Fig. 1.46 Ascending and descending connections of the vestibular nuclei, brainstem, dorsal view (modified from Nieuwenhuys et al. 2008, courtesy of Springer)

The Vestibular Tracts

The axons emanating from the ganglia of the vestibular nerves (Fig. 1.46) project to the ipsilateral vestibular nuclei, a group of four major and several minor nuclei in the rhombencephalon (hindbrain). There they join afferent fibres from the cerebellum, from proprioceptors of the deeper neck region, as well as afferent fibres from the optical system via the superior colliculi. One of their projections is to the ventral posterior nucleus (the somatosensory nucleus) of the thalamus. These projections are bilateral (crossed and not crossed). The thalamus forwards the vestibular information to vestibular areas in the cerebral cortex. They are not as precisely circumscribed as the areas of the other sensory systems and tend to overlap each other.

Ascending fibres of the vestibular nuclei join the medial longitudinal fascicle and enter the interstitial nucleus of Cajal (Nieuwenhuys et al. 2008), which serves as a coordination centre for eye and head movements. Over this route, the vestibular nuclei also project to ipsilateral and contralateral nuclei of ocular muscles: nuclei of the oculomotorius, abducens and trochlear nerve. These nerves stimulate the six external muscles of the eye, located in three perpendicular planes, roughly colinear with the planes of the semicircular canals. Excitatory subunits connect a single semicircular canal to the eye muscles, initiating a compensatory eye movement in the plane of the semicircular canal, whereas their antagonists are inhibited.

The vestibulo-collic reflex produces head movements in the planes of the stimulated canals. More than 30 neck muscles are innervated from the upper cervical cord and receive excitatory or inhibitory inputs, or both, from all six semicircular canals. The motoneurons are contacted by the vestibulospinal system, including lateral, medial and crossed tracts.

Descending fibres form the vestibulospinal tracts and join the reticulospinal tract, by which they reach the motor neurons of skeletal muscles, predominantly activating the extensor and inhibiting the flexor muscles.

One main target of the vestibular tracts is the cerebellum. By mossy fibres, they reach a special region, the vestibular cerebellum, mainly consisting of the flocculonodular lobe, combining the nodulus and the flocculus. The efferent fibres of this region act synergistically on the oculomotor and spinal motor systems to maintain balance in upright movements (Trepel 2004).

1.2.2.8 Neuroanatomical Basics of Language

The cerebrum is divided into four main parts: the frontal lobe is separated from the parietal lobe by the central sulcus and houses capabilities such as planning, motivation, working memory and motor functions including speech production. The parietal lobe is the main sensory part of the brain. The gyri immediately adjoining the central sulcus are the precentral gyrus, origin of the pyramidal tract on the motoric site, and the postcentral gyrus as the primary sensory centre on the parietal side. The parietooccipital sulcus separates the parietal lobe from the occipital lobe, where among others the visual areas are domiciled. The lateral sulcus (or fissura sylvii) separates the temporal lobe on the one hand from the frontal and parietal lobe on the other. The auditory centre is located in the temporal lobe, where acoustic radiation, emanating from the medial geniculate body, terminates.

The whole cerebrum has been mapped by Korbinian Brodmann (1868–1918) according to the cytoarchitectonic patterns of its various parts. These areas are widely used to describe functional compartments of the brain.

An important part involved in language (Fig. 1.47) is Wernicke's area, located in the posterior part of the superior temporal gyrus in Brodmann's area 22 and part of area 39. It is predominant in the left hemisphere of right-handed persons and plays a key role in understanding words. Spoken words arrive at Wernicke's area directly via the auditory cortex in areas 41 and 42 (Shalom and Poeppel 2008). Visual inputs reach this area from the eye via the visual cortices in Brodmann's areas 17, 18 and 19 and the 'read and write centre' in the angular gyrus (Brodmann's area 39). Wernicke's area projects to Broca's area and has connections to the prefrontal cortex by longitudinal association fibres (Friederici 2009).

Vocalising language requires motor outputs from the lower regions of the precentral primary motor cortex (motor areas for the face, mouth, tongue and larynx). The plan and coordination of these motor outputs originate in Broca's area, which lies in the Brodmann's regions 44 and 45. It joins the lower part of the precentral cortex, receives inputs from Wernicke's area via the arcuate fasciculus and projects to the above-mentioned corresponding primary motor areas of both hemispheres (to the contralateral side via the corpus callosum), as well as to the basal ganglia, which are thought to play a role in giving timing cues for the correct motor activity during speech (Fig. 1.47).

Recently, Hickok and Poeppel proposed a dual pathway of language processing (Fig. 1.48): on the basis of the findings that speech recognition is bilaterally organised in the superior temporal gyrus, they postulate a bilateral ventral stream comprising the primary auditory area, Heschl's gyrus, and neighbouring areas of the superior temporal gyrus (including Wernicke's area), adjacent areas of the middle and the inferior temporal gyrus. These areas are important in speech perception. The speech production is generated by a unilateral dorsal stream in the left

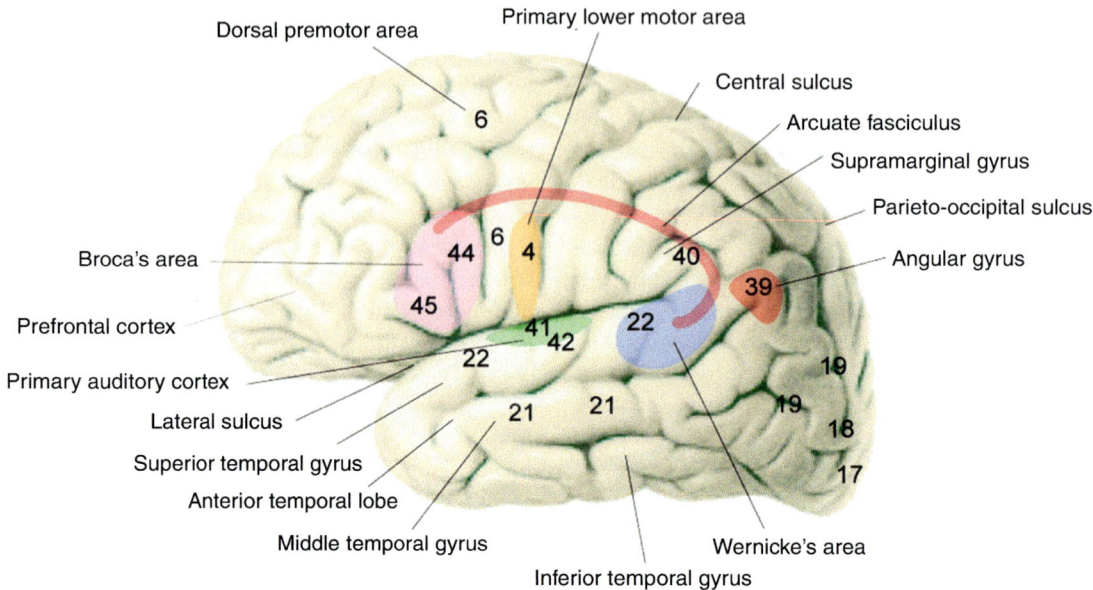

Fig. 1.47 The brain surface; areas active in language (modified from Paulsen et al. 2010, courtesy of Elsevier)

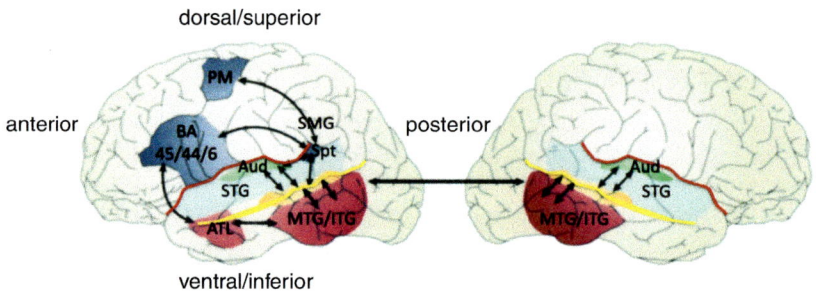

Fig. 1.48 Scheme of the functional anatomy of language processing. Two broad processing streams are depicted, a ventral stream for speech comprehension that is largely bilaterally organised and that flows into the temporal lobe and a dorsal stream for sensory-motor integration that is left-dominant and that involves structures at the parietal-temporal junction and frontal lobe. *ATL* anterior temporal lobe; *Aud* auditory cortex (early processing stages); *BA* 45/44/6 Brodmann's areas 45, 44 and 6; *MTG/ITG* middle temporal gyrus, inferior temporal gyrus; *PM* premotor, dorsal portion; *SMG* supramarginal gyrus; *Spt* Sylvian parietal-temporal region (left only); *STG* superior temporal gyrus; *red line* Sylvian fissure; *yellow line* superior temporal sulcus (STS) (from Hickok 2009, courtesy of Elsevier)

hemisphere including interconnections between the supramarginal gyrus and the dorsal premotor portion (Brodmann's area 6) as well as the area of Broca together with the lower motor gyrus of Brodmann's area 4. The Broca region also connects to the anterior temporal lobe (anterior part of Brodmann's area 21), which is supposed to play a role in processing complex elements of language (Hickok 2009).

1.3 Physics, Acoustics, Psychoacoustics

Kurt Stephan

As phoniatrics is strongly linked to the phenomena of sound and sound perception, a thorough understanding of the nature of sound is essential for interpretation of diagnostic results in phoniatrics as well as for the application of therapeutic approaches to hearing and speech pathologies.

1.3.1 Sound Waves

In contrast to light waves or other electromagnetic waves present in our everyday environment, sound waves are mechanical vibrations of small particles (typically molecules) of a medium (e.g. air, water). Sound waves are created by a vibrating object, called the *sound source*. The vibration of a sound source results in a periodic or aperiodic compression and rarefaction of the particles of the medium, causing local fluctuations of the density that propagate through the medium. Hence, a sound wave can be thought of as a periodic or aperiodic displacement of interacting particles that travel through the medium from one location to another resulting in a transport of energy. If the particles vibrate along the axis of sound propagation, the wave is called *longitudinal*; if they vibrate perpendicular to the axis of propagation, the wave is called *transverse*. The medium can be thought of as the material through which the wave propagates, which can be a gas, a fluid or a solid substance. Without a medium sound cannot be produced.

Sound waves in air and water are always longitudinal, and they travel through the medium at a speed which is specific for the medium. In air the speed of sound at sea level is 340 m/s; in water it is more than four times higher, i.e. 1484 m/s, and in solids it is about 15 times higher. Most often the perception of sound in humans is based on the propagation of sound waves in air.

1.3.2 Physical Properties of Sound

Sound is primarily characterised by wavelength, amplitude and frequency. The wavelength (λ, lambda) is defined as the distance of two successive wave crests or troughs of a sound wave, the amplitude (A) as the maximum deviation from the resting pressure. The frequency (f), which determines the pitch of a tone, is defined as the number of pressure fluctuations per unit time. Frequency, wavelength and sound velocity (c) are related to each other by the following equation (Eq. 1.1):

$$f[\text{Hz}] = c[\text{m/s}] / \lambda[\text{m}] \qquad (1.1)$$

Everyday sounds do not only contain one particular frequency but are rather a mixture or superposition of frequencies and amplitudes with different temporal variation (Fig. 1.49). Only a pure, continuous sine-shaped oscillation is regarded as a pure tone. Sound generated by a musical instrument typically consists of a fundamental frequency (i.e. the lowest tone) and a series of resonant frequencies called *overtones*. The combination of the fundamental and resonant frequencies creates the typical timbre of the instrument, which allows the listener to recognise it. When two tones with very similar frequencies and amplitudes are superimposed, a third tone with a lower frequency is generated.

The relevant measurement for characterising the strength of sound waves is sound pressure (p). It is defined as the local pressure deviation from the ambient atmospheric pressure caused by a sound wave. Its unit is the Pascal [Pa]. Pressure deviations caused by sound waves are very small relative to atmospheric pressure. The human ear is able to perceive them in the range between about 20 µPa (20×10^{-6} Pa) and 20 Pa, where 20 µPa approximately corresponds to the sound pressure at hearing threshold of a 1000 Hz tone. Owing to the huge range of our ear's auditory sensitivity, measurements and calculations in Pa are laborious. For this reason, a more handy measure has been introduced: the *sound pressure level* (SPL) with the unit *decibel* [dB SPL]. The sound pressure level is calculated by a logarithmic transformation of the measured sound pressure according to the formula (Eq. 1.2):

$$L[\text{dB SPL}] = 20 \times \log p / p_0$$
$$\left(\text{with } p_0 = 20\,\mu Pa\right). \qquad (1.2)$$

According to this formula, the hearing threshold for a 1000 Hz tone lies at 0 dB SPL (as measured by a sound level meter). Every increase in sound pressure level by 20 dB indicates an

Fig. 1.49 Time course (upper graphs) and frequency spectra (lower graphs) of typical sound waves: pure tone, 440 Hz, complex tones: superposition of three tones (440, 880 and 1100 Hz), and noise. λ = wavelength. For the noise a wavelength cannot be assigned

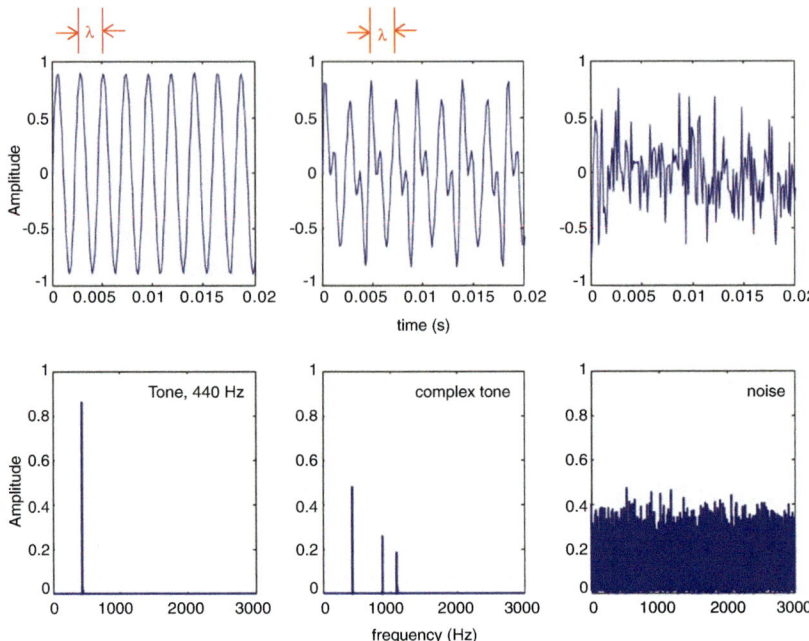

increase in sound pressure by the factor 10. Owing to the logarithmic nature of the dB scale, its values cannot simply be added or subtracted but must be retransformed into Pa before arithmetic operations can be made. By doing so, one finds that doubling the sound pressure of a sound source leads to an increase in SPL of 6 dB.

1.3.3 Propagation of Sound

In gases and liquids, sound propagates as longitudinal waves, whereas in solids transverse propagation of sound waves is also found. It should be noted that propagation of sound does not mean the movement of particles but only transport of energy. During propagation, the waves can be reflected, diffracted or attenuated by the medium. The modalities of sound propagation depend on the properties of the medium through which the sound travels. Additional factors that influence sound propagation are obstacles along the wave's pathway and changes of the type of medium.

The fact that sounds can be heard around corners and barriers involves the mechanisms of *diffraction* and *reflection*. When diffraction occurs, the sound can be thought of being 'bent around'

an obstacle. This effect occurs mainly with low frequencies (for which the wavelength is of the order of the size of the obstacle) and is the reason we hear low frequencies better than high frequencies behind obstacles. With high frequencies (with wavelengths much smaller than the size of the obstacle) the so-called shadow effect occurs, meaning that they appear attenuated behind the obstacle. The shadow effect caused by our head helps our auditory system to recognise the direction from which high-frequency sounds come.

For recognising the direction whence low-frequency sounds originate, our auditory system evaluates the time difference between a sound's arrival at the ipsilateral and the contralateral ear (*inter-aural time difference*).

Another property of a medium that is important for sound propagation is the characteristic acoustic impedance (Z). Z determines how much sound pressure (*p*) is generated by a vibration of molecules of a particular acoustic medium at a given frequency. It is defined as

$$Z = p\,[\mathrm{Pa}]\,/\,v\,[\mathrm{m\,/\,s}] \qquad (1.3)$$

where *v* is the velocity of the sound in the particular medium (Eq. 1.3). The acoustic impedance is particularly relevant for the propagation of sound waves when the medium through which the sound travels is changing, e.g. from air to water. As the acoustic impedance of water is about 3500 times higher than that of air, a large amount of the sound will be reflected at the surface of the water. A similar mismatch of impedances occurs in the human ear when the sound is travelling from the ear canal to the inner ear.

To overcome the huge difference in impedances, impedance-matching is accomplished by the ossicles of the middle ear. This matching, interpreted as 'mechanical amplification with no input of additional energy', ensures that the sound is effectively transmitted from the ear canal to the fluids of the inner ear.

1.3.4 Perception of Sound and Psychoacoustics

The way sound is perceived in humans is described by psychoacoustics (Fastl and Zwicker 2007; Moore 1997). More specifically, psychoacoustics is the scientific field concerned with the psychological and physiological responses associated with sound, including speech and musical stimuli.

The range of frequencies perceived by the human ear reaches from 16 to 20,000 Hz in normal-hearing young individuals. The upper frequency limit of hearing declines with age, an effect called *presbyacusis*.

The human ear is not equally sensitive to all frequencies. Its highest sensitivity lies between 2000 and 5000 Hz where sound pressure levels even below 0 dB SPL can be perceived. As shown in Fig. 1.50, the hearing threshold is strongly dependent on the frequency of sound. In our daily acoustic environment, sound, and also speech in a conversational situation, does not occur at threshold levels but rather at suprathreshold intensities. For such sounds the experienced loudness is a very important subjective quantity.

1.3.5 Loudness

As the human ear is not equally sensitive to all frequencies, two tones are not perceived equally

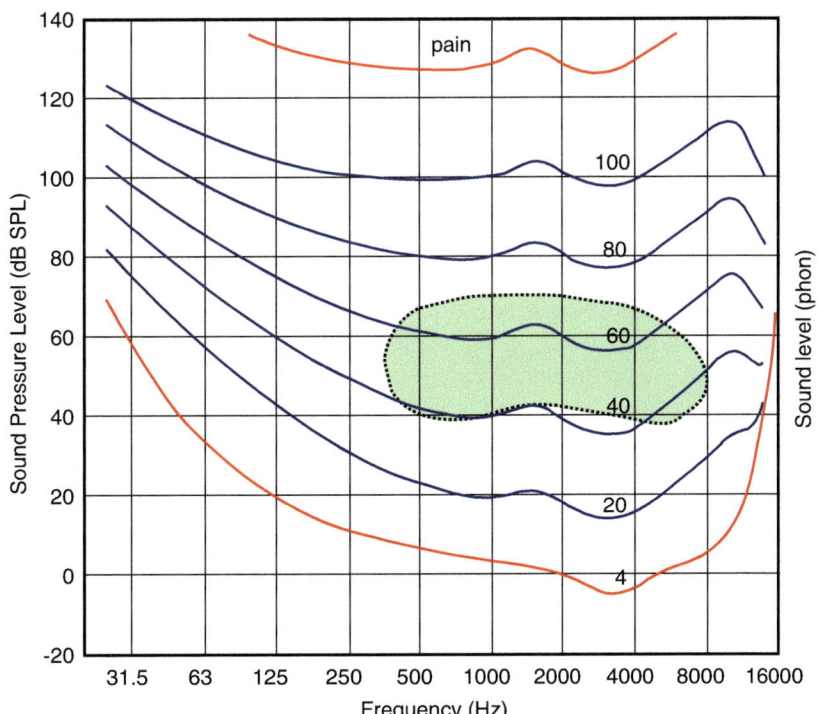

Fig. 1.50 Range of hearing and equal loudness contours for 20, 40, 60, 80 and 100 phon (data from Suzuki and Takeshima 2004, processed and graphic generated by the author). Lowest curve (lower red line): hearing threshold. Also shown is the range of conversational speech (green area) and the threshold of pain (upper red line). The sound pressure level in dB SPL equals the subjective sound level in phon at 1000 Hz

loud when presented at an equal sound pressure level. For instance, if a 1000 Hz tone is presented at a 20 dB level, it is experienced as loud as a 63 Hz tone presented at 60 dB SPL. Subjectively rated equal loudness levels of different tones are reported in specific curves called *isophones* or *equal loudness contours*. The unit of the loudness level of isophones is the phon, where the phon values at 1000 Hz equal the values of dB SPL. Whereas isophones exhibit a very steep dependence on frequency at low sound pressure levels, they show a much flatter dependence at high sound pressure levels.

Another way to judge the intensity of the perceived loudness is by using a 'categorical' scale that encompasses the whole range of categories by which we determine the loudness of everyday sounds. The loudness categories are defined in terms such as 'inaudible', 'very soft', 'soft', 'medium', 'loud' and 'too loud' as a judgement of loudness to stimuli presented at different sound pressure levels. Such scaling is particularly useful for the diagnosis of recruitment (pathological reduction of the auditory dynamic range) and for the fitting of hearing aids and hearing implants.

To account for the different sensitivity of the human ear to different frequencies, especially at low sound levels, an additional scale has been developed, the so-called dB (A) scale. The dB (A) scale weights the sound levels by a filtering function (A-filter), which approximates the sensitivity of the human ear at the isophone curve at 20–40 phon (see Fig. 1.50). By applying this filter function to a measured sound level, the low frequencies and the high frequencies contribute less to the total level of the weighted sound thereby mimicking the loudness perception of the human ear. The dB (A) scale is particularly used in quantifying levels of background noise for acoustic testing and for determining levels of noise exposure in natural or working environments.

1.3.6 Masking of Sound

The perception of sound signals, e.g. tones or speech, is also influenced by the presence of competing noise, an effect called *masking*. Masking plays an important role in everyday listening and in audiometry. Generally, the presence of a masking noise (called *a masker*) raises the hearing threshold of a tone. The masking effect is largest when the frequencies of the signal and of the masker are similar, and it decreases with increasing distance between their frequencies. However, the decrease is not symmetrical with respect to masker frequency: masking is more effective when a low-frequency sound masks a high-frequency signal than vice versa. In this case an effect called *upward spread of masking* occurs. To attain the opposite effect, the masker (i.e. the high-frequency sound) must be of an intense sound level. Owing to the nature of the human cochlea, upward spread of masking is more prominent and is important for understanding speech in noisy environments. It has to be particularly considered for the fitting of hearing aids and hearing implants.

Depending on the masker's frequency spectrum and on its temporal properties (e.g. gaps between sounds), the perception of signals can be influenced in a variety of ways. Masking can also occur in a different temporal relationship from that of the signal: as either simultaneous masking, forward masking or backward masking.

1.3.7 Binaural Hearing

Compared with monaural hearing, binaural hearing allows the auditory system to make better use of the information contained in sounds. Main advantages of binaural hearing are (1) the ability to localise sound sources and (2) the ability to achieve improved speech intelligibility in noise.

1.3.7.1 Localisation
The ability to identify the location or origin of a sound is called sound localisation (Blauert 1996).

Mechanisms involved in sound source localisation include the evaluation of:

- Differences in arrival time of sounds between the right and the left ear (inter-aural time difference, ITD).
- Differences in the levels of high-frequency sounds between the right and the left ear (inter-aural level difference, ILD).
- Asymmetrical spectral reflections from various parts of the bodies, including torso, shoulders and pinnae.

For detecting the spatial origin of low-frequency (about <800 Hz) sound, the auditory system evaluates inter-aural time differences (ITD), e.g. a sound coming from the right side arrives earlier at the right ear than at the left ear. Contrarily, for high frequencies (about >1600 Hz), the inter-aural level differences (ILD) are predominantly evaluated by the brain. The ILDs are mainly due to the head shadow effect, as the level of sound from the right causes a higher sound pressure level on the right ear than on the left ear.

Localisation in the median plane is possible as the human outer ear (pinna and the ear canal) forms acoustic filters that are sensitive to the direction of the incoming sound. Different resonances of these filters cause direction-specific patterns into the frequency responses of the ears, which are evaluated by the brain. The combination of these patterns with other direction-selective reflections at the head, shoulders and torso forms the so-called head-related transfer functions (HRTF) which are specific for each individual. In closed rooms, not only the direct sound from a sound source reaches the ears but also sound that has been reflected from the walls. When localising a sound source under such conditions, the auditory system analyses only the original direct sound (which arrives first at the ear); not the reflected sound (which arrives later). This feature is called the 'law of the first wave front', as the analysis of the reflected sound is suppressed.

1.3.7.2 Speech Intelligibility in Noise

Hearing in noise is one of the more challenging tasks in today's acoustic environment, as background noise is nearly always present in daily listening situations.

The presence of noise may cause substantial masking of acoustic signals and in particular the masking of speech, the most common being the cocktail party effect. For speech understanding in noisy environments, binaural hearing and proper functioning of the inner ear are crucial. The brain's comparison of the right and left auditory inputs will then result in a significant internal noise reduction called *binaural release from masking*.

Speech intelligibility in noise is most often quantified by the *signal-to-noise ratio*, i.e. the ratio between the sound level of the signal (speech) and that of the noise at the point where the listener achieves 50% speech intelligibility. The signal-to-noise ratio is an important measure for assessing the benefit of hearing aids or cochlear implants. Besides advantages of localisation abilities, the improvement of hearing in noise is the main argument for a binaural supply with hearing prostheses.

1.4   Concise Overview of the Physiology of Hearing

Ad Snik

1.4.1   Anatomy and Physiology of the Hearing Organ

The hearing organ, schematically presented in Fig. 1.37 taken from Sect. 1.2, can be subdivided into four parts:

- The external part, comprising the auricle and external auditory canal. This part of the ear collects the airborne sounds and transports these sounds to the entrance of the middle ear, the tympanic membrane.

- The middle ear is an air-filled cavity that comprises the tympanic membrane and (coupled) the middle ear ossicles. The middle ear system transforms the sound waves into mechanical vibrations that are led to the entrance of the inner ear, the oval window.
- The inner ear or cochlea, a fluid-filled, spiral-formed organ that comprises the sensory cells. The mechanical vibrations of the middle ear system are propagated as vibrations through the cochlear fluids. These vibrations activate the sensory cells in the cochlea. In fact, the vestibular system and the cochlea form one organ often referred to as the audiovestibular system. The vestibular system is addressed in Sects. 1.2 and 16.15.
- The auditory neural system that transports the action potentials generated by the activated sensory cells to the brainstem and (sub)cortical auditory areas.

If we look in more detail (Fig. 1.37 from Sect. 1.2), first of all at the outer ear, the auricle or pinna is characterised by certain folds, which play an important part in the processing of high frequencies that we use for localisation of sound sources, in particular in the vertical plane. Furthermore, the auricle is important for separating frontal and rear sources because its shape causes sounds from the front or rear to be diffracted differently, resulting in slight but detectable differences in the frequency spectrum. The tympanic membrane at the end of the external canal has relatively low impedance, comparable to the acoustic impedance of sound in air. As a result, airborne sound waves efficiently vibrate the tympanic membrane. Its low-power but relatively high-amplitude vibrations are transformed into more powerful vibrations with low amplitude, by the ossicular chain system. Thus this system works as an 'impedance' match that effectively transforms the acoustic energy of the airborne sound wave into mechanical energy of the fluid wave in the cochlea, a mechanical amplification procedure that requires no additional energy to perform. The ossicular system is connected to the tympanic membrane via the malleus at one end and to the cochlea at the other. The last ossicle, the stapes, moves pistonwise in the oval window of the cochlea (Slis and Snik 1997a).

The cochlea comprises a spiral-formed twisted canal with approximately 2.5 turns. Figure 1.51 presents schematically the unrolled cochlea. In fact, three different parallel canals can be distinguished, called the scala, the scala media and the scala vestibuli (see Fig. 1.51). Stapes-induced vibrations of the oval window, at the base of the cochlea, cause the fluid in the scala vestibuli to be set into motion, resulting in a longitudinal fluid wave. That motion reaches the top of the cochlea, or the apex, where the scala vestibuli and the scala tympani are connected (illustrated in Fig. 1.51). The longitudinal wave reverses its direction through the scala tympani, towards the second window in the base

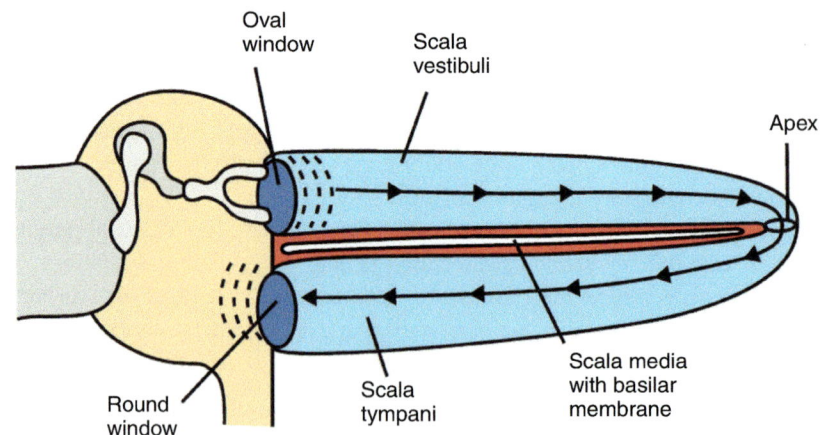

Fig. 1.51 The unravelled cochlea comprising three compartments, the scala vestibuli, the scala tympani and, in between, the scala media with the sensory elements

of the cochlea, the round window. At the round window, the energy of the fluid wave is dissipated at the round window. The third scala is a separated canal in the middle, not connected to the other two scalae. It contains fluid, endolymph, with different ion concentrations than the fluid in the other two scalae, the perilymph. The scala vestibuli is separated from the scala media by a thin, highly mobile membrane, the membrane of Reissner. For the longitudinal waves in the scala vestibuli, mechanically, this membrane does not exist. This means that the longitudinal wave on either side of the (stiffer) membrane between the scala media and scala tympani, the basilar membrane, creates pressure differences over this membrane, causing up-down movements of that membrane. These movements look like a transversal travelling wave. The basilar membrane comprises the sensory elements that are activated by the transversal movements of the membrane. These elements are called the organ of Corti (Slis and Snik 1997b).

At the base of the cochlea, the basilar membrane is relatively thick and narrow. At the apex, the basilar membrane is relatively thin and broad. Between these two extremes, the width of the membrane and its thickness change rather linearly. As a result, the stiffness of the membrane is much higher at the base than at the apex. For high frequencies, the basilar membrane is highly mobile near the base, while for low frequencies, the highest mobility is found near the apex. As a consequence, the mobility of the basilar membrane is frequency-dependent from the base to the apex; when stimulated, the amplitude of the travelling wave will peak at a certain distance from the base, where the distance is determined by the frequency of the sound. This is referred to as tonotopic organisation of the basilar membrane.

The organ of Corti is situated on top of the basilar membrane (see Fig. 1.44 taken from Sect. 1.2), close to the modiolus. Along the full length of the basilar membrane, this organ contains four parallel rows of hair cells, one row of inner hair cells (closest to the modiolus) and three rows of outer hair cells.

Inner and outer hair cells are situated on either side of a rather solid ridge, the tunnel of Corti. Each hair cell is connected to neurons; the inner hair cells mainly to afferent neurons and the outer hair cells mainly to efferent neurons. The differences in anatomy and neural connections suggest that inner hair cells and outer hair cells have different functions. Above the hair cells, the tectorial membrane is situated, which is (only) connected to the cochlear wall near the modiolus. The tips of the cilia of the hair cells are connected to the tectorial membrane, such that they bend when the basilar membrane moves relative to the stiff tectorial membrane. The connection of the cilia to the tectorial membrane is tighter for the outer hair cells than for the inner hair cells (Green 1976).

The endolymph, in the scala media, and the perilymph, in the other two scalae, have different ion concentrations. This causes a potential difference of about 80 mV over the membranes that separate the scala media from the other two scalae, the basilar membrane and membrane of Reissner. This difference in potential is kept constant by ion pumps in the stria vascularis, which covers the outer wall of the scala media. Positively charged ions are pumped from the perilymph to the endolymph. When the cilia of hair cells bend, an influx of positive ions causes depolarisation of the hair cell, which subsequently leads to an action potential in the afferent neuron connected to that hair cell. Inner hair cells are the main sensors. However, only loud sounds stimulate the cilia of the inner hair cells forcefully enough to cause depolarisation. Outer hair cells have another function; apart from sensory properties, they also have motor properties. These cells can amplify the relatively small movements of the basilar membrane caused by soft sounds (the 'active mechanism' or 'cochlear amplifier', which requires the input of additional energy via the efferent neurons), with subsequent sufficiently strong movements of the inner hair cells for depolarisation. These motoric actions of the outer hair cells are controlled by neural feedback loops (Moore 2008) (see Sect. 1.4.3.2) and are the main loci of the non-linearity of the cochlear response.

1.4.2 Perception of Sounds

1.4.2.1 Fundamental Concepts

Our perception of sound is based on logarithmic scales. Concerning loudness, this has led to the introduction of the decibel scale, which is a logarithmic measure of physical sound pressure levels. In pitch perception, we use the octave scale, which is a logarithmic measure of frequency.

Our 'hearing range' is often visualised in a graph of sound pressure levels in decibels (dB) versus frequency in Hertz (Hz) organised into octaves (the interval of one octave represents a doubling of frequency, so that 250 Hz, 500 Hz, 1 kHz and 2 kHz, e.g. are octave steps). Section 1.3 Fig. 1.50 shows the hearing range of a normal-hearing subject, which is determined by the frequency-dependent threshold of hearing (in dB SPL, dB sound level pressure; lower limit) and the loudness discomfort level (also in dB SPL; the blue line marked 100). Adolescents have the best hearing, in a frequency range from 20 Hz to 20 kHz, with a hearing range at 1 kHz from approximately 0 to 110–125 dB SPL. Normal thresholds of hearing differ at each frequency and are worse at the low and high frequencies, as displayed in Sect. 1.3 Fig. 1.50, which shows the standardised normal threshold (the lower red line). For this reason, the hearing thresholds of an individual subject are usually not plotted in dB SPL but in dB HL, or dB Hearing Level, which is relative to the standardised normal-hearing threshold. This standardised normal threshold is 0 dB HL at all frequencies. Thus, hearing thresholds in dB HL are 0 for a normal-hearing person. In clinical practice, however, a normal range of <20 dB HL is typically used. A further decibel scale, dB SL, or dB Sensation Level, is sometimes used, especially in research, to present sounds at a set level above each subject's threshold. Any individual's threshold (in dB SPL or dB HL) can be represented as 0 dB SL. 20 dB SL is therefore 20 dB above the individual's threshold. The loudness discomfort level now equals approximately 100 dB HL for all frequencies. For diagnostic purposes, hearing thresholds and loudness discomfort levels are only measured in the frequency range from 0.25 to 8 kHz. The resulting graph, called an audiogram, is displayed in Fig. 1.52. Note that in an audiogram, hearing levels are presented upside-down. For counselling purposes, the speech dynamic range is indicated, which is the mean sound pressure level of normal conversational speech as a function of frequency, together with its range of 30 dB, expressed in dB HL. During normal running speech, the speech sound levels will be within this area 90% of the time.

1.4.2.2 Air- and Bone-Conduction Stimulation

Normal hearing is based on the perception of air-borne sounds via the outer, middle and inner ear routes. However, a vibrating head (e.g. in an environment with loud sound) also leads to sound perception. The 'normal' route is called air-conduction stimulation, whereas the latter route is bone-conduction stimulation. Stimulation by bone conduction can be demonstrated by placing a vibrating tuning fork anywhere on the skull. The vibrations of the tuning fork induce vibrations of the skull, which are transmitted to the cochlea where they are perceived as sounds. Self-perception of our own voices comes via the 'normal' air-conduction route as well as via bone-conduction (from the vibration of our vocal folds on phonation). Measurements in the cochlea of animals have shown that air-conduction stimulation and bone-conduction stimulation lead to similar movements of the basilar membrane. The mechanism by which the vibrating skull results in fluid waves in the cochlea is complicated. Several factors play a role, such as inertia of the cochlear fluid, compression of the cochlear walls upon the fluid and inertia of the middle ear ossicles, to name the most important ones (Stenfelt and Goode 2005). The relative importance of these factors depends on frequency. Bone conduction can be as much as 50 dB less efficient than air-conduction stimulation. Bone-conduction is more efficient at lower frequencies, explaining why we perceive our own voices to be lower in pitch than others perceive them. During clinical hearing tests in hearing-impaired patients, both stimulation routes are tested, using headphones for the air-conduction route and a bone-

Fig. 1.52 Audiogram format with the speech area indicated in grey (according to Mueller and Killion 1990). The red symbols (open dots) are hearing thresholds of a hearing-impaired patient; the T symbols refer to his loudness discomfort levels

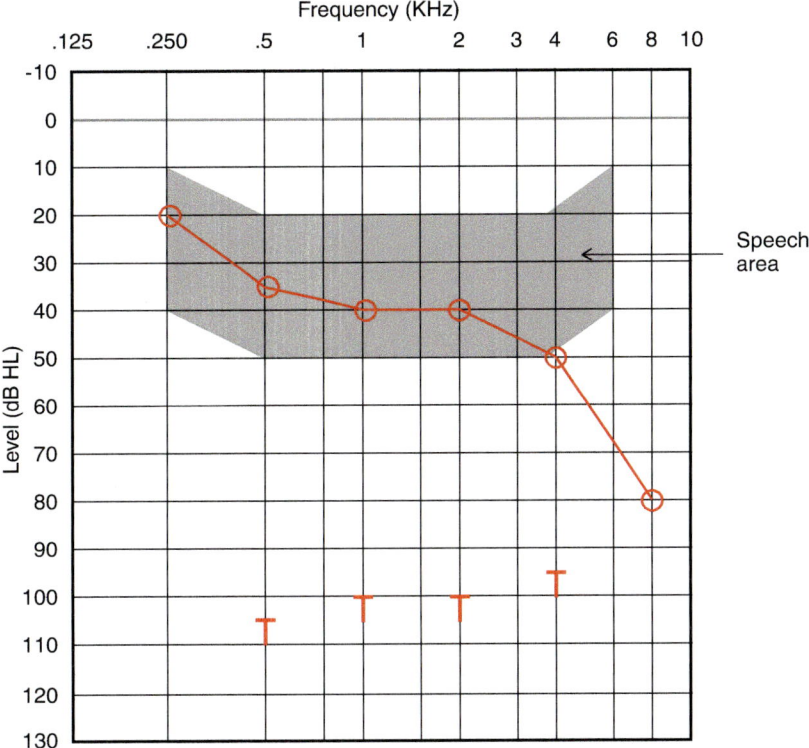

conduction vibrator, placed on the head, to test the bone-conduction route. Owing to calibration, these two routes will show similar hearing thresholds in most hearing-impaired subjects; however, this is no longer the case in patients with an obstructed air-conduction route (e.g. because of absent or fixated middle ear ossicles).

Figure 1.52 shows a patient's hearing thresholds, measured via the air-conduction route. If the cause of the hearing loss is situated in the cochlea (e.g. loss of outer hair cells), then soft sounds are no longer properly detected; however, loud sounds are well perceived by a normal functioning cochlea. This results in a reduced hearing range (or 'dynamic range'). In this case, at 1 kHz, the dynamic range extends from 40 to 100 dB HL. Such a hearing loss is called a sensorineural hearing loss (SNHL). The reduced dynamic range found in SNHL leads to the perceived loudness of a sound growing more rapidly as the level of the sound increases than in normal hearing. This process is called recruitment. If the hearing loss is situated in the middle ear, while the

cochlea is functioning normally, then the thresholds and loudness discomfort level will be shifted equally and the hearing range remains unchanged. Such a hearing loss is referred to as a conductive hearing loss.

1.4.3 Temporal-Spectral Processing

1.4.3.1 Frequency Resolution

Owing to the tonotopic organisation of the basilar membrane, this membrane works as a frequency analyser. A longitudinal wave of a certain frequency leads to maximal membrane motion at a characteristic distance from the oval window. In principle, this enables the separation of simultaneous sounds based on frequency. However, frequency resolution is not perfect. A pure tone will not only excite the basilar membrane at its characteristic point but a certain area around it, the excitation area. The width of excitation areas determines frequency resolution; within such an area, frequency resolution is low; however, between nonoverlapping excitation regions, frequency resolution is optimal (Moore 2008). The 'mechanical' filtering of the basilar membrane seems to be a good explanation for the frequency resolution, as has been reported for loud sounds. Then, typically, excitation areas are approximately one octave. Note that loud sounds, above 60 dB HL, stimulate the inner hair cells directly. For softer sounds, better frequency resolution has been measured. To explain this, a second filter, just for soft sounds, has been postulated, which is based on the (controlled) motoric actions of the outer hair cells.

1.4.3.2 Tuning Curve or Critical Bands and Temporal Resolution

The frequency selectivity of a single auditory neuron, connected to a specific inner hair cell, thus frequency tuned, is quantified by its 'tuning curve'. A tuning curve presents the threshold of activation by sounds of different frequencies. The lowest sound level (threshold) that evokes an action potential occurs at the specific frequency of the inner hair cell, the characteristic frequency (Moore 2008). For frequencies close to that frequency, activation occurs at higher stimulation levels, caused by spread of excitation. Figure 1.53 shows an example. In principle this is a sensitivity curve for that neuron/hair cell. Such a curve can also be determined behaviourally (Slis and Snik 1997b), for example, a psychophysical tuning curve can be obtained by presenting a pure tone at a specific frequency and measuring the

levels required to 'mask' it (i.e. to make the pure tone inaudible) by narrow bandwidth noise centred on that same frequency and then on other surrounding frequencies. The outcome represents the response of the 'auditory filter', a functional conceptualisation of neural tuning curves (Moore 2008). The inverted tuning curve is the critical band for that characteristic frequency and is much more 'sharply tuned' than that reported for loud sounds. The outer hair cells play a role: as previously stated, for soft sounds these cells enable perception of the sound via the inner hair cells by amplification of the movements of the basilar membrane. Inhibition of the motor actions of the outer hair cells occurs, controlled by neural loops; outer hair cells above and below the hair cell with the characteristic frequency are inhibited. This sharpens up the tuning curves.

When outer hair cells are not functional, soft sounds are not perceived, and the louder sounds that are perceived directly by the inner hair cells have poor spectral resolution. This affects speech perception in patients with sensorineural hearing loss to a degree that depends on the severity of the hearing loss. Perception of speech relies on spectral resolution and also on temporal resolution; the shortest perceptible time interval between sounds ('gap detection') is a measure of interest here, indicating, as it does, the listener's ability to distinguish, and therefore more easily process separate speech sounds. For normal-hearing subjects, the gap detection threshold is in the order of a few milliseconds. Temporal resolution varies

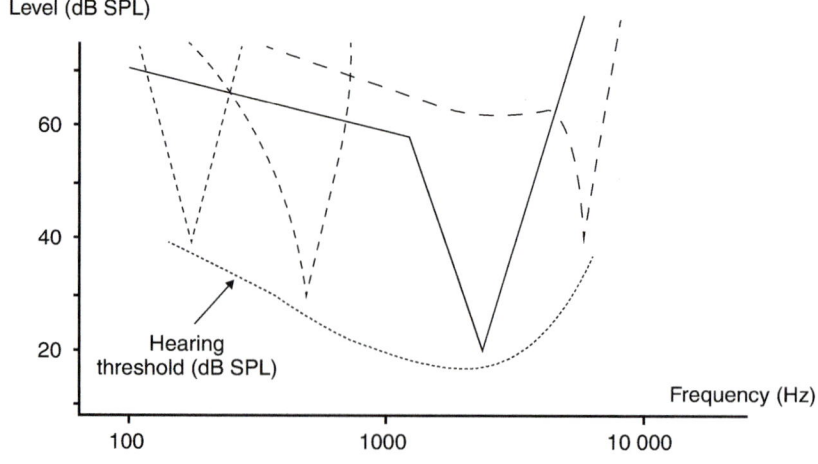

Fig. 1.53 Schematic representation of tuning curves (four) obtained from four different nerves. The lines connect the measured sound pressure levels (in dB SPL) that just resulted in stimulation of the nerve under study (adapted figure from Slis and Snik, 1997b)

according to the spectral content and level and duration of the particular sound stimuli, but no single theory adequately explains how temporal processing occurs (Moore 2008). Temporal resolution plays a role not only in speech processing but also in our ability to localise sounds in space (the inter-aural time difference component of Lord Rayleigh's Duplex theory (Rayleigh 1907)) and our perception of the intensity of sounds shorter than 200 ms (Moore 2008).

See Part IV for further information on the pathology of hearing.

1.5 Principles of Physiology and Biomechanics of Voice: Aerodynamics of Voice

Felix de Jong and Harm K. Schutte

1.5.1 Sound Production

The primary function of the larynx is protection of the lower respiratory tract against the intrusion of foreign bodies. This is clearly seen in the anatomy of the larynx as a functional structure with characteristics of a valve and sphincter. The intralaryngeal musculature, including the thyroarytenoid muscle, is orientated more or less circularly (Harris et al. 1998). This enables active closure of the lower airway.

Sound is produced by a periodic interruption of the expiratory airstream, for which the histoarchitecture of the larynx has evolved into an optimal structure. In Hirano's cover-body theory, the vocal folds consist of five layers: the thyroarytenoid muscle, the vocal ligament with a relatively stiff inner layer and a relatively elastic outer layer, the loose tissue of the Reinke space and the epithelium (Hirano and Kurita 1986; Hirano 1974; Hirano and Kakita 1981). The Reinke space enables the epithelium to move over the vocal ligament. This is a basic condition for the formation of the mucosal wave. In vocal fold pathology, the Reinke space is often affected, resulting into an abnormal mucosal wave (Fig. 1.54).

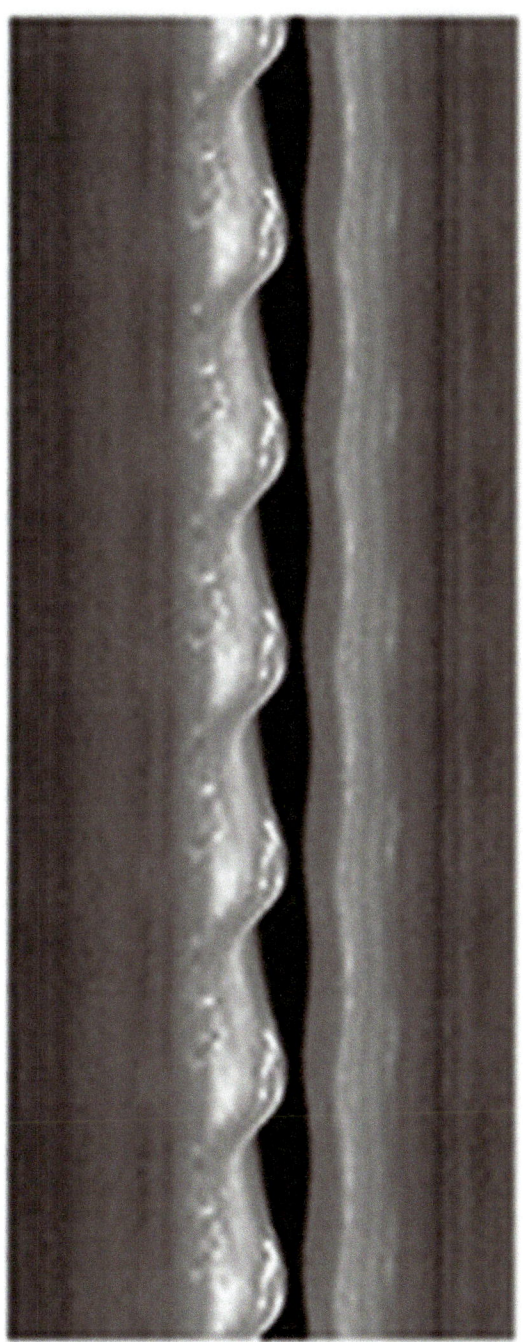

Fig. 1.54 Intracordal fibrosis of the left vocal fold observed by videokymography (courtesy of the author). The mucosal wave is nearly absent. For explanation of the videokymographic registration, see Fig. 1.55. For more information on videokymography, see Schutte et al. (1998)

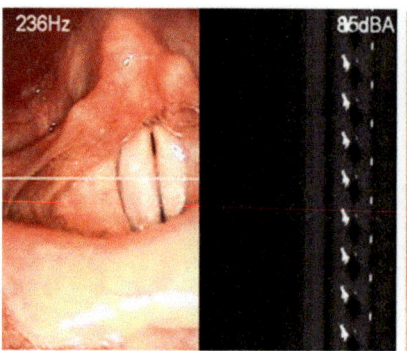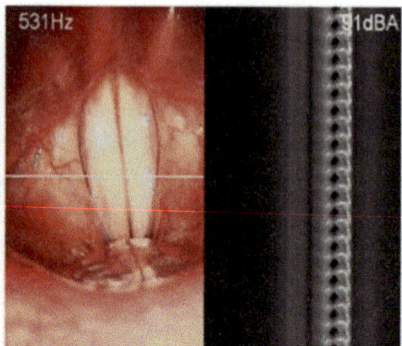

Fig. 1.55 The vibratory pattern of the vocal fold mucosa observed by videokymography (courtesy of the author). The videokymographic picture consists of only one line and is taken at the level of the white line on the white-light picture. This line is written from above to below with a sampling frequency of 7200/s. The amplitude of the chest voice (left) is larger, and glottal closure lasts longer than the falsetto voice (right). It is easy to see that there is a very short closure in the falsetto production

The following description is a simplified version of the mechanism of formation of the mucosal wave. When phonation starts, the vocal folds move from the respiratory position to the phonation position, i.e. medially. When the expiratory air passes through the narrowed glottis, an interaction between the airstream and the vocal fold mucosa occurs. The mucosa is pulled towards the midline by the Bernoulli effect, and the glottis is closed as a consequence. Now the expiratory air stream is stopped and the Bernoulli effect that medialises the mucosa disappears. Subsequently, there is a recoil of the mucosa owing to its inherent elastic forces. The glottis is now open again, and the air can pass, when the cycle starts again (Fig. 1.55).

This causes a periodic interruption of the expiratory air stream that sets the air column vibrating. The frequency of sound is defined as the number of times per second that the expiratory air stream is interrupted by the mucosal wave. Vibrating air with a fundamental frequency between around 20 Hz and 20 kHz is experienced as sound. It should be clear that sound production from the larynx as a sound source cannot be compared to the sound production of a plucked string. Therefore, the term 'vocal fold' is more appropriate than 'vocal cord'. This complex source sound is modified by the selective amplification of the separate harmonics, by the supraglottal resonance cavity into speech or by other vocal expressions.

The development of the mucosal wave pattern is determined by aerodynamic, myoelastic and biomechanical parameters and varies according to the sound intensity and frequency. It is logical that phonation is strongly related to the factors of airflow and subglottal pressure. In phonation there is a complex interaction between aerodynamic parameters and the myoelastic properties and biomechanics that control the degree of adduction and tension of the vocal folds.

Aerodynamic Parameters From the beginning of physiological studies in voice, attention has been paid to these parameters and also to understanding what might happen in voice pathology. Many studies have been performed to measure the rate of airflow and subglottal pressure under several conditions of frequency and sound pressure level. From these studies, it has become clear in general that the relationship between flow and pressure is rather complex. There is a great variety in individual larynges, which makes it difficult to use aerodynamic values for diagnostic purposes. We have also to realise that this complexity of relationship obscures our understanding of the aerodynamic behaviour of the vibrating larynx. Moreover, the relationship between aerodynamics and other parameters is not fully understood.

Assessment of factors other than flow and pressure, such as the acoustics of the vocal tract and the closed quotient of the mucosal wave, is more relevant. In singing pedagogy, these parameters seem to stay central in the process of phonation.

Biomechanical Parameters, Glottal Closure Adequate approximation of the vocal folds is an important condition for the Bernoulli effect. The Bernoulli effect explains how the acceleration of the air particles is related to the air pressure on the walls when the particles are forced to pass a narrowed part of the airway (different diameters of trachea versus glottis). This creates a decrease of the air pressure exercised on the walls of the narrowed passage. Owing to this decrease, the walls (the loosely connected epithelial tissue on the surface of the vocal folds) are sucked inwards, which helps in closing the glottis (more) abruptly. In the formula describing the Bernoulli effect, the distance between the folds is a factor expressed to the fourth power, so the effect is strongest when the vocal folds are near to each other. This is specifically the case at the moments when the vocal folds in the vibratory movements are approximating, which therefore strongly facilitates dynamic closure. The aerodynamic parameters are in equilibrium with the degree of vocal fold closure. With insufficient adduction of the vocal folds, air will escape with insufficient effect on the mucosa (Fig. 1.56).

In most females there is dorsal gap, due to the way the larynx is built, i.e. constitutionally (Fig. 1.57) (Sulter and Albers 1996; Sulter et al. 1995; Schutte et al. 1998).

This dorsal gap is not an abnormality per se but may play an important role in clinical practice. A gap negatively influences voice capacity. The voice may be easily overloaded, which in turn may lead to the formation of nodules on the vocal fold edges, i.e. a clinical issue. If the adduction is too tight, the opening phase of the mucosal wave is too short.

Myoelastic Parameters, Vocal Fold Mucosa The thickness and elastic properties of the vocal fold mucosa depend on the tension and length of the vocal folds. When the thyroarytenoid

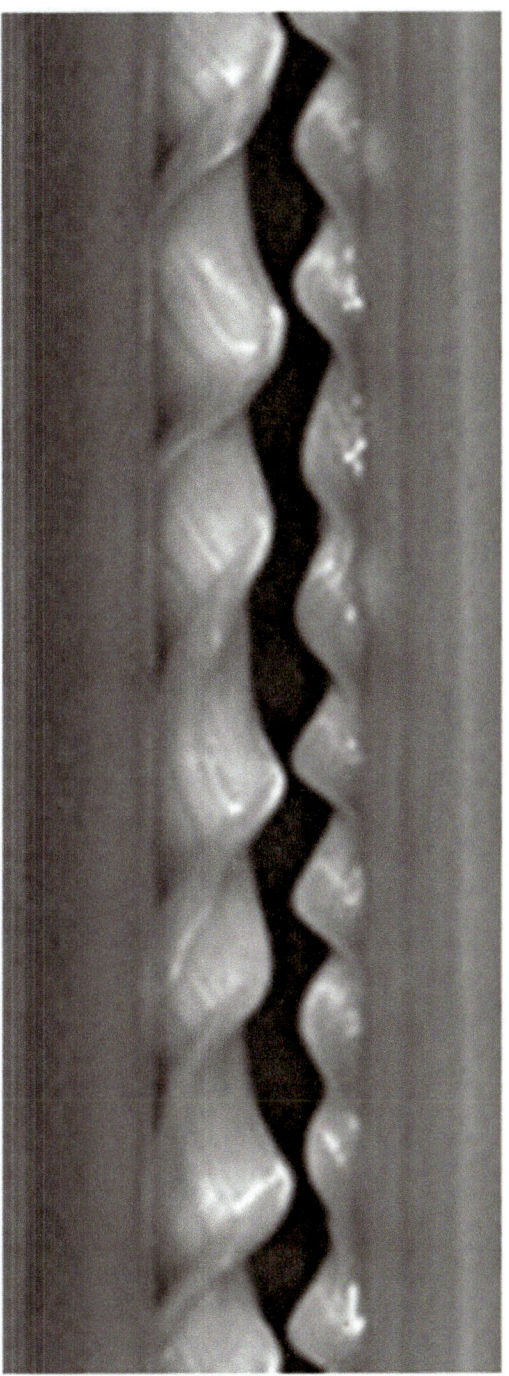

Fig. 1.56 Left laryngeal paralysis observed by videokymography (courtesy of the author). Glottal closure is incomplete. Both vocal folds show an irregular vibration, especially the left, the frequency of which is, additionally, higher than that of the right. This is perceived in the voice (diplophonia) as breathiness and hoarseness. For stroboscopy this means a triggering problem, causing a blurry pattern, by which the image obtained is useless

Fig. 1.57 Incomplete dorsal closure observed by videokymography (courtesy of the author). The videokymographic picture is taken at the level of the white line on the continuous white-light picture. The vibratory pattern shows small amplitude at the level of incomplete closure

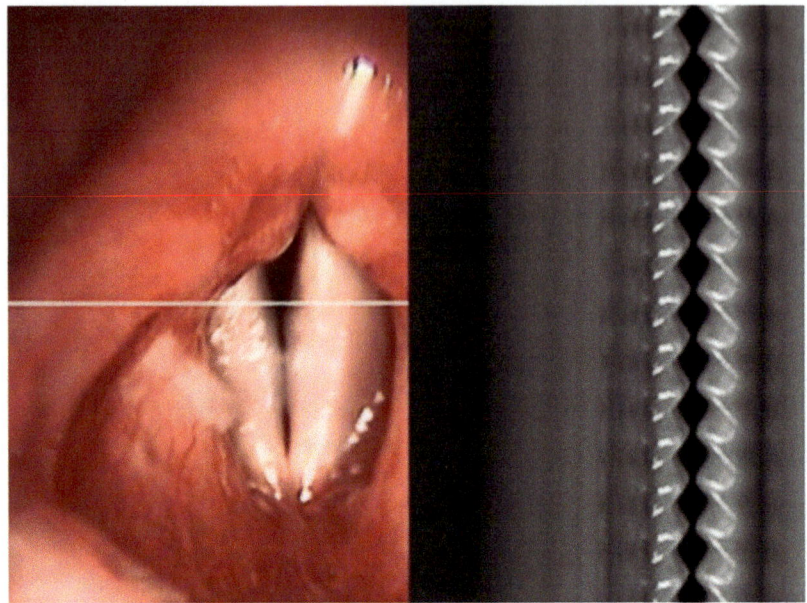

muscle contracts, there is an active tension with shortening of the vocal folds and consequent loosening of the mucosa. Other intrinsic and extrinsic muscles counteract these actions to create adequate balance of the various parameters. When the cricothyroid muscle contracts, there is a stretching and passive increase of the tension of the vocal folds. The mucosa is more tense and thinner.

1.5.2 An Adequate Balance of Parameters

Aerodynamic, myoelastic and biomechanical parameters influence the mucosal wave characteristics in a cooperative way. To create a certain condition regarding frequency and timbre of the source sound, a specific, adequate equilibrium between these parameters is required. The basic glottal sound is complex, comprising a fundamental frequency and harmonics of multiple-integer values of the fundamental. A clear voice sound of a certain vowel is composed of well-defined harmonics with little noise. The abruptness and completeness of the

glottal closure act strongly upon the properties of the harmonics.

Resonator The source sound is modified in the supraglottal resonance cavity. The resonance cavity consists of the hypo-, oro- and nasopharynx. The paranasal sinuses do not contribute to the ultimate sound. The size and form of the resonance cavities are variable, and in this way certain frequencies can be amplified. The selective amplified frequencies or groups of frequencies are called 'formants'. Formants are resonance frequencies of the resonance cavity and are characteristic for different vowels. Formants therefore belong to the vocal tract characteristics, while harmonics are part of the voice source (vocal folds), as is the fundamental frequency.

Registers The main observed difference in vibration pattern of the vocal folds is to be seen in what had been perceived and already described in the seventeenth century, the chest voice and falsetto. In chest voice the vocal fold mucosa is loose and thick and shows, in general, a complete glottal closure during phonation (Fig. 1.55). This is related to a vocal sound with a relatively weak fundamental and a rich series of harmonics. In falsetto the vocal folds are thin and meet each other in the middle only for a short part of the glottal closure, if at all (Fig. 1.55). This leads to a weaker sound with a relatively strong fundamental and only a few harmonics. The difference in perceived sound is determined by this difference.

1.6 Voice and Room Acoustics

Malte Kob

1.6.1 Resonances of Rooms

Like the effect of geometry and colour of a room on its visual impression, the acoustic impression of a room is significantly determined by its shape and the properties of its surfaces. Furthermore, just as the variation of the optimal amount of light and colour in a room reflects its purpose (bedroom, discotheque, museum, office), its optimal acoustic properties strongly depend on its intended use. Whereas rooms for speech performance or measurement require a quiet, 'dry' acoustics, more room support is needed for singers and musicians (Audio Samples 1.1–1.8).

> Ach, ich fühl's, es ist verschwunden
> Ewig hin der Liebe Glück!
> (Ah, I feel it, it has disappeared
> Forever gone love's happiness!)

The voice is provided in four modes:

- Original recording (Audio Sample 1.1 Singing Voice Original)
- A 'dry' room (Audio Sample 1.2 Singing Voice Dry)
- A room with medium reverberation time (Audio Sample 1.3 Singing Voice Medium)
- A 'wet' room with long reverberation time (Audio Sample 1.4 Singing Voice Wet)

The voice is provided in four modes:

- Original recording (Audio Sample 1.5 Running Speech Original)

- A 'dry' room (Audio Sample 1.6 Running Speech Dry)
- A room with medium reverberation time (Audio Sample 1.7 Running Speech Medium)
- A 'wet' room with long reverberation time (Audio Sample 1.8 Running Speech Wet)

The boundaries of (walls, floor, ceiling) and objects in the room (furniture, seats, people) can reflect, diffract or absorb sound that travels against them to different extents. All reflections will cause an increase in sound pressure level in front of the boundary, but resonating structures such as parallel walls not only produce locations with increased sound energy but also those with reduced sound energy (nodes). The amplification effects are called room resonances or room modes. These modes are responsible for the frequency- and location-dependent amplification of sound fields in a room.

A common criterion for a description of the temporal acoustic activity of a room is its reverberation, i.e. the ability to prolong sound input. The character of this prolongation can be described by the reverberation time T_{60}, which represents the time needed for a sound level decay by 60 dB of an interrupted sound source. Optimal values of T_{60} for high speech intelligibility range from 0.5 to 1 s and should be around 1.5 s for chamber music, whereas orchestral music profits from values between 1.5 and 2 s. Church music would profit from values above 3 s. A comprehensive overview of acoustic properties of concert halls can be found in Beranek (2004). Just as for coloured light reflection, the reflected sound is often prolonged differently for low, middle and high frequencies. This is caused by the room shape and the variable absorption characteristics of the room's surfaces.

A special effect can occur if surfaces are arranged such that sound is reflected iteratively between them. This effect is known as flutter echo or ringing resonances and will exhibit a strong colouration of the sound between the surfaces and a prolonged reverberation at distinct frequencies. In most cases, room shapes that can cause such resonances should be avoided.

1.6.2 Excitation of Rooms

As is the case for the importance of light sources in a room, the positioning and number of sound sources play a major role in the ease of voice production and projection. An important part of the sound difference between a baby's cry in a cradle, an opera singer on stage, a single voice and a choir is characterised by the frequency-dependent sound radiation of singers and the ability of the room to amplify or attenuate sound sources with respect to their position in the room.

The directivity of the voice can be compared to that of a loudspeaker: at low frequencies the sound is radiated rather equally in all directions, whereas phonemes with higher frequencies, such as consonants ([ʃ], [z], [f]) and vowels with higher formants ([aː], [ɛː], [iː]), are directed forwards. The efficiency of radiation strongly depends on the extent of mouth opening: a larger opening yields more efficient sound output at higher frequencies and thus a better intelligibility of speech or singing voice (Kob 2001). As a consequence, speech can be understood best when listeners and speakers face each other.

The combination of several voices in an ensemble or choir will produce the 'choir sound': single voices will blend to form a unique sound source to a certain extent. This 'apparent source width' has become another relevant criterion for the characterisation of music ensembles in concert halls (Bradley and Soulodre 1995; Barron 2010).

Acoustic modes represent sound field distributions where locations of strong and weak energy alternate along a direction in space. These distributions also vary with frequency. Owing to the strong reflections at hard walls, the sound pressure is doubled at walls and increased even more in edges and corners of a room. In other locations the sounds can be completely cancelled out. Both conditions might affect the radiation efficiency of speakers and singers, as well as the signal at the ear or microphone at certain frequencies. This effect is most prominent at low fundamental frequencies and in overtone singing. The position of a speaker or singer with respect to the room modes will determine how efficiently the room can accept and transfer the sound that is emitted from the mouth. Thus vocal performance is reduced when voice is generated in a modal node, whereas it is more efficient when the singer is placed at a favourable location that excites many room modes.

1.6.3 Direct Sound vs. Diffuse Sound Field

All rooms can contain three types of sound fields: a direct sound field around the vocalist, a modal sound field given by the room modes and a diffuse sound field. The last is best described by the sound that does not have a specific direction with no temporal or local decay. Consequently, this diffuse sound field must be constant all over the room interior. The room modes show a spatially periodic energy modulation that exhibits maxima of the sound pressure at the walls. These boundaries are therefore beneficial for a good room excitation, but they can also support the direct sound by adding early reflections at the listener's position. The direct sound has a strong dependence on the distance from the voice source. The level will decrease by $1/r^2$ with distance (r). At a certain distance from the voice source, the direct sound level and the diffuse field level will be equal. This distance is called the 'critical distance' (german: 'Hallradius'). Listeners who hear the voice within the critical distance are in the direct sound field; the others are in the diffuse or far field.

Attempts to increase the intelligibility of speech should aim at increasing the critical distance, thus reducing the diffuse sound field or increasing the sound level of the vocalist. An insufficient envelopment of the listener in the diffuse sound field should be countered by increasing reverberation by, e.g. removal of absorbent material or inclusion of electro-acoustic reverberation enhancement systems.

In Fig. 1.58 the different sound paths in a room with a voice source and a listener are illustrated. The balance of direct sound, early reflections and diffuse field has a significant influence on the comfort and performance of a

Fig. 1.58 Sound paths in a room: direct sound, early reflections and diffuse field

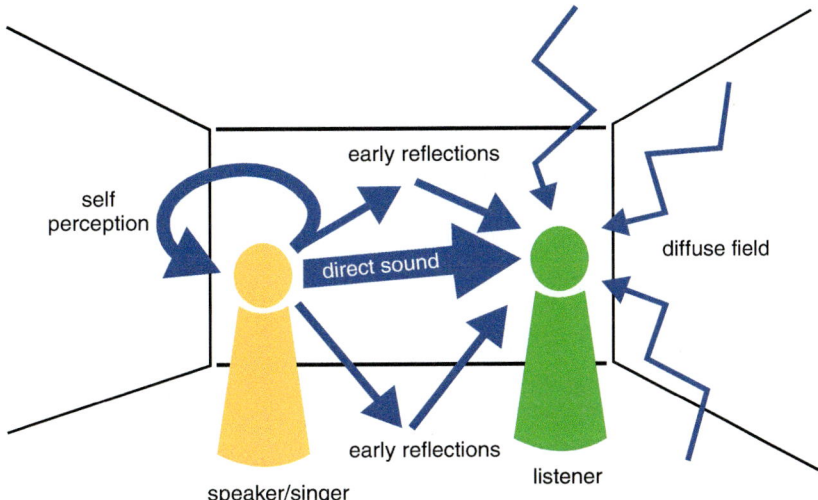

speaker or singer. On the other hand, listeners will experience this balance with respect to speech intelligibility, voice projection and engulfment.

In rooms that are primarily used for speech transmission, the direct sound should dominate over modal resonances and diffuse sound to prevent low and locally changing speech intelligibility. Improved understanding of speech and singing voice can be achieved by supporting early reflections from lateral walls or the ceiling, if these are not too distant.

1.6.4 Feedback Loops of Perception and Production

Perception of one's own voice takes place via air- and bone-borne waves. Healthy singers and speakers will always perceive both waves simultaneously. Room acoustics will only change the properties of the air wave, but this modification can have strong effects. In the case that the voice is produced in the focus of a resonator, the echoes can cause stuttering of a speaker. This effect often occurs when speakers perform under spheres or in front of concave facades.

Another effect of unwanted feedback occurs in rooms with a high diffuse field level, such as classrooms with rigid floors and walls or large windows. Teachers in such rooms will produce not only direct sound but also increase the diffuse field level with their voices. They—but also pupils in private communications—will try to raise their speech level and also pitch to achieve better perception of their speech. This effect is called the Lombard effect. The result is a rather high voice load and a loud learning atmosphere (Kob et al. 2008).

The other important impact of the room on the intelligibility of voice is the presence of reverberation and noise in the room. The first phenomenon is due to the ability of the room to accumulate sound energy, and the presence of noise is due to unwanted sound sources in- or outside the room. Whereas reverberation can be reduced by appropriate installation of absorbers, noise abatement requires improved sound insulation against the surrounding sound sources. The signal-to-noise ratio (SNR) can be a measure to determine the success of insulation against noise.

The signal properties of sound sources—wanted or unwanted—have a significant impact on our hearing. Signals that are similar to the human voice evoke more attention. Whereas this is beneficial for weak voices, e.g. of teachers in noisy environments, it can be a drawback if unwanted voice signals reduce concentration during challenging tasks such as communication.

Rooms used for voice or hearing diagnosis ideally meet these requirements:

- High sound damping at the room boundaries, especially through doors, windows, ventilation and heating systems, to achieve a high signal-to-noise ratio (SNR)
- Negligible room modes and diffuse field to achieve a dry and directive sound field

In addition to these conditions, the analysis of voices should also take into account guidelines for the selection of microphones (Svec and Granqvist 2010).

Guidelines exist for the limit values of some of the above and some other sound parameters for various use cases of rooms, such as classrooms or concert halls. Standards and recommendations are available for the assessment of such values and the scope of their validity:

- Noise criteria (NC) curves according to the American National Standards Institute (ANSI) S12.2 (2008) and ANSI S12.2 (1995) indicate maximum sound pressure values vs. frequency for different room types. These curves (and some other curves with similar meaning) can be easily obtained with modern SPL metres.
- Speech Transmission Index (for Public Address Systems) (STI-PA) according to IEC 60268-16-2011 (2011) indicates a simple speech intelligibility value on a scale from 0 (bad) to 1 (excellent), measured with a loudspeaker that emits a speech-like signal at the sender position and a microphone at the location of the listener. Other indices such as the Room Acoustics Speech Transmission Index (RASTI) give similar values for the intelligibility index between two persons. The Common Intelligibility Scale (CIS) after Barnett and Knight (1995) can be derived from STI using the formula

$$CIS = 1 + \log 10 (STI) \qquad (1.4)$$

- Other indices for description of a method for assessment of the influence of noise on speech intelligibility in communication such as

Speech Intelligibility Index (SIL) or Articulation Index (AI) are available; see, e.g. SS-ISO/TR 3352:1985.

Concerning improvement of classroom acoustics, see Sect. 18.12.

1.7 Voice Ergonomics

Wivine Decoster and Felix de Jong

1.7.1 Health and Ergonomics

The World Health Organization (WHO) presented a definition of health that entered into force on 7 April 1948:

> Health is a state of complete physical, mental and social well-being and not merely the absence of disease or infirmity.
> Preamble to the Constitution of the World Health Organization (1946)

This definition has not changed since then. Diminished health may lead to disability, which is defined by the WHO as

> Disabilities is an umbrella term, covering impairments, activity limitations, and participation restrictions.
> World Health Organization (2015)

Impairment is a problem in bodily function or structure; activity limitation is a difficulty encountered by an individual in executing a task or action; and participation restriction is a problem experienced by an individual in involvement in life situations (International Ergonomics Association 2015). The WHO stresses that disability is not just a health problem:

> It is a complex phenomenon, reflecting the interaction between features of a person's body and features of the society in which he or she lives.

The International Ergonomics Association (IEA) gives a definition of ergonomics:

> Ergonomics (or human factors) is the scientific discipline concerned with the understanding of interactions among humans and other elements of a

system, and the profession that applies theory, principles, data and methods to design, in order to optimize human well-being and overall system performance.
International Ergonomics Association (2015)

This interaction is the core aspect of ergonomics, and the above-mentioned statements indicate the pivotal role of ergonomics in health and disease.

1.7.2   The Domains of Ergonomics

In ergonomics three domains may be distinguished.

Physical Ergonomics In physical ergonomics, the interaction between anatomy, physiology, anthropometry and biomechanics on the one hand, and physical activities on the other, is studied. It encompasses, e.g. work posture, repetitive movements and handling of loads. Problems can lead to musculoskeletal complaints. Adequate design of the workplace is necessary for their prevention; therefore, physical ergonomics is directly associated with occupational safety and health.

Cognitive Ergonomics The subject of cognitive ergonomics is the interaction of individuals and systems of perception, memory, thinking and motoric reactions. A great mental workload may lead to excessive stress and distress. This leads to the advancement of decompensation of the individual.

Organisational Ergonomics The aim of organisational ergonomics is to optimise processes of structure and organisation. Communication, design of workplace and times, teamwork, participative ergonomics, teleworking and quality of care are involved.

These domains are applicable to many aspects of the human body and function (e.g. the back and the voice) and in several contexts (education, arts, health care and management). Voice is typically situated in all three domains.

1.7.3   The Voice Ergonomics Perspective

In the traditional way of handling voice problems, patients apply for (para)medical help when daily activities become dysfunctional or health is challenged. They receive a (combination of) treatment(s) by surgery or medication or receive behavioural training. If necessary, measures are taken to ease the vocal load or to support (partially), replace or compensate for the vocal task. After having obtained the best possible outcome, patients are discharged and should be able to cope vocally with daily life. This course of problem-handling risks temporarily disconnecting the speaker or singer from his living or working environment and hampers reintegration after treatment. Moreover, patients tend to feel dependent on health-care providers.

Voice ergonomics focuses on the interaction between the voice user and his environment by supporting the voice user in optimising this interaction, so integrating the voice use in real-life situations.

For one specific aspect of voice ergonomics, all possible professionals (care givers, scientists, policy-makers, employers) are engaged (doing research, development, treatment, policy) in helping reduce the risk factors for vocal damage in professional users. The main topics are factors of vocal load, efficient voice use, healthy environmental conditions (humidity, air purity), the interrelationship between these aspects and the impact on each individual voice user (Rantala et al. 2012, 2013; Roy et al. 2004; Vilkman 2004). To ensure long-term effects of all these efforts, another aspect is crucial: the voice user himself has to become skillful in fine-tuning his ever-changing vocal behaviour in the ever-changing environmental conditions. To reach this vocal level, he has to be trained in 'voice ergonomic acting'. Here we enter the world of every voice user of any age, gender, occupation or vocal training.

From this perspective, the voice patient is the key person, as an authority not only on his own vocal experiences but also in problem-solving. Analysis of daily vocal interactions reveals six aspects grouped in two dimensions: on the one hand 'the voice', with the aspects (1) anatomy and physiology (how is the voice built? how does it work? how is it influenced?); (2) vocal technique (how do I use the voice?); (3) voice care; and on the other hand 'environment', with the aspects (4) the circumstances (where do I use the voice?); (5) people (who is the audience?); and (6) the message (what and how do I communicate?). All six aspects interact simultaneously and change continuously. If the patient succeeds in managing all these aspects dynamically, a third dimension is realised: the optimal voice (Decoster 2013).

Voice users who act ergonomically can identify these aspects and are aware of this never-ending flow of changing and mutually influencing characteristics. Moreover, they are skillful in rebalancing all aspects in favour of their vocal health. This does not mean that they become self-made voice professionals, but they know that for all of the six aspects, they can rely on specialists: phoniatricians in cases of structural or functional problems, voice therapists for vocal technique and vocal care, engineers for room acoustics (see Sect. 1.6), technicians for audio-visual equipment, etc. all working towards the same voice ergonomic goal.

Phoniatricians who become part of a multidisciplinary ergonomics voice team, like all other team members, use this same ergonomic framework as a reference for their way of acting and decision-making. They negotiate with patients who are unaware of the complexity of their vocal situations about the multitude of facilitating actions. They train patients on how to convert this knowledge into the indispensable skills to handle their vocal tasks even while medical treatment is continuing.

As a consequence of this perspective, the focus for the phoniatrician shifts from the dysfunctional or diseased patient to the competent voice user who (temporarily) seeks medical help.

1.7.4 The Voice Ergonomics Approach

In the voice ergonomic approach, it is essential that each partner of the multidisciplinary team play an equally important role in the care of the voice patient. That means that (1) each specialist in health care, technical equipment, room acoustics, etc. informs himself about the knowledge and skills in the vocally proficient dynamic behaviour of the voice patient; (2) together with the voice patient and his colleagues of the voice ergonomic team, he searches for aspects in the dynamic interaction that could be optimised; (3) he considers how the daily voice use can take advantage of changing aspects within his own speciality; (4) in this approach, he is aware that changes in one aspect of the interaction can influence all others; and (5) hence, he realises that the varieties of vocal behaviour and circumstance need a variety of problem-solving strategies focused on every individual person.

For the phoniatrician, this means that the job is not finished as soon as he diagnoses smooth vocal cords, efficient vocal closure and an 'adapted' voice sound. He will examine the biological, psychological and social aspects; he will assess the variety of vocal influences and circumstances on the voice; he will help to eliminate related barriers, and by asking relevant questions, he will continuously prompt the patient to keep in balance vocal load and vocal capacity in various speaking or singing conditions. In doing so, he enables the patient to become more independent of care givers, at least for those aspects for which the patient himself is able to change the vocal interaction to his benefit. This is the only way to ensure positive long-term effects of medical interventions without relapse, whether with effects on vocal structures and function or not. Obviously, the voice ergonomic phoniatrician improves both his treatment outcomes and the patient's long-term quality of life.

1.8 Basics of Music

Ilter Denizoglu, Cori Casanova, and
Oskar Schindler

1.8.1 General Definitions

Within the framework of sounds in the environment or produced and heard by humans, music has a particular and relevant place. Music can be defined as a rhythmic arrangement of clearly differentiated sounds that seem orderly and meaningful to a listener, a community or, in the large sense, to all human society. For the purpose of this book, occidental music is dominantly considered. The produced or heard formal music is an extremely well-regulated domain in which the elements of acoustic physics and of auditory perception are formalised with precision and also in the written transcription (Table 1.3).

In addition to these elements, we have to consider the contemporary presence of two or more sounds as they overlap or follow one to the other:

- Melody (several successive sounds of different pitch, duration and loudness)
- Meter (groups of sounds of different accent, e.g. waltz, march, etc.)
- Harmony (several sounds/notes sung or played simultaneously)
- Counterpoint, canon, fugue (independent melodic lines heard in accordance when sung or played together)

Three parameters can be distinguished to define singing voice: loudness, frequency and timbre.

Table 1.3 Acoustic and perceptual musical parameters

Acoustic physics (objective)	Auditory perception (subjective)
Frequency	Pitch
Sound pressure	Loudness
Spectrum	Timbre (colours)
Time	Duration
Rhythm	Meter

1.8.1.1 Loudness

The loudness or volume of the sound is a characteristic of music. The music terminology that refers to sound pressure level has its origin mostly in the Italian music terminology that has evolved from the pianissimo (*pp*) to the fortissimo (*ff*), making its way gradually through the piano (*p*), mezzo piano (*mp*), mezzo forte (*mf*) and forte (*f*). There are other terms that refer to a gradual, more or less fast change in loudness (sforzando, crescendo, diminuendo…).

Musicians are exposed to high sound pressure levels in their professional activity: a musician who plays in a symphonic orchestra—and according to the section he is located in—may be exposed to up to 125 dB SPL. The hearing loss from acoustic trauma is one of the more frequent problems among rock musicians or other contemporary genres that use power sound. Tinnitus and hyperacusis are relatively frequent.

According to a study by Jansen et al. (2009) on 241 musicians from five symphony orchestras, 79% complained of hyperacusis, 7% diplacusis, 51% tinnitus and 24% distortion of tones. In a study by Schink et al. (2014), professional musicians had a 57% higher risk of developing tinnitus and a nearly fourfold higher risk of developing hearing impairment in comparison with the general population.

1.8.1.2 Pitch

Like the decibel's relation to loudness, a cent is a ratio between two respective frequencies. The human ear can distinguish a tonal sound with its fundamental frequency, and a musical note corresponds perceptively to the tonal pitch, whether it comes from a human voice or an instrument (Fig. 1.59). Neurologically, the auditory primary and secondary areas are involved in the perception and emission of a musical note. Those auditory areas interact with frontal areas, predominantly from the right hemisphere.

The interval between the first and second harmonics (a doubling in frequency) of the harmonic series is named an octave. When two separate sounds that have this mathematical (onefold) relation in frequency is heard, the human ear tends to hear these two frequencies (i.e. musical

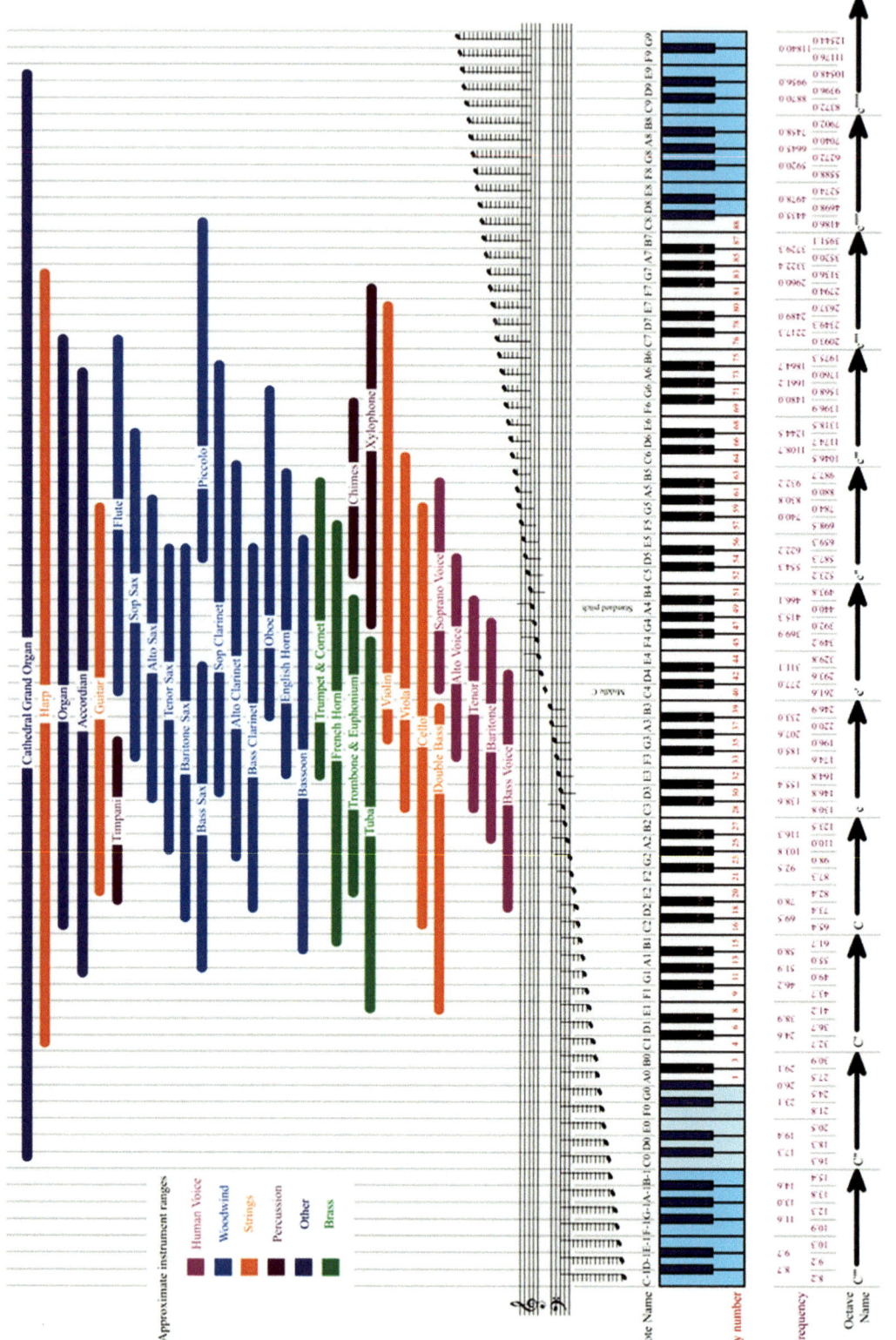

Fig. 1.59 The correlation between the musical note and frequency as well as the frequencies that each instrument can emit. Figure adapted from and with permission of Charles Houghton-Webb and BW Music (2016)

notes) as being essentially 'the same', owing to the closely related harmonic series. The octave relationship is a natural phenomenon that has been referred to as the *basic miracle of music*, which is commonly used in most musical systems (Cooper 1973). There are 12 semitones in an octave, each with 100 cents between its neighbour, which makes 1200 cents in an octave.

The musical notation—the correlation between Hertz and the musical note—may differ from country to country and from culture to culture. In traditional music theory, Latin countries name the musical notes by using the terminology proposed by Guido d'Arezzo (991–1050) as Do, Re, Mi, Fa, Sol, La, Si. Many countries in the world use this system, including Italy, Spain, France and Romania; most Latin-American countries, Greece, Bulgaria, Turkey and Russia; and Arabic-speaking or Persian-speaking countries. However, the Anglo-Saxon countries use different nomenclatures: within the English-speaking and Dutch-speaking world, pitch classes are typically represented by the first seven letters of the Latin alphabet (A, B, C, D, E, F and G), whereas a few European countries, including Germany, adopt an almost identical notation, in which H substitutes for B (Table 1.4). Intervals smaller than a semitone are named 'microtonal intervals'. For example in Turkish classical music, these intervals are known as 'commas' (1/9 of a tone approx.) and are used with a different nomenclature.

Songs are generally composed of certain sets of notes that are known as music scales. Each note in a music scale corresponds to a particular frequency defined by a number. A music scale is in fact a mathematical series (the output of a mathematical function), which spans a single

octave and repeats with the same pattern in other octaves. The music scale is a melodic form constructed from these series of frequencies that divides the octave into a certain number of steps with certain intervals (a recognisable distance between two successive notes of the scale). A specific music scale is defined by an interval pattern and the first note of that specific interval pattern (also known as the *tonic* or first degree of the scale). For example, a C-major scale begins with a C note (tonic of the scale) and has a T-T-S-T-T-T-S pattern (T defines a whole tone while S defines a semitone). There are various scaling systems in different cultures and musical genres that can be described by the content of intervals (e.g. diatonic, chromatic, major, minor, etc.) or by the number of different pitch classes (octatonic, heptatonic, pentatonic, etc.). For example in Turkish classical (traditional) music, the whole note is divided into nine microtone intervals (*commas*), and the music scales are called a *makam*, each of which is formed from a different combination of notes and intervals.

1.8.1.3 Timbre

The recognition of a voice or of the specific timbre of an instrument is found in its harmonic richness. Each note played by an instrument develops or modifies in the resonance structures (the vocal tract in singers or the instrument itself) certain frequencies that are added to the fundamental musical notes and that characterise the instrument timbre or vocal colour.

The peak of a certain harmonics is called formant (F), see Sect. 1.11. While the formants with lower frequencies F1 and F2 are responsible for the voiced vowels and consonants, F3, F4 and F5 are those responsible for the colour, timbre and voice quality. The harmonic is always higher than the fundamental frequency, because vocal colour, as well as tuning in some cases, is involved.

Neurological control The auditory areas of the brain present tonotopy. In other words, the capacity to perceive and analyse each complex sound received through the auditory nerve. Tonotopy allows the perception of the timbre richness of a sound.

Table 1.4 Different naming conventions of pitch notation

Latin	English	German
Do	C	C
Re	D	D
Mi	E	E
Fa	F	F
Sol	G	G
La	A	A
Si	B	H

Fig. 1.60 Graph of intensities and frequencies of speech and music related to the total human hearing range. Copyright © Brüel and Kjær (1984)

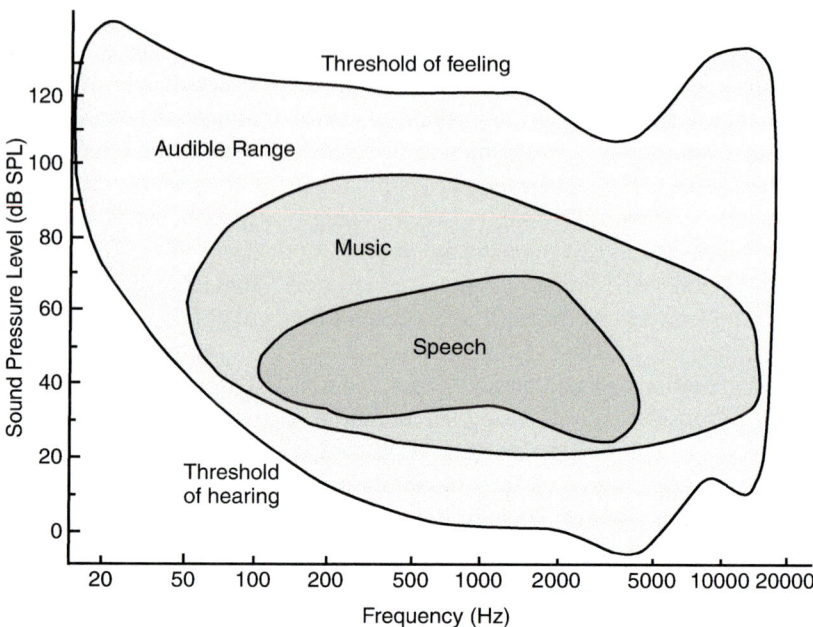

It is important for phoniatricians to take into account the fact that the auditory needs for music are much higher than those for speech, because the quality of music in terms of perception and emission play an important role in the harmonic richness (Fig. 1.60). While an auditory impairment in acute frequencies may have little importance for the understanding or production of speech, it could become highly disabling for an instrument player or a singer.

1.8.1.4 Rhythm

Rhythm is the temporal organisation of sounds and silences that form part of a musical composition.

The capacity to reproduce musical notes temporarily, whether with an instrument or the voice, or following a guideline proposed by the composer or improvisation, not only consists of the auditory perception but also involves the labyrinth responsible for the location in space of the human body, and its psychomotor development.

Binary Rhythm During early childhood, binary rhythm marks the musical development in children. Indeed, as the corporal and vital rhythms (cardiac, respiratory, movement) are binary, the child will walk into the musical rhythm world, hand in hand with these rhythms.

Ternary Rhythm The ternary rhythms (in three tempos, e.g. the waltz), need more psychomotor development, which is achieved with age.

Neurological Control From a neurological point of view, not only the auditory areas take part in the rhythmic perception and production but also the cerebellum, the basal ganglia, the premotor dorsal cortex and the supplementary motor area, which is in charge of the motor control and the temporal cortex area.

1.8.1.5 Tempo

Tempo is the speed or pace of a musical piece. It is defined by number of beats per minute, which is measured by a metronome. Some of the widely used Italian terms indicating the tempo with the beats per minute (bpm) measures are as follows: largo, broadly (40–60 bpm); adagio, slow and stately (literally, 'at ease') (66–76 bpm); andante, at a walking pace (76–108 bpm); moderato, moderately (108–120 bpm); allegro, fast, quickly and bright (120–168 bpm); and presto, very, very fast (168–200 bpm) (Randel 1986).

1.8.2 Basics of Vocal Music: A Muscle-Specific Approach for Phoniatricians

1.8.2.1 Underlying Definitions

Acoustically, vocal music means changing the frequency, amplitude and spectral density (timbre) of, as well as adding noise (i.e. ornaments) to, the singing voice. So-called singing exercises are basics of singing voice therapy procedures that phoniatricians should be familiar with in singing pedagogy.

Vocal Registers From the physio-anatomical aspect vocal registers are simply gears of the larynx governed by different muscle groups that shape the glottal geometry. A vocal register is a range of tones produced by a particular glottal pattern regulated by the source-filter interactions. The vibratory pattern reflects the dynamic glottal geometry, which defines the transformational mode of energy. Although controversy persists, four 'natural' registers are distinguished for a singer: fry, chest, falsetto and whistle. Each register has a particular range of pitches and perceptually characteristic sound properties. The vectorial force distribution alterations of intrinsic (and to some extent, extrinsic) laryngeal muscles define the type of glottal transformation of energy. The thyroarytenoid (TA) muscle is dominant in chest register, whereas the cricothyroid (CT) muscle defines falsetto register by creating passive tension of the vocal ligament. The head (mixed) register is a blended (chest and falsetto) register, which is generally developed by education.

Passaggio The transition zone between two adjacent registers is termed passaggio. In classical singing pedagogy especially, chest and falsetto registers are aimed at being blended by balancing two major pitch mechanisms (TA and CT) in order to create the head register, also known as the mixed register. The result is an even timbre in a wide range of tones without breaks between two registers and a resonant voice throughout the tessitura.

Human Vocal Range/Tessitura Human vocal range depends on the vibration rate of the vocal fold mucosa, which is approximately from 64 to 1046 Hz (four octaves between the notes C2 and C6). By comparison with musical instruments (Fig. 1.59), the so-called middle C (C4: 262 Hz approx.) is in the middle of the vocal range. The lowest sung note of a bass is known as the 'low C' (C2: 65 Hz approx.), whereas the 'high C' (C6: 1046 Hz approx.) is known as the 'soprano C'. These ranges are not definite; tessitura is the vocal range in which sound is musically acceptable by listeners of a particular type of singing. Singers generally tend to sing the high notes at high loudness levels which are known as the 'money notes'. Tessitura may differ among types or genres (even voice subtypes) of singing, and the phoniatrician should assist the singer to find the healthiest way to execute safely the sound that needs to be performed. This is the formula of sustainable professional voice.

The singer must be comfortable in a given tessitura; in other words, tessitura does not define the lowest and highest notes of a singer (as a phonetogram does), rather it is the range of comfortably sung notes on stage. When a singer's vocal range in a phonetogram is larger than the tessitura, the highest and lowest notes in a given song can be interpreted easily, and the performer is then able to express his artistic feelings without thinking of how to execute that note properly. Artistic skills are freed by neuromuscular development, which is the result of exercise, performance and education. A quotation for pianists from Carl Czerny, the well-known composer, pianist and piano teacher, is like the vocalist's dilemma:

> Never must your fingers stand in the way of your artistic interpretation.

The notion of tessitura is related to voice types or the *Fach* system. According to the Fach system, singing voice has been classified according to range, weight and colour, so not only the range plays, but also vocal characteristics play, an important role in classifying voice. Although voice classification is of utmost importance in classical singing because of strict repertoires, it is also useful in contemporary vocal music. Female voices are mainly divided into four types: alto soprano, mezzosoprano, soprano and coloratura soprano. For the male voices bass, baritone, tenor and countertenor are the main types. This classification is also controversial, and several subtypes are defined, and there is even an idea that 'the number of voice types is the same as the number of singers'.

A famous saying that defines the way of being a professional singer explains many things clearly: 'exercise, exercise, exercise'. Exercise is sine qua non for a professional voice user on stage. Sustainability of stage performance requires two main issues: exactness in motor learning and physical fitness. Vocal exercise is important for these two aspects. Exactness in motor learning can be reached by countless repeats and rehearsals. The motor cortex and the vocal end organs will work in concordance after years of education, practice and patience. If the education is based on scientific knowledge, it is easier to reach to a level of adequacy of performance. This approach can be defined as

Conscious preparation to the subconscious.
Stanislavski (2003)

From the physiological aspect, vocal exercises may be classified as follows:

- Onset and damping
- Vocal muscle building exercises
- Vocal tract exercises and formant tuning

1.8.2.2 Onset and Damping
Vocal attack refers to glottal onset for mucosal vibrations. A proper glottal attack is reached by a critical balance between subglottal pressure and glottal resistance. Several types of onsets (i.e. glottal attack) can be distinguished in singing:

- Hard attack: firm glottal closure before transglottal airflow.
- Breathy attack: transglottal airflow before vibratory mucosal contact.
- Attack with glottal fry: starting with a very low frequency known as glottal fry.

- Balanced attack: transglottal airflow drives vocal fold mucosa to vibration simultaneously.

Vocal damping refers to the end of phonation. Especially for hyperfunctional voice disorders, phonation ends with trying hard. For a singer, glottal damping is an important factor for maximum economy on stage as well as a healthy vocal fold mucosa for the next performance.

1.8.2.3 Vocal Muscle Building Exercises
Vocal muscle building exercises can be classified into three subgroups:

- Pitch-based exercises (sostenuto, glissando, portamento, staccato, legato)
- Loudness-based exercises (crescendo, decrescendo, messa di Voce)
- Combined exercises (vocal play, melodies)

Pitch-Based Exercises
Pitch-based exercises develop intrinsic laryngeal muscles selectively, individually or interactively (Fig. 1.61).

Sostenuto Sustaining a selected single tone is termed sostenuto (Fig. 1.62). Vocal quality, tone and the loudness during phonating should not be changed. Breath support is carefully monitored till the end of the phonation. The effort leads the singer to contract the TA and CT muscles isometrically. It is especially good for chest register in the beginning of therapy. As the therapy proceeds and the voice gets better, sostenuto can be used for each note of different registers.

Glissando Gliding voice from one pitch to another is called glissando (Fig. 1.63). It shows the vocal condition throughout the tessitura, so glissando may also be defined as a *vocal stethoscope*. During a glide there are a few tricks: first, the singer must not allow the loudness to increase at the high notes. The passaggio notes will also provide information about the place of the passaggio, the education degree of the singer, register blending quality and even voice type. In this

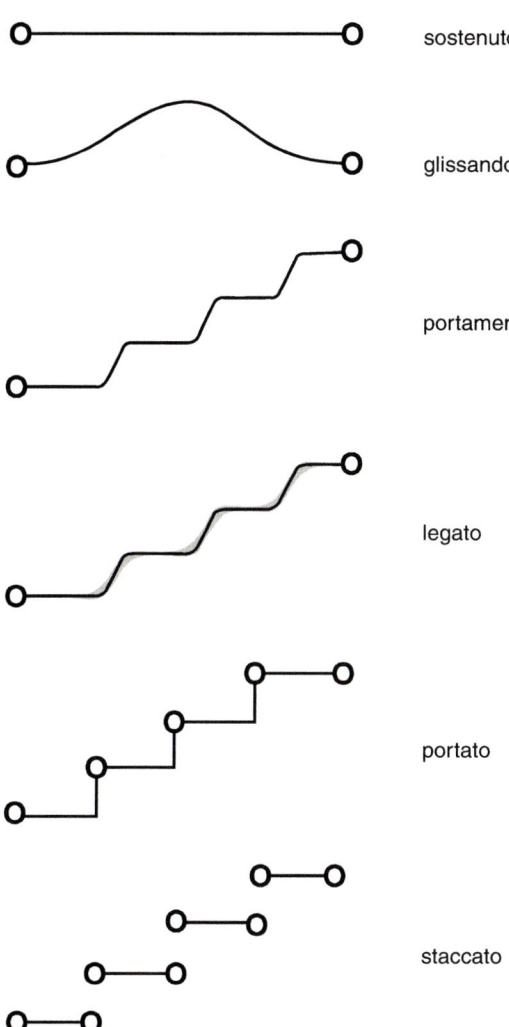

Fig. 1.61 Basic exercises represented by lines

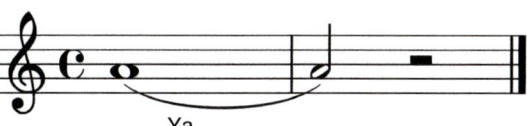

Fig. 1.62 Sostenuto exercise

exercise, interactive TA and CT contraction permits certain vocal registers, through the incremental dominance and transposition of these two muscles.

Legato In legato (Fig. 1.64), distinct tones can be heard, but they are related to a specific connection without a gliding sensation between

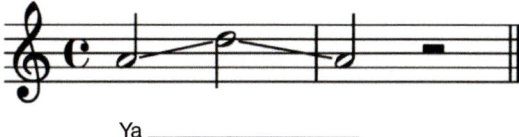

Fig. 1.63 Glissando exercise

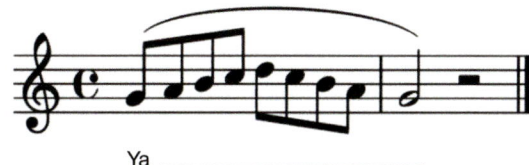

Fig. 1.64 Legato exercise

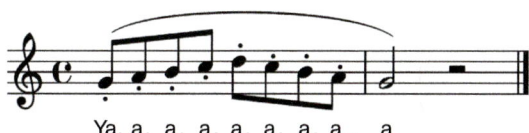

Fig. 1.65 Portamento exercise

them. This is possible with the human vocal instrument. The singer keeps the exact *placement* of the tone by adjusting the correct dominance of CT-TA contraction in the same breath. The transition between the two distinct notes is the result of a perfect balance among the muscles in charge.

Portamento Such exercises may help to develop the transition between TA and CT mechanisms accurately (Fig. 1.65). It is an easier way of applying the legato exercise. In the same breath, two notes are connected by a short glissando. Before separating the breath in portato or staccato, it helps to sustain the vocal pattern in different tones.

Portato This exercise is executed in the same breath, as in portamento, but with vocal pauses between two notes, so that two pitch mechanisms adjust their dominance on the vectorial sum of forces without a soft glide between (Fig. 1.66).

Staccato Unconnected and discontinuous (separated by breath pauses) successive tones are defined as staccato (Fig. 1.67). It increases agility and maintains a crisp, clear onset. A possible

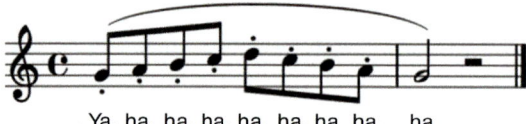

Ya, ha, ha, ha, ha, ha, ha, ha,   ha,

Fig. 1.66 Portato exercise

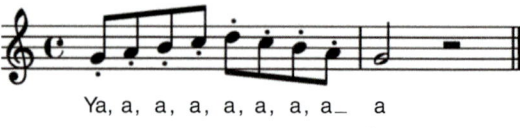

Ya, a, a, a, a, a, a, a_   a

Fig. 1.67 Staccato exercise

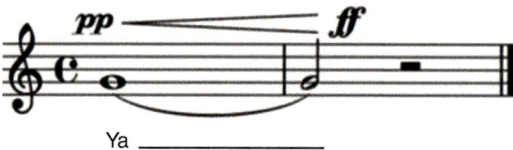

Ya _____

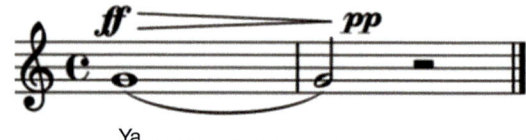

Ya _____

Fig. 1.68 Crescendo (left), decrescendo (right)

muscular mechanism in staccato is the activation of the interarytenoid muscles especially for posterior glottal closure, because the exercise is executed with a breath at each note with the fast activity of the posterior cricoarytenoid muscles.

Loudness-Based Exercises

Loudness-based exercises can be applied at several volume levels in different fashions. Loudness levels or volume of the voice is defined by some abbreviations which refer to the Italian words mentioned above. Intensity of singing voice can be matched with speaking levels between whispering and yelling. Pianississimo (*ppp*) and pianissimo (*pp*) mean soft as a whisper; piano (*p*) for softer than speaking voice; mezzo piano (*mp*) and mezzo forte (*mp*) for a speaking voice; and forte (*f*), fortissimo (*ff*) and fortississimo (*fff*) for loud speaking and yelling.

Loudness-based exercises aim to balance resistance (glottal closure) and power (subglottal pressure). More specifically, they focus on managing the subglottal pressure during singing. The so-called 'diaphragmatic technique' is about the delicate control of the vectorial sum of forces affecting the subglottal pressure. This control starts with inhalation without using the secondary muscles of inspiration (i.e. muscles that interfere with the extrinsic laryngeal muscles). During expiration, by increasing the intrathoracic pressure by the expiratory muscles, the singer should balance the relaxation of diaphragmatic muscle directly and indirectly by major body muscles

concerned with posture that work as 'quasi-antagonists' of the diaphragm. This balance is also known as appoggio (*support*) and reflects the sportive performance and educational level of the vocal performer. *Sforzando* indicates a forceful accent on a note. *Crescendo* means to increase the loudness gradually, whereas *decrescendo* (diminuendo) is decreasing the loudness gradually (Fig. 1.68).

Messa Di Voce An advanced vocal exercise is represented by Messa Di Voce (*placing of voice* in Italian). It involves a gradual crescendo and diminuendo while sustaining a single pitch without changing intonation, timbre, vibrato or pitch. Physically, increasing the subglottal pressure results in an increased transglottal airflow, which in turn causes a pitch elevation. During gradual decrescendo (diminuendo), the pitch tends to decrease to a lower pitch with an opposite physical event. The singer should make glottal resistance, subglottal pressure and filter (i.e. vocal tract) adjustments to execute the messa di voce properly. This is because the messa di voce exercise is an extremely high level of vocal coordination. The exercise can be made more difficult by some modifications such as *Esclamazio viva* and *Esclamazio languida* (Fig. 1.69) that have been described (Reid 1990).

The physiological background is to combine pitch control mechanisms with subglottal pressure changes. The possible mechanism is a muscular adjustment of glottal resistance (especially

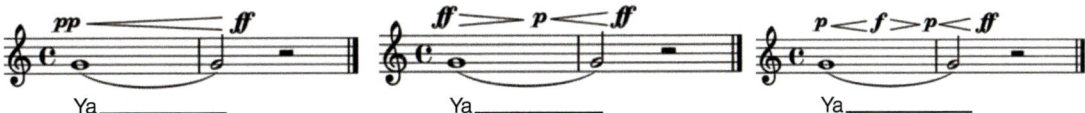

Fig. 1.69 (From left) Messa di Voce, Esclamazio viva and Esclamazio languida

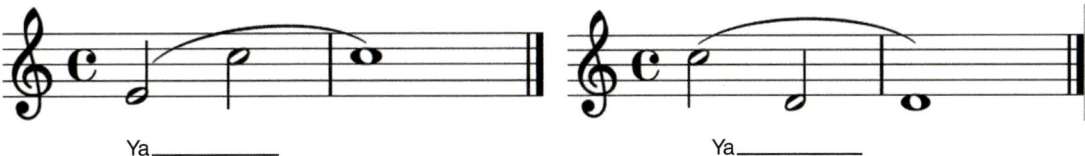

Fig. 1.70 Glissando-sostenuto exercises. Left, ascending scale; right, descending scale

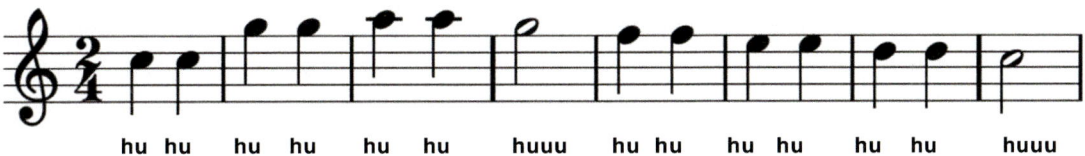

Fig. 1.71 *Twinkle, Twinkle, Little Star* sung without lyrics

between TA and CT) against a changing intensity of subglottal pressure, in order to keep the pitch stable.

Combined Exercises

Different basic exercises can be combined in vocal play of a phrase. In an up-down glissando-sostenuto exercise, in order to provide a firm closure in low pitches, a high pitch can be started and glided to a low pitch without changing the firm closure effect, which ends with a sostenuto at a low pitch. This descending scale exercise may increase TA activity by support of its antagonist, CT. The opposite approach is for descending pitches; starting with a low pitch in modal register can be carried to high pitches to strengthen the CT muscle (Fig. 1.70).

Melodies are like playing chess for the voice system. The singer uses the basic motor schemes, which have been gained before, for new and more complicated tasks. Even a simple 'twinkle twinkle little star' song (Fig. 1.71) sung with a single vowel requires a complex control ability with interactions among glottal resistance, subglottal pressure and the vocal tract.

Tonal exercises containing basic and combined types can be used for warm-up or cool-down processes. The best way for warming up and cooling down is to use tonal exercises instead of singing songs mezza voce. Mezza voce is to sing a song softly (i.e. at half power of the voice), but as in sports physiology, where football players do not play with a *soft* football before the game, they exercise by running or aerobics.

1.8.2.4 Vocal Tract Exercises and Formant Tuning

The spectral distribution of source frequencies depends on the vocal tract resonance characteristics. Formants are resonance frequencies of the vocal tract. When a harmonic is near to or coincides exactly with a formant frequency, the singer is able to produce a louder tone without increasing effort. A soprano can gain up to 30 dB by tuning the first formant (F1) to the fundamental frequency (F0), which is also called as the first harmonic (H1) (Sundberg et al. 2005).

It is also favourable to sing an open vowel at high notes by making small adjustments without changing the linguistic meaning of that given vowel. In order to make a harmonic coincide with a formant, singers use vocal tract reshaping strategies, which is called formant tuning. Vocal tract exercises aim to balance source-filter interactions. These reshaping strategies concern organs (false vocal folds, tongue, soft palate, jaw, lips, aryepiglottic plica and hypopharyngeal walls) that can be consciously adjusted for formant tuning. Mouth opening, velar height and width, tongue position, pharyngeal and epilaryngeal width and vertical larynx position can be reshaped to balance source and filter acoustics. This application is sometimes called a 'covering manoeuvre'. Tuning a specific harmonic to a given formant (H1 and H2 to F1; H2, H3 and H4 to F2) may be used by different voice types. Forward placement of the tongue increases second formant (F2) frequency whereas opening the mouth increases F1 frequency (Fig. 1.72). So when a singer sings

higher notes, the fundamental frequency approaches the F1 frequency. If F0 crosses the F1 frequency, it will not be amplified favourably by the adjacent F1; in order to prevent that crossover, the singer widens the jaw opening, and the F1 is kept somewhat higher than F0 (Sundberg 2003).

Vocal tract reshaping may be defined simply as vowel modification or *aggiustamento* as the musical term in Italian. The art of *aggiustamento* takes years of training and motor learning of absolute execution of each vowel at any given pitch with a definite formant tuning strategy. These strategies are especially used in classical singing but are able to be used in any type of singing. They may be executed in different ways for different purposes. One exercise combines (Fig. 1.73) singing different vowels with different tones so the singer can prepare for the real 'game', by matching the proper formant to the relevant harmonic.

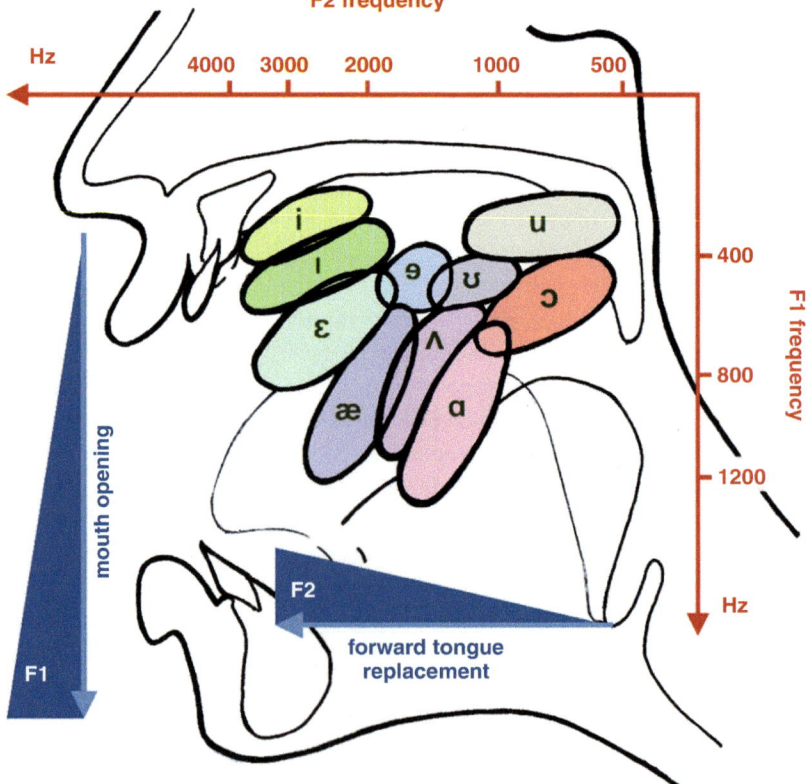

Fig. 1.72 Adjusting the first two formants; forward tongue placement increases F2, mouth opening increases F1 frequencies (the frequency regions for F1 and F2 which result in the 10 English vowels are adapted from Peterson and Barney 1952, with the permission of Acoustical Society of America)

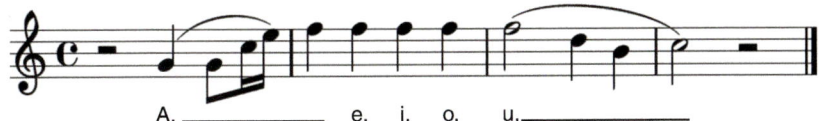

Fig. 1.73 Changing vocal tract shape by using different harmonics with different tones

Lowered Larynx Technique As a formant tuning strategy, the Lowered Larynx Technique (also known as the open throat technique) may also be regarded. It lowers all formants and has several advantages for the classical singer especially.

Singer's Formant Cluster To concentrate harmonic energy around 3 kHz by forming a narrow supraglottal channel that has been defined as the epilaryngeal tube (Titze 2000; Sundberg 1987) is called Singer's Formant Cluster. In other words, the energy of the third, fourth and the fifth formants is concentrated at a specific frequency (the human outer ear canal has a natural resonance frequency around 3 kHz) which makes the singer better heard and understood.

1.8.3 Styles, Genres and Vocal Ornamentation in Singing

The art of singing is possible with any sound regardless of any rules. Vocal artists use various sounds and alterations of sung voice for vocal ornamentation. The most well-known ornamentation is vibrato. Vibrato is generally used as an umbrella term which consists of various types of pulsating changes in voice. This change is generally referred to the pitch alterations, so it can be described in terms of four parameters: pulsation rate, extension of the pitch change, the regularity and the waveform of the undulations (Sundberg 1994). The mechanism is complex; alterations in glottal resistance (Hsiao et al. 1994), vocal tract manoeuvres (supraglottal and articulatory muscle activity, alterations of vertical larynx position) (Sapir and Larson 1993) and management of subglottal pressure-bearing forces (Rothenberg et al. 1988) may be defined as possible factors of rhythmic vocal undulations.

Vibrato Five to seven undulations in fundamental frequency with an extent of about one semitone characterise vibrato. In classical singing especially, vibrato is part of the stage performance that adds colour and variety to vocal perception. It increases lucidity of the vocalist, especially in high tones, and decreases tension in the voice. It is the natural ornament of the singing voice and provides delicate control and perception of the fundamental frequency.

Trillo A fast vibrato that is executed over 8 Hz and extends about two semitones is called trillo.

Wobble A kind of slow oscillation (2–4 Hz) in voice with extension of about three semitones and generally perceived as a shake in the voice is termed wobble.

Tremolo By repetition of the same tone tremolo (occasionally called goat vibrato) differs from the other vocal undulations.

Ventricular folds can be actively used in some singing styles. Vocal ornamentations such as a growl, grunt and scream may be harmful when they are executed improperly during singing. Some styles can use falsetto register (i.e. yodel) intensely or temporarily through the song. Various glottal attacks (breathy, soft, hard, balanced attacks) or fry register are possible to express feelings of the vocal performer on stage. Overtone singing is a specific way of bearing extraordinary sounds for vocal music. The performers re-resonate the sound (e.g. by a reversed tip of tongue) and reinforce a single harmonic sustained over a fundamental pitch.

The singing styles or genres are identified by various factors including culture, registration, ornamentation and vocal timbre (tone colour or quality). In some aspects, singing styles are classified into two groups: classical (opera) and nonclassical or contemporary (pop, rock, jazz, folk, R & B, etc.). No matter what the style is, the vocalists use some basic motor patterns. These basic patterns are well defined by Estill (McDonald Klimek et al. 2005) with specific structural recipes that result in basic voice timbres: speech, sob, falsetto, twang, belt and opera. Speech level singing is possibly the most-used skill all over the world. In other words, it is singing with an everyday speaking voice (i.e. chest register). Sob timbre is a medium-low pitched ranged soft sound with a lowered vertical larynx position. Falsetto is used widely among folk singers, especially in yodelling, as well as in early music. Twang is a popular sound in American country music. It is clearly heard in a noisy environment (it can even be identified as a striking sound) because of the ringing quality (by the narrowing aryepiglottic sphincter and a high larynx). Belted sound of singing (loud, rich with high harmonics, high vertical larynx position) can be found in various contemporary genres and styles especially in musical theatre (i.e. legit). Opera is a well-known style for the open throat technique (comfortably low vertical laryngeal position, epilaryngeal tube, balanced spectral density, a constant sound throughout the tessitura which is rich with both low and high harmonics). Formant tuning (i.e. covering manoeuvre) is a rule of thumb especially in opera performances. The balance of the main pitch mechanisms (i.e. thyroarytenoid and cricothyroid muscles) and tuned source-filter interactions makes it possible to sing high notes safely at high loudness levels (with high subglottal pressures).

Some distinct musical styles may cause slight differences in vocal music. Oratorio is the concert type of opera without theatre, part of it with sacred topics. Cantata, on the other hand, is a short oratorio generally sung by a choir with instrumental accompaniment. Lied (*song* in German) was originally born from setting the romantic German poems to (classical) music. They generally have pastoral and romantic themes and are arranged for a single singer and piano. Singspiel is a genre of opera which is generally characterised by folk-like comic or romantic themes and dominated by spoken dialogues. A cappella is specifically group or solo singing without instrumental accompaniment in which the voice itself may be used as an instrumental sound.

No matter what kind of a musical style or genre is chosen for artistic expressions, the phoniatrician should look for healthy ways for those sounds to be borne in order to provide sustainability in stage performance.

1.8.4 Phoniatrician's Multidimensional Approach for Vocal Pedagogy

Singing as a craft, from a professional aspect of habilitation, has two main dimensions: musical performance and sportive performance. Musical performance is about musical skills and maturity. Time, intonation, sound and expression are the main factors for efficiency and sufficiency in musical performance. But there is another important factor that defines efficiency and sufficiency of a singer: professional sports performance which includes durability, speed and agility, timing/focusing, sustainability, motor learning and practice.

A professional musician, whether a singer or an instrument player, has higher auditory needs than a nonmusician. The frequencies involved in music exceed by far the frequency range implicated in the emission and perception of speech. The phoniatrician who wants to treat professional musicians should have notions about music, as well as its processing at the central and peripheral neurological levels.

A particular topic is represented by music therapy, in which music, especially instrumental music, is employed for education about auditory perception or in the treatment of communication disorders.

The semiformal knowledge of music by phoniatricians is very useful for them and sometimes is also necessary, as in the management of artistic singing or handling music therapy. The musical expertise of a phoniatrician not below the exam level of the sol-fa (solfeggio) of the second year of an academy of music (Conservatory) would be useful, and it is equally desirable for it to include at least an elementary ability to play a musical instrument with notes (e.g. piano, flutes, guitar, xylophone, metallophone). The musical competence of a phoniatrician allows, in a sufficient and precise way:

- A better knowledge of the sounds in their different physical and psychophysical parameters
- A better correlation with acoustic analysis. An adequate evaluation of different sounds (sounds and noises of the environment, extralaryngeal body sounds and noises) and of their different production (sounds and noises of musical instruments or different sources, such as synthesisers)

The application of musical knowledge and ability is strictly applicable to the phoniatric profession in auditory perception rehabilitation, in phonetic-phonologic rehabilitation, in the management of different aspects of the education of prelingual deafness, in music therapy and in the management of the patient with physiological and pathological problems of the singing voice.

Singing voice medicine by phoniatricians is focused on two major areas (as is sports medicine): habilitation and rehabilitation. Habilitation is the process of strengthening and equipping the vocalist to meet very specific and special demands. The habilitation process starts from education (e.g. pedagogical vocology lectures in a conservatory) and then continues with singing voice therapy applications, which may support vocal education. Rehabilitation, on the other hand, is bringing the vocal performer back to a level of adequacy by means of singing voice therapy methods and techniques. Sustainability of the professional vocal performance includes techniques blending voice therapy and singing exercises. Additionally, methods for hearing protection of orchestra musicians, and care of musical performance anxiety (i.e. stage fright), based on knowledge in psychotherapy are other areas of interest for the phoniatrician. A well-known quotation is like the role of the phoniatrician on stage: *the curtain never comes down.*

1.9 Musicians' Medicine

Bernhard Richter and Claudia Spahn

1.9.1 Introduction

The connection between music and medicine is a highly integrated aspect of our culture and reaches far back in our history. In Greek mythology, Orpheus, the most famous singer of ancient times, and Asklepios, the father of medicine, are half-brothers. They share the same father: Apollo, the god of music, art and healing.

For a long time, the main focus of music was its positive effect on health. Thus, in ancient times, listening to and making music, as well as physical activity, were the basic elements of a healthy and balanced development of the body and mind, as described in extenso in Platon's *'Politeia'* (Platon 1998).

First of all, music is a source of joy and health. Today, the positive health effects of music can be measured and proven in scientific studies (Bygren et al. 1996; Kreutz et al. 2004; McDonald et al. 2012). Music can be considered as a powerful salutogenetic factor.

However, owing to the high standards of performance applied to the playing of music, health can also be at risk.

1.9.2 Historical Background

The first sources in the medical literature that refer to questions regarding medical problems of musicians mainly focus on the health problems of wind players. In his treatise on the possible causes of hernias, published in 1486, the physician Giovanni Michele Savonarola, who was teaching in Padua, pointed out that 'trumpeters and flute players' are a professional group especially at risk (cited according to Breuer 1982: 4).

When instrumental practice became specialised and intensified in the course of the nineteenth century, reports on health problems increased. In 1831, after an intensive period of practising the piano, Robert Schumann developed a movement disorder of his right hand which nowadays would be diagnosed as a focal dystonia (Altenmüller and Jabusch 2010). In 1890, Alexander Scriabin had to stop playing the piano with his right hand for several years after injuring it by practising excessively a piano piece by Franz Liszt.

The first textbook addressing 'Musicians' Medicine' was the nineteenth century publication *Ärztlicher Ratgeber für Musiktreibende* (*Medical Guidebook for the Musician*) by Karl Sundelin (1831), Germany.

In the twentieth century, a collection of case reports by Julius Flesch was published as a book entitled *Berufskrankheiten des Musikers* (*Occupational Diseases of the Musician*) (Flesch 1925). At the same time, the Berlin neurologist, music scientist and music critic Kurt Singer, who had been teaching at the 'Staatliche Akademische Hochschule für Musik' since 1923, intended to initiate the integration of the subject 'musicians' medicine' into the music student's study program. In 1926, his monograph *'Die Berufskrankheiten der Musiker'* (*'The occupational diseases of musicians'*) was published (Singer 1926). During the German National Socialism period, these institutional approaches were corrupted owing to Kurt Singer's Jewish roots.

These early approaches notably illustrate the awareness that medical care for elite performers is essential: specialised instrumentalists and singers are continually pushing the limits of the physiological and psychological capability of performance—as are high-performance athletes.

The modern community dedicated to musicians' medicine has different roots in various countries. Important incentives came from the USA. Here, a study of the International Conference of Symphony and Opera Musicians (ICSOM) by orchestral musicians revealing the health implications of playing (Fischbein et al. 1988) and also the cases of famous musicians such as Leon Fleischer and Gary Graffman, who suffered from focal dystonia, caused much concern. As a consequence, 'Performing Arts Medicine' came into existence.

1.9.3 The 'German' Situation

Structurally important contributions also came from Germany: in 1974, the first Chair for the Physiology of Music and Musicians' Medicine was established at the Hanover University of Music, Drama and Media. Further Chairs for Musicians' Medicine followed, e.g. at the Frankfurt University of Music and Performing Arts, as well as at the Hanns Eisler School of Music in Berlin. In 2005, upon foundation of the Freiburg Institute for Musicians' Medicine (FIM) at the Freiburg University of Music, in collaboration with the Albert Ludwigs University and its Medical Centre in Freiburg, two more Chairs for Musicians' Medicine with a focus on preventive and psychosomatic medicine as well as on artistic vocal training were established. In addition, there has been a Chair for Musicians' Medicine at the Dresden University of Music since 2008, and in 2010 a professorship was established at the Cologne University of Music and Dance. Other departments with a focus on musicians' medicine at universities of music exist, for example, in Weimar and in Detmold. Currently, almost all of the German universities of music offer lectures on the topic of musicians' medicine, at least to some extent. The purpose of the subject of musicians' medicine in the study programme at the universities of music is to instruct music students in health topics that will be essential for their future professional life. Here, the physiological and psychological basics of health-preserving techniques for instrument playing and for singing are collectively termed the 'Physiology of Music'.

There are further initiatives for musicians' medicine outside the above-mentioned academic institutions, for example, the Institute for Musicians' Medicine Berlin-Brandenburg, the outpatient facility for musicians at the Düsseldorf University Hospital and the outpatient department for musicians at the University Hospital Münster. Developments in this field are still progressing, so further institutions for musicians' medicine may emerge.

Owing to these wide-ranging activities, Germany has taken a pioneering role in the international context of musicians' medicine in recent years.

The German Association for Music Physiology and Musicians' Medicine (DGfMM) was founded in 1994 with the purpose of professional exchange and training. It associates professional groups working in diagnostics or therapy, including physicians, psychologists, physiotherapists, therapists specialised in body-related methods such as the Feldenkrais and Alexander technique, and speech-language therapists or music teachers who work in the therapy or care of musicians and singers. In recent years, the DGfMM has consistently maintained approximately 400 members (www.dgfmm.org).

1.9.4 The 'International' Situation

Several national associations with a similar focus have been founded worldwide, e.g. in the USA, in Great Britain, France, Switzerland, New Zealand, Taiwan and Austria.

Alongside this international expansion, the scientific journal *Medical Problems of Performing Artists (MPPA)'* was launched in 1985. This journal publishes four issues per year and is multifaceted in its content. It publishes peer-reviewed research papers covering topics including neurological disorders, musculoskeletal conditions, voice and hearing disorders, music performance anxiety, stress, substance abuse, disorders of ageing and other health issues related to the professional requirements of actors, dancers, singers, musicians and other performers. It is now established as an internationally recognised journal with an impact factor of 0.92 and is listed in significant digital databases including MEDLINE and PubMed.

1.9.5 Textbooks

For textbooks on musicians' medicine, comprehensive benchmark publications are now available in different languages. As examples, two significant works are mentioned here: for English-speaking readers the 2010 publication by Sataloff, Brandfonbrener and Ledermann, *'Performing Arts Medicine'* (Sataloff et al. 2010) (already in its 3rd edition); for German-speaking readers the up-to-date textbook *'MusikerMedizin—Diagnostik, Therapie und Prävention von musikerspezifischen Erkrankungen'*, compiled by its editors Spahn, Richter and Altenmüller, published in 2011 (Spahn et al. 2011).

1.9.6 Common Features in Instrumentalists and Singers

The up-to-date modern musicians' medicine comprises the prevention, diagnostics and therapy of health problems that are or may be caused by making music or that may affect the playing of an instrument or singing. Musicians' medicine is equally dedicated to professional musicians and hobby musicians, and it covers care of instrumentalists and singers in a similar setting.

The many common features that arise from the medical treatment of instrumentalists, compared with singers and actors, share a long tradition. For example, in his comprehensive work on occupational medicine published in 1700, *'De morbis atrificum diatriba'*, Bernardino Ramazzini dedicated a whole chapter on the topic *'Krankheiten der Redner, Sänger und anderer dergleichen Leute'* (*'Diseases of speakers, singers and other such people'*) among the latter of which he also included instrumentalists (cited according to Breuer 1982: 17–18).

1.9.7 Health Problems in Instrumentalists and Singers

According to epidemiological studies, the most common causes of medical problems of performing artists—instrumentalists and singers alike—are overuse syndromes, which may lead to a large variety of symptoms such as pain or complaints during the performance or to disabilities for specific playing- or singing-related skills. Detailed descriptions of such problems—including many case reports—can be found in the aforementioned textbooks.

Evaluation of health problems in epidemiological studies shows that besides physical complaints, psychological problems, such as performance anxiety, play an important role in a musician's health (Spahn et al. 2010).

1.9.8 Fields of Medicine Involved

Depending on the health problems presented, very different fields of medicine may be involved in the diagnosis and treatment of musicians.

Currently, there is no medical speciality for musicians' medicine; instead, focused specialisation occurs within existing medical specialities. There is not yet any formal procedure for advanced qualification in musicians' medicine. However, different medical specialisations, for example, psychosomatics, neurology, otorhinolaryngology and orthopaedics, may overlap considerably. There is an especially strong correlation of the speciality of phoniatrics and laryngology, since those working in medical care for singers are required to have knowledge and skills similar to those necessary for the treatment of instrumentalists.

These shared requirements are also emphasised by the fact that among the editors of the above-mentioned textbooks, the authors Bob Sataloff and Bernhard Richter each are specialists with comprehensive experience in the care and cure of professional singers.

1.9.9 Special Requirements

The special requirements of musicians' medicine as described above result in further specific cross-speciality challenges for physicians and therapists when treating musicians. Consequently, knowledge of the working conditions of musicians, as well as the specific psychological and physical requirements for playing an instrument or for singing, is indispensable.

Hence, a close and well-coordinated interaction, as well as an optimised communication between the professional groups involved, is essential for success in the medical treatment of a musician. In order to avoid an incoherent—or even contradictory—outcome when looking at the musician's health problem from different perspectives, the specialised physician in charge is tasked with assembling these 'pieces of the puzzle' into a whole. This also appears to be economically beneficial, as any unnecessary and expensive consultations with other physicians, as well as any non-specific therapies, can be avoided.

Consequently, one of the principal duties of a physician treating a musician is to be the 'interpreter' of the language of the musicians and singers on one hand and of the language of the hitherto involved physicians and therapists on the other. Usually, the people working with a focus on musicians' medicine are practicing musicians themselves or are interested in music and are therefore 'bilingually' competent in the terminology of music as well as of medicine.

1.10 Voice Science and Hygiene in Singing Education

Bernhard Richter and Dirk Mürbe

With regard to the topic of 'how to incorporate fundamentals of a science-based singing pedagogy into a singer's training', three main questions arise:

- What skills are requested from a singer nowadays?
- How should a singer be trained?
- What significance should be given to voice physiology in a singer's training?

The 'market' for artists has been largely globalised. Singers often perform cross-borders, even worldwide. Therefore, each singer is not only required to have very good voice skills, and to deliver a very good artistic performance during his active singing career, but is also required to cope with the challenges of a 'travelling job'. A singer has to be capable of good self-management—mostly without any protection zones to withdraw to—and needs a good awareness of his body and psyche and has to be able to react flexibly to difficult situations. Singers must plan their career well and carefully and consider the profession within the perspective of its life time. This means they need to be aware of the fact that the duration of a singing career is usually limited and that very often a singer's active career is followed by a second career as vocal teacher.

There are neither international nor national regulations for the training of professional singers. The artistic director of a theatre fills the role on the basis of the simple rule of 'who fits best gets the job'—no matter where, by whom or according to which criteria the singer was trained.

So far, there are no reliable data on the question of how many graduates continue seeking a permanent soloist contract. Heiner Gembris and Daina Langner performed a study by investigating the *modus operandi* of the graduates of German universities of music who succeeded in integrating themselves into the (musicians') job market (Gembris and Langner 2005). Half of the 100 singers who participated in the study had, at the beginning of their study, planned to become a soloist. However, after completing their study, only 12% managed to obtain a soloist contract.

By looking at the tradition of vocal pedagogy, we see that initially it was a rather copying-and-mimicking model of education and that the didactics of vocal teaching were predominant. This is visible, for example, in the teaching constellation of masters and students at the Italian 'Conservatoria' in Naples and elsewhere (Haböck 1927).

At that time, the training comprised general instructions in music, including harmony and theory in music, as well as playing an instrument. Furthermore, it included—in part—daily singing lessons given by the vocal teachers who, in turn, had to instruct only a very limited number of students.

Of course, this training system created famous singers. The prime example for this is the still well-known and legendary castrato Farinelli (1705–1782). Farinelli was a student of Nicola Porpora at the *Conservatorio Sant'Onofrio* in Naples, and his debut took place in 1721. Until 1737, he acquired his fame as an opera singer performing at the more important music centres of his time. He experienced his training and active period as a singer in the so-called 'pre-physiological' era, i.e. even before there existed any scientific research on the physiological aspects of voice production (Richter 2013).

In the spirit of the ongoing period of the Enlightenment, these pedagogic procedures gradually changed. As such, approximately 250 years ago, the 'old' Italian school of Johann Friedrich Agricola (1720–1774) was refined in Germany. In 1757, Agricola had presented a translation and supplementation of Pier Francesco Tosi's singing instructions, which had previously been published in 1723 in the Italian language with the title *Opinioni de' cantori antichi, e moderni o sieno osservazioni sopra il canto figurato* (Richter and Seedorf 2003).

Agricola's *Manual of the Singing Art* was written under the influence of the ideas and circumstances of the Enlightenment and was intended to transfer the empirical knowledge of singing teachers of earlier times to a more scientific basis (Agricola 2002). Agricola had become aware of the ongoing French discourse about singing physiology and had studied Ferrein's epochal discovery of vocal fold function in depth (Ferrein 1741).

García the younger, who was one of the early users of a laryngeal mirror in history, followed a similarly enlightened and science-based course (García 1854). He was teaching in France and England and had, even reaching into modern times, significant influence on European vocal pedagogy (Haefliger 1993). Nowadays, a science-based vocal pedagogy largely prevails.

Renate Faltin, Professor for singing at the Berlin University of Music *Hanns Eisler*, comments:

> To be successful, the singing technique has to be adapted to the physiological conditions, independently of the learning method actually being applied (even intuitively-learned singing underlies certain objective principles). In general, many singing teachers convey the technical basics by imaginative pictures, by circumscription, and by

singing demonstrations; they use the student's will of artistic expression as well as predefined pieces of music and interpretations of music to lead the student unnoticeably to technical improvements. This is certainly a method rooted in traditions, i.e., it has proven itself successful. However, there are certain doubts that this method is sufficient nowadays, since, over the past centuries, in all other areas of teaching the methods have been adapted and altered according to technical progress and the latest knowledge, with the aim of faster, more secure and more effective success. Then, why not also in the teaching and learning of singing? There is a need for developing a strategy that, in the first place, provides the students reliable and retrievable knowledge on which they can rely for the whole duration of their professional career.
Faltin (2004)

Here, the question of a teacher's own pedagogical concepts is also important. It could range from the traditional and pure master-student relationship to a teacher-student relationship adopting more modern learning theories and approaches from social psychology.

The renowned German vocal teacher Gerhard Faulstich, Professor at the Hanover University of Music and Theatre, regarding the shared and concurring knowledge of vocal physiology, the bestowed 'knowledge of the singer' and the opinion of different singing schools, reminds us that:

> [...] the willingness of the singer or the singing teacher to incorporate the features they share [...] is an indispensable precondition for a successful implementation.
> Faulstich (2011)

Faulstich draws a parallel between the responsibility of a singing teacher during the practical singing lesson, where often a life-determining course is being set, and the questionable responsibility of a physician. Both of them must be aware of the fact that:

> [his] profession and the responsibility for the patient's or client's body and life (and soul) are intertwined.
> Faulstich (2011)

Since there are neither nationally nor internationally any standardised curricula regarding the study topics for which a singing student has to register, the authors of this section have, together with two well-known professors of singing, developed a model curriculum for the German university system (Richter et al. 2013). This model curriculum includes teaching content that was taught successfully over the course of many years: the curricula of the Studio for Voice Research at the Dresden University of Music, as well as of the Freiburg Institute for Musicians' Medicine at the Freiburg University of Music, both in Germany.

The basis for building this curriculum focused on the study of course content at the other institutions. Here, a paradigm shift has been observed in recent years. While in the past the universities of arts were mostly practice-orientated in their teaching, the modern self-concept—as especially shown by the European-wide Bologna reform of universities—has in recent years also been responding to the need for a science-based approach in German teaching institutions of arts. This becomes visible by the current inclusion of the subject of voice physiology in the curricula of German teaching institutions for singers and actors. In 2012, 50% of the 24 national universities of music in Germany had already integrated the subject of voice physiology into their curricula.

Internationally, there is more diversity regarding the inclusion of the subject of voice physiology. Some professional singers emphasise the importance of teaching units of voice physiology in their curriculum. The renowned singer Renée Fleming, for example, reports on her own education under Beverley Johnson (1904–2001) at the Juilliard School of Music in New York:

> Beverly kept a battered copy of Gray's Anatomy close to her piano among the stacks of scores. She was forever pulling it out to explain something about the mechanism of the voice. 'See that?', she would say, tapping on the page. She would show me a drawing of the pharynx and the larynx, the epiglottis and hard and soft palates, the breath cavities and the diaphragm.
> Fleming (2004)

To facilitate implementation of voice physiology in the curriculum of a university of the arts (or in the curriculum for a bachelor degree in singing), adequate positioning of the subject within a study curriculum is indispensable. 'Adequate' is here defined as the avoidance of the overestimation, as well as the underestimation of vocal physiology, and is a precondition for an innate integration of the subject into active voice pedagogy.

The experiences accumulated since 1959 at the Studio for Voice Research at the Dresden University of Music *Carl Maria von Weber* demonstrate exemplary practice of voice physiology being perceived as one of the contributing elements in a singer's development. Topics within the subject of voice physiology should be closely intertwined with the contents encompassing the subject of singing methods. However, an essential precondition is that the voice physiologist reflects thoroughly the fact that singing cannot be taught by providing theoretical knowledge alone. The teacher giving the individual singing lesson is also required to reinforce the view that the scientific replenishment of the metaphors used in singing pedagogy does not 'disenchant' the voice but that it provides a more efficient design of the arts curriculum.

The most essential basic points of the model curriculum that bear a high practice-related relevance are listed in Table 1.5 below.

At the beginning of the course, there should be an introduction into the physiology and acoustics of the voice. This introduction should portray the meaning, the contextual focus and the interdisciplinary approach of the subject. There is a particular need for an introduction to an effective and comprehensible terminology, which clearly excludes traditional or undefined terms.

Following this basic introduction, the principal elements of voice production, which comprise respiration, phonation (sound production in the larynx) and articulation (sound shaping in the vocal tract), should be outlined. One key aspect related to respiration is to convey knowledge of the respiratory muscles. This leads to an understanding of the respiratory balance and should help the students to classify terminology which is often used, for example, the term 'appoggio' (support).

By conducting simple, practical and surprising experiments (e.g. singing with a burning candle held in front of the mouth without making the flame flicker) may eliminate the overestimated significance of respiratory flow and volume.

Table 1.5 Model curriculum for the subject voice physiology for students of the bachelor course in singing; duration, 1–2 semesters, preferably during the first and second semester (based on the curriculum of the Studio for Voice Research at the Dresden University of Music *Carl Maria von Weber* and of the Freiburg Institute for Musicians' Medicine at the Freiburg University of Music (according to the manual 'Die Stimme' by Bernhard Richter (2013))

Subject	Hours per week
Introduction: the physiology and acoustics of the voice	1
Respiration	6
– Anatomy	
– Physiology	
– Singers' respiration/respiration of lecturers and actors	
Phonation	6
– Anatomy of the larynx	
– Physiology of the larynx	
– Acoustics of the voice source	
– Phonatory aspects of the registers	
Articulation	6
– Anatomy of the vocal tract	
– Physiology of the vocal tract	
– Acoustics of sound modification	
– Articulatory aspects of the registers	
Voice control	4
– Hearing	
– Kinaesthetics, perception of vibration	
– The singer's hearing/room acoustics	
– Vibrato	
Voice categories	3
– Voice types and 'Fach' of classic singing	
– Special characteristics of the speaking voice and of the lecturer's voice	
– Voices of the jazz, rock and pop area	
– Special voice categories (overtone singing, castrates)	
Psychological aspects/stage fright	2
The voice in its life-time perspective	1
Voice strain/voice problems/vocal hygiene/prevention	2

A core element of the lectures will be the sound production in the larynx, i.e. phonation. Here, the focus will not be a comprehensive knowledge of the larynx but of the functional aspects of sound production in the larynx. Accordingly, the description of the laryngeal muscles may remain restricted to different functional muscle groups, for example, the 'opener' and the 'closer' of the glottis.

A prominent concept in singing techniques is that of free, unstrained use of the larynx. Here, it seems to be crucial to familiarise students with the principles of flow phonation: the phonation modus in which the softly contacting vocal folds are brought into vibration with the lowest possible respiratory pressure. This leads to the fundamental understanding that the tight pressing of vocal folds—leading to a raspy voice—and the incomplete closure of the vocal folds, leading to an aspirated voice, cause a higher vocal strain or a constraint of vocal efficiency, respectively.

Despite the lack of clarity regarding the terminology of registers, it is an important aspect and should therefore be included in the voice physiology lectures. The field of register partly belongs to the field of phonation as far as the involvement of muscles and the movements of the vocal folds are concerned.

The resonatory aspects should not be underestimated, since they link into teaching the subjects of acoustics and articulation.

Articulation (sound modification in the vocal tract) can be demonstrated very descriptively and practically during voice physiology lectures. One reason is that the movements of the main 'tools of articulation', i.e. the lips, jaw opening, tongue, palate and larynx, are visible and plausible and can therefore be easily understood by students. The effective teaching of this knowledge might be supported by current scientific publications that visualise (with the MRI-technique) the typical alterations of the vocal tract during singing (Echternach et al. 2012; Mainka et al. 2013; Richter et al. 2017). The typical acoustic phenomena of articulation are also easily analysed and can be demonstrated during lectures in real time by using freely accessible software on a personal computer. Through these tools, the basic singing experience can be demonstrated simply and objectively to new students. The special characteristics of vowel formants should be exemplified and emphasised since they demonstrate that certain vowels within high pitch ranges can no longer be produced 'purely'.

Another key aspect is the visualisation of the capacity of professional singing voices to generate a singers' formant or employ formant tuning.

These insights are usually fascinating for the students and may be introduced during the lecture. Practical exercises in which the students analyse their own voice may deepen the freshly acquired knowledge.

In addition to the above principal components of voice production, voice control is an essential element of voice physiology lectures. Here, a terminological differentiation between auditory voice control (the actual 'hearing') and the kinaesthetic (neuromuscular) voice control is required, since very often this important differentiation is not sufficiently emphasised—either in singing or in pedagogic practice. Teaching basic knowledge of hearing physiology brings with it the preconditions for an understanding of the special characteristics of 'hearing one's own voice'; a topic that has strong relevance for singing as well as for singing pedagogy (Mürbe et al. 2004). The demonstration of kinaesthetic control of the voice is equally important.

Along with the topic of voice control, further basics regarding vibrato in singing and also room acoustics should be included in the lectures.

A physically developing vibrato is always a good indicator of a positive course of a student's career. Noticeable problems with vibrato often indicate at an early stage an undesirable functional development of the voice. Computer-assisted analysing procedures, such as the programme *Madde* (created by Tolvan Data, available for download from www.tolvan.com), can impressively make audible the different aspects of vibrato. Through this, the singer's hearing can be trained and sensitised to the frequency and amplitudes of the vibrato.

The lectures on categorisation of voices should include current findings about the distinction between different voice types and 'Fach'. The holistic approach that should characterise the university's voice training programme includes the demonstration of the particular characteristics of voices of different genres. While in classical singing an aspirated or pressed sound of the voice is only used as an artistic instrument in selected situations, electronically amplified voices in the jazz, pop and rock area usually utilise these techniques more widely for interpretative variety. Hence, an aspirated or pressed sound of the voice may not generally be considered as pathological or artistically inadequate but should be judged according to the intended voice production. Knowledge of special voice categories, such as overtone singing and yodelling, contribute to the student's proficiency and can be demonstrated concretely with modern means of voice analysis such as the programme RTSect (created by Tolvan Data, available for download from www. tolvan.com).

Furthermore, historical and important aspects, for example, the castrate's voice, may be included into this section of the lecture.

Psychological aspects of the voice as well as stage fright are further contents of the voice physiology curriculum unless these topics are already included in other subjects.

Owing to its high relevance to professional practice, a life-time perspective of voice production should be a separate key aspect. Here, the lecture should clearly distinguish between the influence of physiological age in contrast to professional age, i.e. the duration of professional practice.

The complex topics of voice strain, voice failure and their prevention alongside vocal hygiene represent the concluding parts of the curriculum, although voice hygiene and prevention of voice pathology should receive some special attention. However, any overly detailed demonstration of any disease patterns should be avoided since this may be daunting for the students.

A summarised presentation of typical symptoms of short-term or long-term overstress of the voice may be integrated into this part of the curriculum in order to improve the students' reflection of their own voice problems and to facilitate the seeking of medical care at the appropriate time.

1.11   Production, Perception and Acoustics of Speech

Anders Löfqvist

1.11.1   Introduction

Spoken human language communication relies on an acoustic signal that is used to transmit linguistic and paralinguistic information. For producing the signal, an airflow, usually expiratory and created by the lungs, is necessary to drive the vibrations of the vocal folds and also to create transient and noise sources in the vocal tract for voiceless consonants. The linguistic information in the signal consists of the speech sound segments, the vowels and the consonants, and also of the suprasegmental information, intonation, loudness, temporal structure and in some languages tones associated with individual words. The paralinguistic information is in part properties of the signal that are due to the anatomy of the speaker, such as variations in the size of the larynx and the length of the vocal tract from the glottis to the lips; these are partly age-related and due to the growth of the laryngeal and oral structures as a function of age (Fitch and Giedd 1999; Vorperian et al. 2005, 2009).

1.11.2   Speech Production: Statics

The phonological inventory of a language has a limited number of phonemes (categories), vowels and consonants, which varies between languages and usually comprises fewer than 30 items (Ladefoged and Maddieson 1996).

The production of vowel sounds involves the lips, the jaw, the tongue and the velum. They are used to control the acoustic properties of the vocal tract, its acoustic transfer function (Stevens 1998). For vowels produced with vibrating vocal folds, the folds create a periodic acoustic signal with a fundamental frequency determined by the tension and mass of the folds and also by aerodynamic forces, the pressure below the glottis and the airflow through the glottis.

In addition to the fundamental frequency, the source spectrum has a large number of harmonics that are integers of the fundamental. Different vowels are thus produced by moving the tongue in the oral cavity and also by changing the lip opening; in addition, the velum can close the entrance to the nasal cavity to create oral vowels and also open it for nasal vowels.

Some examples of tongue positions for vowels are shown in Fig. 1.74. The tongue contour for the different vowels can be approximated by

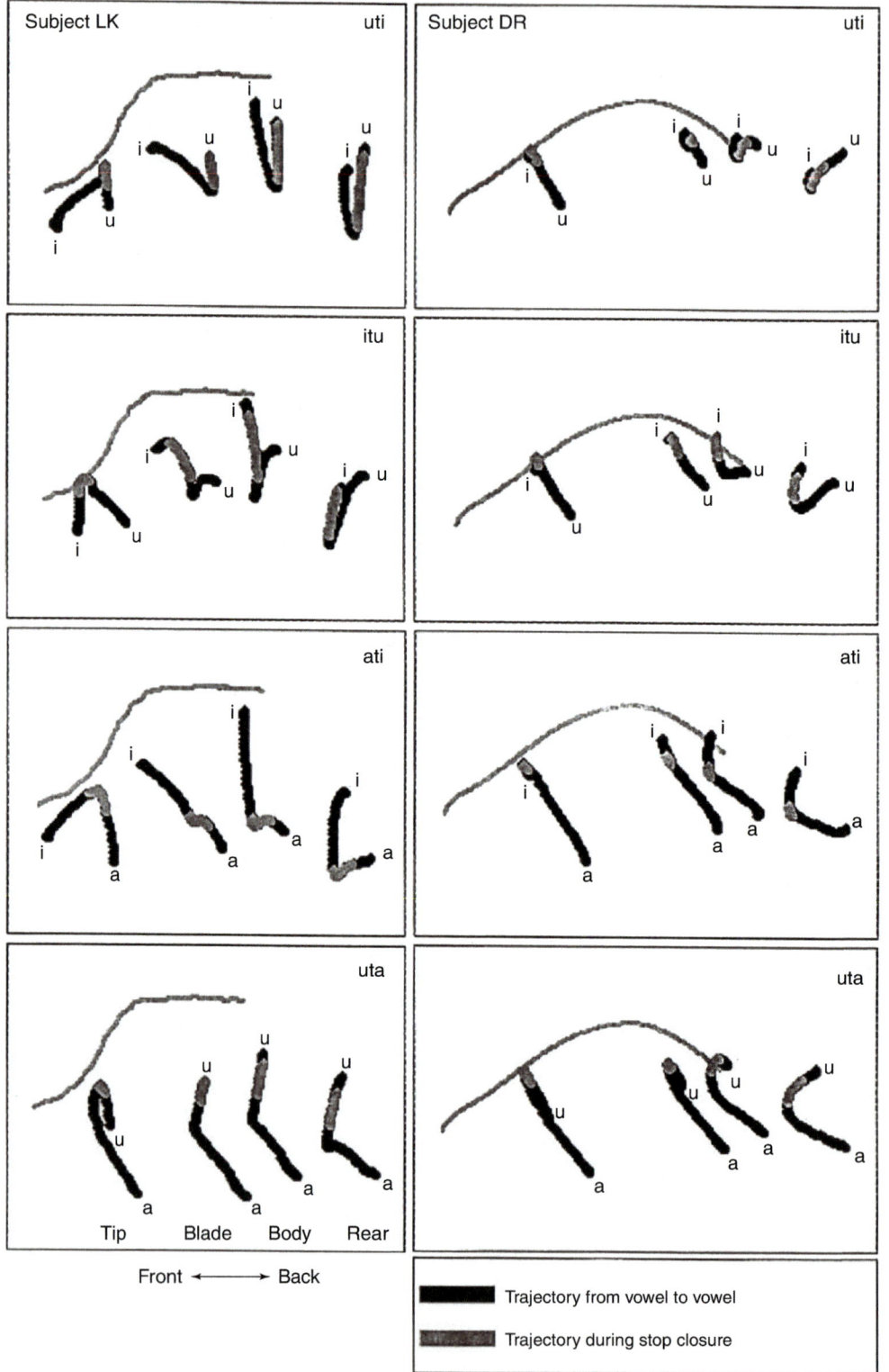

Fig. 1.74 Tongue movements for vowel-consonant-vowel sequences with a voiceless stop /t/ for two speakers. The movement between the two vowels and also the movement during the stop closure are shown. The *line above the tongue* represents an outline of the hard palate

connecting an imaginary line between the four receivers on the tongue. For the vowel /i/, the tongue is positioned forwards and upwards; for the vowel /u/, it is moved backwards; while for the vowel /a/, it is positioned backwards and downwards.

Consonant sounds are produced with a vibrating glottis for voiced consonants or without vibrations for voiceless consonants. There are in theory two ways to suppress the glottal vibrations. The vocal folds can be forcefully adducted, or they can be momentarily abducted, thus opening the glottis and decreasing the velocity of the airflow in the glottis. The latter appears to be widely used in different languages, and the glottal devoicing gesture is temporally coordinated with the oral articulators. It also appears that the cricothyroid muscle is activated to increase the longitudinal tension of the folds and assist in suppressing the vibrations.

Consonants can be produced with a complete closure of the vocal tract for stop consonants or with a small channel between the tongue and the teeth or the hard palate, between the lips or between the lower lip and the upper incisors for fricative consonants. During a complete closure of the oral cavity, the velum can be lowered so that the acoustic signal can pass through the nasal cavity, thus making nasal consonants. For another class of consonant sounds, the laterals, the anterior middle part of the tongue is in contact with the hard palate, while there is free passage at the sides of the tongue. Finally, rhotic sounds are made by increasing the air pressure from the lungs so that a part of the vocal tract can vibrate, driven by the aerodynamics, such as the tongue tip or the uvula.

For consonants, there is contact between the lips or between the tongue and the hard palate. Consonant sounds can thus have different places of articulation depending on where the contact is. If the contact is between the lips, the sound is labial. Different parts of the tongue, such as the tip, the blade, the body and the root are used to produce apical, laminar, velar and pharyngeal consonants. The place of the contact between the tongue and the hard palate can also be used for classification, such as dentals, alveolars, palatals, velars, uvulars, velar, pharyngeal and laryngeal consonants.

Different languages use different combinations of place of articulation, consonant type and voicing to create their sound systems (Ladefoged and Maddieson 1996).

1.11.3 Speech Production: Dynamics

The classification of consonants in terms of their manner and place of articulation is basically a static, idealised, description of how they are produced. In running speech, the movements of articulators are influenced by a number of factors so that articulators most often do not reach and maintain some ideal static configuration (Löfqvist 2010). In fact, in running speech articulators may slow down, but they never stop completely. Figure 1.75 shows an example.

This figure shows articulatory movements for four speakers during the production of a sequence of the vowel /a/, followed by a velar stop consonant, followed by the vowel /a/ again. The records were obtained by articulography, which tracks the movement of receivers attached to different oral structures; the grey line shows the outline of the hard palate (this was obtained by having the subject move the tongue tip along the palate and is thus only an approximation). One salient property of the movement of the rearmost receivers on the tongue is that they do not move in straight lines from the position for the first vowel to the point of contact between the tongue and the palate and then back to the vowel position. Rather, they loop around in a counterclockwise trajectory (this depends on the coordinate system used) which is a very common finding. The most probable reason for this pattern is that it follows from a principle that minimises a cost function such as the jerk (third derivative of position) or speed. The looping patterns thus avoid successive accelerations and decelerations of the tongue. It is also evident from this figure that the tongue dorsum moves continuously during the consonant closure, sliding along the palate. Figure 1.74 shows tongue movements for sequences of vowels flanking a dental stop consonant /t/. This stop

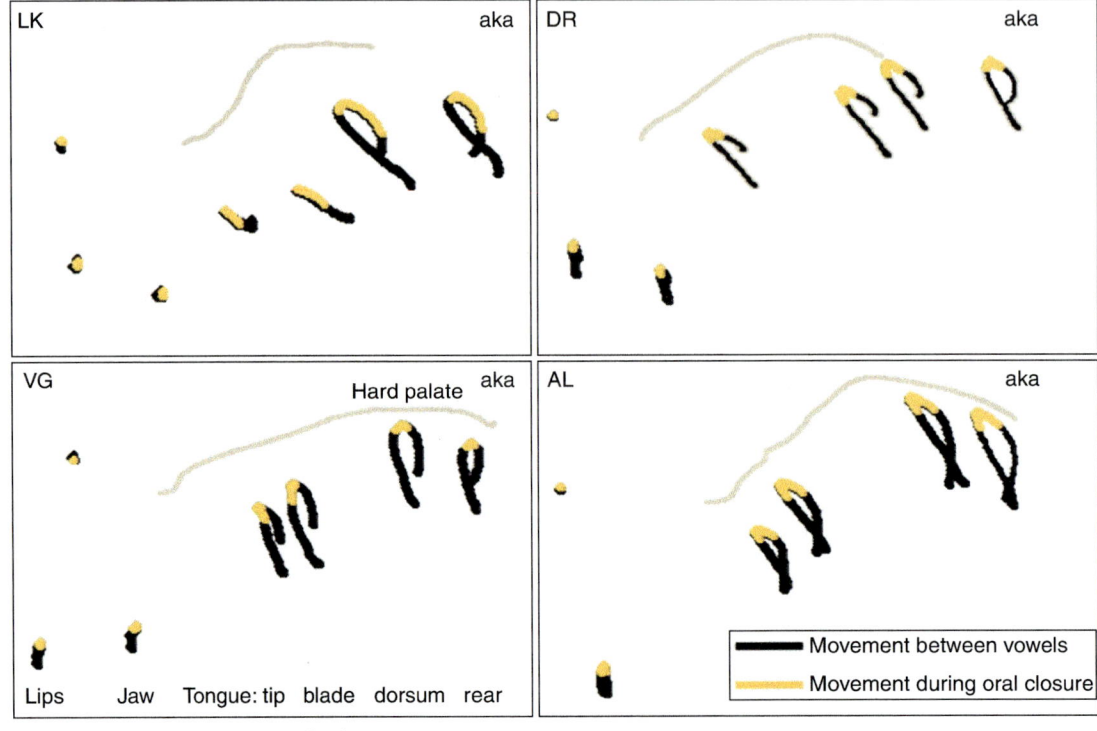

Fig. 1.75 Tongue movements during the sequence /aka/ for four speakers. The movement between the two vowels and the movement during the stop closure are shown. All movements are counterclockwise. The *grey line* at the top in each panel is an outline of the hard palate

requires contact between the tongue tip and the anterior part of the palate. The posterior part of the tongue assists in making the contact between the tip and the palate. The patterns of tongue control are speaker-dependent. This is illustrated by the top four panels in Fig. 1.74. Here, the speaker in the left column moves the posterior part of the tongue, blade, body and rear, down and up for the consonant, but such a movement is not shown by the speaker in the right column. Since there is a limited number of speakers who have been recorded during speech, the nature of such different individual tongue movement strategies is not well understood.

Whenever two articulators meet, at least one of them is made of soft tissue. Thus, they can meet at high velocities. A good example of this is the making of the oral closure for bilabial stop and nasal consonants. Here, the lips meet moving at almost their peak velocities, resulting in an air-tight closure due to tissue compression and also mechanical interactions between the lips, with the lower lip pushing the upper lip upwards owing to its higher velocity and mass. This control mechanism can be described as a virtual target so that the lips would have to pass beyond each other to reach it. Such a control ensures that the lips meet irrespective of their starting positions for the closing movement (Löfqvist 2010).

Another phenomenon in running speech is that adjacent speech segments influence each other and modify their static properties. This is referred to as coarticulation. For example, if the voiceless fricative /s/ is followed by a vowel produced with lip rounding, the lips begin to round during the fricative, since its production does not in itself involve the lips. The effect of lip rounding is a lowering of the noise spectrum of the fricative.

Finally, in running speech, segments may be completely left out or very much reduced, only leaving a small trace in articulation. Such reduction phenomena are governed by intonation and by predictability from contextual factors.

1.11.4 Speech Acoustics

The vibrating vocal folds produce a source signal with a fundamental frequency and a set of higher harmonics that are multiples of the fundamental frequency (Stevens 1998).

The number and amplitude of the higher harmonics in the source signal depend on the mode of the glottal vibrations. These properties are related to the tilt of the source spectrum, i.e. how rapidly the amplitude of the harmonics decreases with frequency. A standard value of the tilt is often given as −12 dB/octave, meaning that the difference in amplitude between two harmonics one octave apart in frequency is 12 dB. This is a conventional and arbitrary value; however, it differs between speakers and also within a speaker, since the source spectrum is continuously changing in running speech owing to linguistic factors such as stress and intonation and also at transitions between voiced and voiceless sounds. The source spectrum is determined by the source pulse, the airflow through the glottis during a single glottal period. The characteristics of the source pulse depend on the subglottal pressure created by the lungs, the size of the glottal opening and the degree of adduction and tension of the vocal folds. One important property of the source pulse is how fast the airflow decreases at glottal closure; the flow doesn't necessarily reach zero in normal voices, since many such voices have a posterior glottal chink. The general rule is that the faster this decrease is, the less is the tilt of the source spectrum. Thus, a pressed voice with a high degree of glottal adduction results in a source spectrum with a low tilt, whereas a breathy voice with a low degree of adduction has a steeper tilt. The former voice is thus in a sense more sonorous, but not necessarily more efficient.

Figure 1.76 shows four simulated source pulses and their spectra.

The main difference between the pulses is in the decrease of the airflow at glottal closure. It decreases more rapidly from top to bottom and is thus fastest in the bottom pulse. From comparison of the four source spectra, it is apparent that the tilt is highest in the top spectrum and lowest in the bottom spectrum. The spectrum at the top only has frequency components up to around 2 kHz, while the bottom one has frequency components up to almost 4 kHz. The two spectra in between have successively lower tilts. The bottom pulse and spectrum are examples of a more pressed phonation. The top pulse is characteristic of a more breathy phonation. It is, however, important to note that these simulated pulses have no DC air flow, a continuous airflow during the whole glottal pulse that can occur owing to an incomplete glottal closure.

The source signal is modified by the filter function of the vocal tract (Stevens 1998). This results in a redistribution of the energy in the signal due to resonances in the vocal tract. The acoustic transfer function of the vocal tract depends on the resonance properties of the tract because of a standing wave pattern. When the signal from the glottis reaches the mouth opening, a wave is reflected back into the tract; at the glottis another reflection occurs. The standing wave can be described in terms of sound pressure and sound velocity. The reflection at the glottis is associated with a pressure maximum and a velocity minimum. The opposite holds at the lip opening. The frequency of the standing wave depends on the distance between the lips and the glottis and is subject to the pressure and velocity conditions between them. The lowest resonance frequency of the tract open at the lips has one pressure maximum and one pressure minimum and is equal to one quarter of a wavelength. Additional resonances occur for odd-numbered waves. Assuming the length of the vocal tract to be approximately 17.5 cm, and the speed of sound about 350 m/s, the lowest resonance of vocal tract without constrictions is about 500 Hz, calculated from

$$c = f^* \lambda \qquad (1.5)$$

(speed of sound c, frequency f, wavelength λ).

96

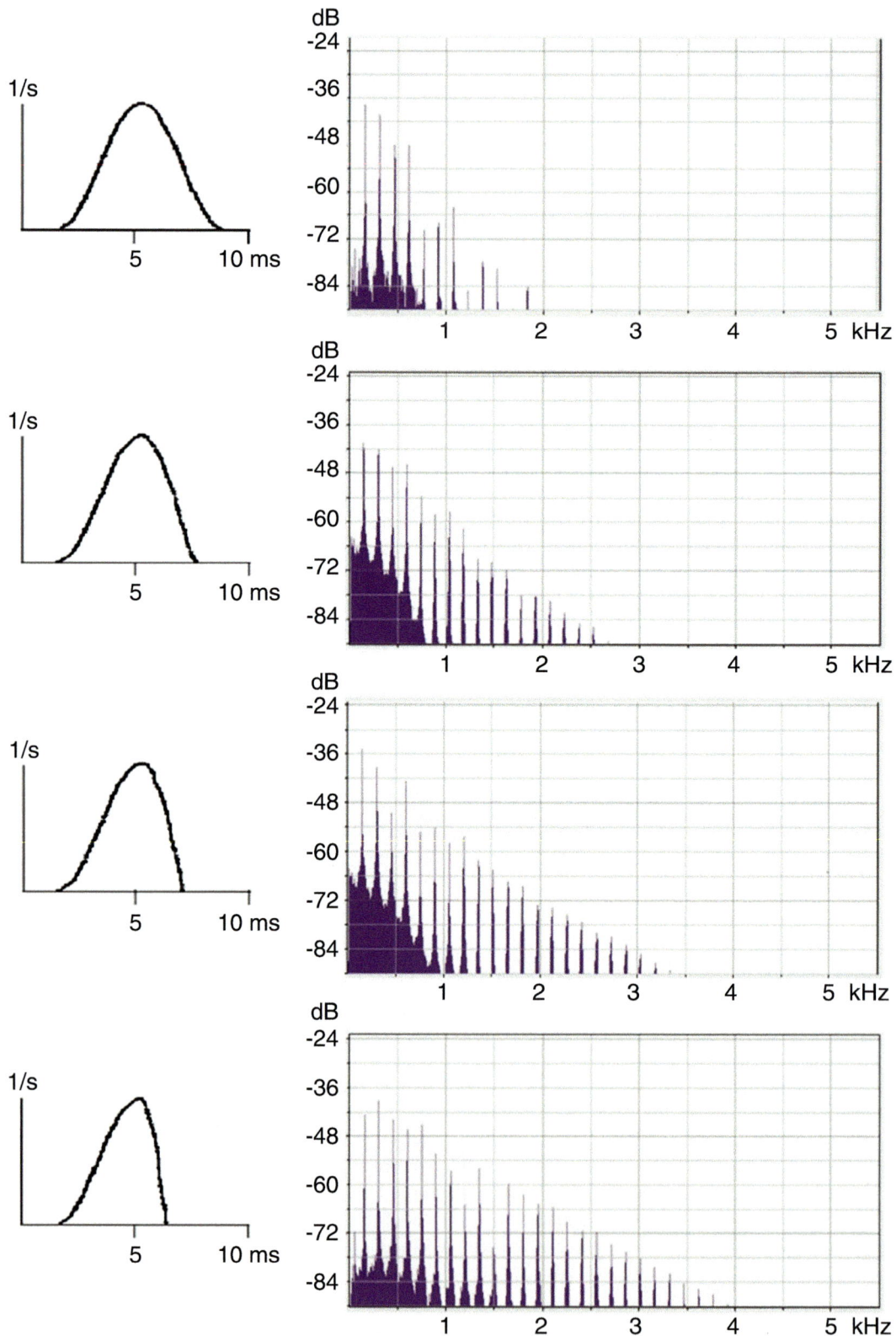

Fig. 1.76 The left column shows four simulated glottal pulses. Their spectra are shown in the right column

Fig. 1.77 X-ray images and schematic cavity configurations for two vowels

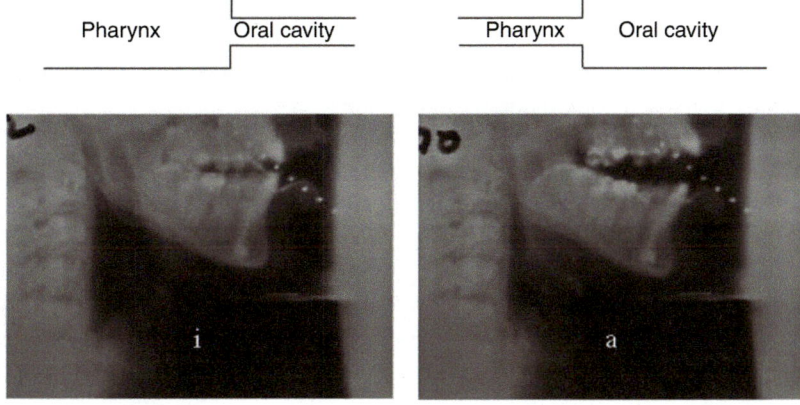

| Pharynx | Oral cavity | | Pharynx | Oral cavity |

The next two resonances would appear at 1500 and 2500 Hz, which correspond to a neutral vowel. By moving the tongue and making constrictions in different parts of the vocal tract and controlling the size of the constriction, a speaker produces the different vowel sounds in the language. The cross-sectional area of the vocal tract from the glottis to the lips is called the area function, and this determines the acoustic transfer function of the vocal tract.

Each vowel is thus characterised by specific resonances of the vocal tract, and a spectral analysis will reveal them as formants, i.e. a group of harmonics amplified by the vocal tract resonances. The formants, usually abbreviated by the symbol 'F', are numbered in increasing frequency, i.e. F1, F2, F3 and F4. There are many vocal tract resonances, arising from the transfer function of the vocal tract, but their amplitude depends on the source spectrum; the higher formants have no acoustic energy, since the source spectrum has a finite number of harmonics. Therefore, one is usually only interested in the formants that can be measured, but the selection depends on the purpose of the analysis. For an ideal vocal tract with hard walls and thus without losses, the bandwidth of the formants would be very narrow. A real vocal tract has of course no rigid walls, so there are losses due to wall vibrations.

At transitions between vowels and consonants, the acoustic transfer function changes, and these changes cause the vowel formants to vary, i.e. the formants change, and these changes are known as formant transitions.

Figure 1.77 shows X-ray pictures and simplified vocal tract configurations for two vowels that have opposite configurations of the vocal tract. For the vowel /i/, the tongue is moved upwards and forwards, resulting in a large cavity in the pharynx. On the other hand, the vowel /a/ has the tongue moved downwards and backwards, resulting in a large cavity in the mouth.

Voiceless consonants are produced without vocal fold vibrations. The open glottis allows a buildup of oral air pressure behind a closure or a narrow channel. For these sounds, the noise source is located in the vocal tract and can be continuous, for fricatives, or transient, for stop consonants.

For fricative consonants, a small channel or slit is made between a part of the tongue and the palate. The noise source for a fricative is governed by the interaction between the geometric properties of the channel and the air passing through the channel (Shadle 2010). Under some conditions, turbulent flow occurs resulting in turbulent noise. The presence of turbulence is determined by Reynolds number:

$$\mathrm{Re} = VD / v = UD / Av \qquad (1.6)$$

(velocity V, cross-sectional dimension of the channel D, volume flow U, cross-sectional area A, kinematic viscosity of the fluid v).

The flow through the channel is regulated by the pressure drop across the channel, which depends on the expiratory lung pressure.

Stop consonants are made with a momentary complete closure of the vocal tract and a raised velum, so that no air can escape through the nose; the result is a buildup of the pressure in the oral cavity behind the closure. At the release of the consonant, a transient noise burst occurs followed by a very brief period of fricative noise due to turbulence as the oral constriction is increased (Stevens 1998). In some languages, voiceless stops have a brief period of aspiration noise after the release of the oral closure. This aspiration noise is created in the glottis. During the stop closure, the glottis is opened, and at the oral release, the glottis is still open and in the process of closing. The duration of the aspiration period can differ between languages. A common measure of this period is the voice onset time (VOT), which is measured as the interval between the oral release for the stop and the onset of glottal vibrations for a following sound. The control of different types of aspiration in stop consonants depends on the timing between the oral closing and opening movements and the laryngeal devoicing gesture.

1.11.5 Speech Perception

As noted above, in running speech many segments are heavily reduced or completely omitted, but speech is usually understood in spite of these changes. Another factor with implications for both speech acoustics and speech perception is illustrated in Fig. 1.78.

This figure plots the lower two formants of three vowels for three different age groups. An examination of the formant frequencies as a function of age shows that they decrease in the order 5 years, 10 years and adults. The reason is that the vocal tract grows in the same order, and a longer vocal tract has lower resonant frequencies than a shorter one (Fitch and Giedd 1999; Vorperian et al. 2005, 2009).

Thus, the formant frequencies of a given vowel differ between speakers of different ages. Also mentioned above were mutual influences between segments in articulation. As a

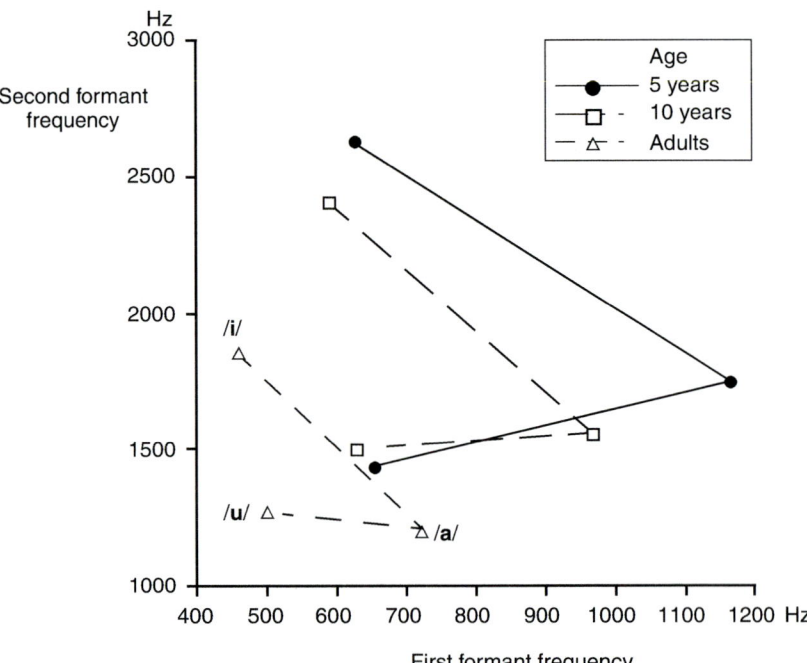

Fig. 1.78 The first two formant frequencies of three vowels as a function of age (data from Lee et al. 1999)

consequence of these and other factors, there can be no invariant acoustic properties of speech sounds. Rather, their properties vary with a

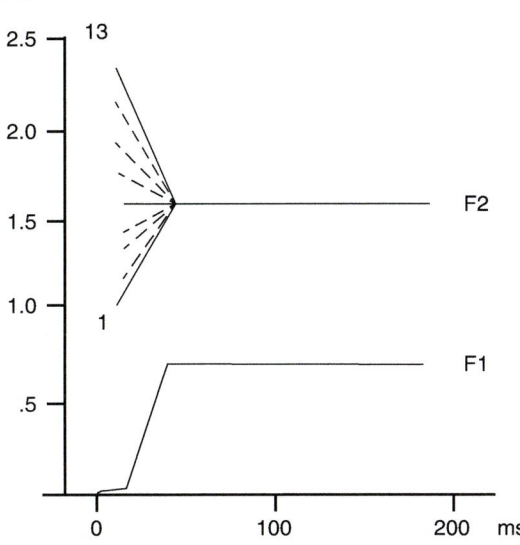

Fig. 1.79 Stimulus set for categorical perception. The stimuli consist of an initial vowel transition and the first and second formants for the vowel /a/. The second formant transition in stimulus #1 is rising, while the F2 transition in stimulus #13 is falling. The stimuli in between have different directions of the formant transition and thus form a continuum of transitions between stimulus #1 and #13

number of factors, and some segments may even be lacking from running speech. However, speech is still understood and fulfils its communicative function. One reason is that there is structure at many levels, phonotactic, morphological, syntactic, semantic and contextual. Thus, it is not necessary to have all the segments for the words to be understood.

One feature of speech perception that has received considerable attention over the years is what is known as categorical perception. A typical stimulus set used in experiments of categorical perception is shown in Fig. 1.79 for synthetic consonant-vowel syllables.

The difference between the individual stimuli is the extent and direction of the second formant transition; the vowel is /a/. In stimulus #1, the second formant is rising from a low-frequency value, while for stimulus #13, it is falling from a high frequency. The change in the first formant is identical across all stimuli. The stimulus set thus forms a continuum of changes in the second formant transition. The results of an identification experiment using this stimulus set are shown in Fig. 1.80.

In such an experiment, participants are asked to identify the initial consonant; the vowel is identified as /a/ (with only two formants and the

Fig. 1.80 Results from an identification experiment using the stimuli shown in Fig. 1.79. The numbers on the *x*-axis represent the stimuli shown in Fig. 1.79. The *y*-axis shows the identification score for each stimulus. For example, stimuli #1–6 are perceived as a labial consonant /b/, while stimuli #10–13 are perceived as a velar consonant /g/

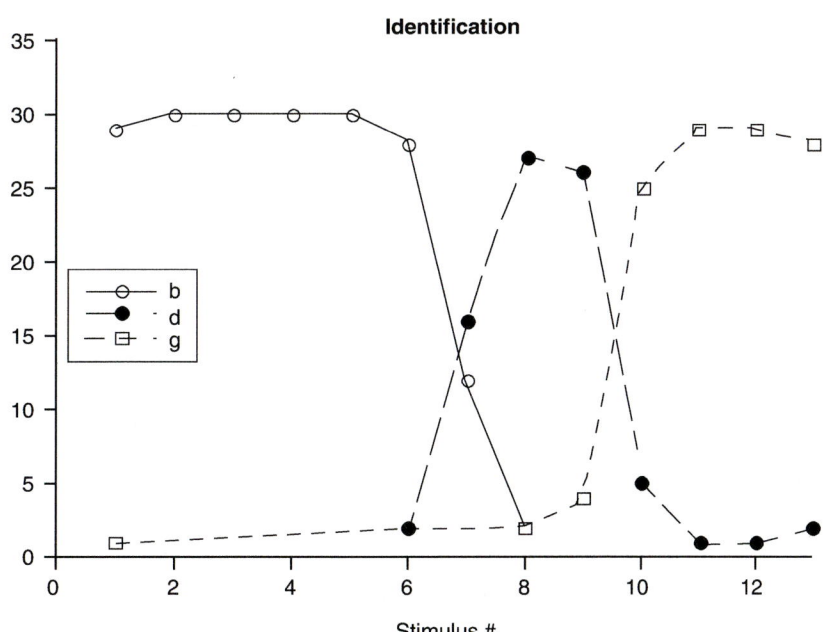

variations in the transition of the second formant shown in Fig. 1.79, this only works for this particular vowel). The results of the identification experiment show that stimuli 1–6 are perceived as a labial consonant, stimuli 7–9 as a dental and stimuli 10–13 as a velar consonant. It is also evident that there are abrupt changes in the response pattern between categories; there appears to be a category boundary at stimulus #7 and another at #10. Another property of categorical perception is that in a discrimination experiment with the same stimulus set, listeners are much better at discriminating between stimuli that cross a category boundary. That is, discrimination is better for stimuli 2 and 8 which span a category boundary than between 2 and 3.

One contentious issue in speech perception is the nature of what is being perceived. There are currently at least two opposing views. Some argue that speech perception follows general principles of auditory perception (Dahan and Magnuson 2011; Diehl et al. 2004; Samuel 2011). However, some argue that speech perception is rather like visual perception. Here, most likely no one would argue that we 'perceive' the light but rather the object structuring the light. Accordingly, the argument is that we perceive the articulatory movements that shape the acoustic speech signal (Galantucci et al. 2006).

1.12 Articulatory Models

Peter Birkholz and Christiane Neuschaefer-Rube

1.12.1 Introduction

Articulatory models are used to study different functions of the articulatory system. With regard to speech production, they are called vocal tract models. The earliest vocal tract models were manually operated mechanical devices. The first fully functional speaking machine for generating connected utterances was constructed and demonstrated by Wolfgang von Kempelen in 1791 (von Kempelen 1791) and a replica of it is shown in Fig. 1.81. For producing voiced sounds, it used bellows to supply air to a reed, which excited a rubber tube resonator that was varied in shape with one hand. Consonants could be produced by means of four separate constricted passages that were controlled with the fingers of the other hand. Further mechanical speaking machines were constructed, for example, by Alexander Graham Bell in the latter 1800s and Riesz in 1937 (cf. Flanagan 1965). With the advance of digital computer technology, the first computer-implemented models of the vocal tract were developed in the 1970s. Today, a wide variety of computer models of the articulatory system exists. However, the interest in mechanical analogues of the vocal system continues today, and one of the more advanced computer-controlled mechanical models is the 'WASEDA talker', which was developed at Waseda University in Tokyo, Japan.

- Hallo. Wie geht es Dir? (Hello. How are you?) (Audio Sample 1.9 Example-Hallo)
- Lea und Doreen mögen Bananen (Lea and Doreen like bananas) (Audio Sample 1.10 Example Lea-und-Doreen)

The articulatory system can be modelled at different levels of detail. With regard to speech production, it is mainly the shape of the vocal tract that matters, because it determines the acoustic resonances. Therefore, many articulatory models simulate how the vocal tract shape is varied by the articulators, but do not bother with the biomechanics of the tissue. These models are used, for example, as tools for education, to study articulatory-acoustic relations and as visual feedback in speech training systems.

- A very popular round: 'Dona nobis pacem' sung by two voices, tenor and bass, in canon (Video 1.1 dona-nobis-pacem created by Peter Birkholz)
- Salvete. This music video was created for the opening ceremony of the 27th Annual Meeting of the German Society of Phoniatrics and Pedaudiology (DGPP) 2010, held at RWTH Aachen University, by Peter Birkholz using Vocal Tract Lab (www.vocaltractlab.de). The

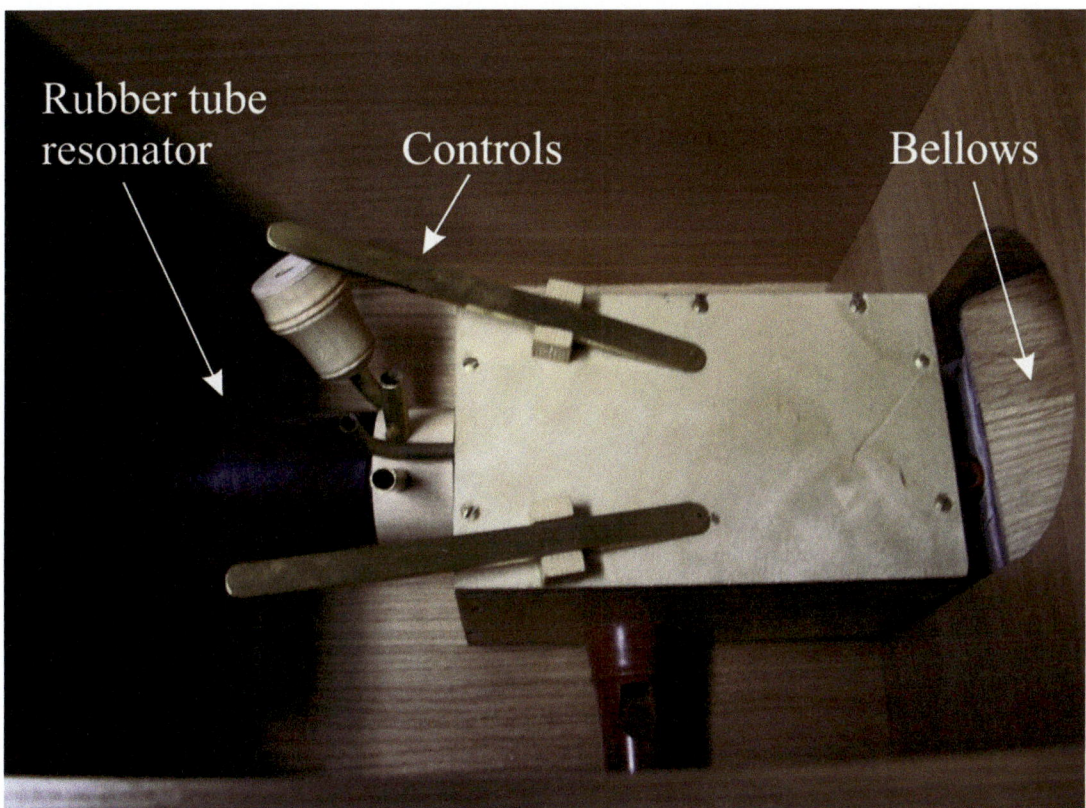

Fig. 1.81 Replica of the mechanical speaking machine of Wolfgang von Kempelen, rebuilt at Saarland University, Germany. Photo courtesy of Fabian Brackhane and Jürgen Trouvain

song is based on the well-known 'Canon in D' by Pachelbel (1653–1706) with customised Latin lyrics. The instrumental accompaniment was created by using the software FRINIKA (Video 1.2 salvete-pachelbel)

In contrast, biomechanical models of the articulatory system are more detailed than 'shape models', as they physically simulate the anatomical structure of hard and soft tissue components and their interactions. These models are controlled with simulated muscle forces and do not only allow the study of speech production but also the other important functions of mastication and swallowing. Although they are mostly still at the research stage, for the future they hold a great potential to enhance our limited understanding of dysfunctions such as speech disorders, swallowing disorders and functional articulatory deficits following surgery.

1.12.2 Classification of Articulatory Models

Computer models of the articulatory system can be roughly arranged into three major classes, namely, geometrical, statistical and biomechanical. The models in each class can be further subdivided into two-dimensional (2D) and three-dimensional (3D) models. While the 3D models define the full 3D structure of the system, the 2D models are limited to a representation in the midsagittal plane. All models have in common the representation of the momentary state of the articulatory system in terms of a number of control parameters, but the kind of parameters depends on the model class.

1.12.2.1 Geometrical Models
Geometrical models describe the vocal tract shape by a number of defined parameters that specify

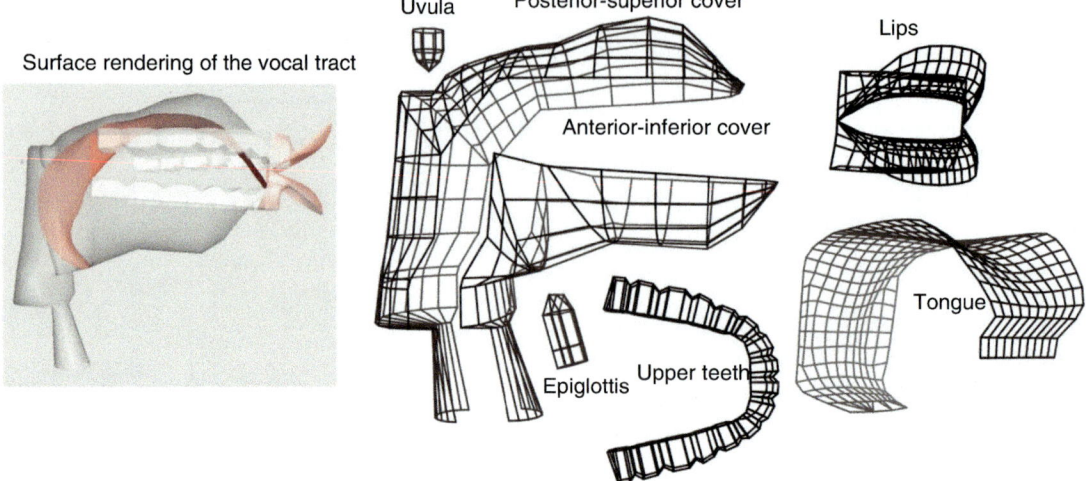

Fig. 1.82 Surface rendering and wireframe models of the parts of the 3D geometrical vocal tract model of Birkholz (2013a)

the shape and position of the articulators. The parameters are assumptions about the degrees of freedom of the articulatory system, based on observations. They are defined so as to permit the necessary flexibility to reproduce the variety of natural vocal tract shapes, while preventing shapes that would violate the structural constraints of human anatomy. Typical parameters of such models are, for example, the degree of lip protrusion, the degree of lip opening, the vertical position of the hyoid and the extent of the velopharyngeal opening. One of the more influential 2D articulatory models was presented by Mermelstein (1973). It defines the vocal tract outline in the midsagittal plane, on the basis of a set of ten parameters, which indicate the positions of the jaw, tongue body, tongue tip, lips, velum and hyoid. As in most other models of that time, it was derived from X-ray tracings of the vocal tract. The purpose of the model was the study of speech production. Therefore, the cross-sectional area function of the system had to be estimated from the dimensions in the midsagittal plane. This estimation process, owing to the missing third dimension, is one of the major limitations of 2D articulatory models for speech production.

A 3D geometrical model for speech synthesis was developed by Birkholz (2013a). It comprises a number of geometrical surfaces for individual parts of the vocal tract whose shape is defined by 23 control parameters (Fig. 1.82). Together these surfaces form the boundary of the vocal tract. Given the full 3D shape of the vocal tract, its cross-sectional area for the acoustic simulation can be estimated much more accurately than from 2D models. The basic anatomical dimensions and the mapping from parameter values to surface shapes were based on a corpus of magnetic resonance imaging (MRI) data. Because MRI produces very detailed images of the vocal tract and is without any known harmful effects on the subject, it has become the preferred method to obtain detailed 3D data for the construction of articulatory models.

1.12.2.2 Statistical Models

In contrast to geometrical models, statistical articulatory models are based on statistical analysis of observed articulations. The basic idea is to represent the observed shape of the vocal tract, or of individual articulators, as the weighted sum of a small number of linear (shape) components. The weights of the components are the control parameters of the model. The components are determined by a factor analysis technique that exploits correlations among the set of observed shapes. Such factor analysis techniques are, for example, principal component analysis (PCA), guided PCA, arbitrary factor analysis, parallel factor analysis (PARAFAC) and linear component analysis (LCA) (Engwall 2003). While PCA and PARAFAC are optimal, in the sense that they explain the variance in the observations with the smallest possible number of components, they do not guarantee that the components can be interpreted in articulatory terms. Therefore, the other types of factor analysis are preferred in the construction of articulatory models.

A widely used 2D statistical model of the vocal tract was introduced by Maeda (1990). To create the model, he applied arbitrary factor analysis to the vocal tract outlines of roughly 1000 frames of cine-radiographic data corresponding to 10 French sentences uttered by two speakers. This allowed the modelling of the observed variation in tongue shape with only four components, which were interpreted in articulatory terms as mandibular position, tongue dorsum position, dorsal shape and tongue tip position. The entire vocal tract configuration could be described with reasonable accuracy with as few as seven parameters.

A detailed statistical 3D model of the tongue was constructed by Engwall (2003). It was based on the tongue shapes of 44 natural articulations of one individual measured with 3D MRI. The data were analysed with linear component analysis to obtain a set of six control parameters for the tongue. This tongue model was complemented with graphical representations of the other parts of the vocal tract and the face and used in a computer-based speech training system as described further below.

1.12.2.3 Biomechanical Models

Common to both geometrical and statistical articulatory models is that they only model the shape of the articulators, but do not model the biomechanics of the tissue. As a consequence, both types of model can potentially generate articulations that are physically impossible, for example, when extreme values of different control parameters are combined. In contrast, biomechanical articulatory models generate vocal tract shapes

by physically simulating the deformation and movement of the actual tissue. Therefore, most of them use the finite element method (FEM) to model the anatomical structures. With this method, the tissue is divided into a number of small connected elements, for example, triangles in the 2D domain or tetrahedrons in the 3D domain. The deformation of these elements is then calculated on the basis of the internal and external forces acting on the elements and their elastic properties. External forces include the forces of simulated muscles, which are the control parameters of this type of model.

An example of a 2D FEM model of the tongue for the study of speech motor control is that of Payan and Perrier (1997), which simulates the forces of seven muscles: the anterior and posterior parts of the genioglossus, the styloglossus, the hyoglossus, the verticalis and the superior and inferior parts of the longitudinalis. The most comprehensive 3D FEM model of the whole jaw-tongue-hyoid complex developed so far has been created by Stavness et al. (2011) and is illustrated in Fig. 1.83. It allows the muscle-driven physical simulation of both the hard and soft tissue components and realistically accounts for their interconnections.

Although biomechanical models allow the most realistic simulation of the articulatory system, they are very challenging to create. Furthermore, these models are hard to validate, because this would require the simultaneous measurement of muscle forces and vocal tract shapes of humans. Finally, the precise temporal control of the models for the execution of specific functions, such as speaking or swallowing, remains a major challenge owing to the large number of muscle input degrees of freedom.

1.12.3 Application of Articulatory Models

Articulatory models are applied in multiple specialities such as phoniatrics, phonetics and speech technology. In phoniatrics, the application of these models is still mostly at the very beginning. One of the more promising applications of

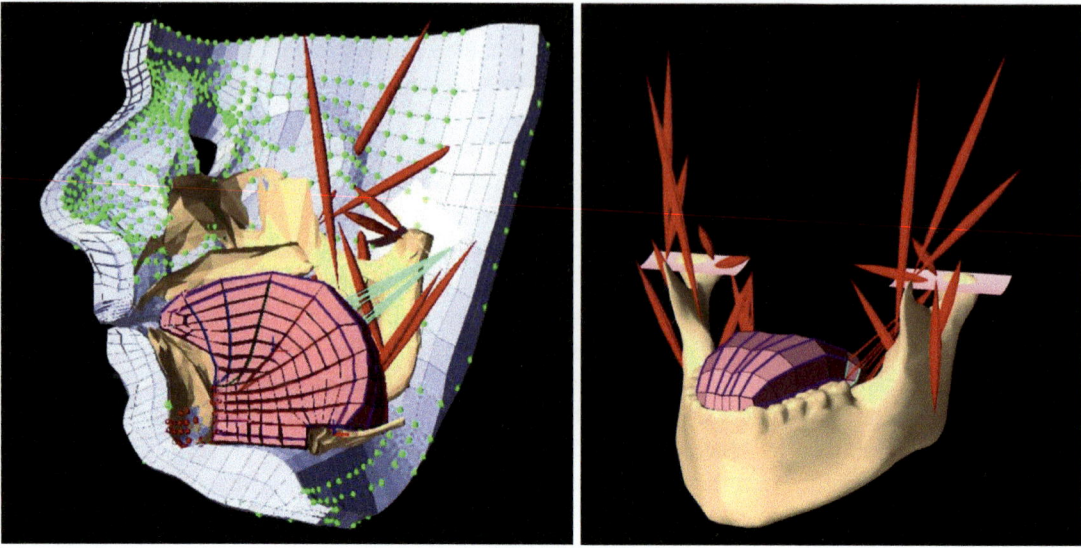

Fig. 1.83 Two views of a muscle-controlled, combined jaw-tongue-hyoid finite element model of the articulatory system. The red lines show the extrinsic muscles. Courtesy of Ian Stavness (Lloyd et al. 2012)

biomechanical models of the articulatory system is in the prediction of functional side effects of vocal tract surgery, for example, of oncologic tongue, velum or jaw resection, cleft palate surgery and surgery in snoring medicine. Despite advanced surgical reconstructions after resection of oral or pharyngeal tumours, many patients suffer from speech and swallowing problems afterwards. In principle, biomechanical models of the vocal tract could be used to mimic the surgical treatment virtually. This would allow the prediction and visualisation of the surgical results in terms of speech and swallowing functions and facilitate individual therapeutic decisions. However, these applications are still underdevelopment. Furthermore, biomechanical models could enhance our understanding of the dysfunctions of obstructive sleep apnea and swallowing disorders.

Another application of vocal tract models in phoniatrics is to provide patients with model-based visual biofeedback of their articulatory and swallowing movements. For example, hearing-impaired children can improve their own pronunciation when they are shown how their own articulation deviates from the correct articulation. For this, the vocal tract state of the patient has to be estimated in real-time from sensory data and to be shown as an animation model on a computer screen for immediate feedback. Engwall et al. (2006) developed the computer-based speech training system ARTUR for patients with speech, language or hearing disorders. This system detects the pronunciation of patients on the basis of the audio signal and simultaneously records video images of the lips. A statistical vocal tract model (Engwall 2003) in combination with a face model is used to give the patient visual feedback of his articulation and provide suggestions on how to improve his articulation (Fig. 1.84). While ARTUR estimates the vocal tract state indirectly from the patients' speech signal and lip shape, there are also more direct methods to measure articulation in real-time. For example, Preuß et al. (2013) recently proposed a method where the user wears a thin acrylic pseudo-palate (similar to a dental brace) populated with optical distance sensors in his mouth to measure the position of the lips and the anterior tongue. These data are used to control an animated reference model of the vocal tract. Although still under development, this method is very promising for real-time feedback of articulation in speech therapy as well. Owing to the direct and instantaneous measurement and visualisation of

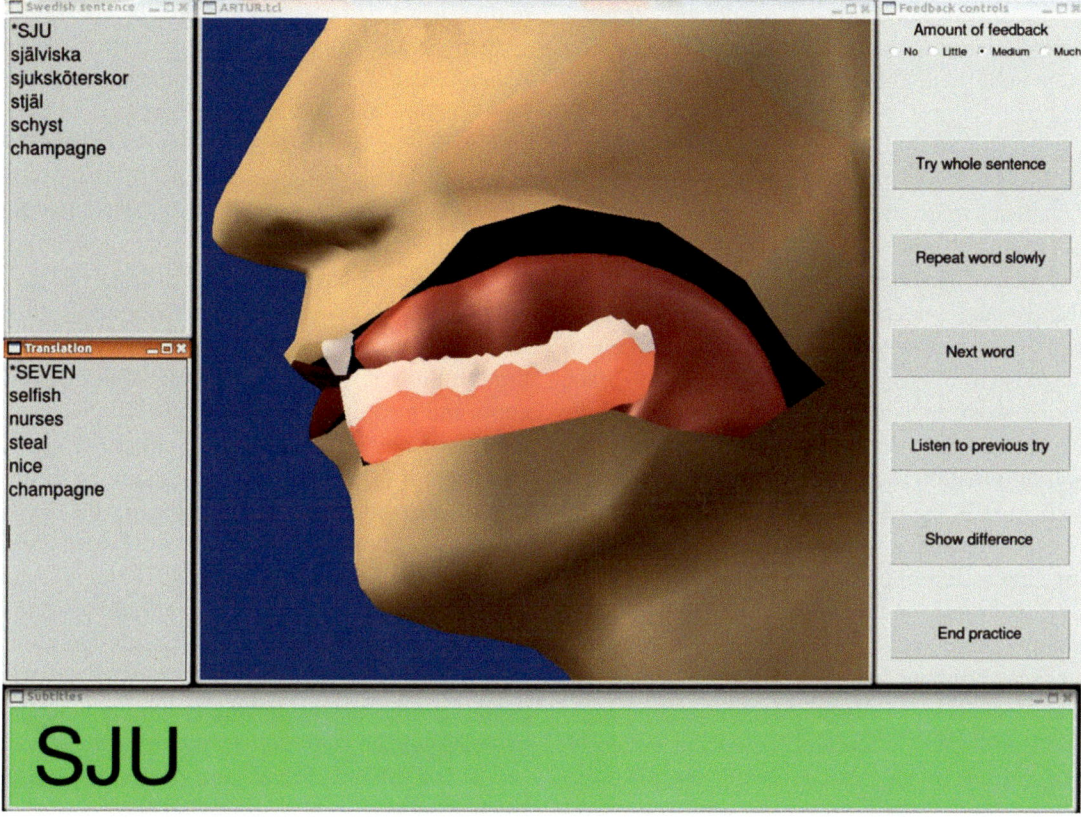

Fig. 1.84 The user interface of the speech training system ARTUR giving articulatory feedback. The main panel shows a cutaway rendering of the vocal tract, and the bottom panel shows the current training word. Courtesy of Olov Engwall (2005)

articulation, it is also considered as a feedback method in the therapy of dysphagia.

Besides these direct applications, vocal tract models can also be used in research on speech acquisition. For example, Kröger et al. (2009) proposed a comprehensive computer-implemented model to simulate how children learn to speak, by simulating the neural mechanisms in combination with a model of the vocal tract. Speech acquisition models are not only used to put theories of speech production and perception to the test, but also to enhance our understanding of speech and language disorders based on neural defects.

Beyond the phoniatric applications of articulatory models presented above, they are used as educational instruments, as modules in articulatory speech synthesis (Birkholz 2013a, b), and as

tools to study the evolution of speech (de Boer and Fitch 2010).

1.13   Linguistics, Neurolinguistics and Neuropsychology

Lisa Bartha-Doering and Christian Dobel

1.13.1 Introduction to Neurolinguistics

Neurolinguistics is the study of the relationship between language and the brain and is focused on the neural mechanisms that underlie language acquisition and processing. The roots of neurolinguistics lie in clinical neurology and date back to the late nineteenth century, when detailed descriptions of language deficits following brain injury were published. This traditional approach of clinical-pathological correlations was extended by the development of modern imaging techniques such as positron emission tomography (PET) and functional magnetic resonance imaging (fMRI), as well as time-sensitive electrophysiological techniques including electroencephalography (EEG) and magnetoencephalography (MEG), which are able to provide activation patterns of language processing even in the healthy brain. Much work in neurolinguistics is informed by psycholinguistic models of language structure and information processing. However, today neurolinguistics is an interdisciplinary field with researchers from a variety of backgrounds including linguistics, phoniatrics, psychology, philosophy, neurology, neuroanatomy, neurophysiology, neurobiology, artificial intelligence and computer science, bringing along a variety of techniques and concepts.

Neurolinguistic research is carried out in all major areas of linguistic components, including phonology, morphology, syntax, semantics, prosody and pragmatics, and covers all language functions such as comprehension, naming, repetition, reading and writing. Neurolinguistic research areas include studies on the localisation of language functions and components, the time course of language information processing, the identification of brain structures related to (first and second) language acquisition, developmental language disorders and dyslexia, language deficits following acquired (neurological) disorders and the contribution of all this knowledge to language therapy in children and adults.

1.13.2 Language Components

Different language components are used to understand and produce language. While these components are closely interconnected, each one has its own developmental periods and is thought to have its own neural substrates. The *phonetic system* deals with all possible sounds that the human vocal apparatus can produce. The sound system of an individual language is called the *phonological system*. It involves the rules about the structure and sequence of language sounds and includes an inventory of a distinct number of sounds and their features.

The meaning of words is organised by the *semantic system*. This system relates a vocabulary of signs (spoken, written or signed) to specific meanings. A single sign connected to a meaning is called a *lexeme*. The systematic organisation of words connected to specific concepts and meanings forms the *mental lexicon*.

The *syntactic system* relates to the structure of language. It organises the combination of meaningful elements within a language, the *morphemes*, into utterances. This involves word order and sentence structure. The rules for the internal structure of words are called *morphology*; the rules of the internal structure of phrases and sentences are called *syntax*.

The *pragmatic system* deals with the practical use of language and involves the rules for appropriate and effective communication. This use is often directed by the culture and the context of use. Using language for greeting, changing language for talking differently and following rules such as turn taking are skills involved by the pragmatic system.

1.13.3 Localisation of Language Functions in the Brain

1.13.3.1 The Classic View

In 1861, Paul Broca started the process of identifying the parts of the brain that are involved in language (Broca 1861). The French neurosurgeon examined the brain of a recently deceased patient who had been unable to speak but could understand spoken language. At autopsy, Broca found an extensive lesion in the left inferior frontal cortex. In the next years, Broca studied eight other patients, all of whom had similar language deficits caused by lesions in their left frontal hemisphere. This led him to identify, for the first time, the existence of a *language centre* in the posterior portion of the frontal lobe of the left hemisphere, now often referred to as *Broca's area.*

Ten years later, Carl Wernicke, a German neurologist, discovered that damage to a different part of the brain also caused language problems (Wernicke 1874). This area of the brain, which was later called *Wernicke's area*, was located in the posterior portion of the temporal lobe, the superior temporal gyrus. Wernicke's patients with a lesion at this location displayed a severe disorder of speech comprehension and an inappropriate use of words in language production. Wernicke developed the idea that many language functions resulted from connecting various brain components.

In 1884, Lichtheim further developed this model which is now known as the Wernicke-Lichtheim or connectionist model (Lichtheim 1884, see Fig. 1.85).

This model was both neuroanatomical and functional in its basis. It proposed that Broca's and Wernicke's areas form a triangle with a third area which Lichtheim called the *concept centre.*

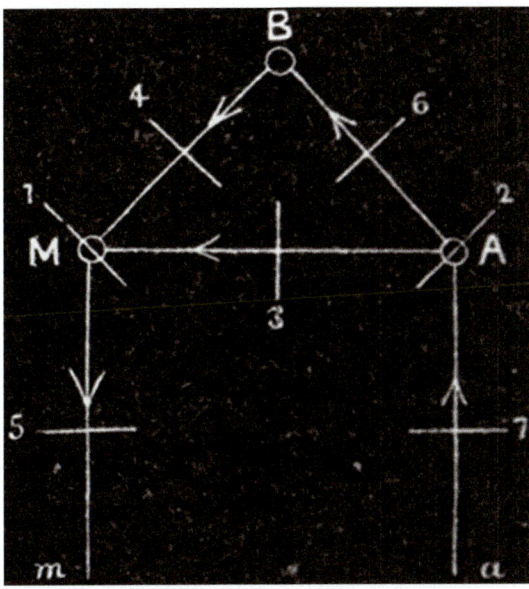

Fig. 1.85 Lichtheim model. From Compston A, From the Archives, Brain (2006), 129(6):1347–1350 by permission of Oxford University Press. *a* auditory speech input, *A* centre for auditory word representations, *m* motor speech input, *M* centre for motor word representations, *B* centre for object concepts

Broca's area was involved in speech production, while Wernicke's area contained the memory traces of the auditory forms of words with the primary function of perception of speech, with the arcuate fasciculus forming a connection between them both. The concept centre, Lichtheim hypothesised, stored word meanings and facilitated auditory comprehension. This classic model predicted the linguistic consequences of damage to various brain regions of the left hemisphere and served as the foundation for classifying different types of acquired language disorders, the *aphasias*. This connectionist model remained the primary framework for understanding aphasia.

1.13.3.2 Modern Neurobiological Models of Language

In the last 20 years, modern brain imaging techniques and an increase of interdisciplinary neuroscience research connecting linguistics, cognitive psychology, medicine and computational modelling have challenged the classic view. Today, non-invasive functional brain imaging makes it possible to study activation of brain areas associated with language processing in healthy subjects and patients while they perform language tasks. These studies have confirmed the importance of Broca's and Wernicke's areas for language while also identifying them as part of a broader network of connected brain areas that contribute to language processing.

Built on earlier theories such as those introduced above, the dual stream model of language processing by Hickok and Poeppel (2004) suggests two functionally distinct neural networks that process language information. Early stages of speech processing involve the middle to posterior portions of the superior temporal sulcus bilaterally with a weak left-hemisphere dominance. Subsequently, the system diverges into two streams, a dorsal pathway that projects towards the inferior parietal and posterior frontal lobe regions that maps sensory or phonological representations onto articulatory motor representations (such as in repetition) and a ventral pathway that projects to the middle and inferior

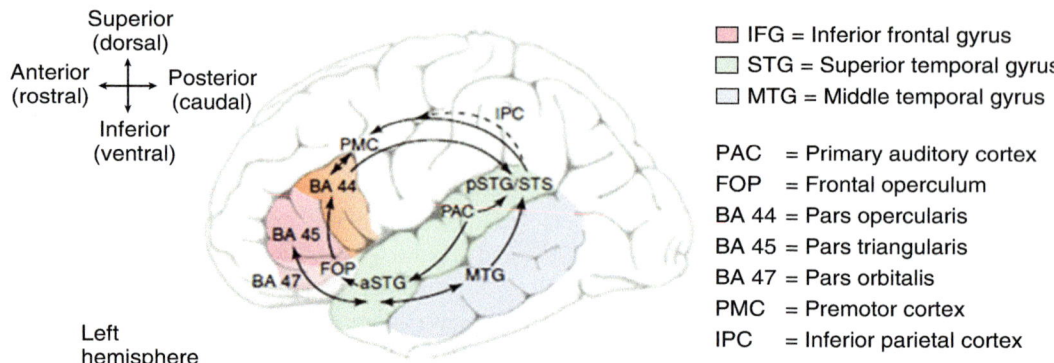

Fig. 1.86 The dynamic dual pathway model of auditory language comprehension. Reprinted from TRENDS in Cognitive Sciences, 16/5, Friederici (2012), the cortical language circuit: from auditory perception to sentence comprehension, 262–268, Copyright 2012 with permission from Elsevier

temporal cortices that maps sensory or phonological representations onto lexical conceptual representations (such as in language comprehension).

With a more specific focus on syntax, the dynamic dual pathway model of auditory language comprehension by Friederici and Alter (2004, see Fig. 1.86) explains syntactic and semantic information as primarily processed in a left hemispheric temporo-frontal pathway, including distinct circuits for syntactic and semantic information. In contrast, sentence level prosody is considered to be processed in a temporo-frontal pathway in the right hemisphere.

Stimulus properties and processing demands are responsible for the relative lateralisation of these functions. Furthermore, the integrative speech processing framework by Kotz and Schwartze (2010) links cortical speech processing networks to subcortical structures by incorporating cerebello-thalamo-cortical and cortico-striato-thalamo-cortical circuits.

Overall, on the basis of clinical and experimental findings, modern neurobiological models of language draw a picture of a wide network of interconnected cortical and subcortical areas being responsible for language processing (for further reading see Hickok and Small 2015).

1.13.4 Development of Language Localisation

Anatomical data demonstrate that structural brain asymmetries are already present prenatally and point towards a genetic underpinning of the left hemispheric language lateralisation bias (Kasprian et al. 2011). Correspondingly, there is evidence from functional imaging studies that left hemispheric dominance for language already exists in neonates and 3-month-old infants (Dehaene-Lambertz et al. 2002). Throughout childhood, the brain develops and matures, including myelination and changes in cortical thickness, white matter volumes and volumes of subcortical structures. Brain areas and circuits become increasingly specialised in developing and processing specific language functions, depending on the individual linguistic demands. Studies have for instance shown that the processing of phonemes becomes increasingly left lateralised in brain development, whereas prosody detection becomes more lateralised towards the right hemisphere with age. These findings are in line with studies illustrating the increasingly specific phonemic repertoire during development: whereas newborns are able to distinguish all of the world's phonemes, they lose this ability during the first years of life but become more and more tuned to the specifics of their mother tongue. Hereby, the linguistic status of the sounds

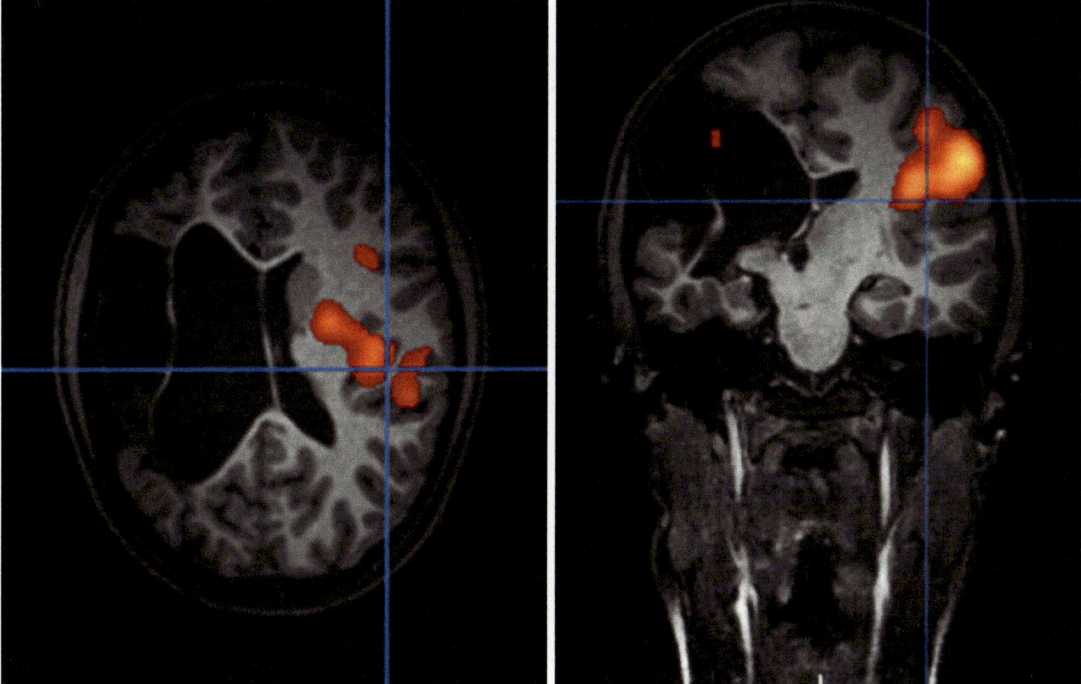

Fig. 1.87 fMRI images showing language reorganisation towards the right hemisphere in left paediatric stroke

seems to be critical in the determination of lateralisation, as the same sound can be processed unilaterally or bilaterally, depending on whether it belongs to the phonemic repertoire of the environmental language.

Furthermore, structural changes can influence localisation and processing of language. In this regard, there is a widely held belief that lesions originating from the prenatal period, or lesions acquired during the first years of life, rarely result in obvious language deficits. This sparing of language functions after early lesions has been attributed to the remarkable plasticity of the immature brain. Indeed, some studies with functional imaging have supported this view by describing a right hemispheric activation in paediatric stroke patients that mirrors the typical left hemispheric activation pattern in healthy subjects (Tillema et al. 2008; for an example of right lateralised language following paediatric stroke, see Fig. 1.87).

However, other reports have described several examples in which organisation of language following left hemispheric injury occurs in the ipsilateral hemisphere (Liegeois et al. 2004). There is also discussion on the influence of lesion size, underlying pathology and lesion localisation, most importantly lesion involvement of typical language areas, on language localisation.

Thus, the relation of brain maturation and the development of cognitive functions are a dynamic and interactive process, and later aspects of development may shape the system and use distributed networks with increasing efficiency. Functional studies of the relationship between maturation of the brain and cognitive development have stressed both progressive and regressive neural mechanisms of change, that is, brain regions becoming increasingly or decreasingly involved in cognition with age (Brown et al. 2005).

1.13.5 Neuropsychological Aspects of Language

With an emphasis on clinical and experimental investigations, neuropsychology covers the complex interaction of memory, visuo-perception, auditory perception, attention, practice and language and its relationship to the brain. In this sense, the focus of neurolinguistics is part of the broader neuropsychological research field. Although it might be useful to isolate processes in order to study them, language is neither anatomically nor conceptually an isolatable system. Leaving aside the discussion on modularity of language, the examination of language functions requires a basic understanding of language-associated cognitive processes. If a child has a reduced auditory short-term memory, it will not be able to understand long sentences. If a patient suffering from frontotemporal dementia is not able to modify ongoing behaviour, he will produce errors in naming or generating words. In these cases, the neurolinguistic interpretation of language deficits is tremendously dependent on the knowledge of associated cognitive deficits.

Cognitive functions closely connected to language functions comprise mnestic functions including the verbal short-term and long-term memory, particularly semantic memory, as well as frontal-executive functions including attention, inhibition, mental flexibility and task switching. Furthermore, motor and visuo-perceptual deficits often accompany language disorders and have to be recognised for adequate neurolinguistic assessment. Because of their marked importance for language functioning, the next two subsections are dedicated to the relationship of memory and frontal-executive functions to language. Readers further interested in cognitive functions closely related to language are referred to Mariën and Abutalebi (2008).

1.13.5.1 Language and Memory

The differentiation of multiple memory systems has been demonstrated in functional, as well as in neuroanatomical, studies of clinical and non-clinical populations (Gathercole et al. 2004). Auditory short-term memory, the capacity to retain auditory information for a short period of time, is a key capacity in language acquisition and processing. It can be defined as the small amount of information that can be kept in an accessible state in order to be used in ongoing

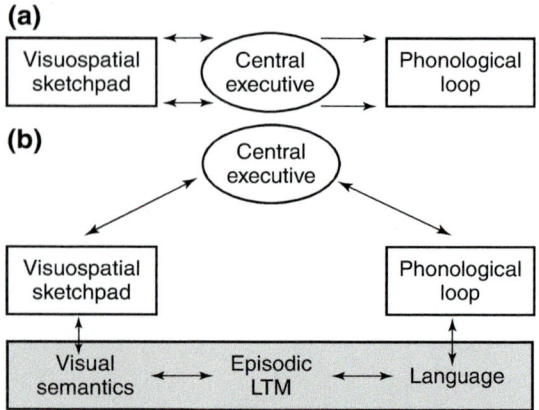

Fig. 1.88 Reprinted from Trends in Cognitive Sciences, 4/11, Baddeley (2000), The episodic buffer: a new component of working memory? 417–423, Copyright 2000 with permission from Elsevier

cognitive tasks. According to Baddeley's working memory model, a central executive acts as a supervisory system and controls the information flow to and from three systems: the phonological loop, the visuospatial sketchpad and the episodic buffer (Baddeley and Hitch 1974, see Fig. 1.88).

The phonological loop deals with sound and phonological information. It involves a short-term phonological store with auditory memory traces that are subject to rapid decay and an articulatory rehearsal component (or *articulatory loop*) that can revive the memory traces. The episodic buffer is believed to link information across domains to form integrated units of visual, spatial and verbal information with time sequencing, such as the memory of TV news.

Although different models of short-term memory are available (see for instance Cowan 2005), there is no doubt about the importance of an adequate short-term memory capacity for intact language functioning. Auditory short-term memory is involved in learning new words, processing grammatical information and sentence comprehension. Deficits in auditory short-term memory have been found in children with developmental language disorders and dyslexia (Smith-Spark and Fisk 2007). Auditory short-term memory impairment has been proven to be a marker of specific language impairment and a cognitive predictor of language outcome in children with specific language impairment (Conti-Ramsden and Hesketh 2003). Furthermore, several acquired language disorders, most prominently conduction aphasia, have been shown to be associated with a profound impairment of short-term memory (Caplan et al. 2013).

Long-term memory is usually divided into two further main memory types: declarative and procedural memory. The *declarative memory system* ('knowing what') is the memory of facts and events. It binds different and arbitrarily related representations or perceptual experiences that are explicitly and consciously stored and retrieved. It is therefore sometimes referred to as explicit memory. Declarative memory can be further subdivided into semantic memory and episodic memory. *Semantic memory* represents the knowledge about facts, which is independent of personal experience, for instance, the capital cities of a geographical region. The semantic memory system includes world knowledge, object knowledge, language knowledge and conceptual priming. Episodic memory is the memory of autobiographical events including times, places, associated emotions and other contextual knowledge, for instance, the memories of the first holidays at the seaside.

The *procedural memory system* ('knowing how') is involved in the acquisition and retrieval of habits, motor and cognitive skills (for instance, driving a car). Unlike declarative memory, encoding and retrieval via the procedural system can occur without awareness. Procedural memories are typically acquired through repetition and practice. Procedural memory is therefore sometimes referred to as implicit memory.

A range of studies in animals and humans suggests that declarative and procedural memories are composed of a network of interconnected brain structures, though dependent on mostly distinct substrates. New memories are consolidated in the hippocampus and associated medial temporal lobe structures. Over the years, these memories increasingly rely on neocortical structures, particularly in the temporal lobes where declarative memories are closely related to the ventral stream. Furthermore, the inferior frontal lobes play a role in selection and retrieval of declarative memories. In contrast, procedural memories are rooted in circuits involving the basal ganglia with the nucleus caudatus and frontal regions. Furthermore, inferior parietal and superior temporal regions as well as the cerebellum are part of the procedural memory network (Ullman 2013).

The acquisition, representation and processing of language seemingly requires both procedural and declarative memory systems (Bates 2004). For instance, the procedural memory system seems to play a role in learning and storing regularities about the phonology of incoming speech (Saffran et al. 1996). Procedural memory is furthermore considered to support the acquisition and storage of grammatical forms, which are mainly rule-based, whereas irregular grammatical forms (e.g. *come–came*), given their arbitrary relationship, are proposed to be acquired and stored by the declarative memory system. Most importantly, declarative memory, especially semantic memory, is argued to be involved in learning and storing of lexical items (Naigles 2002). It includes memories for

> words and other verbal symbols, their meaning and referents, about relations among them, and about rules, formulas, and algorithms for manipulating them.
> Tulving (1972)

Thus, semantic memory plays a crucial role in language acquisition and processing. The independent functioning of different memory and language systems has been reported in clinical populations. Evidence suggests that semantic dementia, Alzheimer's disease and amnesia each affect semantic memory functions and lexical functions similarly, while leaving grammatical knowledge and procedural memory largely intact (Ullman 2008). On the other hand, autism, Parkinson's disease and Tourette syndrome are reported to involve syntactic deficits and procedural memory deficits, whereas declarative memory and lexical functions are often spared.

Overall, different memory systems are important for adequate language acquisition and use, and knowledge of the relationship of language and memory is tremendously important for satisfactory diagnosis and therapy of language (and memory) disorders.

1.13.5.2 Language and Executive Functions

Executive functioning refers to the 'command and control' functions of the prefrontal cortex and related subcortical structures. Executive functions comprise attention regulation, including detection, vigilance, control of distractibility and shifting attention. Furthermore, planning, goal setting and monitoring, mental flexibility, fluency, abstract reasoning and concept formation, as well as problem-solving and judgement, are part of the frontal-executive system. In addition, maintaining self-awareness and identity, behavioural regulation, mood modulation and emotional regulation are regarded as frontal-executive functions. These processes are required for conscious control of thought, emotion and action and are important for adequate language acquisition and communication (Elliott 2003).

Because executive functions integrate information at higher levels across different cognitive domains, damage to the executive system typically affects the ability to organise and regulate multiple information types and behaviour. Thus, the loss of executive functioning results in a cluster of deficits. Combinations of language impairment and executive deficits are observed in a variety of diseases including neurodevelopmental disorders such as attention deficit hyperactivity disorder and autism, stroke, tumour, multiple sclerosis, herpes simplex encephalitis and dementia, the foremost being frontotemporal dementia (Eslinger 2008). Language stereotypes, perseverations, echolalia, concreteness, comprised verbal flexibility, reduction of speech output and mutism are typical signs of executive dysfunction affecting language.

In sum, language cannot be seen as an isolated system; various cognitive functions are closely related to the language system. Thus, for an adequate understanding and testing of language functioning, knowledge of cognitive abilities, including mnestic and executive functions, is extremely important. Therefore, the support of an interdisciplinary team of neuropsychologists and neurolinguists in the diagnosis of language and associated cognitive functions is highly desirable.

1.14 Basics of Speech and Language Therapy in Children

Michèle Kaufmann-Meyer

1.14.1 Introduction

The modern world places great emphasis on communication. Opportunities to travel to and live in different places require us to communicate within complex cultural and linguistic environments. This can be hugely beneficial for children and families but can also be a burden, presenting added difficulties or obstacles for children with speech, language or communication difficulties. The fast pace of modern society challenges the existing understanding of language development. Social and professional awareness of speech and language difficulties has increased as a result of these issues, and speech and language therapy must attempt to take such factors into account.

1.14.2 Speech and Language Development: Between Norms and Individuality

Timetables (see Sect. 11.3 for details) describing the natural course of general and language development are often suggested in summary tables and reports on cognitive processes. These templates suggest clear milestones for mastering expressive and receptive language skills, from babbling and first words to the formation of sentences for each language. The foundations of a child's linguistic knowledge are laid during the first 5 years of life. Phonemic, lexical, syntactic and prosodic abilities are all developed during this time (Karmiloff and Karmiloff-Smith 2003; Brigaudiot and Danon-Boileau

2002; Nicolosi et al. 2003; Kannengießer 2009); the bases of non-verbal communication, such as joint attention and reciprocity, have been laid in the preverbal stage (Bruner 1987; Guidetti 2003). Comparisons of early language acquisition across 18 languages by using the CDI-parental questionnaire (The MacArthur-Bates Communicative Development Inventories: Fenson et al. 2007) show similarities across languages for early language development. The rate of lexical acquisition varies enormously in individuals but should positively accelerate in the second year of life. The strong relationship between vocabulary production and later grammatical development can be shown across languages. (For an overview on crosslinguistic comparison of CDI-Studies for 18 languages, see Bleses et al. 2008.) Crosslinguistic trends in children's speech acquisition have been summarised by McLeod (2007).

Language development is, however, far from complete by the age of five. Skills such as literacy (related to the needs of a society for reading and writing abilities) and narrative development continue to develop, thus establishing a more structured and formal approach to language.

1.14.3 Diagnostics

It is, however, important to recognise that these milestones and templates provide only a general, normalised overview of language development. In the multicultural real world each child's language development proceeds at a different rate and is influenced by numerous intrinsic and extrinsic factors. There is a fundamental link between our speech and language ability and our social experience, so that such issues as gender and the specifics of the communication and linguistic environment (e.g. bi- or multi-lingualism) exert a strong influence on the process of language development.

The ICF-CY (International Classification on Functioning, Disability and Health—Child and Youth version, WHO 2007) provides a formal framework for the classification of health and functioning that should underlie the assessment of speech and language skills. It takes a biopsychosocial approach (i.e. incorporating biological, psychological and social factors) and focuses on the child's capabilities and strengths, rather than on his or her health condition or any developmental delay. Figure 2.1 taken from Sect. 2.1 (The interactions between the components of the International Classification of Functioning) shows how any health condition comprises underlying body functions and structures, activities and participatory abilities, which in turn affect and are affected by environmental and personal factors (ICF-CY, WHO 2002, 2007).

Modern professionals working in this area are confronted with diverse and complex situations and must attempt to incorporate such considerations into assessment, diagnosis and treatment plans.

This can be achieved by building for each individual child a 'developmental profile', which should be holistic in its scope and include information on the child's cognitive skills, hearing status, language comprehension, language production, communication modes and abilities, motor speech ability, social behaviour, family and contextual factors, socio-economic situation, the existence of support by other specialists (such as physiotherapists or occupational therapists), scholastic demands and the parents' needs.

The assessment of speech and language development is a multidisciplinary task, and a clear diagnosis can only be made when hearing ability and general and non-verbal developmental status are incorporated. Methods include screening (such as observation and the use of parents' descriptions and interviews) and standardised normative tests. Good testing of speech and language ability should include at least age-appropriate assessments of language comprehension and speech production. Investigation of each linguistic component (semantic-lexical, syntactic-morphological, phonetic-phonological, communicative-pragmatic), speech-motor function (including oral motor and speech motor function, feeding/eating and swallowing) and the verbal short-term memory buffer is essential (overviews of these issues can be found in the following texts:

Nicolosi et al. 2003; de Langen-Müller et al. 2011; Bleses et al. 2008; Kannengießer 2009; Charles Sturt University 2015).

All test results, including assessments of the child's hearing ability and general development, must be interpreted as a whole. Such interpretation should also take the child's individual personal and social situation into account.

1.14.4 Therapy

The outcome of this multidimensional approach should be an appropriate diagnosis of the speech or language disorder or delay and should help to identify the initial focus of treatment. In addition, the ICF-CY (WHO 2007) details the broad consequences of a child's limited communication skills on activities and participation.

Consideration of the main principle of the ICF-CY (WHO 2007), which is to ensure the best possible ability for social participation and quality of life, can help establish the framework for such a therapeutic plan and treatment. The evidence base underlying the various treatment approaches must also be incorporated when identifying the best approach (see Sect. 2.3 for more details).

Therapeutic approaches to speech and language disorders can have the following characteristics:

- Family-centred approaches, including parental training
- Individual or group therapy
- Directive therapy (typically for children older than 3 years), in which rules and exercises to support correct language usage are employed
- Non-directive therapy (typically for children younger than 3 years), in which situational learning takes place by using models or indirectly focusing on particular language structures, for example, focused stimulation in late talker therapy

To meet the requirements of bi- and multilingual socialisation of children, the International Expert Panel on Multilingual Children's Speech has prepared a position paper for professionals in this field (McLeod 2014).

Once the necessity of speech, language or communication therapy has been demonstrated, it should be implemented as soon as possible, in order to avoid negative consequences for the child's further development and his or her academic skills. An individual therapy plan must be developed according to the child's individual needs and circumstances. This is best done within a multidisciplinary team. The therapeutic work itself needs to be carried out by those with expertise in speech, language and feeding/eating disorders, such as logopedists, speech and language pathologists, and speech and language therapists.

Most services have multidisciplinary teams within which assessment and treatment of speech, language, communication and swallowing disorders can take place. These networks enable collaboration between all professionals involved in the child's management as well as parents/carers and other significant members of the child's social environment. Referrals for further specialist investigation or care can also be easily carried out through such teams.

Speech and language therapy should include setting clear therapeutic goals, guided by the above assessment. New goals should be set as the child's abilities develop over time. This goal setting must be guided by frequent evaluations, which should include observation and standardised normative testing, in order to monitor the progress of language and communication abilities and assess whether previous goals have been reached. Information on the child's social environment is again important to consider when setting new goals.

1.14.5 Work with the Parents/Carers

Experts in language and speech development acknowledge the crucial role that parents and carers play as both the primary source of information for the clinician and also as the child's main support resource. The feelings of the parents/carers and their understanding of the situation will strongly influence the course of any assessment or therapy because they are the primary reference people in the child's life. Any intervention should therefore ensure that the requirements of the parents/carers are met and, ideally, work together with them to make the most of their positive influence on the child. Interventions must, at least, have the clear consent of parents/carers.

Working with the parents should include all actions that are to be taken to support the process of enhancing the speech and language development of the child. For this, parents need information about the diagnosis, the specific speech and language disorder of their child and the approach and goals of therapy, including training or advice on language-enhancing parent behaviour (Schneider and Lüdemann 1998).

The specifics of the roles that parents and carers play in their child's therapy depend upon the age of the child and the nature of the speech/language disorder. The role itself will change over time. Activities with parents that reach beyond just giving specific information include parental training, advising parents on how to support the child's exercises at home and counselling:

- Parental training: parents reflect and train their child's behaviour for daily communication, which is known to be crucial in enhancing language development (e.g. responsiveness, corrective and expanding feedback techniques, turn taking, dialogic book reading), and adapt it to the abilities of the child. In early interventions of speech and language disorders or delayed language development, family-centred approaches focus on teaching parents of young children to apply language facilitation strategies in everyday contexts (e.g. the 'It Takes Two to Talk', Girolametto and Weitzman 2006). Brief interventions for the parents, which last approximately 10–14 sessions and have the clear focused goal of enhancing parental behaviour, are most effective (for an overview, see Brady et al. 2009 or Bakermans-Kranenburg et al. 2003).
- Advising parents on how to support the child's exercises at home by remaining in the role of the parent and not taking on the role of co-

therapist: parents carry out at home exercises that have been given by the therapist to enhance training frequency. The parental adaptation of the role of a co-therapist is no longer recommended and is viewed very critically these days, especially regarding toddlers and young children. The modern paradigm of parental support underlines the need for empowerment and a good and natural relationship between parents and child (Sarimski et al. 2013).

- Counselling:

Parents' feelings and attitudes towards their child and the disorder itself are reflected in their behaviour. Changes in behaviour can occur through insight into these interdependent factors.
Schneider and Lüdemann (1998, translated)

1.14.6 Monitoring the Progress and Termination of Therapy

Intermediate assessment and the resulting documentation of progress and remaining deficits should contribute to any decision about prolonging, temporarily interrupting or ending speech therapy.

A temporary interruption of therapy can have a very beneficial outcome, by allowing the child time to internalise certain language processes.

As all relationships based on mutual trust, the end of therapy must be transparently planned for parents and the child.

1.15 Introduction to Brain Imaging and its Application in Phoniatric Sciences

Christian Dobel, Ken Roßlau, and Christo Pantev

1.15.1 Introduction to Brain Imaging Methods

Cognitive neuroscience constitutes an interdisciplinary approach to investigate cognitive functions such as perception, language or emotion with neuroscientific methods. These methods allow the measurement and description of brain functions with high resolution in time or space. They encompass animal, lesion, brain-stimulation and brain imaging studies. Regarding higher complex functions such as language, the birth of the field was dominated by lesions studies (e.g. aphasia; for an introduction into these fields, see, e.g. Sect. 1.13). These had a large impact on theories about normal cognitive functioning. The advent and wide availability of non-invasive brain imaging methods made it possible to investigate the functioning of both normal and impaired brain functions. The functional imaging of language functions and structural descriptions of language-relevant regions in both adults and children has become almost a standard procedure (see Sect. 11.16 and in Vol. 2 Part V). Similarly, articulatory processes and speech impairments are investigated by using dynamic methods (see Vol. 2, Part I). While structural and functional imaging has an established role in the phoniatric sciences spanning such diverse fields as imaging of ear malformations, tumours (see Sect. 16.21), the vocal tract (see contribution in Sect. 6.9) as well as stuttering (see Vol. 2, Part II), other approaches still await a broad neuroscientific approach. Combining behavioural paradigms and measures with brain imaging, these methods allow the investigation, monitoring and mapping of brain functions with high sensitivity in time and space. Methods such as functional magnetic resonance imaging (fMRI) and electroencephalography (EEG) are common in almost all clinical settings because they are the foundation of clinical application and are used in standardised and daily practice. Others, such as magnetoencephalography (MEG) and positron emission tomography (PET), depend on an interdisciplinary team and on highly trained scientists for the recording and analysis of the data. These methods have in common their permitting the measurement of brain activity in a spontaneous manner, i.e. without external input, but also in response to the stimulation of one or several senses, in a systematic fashion. The differences between the methods are the conditions for their application, what they measure and what conclu-

sions can be drawn from them. Anticipating later conclusions, we should like to stress the importance of corroborating findings from different methods both behavioural and neurophysiological.

With regard to application, EEG is the most common and available in all ENT departments. Strictly speaking, brain-evoked response audiometry (BERA) and cerebral-evoked response audiometry (CERA) do not count as brain imaging owing to their low sensor density, but they have already been established methods to describe neurophysiological processes with high sensitivity in time for about two decades (see Sect. 16.11). BERA is used as a routine method for the diagnosis of hearing impairment in children as well as in adults. This method allows the investigation of the functioning of very early hearing ability (~10–20 ms after tone presentation) at the brainstem level. For this approach only a few electrodes (3–4) are necessary, and an explicit response of the subject is not required. In fact, in infants it is performed while they sleep, in order to avoid movement artefacts. Measurements including those from electrode positioning usually take no longer than 45 min. Using more electrodes and more complex stimulation gives the possibility of investigating higher levels of auditory processing (>100 ms), including speech perception at the most advanced processing stage. Mounting electrode caps with, e.g. 64 electrodes (Fig. 1.89) takes about 30 min and is often exhausting for children and patients (Picton et al. 2000). The main advantage of EEG is its wide availability, the establishment and comparability of several stimulation and analysis procedures (e.g. for the BERA) and its high ability to monitor brain functions with high sensitivity in time, i.e. in the range of milliseconds. Disadvantages are the laborious nature of electrode placement and the only moderate ability to determine the origin of a brain signal.

EEG and MEG measure online the activity of cell assemblies encompassing at least around 10,000 cells firing in synchrony. In contrast to EEG, typical MEG systems possess a much larger number of sensors covering the head and extending to inferior parts (Fig. 1.90).

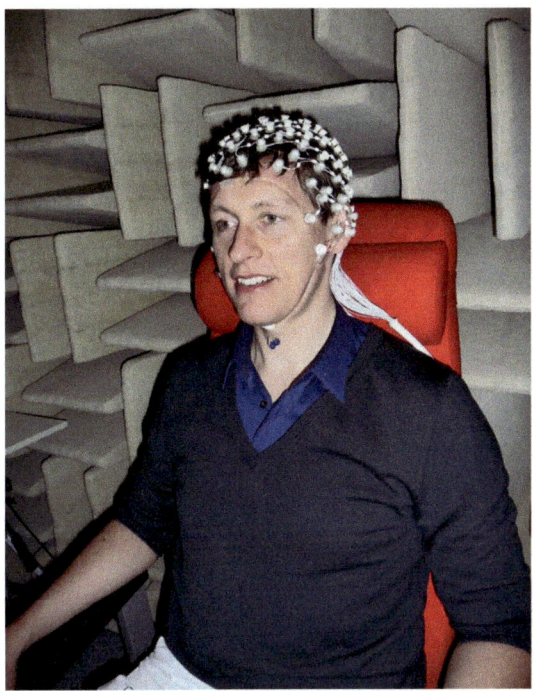

Fig. 1.89 Application of the EEG-Cap

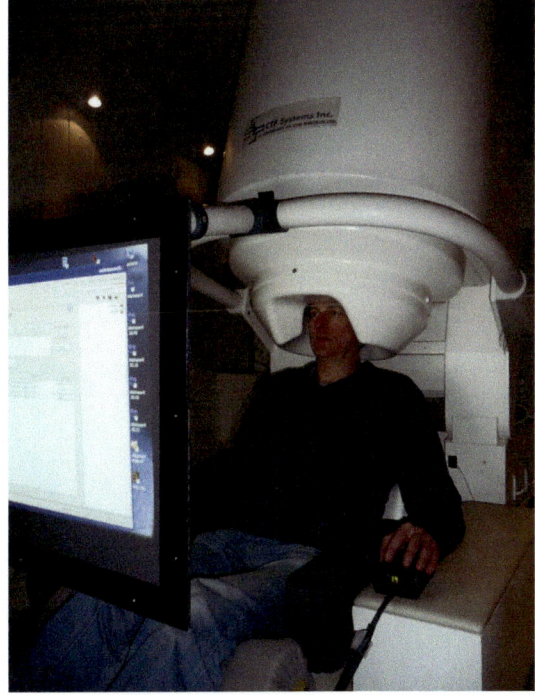

Fig. 1.90 Application during MEG measurement

The high density of sensors and the high coverage of the scalp with sensors allow the calculation of mathematical solutions to determine the neurophysiological generators of a signal. Even though this is often done in high-density EEG measurements as well, the confidence in MEG results is higher, because the electromagnetic brain signal is not distorted by the surrounding brain tissue, the skull and the scalp. The sensitivity in time is in the range of milliseconds and in space of cm^2, depending on the strength and complexity of the signal. MEG measurements can be initiated after very little preparation time usually not longer than 5–10 min (Gross et al. 2013). Because EEG and MEG record signals that are generated by the working brain, both are completely non-invasive methods that can be used as often and long as necessary and applicable. As no electrodes and sensors are attached for MEG, this is even less intrusive for participants. The drawback is that it must be assured that the head stays in a fixed position in the dewar device or that its position is at least monitored.

While these methods measure ongoing activity of cell assemblies, fMRI registers the amount of oxygenated blood in a specific region (the so-called BOLD response). The spatial sensitivity is very high, in the range of a few mm^3, but the resolution in time (6–10 s) is low. It is generally considered to be a more or less non-invasive technique (at least for field strengths between 1.5 and 3 T). The scanners produce considerable noise, and the measurement itself is often exhausting for patients and especially children, because the head space is very confined and restrictive (Schad 2002).

In contrast to these methods, PET is considered an invasive technique, because it measures gamma rays emitted by positron-emitting tracers that are injected or inhaled before measurement. The gamma ray-emitting radionuclei are attached to biologically active molecules, such as fludeoxyglucose (FDG). This is chemically similar to glucose and provides an index of metabolic activity by its uptake.

All of these methods allow the monitoring of spontaneous activity (i.e. when participants are in repose) but also in response to specific stimuli such as tones or pictures. This approach calls for experimental stimuli that are carefully selected and controlled. Depending on the design employed, the number of different stimuli within one experimental condition can be highly variable, with at least two different stimuli (e.g. a high and a low tone for two conditions). Very often the participants have to give a manual response to the stimuli, e.g. via button pressing. Nevertheless, brain activity can be also measured without such overt responses, for example, if participants are too young or their responses impaired.

In recent years several methods have been introduced that allow the stimulation of specific brain regions from the scalp. This is done by either introducing a strong electric current (as in transcranial direct current stimulation, tDCS) or a magnetic field (as in transcranial magnetic stimulation, TMS). It is highly interesting to combine these approaches with brain imaging and behavioural measures, because it allows the determination of the causal role of specific regions in cognitive and neural processing.

1.15.2 Possible Applications in a Phoniatric Setting

BERA and CERA are standard methods for measuring objective hearing thresholds, especially in young children (1 month to 5 years), because other audiometric, subjective measurements are not reliable enough to serve for diagnostic purposes. The other methods, introduced above, are suited to investigation of higher processing levels of auditory and language functions. As mentioned above, brain imaging methods do not necessarily involve overt responses by participants, and so brain activity evoked by complex auditory and verbal material can be measured, e.g. in children with specific language impairment, in patients with hearing impairments or in patients who have received a cochlear implant (e.g. Ortmann et al. 2013). This allows, for example, the measurement of dysfunctional brain activity in response to simple tones, in comparison with that to speech sounds such as phonemes and syllables. EEG and MEG allow the monitoring of such dysfunctional processes over time. Because a wealth of literature on the hierarchy of auditory processing exists, this approach is especially suitable for researchers with an interest in cognitive processes. In combination with source analyses, these data additionally allow the determination of the neural generators. From fMRI the investigator can tell with high confidence which neural networks are impaired. As a major advantage of these methods, the development of diseases can be measured over time as well as how the diseases respond to therapeutic treatments. The behavioural measures are good indicators of whether a treatment is effective at an overt level, and the neurophysiological measurements are an indication for researchers and practitioners of what the underlying mechanisms are. This combination helps to develop more effective therapeutic approaches. Phoniatric areas in which such an approach has been successfully taken involve stuttering (see Vol. 2, Part II), processing of music in professional musicians (e.g. Rosslau et al. 2016) and persons learning musical abilities (e.g. Herholz et al. 2015) as well as dyslexia (for an overview, see, e.g. Johnson and de Haan 2015). A classic phoniatric domain, but in combination with neuroscience as a still emerging field, constitutes the processing and perception of voice (Zäske et al. 2014). Here, as mentioned above, monitoring the course of treatment will advance our understanding of the neurophysiology of voice alterations, e.g. after hormonal treatment (e.g. Deuster et al. 2016).

References

Agricola JF (2002) Anleitung zur Singkunst. In: Seedorf T (ed) Bärenreiter, Kassel. Reprint of the edition 1757

Ahmad SM, Soliman A (2007) Congenital anomalies of the larynx. Otolaryngol Clin N Am 40(1):177–191

Altenmüller E, Jabusch HC (2010) Focal dystonia in musicians—phenomenology, pathophysiology, triggering factors, and treatment. Med Probl Perform Art 25(1):3–9

American National Standards Institute (1995) ANSI S3.2-1989 (R 1995) Method for measuring the intelligibility of speech over communications systems

American National Standards Institute (2008) ANSI S12.2-2008: criteria for evaluating room noise

am Zehnhoff-Dinnesen A, Zorowka P, Kanoika N et al (2016) Status of phoniatrics in the different countries on basis of national UEP coordinators' reports. In: Paper presented at 28th UEP Congress and 22nd SOMEF Congress, Congress Center Bizkaia Aretoa, Bilbao, Spain, 29 September-1 October 2016

Ashmore J (2008) Cochlear outer hair cell motility. Physiol Rev 88(1):173–210

Baddeley A (2000) The episodic buffer: a new component of working memory? Trends Cogn Sci 4(11):417–423

Baddeley A, Hitch GJ (1974) Working memory. In: Bower GH (ed) The psychology of learning and motivation. Academic Press, New York, pp47–89

Bakermans-Kranenburg MJ, Van Ijzendoorn MH, Juffer F (2003) Less is more: meta-analyses of sensitivity and attachment interventions in early childhood. Psychol Bull 129(2):195–215

Barnett PW, Knight RD (1995) The common intelligibility scale. Proc I O A 17(7):201–206

Barron M (2010) Auditorium acoustics and architectural design, 2nd edn. Spon Press, Oxfordshire

Bates EA (2004) Explaining and interpreting deficits in language development across clinical groups: where do we go from here? Brain Lang 88(2):248–253

Bellis TJ (1997) Understanding auditory processing disorders in children. American Speech-Language-Hearing Association. http://www.asha.org/public/hearing/Understanding-Auditory-Processing-Disorders-in-Children. Accessed 2 Feb 2015

Benninghoff A, Drenckhahn D (2003) Anatomie Bd. 1. Elsevier GmbH Urban & Fischer, München

Benninghoff A, Drenckhahn D (2004) Anatomie Bd. 2. Elsevier GmbH Urban & Fischer, München

Beranek LL (2004) Concert halls and opera houses: music, acoustics and architecture, 2nd edn. Springer, Heidelberg

Birkholz P (2013a) Modeling consonant-vowel coarticulation for articulatory speech synthesis. PLoS One 8:e60603. https://doi.org/10.1371/journal.pone.0060603

Birkholz P (2013b) VocalTractLab. www.vocaltractlab.de. Accessed 7 Dec 2016

Blauert J (1996) Spatial hearing—Revised edition: the psychophysics of human sound localization. The MIT Press, Cambridge

Bleses D, Vach W, Slott M et al (2008) Early vocabulary development in Danish and other languages: a CDI-based comparison. J Child Lang 35(3):619–650

Blitzer A, Brin MF, Fahn S et al (1986) Botulinum toxin (Botox) for the treatment of "spastic dysphonia" as part of a trial of toxin injections for the treatment of other cranial dystonias (letter). Laryngoscope 96:1300

Böhme G (2001) Sprach-, Sprech-, Stimm- und Schluckstörungen, vol 2: Therapie. Urban & Fischer, München

Böhme G (2003) Sprach-, Sprech-, Stimm- und Schluckstörungen, vol 1: Klinik. Urban & Fischer, München

Bradley JS, Soulodre GA (1995) The influence of late arriving energy on spatial impression. J Acoust Soc Am 97(4):2263–2271

Brady N, Warren SF, Sterling A (2009) Interventions aimed at improving child language by improving maternal responsivity. Int Rev Res Ment Retard 37:333–357

Breuer R (1982) Berufskrankheiten von Instrumentalmusikern aus medizinhistorischer Sicht (vom 15. Jahrhundert bis 1930). Inaugural-Dissertation zur Erlangung des Doktors der Medizin. Johannes-Gutenberg-Universität Mainz, Mainz

Brigaudiot M, Danon-Boileau L (2002) La naissance du langage dans les deux premiüres annöes. Presse Universitaires du France, Paris

Broca P (1861) Remarques sur le siège de la faculté du langage articulé, suivies d'une observation d'aphémie (perte de la parole). Bull Soc Anat Paris 6(36):330–357

Brown TT, Lugar HM, Coalson RS et al (2005) Developmental changes in human cerebral functional organization for word generation. Cereb Cortex 15(3):275–290

Brüel and Kjær (1984) Measuring sound. Nærum

Bruner J (1987) Comment les enfants apprennent à parler. (Children's talk, learning to use language). Retz, Paris

Bygren LO, Konlaan BB, Johansson SE (1996) Attendance at cultural events, reading books or periodicals, and making music or singing in a choir as determinants for survival: Swedish interview survey of living conditions. Br Med J 313(7072):1577–1580

Caplan D, Michaud J, Hufford R (2013) Short-term memory, working memory, and syntactic comprehension in aphasia. Cogn Neuropsychol 30(2):77–109

Charles Sturt University (2015) Multilingual children's speech. http://www.csu.edu.au/research/multilingual-speech. Accessed 9 Sept 2015

Chomsky N (1965) Aspects of the theory of syntax. MIT Press, Cambridge

Clark GM (2003) Cochlear implants: fundamentals and applications. Springer, New York

Clark GM, Pyman BC, Bailey QR (1979) The surgery for multiple-electrode cochlear implantations. J Laryngol Otol 93(3):215–223

Conti-Ramsden G, Hesketh A (2003) Risk markers for SLI: a study of young language-learning children. Int J Lang Comm Disord 38(3):251–263

Cooper P (1973) Perspectives in music theory: a historical—analytical approach. Mead Dodd, New York, p 16

Cowan N (2005) Working memory capacity. Psychology Press, New York

Czermak N (1863) Der Kehlkopfspiegel und seine Verwerthung für Physiologie und Medizin. Engelmann, Leipzig

Dahan D, Magnuson J (2011) Spoken word recognition. In: Traxler M, Gernsbacher M (eds) Handbook of psycholinguistics, 2nd edn. Academic Press, New York, pp 249–283

De Boer B, Fitch WT (2010) Computer models of vocal tract evolution: an overview and critique. Adapt Behav 18(1):36–47

de Langen-Müller U, Kauschke C, Kiese-Himmel C et al (eds) (2011) Diagnostik von Sprachentwicklungsstörungen (SES), unter Berücksichtigung umschriebener Sprachentwicklungsstörungen (USES). Guidelines of the "Deutsche Gesellschaft für Phoniatrie und Pädaudiologie e.V." (DGPP) and "Deutsche Gesellschaft für Kinder- und Jugendpsychiatrie, Psychosomatik und Psychotherapie" (DGKJP). Arbeitsgemeinschaft der Wissenschaftlichen Medizinischen Fachgesellschaften e.V. (AWMF), Register-Nr. 049/006. http://www.dgpp.de/cms/pages/de/profibereich/konsensus.php#3. Accessed 13 Aug 2015

De Vincentiis M (ed) (2001) Deglutologia. Omega Edizione, Torino

Decoster W (2013) Ontknoop je stem. School of Education. http://associatie.kuleuven.be/schoolofeducation/projecten/ontknoopjestem. Accessed 14 Apr 2015

Dehaene-Lambertz G, Dehaene S, Hertz-Pannier L (2002) Functional neuroimaging of speech perception in infants. Science 298(5600):2013–2015

Deuster D, Di Vincenzo K, Szukaj M et al (2016) Change of speech fundamental frequency explains the satisfaction with voice in response to testosterone therapy in female-to-male gender dysphoric individuals. Eur Arch Otorhinolaryngol 273(8):2127–2131

Diehl R, Lotto A, Holt R (2004) Speech perception. Ann Rev Psychol 55:149–179. https://doi.org/10.1146/annurev.psych.55.090902.142028

Echternach M, Markl M, Richter B (2012) Dynamic real-time magnetic resonance imaging for the analysis of voice physiology. Curr Opin Otolaryngol Head Neck Surg 20(6):450–457

Elliott R (2003) Executive functions and their disorders. Br Med Bull 65(1):49–59

Engwall O (2003) Combining MRI, EMA and EPG measurements in a three-dimensional tongue model. Speech Commun 41(2–3):303–329

Engwall O (2005) ARTUR—the articulation TUtoR. http://www.speech.kth.se/multimodal/ARTUR/. Accessed 17 Dec 2016

Engwall O, Bälter O, Öster AM et al (2006) Designing the user interface of the computer-based speech training system ARTUR based on early user tests. J Behav Inform Tech 25(4):353–365

Eslinger P (2008) The frontal lobe. Executive, emotional, and neurological functions. In: Marien P, Abutalebi J (eds) Neuropsychological research: a review. Psychology Press, Hove, East Sussex, pp 379–408

Faltin R (2004) Singen lernen? Aber logisch! Von der Technik des klassischen Gesanges, 4th edn. Wißner, Augsburg

Fastl H, Zwicker E (2007) Psychoacoustics facts and models, 3rd edn. Springer, Berlin

Faulstich G (2011) Singen lehren - Singen lernen, 7th edn. Wißner, Augsburg

Felsenfeld S (2002) Finding susceptibility genes for developmental disorders of speech: the long and winding road. J Commun Disord 35(4):329–345

Fenson L, Marchman VA, Thal DJ et al (2007) The MacArthur Communicative Development Inventories: user's guide and technical manual, 2nd edn. Paul H. Brookes Publishing Co, Baltimore

Ferrein A (1741) De la formation de la voix de l'homme. Histoire de l'Académie Royale des Sciences de l'Année 1741. Archives de l'Académie des Sciences, pp 409–432. http://gallica.bnf.fr. Accessed 24 Apr 2015

Fettiplace R, Hackney CM (2006) The sensory and motor roles of auditory hair cells. Nat Rev Neurosci 7(1):19–29

Fischbein M, Middelstadt SE, Ottati V et al (1988) Medical problems among ICSOM musicians: overview of a national survey. Med Probl Perform Art 3(1):1–8

Fitch T, Giedd J (1999) Morphology and development of the human vocal tract: a study using magnetic resonance imaging. J Acoust Soc Am 106(3 Pt 1):1511–1522. https://doi.org/10.1121/1.427148

Flanagan JL (1965) Speech analysis, synthesis and perception. Springer, Berlin

Fleming R (2004) The inner voice: the making of a singer. Penguin Books, New York

Flesch L (1925) Berufskrankheiten des Musikers. Niels Kampmann, Celle

Friederici AD (2009) Pathway to language: fiber tracts in the human brain. TiCS 13(4):175–181

Friederici AD (2012) The cortical language circuit: from auditory perception to sentence comprehension. Trends Cogn Sci 16(5):262–268

Friederici AD, Alter K (2004) Lateralization of auditory language functions: a dynamic dual pathway model. Brain Lang 89(2):267–276

Friedrich G, Bigenzahn W, Zorowka P (2013) Phoniatrie und Pädaudiologie, 5th edn. Median-Verlag, Heidelberg

Fröschels E (1913) Lehrbuch der Sprachheilkunde. Deuticke, Leipzig

Galantucci B, Fowler C, Turvey M (2006) The motor theory of speech perception reviewed. Psychon Bull Rev 13(3):361–377. https://doi.org/10.3758/BF03193857

García M (1854) Observations on the human voice. Proc R Soc Lond 7:399–410

Gathercole SE, Pickering SJ, Ambridge B et al (2004) The structure of working memory from 4 to 15 years of age. Dev Psychol 40(2):177–190

Gembris H, Langner D (2005) Von der Musikhochschule auf den Arbeitsmarkt. Erfahrungen von Absolventen, Arbeitsmarktexperten und Hochschullehrern. Wißner, Augsburg

Girolametto L, Weitzman E (2006) It takes two to talk®—the Hanen program® for parents: early language intervention through caregiver training. In: McCauley R, Fey M (eds) Treatment of language disorders in children. Brookes Publishing, Baltimore, pp 77–104

Graham A (2001) The development and evolution of the pharyngeal arches. J Anat 199(Pt 1–2):133–141

Green DM (1976) An introduction to hearing. Lawrence Erdbaum Ass., New York

Gross J, Baillet S, Barnes GR et al (2013) Good practice for conducting and reporting MEG research. NeuroImage 65:349–363

Guidetti M (ed) (2003) Pragmatique et psychologie du développement. Belin Sup Psychologie, Paris

Gutzmann H (1912) Sprachheilkunde. Kornfeld, Berlin

Haböck F (1927) Die Kastraten und ihre Gesangskunst: Eine gesangsphysiologische, kultur- und musikhistorische Studie. Deutsche Verlagsanstalt, Berlin

Haefliger E (1993) Die Singstimme. Schott, Mainz

Harris TM, Harris S, Rubin JS et al (1998) The voice clinic handbook. Whurr Publishers Ltd, London

Herholz SC, Coffey EB, Pantev C et al (2015) Dissociation of neural networks for predisposition and for training-related plasticity in auditory-motor learning. Cereb Cortex 26(7):3125–3134

Hickok G (2009) The functional neuroanatomy of language. Phys Life Rev 6(3):121–143

Hickok G, Poeppel D (2004) Dorsal and ventral streams: a framework for understanding aspects of the functional anatomy of language. Cognition 92(1–2):67–99

Hickok G, Small S (eds) (2015) Neurobiology of language. Academic Press, London

Hirano M (1974) Morphological structure of the vocal cord as a vibrator and its variations. Folia Phoniatr (Basel) 26(2):89–94

Hirano M (1975) Phonosurgery—basic and clinical investigations. Official report, 76th Annual Convention ORL Society of Japan, Nara

Hirano M, Kakita Y (1981) Cover-body theory of vocal fold vibration. In: Daniloff RG (ed) Speech science. College Hill Press, San Diego, pp 1–46

Hirano M, Kurita S (1986) Histological structure of the vocal fold and its normal and pathologic variations. In: Kirchner JA (ed) Vocal fold histopathology, a symposium. College-Hill Press, San Diego, pp 17–24

Hirschberg J (ed) (1997) Cleft palate and velopharyngeal insufficiency. Folia Phoniatr Logop 49, special edition

Hirschberg J, Hacki T, Mészáros K (eds) (2013) Foniátria és társtudományok (Phoniatrics and associated disciplines). Eötvös, Budapest

Hsiao TY, Solomon NP, Luschei ES et al (1994) Modulation of fundamental frequency by laryngeal muscles during vibrato. J Voice 8(3):224–229

Husson R (1950) Thèse de doctorat des sciences: étude des phénomènes physiologiques et acoustiques de la voix chantée. Éditions de la Rev Sc, Paris

IEC 60268-16-2011 (2011) Sound system equipment—Part 16: objective rating of speech intelligibility by speech transmission index

International Ergonomics Association (2015) Definition and domains of ergonomics. http://www.iea.cc/whats/index.html. Accessed 14 Apr 2015

International Federation of Oto-Rhino-Laryngological Societies (1986) Phoniatrics, a subspeciality of otolaryngology. IFOS Newsletter, December 1986

International Federation of Oto-Rhino-Laryngological Societies (1993) Paper on basic phoniatric education in the frame of ENT-training programs. IFOS Newsletter, Autumn 1993

Isshiki N (1989) Phonosurgery. Springer, Tokyo

Jansen EJM, Helleman HW,·Dreschler WA et al (2009) Noise induced hearing loss and other hearing complaints among musicians of symphony orchestras. Int Arch Occup Environ Health 82(2):153–164

Jette ME, Thibeault S (2011) Morphology of vocal fold mucosa: histology to genomics. In: Colton R et al (eds) Understanding voice problems: a physiological perspective for diagnosis and treatment. Lippincott Williams & Wilkins, Philadelphia

Johnson MH, de Haan M (2015) Developmental cognitive neuroscience: an introduction. Wiley Blackwell, Chisester

Kannengießer S (2009) Grundlagen, Diagnostik und Therapie. Elsevier Urban Fischer, Munich

Karmiloff K, Karmiloff-Smith A (2003) Comment les enfants entrent dans le langage. Retz, Paris

Kasprian G, Langs G, Brugger PC et al (2011) The prenatal origin of hemispheric asymmetry: an in utero neuroimaging study. Cereb Cortex 21(5):1076–1083

Kemp DT (2007) Otoacoustic emissions: concepts and origins. In: Fay D, Popper A (eds) Springer handbook of auditory research. Springer, New York, pp 1–38

Kliegman RM, Nelson WE (2007) Nelson textbook of pediatrics. Elsevier, Amsterdam

Klinger M, Schramm U (2001) In: Bock R et al (eds) Virtuelle Mikroskopie. Universität des Saarlandes, Homburg. www.mikroskopie-uds.de. Accessed 2 Feb 2017

Kob M (2001) Physical modelling of the singing voice. PhD Dissertation, RWTH Aachen, Aachen

Kob M, Behler G, Kamprolf A et al (2008) Experimental investigations of the influence of room acoustics on the teacher's voice. Acoust Sci Technol 29(1):86–94

Kotz SA, Schwartze M (2010) Cortical speech processing unplugged: a timely subcortico-cortical framework. Trends Cogn Sci 14(9):392–399

Kreutz G, Bongard S, Rohrmann S et al (2004) Effects of choir singing or listening on secretory immunoglobulin A, cortisol, and emotional state. J Behav Med 27(6):623–635

Kröger BJ, Kannampuzha J, Neuschaefer-Rube C (2009) Towards a neurocomputational model of speech production and perception. Speech Commun 51(9):793–809

Kußmaul A (1877) Die Störungen der Sprache. Vogel, Leipzig

Ladefoged P, Maddieson I (1996) The sounds of the world's languages. Blackwell, Oxford

Lai CSL, Fisher SE, Hurst JA et al (2001) A forkhead-domain gene is mutated in a severe speech and language disorder. Nature 413:519–523

Lee S, Potamianos A, Narayanan S (1999) Acoustics of children's speech: developmental changes of temporal and spectral parameters. J Acoust Soc Am 105(3):1455–1468

Lichtheim L (1884) Die verschiedenen Symptomenbilder der Aphasie. Arch Psychiatr Nervenkr 15:822–828

Liegeois F, Connelly A, Cross JH et al (2004) Language reorganization in children with early-onset lesions of the left hemisphere: an fMRI study. Brain 127(Pt 6):1229–1236

Lloyd JE, Stavness I, Fels S (2012) ArtiSynth: a fast interactive biomechanical modeling toolkit combining multibody and finite element simulation. In: Soft tissue biomechanical modeling for computer assisted surgery. Springer, Berlin, pp 355–394. http://artisynth. magic.ubc.ca/artisynth/. Accessed 17 Dec 2016

Löfqvist A (2010) Theories and models of speech production. In: Hardcastle W et al (eds) The handbook of phonetic sciences, 2nd edn. Blackwell, Oxford, pp 353–377

Luchsinger R, Arnold GE (1970) Handbuch der Stimm- und Sprachheilkunde, 3rd edn. Springer, Wien

Maeda S (1990) Compensatory articulation during speech: evidence from the analysis and synthesis of vocal-tract shapes using an articulatory model. In: Hardcastle WJ, Marchal A (eds) Speech production and speech modelling. Springer, Dordrecht

Mainka A, Poznyakovskiy A, Platzek I et al (2013) Supraglottische Konfiguration beim klassischen Gesang: eine MRT-basierte Fallstudie. In: Gross M, Schönweiler R (eds) Aktuelle phoniatrisch-pädaudiologische Aspekte, vol 21, pp 88–90

Mariën P, Abutalebi J (2008) Neuropsychological research. A review. Psychology Press, Hove

McDonald Klimek M, Obert K, Steinhauer K (2005) The Estill Voice Training System: Level two, Figure combinations for six voice qualities (workbook). Estill Voice Training Systems International, LLC. ISBN 0-9764816-1-8

McDonald R, Kreutz G, Mitchell L (2012) Music, health and wellbeing. Oxford University Press, Oxford

McLeod S (ed) (2007) The international guide to speech acquisition. Thomson Delmar Learning, Clifton Park

McLeod S (2014) Resourcing speech-language pathologists to work with multilingual children. Int J Speech Lang Pathol 16(3):208–218

Mermelstein P (1973) Articulatory model for the study of speech production. J Acoust Soc Am 53(4):1070–1082

Moore BCJ (1997) An introduction to the psychology of hearing, 6th edn. Emerald, Bingley

Moore BCJ (2008) An introduction to the psychology of hearing, 5th edn. Academic Press, San Diego

Moore KL, Persaud TVN (2003) Embryologie. Elsevier GmbH Urban & Fischer, München

Mueller G, Killion M (1990) An easy method for calculating the articulation index. Hear J 43(9):14–17

Müller J (1839) Über die Compensation der physischen Kräfte am menschlichen Stimmorgan. Hirschwald, Berlin

Mürbe D, Pabst F, Hofmann G et al (2004) Effects of a professional solo singer education on auditory and kinesthetic feedback: a longitudinal study of singers' pitch control. J Voice 18(2):236–241

Naigles LR (2002) Form is easy, meaning is hard: resolving a paradox in early child language. Cognition 86(2):157–199

Nicolosi L, Harryman E, Kresheck J (2003) Terminology of communication disorders, 5th edn. Lippincott Williams & Wilkins, Philadelphia

Nieuwenhuys R, Voogd J, van Huijzen C (2008) The human central nervous system. Springer, Heidelberg

Obrębowski A, Tarkowski Z (2003) Zaburzenia procesu komunikatywnego. Orator, Lublin

Ortmann L, Knief A, Deuster D et al (2013) Neural correlates of speech processing in prelingually deafened children with cochlear implants. PLoS One 8(7):e67696. https://doi.org/10.1371/journal.pone.0067696

Paulsen F, Waschke J, Sobotta BA (2010) Atlas der Anatomie des Menschen, 23rd edn. Elsevier GmbH, Urban & Fischer, München

Payan Y, Perrier P (1997) Synthesis of VV sequences with a 2D biomechanical tongue model controlled by the equilibrium point hypothesis. Speech Commun 22(2–3):185–205

Perelló J (1977) Lexikon de communicologia. Augusta, Barcelona

Perelló J (1982) The history of IALP 1924–1982. Augusta, Barcelona

Peterson GE, Barney HL (1952) Control methods used in a study of the vowels. J Acoust Soc Am 24(2):175–184. https://doi.org/10.1121/1.1906875

Picton TW, Bentin S, Berg P et al (2000) Guidelines for using human event-related potentials to study cognition: frecording standards and publication criteria. Psychophysiology 37(2):127–152

Platon (1998) Der Staat. Deutscher Taschenbuch Verlag, München

Preuß S, Neuschaefer-Rube C, Birkholz P (2013) Real-time control of a 2D animation model of the vocal tract using optopalatography. In: Proceedings of the Interspeech 2013, Lyon, France, pp 997–1001

Pruszewicz A (ed) (1992) Foniatria kliniczna. Państwowy Zakład Wydawnictw Lekarskich, Warszawa

Randel D (1986) The New Harvard dictionary of music. Harvard University Press, Tempo

Rantala LM, Hakala S, Holmqvist S et al (2012) Connections between voice ergonomic risk factors and voice symptoms, voice handicap, and respiratory tract diseases. J Voice 26(6):819.e13–819.e20

Rantala LM, Hakala S, Holmqvist S et al (2013) Connections between voice ergonomic risk factors in classrooms and teachers' voice production. Folia Phoniatr Logop 64(6):278–282

Rayleigh L (1907) On our perception of sound direction. Philos Mag 13(74):214–232

Reid C (1990) Bel Canto principles and practices. 5th printing. Joseph Patelson Music House, New York, p 100

Richter B (2013) Historische Vorbemerkungen. In: Richter B (ed) Die Stimme. Henschel Verlag, Leipzig

Richter B, Seedorf T (2003) Befragung stummer Zeugen: Gesangshistorische Dokumente im deutenden Dialog zwischen Musikwissenschaft und moderner Gesangsphysiologie. Basler Jahrbuch für historische Musikpraxis XXVI 2002, Amadeus Verlag, Winterthur, pp 173–186

Richter B, Mürbe D, Schmid B et al (2013) Stimmphysiologie in der Ausbildung von Sängern und Schauspielern. In: Richter B (ed) Die Stimme. Henschel Verlag, Leipzig

Richter B, Echternach M, Traser L, Burdumy M, Spahn C (2017) The voice—insights into the physiology of singing and speaking. Helblingen, Esslingen. DVD-ROM

Rieber RW, Fröschels E (1966) An historical review of the European literature in speech pathology. In: Rieber RW, Brubaker RS (eds) Speech pathology. North-Holland Publ, Amsterdam

Rosslau K, Herholz SC, Knief A et al (2016) Song perception by professional singers and actors: an MEG study. PLoS One 11(2):e0147986. https://doi.org/10.1371/journal.pone.0147986

Rothenberg M, Miller D, Molitor R (1988) Aerodynamic investigation of sources of vibrato. Folia Phoniatr (Basel) 40(5):244–260

Roy N, Merrill RM, Thibeault S et al (2004) Prevalence of voice disorders in teachers and the general population. J Speech Lang Hear Res 47(2):281–293

Rutter MJ, Dickson JM (2014) Embryology of the larynx. In: Elden LM, Zur KB (eds) Congenital malformations of the head and neck. Springer, New York

Saffran JR, Aslin RN, Newport EL (1996) Statistical learning by 8-month-old infants. Science 274(5294):1926–1928

Samuel AG (2011) Speech perception. Ann Rev Psychol 62:49–72. https://doi.org/10.1146/annurev.psych.121208.131643

Sapir S, Larson KK (1993) Supralaryngeal muscle activity during sustained vibrato in four sopranos: surface EMG findings. J Voice 7(3):213–218

Sarimski K, Hintermair M, Lang M (2013) Familienorientierte Frühförderung von Kindern mit Behinderung. Ernst Reinhardt Verlag, Munich

Sataloff RT, Brandfonbrener AG, Lederman RJ (eds) (2010) Performing arts medicine, 3rd edn. Science & Medicine, Narberth, PA

Schad LR (2002) Functional magnetic resonance tomography (fMRI). 1: basic principles and measuring techniques. Radiologe 42(8):659–666; quiz 667–669

Schindler O, Schindler A (2001) Fisiologia della communicazione umana. Omega Edizione, Torino

Schindler O, Schindler A, Wendler J (2014) Dysphasien. In: Wendler J, Seidner W, Eysholdt U (eds) Lehrbuch der Phoniatrie und Pädaudiologie, 5th edn. Thieme, Stuttgart

Schink T, Kreutz G, Busch V et al (2014) Incidence and relative risk of hearing disorders in professional musicians. Occup Environ Med. https://doi.org/10.1136/oemed-2014-102172. Accessed 31 May 2016

Schneider P, Lüdemann D (1998) Logopädische Elternberatung bei Kommunikationsstörungen. In: Böhme G (ed) Sprach-, Sprech-, Stimm- und Schluckstörungen. Band 2. Therapie. Springer, Berlin, pp 36–48

Schönweiler R, Nickisch A, am Zehnhoff-Dinnesen A et al (2012) Auditive Verarbeitungs- und Wahrnehmungsstörungen—Vorschlag für Behandlung und Management bei AVWS. Leitlinien der Deutschen Gesellschaft für Phoniatrie und Pädaudiologie (Auditory processing and perception disorders: proposed treatment and management: guidelines of the German Society for Phoniatrics and Pedaudiology). HNO 60(4):359–368

Schutte HK (1992) The efficiency of voice production. Singular Publishing Group, Inc, San Diego

Schutte HK, Svec JG, Sram F (1998) First results of clinical application of videokymography. Laryngoscope 108(8 Pt 1):1206–1210

Sedlacek E, Sedlacek K (1973) Zum 80. Geburtstag von Prof. Miloslav Seeman. Folia phoniat 25:1–8

Seeman M (1955) Poruchy détski reči. Státni zdravotnické nakladalstvi, Praha

Shadle C (2010) The aerodynamics of speech. In: Hardcastle W et al (eds) The handbook of phonetic sciences, 2nd edn. Blackwell, Oxford, pp 39–80

Shalom DB, Poeppel D (2008) Functional anatomic models of language: assembling the pieces. Neuroscientist 14(1):119–127

Sidrah M, Ahmed BS, Ahmed MS et al (2007) Congenital anomalies of the larynx. Otolaryngol Clin N Am 40:177–191

Singer K (1926) Die Berufskrankheiten der Musiker. Max Hesses Verlag, Berlin

Slis IH, Snik AFM (1997a) Anatomie van het gehoororgaan. In: Peters HFM (ed) Handboek stem- spraaktaalpathologie. Bohn, Stafeu and Van Loghum, Houten, pp 51–56

Slis IH, Snik AFM (1997b) Werking van het gehoororgaan. In: Peters HFM (ed) Handboek stem- spraaktaalpathologie. Bohn, Stafeu and Van Loghum, Houten, pp 298–306

Smith-Spark JH, Fisk JE (2007) Working memory functioning in developmental dyslexia. Memory 15(1):34–56

Spahn C, Echternach M, Zander MF et al (2010) Music performance anxiety in opera singers. Logoped Phoniatr Vocol 35(4):175–182

Spahn C, Richter B, Altenmüller E (eds) (2011) MusikerMedizin: Diagnostik, Therapie und Prävention von musikerspezifischen Erkrankungen. Schattauer Verlag, Stuttgart

Speckmann EJ, Hescheler J, Köhling R (2013) Physiologie, 6th edn. Elsevier GmbH, Urban & Fischer, München

SS-ISO/TR 3352:1985 (1985) Acoustics—assessment of noise with respect to its effect on the intelligibility of speech

Stanislavski C (2003) An actor prepares (translated by Reynolds Hapgood E.). A theatre arts book. Routledge, New York, pp 14–15

Stavness I, Lloyd JE, Payan Y et al (2011) Coupled hard–soft tissue simulation with contact and constraints applied to jaw-tongue-hyoid dynamics. Int J Numer Meth Biomed Eng 27(3):367–390

Stenfelt S, Goode R (2005) Bone-conduction sound, physiological and clinical aspects. Otol Neurotol 26(6):1245–1261

Stevens K (1998) Acoustic phonetics. MIT Press, Cambridge, MA

Sulter AM, Albers FW (1996) The effects of frequency and intensity level on glottal closure in normal subjects. Clin Otolaryngol 21(4):324–327

Sulter AM, Schutte HK, Miller DG (1995) Differences in phonetogram features between male and female subjects with and without vocal training. J Voice 9(4):363–377

Sundberg J (1987) The science of singing voice. North lllinois University Press, Dekalb, IL

Sundberg J (1994) Acoustic and psychoacoustic aspects of vibrato. KTH, STL-QPSR 35(2–3):45–68

Sundberg J (2003) Research on the singing voice in retrospect. Speech, Music and Hearing, KTH, Stockholm TMH-QPSR 45(1):11–22

Sundberg J, Fahlstedt E, Morell A (2005) Effects on the glottal voice source of vocal loudness variation in untrained female and male voices. J Acoust Soc Am 117(2):879–885

Sundelin K (1831) Ärztlicher Ratgeber für Musiktreibende. Gröbenschütz und Seiler, Berlin

Suzuki Y, Takeshima H (2004) Equal-loudness-level contours for pure tones. J Acoust Soc Am 116(2):918–933

Svec JG, Granqvist S (2010) Guidelines for selecting microphones for human voice production research. Am J Speech Lang Pathol 19(4):356–368

ten Donkelaar HJ (2011) Clinical neuroanatomy. Springer, Heidelberg

Tillema JM, Byars AW, Jacola LM et al (2008) Cortical reorganization of language functioning following perinatal left MCA stroke. Brain Lang 105(2):99–111

Titze IR (2000) Acoustic interpretation of resonant voice. J Voice 15(4):519–528

Trepel M (2004) Neuroanatomie. Elsevier GmbH Urban & Fischer, München

Tulving E (1972) Episodic and semantic memory. In: Tulving E, Donaldson W (eds) Organization of memory. Academic Press, New York, pp 381–403

Türck L (1860) Praktische Anleitung zur Laryngoskopie. Braumüller, Wien

Ullman MT (2008) The role of memory systems in disorders of language. In: Stemmer B, Whitaker HA (eds) Handbook of the neuroscience of language. Elsevier Ltd, Oxford, pp 189–198

Ullman MT (2013) Declarative/procedural model of language. In: Pashler H (ed) Encyclopedia of the mind. Sage, Los Angeles, pp 224–226

van den Berg JW (1958) Myoelastic-aerodynamic theory of voice production. J Speech Hear Res 1(3):227–244

Vasilenko JS (2002) Golos. Energoistad, Moscow

Vilkman E (2004) Occupational safety and health aspects of voice and speech professions. Folia Phoniatr Logop 56(4):220–253

Vilkman E, Wellens W, Neuschaefer-Rube C et al (2010) Logbook Phoniatrics UEMS 2010. http://www.phoniatrics.eu/uep/education/logbook-phoniatrics-uems-2010/index.html. Accessed 2 Feb 2015

von Bruns V (1862) Die erste Ausrottung eines Polypen in der Kehlkopfshöhle. Laupp'sche Buchh, Tübingen

von Bruns V (1873) Die Laryngoskopie und die laryngoskopische Chirurgie, 2nd edn. Laupp'sche Buchh, Tübingen

von Helmholtz H (1859) Ueber die Klangfarbe der Vocale. Ann Phys 184(10):280–290

von Kempelen W (1791) Mechanismus der menschlichen Sprache nebst der Beschreibung seiner sprechenden Maschine. Degen, Wien

von Leden H (1981) From Galen to Gutzmann. HNO-Praxis 6:175–178

von Leden H (1997a) A cultural history of the larynx and voice. In: Sataloff RT (ed) Professional voice, the science and art of clinical care, 2nd edn. Singular Publishing Group, San Diego, pp 7–86

von Leden H (1997b) The history of phonosurgery. In: Sataloff RT (ed) Professional voice, the science and art of clinical care, 2nd edn. Singular Publishing Group, San Diego, pp 561–580

Vorperian H, Kent R, Lindstrom M et al (2005) Development of vocal tract length during early childhood: a magnetic resonance imaging study. J Acoust Soc Am 117(1):338–350. https://doi.org/10.1121/1.1835958

Vorperian H, Wang S, Chung M et al (2009) Anatomic development of the oral and pharyngeal portions of the vocal tract: an imaging study. J Acoust Soc Am 125(3):1666–1678. https://doi.org/10.1121/1.307558

Wendler J (ed) (1980) Festschrift zu Ehren von Hermann Gutzmann sen. Humboldt-Univ, Berlin

Wendler J (2010) In memoriam: Aatto Sonninen. J Voice 24(1):1. https://doi.org/10.1016/j.jvoice.2009.06.006

Wendler J (2012) UEP from yesterday up until today—looking back at 40 years between crisis and success. Paper presented at the XXIII UEP Congress, Lund, 12–14 May 2011. http://www.phoniatrics.eu/uep/inside_uep/. Accessed 24 Nov 2016

Wendler J, Wellens W (eds) (1983) Ann Bull UEP 1:27–30

Wendler J, Seidner W, Eysholdt U (eds) (2005) Lehrbuch der Phoniatrie und Pädaudiologie, 4th edn. Thieme, Stuttgart

Wernicke C (1874) Der aphasische Symptomencomplex: Eine psychologische Studie auf anatomischer Basis. Cohn und Weigert, Breslau

World Health Organization (1946) Preamble to the constitution of the World Health Organization as adopted by the International Health Conference, New York, 19–22 June, 1946; signed on 22 July 1946 by the representatives of 61 States (Official Records of the World Health Organization, No. 2, p 100) and entered into force on 7 April 1948. http://www.who.int/about/mission/en/. Accessed 1 Dec 2017

World Health Organization (2002) Towards a common language for functioning, disability and health. http://www.who.int/classifications/icf/icfbeginnersguide.pdf. Accessed 24 Jul 2017

World Health Organization (2007) International Classification of Functioning, Disability and Health for Children and Youth (ICF-CY). http://apps.who.int/bookorders/anglais/detart1.jsp?codlan=1&codcol=15&codcch=716. World Health Organization, Geneva. Accessed 13 Aug 2015

World Health Organization (2015) Disabilities. http://www.who.int/topics/disabilities/en/. Accessed 14 Apr 2015

Zäske R, Volberg G, Kovács G et al (2014) Electrophysiological correlates of voice learning and recognition. J Neurosci 34(33):10821–10831. https://doi.org/10.1523/JNEUROSCI.0581-14.2014

Zilles K, Tillmann BN (2010) Anatomie. Springer, Heidelberg

Healthcare

2

Ojan Assadian, Peter Matulat, Katrin Neumann,
Antonio Schindler, and Erkki Vilkman

2.1 WHO Classification of Diagnosis and Functioning

Antonio Schindler and Peter Matulat

2.1.1 Diagnosis and Classification Systems

Diagnosis is the determination of a disease by the summary assessment of the collected findings. Diagnosis is the central point in clinical practice, as it allows the treatment to be decided upon and the prognosis of a given disease or disorder to be predicted. The path to diagnosis, diagnostics, typically ends with disease or disorder being named according to disease classification systems. Classifications and uniform terminology are also important for science, as they allow for the aggregation of data from different sources (World Health Organization 2017a). The World Health Organization (WHO) has developed a family of classifications, the International Statistical Classification of Diseases and Related Health Problems (ICD) (World Health Organization 1992); the International Classification of Functioning, Disability and Health (ICF) (World Health Organization 2001); and the International Classification of Functioning, Disability and Health: Children and Youth Version (ICF-CY) (World Health Organization 2007a), in order to provide a framework to encode a wide range of information about health, diagnosis, functioning and disability in adults and children. In the field of mental illness, an alternative classification system is found in the Diagnostic and Statistical Manual of Mental Disorders (DSM V) (American

O. Assadian
Landesklinikum Neunkirchen, Neunkirchen, Austria
e-mail: o.assadian@hud.ac.uk

P. Matulat
Clinic of Phoniatrics and Pedaudiology, University
Hospital Münster, Münster, Germany
e-mail: matulat@uni-muenster.de

K. Neumann
Department of Phoniatrics and Pediatric Audiology,
ENT Clinic, St. Elisabeth Hospital, University of
Bochum, Bochum, Germany
e-mail: Katrin.neumann@rub.de

A. Schindler
Department of Surgical Sciences, University of Turin,
Turin, Italy
e-mail: antonio.schindler@unimi.it

E. Vilkman
Department of Otolaryngology and
Phoniatrics – Head and Neck Surgery,
Helsinki University Hospital,
Helsinki, Finland
e-mail: Erkki.Vilkman@hus.fi

© Springer-Verlag GmbH Germany, part of Springer Nature 2020
A. am Zehnhoff-Dinnesen et al. (eds.), *Phoniatrics I*, European Manual of Medicine,
https://doi.org/10.1007/978-3-662-46780-0_2

Table 2.1 Chapter numbers and titles in ICD-10 Version 2016 (World Health Organization 2016)

Chapter	Title
I	Certain infectious and parasitic diseases
II	Neoplasms
III	Diseases of the blood and blood-forming organs and certain disorders involving the immune mechanism
IV	Endocrine, nutritional and metabolic diseases
V	Mental and behavioural disorders
VI	Diseases of the nervous system
VII	Diseases of the eye and adnexa
VIII	Diseases of the ear and mastoid process
IX	Diseases of the circulatory system
X	Diseases of the respiratory system
XI	Diseases of the digestive system
XII	Diseases of the skin and subcutaneous tissue
XIII	Diseases of the musculoskeletal system and connective tissue
XIV	Diseases of the genitourinary system
XV	Pregnancy, childbirth and the puerperium
XVI	Certain conditions originating in the perinatal period
XVII	Congenital malformations, deformations and chromosomal abnormalities
XVIII	Symptoms, signs and abnormal clinical and laboratory findings, not elsewhere Classified
XIX	Injury, poisoning and certain other consequences of external causes
XX	External causes of morbidity and mortality
XXI	Factors influencing health status and contact with health services
XXII	Codes for special purposes

Psychiatric Association 2013). It corresponds to Chap. 5 (see Table 2.1) of the ICD-10, pursues a descriptive approach and takes gender-specific differences into account.

2.1.2 International Statistical Classification of Diseases and Related Health Problems (ICD)

The most commonly used nosological framework for the classification of diagnoses, disorders and health conditions is the International Statistical Classification of Diseases and Related Health Problems (ICD), which includes codes for diseases, signs and symptoms, findings, social

circumstances, and related external causes and factors. Some significantly extended country-specific versions exist. ICD-10 Version 2016 is currently being revised and is intended to be replaced by ICD-11 (World Health Organization 2017b) in the mid-2018.

ICD-10 aims to list clinical conditions (diseases and symptoms) according to a framework of organ-specific similarities in symptoms and findings. It is used worldwide to code medical diagnosis and represents the basis of the reimbursement system in the majority of countries. ICD-10 is divided into 27 chapters (see Table 2.1).

Codes interesting for phoniatricians are compiled in Table 2.2.

2.1.3 International Classification of Functioning, Disability and Health (ICF) and the Children and Youth Version (ICF-CY)

The International Classification of Functioning, Disability and Health (ICF) and the ICF-CY were officially endorsed in 2001 and 2007 (World Health Organization 2001, 2007a).

The ICF and ICF-CY are nowadays considered the most relevant classifications. The ICF and ICF-CY serve a uniform and standardised language for the description of functional health, disability, social impairment and a person's associated environmental factors.

The children and youth version of the ICF (ICF-CY) was developed to take into account that:

> The manifestations of disability and health conditions in children and adolescents are different in nature, intensity and impact from those of adults.
> World Health Organization (2007a)

According to Illum and Gradel (2015), the ICF-CY is a helpful tool for the assessment of functioning in children with various disabilities.

The ICF and ICF-CY provide a classification system with three levels: impairments, disabilities and handicaps. An impairment is primarily a problem of body function and structure (a definition that is shared with the ICD). The term 'disabilities'

Table 2.2 ICD-10 codes compiled for phoniatricians by Muhittin Demir, Barbara Arnold, Rainer Schönweiler, Dirk Deuster, Peter Matulat and Antoinette am Zehnhoff-Dinnesen (World Health Organization 2016)

Class title	Code
I Certain infectious and parasitic diseases	*A00-B99*
I-Other viral diseases	B25-B34
Cytomegaloviral disease	B25
Cytomegaloviral disease, unspecified	B25.9
II Neoplasms	*C00-D48*
II-Malignant neoplasms	C00-C97
Malignant neoplasm of lip	C00
Malignant neoplasm of base of tongue	C01
Malignant neoplasm of other and unspecified parts of tongue	C02
Malignant neoplasm of gum	C03
Malignant neoplasm of floor of mouth	C04
Malignant neoplasm of palate	C05
Malignant neoplasm of other and unspecified parts of mouth	C06
Malignant neoplasm of tonsil	C09
Malignant neoplasm of oropharynx	C10
Malignant neoplasm of nasopharynx	C11
Malignant neoplasm of piriform sinus	C12
Malignant neoplasm of hypopharynx	C13
Malignant neoplasm of other and ill-defined sites in the lip, oral cavity and pharynx	C14
Malignant neoplasm of larynx	C32
Malignant neoplasm: Glottis	C32.0
Malignant neoplasm: Supraglottis	C32.1
Malignant neoplasm: Subglottis	C32.2
Malignant neoplasm: Laryngeal cartilage	C32.3
Malignant neoplasm: Overlapping lesion of larynx	C32.8
Malignant neoplasm: Larynx, unspecified	C32.9
V Mental and behavioural disorders	*F00-F99*
V-Mood [affective] disorders	F30-F39
V-Neurotic, stress-related and somatoform disorders	F40-F48
Dissociative motor disorders	F44.4
Dissociative anaesthesia and sensory loss	F44.6
Other dissociative [conversion] disorders	F44.8
Dissociative [conversion] disorder, unspecified	F44.9
Other somatoform disorders, e.g. globus hystericus	F45.8
V-Behavioural syndromes associated with physiological disturbances and physical factors	F50-F59
V-Disorders of adult personality and behaviour	F60-F69
Gender identity disorders	F64
Transsexualism	F64.0
Dual-role transvestism	F64.1
Gender identity disorder of childhood	F64.2
Other gender identity disorders	F64.8
Gender identity disorder, unspecified	F64.9
V-Mental retardation	F70-F79
Mild mental retardation	F70
Mild mental retardation: With the statement of no, or minimal, impairment of behaviour	F70.0
Mild mental retardation: Significant impairment of behaviour requiring attention or treatment	F70.1
Mild mental retardation: Other impairments of behaviour	F70.8
Mild mental retardation: Without mention of impairment of behaviour	F70.9
Moderate mental retardation	F71

(continued)

Table 2.2 (continued)

Class title	Code
Severe mental retardation	F72
Profound mental retardation	F73
Unspecified mental retardation: With the statement of no, or minimal, impairment of behaviour	F79.0
V-Disorders of psychological development	F80-F89
Specific developmental disorders of speech and language	F80
Specific speech articulation disorder	F80.0
Expressive language disorder	F80.1
Receptive language disorder	F80.2
Acquired aphasia with epilepsy [Landau-Kleffner]	F80.3
Other developmental disorders of speech and language	F80.8
Developmental disorder of speech and language, unspecified	F80.9
Specific developmental disorders of scholastic skills	F81
Specific reading disorder	F81.0
Specific spelling disorder	F81.1
Specific disorder of arithmetical skills	F81.2
Mixed disorder of scholastic skills	F81.3
Other developmental disorders of scholastic skills	F81.8
Developmental disorder of scholastic skills, unspecified	F81.9
Specific developmental disorder of motor function	F82
Mixed specific developmental disorders	F83
Pervasive developmental disorders	F84
Childhood autism	F84.0
Atypical autism	F84.1
Rett syndrome	F84.2
Other childhood disintegrative disorder	F84.3
Overactive disorder associated with mental retardation and stereotyped movements	F84.4
Asperger syndrome	F84.5
Other pervasive developmental disorders	F84.8
Pervasive developmental disorder, unspecified	F84.9
V-Behavioural and emotional disorders with onset usually occurring in childhood and adolescence	F90-F98
Hyperkinetic disorders	F90
Disturbance of activity and attention	F90.0
Hyperkinetic conduct disorder	F90.1
Other hyperkinetic disorders	F90.8
Hyperkinetic disorder, unspecified	F90.9
Conduct disorders	F91
Conduct disorder confined to the family context	F91.0
Mixed disorders of conduct and emotions	F92
Emotional disorders with onset specific to childhood	F93
Social anxiety disorder of childhood	F93.2
Disorders of social functioning with onset specific to childhood and adolescence	F94
Elective mutism	F94.0
Other childhood disorders of social functioning	F94.8
Childhood disorder of social functioning, unspecified	F94.9
Tic disorders	F95
Combined vocal and multiple motor tic disorder [de la Tourette]	F95.2
Nonorganic enuresis	F98.0
Nonorganic encopresis	F98.1
Feeding disorder of infancy and childhood	F98.2
Pica of infancy and childhood	F98.3
Stereotyped movement disorders	F98.4
Stuttering [stammering]	F98.5

Table 2.2 (continued)

Class title	Code
Cluttering	F98.6
Unspecified behavioural and emotional disorders with onset usually occurring in childhood and adolescence	F98.9
VI Diseases of the nervous system	*G00-G99*
VI-Extrapyramidal and movement disorders	G20-G26
Dystonia	G24
Idiopathic familial dystonia	G24.1
Idiopathic nonfamilial dystonia	G24.2
Spasmodic torticollis	G24.3
Idiopathic orofacial dystonia	G24.4
Blepharospasm	G24.5
Other dystonia	G24.8
Dystonia, unspecified	G24.9
VI-Episodic and paroxysmal disorders	G40-G47
Epilepsy	G40
Generalised idiopathic epilepsy and epileptic syndromes	G40.3
Other epilepsy	G40.8
Epilepsy, unspecified	G40.9
VI-Polyneuropathies and other disorders of the peripheral nervous system	G60-G64
Hereditary motor and sensory neuropathy	G60.0
Hereditary and idiopathic neuropathy, unspecified	G60.9
VIII Diseases of the ear and mastoid process	*H60-H95*
VIII-Diseases of external ear	H60-H62
Otitis externa	H60
Other infective otitis externa	H60.3
Cholesteatoma of external ear	H60.4
Acute otitis externa, noninfective	H60.5
Other otitis externa	H60.8
Otitis externa, unspecified	H60.9
Impacted cerumen	H61.2
Acquired stenosis of external ear canal	H61.3
Other specified disorders of external ear	H61.8
Disorder of external ear, unspecified	H61.9
VIII-Diseases of middle ear and mastoid	H65-H75
Nonsuppurative otitis media	H65
Acute serous otitis media	H65.0
Other acute nonsuppurative otitis media	H65.1
Chronic serous otitis media	H65.2
Chronic mucoid otitis media	H65.3
Other chronic nonsuppurative otitis media	H65.4
Nonsuppurative otitis media, unspecified	H65.9
Suppurative and unspecified otitis media	H66
Acute suppurative otitis media	H66.0
Chronic tubotympanic suppurative otitis media	H66.1
Chronic atticoantral suppurative otitis media	H66.2
Other chronic suppurative otitis media	H66.3
Suppurative otitis media, unspecified	H66.4
Otitis media, unspecified	H66.9
Eustachian salpingitis and obstruction	H68
Eustachian salpingitis	H68.0
Obstruction of Eustachian tube	H68.1

(continued)

Table 2.2 (continued)

Class title	Code
Eustachian tube disorder, unspecified	H69.9
Mastoiditis and related conditions	H70
Acute mastoiditis	H70.0
Chronic mastoiditis	H70.1
Cholesteatoma of middle ear	H71
Perforation of tympanic membrane	H72
Central perforation of tympanic membrane	H72.0
Attic perforation of tympanic membrane	H72.1
Other perforations of tympanic membrane	H72.8
Other disorders of tympanic membrane	H73
Acute myringitis	H73.0
Chronic myringitis	H73.1
Disorder of tympanic membrane, unspecified	H73.9
Other disorders of middle ear and mastoid	H74
Tympanosclerosis	H74.0
Adhesive middle ear disease	H74.1
Discontinuity and dislocation of ear ossicles	H74.2
Other acquired abnormalities of ear ossicles	H74.3
Polyp of middle ear	H74.4
Disorder of middle ear and mastoid, unspecified	H74.9
VIII-Diseases of inner ear	H80-H83
Otosclerosis	H80
Cochlear otosclerosis	H80.2
Otosclerosis, unspecified	H80.9
Disorders of vestibular function	H81
Other peripheral vertigo	H81.3
Vertigo of central origin	H81.4
Disorder of vestibular function, unspecified	H81.9
Other diseases of inner ear	H83
Labyrinthitis	H83.0
Labyrinthine fistula	H83.1
Noise effects on inner ear	H83.3
VIII-Other disorders of ear	H90-H95
Conductive and sensorineural hearing loss	H90
Conductive hearing loss, bilateral	H90.0
Conductive hearing loss, unilateral with unrestricted hearing on the contralateral side	H90.1
Conductive hearing loss, unspecified	H90.2
Sensorineural hearing loss, bilateral	H90.3
Sensorineural hearing loss, unilateral with unrestricted hearing on the contralateral side	H90.4
Sensorineural hearing loss, unspecified	H90.5
Mixed conductive and sensorineural hearing loss, bilateral	H90.6
Mixed conductive and sensorineural hearing loss, unilateral with unrestricted hearing on the contralateral side	H90.7
Mixed conductive and sensorineural hearing loss, unspecified	H90.8
Ototoxic hearing loss	H91.0
Presbycusis	H91.1
Sudden idiopathic hearing loss	H91.2
Deaf mutism, not elsewhere classified	H91.3
Other specified hearing loss	H91.8
Hearing loss, unspecified	H91.9
Otalgia and effusion of ear	H92
Otalgia	H92.0

Table 2.2 (continued)

Class title	Code
Otorrhoea	H92.1
Otorrhagia	H92.2
Tinnitus	H93.1
Other abnormal auditory perceptions	H93.2
Disorders of acoustic nerve	H93.3
X Diseases of the respiratory system	*J00-J99*
X-Acute upper respiratory infections	J00-J06
Acute nasopharyngitis [common cold]	J00
Acute sinusitis	J01
Acute maxillary sinusitis	J01.0
Acute frontal sinusitis	J01.1
Acute ethmoidal sinusitis	J01.2
Acute sphenoidal sinusitis	J01.3
Acute pansinusitis	J01.4
Other acute sinusitis	J01.8
Acute sinusitis, unspecified	J01.9
Acute pharyngitis	J02
Acute tonsillitis	J03
Acute laryngitis and tracheitis	J04
Acute laryngitis	J04.0
Acute tracheitis	J04.1
Acute laryngotracheitis	J04.2
Acute obstructive laryngitis [croup] and epiglottitis	J05
Acute obstructive laryngitis [croup]	J05.0
Acute epiglottitis	J05.1
X-Other diseases of upper respiratory tract	J30-J39
Vasomotor and allergic rhinitis	J30
Vasomotor rhinitis	J30.0
Allergic rhinitis due to pollen	J30.1
Other seasonal allergic rhinitis	J30.2
Other allergic rhinitis	J30.3
Allergic rhinitis, unspecified	J30.4
Chronic rhinitis, nasopharyngitis and pharyngitis	J31
Chronic rhinitis	J31.0
Chronic nasopharyngitis	J31.1
Chronic pharyngitis	J31.2
Chronic sinusitis	J32
Chronic maxillary sinusitis	J32.0
Chronic frontal sinusitis	J32.1
Chronic ethmoidal sinusitis	J32.2
Chronic sphenoidal sinusitis	J32.3
Chronic pansinusitis	J32.4
Other chronic sinusitis	J32.8
Chronic sinusitis, unspecified	J32.9
Nasal polyp	J33
Polyp of nasal cavity	J33.0
Polypoid sinus degeneration	J33.1
Other polyp of sinus	J33.8
Nasal polyp, unspecified	J33.9
Other disorders of nose and nasal sinuses	J34
Abscess, furuncle and carbuncle of nose	J34.0

(continued)

Table 2.2 (continued)

Class title	Code
Cyst and mucocele of nose and nasal sinus	J34.1
Deviated nasal septum	J34.2
Hypertrophy of nasal turbinates	J34.3
Other specified disorders of nose and nasal sinuses	J34.8
Chronic diseases of tonsils and adenoids	J35
Chronic tonsillitis	J35.0
Hypertrophy of tonsils	J35.1
Hypertrophy of adenoids	J35.2
Hypertrophy of tonsils with hypertrophy of adenoids	J35.3
Other chronic diseases of tonsils and adenoids	J35.8
Chronic disease of tonsils and adenoids, unspecified	J35.9
Chronic laryngitis and laryngotracheitis	J37
Chronic laryngitis	J37.0
Chronic laryngotracheitis	J37.1
Diseases of vocal cords and larynx, not elsewhere classified	J38
Paralysis of vocal cords and larynx	J38.0
Polyp of vocal cord and larynx	J38.1
Nodules of vocal cords	J38.2
Other diseases of vocal cords	J38.3
Oedema of larynx	J38.4
Laryngeal spasm	J38.5
Stenosis of larynx	J38.6
Other diseases of larynx	J38.7
Other diseases of upper respiratory tract	J39
Upper respiratory tract hypersensitivity reaction, site unspecified	J39.3
X-Chronic lower respiratory diseases	J40-J47
Asthma	J45
Predominantly allergic asthma	J45.0
Nonallergic asthma	J45.1
Mixed asthma	J45.8
Asthma, unspecified	J45.9
XI Diseases of the digestive system	*K00-K93*
XI-Diseases of oral cavity, salivary glands and jaws	K00-K14
Dentofacial anomalies [including malocclusion]	K07
Major anomalies of jaw size	K07.0
Anomalies of jaw-cranial base relationship	K07.1
Anomalies of dental arch relationship	K07.2
Anomalies of tooth position	K07.3
Malocclusion, unspecified	K07.4
Dentofacial functional abnormalities	K07.5
Temporomandibular joint disorders	K07.6
Other dentofacial anomalies	K07.8
Oral mucositis (ulcerative)	K12.3
XI-Diseases of oesophagus, stomach and duodenum	K20-K31
Gastro-oesophageal reflux disease	K21
Gastro-oesophageal reflux disease with oesophagitis	K21.0
Gastro-oesophageal reflux disease without oesophagitis	K21.9
Achalasia of cardia	K22.0
Ulcer of oesophagus	K22.1
Dyskinesia of oesophagus	K22.4
Barrett oesophagus	K22.7
Gastritis, unspecified	K29.7

Table 2.2 (continued)

Class title	Code
Functional dyspepsia	K30
XII Diseases of the skin and subcutaneous tissue	*L00-L99*
Chronic radiodermatitis	L58.1
Disorder of skin and subcutaneous tissue related to radiation, unspecified	L59.9
XVI Certain conditions originating in the perinatal period	*P00-P96*
XVI-Foetus and newborn affected by maternal factors and by complications of pregnancy, labour and delivery	P00-P04
Foetus and newborn affected by maternal conditions that may be unrelated to present pregnancy	P00
Foetus and newborn affected by maternal complications of pregnancy	P01
Foetus and newborn affected by complications of placenta, cord and membranes	P02
Foetus and newborn affected by other complications of labour and delivery	P03
Foetus and newborn affected by noxious influences transmitted via placenta or breast milk	P04
XVI-Disorders related to length of gestation and foetal growth	P05-P08
Slow foetal growth and foetal malnutrition	P05
Disorders related to short gestation and low birth weight, not elsewhere classified	P07
Extremely low birth weight	P07.0
Other preterm infants	P07.3
XVI-Disorders related to length of gestation and foetal growth, different types of birth trauma	P10-P15
XVI-Infections specific to the perinatal period	P35-P39
Congenital rubella syndrome	P35.0
Congenital cytomegalovirus infection	P35.1
Congenital herpesviral [herpes simplex] infection	P35.2
Bacterial sepsis of newborn	P36
Congenital tuberculosis	P37.0
Congenital toxoplasmosis	P37.1
XVI-Other disorders originating in the perinatal period	P90-P96
Congenital hypertonia	P94.1
Congenital hypotonia	P94.2
Disorder of muscle tone of newborn, unspecified	P94.9
XVII Congenital malformations, deformations and chromosomal abnormalities	*Q00-Q99*
XVII-Congenital malformations of the nervous system	Q00-Q07
Microcephaly	Q02
Congenital hydrocephalus	Q03
Other congenital malformations of brain	Q04
Spina bifida	Q05
Other congenital malformations of nervous system	Q07
XVII-Congenital malformations of eye, ear, face and neck	Q10-Q18
Congenital malformations of ear causing impairment of hearing	Q16
Congenital absence of (ear) auricle	Q16.0
Congenital absence, atresia and stricture of auditory canal (external)	Q16.1
Absence of Eustachian tube	Q16.2
Congenital malformation of ear ossicles	Q16.3
Other congenital malformations of middle ear	Q16.4
Congenital malformation of inner ear	Q16.5
Congenital malformation of ear causing impairment of hearing, unspecified	Q16.9
Other congenital malformations of ear	Q17
Accessory auricle	Q17.0
Macrotia	Q17.1
Microtia	Q17.2
Other misshapen ear	Q17.3

(continued)

Table 2.2 (continued)

Class title	Code
Misplaced ear	Q17.4
Prominent ear	Q17.5
Sinus, fistula and cyst of branchial cleft	Q18.0
Preauricular sinus and cyst	Q18.1
Other branchial cleft malformations	Q18.2
Webbing of neck	Q18.3
Macrostomia	Q18.4
Microstomia	Q18.5
Macrocheilia	Q18.6
Microcheilia	Q18.7
Other specified congenital malformations of face and neck	Q18.8
Congenital malformation of face and neck, unspecified	Q18.9
XVII-Congenital malformations of the respiratory system	Q30-Q34
Congenital malformations of nose	Q30
Congenital malformations of larynx	Q31
Web of larynx	Q31.0
Congenital subglottic stenosis	Q31.1
Laryngeal hypoplasia	Q31.2
Laryngocele	Q31.3
Congenital laryngomalacia	Q31.5
Other congenital malformations of larynx	Q31.8
Congenital malformation of larynx, unspecified	Q31.9
XVII-Cleft lip and cleft palate	Q35-Q37
Cleft palate	Q35
Cleft hard palate	Q35.1
Cleft soft palate	Q35.3
Cleft hard palate with cleft soft palate	Q35.5
Cleft uvula	Q35.7
Cleft palate, unspecified	Q35.9
Cleft lip	Q36
Cleft lip, bilateral	Q36.0
Cleft lip, median	Q36.1
Cleft lip, unilateral	Q36.9
Cleft palate with cleft lip	Q37
Cleft hard palate with bilateral cleft lip	Q37.0
Cleft hard palate with unilateral cleft lip	Q37.1
Cleft soft palate with bilateral cleft lip	Q37.2
Cleft soft palate with unilateral cleft lip	Q37.3
Cleft hard and soft palate with bilateral cleft lip	Q37.4
Cleft hard and soft palate with unilateral cleft lip	Q37.5
Unspecified cleft palate with bilateral cleft lip	Q37.8
Unspecified cleft palate with unilateral cleft lip	Q37.9
XVII-Congenital malformations and deformations of the musculoskeletal system	Q65-Q79
Other congenital deformities of skull, face and jaw	Q67.4
Congenital musculoskeletal deformities of head, face, spine and chest	Q67
Facial asymmetry	Q67.0
Plagiocephaly	Q67.3
Other congenital malformations of skull and face bones	Q75
Hypertelorism	Q75.2
Mandibulofacial dysostosis (Franceschetti, Treacher Collins)	Q75.4
Congenital malformation of skull and face bones, unspecified	Q75.9
XVII-Other congenital malformations	Q80-Q89

Table 2.2 (continued)

Class title	Code
Neurofibromatosis (non-malignant)	Q85.0
Tuberous sclerosis	Q85.1
Other phakomatoses, not elsewhere classified	Q85.8
Congenital malformation syndromes due to known exogenous causes, not elsewhere classified	Q86
Foetal alcohol syndrome (dysmorphic)	Q86.0
Foetal hydantoin syndrome	Q86.1
Dysmorphism due to warfarin	Q86.2
Other congenital malformation syndromes due to known exogenous causes	Q86.8
Other specified congenital malformation syndromes affecting multiple systems	Q87
Congenital malformation syndromes predominantly affecting facial appearance	Q87.0
Congenital malformation syndromes predominantly associated with short stature	Q87.1
Congenital malformation syndromes predominantly involving limbs	Q87.2
Congenital malformation syndromes involving early overgrowth	Q87.3
Marfan syndrome	Q87.4
Other congenital malformation syndromes with other skeletal changes	Q87.5
Other specified congenital malformation syndromes, not elsewhere classified	Q87.8
Situs inversus	Q89.3
XVII-Chromosomal abnormalities, not elsewhere classified	Q90-Q99
Down syndrome	Q90
Trisomy 21, meiotic nondisjunction	Q90.0
Trisomy 21, mosaicism (mitotic nondisjunction)	Q90.1
Trisomy 21, translocation	Q90.2
Down syndrome, unspecified	Q90.9
Edwards syndrome and Patau syndrome	Q91.-
Deletion of short arm of chromosome 4	Q93.3
Deletion of short arm of chromosome 5	Q93.4
Turner syndrome	Q96
Klinefelter syndrome karyotype 47,XXY	Q98.0
Chimera 46,XX/46,XY	Q99.0
46,XX true hermaphrodite	Q99.1
Fragile X chromosome	Q99.2
XVIII Symptoms, signs and abnormal clinical and laboratory findings, not elsewhere classified	*R00-R99*
XVIII-Symptoms and signs involving the digestive system and abdomen	R10-R19
Heartburn	R12
Dysphagia	R13
XVIII-Symptoms and signs involving the nervous and musculoskeletal systems	R25-R29
Abnormal head movements	R25.0
Tremor, unspecified	R25.1
Fasciculation	R25.3
Other and unspecified abnormal involuntary movements	R25.8
Immobility(bedfast, chairfast)	R26.3
XVIII-Symptoms and signs involving speech and voice	R47-R49
Speech disturbances, not elsewhere classified	R47
Dysphasia and aphasia	R47.0
Dysarthria and anarthria	R47.1
Other and unspecified speech disturbances	R47.8
Dyslexia and other symbolic dysfunctions, not elsewhere classified	R48
Dyslexia and alexia	R48.0
Agnosia	R48.1
Apraxia	R48.2
Other and unspecified symbolic dysfunctions	R48.8

(continued)

Table 2.2 (continued)

Class title	Code
Voice disturbances	R49
Dysphonia	R49.0
Aphonia	R49.1
Hypernasality and hyponasality	R49.2
Other and unspecified voice disturbances	R49.8
XVIII-General symptoms and signs	R50-R69
Headache	R51
Other chronic pain	R52.2
Enlarged lymph nodes, unspecified	R59.9
Delayed milestone	R62.0
Other lack of expected normal physiological development	R62.8
Feeding difficulties and mismanagement	R63.3
Abnormal weight loss	R63.4
Nonspecific symptoms peculiar to infancy (excessive crying of infant)	R68.1
Dry mouth, unspecified	R68.2
XIX Injury, poisoning and certain other consequences of external causes	S00-T98
XIX-Injuries to the neck	S10-S19
Contusion of throat	S10.0
XIX-Burns and corrosions confined to eye and internal organs	T26-T28
Burn of larynx and trachea	T27.0
Burn involving larynx and trachea with lung	T27.1
Burn of mouth and pharynx	T28.0
Burn of oesophagus	T28.1
Corrosion of mouth and pharynx	T28.5
Corrosion of oesophagus	T28.6
XXI Factors influencing health status and contact with health services	Z00-Z99
XXI-Persons encountering health services in circumstances related to reproduction	Z30-Z39
Twin, born in hospital	Z38.3
XXI-Persons encountering health services for specific procedures and healthcare	Z40-Z54
Adjustment and management of implanted hearing device	Z45.3
Fitting and adjustment of hearing aid	Z46.1
Surgical follow-up care, unspecified	Z48.9
XXI-Persons with potential health hazards related to socioeconomic and psychosocial circumstances	Z55-Z65
Acculturation difficulty	Z60.3
XXI-Persons encountering health services in other circumstances	Z70-Z76
Tobacco use	Z72.0
Alcohol use	Z72.1
XXI-Persons with potential health hazards related to family and personal history and certain conditions influencing health status	Z80-Z99
Family history of deafness and hearing loss	Z82.2
Family history of congenital malformations, deformations and chromosomal abnormalities	Z82.7
Family history of other disabilities and chronic diseases leading to disablement, not elsewhere classified	Z82.8
Personal history of malignant neoplasm of other respiratory and intrathoracic organs	Z85.2
Personal history of certain conditions arising in the perinatal period	Z87.6
Acquired absence of part of head and neck	Z90.0
Personal history of irradiation	Z92.3
Tracheostomy status	Z93.0
Gastrostomy status	Z93.1
Presence of otological and audiological implants	Z96.2
Presence of external hearing aid	Z97.4

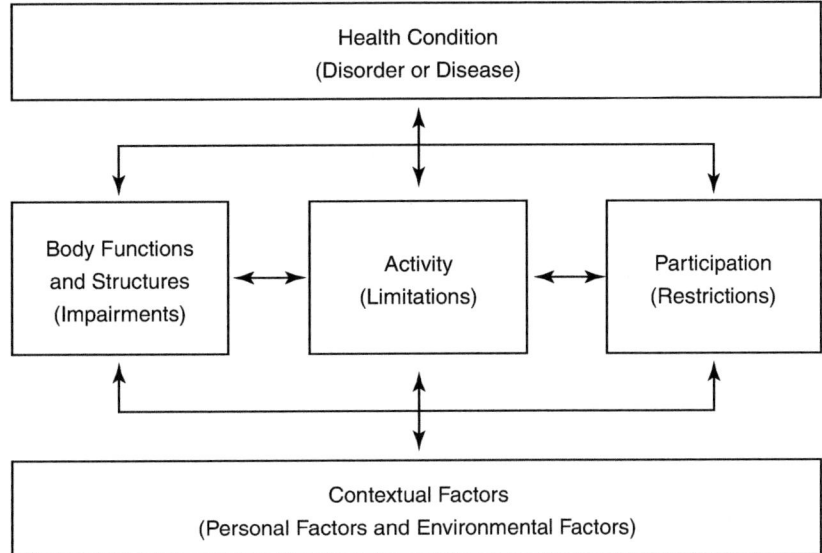

includes impairments, activity limitations and participation restrictions. 'Handicap' refers to the result when an individual with an impairment or disability cannot fulfil a normal life role. 'Handicapped' is, however, not a medical term; it reflects the interaction between the individual's impairments and the social environment. The primary goals of the ICF and ICF-CY are the social participation of the handicapped person. They are not primarily deficit-orientated.

Functioning is described from the perspective of the body, the person and the society. Interactions between the components of the ICF/ICF-CY are described in a dual model as shown in Fig. 2.1. This model differentiates between two parts that make up the health condition: functioning and disability and contextual factors.

Functioning and disability includes the body component (including the physiological and psychological functions of body systems and anatomical structures) on the one hand and activity and participation on the other. Activity is here defined as action of an individual and participation as involvement in a life situation. Activity limitations and participation restrictions are possible results of difficulties at the person level.

Environmental factors and personal factors (personal factors are not classified in ICF and ICF-CY) are independent but influence all other components of the concept.

In contrast to the biomedical model, as a biopsychosocial model, the ICF and the ICF-CY can describe the effects of health problems—as described in the ICD—on functional health. They complement the ICD.

The ICF and ICF-CY use a mono-hierarchically nested structure with alphanumeric codes. Body Functions (b), Body Structures (s), Activity and Participation (d) and Environmental Factors (e) are the 'chapter headings' of the first level and define the first letter of the alphanumeric code. The next level(s), which define(s) the later digits in the alphanumeric code, include sub'chapters', group headings where appropriate and additional detail.

The coding also allows the addition of one number, called a qualifier, that indicates the extent of the individual's impairments and the extent of his participation restrictions or activity limitations. In the case of environmental factors, the qualifier can be used to denote either a facilitator or a barrier: the + sign denoting a facilitator, while the decimal point alone denotes a barrier. The qualifier can have a value ranging from 1 to 4, corresponding to mild (1), moderate (2), severe (3) or complete (4) impairment, limitation, restriction, barrier or facilitator for each ICF/ICF-CY category.

2.1.4 Coding Examples

Aphasia The following example will clarify the coding system. A patient with severe Broca's aphasia following a small frontal ischemic stroke cannot produce verbal messages and sustain a conversation, uses a communication board to express himself and has lost his job. The application of the ICF in this case will be b16710.3 (severe impairment in the expression of spoken language), s11000.1 (mild impairment of the frontal lobe), d330.3 (severe difficulty in speaking), d3501.4 (complete difficulty in sustaining a conversation), e1251. + 3 (communication board as substantial facilitator) and e5902.4 (lack of labour and employment policies as complete barrier) (World Health Organization 1992).

Stuttering The following example will clarify the difference between ICD and ICF. A 10-year-old child is assessed by a phoniatrician because of stuttering. During the assessment the rhythm of speech is impaired, and speech is characterised by impairment in the flow of speech with involuntary repetitions and prolongations of sounds. The child is severely impaired in reading aloud in the classroom and is limited in conversations with her peers. In this case the ICD code is F98.5, stuttering. The ICF coding will be b330.3 (severe impairment in fluency and rhythm of speech), d166.3 (severe limitation in school reading) and d.350.3 (severe limitation in conversation).

2.1.5 ICF and ICF-CY in Communication Disorders

During the development of the ICF and ICF-CY, concepts of structure and the organisation of information regarding the individuals and their needs were developed by various professional groups for various disciplines within medicine, early intervention, rehabilitation and education. In many cases, checklists and questionnaires summarising the essential codes for the area of interest were developed.

The WHO has even published a checklist with essential categories, which is:

> a practical tool to elicit and record information on the functioning and disability of an individual.
> World Health Organization (2007b)

The ICF and ICF-CY are helpful frameworks providing an internationally uniform description of communication problems (Schindler et al. 2002; Threats 2006). Washington (2007) shows that the framework is not only suitable for describing children with specific language impairment (SLI) but can also be used for the management and control of the therapeutic outcome in these children. Application of these frameworks in the treatment of stuttering has been described by Yaruss (2007). The significance of this approach for communication disorders following traumatic brain injury was investigated by Larkins (2007).

ICF core sets for various diseases, e.g. hearing loss, have been recorded and are available for individual compilation (ICF Research Branch 2013). The Canadian guidelines for investigation and treatment on auditory processing disorders in children and adults explicitly use this conceptual framework (The Canadian Interorganizational Steering Group for Speech Language Pathology and Audiology 2012).

The American Speech-Language-Hearing Association (2017) briefly described the functional targets for a number of diseases (e.g. apraxia of speech, aphasia, dysarthria, SLI, swallowing, tinnitus, voice) on the basis of the ICF and ICF-CY.

2.2 Legislative Aspects

Erkki Vilkman

2.2.1 Introduction

According to the World Health Organization constitution:

> Governments have a responsibility for the health of their peoples, which can be fulfilled only by the provision of adequate health and social measures.
> World Health Organization (2006)

The Treaty on the Functioning of the European Union (European Union 2007) puts much emphasis on human health protection in all Union policies and activities:

> Union action, which shall complement national policies, shall be directed towards improving public health, preventing physical and mental illness and diseases, and obviating sources of danger to physical and mental health. Such action shall cover the fight against the major health scourges, by promoting research into their causes, their transmission and their prevention, as well as health information and education, and monitoring, early warning of and combating serious cross-border threats to health.

2.2.2 Healthcare

In Europe there is large variation in how the healthcare system is arranged. In general, the system is publicly funded by taxes with varying degrees of support by private insurances (World Health Organization 2010).

The Consolidated version of the Treaty on the Functioning of the European Union (2008) stipulates, for instance, that each member state arranges adequate healthcare to its citizens (European Union 2007).

The directive on patients' rights in cross-border healthcare (European Parliament of the Council and the European Union 2011) defines in more detail the rights of EU citizens to seek treatment in an EU country other than the one the patient is insured in. EU citizens while travelling for any reason within the EU (in this case the 28 EU member states and Iceland, Liechtenstein, Norway and Switzerland) have the right to any medical treatment in acute situations. In acute cases the European Health Insurance Card ensures that the costs of the treatment are covered.

When living in an EU country other than the country where the person is insured, the basic principle is the same as for acute illness; however, as the healthcare and social security systems vary from country to country, the arrangements will vary accordingly.

Similarly, an EU citizen can seek planned medical treatment in another EU country on the same terms and at the same cost as for people living in that country. However, some countries may restrict access to some types of healthcare, for instance, if demand for treatment is higher than their capacity to provide it. The patient may be entitled to receive some or all of the costs covered, depending on the insurance rules and regulations of the patient's native country. The national health insurer cannot refuse to cover the costs if the specific treatment that the patient needs is unavailable in the home country, but is covered by the statutory health insurer, and if the patient cannot get the treatment needed without undue delay in the home country. In principle, the treatment costs will be covered only if the law in the country where the patient is insured recognises the treatment.

2.2.3 Rehabilitation

The global legislative basis of rehabilitation is the United Nations Convention on the Rights of Persons with Disabilities (United Nations 2006), which is ratified by the EU. According to the UN convention, the countries that have ratified the convention:

> shall take effective and appropriate measures, including through peer support, to enable persons with disabilities to attain and maintain maximum independence, full physical, mental, social and vocational ability, and full inclusion and participation in all aspects of life.
> United Nations, UN Convention, Article 26 (2006)

To meet this goal, the countries have to arrange:

> habilitation and rehabilitation services and programmes, particularly in the areas of health, employment, education and social services.
> United Nations (2006)

The rehabilitation has to be started as early as possible and should be based on evaluations made by a multidisciplinary team. Further, the same article stresses the necessity of continuous training of the staff working in the field. Finally, the use of adequate assistive devices and technologies has to be promoted by the countries ratifying the convention.

In addition, the EU Commission has formulated a disability strategy for the years 2010–2020 (EU Commission 2003a). The Commission stresses, for instance, that people with disabilities are entitled to 'affordable quality health and rehabilitation services'. The WHO framework International Classification of Functioning, Disability and Health (World Health Organization 2001, see Sect. 2.1) can be used as a platform for estimating health and disability at the individual and population levels.

For phoniatric patients, the rehabilitation and its arrangements can be taken care of by many professional groups of varying educational background. In many countries the term medical rehabilitation is used when professionals approved by law provide the rehabilitation. Such professionals are, besides physicians, for instance, (neuro)psychologists, speech and language therapists, logopedists, physiotherapists, social workers and occupational therapists. In Europe much effort is put in unifying the educational programmes in these professional groups.

Within child phoniatrics the habilitation and rehabilitation services provided by professionals of (special) education in kindergartens and schools are of paramount importance.

2.2.4 Occupational Safety and Health (OSH)

The Consolidated version of the Treaty on the Functioning of the European Union (2008) (European Union 2007) states that the EU supports the activities of its member states in improving the working environment to protect workers' health and safety (Article 153). The issue is addressed in more detail in the European Framework Directive on Safety and Health at Work (European Council 1989). The Framework Directive covers all kinds of work and not only technical safety but also general prevention of ill health. The employer has the responsibility to take adequate preventive measures to make work healthier and safer. This should be a part of general management processes. The key element of the Directive is risk assessment, which includes such principles as hazard identification, worker participation, introduction of adequate measures with the priority of eliminating risk at source, documentation and periodical reassessment of workplace hazards.

For phoniatrics it seems that environmental noise as a risk factor for occupational inner ear damage is well understood and covered in the work of European Agency for Safety and Health at Work (e.g. Schneider et al. 2005) as well as in working life. For European OSH legislation, occupational voice disorders would be covered under the general requirements of the framework directive (European Council 1989) to assess risks and put in place prevention measures. General duties to provide information and training for workers would also apply. At present, however, occupational voice problems of teachers, for instance, are just briefly addressed in reports by European Agency for Safety and Health at Work (European Agency for Safety and Health at Work's Topic Centre OSH 2013; Schneider et al. 2005). Occupational voice problems are compensated for as occupational diseases in some EU countries (EU Commission 2003b).

A European schedule of occupational diseases lists 'Hypoacousis or deafness caused by noise' (number 503) and 'Nodules on the vocal chords caused by sustained work-related vocal effort' (number 2.503) (EU Commission 2003c). The International Labour Organization has also created a similar list (International Labour Organization 2010).

2.3   Investigating Effectiveness of Treatment and Rehabilitation of Communication and Swallowing Disorders

Katrin Neumann

2.3.1   The Problem of Evidence-Based Treatment in Communication and Swallowing Disorders

Evidence-informed healthcare encompasses the use of the best available, i.e. least biased and most trustworthy, evidence in decision-making for treatments in order to ensure ethical and accountable practice, protect patients from incompetence and other risks and gain the best patient outcomes (McCormack et al. 2013). It has become fundamental to medical practice. It aims at overcoming the gap between what is known and what is consistently done. Unfortunately, for a long time, professionals and policymakers have largely ascribed only secondary importance to the use of evidence reviews in the implementation of treatments (Grimshaw et al. 2012). This also holds true for therapies of communication and swallowing disorders. Behavioural speech, language and voice therapies are often lengthy and frequently, if not predominantly, with no or only low necessity to provide evidence of the effectiveness of the therapy.

Since the advent of evidence-based medical practice in the 1990s, it has become increasingly important to search for the fulfilment of its criteria for specific therapies. This is laudable but has been accompanied by two shortcomings in the field of communication disorders: (1) Many therapies are believed by therapists to be evidence-based but have never strictly been proven to be that and (2) therapists have often argued that their behavioural treatments are too individual-specific for the application of evidence-based principles.

Even if this belief has been more or less overcome, in daily practice the effect of such therapies is often described only verbally without the use of repeated and multidimensional outcome measures.

However, as has been shown for other behavioural treatments such as psychotherapy, the evaluation of the effectiveness of a behavioural therapy from the impression of the therapist himself usually overestimates the therapeutic effect. Patients also tend to evaluate a short-term therapy effect positively because they have expended effort, cost and time, and they want to believe in an effect of the chosen therapy. However, from a more retrospective point of view, they often allocate no or only a short-term effect to a treatment. The most reliable persons to ask are relevant others such as relatives or friends. They often evaluate a treatment effect more unaffectedly than the therapists or the patient (Dineen 1998).

2.3.2   Evidence-Based Medicine and Evidence-Informed Healthcare

Evidence-based medicine (EBM) has been defined by Sackett and coworkers as the:

> conscientious, explicit and judicious use of current best evidence in making decisions about the care of individual patients.

It mathematically estimates the risks of benefit and harm, coming from high-quality research on population samples, to provide information for clinical decision-making for diagnosis and treatment of patients. The outcome of such studies is the development of an evidence-based practice that aims at the generalisation of medical procedures.

For this, medical professionals have to integrate the best available research evidence with their individual clinical expertise and the values and expectations of their patients. The consideration of the patients' expectations meets the fact that the effectiveness of healthcare also depends on individual factors such as quality-of-life and value-of-life judgments. Examples of such measures in communication disorders are the Voice Handicap Index (VHI) for voice disorders and quality-of-life questionnaires for the rehabilitation of hearing-impaired children fitted with cochlear implants or hearing aids. In controlled experimental settings, such factors frequently show unexpected results. For example, the VHI in patients after a laryngectomy has been shown to be less high than that for spasmodic dysphonia (Moerman et al. 2008). Hence, the application of available evidence depends on personal, political, cultural, religious, ethical, economic and aesthetic values. This has brought about a shift from the original term 'evidence-*based* medicine' to 'evidence-*informed* healthcare'.

The US Preventive Services Task Force has developed the following widely used ranking system to describe the evidence of the effectiveness of therapies or screenings:

- Level I: Evidence obtained from at least one properly designed randomised controlled trial.
- Level II-1: Evidence obtained from well-designed controlled trials without randomisation.
- Level II-2: Evidence obtained from well-designed cohort or case-control analytical studies, preferably from more than one Centre or research group.
- Level II-3: Evidence obtained from multiple time-series designs with or without the intervention. Dramatic results in uncontrolled trials might also be regarded as this type of evidence.
- Level III: Opinions of respected authorities, based on clinical experience, descriptive studies or reports of expert committees.

The implementation of evidence-informed healthcare is an ongoing process that requires increasingly detailed description of interventions, the use of outcome measures, the outline of a treatment context and of the intensity and the levels at which interventions are implemented (McCormack et al. 2013). As platforms of the

required knowledge, scientific societies and expert groups have elaborated guidelines, position papers and other publications with recommendations on evidence-based procedures and interventions in their fields, weighting the risks versus benefits of specific services. These guidelines need periodical updates.

EBM uses techniques from science, engineering and statistics. Important tools are systematic reviews of the medical literature, meta-analyses, risk-benefit analyses and randomised controlled trials (RCTs).

Systematic Reviews Literature reviews that provide an exhaustive summary of current literature relevant to a research question in order to identify, appraise, select and synthesise all high-quality research evidence relevant to that question are called systematic reviews. They start with a thorough search of the literature for relevant publications and have to list the databases and citation indexes searched, such as PubMed, Embase, the Cochrane Library, ISI Web of Knowledge and Conference Proceedings Citation Index—Science (CPCI-S), as well as any hand-searched journals or additional literature, in its methods section. The titles and the abstracts of the articles identified for a research question are screened according to predefined criteria for eligibility and relevance. Each included study may be assigned an objective assessment of methodological quality, for example, according to the quality standards of Cochrane collaboration.

Systematic reviews often use statistical techniques such as meta-analysis to combine results of the eligible studies. They score the levels of evidence as described above related to the methodology used. A central part is the application of critical appraisal methods, i.e. of explicit, transparent methods to assess the data in published research, applying the rules of evidence to factors such as internal validity, adherence to reporting standards, conclusions and generalisability.

Meta-Analysis As many as possible, high-quality studies representing the current knowledge on a topic are screened by a meta-analysis to investigate a specified effect of a procedure. Each of the studies included in the final analysis reveals a certain contribution. In a simple meta-analysis, a common statistical measure applicable to all involved studies is identified, such as an effect size or a p-value, and a weighted average of that common measure is calculated by involving the sample sizes of the individual studies and possibly other factors, such as study quality. Thus, a meta-analysis performs 'a study on studies'; it aggregates information in order to achieve a higher statistical power (meaningfulness) for a research question of interest. Meta-analyses should elucidate why trial results differ, improve research and editorial standards by calling attention to the strengths and weaknesses of the research in an area and give practitioners a more objective view of the research literature.

One of the main fields where meta-analyses are performed is the evaluation of medical treatment effects. Here, the magnitude of a therapy effect obtained in a 'treatment situation' compared with a 'comparator situation' is quantified on the basis of a literature review. The studies are collapsed, their results are coded and the effect size of a treatment related to a defined outcome criterion is calculated by representing the difference in mean values between the study group and its comparator group. The effect size is a parameter that measures the extent of a change caused by an intervention. For example, there might be a significant difference between the outcomes of two treatments. This, however, does not give information on how much one treatment is more effective than the other; the latter is expressed by the effect size. A frequently used effect size is Cohen's d (Cohen 1988). It is considered to be small between 0.2 and 0.5, average between 0.5 and 0.8 and large above 0.8. An effect size that is calculated by comparing the pre- and post-treatment scores tends to produce a higher value than the comparison of active treatment versus a control situation because a placebo effect needs to be taken into consideration.

There are some usual criticisms uttered about systematic reviews and meta-analyses, that they sometimes fail to reflect the real-world interaction between evidence and action, and furthermore that they may have limited relevance or applicability and create potentially inappropriate over-reliance on their outcomes that could discourage innovation (Grimshaw et al. 2012; McCormack et al. 2013). Systematic reviews typically focus on the minimisation of bias. This often comes at the expense of the details related to the complexity and context of treatments bearing the danger of oversimplified and misleading interpretations. Therefore, explanatory approaches and refined models that investigate how certain therapy programmes work seem to be favourable. Because decisions need to be made about which interventions shall be implemented and how, even with a limited evidence base, there has been a call for the inclusion of broader types of evidence. Contemporary evidence-informed decision-making models advocate a combination of research evidence and clinical expertise, patient preferences and values and available resources (McCormack et al. 2013).

For example, over the past decade, mild and moderate temporary hearing loss of less than 40 dB, caused by otitis media with effusion (OME), has gained increasing attention. It is acknowledged that a prolonged hearing loss of 20 dB or even less may distort language development, necessitating treatment. However, systematic reviews and meta-analyses on the causal effects of OME on developmental language disorders have not confirmed this observation. They have been criticised because of systematic errors and because they are hardly generalisable for children with increased risk for language-relevant comorbidities. However, over time, subsequent reviews on this issue have been more cautious in their interpretations, included more complex outcome variables and considered more subgroup and contextual information.

A Cochrane review on the effect of grommets in children with OME (Lous et al. 2005) again did not show a noteworthy long-term effect on language development and other outcome variables, and the effect of grommets seemed to be small, in particular for facing potentially adverse effects. However, according to their cautious interpretation, the authors recommended an initial period of watchful waiting as appropriate management strategy for most children with OME. Because no evidence was available for subgroups of children with speech or language delays, with behavioural and learning problems or with clinical syndromes, practitioners were recommended to make treatment decisions for such children on the basis of other evidence and indications of disability related to hearing impairment. Furthermore, the authors identified a need for the determination of the most suitable variables, including more complex parameters such as measures of speech-in-noise and binaural hearing, and appropriate 'softer' outcomes to be the subject of interaction tests. The increasing knowledge gained on the consequences of OME and its treatment is a positive example on modern evidence-informed decision-making based on combined research evidence and clinical expertise.

Meta-analyses and systematic reviews have sometimes revealed conflicting and contradictory findings. However, their advantage is that all steps are clearly described, making the decision-process transparent, and errors may be prevented by thoughtful planned and interpreted analyses. This clearly overcomes the 'scientific nihilism' of eminence- and opinion-based evaluations of therapies and procedures.

Randomised Controlled Trial (RCT) An RCT is a defined design of a medical study and counts as the golden standard of a clinical trial. Clinical trials are prospective biomedical or behavioural studies on human subjects performed in order to answer specific research questions about biomedical or behavioural interventions, vaccines, dietary changes or devices, generating safety and efficacy information. An RTC tests the effectiveness or efficacy of different types of medical intervention within a cohort, a population of patients. Its main principle is to allocate patients randomly to one (or more) group(s) receiving either a specific treatment or an alternative treatment. The groups undergo therapy in exactly the same way with respect to procedures, tests, outpatient visits and follow-up calls, only differing in the essentials of the treatments under comparison.

2.3.3 Applications of EBM for Communication and Swallowing Disorders

Because randomised controlled trials are often difficult to perform for behavioural speech, language, voice and swallowing therapies, for example, owing to problems in establishing a control group with a long waiting period, and because procedures such as double-blinding are not feasible owing to the necessary interaction between therapist and patient, less rigorous study designs have to be accepted. Commonly, in clinical research methodological lax studies show better treatment effects than more strict ones and include a considerable bias. Nevertheless, the proof of effectiveness for the mentioned behavioural therapies is also required. This should be a precondition for the reimbursement of therapy costs by health insurance or governmental institutions. Patients are entitled to receive the best available and most effective treatment according to the current state of the art. However, in practical clinical life, the need or the voluntary obligation for provision of evidence of the effectiveness of an offered therapy is the exception rather than the rule. Nevertheless, it should become a regular constituent of daily routine.

Some major principles for calling a therapy effective and successful have been established for stuttering therapy and may also be extrapolated for other behavioural therapies of speech, language, voice and swallowing:

- A validation must have been performed with a sufficiently large and representative sample of treated subjects.
- Objective and eventual semi-objective criteria of the therapy success have to be available (e.g. for voice therapy, the results of an acoustic analysis and perceptual ratings by independent examiners. A subjective evaluation of the therapy outcome by the patient or the therapist alone is not sufficient).
- Repeated measures with valid and standardised tests or sufficient long voice/language samples of high-quality recordings are required.

- Evidence has to be revealed of a transfer of an improved voice/speech/language/communication mode to situations outside of the therapy situation.
- Evidence for the stability of a long-term benefit from the treatment has to be given. A period of 12 months after the last therapeutic intervention counts as minimum here; more favourable is a period of 18 months or 2 years.
- It has to be ensured by the involvement of sufficient control groups or conditions in the validation study of the therapy, that a reduction of symptoms is a consequence of the therapeutic intervention.
- The speech/language or voice of treated patients should sound natural and occur spontaneously after the treatment. This might hold true for voice disorders or speech fluency disorders. For other diseases such as aphasia, this criterion cannot always be fulfilled.
- A treated patient should be able to speak unworriedly, without the necessity of a continuous self-management of his or her vocalisation/communication.
- The treatment should not only improve speech/language/voice/speech fluency or communication in general but should also reduce the anxiety of speaking and should influence the expectations and self-esteem of a patient in a positive way.
- A reported success of a therapy must not be blown up by non-detected or non-reported drop-outs.
- The therapeutic method has to function with every qualified therapist, even if he or she has no special status, prestige or suggestive qualities.
- The method has to be successful even if it is not new and if the initial enthusiasm for it has gone.

For a therapy study, it is essential to choose an unbiased, representative sample, facing the fact that study samples on communication disorders are often relatively small and clinically based (as opposed to *population-based samples*).

Evidence-based medical progress requires the manual-accordant performance of standardised treatment methods (Euler et al. 2014). This is the only way to make different methods comparable or to make treatments that use the same method but are performed at different sites comparable. It also leaves the opportunity open for further systematic development of the treatment protocol. This rule is applicable for (1) specific therapy protocols, (2) single components of treatment or assessment and (3) general therapy concepts. So far, subjective-eclectically composed therapies constitute the mass rather than the exception in many European countries' scene of behavioural therapies of communication disorders. They may be effective in single cases or for specific therapists; however, this can neither be generalised, because of their lack of evidence, nor does it contribute to the cumulative increase of scientific knowledge.

In clinical routine, a meticulous and objective evaluation of the treatment success is time-consuming, costly and elaborate. Therefore, the provision of continuously updated information on evidence-based and standardised treatment concepts by manuals and guidelines, based on systematic reviews and meta-analyses, is one of the main tasks of professionals working in treatment research. On the other hand, the access and practical application of this information by the therapists is inevitable.

The field of treatment of communication disorders is characterised by large diversity. Consequently, some treatments applied traditionally may have no significant positive long-term effect. For example, in *stuttering therapy* it has been shown recently that the treatment most often prescribed in Germany, namely, a weekly session of individual treatment by a therapist, usually with an assorted package of mostly individually composed components, is of limited effectiveness (Euler et al. 2014). For other treatments there are not enough high-quality studies available to provide evidence of their effectiveness. This is, for example, the outcome of a systematic Cochrane review on the *application of botulinum toxin therapy for spasmodic dysphonia*, even if it seems to be counter-intuitive (Watts et al. 2006). These examples point once more to the necessity of performing high-quality studies if an intervention has the potential to become state of the art.

It is an important task of treatment research not only to add new procedures but also to delete those that have not been proven to be effective. Systematic reviews and meta-analyses are most helpful in verifying some kinds of intervention and falsifying others. For example, a systematic review on the effect of *different management strategies for dysphagic stroke patients* revealed that acupuncture, drug therapy, neuromuscular electrical stimulation, pharyngeal electrical stimulation, physical thermal or tactile stimulation, transcranial direct current stimulation and transcranial magnetic stimulation each had no significant effect on case fatality or the association of death and nonoral nutrition. However, behavioural interventions and acupuncture reduced dysphagia, and pharyngeal electrical stimulation reduced pharyngeal transit time. Moreover, compared with nasogastric tube feeding, percutaneous endoscopic gastrostomy (PEG) reduced treatment failures and gastrointestinal bleeding and led to higher feed delivery and albumin concentration, whereas nutritional supplementation was associated with reduced pressure sores and increased energy and protein intake (Geeganage et al. 2012).

As found for systematic reviews and meta-analyses on behavioural therapies of communication disorders, acceptable methodological criteria or sample sizes are often fulfilled only by a small minority of published studies. Thus, more research with sufficient methodology and large enough sample sizes to evaluate treatment effects reliably is necessary.

Some constituents of behavioural therapies of communication disorders have been shown to be efficient for specific disorders, for example, *prolonged speech for stuttering therapy* (Bothe et al. 2006; Euler et al. 2014). Others seem to be effectively applicable, such as intensive therapies, group therapies, management by programmed steps, practising of transfer into everyday life situations and of self-evaluation and the use of behaviour-dependent maintenance programmes, but a confirmation by systematic reviews and meta-analyses is often lacking.

For the treatment of *developmental disorders of speech and language*, a systematic review by Law et al. (2003) suggested that speech and language therapy is effective for children with phonological or vocabulary difficulties but that there is less evidence that interventions are effective for children with receptive difficulties. Mixed findings were reported concerning the effectiveness of expressive syntax interventions. No differences were shown between clinician-administered intervention and intervention implemented by trained parents, and studies did not reveal a difference between the effects of group and individual interventions. The use of normal language peers in therapy was described to have a positive effect on therapy outcome (Law et al. 2003). By contrast, a meta-analysis of Nelson et al. (2006) showed improvements for additional treated domains, including articulation, phonology, expressive and receptive language, lexical acquisition and syntax among children in all age groups studied and across multiple therapeutic settings. In general, studies of interventions of developmental language disorders are reported to be heterogeneous (Law et al. 2003; Nelson et al. 2006) and small, seem to be biased by plateau effects and report only short-term outcomes, which make interventions hardly comparable and generalisable (Nelson et al. 2006).

For *swallowing disorders*, an example for verification and falsification of different kinds of intervention by a systematic Cochrane review is given above (Geeganage et al. 2012). In particular neurogenically caused swallowing disorders are well examined by high-quality studies.

For the treatment of *voice disorders*, a Cochrane review on the effectiveness of therapies of functional voice disorders revealed that neither direct voice therapies nor indirect therapies alone were successful in the long run. Instead, the combination of direct and indirect therapy constituents has been shown to be effective (Ruotsalainen et al. 2007). This insight seems somewhat too unspecific to be helpful and is caused by the low quality of the contributing studies.

A manual-faithful procedure for the outcome assessment of voice therapies has been developed by the European Laryngological Society (ELS) as a multidimensional protocol. This protocol comprises five dimensions: perceptual voice evaluation, videostroboscopy, acoustic analysis, aerodynamic analysis and subjective rating by the patient using the Voice Handicap Index. Its validation in a retrospective multicentre study revealed largely satisfactory results for the validity, practicability and applicability of the ELS protocol for all 'common' voice disorders, but not for extreme voices such as substitution voices or spasmodic dysphonia. The five dimensions proved to be not redundant and were able selectively to differentiate pre-post changes among various aetiologies of voice disorders, various types of treatment and between genders (Dejonckere et al. 2001).

Systematic reviews and meta-analyses in the field of *hearing disorders* reflect clearly the restrictions of the applied methods but also the often too enthusiastic view of professionals on new, quickly developing technologies. Outcomes of those reviews are often counter-intuitive and disappointing, and authors usually complain about methodological flaws such as heterogeneity of studies restricting or preventing proper interpretation. For example, Vlastarakos et al. (2010) ran a systematic review and a meta-analysis on the effect of cochlear implantation in children under the first year of age and reported hardly generalisable outcomes for 10 of 125 identified children, and only 4 children showed a better outcome than children implanted under the age of 2 years. On the other hand, the examples of reviews on OME mentioned above demonstrate how the outcome of treatment studies may be improved by better suited outcome variables, a more integrated view on the results and their careful interpretation.

A good example of such an integrated view is intervention of stroke-induced *aphasia*. Here the authors of a systematic review found modest evidence for intensive treatment and constraint-induced language therapy on measures of language impairment and communication activity/participation and recommended the use of this knowledge in conjunction with clinical expertise and the client's individual values (Cherney et al. 2008).

For stuttering therapy it has been shown recently that fluency-shaping or stuttering-modification approaches, preferably with an intensive time schedule and in group sessions, were effective showing high effect sizes (Euler et al. 2014). Similar outcomes have been shown for *voice therapies of functional dysphonia*, where high satisfaction, greater attendance rates and significant improvements were found after treatment in intensive groups compared with conventional standard therapy once a week (Wenke et al. 2014). For stuttering, computer-based fluency biofeedback therapies, performed as 2- to 3-week intensive courses with a structured maintenance programme, have been shown to be effective (Cherney et al. 2008; Euler et al. 2014). The Australian Lidcombe therapy programme of stuttering in children is also a good example of an evidence-based intervention (Lattermann et al. 2008; Onslow 2015). Here, a consortium constantly evaluates components of the therapy, keeps the manual-faithful application of the programme under surveillance, assesses its long-term outcome and constantly refines and evaluates the treatment. A transfer of the knowledge from these commendable therapy concepts to interventions in other communication disorders appears useful.

2.4 Principles of Sterilisation and Disinfection of Medical Devices in Phoniatrics

Ojan Assadian

2.4.1 Transmission of Pathogens in Healthcare Settings

During diagnostic procedures or treatment in ear-nose-throat practice, patients can be exposed to a variety of exogenous microorganisms (bacteria, viruses, fungi and protozoa) from other patients, healthcare personnel or visitors. Other reservoirs include residual bacteria on the patient's skin, mucous membranes or respiratory tract and inanimate environmental surfaces or objects that have been linked to transmission of infection, such as adjacent and multiply touched surfaces, medical equipment or medications.

Without exception, transmission of infection requires the presence of three elements: a source, a susceptible target and a pathway for the transmission of microorganisms from the source to the target. The pathway can be direct or indirect. While the most important mode of transmission is probably by the hands of medical staff, contaminated and incorrectly reprocessed medical devices are important vehicles for indirect transmission of pathogens from one source to a new target. Indeed, a thorough review of more than 1000 outbreaks concluded that 12% of these had been caused by contaminated medical equipment (Gastmeier et al. 2005).

In view of this, it is not surprising that even unusual infections, such as an outbreak of otitis media caused by *Mycobacterium chelonae*, have occurred, transmitted through inadequately cleaned and disinfected otological instruments (Lowry et al. 1988). Outbreaks such as this highlight the need for adequate reprocessing of medical devices between examinations to prevent the transmission of microorganisms to patients.

2.4.2 Principles of Reprocessing of Medical Devices

Cleaning, disinfection and sterilisation of reusable medical devices are cornerstones of infection prevention and control in healthcare settings. Together, they are summarised under the term 'reprocessing'. Cleaning is the removal of all foreign material, such as dirt and organic material from a medical device. Cleaning generally removes rather than kills microorganisms. It is accomplished with water, detergents and mechanical action. The terms 'decontamination' and 'sanitation' may sometimes be used for this process. Sterilisation is the complete elimination of all forms of microorganisms, while disinfection eliminates chiefly all pathogenic microorganisms, with the exception of bacterial spores.

Either physical or chemical processes, or a combination of both, can achieve sterilisation. Pressured steam, dry heat and low temperature sterilisation processes (ethylene oxide gas, formaldehyde or plasma sterilisation) and liquid chemicals are the principal sterilising agents used today.

Disinfection is generally accomplished by the use of liquid chemicals or low-level physical processes. The efficacy of disinfection is affected by a number of factors, each of which may nullify or limit the efficacy of the process. Some of the factors that have been shown to affect disinfection efficacy are the previous cleaning of the object, the organic load on the object, the type and level of microbial contamination, the concentration of and exposure time to the germicide, the physical configuration of the object (e.g. crevices, hinges, lumina) and the temperature and pH of the disinfection process.

Furthermore, disinfection may be subdivided into high-level, intermediate-level and low-level disinfection. High-level disinfection methods destroy vegetative bacteria, mycobacteria, fungi and enveloped (lipid) and non-enveloped (nonlipid) viruses, but not necessarily bacterial spores. It is important to bear in mind that soiled instruments must be thoroughly cleaned before any disinfection process; otherwise organic residues may interfere with the disinfection process. Intermediate-level disinfection kills vegetative bacteria, most viruses and most fungi, but not resistant bacterial spores. Low-level disinfection kills most vegetative bacteria and some fungi as well as enveloped (lipid) viruses (e.g. hepatitis B, C, *hantavirus* and *HIV*). Low-level disinfection does not kill mycobacteria or bacterial spores. This method is typically used to clean environmental surfaces. Regrettably, there is no universally applicable reprocessing method. Selection of the method depends on a risk assessment, the expected microorganisms on an instrument and the physical properties of the instrument, such as potential for corrosion or instability to heat. The antimicrobial capacity reprocessing methods are summarised in Table 2.3.

In general, methods able effectively to kill microorganisms in Categories A (vegetative bacteria, fungi and enveloped virus) and B (*Mycobacterium sp.*, non-enveloped virus) are regarded as disinfection processes. They are ineffective against bacterial spores or protozoal cysts (Category C, spores of *Clostridium perfringens* Category D). Only sterilisation methods are able to kill bacterial spores.

Not all medical devices need to be sterilised. Unfortunately, this aspect is rarely considered, and substantial financial resources are wasted every year in practitioner's offices and hospitals because little attention is given to simple infection control principles for deciding the correct reprocessing method of medical devices.

Depending on the anatomical region of a patient's body, they may need to be cleansed, disinfected or sterilised (Table 2.4).

Table 2.3 Categories of microorganisms ranked from A to D in decreasing order of their susceptibility to destruction

A Fungi (*Candida* species, *Cryptococcus* species, *Aspergillus* species, dermatophytes)
Vegetative bacteria (*Staphylococcus aureus*, *Salmonella typhi, Pseudomonas aeruginosa*, coliforms)
Enveloped viruses (*herpes simplex virus, varicella-zoster virus, cytomegalovirus, measles virus, mumps virus, rubella virus, influenza virus, respiratory syncytial virus, hepatitis B and C viruses, hantavirus and human immunodeficiency virus*)

B Mycobacteria (*M. tuberculosis, M. avium-intracellulare, M. chelonae*)
Non-enveloped viruses (*coxsackievirus, poliovirus, rhinovirus, Norwalk-like virus, hepatitis A virus*)

C Bacterial spores (*B. subtitles, B. anthracis, C. tetani, C. difficile, C. botulinum*)
Protozoa with cysts (*Giardia lamblia, Cryptosporidium parvum*)

D Spores of *Clostridium perfringens*

The method of reprocessing depends on the category of a medical device, which can be non-critical, semi-critical or critical (Rutala 1996; Rutala and Weber 2013). Medical devices that will enter sterile tissue, the vascular system or the inner ear are considered 'critical' and must be sterile when used on a patient. Examples include, but are not limited to, surgical ear, nose and throat instruments, implants, intravenous fluids or needles used for administration of i.v. fluids. Critical items must be sterilised.

'Semi-critical' medical devices are objects that come in contact with mucous membranes or with non-intact skin. Most instruments used in the ear, nose and throat belong to this category. Such instruments must be free of all pathogenic microorganisms; however, bacterial spores or non-pathogenic microorganisms such as the typical microbial flora of healthy hands may be present. Intact mucous membranes are, to a certain extent, more resistant to infection by common bacterial spores or bacteria found in the environment yet are susceptible to other organisms, such as *Staphylococcus aureus*, pathogenic streptococci, tubercle bacilli or viruses. Respiratory therapy equipment, laryngoscopes, endoscopes or specula are typical ear, nose and throat instruments included in this category. Semi-critical medical devices require adequate disinfection. Legally, it must be noted that medical devices labelled 'single-use' disposables by the manufacturer must not be reprocessed.

Finally, medical devices that only come in contact with intact skin are considered to be 'noncritical'. Such medical devices require thorough cleaning or low-level disinfection. Examples include, but are not limited to, bedpans, stethoscopes, blood pressure cuffs, crutches, bed rails, linens and furniture.

Table 2.4 Classification scheme for medical devices (modified according to Rutala 1996)

Classification		Example	Reprocessing method
Critical instruments	Penetrate sterile tissue, enter sterile anatomic regions or contact patient's blood	Implants, i.v. Catheters, biopsy forceps, scalpels	Sterilisation
Semi-critical instruments	Contact mucous membranes or non-intact skin	Rhino-laryngoscopes, nasopharyngeal laryngoscopes, blades and handles of rigid endoscopes	Disinfection
Noncritical instruments	Only contact intact skin	Blood pressure cuffs, stethoscopes, bedpans, examination beds	Cleaning

2.4.3 Legal Aspects of Reprocessing and European Directives

For many decades a simple strategy was followed: manufacturers of medical devices had optimised their product for the intended application without paying any consideration to its ability to be reprocessed. Medical practitioners purchased such instruments and cleaned and reprocessed them 'as well as possible' in good faith that the method applied would 'do the job'. With the latest publication of the European Council's Directive 93/42/EEC in 1993 (European Commission 1993), which—among others—is also the basis for reprocessing of medical devices, this situation has changed.

Annex I, clause 8.1 clearly stipulates that:

> ... medical devices ... must be designed and manufactured in such a way that, when used under the conditions and for the purposes intended, they will not compromise the clinical condition or the safety of patients, or the safety and health of users or, where applicable, other persons, provided that any risks which may be associated with their intended use constitute acceptable risks when weighed against the benefits to the patient and are compatible with a high level of protection of health and safety.

The meaning of this sentence is that an instrument must be designed and operated in such a manner that any risk is reduced to the minimum, including the risk of transmission of microorganisms.

For both users and manufacturers, clause 13.6 (h) may be most important: this section dictates that any reusable medical device must come with appropriate instructions for use, which must contain information on:

> ... the appropriate process to allow reuse, including cleaning, disinfection, packaging and, where appropriate, the method of sterilisation ... and the number of times of reuse.

While this regulation generally is a major step forward towards increased patient safety, new challenges pertaining to correct reprocessing of medical devices have emerged. First, medical practitioners might not reprocess their instruments by following empirically implemented methods, and health authorities must check whether reprocessing follows scientifically accepted and validated methods. Sometimes, this may cause difficulties, since there may be debate on the methods used, and this requirement is always associated with increased costs for healthcare providers, owing to investment in cleaning/disinfecting machines or autoclaves.

Second, the European Council has made it very clear that the manufacturer of medical devices has equal obligations in this context and must provide appropriate instructions for use, including reprocessing of reusable instruments. By looking into most instructions for the use of any type of medical device, it quickly becomes apparent that even two decades after stipulation of the European Council's Directive 93/42/EEC (European Commission 1993), most medical device manufacturers seem to be unaware of their duty to provide adequate information on reprocessing. The example of a medical device used in phoniatrics, a video-fibre laryngoscope, highlights the current difficulties: under the chapter 'cleaning/safety' the manufacturer states:

> To make the unit sanitary, you need to take a soft cloth and a mild soap detergent. Wipe down the entire unit and make sure every part is cleaned. As long as the unit is in good working condition and not damaged this procedure shall be sufficient. If you are concerned about infection, it is recommended not to consider re-using the unit.

Clearly, such instructions for use are legally safe for the manufacturer, however, not truly helpful for users. Matters have become even more complex. If a medical practitioner were to decide to reprocess this device differently from the provided instruction, the user would immediately lose the equipment's warranty.

However, it is important to keep in mind that the EC Directive 93/42/EEC stipulated only general principles, which had to be translated into national law by the various European Union's member states. Therefore, a number of differences and variations exist within the European Union, which are impossible to discuss in detail within a book section. Medical practitioners or medical administrators in charge of managing their medical institutions are, therefore, advised to seek information for reprocessing medical devices according to the national laws and regulations of their own state.

It seems that while medical practitioners, medical societies and representing associations are currently discussing how reprocessing should be performed and financed in economically difficult times, one important partner in this matter is overlooked: the manufacturer, who is required to provide adequate information on his product. Therefore, before the next expensive medical device is purchased, the user should specifically ask the manufacturer if the device is intended for reuse, and which specific methods for reprocessing should be applied. If phrases such as 'mild detergent', 'soft cloth' or 'do not use the following' are depicted in a medical device's instructions for use, without specifically stating applicable methods, the user may consider looking for an alternative on the European market or should consult experts from their own central sterile service department, if available.

References

American Psychiatric Association (ed) (2013) Manual of mental disorders, 5th edn. American Psychiatric Association, Arlington

American Speech-Language-Hearing Association (2017) Functional goal writing using ICF. Available via http://www.asha.org/slp/icf/. Accessed 24 July 2017

Bothe AK, Davidow JH, Bramlett RE et al (2006) Stuttering treatment research 1970-2005: I. Systematic review incorporating trial quality assessment of behavioral, cognitive, and related approaches. Am J Speech Lang Pathol 15(4):321–341

Cherney LR, Patterson JP, Raymer A et al (2008) Evidence-based systematic review: effects of intensity of treatment and constraint-induced language therapy for individuals with stroke-induced aphasia. J Speech Lang Hear Res 51(5):1282–1299

Cohen J (1988) Statistical power analysis for the behavioral sciences, 2nd edn. Lawrence Erlbaum, Hillsdale

Dejonckere PH, Bradley P, Clemente P et al (2001) A basic protocol for functional assessment of voice pathology, especially for investigating the efficacy of (phonosurgical) treatments and evaluating new assessment techniques. Guideline elaborated by the Committee on Phoniatrics of the European Laryngological Society (ELS). Eur Arch Otorhinolaryngol 258(2):77–82

Dineen T (1998) Manufacturing victims. Robert Davies Multimedia Publishing, Bel Air

EU Commission (2003a) European disability strategy 2010-2020, SEC(2010) 1323, SEC(2010) 1324

EU Commission (2003b) Report on the current situation in relation to occupational diseases' systems in EU Member States and EFTA/EEA countries, in particular relative to Commission Recommendation 2003/670/EC. EU 2013

EU Commission (2003c) Commission recommendation of 19 September 2003 concerning the European schedule of occupational diseases (Text with EEA relevance) (notified under document number C(2003) 3297). OJEU L 238 vol 46, pp 28–34. Available via http://eur-lex.europa.eu/legal-content/EN/TXT/PDF/?uri=CELEX:32003H0670&from=EN. Accessed 21 Dec 2016

EU European Council (1989) Directive on the introduction of measures to encourage improvements in the safety and health of workers at work. 89/391/EEC

EU European Council (1993) Directive 93/42/EEC of 14 June 1993 concerning medical devices. Available via http://www.mdss.com/pdf/MDD93_42EEC.pdf. Accessed 7 April 2019

Euler HA, Lange BP, Schroeder S et al (2014) The effectiveness of stuttering treatments in Germany. J Fluen Disord 39(1):1–11

European Agency for Safety and Health at Work's Topic Centre OSH (2013) Occupational safety and health and education: a whole-school approach. Publications Office of the European Union, Luxembourg

European Parliament and the Council of the European Union (2011) Directive on the application of patients' rights in cross-border healthcare. 2011/24/EU. Available via http://eur-lex.europa.eu/legal-content/EN/TXT/?uri=celex%3A32011L0024. Accessed 21 Dec 2016

European Union (2007) The treaty on the functioning of the European Union. 9.5.2008 EN Official Journal of the European Union C 115/47. Consolidated version of the Treaty on the Functioning of the European Union, 13 December 2007, 2008/C 115/47″. Available via http://www.refworld.org/docid/4b17a07e2.html. Accessed 21 Dec 2016

Gastmeier P, Stamm-Balderjahn S, Hansen S et al (2005) How outbreaks can contribute to prevention of nosocomial infection: analysis of 1,022 outbreaks. Infect Control Hosp Epidemiol 26(4):357–361

Geeganage C, Beavan J, Ellender S et al (2012) Interventions for dysphagia and nutritional support in acute and subacute stroke. Cochrane Database Syst Rev (10):CD000323. Accessed 1 May 2016

Grimshaw JM, Eccles MP, Lavis JN et al (2012) Knowledge translation of research findings. Implement Sci 7(1):50–57

ICF Research Branch (2013) ICF-based documentation tool. Available via http://www.icf-core-sets.org. Accessed 24 July 2017

Illum ON, Gradel KO (2015) Assessing children with disabilities using WHO International Classification of Functioning, Disability and Health Child and Youth

Version Activities and Participation D Codes. Child Neurol Open 2(4):1–9

International Labour Organization (2010) ILO list of occupational diseases (revised 2010). Available via http://www.ilo.org/safework/info/publications/WCMS_125137/lang%2D%2Den/index.htm. Accessed 21 Dec 2016

Larkins B (2007) The application of the ICF in cognitive-communication disorders following traumatic brain injury. Semin Speech Lang 28(4):334–342

Lattermann C, Euler HA, Neumann K (2008) A randomised control trial to investigate the impact of the Lidcombe Program on early stuttering in German-speaking preschoolers. J Fluen Disord 33(1):52–65

Law J, Garrett Z, Nye C (2003) Speech and language therapy interventions for children with primary speech and language delay or disorder. Cochrane Database Syst Rev (3):CD004110. Accessed 1 May 2016

Lous J, Burton MJ, Felding JU et al (2005) Grommets (ventilation tubes) for hearing loss associated with otitis media with effusion in children. Cochrane Database Syst Rev (1):CD001801. Accessed 1 May 2016

Lowry PW, Jarvis WR, Oberle AD et al (1988) Mycobacterium chelonae causing otitis media in an ear-nose-and-throat practice. N Engl J Med 319(15):978–982

McCormack B, Rycroft-Malone J, Decorby K et al (2013) A realist review of interventions and strategies to promote evidence-informed healthcare: a focus on change agency. Implement Sci 8(1):107

Moerman MBJ, Dejonckere PH, Lieftink AF (2008) Comparación de los trastornos de la voz con el Voice Handicap Inventory Index (Comparing voice pathologies with the Voice Handicap Index: Is a weighting factor required?) Sociedad Iberoamericana de Informacion Cientifica 20.03.2008. Salud(i)Ciencia 16:407–410

Nelson HD, Nygren P, Walker M et al (2006) Screening for speech and language delay in preschool children: systematic evidence review for the US Preventive Services Task Force. Pediatrics 117(2):e298–e319

Onslow M (2015) Stuttering and its treatment: eleven lectures. Available via http://sydney.edu.au/health-sciences/asrc/docs/eleven_lectures.pdf. Accessed 6 May 2015

Ruotsalainen JH, Sellman J, Lehto L et al (2007) Interventions for treating functional dysphonia in adults. Cochrane Database Syst Rev (3):CD006373. Accessed 1 May 2016

Rutala WA (1996) APIC guideline for selection and use of disinfectants. Am J Infect Control 24(4):313–342

Rutala WA, Weber DJ (2013) New developments in reprocessing semicritical items. Am J Infect Control 41(5 suppl):S60–S66

Schindler A, Manassero A, Dao M et al (2002) The β-2 draft of the international classification of impairment, disabilities and handicap. Application to communication disorders. Eur Medicophys 38(3):123–129

Schneider E, Paoli P, Brun E (2005) Noise in figures. European Agency for Safety and Health at Work, Office for Official Publications of the European Communities, Luxembourg

The Canadian Interorganizational Steering Group for Speech Language Pathology and Audiology (2012) Canadian guidelines on auditory processing disorder in children and adults: assessment and intervention. Available via http://www.ooaq.qc.ca/publications/doc-documents/Canadian_Guidelines_EN.pdf. Accessed 24 July 2017

Threats TT (2006) Towards an international framework for communication disorders: use of the ICF. J Commun Disord 39(4):251–265

United Nations (2006) Convention on the rights of persons with disabilities and optional protocol. Available via https://www.un.org/development/desa/disabilities/convention-on-the-rights-of-persons-with-disabilities.html. Accessed 21 Dec 2016

Vlastarakos PV, Proikas K, Papacharalampous G et al (2010) Cochlear implantation under the first year of age - the outcomes. A critical systematic review and meta-analysis. Int J Pediatr Otorhinolaryngol 74(2):119–126

Washington KN (2007) Using the ICF within speech-language pathology: application to developmental language impairment. Adv Speech Lang Pathol 9(3):242–255

Watts C, Nye C, Whurr R (2006) Botulinum toxin for treating spasmodic dysphonia (laryngeal dystonia): a systematic Cochrane review. Clin Rehabil 20(2):112–122

Wenke RJ, Stabler P, Walton C et al (2014) Is more intensive better? Client and service provider outcomes for intensive versus standard therapy schedules for functional voice disorders. J Voice 28(5):652.e31. pii: S0892-1997(14)00039-3

World Health Organization (1992) International statistical classification of diseases and related health problems, 10th Revision (ICD-10). WHO, Geneva

World Health Organization (2001) International classification of functioning, disability and health. Available via http://apps.who.int/gb/archive/pdf_files/WHA54/ea54r21.pdf?ua=1. Accessed 2 Dec 2017

World Health Organization (2002) Towards a common language for functioning, disability and health. Available via http://www.who.int/classifications/icf/icfbeginnersguide.pdf. Accessed 24 July 2017

World Health Organization (2006) Constitution of the World Health Organization. Basic documents (45 ed Supplement). WHO, Geneva

World Health Organization (2007a) International classification of functioning, disability, and health: children and youth version (ICF-CY). WHO, Geneva

World Health Organization (2007b) ICF Checklist: version 2.1a, clinician form. Available via http://www.who.int/classifications/icf/training/icfchecklist.pdf. Accessed 24 July 2017

World Health Organization (2010) The world health report - health systems financing: the path to universal coverage. WHO, Geneva

World Health Organization (2016) ICD-10: 2016 International statistical classification of diseases and related health problems, 10th Revision. Available via http://apps.who.int/classifications/icd10/browse/2016/en. Accessed 22 Nov 2017

World Health Organization (2017a) Classifications and standards. Available via http://www.who.int/research-observatory/classifications/en/. Accessed 24 July 2017

World Health Organization (2017b) The 11th revision of the International Classification of Diseases (ICD-11). Available via http://www.who.int/classifications/icd/revision/en/. Accessed 24 July 2017

Yaruss JS (2007) Application of the ICF in fluency disorders. Semin Speech Lang 28(4):312–322

Basics of Related Medical Disciplines

3

Hanno J. Bolz, Tiemo Grimm, Gereon Heuft,
Christian Postert, Georg Romer, Eva Seemanova,
Esther Strittmatter, Dagmar Weise,
and Klaus Zerres

3.1 Basics of Genetics and the Clinical Impact of Genetic Testing in Patients with Hearing Impairment

Hanno J. Bolz

3.1.1 Prevalence and Genetic Heterogeneity

Hearing impairment is the most common sensory disorder, affecting approximately 1 in 500 newborns. In developed countries, most cases of early-onset hearing loss are of genetic origin. The complexity of hearing is reflected by the extensive

H. J. Bolz
Senckenberg Centre for Human Genetics,
Frankfurt am Main, Germany
e-mail: h.bolz@senckenberg-humangenetik.de

T. Grimm
Department of Human Genetics, Biocenter,
University of Würzburg, Würzburg, Germany
e-mail: tgrimm@biozentrum.uni-wuerzburg.de

G. Heuft
Department of Psychosomatics and Psychotherapy,
University Clinic Münster, Münster, Germany
e-mail: gereon.heuft@ukmuenster.de

C. Postert
Department of Applied Health Sciences, University
of Applied Health Science, Bochum, Germany
e-mail: Christian.Postert@hs-gesundheit.de

G. Romer
Klinik für Kinder- und Jugendpsychiatrie,
-psychosomatik und –psychotherapie,
Univeritätsklinikum Münster, Münster, Germany
e-mail: sekre.romer@ukmuenster.de

E. Seemanova
Department of Child Neurology, 2nd Medical School
of Charles University Prague,
Prague, Czech Republic
e-mail: Eva.seemanova@lfmotol.cuni.cz

E. Strittmatter
Health Care Centre Walstedde Day Hospital,
Drensteinfurt, Germany
e-mail: esther.strittmatter@web.de

D. Weise
Abteilung Neuropädiatrie, Universitätsmedizin
Göttingen, Göttingen, Germany
e-mail: dweise@med.uni-goettingen.de

K. Zerres
Institute of Human Genetics, University Clinic
RWTH Aachen, Aachen, Germany
e-mail: kzerres@ukaachen.de

© Springer-Verlag GmbH Germany, part of Springer Nature 2020
A. am Zehnhoff-Dinnesen et al. (eds.), *Phoniatrics I*, European Manual of Medicine,
https://doi.org/10.1007/978-3-662-46780-0_3

genetic heterogeneity of deafness (http://hereditaryhearingloss.org), with about a hundred known causative genes and probably many more to be identified. In 70% of hearing-impaired neonates, the sensory deficit is non-syndromic (non-syndromic hearing loss, NSHL) (Hilgert et al. 2009; Parker and Bitner-Glindzicz 2015; Van Camp and Smith 2015). Deafness is also part of several hundred syndromes.

3.1.2 Modes of Inheritance

All Mendelian traits can be observed. Regarding the non-syndromic forms of hearing loss, autosomal recessive inheritance (autosomal recessive non-syndromic hearing loss, ARNSHL) is most common, accounting for approximately 80% of cases. In individuals with ARNSHL, both copies (alleles) of the underlying gene are mutated, while the parents are healthy mutation carriers (heterozygosity, the mutation is present in only one copy of the gene; Fig. 3.1a). The risk for hearing loss in children of such carrier parents is 25%. Depending on the size of the family, hearing loss may occur sporadically ('simplex patients') or in several siblings at the most, but usually not 'vertically' in subsequent generations. ARNSHL is particularly common in countries with high rates of parental consanguinity (e.g. North African and Middle East countries).

Approximately 20% of patients have autosomal dominant non-syndromic hearing loss (ADNSHL), which is typically post-lingual and progressive. In ADNSHL, hearing loss already occurs when only one allele carries the mutation

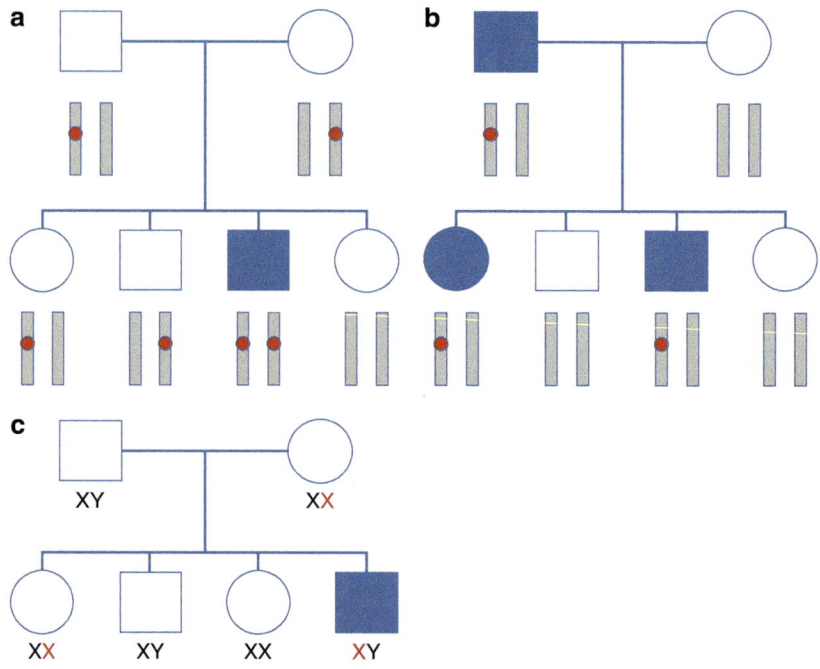

Fig. 3.1 Mendelian modes of inheritance observed in hearing loss. (**a**) Autosomal recessive; (**b**) autosomal dominant; (**c**) X-linked inheritance. Circles, female individuals; squares, male individuals. Horizontal connections indicate partnerships. Symbols of children are horizontally arranged below the parents. Solid symbols, affected individuals. Open symbols, unaffected individuals. Grey bars below individuals in A and B represent the two copies of autosomal deafness genes. 'X' and 'Y' in C stand for the sex chromosomes. Red dots and red X indicate presence of deafness-causing mutation

(Fig. 3.1b). The recurrence risk for offspring of affected persons is 50%.

X-linked hearing loss (XNSHL) is caused by mutations on the X chromosome and therefore primarily affects males; heterozygous (female) carriers usually have normal hearing. XNSHL is very rare (<1%) (Fig. 3.1c).

Moreover, hearing loss may—very rarely—result from mutations of mitochondrial DNA. Because mitochondria are exclusively inherited maternally, transmission occurs only through affected females whose children will all be affected.

3.1.3   Molecular Genetic Testing

Conventional DNA Sequencing (Sanger Sequencing) Because of the extensive genetic heterogeneity of hearing impairment, the identification of the causative mutation in patients has been the exception until recently. The exons are the protein-coding parts of genes and harbour more than 80% of disease-causing mutations, and they therefore represent the regions of primary diagnostic interest. Because they are interrupted by the non-coding introns, genetic testing has so far required the laborious individual amplification and conventional sequencing ('Sanger sequencing') of all exons of a gene of interest. For all currently known deafness genes, this amounts to more than 1500 exons, and

comprehensive genetic analysis has therefore not been possible so far.

3.1.4   High-Throughput Sequencing (Next-Generation Sequencing): A Breakthrough in Diagnostics

Bypassing the Bottleneck of Conventional Sequencing With the advent of next-generation sequencing (NGS), a term being applied for various high-throughput DNA sequencing technologies (van Dijk et al. 2014), deafness genes have finally become accessible to comprehensive analysis and routine testing (Rehm 2013). In short, NGS allows simultaneous targeted sequencing of all genes of interest ('gene panels': up to hundreds or even thousands of genes, depending on the applied technology and the capacity of the respective NGS platform) in many patients. Basically, the genes of interest (in most cases, only their exons; see above) are captured by hybridisation with synthetic oligonucleotides from the patient's fragmented genome (which is present 'in a few copies' after DNA extraction from peripheral blood), followed by amplification and massively parallel sequencing. Samples from many patients can be pooled owing to the use of sequence barcodes ligated to the fragments (Fig. 3.2). On a platform with sufficient capacity, all deafness genes can be sequenced in multiple

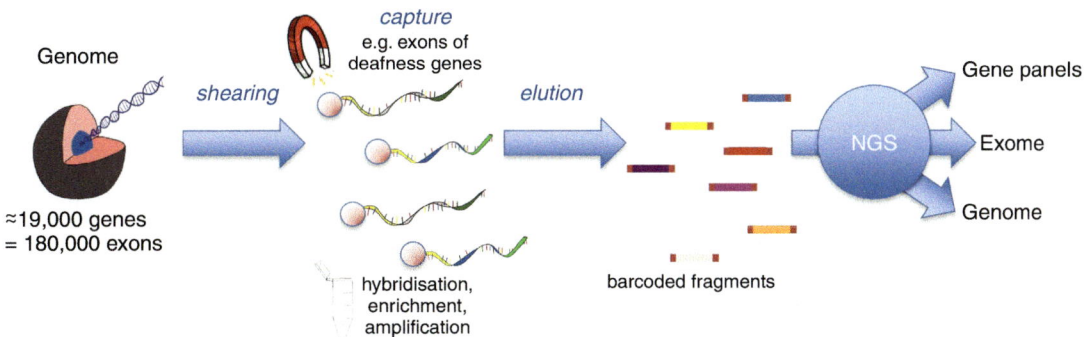

Fig. 3.2 Workflow scheme of next-generation sequencing (NGS)

patients (often 24 patients, depending on the applied barcodes) simultaneously.

Dramatically Increased Diagnostic Yield NGS has begun to transform not only the field of medical genetics but medicine as a whole. In our experience, targeted NGS of all known deafness genes, including those for the clinically most important and prevalent syndromes, identifies the molecular basis of the sensory deficit in more than 60% of the patients (in both autosomal dominant and autosomal recessive forms).

With NGS increasingly being applied for genetic diagnostics of hearing loss, the true distribution of mutations across the genes is now becoming known. This in turn helps in prioritising genes when carrying out genetic testing via conventional (Sanger) sequencing—which is important because not every laboratory can afford

the expensive NGS infrastructure and because healthcare providers do not yet generally reimburse NGS-based testing.

Quantification of NGS Data Uncovers Hidden Structural Mutations To obtain reliable results, every nucleotide of a deafness gene is sequenced repetitively—resulting in a high coverage consisting of multiple sequence reads (Fig. 3.3). In analyses based on PCR amplification followed by Sanger sequencing, large structural mutations—for example, whole-exon deletions—cannot be detected if present on only one of the two gene copies: in such cases, PCR amplicons and (normal) sequences are derived from the exon of the unaffected gene copy. Quantitative analyses to detect deletions or duplications of one or more exons have so far depended on the commercial availability of MLPA kits (MLPA, multiple ligation-dependent

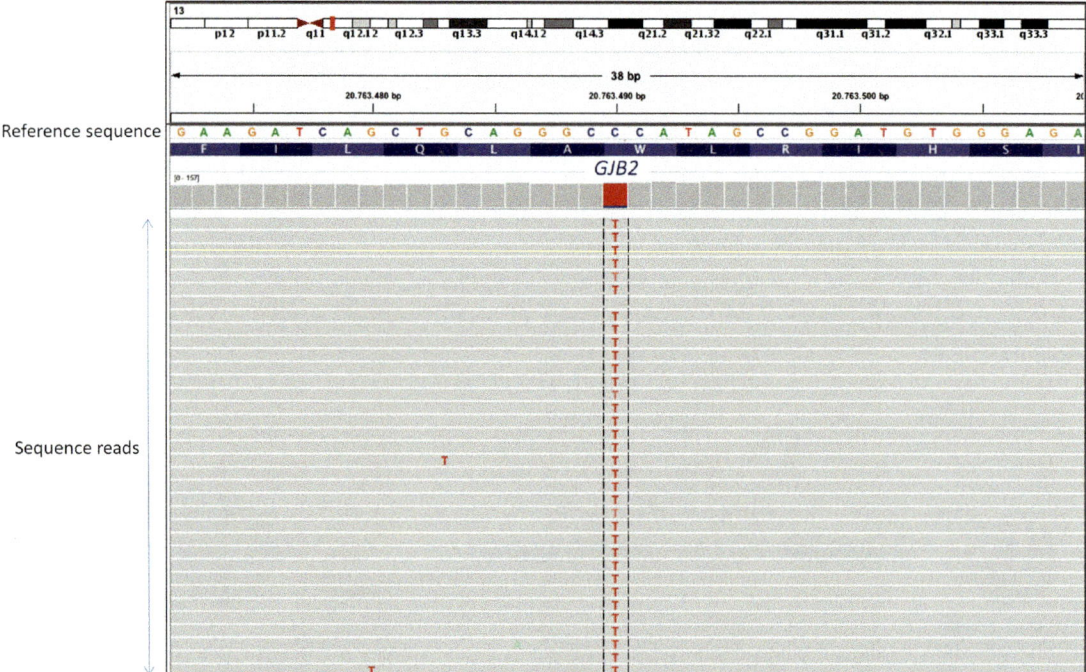

Fig. 3.3 A Schematic representation of the mapped sequencing reads (reverse strand) visualised with the Integrative Genomics Viewer (IGV) for a patient with non-syndromic deafness due to a *homozygous* nonsense mutation (p.Trp77*) of the *GJB2* gene. The c.231G > A mutation (C > T on the reverse strand displayed here) is present in virtually all reads covering this region of the gene

probe amplification, a variation of the PCR method that measures the copy number of the exons of a target gene). Because MLPA kits exist for only a small fraction of known deafness genes and MLPA analyses are usually carried out gene-by-gene, this method is not suited for comprehensive genetic diagnostics in hearing loss patients.

In contrast, quantification of NGS reads can be implemented into bioinformatic pipelines and may reliably detect structural mutations (Eisenberger et al. 2013) in all deafness genes present in the panel: heterozygous loss of one (or multiple) exons results in a reduction of generated sequence reads, corresponding to approximately 50% of the expected number (Fig. 3.4), while a homozygous deletion results in a failure to generate reads.

3.1.5 The Relevance of an Early Genetic Diagnosis in Hearing Loss: The Role of NGS

Although the identification of the genetic basis of the hearing deficit is still the exception in most patients, it is crucial, especially in newborns and infants, to provide effective medical care for several reasons.

Identification of Syndromes Before Manifestation of Extra-cochlear Symptoms Without a genetic diagnosis, children with hearing loss of then unknown aetiology should, in their first decade of life, regularly be investigated by different specialists, at least including ophthalmologists (for Usher syndrome), cardiologists (for Jervell and Lange-

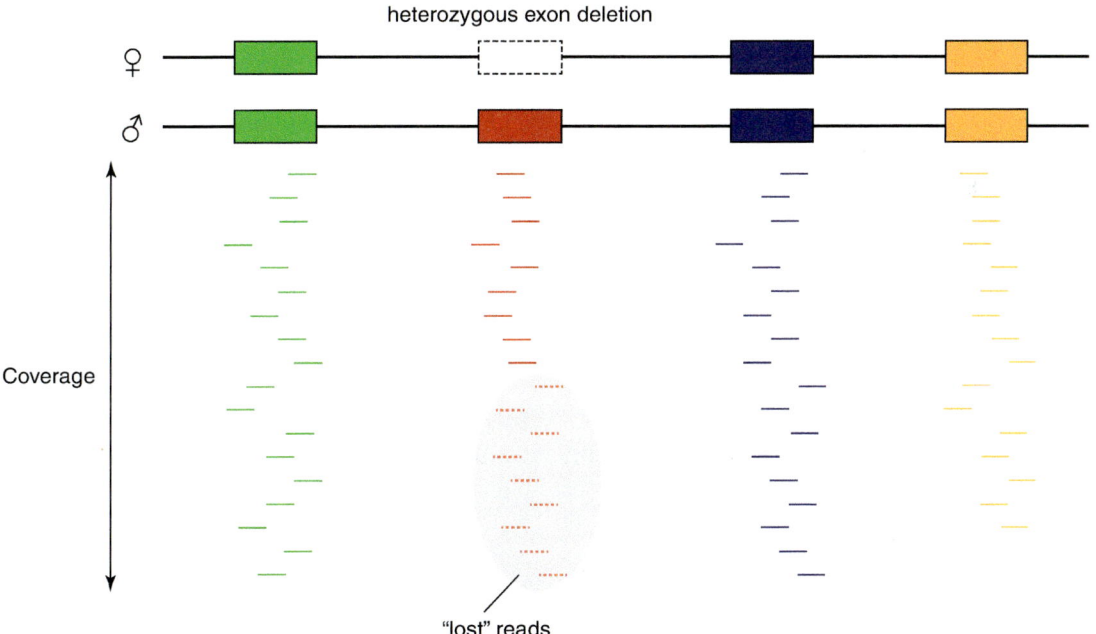

Fig. 3.4 Quantitative readout of NGS data. Unlike Sanger sequencing, NGS is capable of unmasking large structural mutations such as deletions of one or several exons. Every cell contains two copies of every autosomal gene, a maternal and a paternal copy. Boxes represent the exons that undergo targeted enrichment. The coverage, consisting of sequenced reads that redundantly cover every exonic position, is shown below. In this example, the red exon is deleted on the maternal gene copy. As a consequence, only about half of the normal read number will be generated for the red exon, compared with the respective exon in control samples and to the neighbouring exons. The bioinformatic pipeline can reliably detect the ~50% reduction of NGS reads in such patients

Nielsen syndrome), nephrologists (for Alport syndrome) and endocrinologists (for Pendred syndrome). This results in significant economic costs for the healthcare system but also in a considerable psychological burden for the patients and their parents.

If a mutation is found in a 'non-syndromic gene', there is no need for comprehensive follow-up by other medical disciplines. On the other hand, if the mutation predicts syndromic hearing loss, the parents know which specialist (besides the paedaudiologist) should be consulted:

- About 10% of children with apparently non-syndromic congenital or early-onset hearing loss have Usher syndrome and develop retinal degeneration at an older age (in the first decade in Usher syndrome type 1 or in the second decade in type 2). The identification of mutations in an Usher syndrome gene thus predicts severe visual impairment (potentially ending up in blindness) with currently no therapeutic option and therefore is important information for the parents when considering cochlear implantation versus hearing aids.

- Another important example is Jervell and Lange-Nielsen syndrome (JLNS), a condition resulting from mutations in the genes *KCNQ1* and *KCNE1*: JLNS patients initially appear to have non-syndromic hearing loss. Often, the first clinical manifestation of the accompanying arrhythmia is sudden cardiac death. This may affect several children in a family before it is realised that deafness in such families signals the risk of sudden death. Thus, the identification of *KCNQ1/KCNE1* mutations by comprehensive NGS-based testing of deafness genes in newborns with hearing loss must result in follow-up by a cardiologist, which is potentially life-saving. Importantly, the overall prevalence of JLNS is low but higher in populations where consanguinity is common. In view of increasing migration from Middle East countries into Europe, paedaudiologists should be aware of this syndrome.

- Patients with apparently recessive non-syndromic hearing loss may have mutations in

SLC26A4, the gene associated with Pendred syndrome. These patients may develop (or already have) goitre with hypothyroidism, requiring levothyroxine treatment to ensure normal somatic and mental development. Moreover, the patients usually have enlarged vestibular aqueducts and endolymphatic sacs and anatomical abnormalities of the cochleae (Mondini dysplasia). They should therefore avoid activities that can lead to minor head trauma (e.g. contact sports, etc.).

Disentanglement of Complex Genetic Causes Disease may be due to mutations in more than one gene, especially in offspring of consanguineous partnerships. For example, deaf-blindness is not always caused by mutations in one of the Usher syndrome genes. It may also reflect an overlap of non-syndromic deafness and non-syndromic retinal degeneration, resulting from independent mutations of a deafness gene (e.g. *OTOA*) on one hand and a retinal dystrophy gene (e.g. *NR2E3*) on the other—together mimicking a syndromic condition. Disentangling such constellations has a major impact on genetic counselling. In the given example, instead of an Usher syndrome recurrence risk of 25% for further offspring, there are separate recurrence risks: 25% for either deafness or retinal degeneration and 6.25% for the combination of both (presenting like Usher syndrome).

Identification of Potentially Treatable Conditions Mutations in PEX genes cause peroxisome biogenesis disorders (PBD), including Refsum syndrome, a metabolic condition very similar to Usher syndrome. Comprehensive NGS-based panel analysis may identify the Refsum syndrome patients among those with apparent Usher syndrome (Zaki et al. 2016). Importantly, and in contrast to Usher syndrome and other deaf-blindness disorders, therapeutic options do exist for patients with mild PBD, who may benefit from a phytanic acid-restricted diet and extracorporeal lipid apheresis (Kohlschütter et al. 2012; Baldwin et al. 2010; Ruether et al. 2010).

3.1.6 Newborn Hearing Screening Should Be Supplemented by Comprehensive Genetic Testing

In view of the impact that an early genetic diagnosis has on the clinical management of patients and with the availability of comprehensive genetic testing with NGS of large gene panels, such genetic analyses should become part of the diagnostic workup in newborns and infants who fail hearing screening.

3.2 Genetic Counselling

Tiemo Grimm, Eva Seemanova, and Klaus Zerres

3.2.1 Introduction

The expanding knowledge in human genetics has led to practical applications at an increasing rate in genetic counselling. Conventional and invasive diagnostic procedures have been complemented or entirely replaced by genetic testing. DNA tests allow the prediction of diseases and the modification of risk figures. With increasing numbers of both diagnostic and predictive genetic tests available, genetic counselling is becoming more important in clinical practice.

Genetic counselling is an important area of applied human genetics. Patients request advice or are referred by their physicians for counselling in order to understand biological facts, medical implications and recurrence risks of genetic diseases (Fletcher et al. 1985; Fuhrmann and Vogel 1983; Harper 2010; Resta 2006; Speicher et al. 2010).

3.2.2 Definition of Genetic Counselling

Genetic counselling refers to the totality of activities that:

- Establish the diagnosis.
- Assess the recurrence risk.

- Communicate the likelihood of recurrence to the patient and family.
- Provide information regarding the many problems raised by the disease and its natural history, including the potential medical, economic, psychological and social burdens.
- Provide information regarding potential reproductive options, including prenatal diagnosis.
- Provide referral of patients to appropriate specialists.

The range of problems and questions arising during genetic counselling covers a wide area. Generally, not all patients and families turn out to have classical genetic illnesses, such as monogenic diseases or chromosomal aberrations. Many consultations deal with various birth defects, mental retardation, delayed development, dysmorphic-looking children, short stature and similar problems that may or may not have a genetic cause.

3.2.3 Indications of Genetic Counselling

Important questions in genetic counselling are as follows:

Birth of a Child with a Congenital or Developmental Disorder If a child with birth defects or developmental delay is born to healthy parents, the most common question concerns the risk to any other of their children.

A Parent Is Affected The illness of a parent is a frequent concern leading to the question of recurrence risk in the parents' children. If the person consulting is affected or even pregnant, the question of the impact of pregnancy on the course of the disease is another important issue.

Diseases or Developmental Disorders in Relatives of an Affected Person As a rule, this situation requires communication with multiple members of a family. Careful pedigree analysis and risk calculations frequently yield relatively low risks. The issue of predictive testing for late-onset diseases in unaffected but at-risk family members must be considered carefully.

Age Risks Owing to an increasing number of pregnancies in women of advanced age in Western societies, the demand for counselling in this topic is increasing. Most consultants are aware that increased maternal age increases their risk of having a child with a chromosomal disorder. Elevated paternal age increases the risk of point mutations, but this risk is relatively low (1% or less).

Teratogenic or Mutagenic Effects A child's exposure to exogenous factors such as drugs, radiation, alcohol or prenatal infections during pregnancy (teratogenic risks) is a frequent indication for genetic counselling. Potential risks for adverse effects, however, are often overestimated. The number of drugs with proven teratogenic or mutagenic effects is rather small (Shepard and Lemire 2010).

A history of drug and alcohol consumption should be carefully evaluated and discussed. Prenatal infections represent complex situations that require interdisciplinary management.

Consanguinity First cousins and more remote relatives who contemplate marriage occasionally ask for advice about the risks of having children with inherited diseases. Consanguinity definitely increases the risks of disease caused by homozygosity of recessive genes, but the absolute risks are relatively low. It has been estimated that the rate of various diseases, birth defects and mental retardation among offspring of first-cousin matings is at most twice the background rate faced by any given couple. These risks are even lower for more remote consanguinity and thus are difficult to separate from the population background rate for such disorders.

3.2.4 Genetic Diagnosis

Accurate diagnosis of a genetic disease by the use of all the modalities of modern medicine is the cornerstone of genetic counselling. Diagnostic accuracy is emphasised since similar phenotypes may sometimes have different modes of inheritance or may not be inherited at all. The family history is important because a clear-cut pattern of inheritance such as in autosomal dominant traits often provides the basis for counselling when a definitive diagnosis may not be clear. Previous medical and hospital records are helpful in arriving at a correct diagnosis. Since many genetic diseases are associated with somewhat characteristic facial features, inspecting photographs of family members may be helpful. Chromosomal examinations in addition to array CGH analysis are frequently required in the diagnosis of complex birth defects. Since many genetic diseases are rare, even trained medical geneticists and specialists in a given field of medicine may have difficulty in arriving at an accurate diagnosis. They cannot be equally knowledgeable about all genetic diseases in every area of medicine but do need to be aware of recent monographs and computerised expert systems to establish the appropriate diagnosis. The Catalogue of Mendelian Traits in Man by McKusick and its computerised version OMIM are helpful (OMIM et al. 2016).

A definitive clinical diagnosis often cannot be made even by experienced specialists owing to the enormous complexity of development and its possible perturbation by frequently unknown genetic, epigenetic and environmental factors. Fewer diagnostic uncertainties occur with monogenic diseases than with various birth defects. However, even in this area, the growth of the McKusick catalogue over the years (i.e. from 866 definitive loci in 1971 to more than 15,000 definitive loci in November 2016 (OMIM et al. 2016)) attests to the rapid expansion of knowledge in this field.

3.2.5 Molecular Diagnosis

As more genes are being cloned and the molecular nature of mutations causing disease becomes known, direct DNA diagnosis of genetic disease is increasingly possible. Unlike indirect diagnosis from the use of linked DNA markers, a family study is not required for direct genetic testing. However, the exact nature of the mutation to be detected must usually be known. It is good practice to isolate and store DNA from patients with genetic diseases for appropriate future study. The resultant information may be of great help in counselling family members in the future.

Many diseases such as hearing loss and language delay are genetically heterogeneous with many different disease-causing genes. With increasing identification of disease-causing genes in combination with improving novel sequencing techniques such as exome analysis or panel diagnostics, the analysis of many candidate genes in a single step allows the disclosure of the underlying genetic defect in an increasing number of affected families.

3.2.6 Multifactorial Disorders

Genetic advice on multifactorial conditions such as birth defects or common diseases of late onset lacks the precision that can be achieved when counselling patients with Mendelian disorders. Empirical risk figures, based on the frequency of recurrence of the disease in many affected families, need to be used. These recurrence risks are usually lower than those in the Mendelian diseases and range from 3 to 5% for many common birth defects, such as neural tube defects, cleft lip and cleft palate (Fig. 3.5).

In contrast to that of monogenic disorders, the risk in multifactorial disorders increases with an increasing number of affected relatives, with increasing severity of the disease, and is usually negligible for distant relatives.

Careful search for the rare monogenic variety of a disease that appears multifactorial must always be kept in mind.

Transmitted chromosomal abnormalities, such as translocations, do not segregate by Mendelian ratios, and counselling must be based on empirical risk figures.

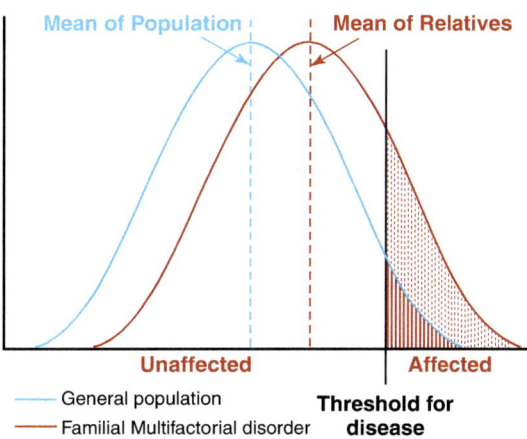

Fig. 3.5 Threshold model for multifactorial (disease) traits. For multifactorial conditions, it is postulated that there is a liability threshold. People whose liability is above this will manifest the disease. A certain combination of genetic and environmental factors, which add together, is needed in order for a person to be affected with a multifactorial condition. Left curve, distribution of liability in the general population; right curve, in relatives of affected individuals, according to the multifactorial threshold model

3.2.7 Recurrence Risk

Genetic risks in Mendelian diseases are clearly defined and depend upon the specific mode of inheritance (Fuhrmann and Vogel 1983; Harper 2010; Speicher et al. 2010). The actual clinical risks to the patient, particularly in autosomal dominant inheritance, depend upon variable penetrance and expression, especially in late-onset disorders. Patients are more interested in the actual recurrence risk of the clinical feature than in the formal genetic risks alone. In diseases with decreased penetrance, the actual recurrence risk is lower than the formal risk of genetic transmission. For example, an offspring's risk of an autosomal dominant disease with 70% penetrance is 35% rather than 50% ($0.5 \times 0.7 = 0.35$). The risk declines with late-onset diseases, as a person remains unaffected beyond the age at which the disease first becomes manifest. McKusick's catalogue is available as a computerised data base online (OMIM) and is updated frequently (OMIM et al. 2016).

3.2.8 Communication and Support

The meaning of genetic risks must be conveyed in terms that can be understood by patients. The probability that 3–4% of all children of healthy parents are born with birth defects or possible genetic diseases should be communicated as a baseline risk figure that applies to the general population. There may be problems in communicating the extent of uncertainty. For example, with a sporadic case of a non-diagnosable disorder, the risk might be zero if the disease is non-genetic, 2–3% if there is a multifactorial aetiology, and 25% if it is caused by an autosomal recessive trait. It must be emphasised that the individual risk of a specific family can differ significantly from the empirical risk figure available for this constellation. Empirical risk figures include families with individual higher as well as lower risks that require special explanation in genetic counselling.

The physical as well as emotional burden of the disease must be discussed. It is well known that very severe but invariably fatal conditions in early life often carry a less severe burden to the family than those associated with chronic or slowly progressive diseases. Since problems may be complex and may prove to be emotionally difficult for the patient, it may be necessary to have several counselling sessions. In any case, the counsellor should provide a written summary of the counselling session by using lay language.

3.2.9 Directive Versus Non-directive Genetic Counselling

The practice of medical genetics clearly has evolved in the direction of non-directive counselling. Non-directive genetic counselling mirrors the trend to increasing patient autonomy. Since each family is unique and reactions to risks vary, non-directive counselling fosters mature decision-making. However, absolutely neutral advice is rarely possible or even desirable. The person or family requesting advice usually wants and needs more than a computer-like professional who only dispenses facts. The counsellor may unconsciously emphasise the more positive or the more frightening aspects of a given disease. These feelings tend to affect the counselling process directly or indirectly, often by nonverbal clues. Not all couples have the necessary educational background and social or emotional maturity to make fully informed decisions. In addition, many couples expect the medical geneticist, whom they consider an experienced expert on their disease, to assist them in arriving at a decision they can live with. 'What would you do if you were in our position?' is a frequent question from those counselled, regardless of background. However, since a couple's economic situation, religious affiliation and cultural background may differ substantially from that of the counsellor, the counsellor's choice for his or her own circumstances is usually not appropriate. Reproductive decisions differ widely among individual couples even if the genetic facts and the disease burden are identical.

3.2.10 Conclusions

Knowledge of human genetics can be applied to genetic counselling of individuals and families at risk of hereditary anomalies and diseases. Genetic counselling refers to the sum of activities that (a) establish the diagnosis of such diseases, (b) assess the recurrence risk, (c) communicate to the client and family the chance of recurrence and (d) provide information regarding the many problems raised by the disease, including natural history and variability of the disease. Formal methods applied in risk assessment include the use of genetic algorithms, statistical considerations and empirically derived risk estimates if the mode of inheritance is unknown. An increasing number of underlying gene defects can be diagnosed at the DNA level, thus allowing a precise assessment of genetic risks for members of affected families. Genetic counselling is not merely concerned with scientific issues that are at the root of genetic disease. It must provide understanding and empathy for the clients' concerns, and it must deal appropriately with the many psychological aspects of the process. As such, genetic counselling is an important part of comprehensive medical care (Fletcher et al. 1985; Resta 2006).

Remark This section is based on a more detailed book chapter (Grimm and Zerres 2010).

3.3 Neuropaediatric Approaches to a Child with Suspected Language Disorder

Dagmar Weise

3.3.1 Introduction

Developmental disorders in children are often accompanied by language disorders. Such language disorders can have structural, functional or psychological causes. They can also be a consequence of complex disorders with impaired sensomotoric and cognitive abilities.

The development of language is based on a number of capabilities of the central nervous system. It depends on an intact primary and secondary auditory pathway, the sensomotoric development of the speech organs and the integrity and proper functioning of various structures of the cerebral cortex and their neural connections.

Individual language development begins around the 28th week of gestation. At this point, hearing organs and their neuronal structures are fully grown and fully functional. Children are therefore born with an auditory memory and can recognise their mother's language and its prosody. The first months of a child's life are the most sensitive period in the development of language. Despite the great variability of normal language development (Nass and Trauner 2012), the first indicators of a delay in language development can be seen within the first 2 years of life (Table 3.1).

Table 3.1 Early indicators of language delay or communication disorder

Lack of consonant and vowel utterances	By 10 months of age
Lack of pointing	By 18 months of age
Fewer than 50 words	By 2 years of age
No two-word combinations	By 2 years of age

Table 3.2 Differential diagnosis of developmental language disorder

- Hearing impairment
- Intellectual disability
- Oral motor dysfunction
- Autistic spectrum disorder
- Selective mutism
- Landau Kleffner syndrome/epileptic encephalopathy
- Environmental deprivation

3.3.2 Diagnosis

Developmental language and speech disorders are described in ICD-10 and are classified as follows:

- Articulation disorder
- Disorder of expressive language
- Disorder of receptive language

These specific language impairments must be differentiated from:

- Language impairments due to the environment
- Secondary language impairments

Secondary language impairments occur in hearing disorders, intellectual disability, autism, selective mutism and other psychiatric disorders, as well as in many neuropaediatric diseases such as cerebral palsy, metabolic and genetic disorders and epileptic encephalopathies (Table 3.2).

If an age-appropriate language development does not occur around the age of 2 years, a phoniatric exploration including a hearing test should be performed. For those children who are suspected of having a developmental disorder other than a sole developmental speech-language disorder, for example, an autism spectrum disorder, epilepsy, primary ciliary dyskinesia, a syndrome, or a metabolic or a neurodevelopmental disorder, a paediatric examination including a broad developmental screening test (e.g. Denver Developmental Screening Test; Frankenburg et al. 1992) and maybe neuropaediatric, genetic, cognitive, electro-physiological, metabolic, radiological, psychological or other specific tests are indicated (Table 3.3). The development of these children has to be carefully observed at least until their third year of life (Rescorla et al. 1997). A developmental speech-language disorder that persists at 3 or 4 years of age is an indication for a speech-language therapy. Parent training and early language therapy are effective in improving the language skills of late talkers at

ages 2–3. Further assessment and treatment depend on the individual child's history and the results of the above-mentioned tests.

EEG investigation is often worthwhile, even without clinically evident *cerebral seizures* (Billard et al. 2009). Subclinical seizures or epileptiform discharges in EEG without cerebral seizures, especially with transition into nonconvulsive status epilepticus during sleep, can cause language disorders (Overvliet et al. 2010). This should be considered in the presence of the following clinical findings, and a sleep EEG should be performed:

- Language regression
- Verbal auditory agnosia

Some *genetic syndromes* (Table 3.4) are accompanied by various language and speech disorders. Suspected diagnoses for several of these syndromes are based on specific dysmorphias (Goorhuis-Brouwer et al. 2003). Cytogenetic and molecular genetic investigations can confirm or rule out such suspicions and enable genetic counselling.

A number of *metabolic disorders* can initially present as a developmental language disorder. Mitochondrial respiratory chain defects, organic acidurias and disorders of creatine biosynthesis (Vodopiutz et al. 2007) especially are found within the first years of life. The lysosomal storage diseases mucopolysaccharidosis type III (Sanfilippo syndrome) (Cleary and Wraith 1993) or the juvenile progressive form of Tay-Sachs disease (Fernandez-Filho and Shapiro 2004) can also be mistaken as a developmental language disorder. A metabolic

Table 3.3 Evaluation of a child with a suspected language disorder

Methods	Recommended age for investigation (years)
• Complete neurodevelopmental and family history	2
• Detailed neurological examination including social interaction and communicative behaviour	2
• Hearing test	2
• Developmental screening test, e.g. *Denver Developmental Screening Test* (DDST), 0–6 years (Frankenburg et al. 1992)	2
• Psychometric testing to establish general cognitive function, e.g. *Snijders-Oomen Nonverbal Intelligence Test—Revised* (SON-R), 2½–7 years (Tellegen et al. 1998)	3
• Depending on history and examination, other tests to consider:	2–4
EEG – Sleep EEG – Genetic studies: karyotype, fragile X study, array CGH – Metabolic screening: urinary analysis of organic acids, creatine and guanidine acetate, mucopolysaccharides and oligosaccharides. Blood lactate, specific enzyme activities in leukocytes – MRI of the brain	

Table 3.4 Genetic syndromes known to be associated with language delay/impairment

- Fragile X syndrome
- Klinefelter syndrome
- Trisomy 21
- Angelman syndrome
- Smith-Magenis syndrome
- Rett syndrome
- Velocardiofacial syndrome
- Prader-Willi syndrome

screening test and specific determination of enzyme activity in leukocytes or on dried bloodspot cards (Table 3.3) should be performed in cases of clinical suspicion.

If clear neurological deficits or pathological EEG findings are reported, a cranial MRI scan is required in order to identify *structural changes in the brain*. Neuronal migration disorders (Guerreiro et al. 2002), congenital bilateral peri-sylvian syndrome (Brandao-Almeida et al. 2008; Nevo et al. 2001) and a neurocutaneous syndrome, such as tuberous sclerosis, are clinical entities that can be detected.

3.3.2.1 Neurophysiological Studies in a Child with a Global Developmental Disorder

Electroencephalography (EEG)
Method Fluctuations in field potentials caused by activity in the underlying brain structures can be recorded on the scalp. The majority of the activity which can be ascertained on EEG is derived from postsynaptic potentials, which are summed as field potentials over the cerebral cortex. With a defined distribution of electrodes covering the four areas of the brain (frontal, parietal, temporal and occipital regions), the multiline graphical plot of the EEG can display a topographical structure.

Cortical potentials are susceptible to internal as well as external influences, so monitoring conditions must be clearly defined and followed. Photostimulation, hyperventilation and sleep deprivation are used as provocation methods.

Indications EEG is indicated in the following cases:

- Identification of electrical patterns typical of epilepsy, such as spikes and sharp-waves that are important for diagnosis, classification and observation of children who suffer from epileptic seizures
- Searching for focal disorders as evidence of brain area-related dysfunction
- Change in background activity as a sign of globally impaired brain function, such as

toxic-metabolic or inflammatory changes in the brain
- Assessment of bioelectrical maturation

Limitations Arguments for limitations of this method are:

- Interpretation of the EEG is much more difficult in children than adults. Alongside the specific challenge of complying with the monitoring conditions, particular sharp-waves and rhythmic waves, especially related to tiredness, falling asleep or sleeping, are present in healthy children, which could be misinterpreted as epileptiform patterns
- Because of the spatial separation between the scalp and the cortex, within which various conducting media lie (skin, bone, meninges, vessels, fluid):
  - Definite topographical mapping of EEG potentials is not possible
  - Epilepsy cannot be ruled out, even in the absence of patterns that are typical of epilepsy

Visually Evoked Potentials (VEP)
Method Light stimuli on the retina generate potentials that are transferred along the optic nerve, optic chiasma, lateral geniculate body and Gratiolet line of sight to area 17 (area striata) of the occipital lobe (the primary visual cortex). By an averaging technique, a summation of numerous evoked potentials can be recorded over the scalp. Older children are required to fixate on the centre of a rapidly reversing chessboard pattern shown on a screen. Newborns and infants receive retinal stimulation via LED-light-flash glasses.

The VEP curves that are measured by using either of these two stimulation methods correspond to cortical potentials with age-related, relatively constant latencies and amplitudes.

Indications VEP are indicated in disorders of the visual pathway between the retina and visual cortex, which can change VEP curves:

- Disorders of the myelin sheath lead to a prolonged latency of the VEP

- Axonal damage to the optic nerve leads to a more or less pronounced reduction in VEP amplitude
- No VEP is found in cortical blindness
- In certain forms of neuronal ceroid lipofuscinosis, high-amplitude short-latency VEP at the beginning of the disease, or the loss of VEP in a later stage, can give a clue to this group of diseases

VEP testing should be considered in the following clinical settings: optic neuritis, in isolation or as part of multiple sclerosis; leukoencephalopathy; tumour of the visual pathway (optic glioma as part of neurofibromatosis type 1, craniopharyngioma, etc.); papilloedema as part of cerebral phantom tumour; optic atrophy; cortical blindness; and neuronal ceroid lipofuscinosis.

Limitations Arguments for limitations of this method are:

Noncompliance with the measurement conditions can easily lead to measurement errors. The informative value of the investigation can therefore be limited in children.

Somatosensory Evoked Potentials (SSEP)

Method Through repeated suprathreshold sensitive skin stimulation with a defined square pulse of very short duration, sensitive or sensory neural action potentials can be triggered, which are transmitted to the central nervous system. The afferents in the neural pathways begin in free nerve endings or in special receptor organs in the skin, following the sensitive parts of the nerves through the dorsal root of the equilateral posterior funiculus in the spinal cord (spinothalamic tract) through the cuneate nucleus (upper extremity) or the gracile nucleus (lower extremity) into the medulla oblongata and, after crossing in the pons, through the medial lemniscus to the thalamus. Onward transmission of the signal takes place after switching to the second central neuron over thalamocortical pathways passing through the internal capsule into the sensory postcentral region.

According to the somatotopic structure of the cortex, the SSEP are recorded over the contralateral scalp in reference to the area of stimulation. The choice of nerve to be stimulated (e.g. the median nerve in the area of the wrist or the tibial nerve in the area of the ankle) depends upon the clinical issue that is investigated.

Owing to increasing myelinisation and fibre thickness of the conducting nerves and maturation of the synapses in the developing child, the spinal and central conduction time decreases from birth until the sixth to eighth year of life. At the same time, the latency of the SSEP increases because of increasing body length. Age and body-length-related reference values should be applied to the child being investigated.

Indications SSEP are indicated in the following cases:

- Diseases of the peripheral nervous system (sensory polyneuropathy, entrapment syndrome, polyradiculitis, plexus/nerve root affection)
- Diseases of the spinal cord (myelitis, spinocerebellar ataxia, tumour, vascular changes, tethered cord)
- Diseases of the central nervous system (leukoencephalopathy, tumour)
- Forms of neuronal ceroid lipofuscinosis (as in VEP, some high-amplitude, short-latency SSEP, also loss of SSEP)

Limitations Arguments for limitations of this method are:

- Only fast-conducting nerve fibres are stimulated (tactile sensitivity and proprioception)
- Disorders of pain or temperature sensitivity are not registered

Motor Electroneurography

Method The stimulation of a motor nerve triggers a muscle action potential (MAP). The nerve conduction velocity (NCV) of the stimulated nerves is calculated from the distance between a distal and proximal site of stimulation and their difference in latencies to the site of measurement—defined by MAP. The NCV of peripheral nerves, with their variously structured fibres, depends upon the thickness of the myelin sheath, fibre cross section and body temperature. The myelination of peripheral nerves undergoes a developmental process that begins in the 15th week of gestation and can extend up until the fifth year of life, depending on the type of nerve fibre.

The most important parameters when analysing neurography traces are latency (which is an indicator of myelin sheath function) and amplitude (which provides information about the axonal integrity of the nerve fibres). Age-related reference values exist for NCV, distal latency and amplitude of the MAP.

Indications Motor electroneurography is indicated in the following cases:

- Demyelinating and axonal neuropathy
- Axonal lesions
- Entrapment syndrome
- Leuko-encephalopathy with involvement of the peripheral nervous system

Limitations Arguments for limitations of this method are:

Stimulation must be at a supramaximal level; otherwise the detected NCV will be too slow. Full cooperation of the child is therefore necessary.

3.3.2.2 Neurometabolic Studies in a Child with a Global Developmental Disorder

Basic Laboratory Studies

Blood Full blood and differential leukocyte count (looking for vacuolated lymphocytes), glucose, pH and blood gases, lactate, sodium, potassium, calcium, phosphate, alkaline phosphatase, transaminases, creatine kinase, creatinine, uric acid, homocysteine, iron, ferritin, thyroid-stimulating hormone (TSH), free triiodothyronine (fT3), free thyroxine (fT4) and very-long-chain fatty acids. If neonatal metabolic screening has not been done: amino acids and

acylcarnitines in tandem mass spectrometry, biotinidase.

Urine Organic acids, creatine and guanidinoacetate.

Further Tests According to Clinical Findings

- Microcephaly: toxoplasmosis and CMV serology, possibly also CMV DNA analysis (PCR) on postpartum preserved dried blood spot card if necessary. In girls one should consider a genetic investigation for Rett syndrome
- Dysmorphia: isoelectric focusing of transferrins (congenital disorder of glycosylation (CDG syndrome)), copper/ceruloplasmin (Menkes disease) and 7-dehydrocholesterol (Smith-Lemli-Opitz syndrome). Genetic investigations such as chromosome analysis, fragile X syndrome investigation and array comparative genomic hybridisation (aCGH). Targeted genetic investigation for suspected monogenetic disease. Oligosaccharides/mucopolysaccharides in urine
- Autistic behaviour: purine and pyrimidine metabolites in urine
- Cherry-red spot fundus: specific determination of enzyme activity in leukocytes or on dried blood spot cards (GM1 and GM2 gangliosidosis, Niemann-Pick disease)
- Cerebral seizures: investigation of enzyme activity PPT1, TPP1 on the dried blood spot card for infantile or late-infantile neuronal ceroid lipofuscinosis

3.3.3   Further Diagnostic Procedures

Whether and to what extent a child with a developmental language disorder requires further diagnostic tests should be guided by the following questions:

- Are other components of the child's development affected?
- Is there a *delay* or *loss* of age-appropriate language skills?

Table 3.5 Differential diagnosis of developmental delay

Predominant speech delay
- Hearing impairment
- Congenital bilateral perisylvian syndrome
- Infantile autism

Predominant motor delay
- Neuromuscular disorder
- Cerebral palsy
- Ataxia, e.g. in congenital cerebellar malformation

Global developmental delay
- Cerebral malformation
- Intrauterine infection
- Genetic disorder
- Perinatal asphyxia
- Progressive disease of the nervous system, initial presentation

Table 3.6 Differential diagnosis of progressive disease of the nervous system

Onset before 2 years of age

Disorders of amino acid metabolism

Disorders of creatine biosynthesis

Disorders of lysosomal enzymes

Carbohydrate-deficient glycoprotein syndromes

Mitochondrial disorders

Genetic disorder
- Rett syndrome

Neurocutaneous syndrome
- Tuberous sclerosis

Disorders of grey matter

Disorders of white matter

Onset after age 2 years

Infectious disease
- Subacute sclerosing panencephalitis

Disorders of lysosomal enzymes

Disorders of grey matter

Disorders of white matter

Delayed achievement of developmental milestones is one of the more common problems evaluated by child neurologists (Shevell et al. 2003). The question 'Is the development delayed or regressing?' is sometimes difficult to answer, especially in infants. Even in static encephalopathies, new symptoms, such as seizures, may occur as the child gets older, and delayed acquisition of milestones without other neurological deficits is sometimes the initial feature of progressive disorders. However, once it is clear that previously achieved milestones have been lost or that focal neurological deficits are evolving, a progressive disease of the nervous system is a consideration (Pina-Garza 2013) (Tables 3.5 and 3.6).

Case Study 3.1

A 3-year-old girl presents at the neuropaediatric outpatient department because of a severe language delay. She cannot speak any words except 'mama' and 'baba', but she can vocalise a few vowels. The parents describe excessive drooling and an inability to chew and swallow solid food. She occasionally chokes on solid food and also on fluids (Fig. 3.6).

The girl is the second child of healthy, nonconsanguineous parents. Her brother, who is 10

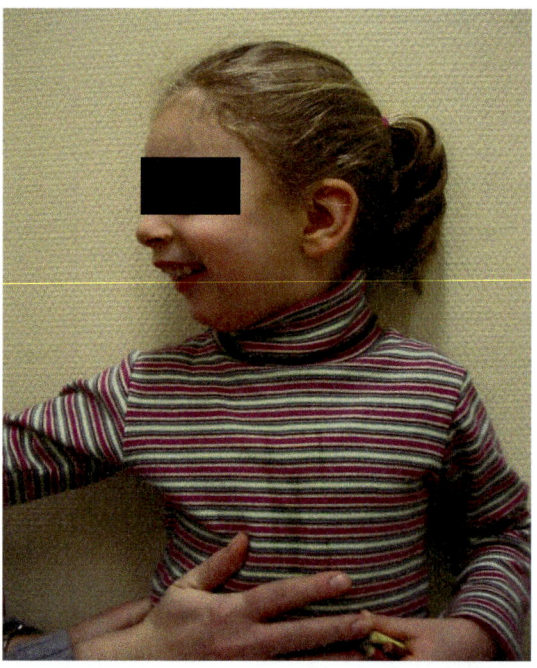

Fig. 3.6 A girl with a severe disorder of expressive language development. Retrogenia. Flecks of saliva on her jumper. Photo at age of 4.5 years with kind permission from the parents

years older, is healthy and normally developed. Pregnancy and birth were uneventful. The gross motor developmental milestones were adequately achieved. No severe illness is on record. Hearing test results were normal.

On examination the girl is friendly but shy, with no verbal communication. There is obvious orofacial hypotonia with lack of mouth closure and constant drooling, retrogenia, high-arching palate and no midline defects. The movements of the tongue are limited, resembling oral dyspraxia. On complete neurological examination, no further deficits were observed.

Laboratory Cytogenetic studies and CGH array excluded chromosomal abnormalities, microdeletions and duplications.

EEG Normal

Brain Imaging Magnetic resonance imaging showed bilateral perisylvian polymicrogyria, especially in the frontal and temporal operculum (Fig. 3.7).

Diagnosis Worster-Drought syndrome (Worster-Drought 1974).

Treatment Speech therapy, orthodontic treatment and psychological support. Technical devices for communication were very helpful. To suppress excessive drooling, one can give cholinergic agents or inject botulinum toxin in the salivary glands.

Conclusion The girl presented with a severe expressive language disorder, oral motor dysfunction with dysphagia and dysarthria. This is a typical clinical picture of the Worster-Drought syndrome or Foix-Chavany-Marie syndrome, a suprabulbar palsy caused by bilateral lesions of the anterior operculum (Christen et al. 2000). The aetiology can be cortical malformation, post-infectious residual damage, epileptic discharges or ischaemia in the region of the operculum, i.e. the cortex of the perisylvian fissure (Suresh and Deepa 2004). The MRI of the brain showed bilateral perisylvian polymicrogyria, which is the

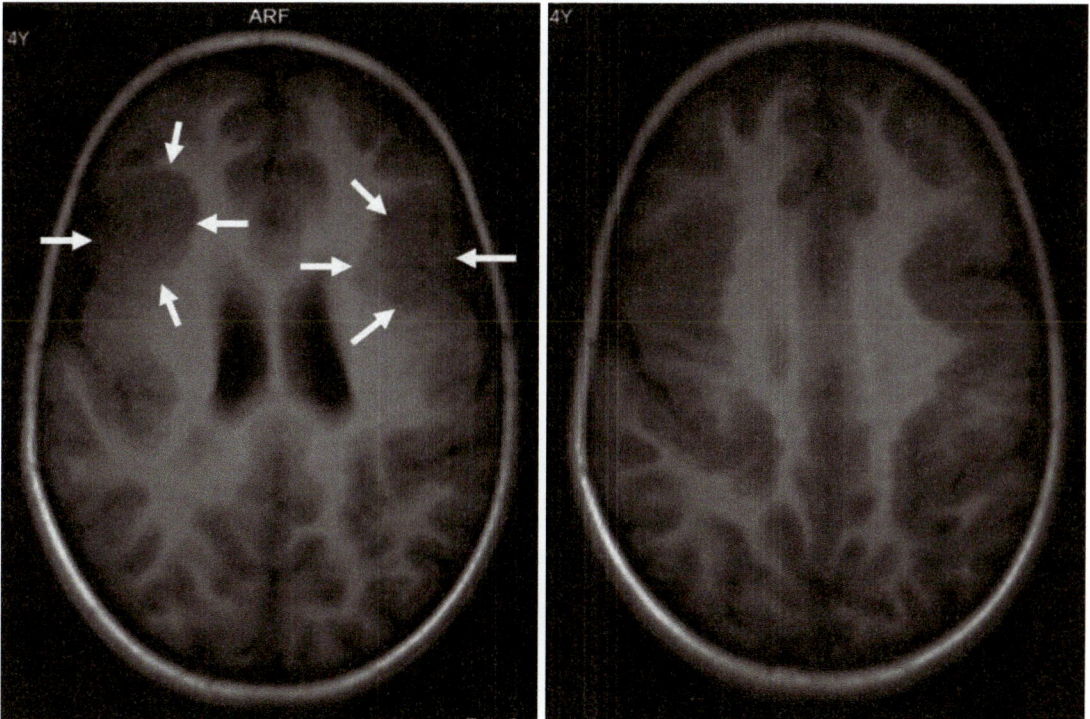

Fig. 3.7 Axial T1-weighted MRI of the 4-year-old girl, showing a bilateral perisylvian polymicrogyria, indicated by arrows

most common congenital malformation found in this syndrome, also known as congenital bilateral perisylvian syndrome (Nevo et al. 2001). Patients very often present with epileptic seizures.

This case emphasises the need for brain imaging in children with severe expressive language impairment not explained by a previously known neurological condition such as cerebral palsy. The treatment requires a long-term multidisciplinary approach, and technical communication devices are often needed.

Case Study 3.2

A 6-year-old boy is sent to the neuropaediatric department for further diagnostic procedures. Parents and teachers complain about very fluctuating receptive language ability, with periods in which the boy does not understand spoken language and has to use signs and gestures for communication.

The boy is the first child of healthy, non-consanguineous parents. Pregnancy was normal, and birth in the 40th week of gestation was by Caesarean section because of prolonged labour. There were no perinatal complications for the child. Developmental milestones were adequately achieved in infancy, with independent walking at 12 months of age, first words spoken at 12 months and two-word sentences at 24 months. At 2.5–3 years of age, the boy was considered to have a delay in his expressive language abilities with dyslalia and stuttering. He later developed periods of impaired speech comprehension lasting 2–3 weeks. His stuttering worsened at the same time. Speech therapy started at 4 years of age, but the fluctuating symptoms recurred. A few months before consulting the neuropaediatric department, a severe aggravation with complete loss of speech comprehension prompted a thorough hearing test. An auditory agnosia was stated as a probable cause.

At 4 years of age, an adenotomy was performed, but there were no other illnesses or operative procedures. The boy attends a special school for children with language disorders.

On *examination* the boy is friendly but does not speak. He does not seem to understand simple verbal commands. He communicates with his mother by using sign language, whereas, while making mental calculations, he talks to himself in an incomprehensible language. The complete neurological examination is normal, no cranial nerve dysfunction. No dysmorphic features.

Laboratory Normal karyotype and no fragile X genotype.

EEG Focal epileptiform discharges over the central and temporal region shifting from left to right, or bilaterally. Continuous sharp-waves during sleep, i.e. non-convulsive status epilepticus during sleep (Fig. 3.8).

Brain Imaging Normal MRI.

Diagnosis Landau Kleffner syndrome (Landau and Kleffner 1957).

Treatment Anticonvulsive treatment with sultiame and clobazam. Recovery of language comprehension and intelligible speech. Disappearance of epileptiform discharges on EEG (Fig. 3.9). The treatment was continued until the beginning of puberty (at age 13). One year later, he has not had a recurrence of auditory agnosia or speech problems. The EEG was normal.

Conclusion The boy suffered from acquired aphasia due to subclinical seizures. The main symptom was auditory agnosia, which was caused by impaired cortical processing of auditory signals due to epileptiform discharges. The aetiology of Landau Kleffner syndrome is unknown, but this epilepsy syndrome is thought to belong to the group of benign partial epilepsies of childhood (Deonna and Roulet-Perez 2010; Deonna et al. 1993; Lillywhite et al. 2009). Seizures and epileptiform discharges on EEG disappear with puberty (Liukkonen et al. 2010).

This case highlights the importance of the EEG in the examination of children with language disorders, especially where there is a loss of age-appropriate language skills, clinical signs of auditory agnosia and acquired aphasia. Brain imaging should be conducted to exclude a tumour or malformations, as these could equally cause the above-mentioned symptoms.

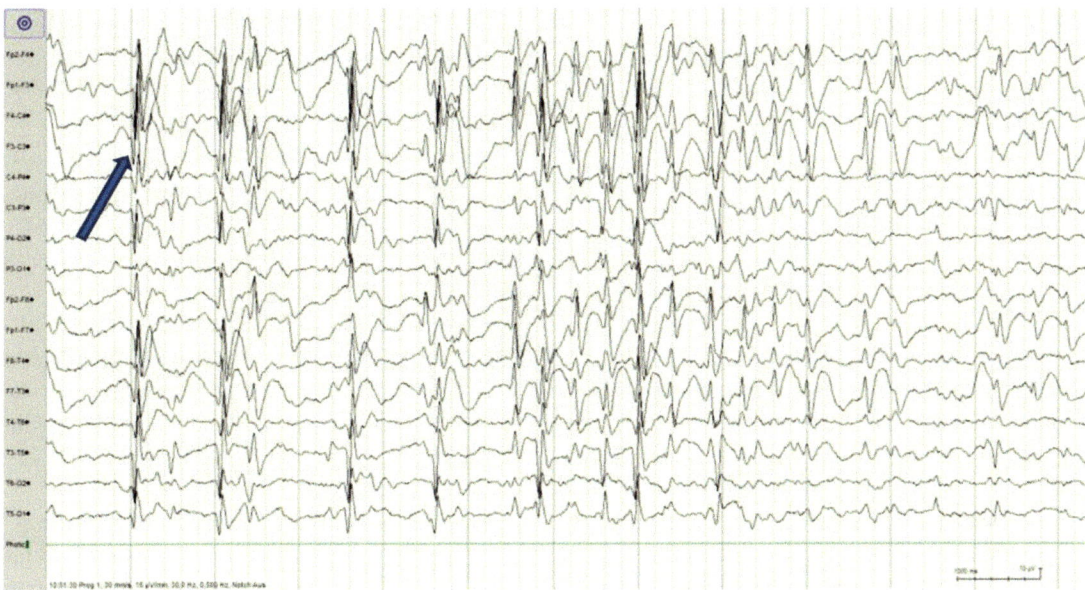

Fig. 3.8 Sleep-EEG monitoring of a 6-year-old boy with almost continuous tracing of high-amplitude sharp-slow-wave complexes over the left fronto-centro-temporal region with rapid transmission to the opposite side (arrow). Bioelectrical status epilepticus in sleep

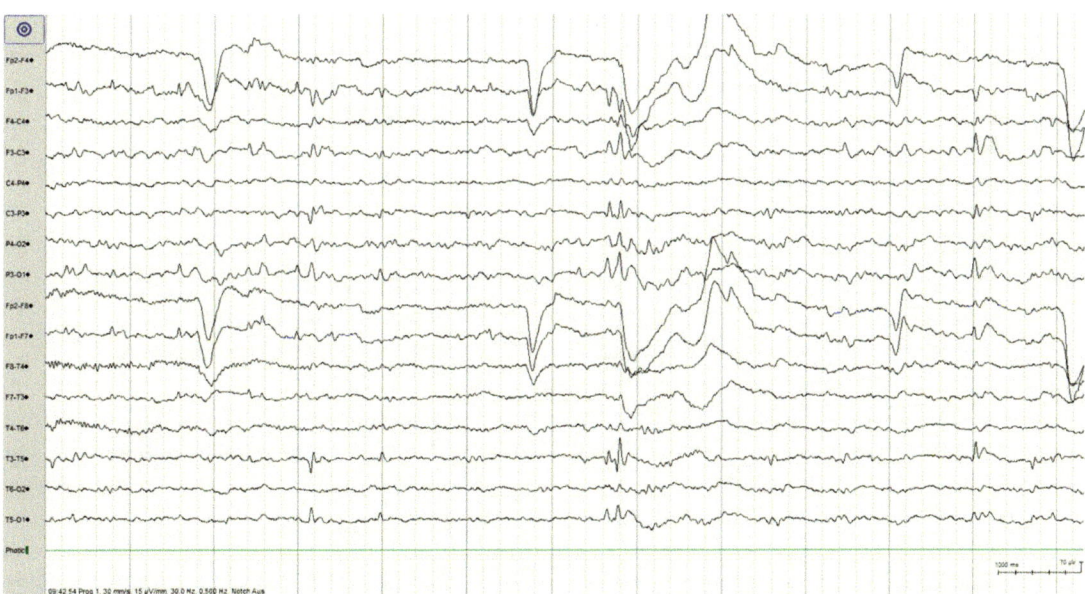

Fig. 3.9 Sleep-EEG trace of the 6-year-old boy 2 weeks later on anticonvulsive therapy with sultiame. Occasional sharp-wave complexes over the left fronto-centro-temporal region

3.3.4 Treatment

There are two categories of intervention for cases of language disorders:

- Language support
- Disorder-specific language therapy

These categories have different indications.

Language Support This term encompasses all procedures both within and outside of the family which are empirically stimulating and important for language development: from frequent verbal interaction (e.g. regular comments from adults regarding the child's activities—parallel talking), looking at picture books together and describing what is portrayed, reading out loud, rhyming games and singing with children, avoiding extensive exposure to television and other media with which the child cannot interactively communicate (Chonchaiya and Pruksanonda 2008) up to the provision of an increased language input or implementation of programmes promoting language development in child daycare centres. All of these are primary and secondary preventive procedures with an educational emphasis.

Language Therapy A medical intervention to treat defined developmental speech-language disorders is called language therapy. These disorders include specific developmental speech-language disorders and speech-language disorders associated with a comorbidity such as hearing impairment. Furthermore, language therapy for children encompasses acquired language disorders such as dysarthria due to cerebral palsy or aphasia.

Therapy of developmental speech-language disorders should start around 3–4 years of age at latest. Systematic reviews, meta-analyses and randomised controlled trials have shown that parent-centred approaches and child-centred interventions are highly effective in improving the language skills and further language development of late talkers at ages 2–3 (Buschmann et al. 2009; Cable and Domsch 2011; Roberts and Kaiser 2011, 2015; Robertson and Weismer

1999). There is good evidence that late talkers benefit from a parent's training how to communicate with the child (Buschmann et al. 2009; Roberts and Kaiser 2011). For late talkers with receptive deficits or additional risk factors such as familial disposition for language disorders, low parental level of education or weak nonverbal abilities, eventually, in addition to parent's training, a child-centred early language therapy should start in the third year of life. Early language therapy has been shown to stimulate the development of the vocabulary, increases the child's motivation to speak and facilitates the acquisition of syntactic structures.

Language therapy is the domain of logopaedics/speech-language therapists and phoniatricians and is usually tailored to the individual based on her or his specific profile and severity of the disorders according to the test results. Particular treatment forms may target oral motor disorders such as orofacial stimulation according to Castillo-Morales (Limbrock et al. 1993).

3.4 Basics of Psychosomatic Medicine

Gereon Heuft

3.4.1 Epidemiological and Public Health Importance of Psychological Disorders

Psychological and psychosomatic disorders are quite frequent in the general population. As the prevalence and incidence are usually even higher in the context of an inpatient or outpatient treatment setting, the specialist in phoniatrics should know that there is a high probability of his patients suffering from an additional comorbid psychological disorder.

Thus, Wittchen et al. (2011) found the 1-year prevalence of psychological disorders across all ages in the EU to be 38.2%. This prevalence, with the exception of increasing dementia, has remained unchanged since 2005. The disease burden has a huge impact, not only on disability periods and early retirements but also by reducing the quality of life for people with somatic diseases (such as diabetes mellitus or coronary heart disease) and increasing the associated costs and mortality (Zipfel et al. 2002; Hochlehnert et al. 2007; Beutel and Schulz 2011). Rozanski et al. (2005) showed that the level of depression as measured by the Beck Depression Inventory (BDI; Hautzinger et al. 1994) was an essential determining factor in the survival of patients after a heart attack.

In 2011, after injuries and their consequences (14.3%), diseases of the respiratory system (15.8%) and diseases of the musculoskeletal system (21.7%), psychological disorders (12.1%) represented the fourth-largest proportion of days of work disability (DAK 2011). On days of work disability due to the disorders of the musculoskeletal system, 7.1% of patients suffered from back pain. It is very likely that a proportion of people in this group suffered from somatoform (pain) disorders, thus including a group of psychological disorders. Among people who had suffered an accident or other serious illnesses, many require additional psycho-traumatological, psycho-oncological, etc. (co-)treatment, even though these secondary psychological diagnoses were not part of the primary diagnosis. The average duration of a disability due to mental illness was 28.9 days, whereas those with musculoskeletal disorders were work-disabled on average for 17.2 days, and those with disorders of the respiratory system were unable to work on average for 6.3 days. Thus, while other types of diseases occur frequently causing disability, mental illness is often associated with a longer period of work disability.

According to epidemiological studies, psychological disorders are not only among the more common types of disease but also the more expensive. According to Wittchen et al. (2011), overall:

> the social burden of mental disorders—as measured by the indicator "adjusted life years (DALYs)" of the World Health Organization—is far greater than that of any other disease group (cancer, heart disease, etc.).

Therefore, timely and high-quality diagnosis and treatment is needed to prevent their exacerbation, their becoming chronic and the use of inadequate therapies of the psychological disorders.

Interim conclusion: it is absolutely essential that all physicians have basic psychosomatic competence at the interface of somatic differential diagnosis and therapy, somato-psychological, psychosomatic and psychotherapeutic (co-)treatments. Each specialist in phoniatrics should also be aware that among his patients, the burden of psychological or psychosomatic illnesses described here is present as comorbidity, independent of the underlying somatic disease.

Therefore, some suggestions are made here as to how a specialist in phoniatrics can detect a possible psychological comorbidity in his patients during consultation and what interventions he himself can initiate and implement. In the next subsection, interactions between somatically defined diseases and the psychological state of the patient will be explained.

3.4.2 Basic Psychosomatic Competence of a Specialist in Phoniatrics

An important clue to a psychological (co)morbidity can be a discrepancy between phoniatric findings and the patient's condition: the patient's suffering cannot be identified from the somatic findings alone. For the specialist in phoniatrics, the question becomes important as to what else causes depression in the patient or what else is worrying him. The doctor can develop a feeling of being unable to help the patient sufficiently. This feeling can go so far that in his countertransference, the doctor feels helpless towards the patient or even begins to develop feelings of aversion to him. 'Balint groups', in which mutual trust is developed through regular meetings in a constant circle of colleagues, are a proven training ground for a specialist in phoniatrics to be trained in becoming aware of those feelings that may offer important diagnostic clues. A Balint group could become the role of a psychosomatic ground and is ideally interdisciplinary, with the different disciplines mutually complementing their expertise. In the Balint group, the treatment reality of the patient is often reflected—the distressed patient also consults, in addition to his family doctor, a variety of medical specialists for his 'inexplicable' symptoms.

In addition, for many years physicians of all somatic disciplines in Germany have been offered an additional qualification in basic psychosomatic care via the Medical Council. This very successful training concept includes a total of 80 h of instruction: 20 h of theory, supplemented with 60 h of intensive training in physician-patient dialogues, including roleplaying, etc. The curriculum is designed to enable physicians to recognise psychological comorbidities on the basis of identification of criteria and training in countertransference perception, as well as successfully to intervene verbally in milder disorders, such as those within the context of a patient's coping with physical disorders. Physicians also acquire differential diagnostic skills to recognise complex psychological disorders and to make appropriate referrals to specialists (in psychosomatic medicine and psychotherapy or psychiatry). A basic training of phoniatricians in psychosomatics is desirable.

Below, the frequent psychological or psychosomatic disorders that a specialist in phoniatrics should be able to recognise are discussed (for additional information, see Eckhardt-Henn et al. 2009).

3.4.3 Interactions Between Somatic Disease and Psychological State

The term somato-psychological disorder is used in the context of a patient whose primary complaint is some organic disease but who has difficulties coping with it (e.g. vocal fold paralysis due to recurrent nerve palsy). If no additional comorbidities are present in the patient's case history but the phoniatrician finds it necessary to have more intensive dialogue in order to help the patient cope successfully with his illness, the short-term psychological disorder is diagnosed as acute stress disorder (ICD-10: F43.0). If the somato-psychological-dependent stress lasts for several weeks or months, there is an adjustment disorder, in the sense of a disease-coping process, termed earlier as ICD-10: F43.2. These two disorders may already be so severe that they lead to work disability.

With increasing severity, a long-lasting adjustment disorder can meet the criteria of a major depressive episode (ICD-10: F32.0). When psychological disorders triggered by somatic diseases become chronic, they can develop into a severe recurrent depressive disorder (major depression) (ICD-10: F33.2). Other common psychological disorders that may be induced by systemic diseases belong to the spectrum of anxiety disorders (ICD-10: F40ff). Within the group of patients with anxiety disorders, those with hypochondriac disorders must be differentiated from others (ICD-10: F45.2). These patients fear that they suffer from some organic illness without having any serious somatic disease or without having survived some previous somatic illness. These body-related anxieties lead those affected to consult physicians frequently with the request for repeated physical examinations in order that they may experience 'calming' of their fears. Unfortunately, this often does not last long, so that the patients feel that they 'must' consult the physicians once again.

Patients who were already suffering from a psychological or psychosomatic disorder under the burden of morbidity as described in Sect. 3.4.1 before they developed a phoniatric somatic disease have basically greater difficulties coping with the emerging somatic illness because of their increased psychological vulnerability. The interactions between the psychological and the somatic aspects can reinforce each other negatively to such an extent that a clearly increased mortality has been demonstrated for some of these interactions (e.g. cardiovascular disease and depression). Basically, this is also conceivable for phoniatric disorders, but as yet there are no studies available on it.

3.4.4 Dissociative Motor Disorders

Psychogenic aphonia is a very common psychosomatic disorder within the field of phoniatrics. It is defined by the WHO nomenclature as dissociative movement disorder (ICD-10: F44.4). Dissociative motor disorders are generally related to the striated muscles. 'Pseudoneurological phenomena' can manifest themselves all over the body, e.g. as abasia, astasia or flaccid paresis. The motor symptoms correspond to a dysfunction of the voluntary muscles for which no organic basis can be identified. From a communication theory point of view, the symptoms often have the character of body language ('I have lost my voice'). From the point of view of psychodynamics, the symptoms represent a symbol and an effort at compromise in solving an unconscious conflict. It is conceivable, for example, that by a psychogenic aphonia, more aggressive verbal utterances can be 'avoided'.

In addition to the dissociative movement disorders, rare dissociative sensibility and sensation disorders (ICD-10: F44.6) have been described. Psychogenic deafness is recognised as one form of these diseases in phoniatrics. A conceivable combination of psychogenic hearing impairment on the one hand, and sensorineural hearing loss on the other, makes differential diagnosis particularly difficult. In investigations by expert consultants, the question sometimes arises, for example, whether the extent of hearing loss induced by a 'noise trauma' is exclusively of somatic origin. Especially in those cases where the symptoms of hearing loss can also be used to avoid conflict, the somatic hypothesis provides the patient with an exculpatory disease model. That is, the patient's hearing is particularly 'bad' just when there is a discussion of topics that are stressful for him. When there are legal disputes over compensation (for pain and suffering or pension) after an acoustic trauma, the dissociative aspects of hearing loss may also become extensive enough so as to be hugely relevant.

3.4.5 Relevant Possibilities for Intervention in the Phoniatrician-Patient Relationship

Basically, the specialist in phoniatrics should be aware that there is absolutely no affect in human beings that do not have, at the same time, a somatic co-reaction as a result and vice versa; each somatic disease demands a psychological coping capacity to a greater or lesser extent. There is thus in every patient an inseparable somato-psychological-psychosomatic dynamics, which plays a decisive part in shaping the doctor-patient relationship.

If the phoniatrician can communicate to his patients at the very beginning of the physician-patient encounter, 'We are following the principles of modern medicine, which take into account both the somatic and possible psychological interactions at the same time, which should be of benefit for you', he facilitates from the outset his access to the patient, for example, when he has to get more details of his medical history. Thus, when he asks additional questions to obtain a fuller picture of his medical history, 'When the complaints started 3 months ago, what was your situation in your personal and professional life?', there is no need for the phoniatrician to give time-consuming explanations to the patient, namely, that he is trying to establish the triggering causes of the symptoms. The patient feels that the phoniatrician is interested in him as a person and would like to bring to light the cause of his symptoms in order to be able to provide appropriate treatment.

The perception of one's own countertransference, that is, the feelings that the patient triggers in his counterpart because of the intrapsychic dynamics, is often the key to understanding the treatment relations experienced as being conflict-laden. Thus, when a patient is fearful and clinging, the doctor develops the feeling: 'How can I get rid of this patient?' Instead of trying to achieve 'pseudo-relaxation' of the situation in an unreflected fashion, such as by prescribing a medication of whose efficacy he himself is not convinced, he could learn to formulate the issue as follows: 'Could it be that they are worried that I do not care enough about them and their illness? What can I do now that they leave this session today as relaxed as possible?' Thus, the feeling of the patient is authentically addressed, and at the same time, the conflict does not worsen. Even though a (pseudo)solution is not offered immediately—a 'solution' that in retrospect might turn out to be disappointment—a surprising relaxation in the doctor-patient interaction can often be achieved by such interventions.

In addition to obtaining the biographical case history, more helpful interview techniques can be learned by the phoniatrician such as asking circular questions: 'If your wife were here now, how would she describe your situation?' This question allows the patient to describe how his illness is dealt with at home without having to say that the descriptions of his illness by family members are correct: 'My wife says I always get upset so very fast, but I myself do not see the situation in this way'. This enables one to get a 'case history from a third person' without family members being present. Depending on the answers, it might be useful to stimulate a real pair dialogue. The phoniatrician can, of course, reach this advanced psychological diagnosis in cooperation with a medical or a psychological psychotherapist: 'I note in our conversation that there is some substantial burden which could have an impact on your voice; I suggest that we additionally take into account this important aspect, in that you have a consultation with Dr. X and get back to me as soon as possible with the results'.

Either the phoniatrician decides to acquire an additional qualification in psychosomatic primary care, to be able to recognise and diagnose by himself psychological comorbidities and dissociative disorders with greater certainty, or he works together with medical and psychological psychotherapist consultants. In either case he should basically be able to recognise the relationships and disease patterns described here, in order not to make false differential diagnoses and to avoid causing unnecessary suffering to the patient. If the patient is already under psychiatric or psychotherapeutic treatment because of his psychological comorbidity, with the patient's consent, the phoniatrician should establish a consultative contact with those treating him.

In the following, two case studies in psychosomatic medicine and psychotherapy are presented:

Case Study 3.3

A 53-year-old patient had been diagnosed with a vocal fold carcinoma 1 week earlier. His family noticed that he had been clearing his throat quite often within the previous few months, and he had noticed a progressive hoarseness in his voice within the previous 6 weeks. He had been very busy in his work as an executive, so he postponed a physical investigation to go on holiday. After receiving the diagnosis, he began to feel guilty and felt he had probably gone to the doctor 'too late'. In addition he began to fear the upcoming operation. He felt more and more oppressed by worries about his occupational and personal future: he could not afford to stay away from work for long, and he anticipated financial difficulties related to paying off a loan for his house if the illness were to persist for a long time.

Diagnosis and Differential Diagnosis The patient is clearly stressed by the recent carcinoma diagnosis. Since psychosomatic intervention is necessary, an acute stress disorder (ICD-10: F43.0) is diagnosed. If the symptoms were to last more than 2 or 3 weeks, an adjustment disorder (ICD-10: F43.2) would be diagnosed. In both cases, immediate psychosomatic co-treatment either by a somatic physician or by a psycho-oncologically trained psychosomatic medical expert is appropriate.

Differential diagnosis should clarify whether at least two or three of the main criteria of a depressive episode are met (ICD-10: F32.0). As the patient does not have low drive and does feel hopeless about his future outlook, he does not meet the criteria of having a depressive disorder. Furthermore he demonstrates no convincing suicidal ideation. The criteria of an autonomous anxiety disorder are also not met because the patient's anxiety is only related to his disease process.

Other psychological comorbidity or disease was definitively ruled out from the history of this otherwise healthy patient.

Procedure and Progress The patient obtained detailed information from in-depth discussions with somatic physicians and was therefore able to reduce his anxiety. Five psycho-oncological treatments with a medical expert in psychosomatic medicine and psychotherapy were undertaken before and after the operation, which helped the patient to understand the process of acute disease and reduce his feelings of guilt. It was agreed that he would contact us for psychosomatic co-treatment in future if he experienced psychic distress again. Psychopharmacological medication was not necessary.

Case Study 3.4

A 58-year-old female patient attended the phoniatrics clinic as an emergency patient. She had suddenly become unable to speak 2 days earlier. She had only been able to whistle and was therefore unfit for her work as a teacher. Despite this being an 'emergency situation', the patient seemed to be only a little distressed, and when taking her history, she sometimes cheerfully shrugged her shoulders: she did not know where this could come from either!

Diagnosis and Differential Diagnosis Presuming that all somatic results are within normal limits, the diagnosis is almost certainly a dissociative movement disorder (ICD-10: F44.4). Dissociative movement disorders fundamentally concern the voluntary musculature and present as 'pseudo-neurological phenomena'. Because patients are often surprisingly unconcerned, the phenomenon is known as 'belle indifférence'. This, in combination with an underlying neurotic conflict, points towards primary morbid gain. Thereby the symptoms are unconsciously motivated by potential decrease of the intrapsychic conflict.

The detailed biographical history brought to light that the patient has always been sensitive to hurtful words or slights. She was recently faced with a new school principal who was almost 20 years younger than she and talked about his plans regarding the conceptual development of the school mainly to her younger colleagues. One week before her symptoms began, she had to defend herself to the new principal for giving a student bad grades after his parents had filed a complaint to the school management. She then lost her voice.

Course of Treatment A consultation and examination was immediately begun in the outpatient Clinic for Psychosomatics and Psychotherapy. After the patient was able to recognise the situation that caused her illness (defending herself to the principal), further clarification of her psychological vulnerability could follow. Working together with the patient, it was revealed that, as the middle sister of 3, she never felt valued in her parental home. She experienced this repetitive dysfunctional pattern throughout her adult life, but it had been compensated for by the high esteem in which she was held by the former school principal and the parents of her students. Since the new management has been in charge, she has been thrown into an offside position, at least from a subjective point of view, which had worsened her sensitivity for hurtful words or slights. The dissociative aphonia presents a suboptimal 'solution' in terms of a primary morbid gain used in order to step out of the conflict situation by rendering her unable to work.

Over 25 sessions in the framework of psychodynamic psychotherapy, the patient managed successfully to work on her repetitive dysfunctional conflict of self-confidence, and her voice returned to the extent that she could return to work. At the same time, she worked on reducing her dependence on others' esteem in her working life by strengthening her private relationships as a source of esteem.

3.5 Basics of Child and Adolescent Psychiatry: Attention-Deficit/Hyperactivity Disorder

Esther Strittmatter and Georg Romer

3.5.1 Introduction

Parents of children with psychiatric disorders may initially consult a phoniatrician/paedaudiologist owing to anomalies in communication resembling developmental disorders of speech and language, hearing impairment or perception disorders. Therefore, knowledge about the most common diseases in child and adolescent psychiatry is essential for early recognition and therapy of affected children. Marked inattention/hyperactivity may hint at an attention-deficit/hyperactivity disorder; verbal and nonverbal impairment in communication and in social interaction at an autism spectrum disorder; and consistent failure to speak in unfamiliar public settings combined with social phobia at selective mutism.

Phoniatricians/paedaudiologists should be alert to psychiatric disorders such as differential diagnoses of a delay in hearing or speech/language development and immediately refer affected children to a child and adolescent psychiatrist. Early detection improves the effectiveness of therapeutic options and prevents secondary comorbidities and significant social, occupational and academic impairment.

Similarly, children with psychiatric disorders should be referred to phoniatricians/paedaudiologists to exclude hearing impairment and to give support in improving speech/language development.

In this Sect. 3.5 and the following Sects. 3.6 and 3.7, some of the more relevant disorders in child and adolescent psychiatry are presented.

3.5.2 Prevalence of Attention-Deficit/Hyperactivity Disorder (ADHD)

As the name of the disorder indicates attention-deficit/hyperactivity disorder (ADHD) presents as a pattern of persistent inattention or hyperactivity and impulsivity that interferes with functioning or development. ADHD is one of the more common disorders in child and adolescent psychiatry. Meta-analysis suggests a pooled prevalence of 5.3% in children and adolescents (Polanczyk et al. 2007) and 2.5% in adults (Simon et al. 2009). The prevalence of ADHD seems to have been stable over the past three decades (Polanczyk et al. 2014). Males are more often affected than females with a male-to-female sex ratio of 2.4:1 in population studies and 4:1 in clinical studies (Polanczyk et al. 2007). Often, comorbid disorders (e.g. oppositional defiant and conduct disorder, anxiety disorders, depressive disorders) occur in individuals with ADHD (Steinhausen et al. 2006). While only 15% of the children with ADHD meet full diagnostic criteria at the age of 25 years, approximately two-thirds will have persistent functional impairment into adulthood (Faraone et al. 2006).

3.5.3 Symptomatology

The core symptoms of ADHD are inattention or hyperactivity-impulsivity (American Psychiatric Association 2013). Typically, the symptoms start in early childhood. However, because of the high variability in behaviour in young children, a valid diagnosis is difficult before the age of 4 years. In preschool children the main manifestations are excessive motor activity and shorter playing time. Sometimes these children are greater risk-takers than their peers and are thus more likely to injure themselves. When their elementary schooling begins, their inattention becomes often more apparent. Often ADHD is associated with learning disorders and poorer academic achievement. Furthermore, impulsive behaviour, affective instability and motor hyperactivity can lead to conflict with parents, teachers and peers. In adolescents hyperactive symptoms manifest as inner restlessness, while inattention persists and is often accompanied by poor planning abilities. School failure and peer rejection may lead to low self-esteem, social disability and secondary comorbidities (e.g. substance abuse). For an overview the main DSM-5 diagnostic criteria are summarised in Table 3.7. They are further exemplified in the case report.

Case Study 3.5

On the advice of the child and adolescent psychiatrist, Mrs. Schmidt presents with her 9-year-old son Kevin to the phoniatrician for the purpose of excluding sound conduction and per-

Table 3.7 DSM-5 diagnostic criteria for ADHD (modified from American Psychiatric Association 2013)

Inattention	Hyperactivity-impulsivity
(a) Fails to give close attention, makes careless mistakes	(a) Fidgets with or taps hands or feet or squirms in seat
(b) Has difficulty sustaining attention	(b) Leaves seat in situations when remaining seated is expected
(c) Does not seem to listen	(c) Often runs about or climbs in inappropriate situations (in adolescents/adults: feeling restless)
(d) Fails to finish tasks (e.g. schoolwork)	(d) Unable to play quietly
(e) Has difficulty organising tasks and activities	(e) Often 'on the go', acting as if 'driven by a motor'
(f) Avoids or is reluctant to engage in tasks that require sustained mental effort	(f) Talks excessively
(g) Often loses things	(g) Blurts out an answer before a question has been completed
(h) Easily distracted by extraneous stimuli	(h) Has difficulty waiting his or her turn
(i) Forgetful in daily activities	(i) Often interrupts or intrudes on others

Six or more of the preceding symptoms have been present for at least 6 months

Yes   yes

Yes   yes

Predominantly inattentive presentation   **Combined presentation**   **Predominantly hyperactive/impulsive presentation**

Predominantly inattentive presentation   **Combined presentation**   **Predominantly hyperactive/impulsive presentation**

ception disorders. In the waiting room, Kevin is disturbing the other patients by his antics. On entering the doctor's room, Kevin begins to explore his surroundings and without permission starts to finger the doctor's instruments and a personal family picture. When Mrs. Schmidt tells Kevin to sit down, he doesn't appear to hear her. In order to conduct a conversation with the doctor, Mrs. Schmidt takes out a Gameboy to occupy Kevin. Immediately Kevin sits down and begins to play. Mrs. Schmidt complains to the doctor that he often disturbs lessons with his fidgeting, inability to sit still and by leaving his seat. Because Kevin cannot concentrate for more than a few minutes, he does not complete schoolwork (or homework). Furthermore he frequently mislays or loses his school materials. Kevin is often embroiled in conflict with his peers and his mother. At home his room looks a mess. While Kevin is reluctant to do homework or schoolwork, he can play videogames for hours.

3.5.4 Aetiology and Developmental Psychopathology

In 2013, the American Psychiatric Association (APA) has reconceptualised ADHD as a neurodevelopmental disorder in the fifth edition of the *Diagnostic and Statistical Manual of Mental Disorders* (DSM-5) (American Psychiatric Association 2013). ADHD is caused multifactorially. Studies on twins indicate a heritability of ADHD of 70–80% (Larsson et al. 2014). The interaction of several genetic and environmental risk factors leads to epigenetic changes and dysregulation of dopaminergic, noradrenergic and serotonergic monoamine systems. Structural and functional brain imaging studies have shown an under-activation and lower connectivity in frontal, striatal, limbic and cerebellar pathways. Furthermore, total brain volume is 3–5% smaller than normal. The described abnormalities result in a wide range of neurocognitive impairments (e.g. dysregulation of information processing, attention, inhibitory control and reward), which is consistent with the heterogeneity of the disorder (for elaborated review, see Faraone et al. 2015).

3.5.5 Differential Diagnosis

For differential diagnosis, oppositional defiant disorder, specific learning disorder, tic disorders, intellectual disability, reactive attachment disorder, anxiety disorders, depressive disorders and personality disorders should be considered. However, 60–85% of the patients have at least one of the mentioned disorders as a coexisting condition (Steinhausen et al. 2006).

3.5.6 Diagnostics and Treatment

The diagnosis relies on clinical symptoms reported by the patient, the parents or other informants (e.g. teachers). Thus, a structured clinical interview remains the 'gold standard' for diagnosis. The diagnostic criteria are listed in Table 3.7. According to the International Classification of Diseases (ICD-10), the age of onset has to be below 7 years. In contrast, DSM-5 has increased the age of onset from 7 years to 12 years. Validated rating scales help to assess quantitatively the behaviour in different contexts (e.g. at home and at school). A physical examination and laboratory tests should be performed to exclude somatic disorders. Furthermore, impaired hearing (e.g. disturbances of sound conduction and perception) and impaired vision should be excluded.

Although ADHD cannot be cured, several evidence-based treatments exist to reduce impairment and improve quality of life. Meta-analysis has shown that stimulants (methylphenidate, amphetamine) and non-stimulants (atomoxetine, guanfacine) effectively reduce the ADHD core symptoms inattention and hyperactivity-impulsivity (Faraone et al. 2015). In most cases medications are well tolerated, and adverse events are manageable (Cortese et al. 2013). Non-pharmacological treatment approaches (e.g. cognitive behavioural therapy, parent training,

parent-child interaction therapy, school-based approach) mainly help to prevent or to improve secondary comorbidities and aim at ameliorating quality of life (Faraone et al. 2015; Sonuga-Barke et al. 2013).

3.5.7 Summary and Clinical Implications

ADHD is a common and impairing disorder in children and adolescents. Each ear, nose and throat specialist/phoniatrician/paedaudiologist should be alert to the disorder when a child presents for the differential diagnosis of an auditory disorder. Children with marked inattention or hyperactivity-impulsivity should be referred to a child and adolescent psychiatrist, as effective treatment options exist that can ameliorate the course of the disease and prevent secondary comorbidities.

3.6 Basics of Child and Adolescent Psychiatry: Autism Spectrum and Pervasive Developmental Disorders

Christian Postert

3.6.1 Introduction

The term autism is derived from the Greek word *autos* implying here a self-closed individual who is isolated from social relations. Autism spectrum disorders (ASD) are categorised in the International Statistical Classification of Diseases and Related Health Problems (ICD-10) as pervasive developmental disorders that are behaviourally characterised by:

(a) Persistent qualitative impairment in both verbal and nonverbal communication
(b) Persistent qualitative impairment in social interaction
(c) Restricted and repetitive patterns of behaviour and interests

As impairment in communication and in social interaction are closely interrelated and their severity highly correlated, (a) and (b) have been merged into one domain in the *Diagnostic and Statistical Manual of Mental Disorders* (DSM-5). Current prevalence rates indicate that autism spectrum disorders are frequent in the population as they occur in 1 in 68 births, or 14.7 children per 1000. Boys are five times more prone to the disorder than girls (Centers for Disease Control and Prevention 2014).

Research strongly suggests that impaired understanding of other minds (also called 'Theory of Mind' or 'Mentalising') is a common feature of people with ASD that may help to explain some, but not all, of the ensuing socio-communicative impairment (Boucher 2012). Autism spectrum disorders represent only the severe end of a continuous distribution of social communication skills in the general population. Individuals affected differ widely in the severity of symptoms and their impairment, and there is an arbitrary nature to diagnostic cut-offs in this spectrum (Constantino and Charman 2015).

Various subtypes of the autism spectrum are subsumed in the ICD-10 under the heading of Pervasive Developmental Disorders. Asperger syndrome calls attention to the fact that significant social impairment may occur in individuals without language or intellectual delays. Rett syndrome and childhood disintegrative disorder share several symptoms with autism but may have unrelated causes. Pervasive developmental disorders not otherwise specified (PDD-NOS, also called atypical autism) are diagnosed when the criteria are not met for a more specific disorder. However, in most recent research, it has become increasingly apparent that these diagnostic subtypes are not reliable across clinicians or time (Lord and Jones 2012). Consequently, the various pervasive developmental disorders were consolidated in DSM-5 into a single umbrella diagnosis of autism spectrum disorder (ASD) that is only differentiated by dimensions of severity and associated features (i.e. known genetic disorders, epilepsy and intellectual disability). The current ICD-11 Beta Draft (World Health Organization 2016a, b) also follows this categorisation.

3.6.2 Symptomatology

ASD may be typically identified before the age of 2 (Fakhoury 2015). Individual profiles differ markedly in the number and quality of symptoms displayed but are relatively stable from 2 years onwards (Constantino and Charman 2015). Symptomatology may also vary as a function of environmental demands at home, in school or within peer groups. The spectrum ranges from severe impairment in nonverbal individuals locked into various types of repetitive behaviour to verbal high-functioning individuals with normal intelligence but distinctly odd social interaction and communication.

Early ASD symptomatology may include children who:

- Do not point things out to create joint attention.
- Do not share emotions with other persons.
- Do not babble in early infancy, remain nonverbal later on or are characterised by a strikingly monotonous tone of voice.
- Do not use facial expressions or gestures to compensate for language deficits.
- Do not use toys or dolls in pretend play.

Children with ASD may show:

- Hypersensitivity to touch, noise, light or smell
- Delayed fine motor skills
- Unusual attachment to objects, with highly repetitive play
- Rigidity in repetitive action sequences and a preoccupation with tactile or olfactory qualities of objects
- Highly peculiar special interests and unusual obsessions, compulsions and stereotypes
- Over-concrete thinking leading to difficulty in the pragmatic understanding of literary and metaphorical expressions

Co-occurring epilepsy and psychiatric disorders are frequent and may include anxiety, ADHD or depression and symptoms such as self-injurious behaviour or aggression.

Case Study 3.6

Leo was referred to the phoniatrician for evaluation of hearing and of communication delays. At 2 years he is still nonverbal and rarely responds to his name being called. His parents report that he is preoccupied with the texture, smell and size of toys and other objects and orders them according to size, but not to their function. He does not point to objects of desire or share his emotions or intentions with his family. In kindergarten, he is alone most of the time, does not engage in symbolic play and exhibits a persistent lack of social interest and reciprocity. In interaction with the phoniatrician, he shows poor eye contact and seems to be more disinterested than shy or anxious.

3.6.3 Aetiology and Developmental Psychopathology

We do not yet understand the causes of ASD despite knowing about the genetic roots of ASD interacting with environmental factors. There may be hundreds of different aetiologies underlying the manifestation of ASD (Lord and Bishop 2015; Mandy and Lai 2016). Research suggests that several hundred different genes are probably involved as risk factors for autism. Many of the genetic variants associated with ASD have also been strongly implicated in other neuropsychiatric disorders, such as ADHD, schizophrenia, epilepsy and intellectual disability. Each gene can only account for a tiny elevation for risk in ASD (odds ratios between 1.0 and 1.2) (Constantino and Charman 2015). Phenotypic expression of these genetic influences varies according to intervening influences from the intrauterine environment and early life experiences, for example, infectious diseases or serious medical complications during the neonatal period (Constantino and Charman 2015). Severe early deprivation in parent-child interaction may influence the probability of manifesting a full ASD phenotype from a prodromal phase (Mandy and Lai 2016).

3.6.4 Differential Diagnosis

At first sight, some other diseases may give the impression of similar clinical phenomena. Children with social phobia and anxiety may be shy and withdrawn or even cease to speak in unfamiliar environments, as in the case of selective mutism. However, they are only socially inhibited, not disabled, and their parents report uninhibited communicative and social skills in familiar contexts. In children with language and social delays, it may be difficult to assess whether this impairment can be accounted for by hearing loss or by an ASD diagnosis. Every child with language delays should be screened for ASD and vice versa.

3.6.5 Diagnostics and Treatment

Early diagnosis and treatment are important, as the appropriate behavioural therapies may significantly affect the prognosis. However, there is no laboratory test or specific neural signature for ASD available (Constantino and Charman 2015). The diagnosis of ASD is based on a purely behavioural description of a constellation of symptoms. Families usually take time to recognise that a child is persistently unable to meet the demands of its social environment. Therefore, the average age of diagnosis is often delayed to 3–6 years of age with the risk of missing a critical window for early ASD interventions.

Parents of children with ASD often notice developmental problems in their children as early as 12 months of age and most often express concerns of hearing and vision. Later on, many children with ASD may come into phoniatric or paediatric consultation as the first point of contact, owing to language developmental delay. Therefore, phoniatricians may play an important role in the early recognition of ASD. The *Modified Checklist for Autism in Toddlers, Revised* (M-CHAT-R) can be used as an effective and useful online tool for screening 18- to 24-month-old children that relies on the parent's report. It is easily available through the Autism Speaks website (Robins et al. 2016).

If the screening is positive, further evaluation of the child should be conducted by a child psychiatrist, psychologist, paediatrician or child neurologist with expertise in diagnosing ASD. Appraisal of symptoms requires obtaining information from multiple sources by interviewing parents, caregivers and teachers (Constantino and Charman 2015). Several diagnostic tools have been developed for the evaluation of the behavioural characteristics of children with ASD. The most common one for the direct assessment of the child is the *Autism Diagnostic Observation Schedule* (ADOS-2), involving a variety of play-based imaginative activities and social tasks. It is commonly used as a gold standard in combination with the *Autism Diagnostic Interview—Revised* (ADI-R), a semi-structured interview conducted with the parents on the child's development in language, social skills, behaviour and cognition (Lord et al. 1994; Fakhoury 2015).

The aetiological heterogeneity presents a substantial obstacle to the development of therapies. However, new well-designed randomised controlled trials are providing increasing support for early and intensive behavioural interventions including picture-based communication systems (Constantino and Charman 2015). Approaches that help to develop specific parenting strategies may improve parent-child interaction and lead to better language comprehension and reduction in autism severity; however, this factor still has to be further investigated as effect sizes of present studies are still small (Oono et al. 2013).

3.6.6 Summary and Clinical Implications

Autism spectrum disorders are frequent and come with substantial impairments in social interaction and communication as well as episodes of excessive repetitive behaviour. The variability of symptoms corresponds to a wide variety

of genetic and environmental factors that interact in the developmental trajectories to the full manifestation of the spectrum disorder. In the clinical management of individuals with ASD, hearing evaluations can be challenging owing to a frequent hypersensitivity to touch, sound and light. Unfamiliar healthcare settings with crowded waiting rooms and long waiting times are especially demanding for these children. Parents usually know very well how to manage their child and can be a very helpful resource for smoothing stressful situations, for example, using headphones in cases of ear sensitivity. Planning early clinical appointments with some extra time and involving parents and communication devices, such as picture-based systems or comfort items, during the visit may ease necessary clinical procedures, such as taking an audiogram (Biyani et al. 2015).

3.7 Basics of Child and Adolescent Psychiatry: Selective Mutism

Christian Postert

3.7.1 Introduction

Selective mutism (SM) is characterised by a consistent failure to speak where speech is expected, especially in unfamiliar public settings such as in school, despite fluency with the given language. In familiar settings such as at home, speaking is not compromised in SM. Prevalence rates for SM range from 0.18 to 1.9%. Girls tend to be more prone to SM than boys (Muris and Ollendick 2015; Scott and Beidel 2011). The *Diagnostic and Statistical Manual of Mental Disorders* (DSM-5) lists SM among the anxiety disorders, as social anxiety is a prominent symptom in many children with SM (Keeton and Crosby Budinger 2012). SM comes with significant social, occupational and academic impairment over extended periods of time and needs early and intensive child psychiatric intervention.

3.7.2 Symptomatology

Symptoms are usually obvious already at preschool age but become manifest and severely interfering in daily function when children enter elementary school and meet the challenge of speaking in a novel social setting. Many children are initially anxious and shy when confronted with entering school for the first time but regain their balance and start to speak in school after a few weeks. Therefore, the diagnosis of SM is not made during the first month after school enrolment.

Longitudinal research shows that total absence of speech in unfamiliar situations has a mean duration of 8 years in SM and usually dissipates or disappears then. However, until then, significant social, occupational and academic impairment occurs, and associated symptoms such as anxiety or problems in school performance tend to persist for even longer periods of time (Muris and Ollendick 2015).

Case Study 3.7

When 6-year-old Sophia enters the consultation room with her mother, she shies away from contact, hides behind her mother and avoids eye contact. Her mother appears distressed and frustrated by the child's mutism but seems to be used to respond quickly on behalf of the child. Symptoms did not come to attention until Sophia entered school. Teachers report that Sophia has not spoken in school since school enrolment 6 months ago. Whereas Sophia hesitantly accepts assigned tasks, she does not interact with other children in a larger group and does not respond verbally to teachers' questions. In school, she only whispers to a close girlfriend she still knows from kindergarten; if other children get in touch with her, she turns away in most cases. Whereas she is delighted to chat with her family members when being alone with them, she anxiously falls silent even in the presence of distant family members or in public events such as church meetings.

3.7.3 Aetiology and Developmental Psychopathology

The majority of data derive from small-scale samples that may not be representative for all children affected by SM (Viana et al. 2009; Hua and Major 2016). Therefore, the exact aetiological pathways of SM are not yet known. However, available evidence suggests that SM originates from the interplay of several temperamental, neurodevelopmental and environmental risk factors. Behavioural inhibition as a temperamental trait is often found among children with SM who show persistent and avoidant fearfulness when confronted with unfamiliar persons and situations (Muris and Ollendick 2015). Neurodevelopmental factors such as language and speech problems may contribute to the development of SM, especially if the anticipation of embarrassment in public speech situations leads to persistent avoidance behaviour. Silence may be used here as a means to conceal developmental delays. Environmental factors such as family dysfunction, stressful life events, immigrant status, bilingualism and parental control contribute to the stress experienced by affected children and to the manifestation of symptoms (Muris and Ollendick 2015).

3.7.4 Differential Diagnosis

As SM may be seen as an extreme and early variant of social phobia that manifests especially in speech situations, there is considerable overlap with the symptoms of social phobia and other anxiety disorders (Keeton and Crosby Budinger 2012). Children with autism spectrum disorders and SM may both be nonverbal in the clinical consultation. However, in many cases of autism spectrum disorders, there is an inability to communicate appropriately irrespective of context. In SM, there is only an inhibition to speak in public situations, whereas in familiar context at home, parents report unrestricted verbalisation. SM must be distinguished from temporary speech avoidance manifesting in children who learn a second language in which they are not yet fluent.

3.7.5 Diagnostics and Treatment

Diagnosis of SM requires a comprehensive and multimodal evaluation involving audiology, child psychiatry and psychology and speech/language pathology. For a diagnosis of SM according to DSM-5 and the current ICD-11 Beta Draft (World Health Organization 2016a, b), the symptoms must be present for at least 1 month (excluding the very first month of school attendance) and involve significant impairment in social, occupational and academic function.

Several randomised controlled studies with rather small sample sizes have supported the efficacy of cognitive behavioural therapy in the treatment of SM. Therapy effects are greater in younger children, underscoring the necessity of early diagnosis and intervention (Hua and Major 2016; Wong 2010). Treatment involves systematic reinforcement of speech behaviour and assisting the child to a gradual exposure to increasingly difficult speech situations while learning to cope with negative emotions such as embarrassment (Muris and Ollendick 2015). This approach is complemented by social skills training to improve both verbal and nonverbal social competence and family therapeutic interventions to screen for and ameliorate stress from biographical or relational factors in the family. Counselling of the parents and teachers is especially important to help them to manage the child's distress and its avoidance behaviour effectively. Data suggest that selective serotonin reuptake inhibitors (SSRIs) such as fluoxetine may be a psychopharmacological complement to therapies for those who do not respond sufficiently to psychosocial treatment alone (Muris and Ollendick 2015). Comorbid language problems may need logopaedic interventions in order to improve language function. If treatment succeeds and the child starts to speak in unfamiliar settings, further therapeutic attention has to be paid to persisting social anxiety that is common among these children.

3.7.6 Summary and Clinical Implications

Social anxiety and the avoidance of unfamiliar speech situations in which embarrassment may occur are at the core of SM. When children appear shy, anxious and withdrawn and remain mute in the clinical encounter, attention should be given to their ability to speak at school or in unfamiliar social situations. If parents or teachers report mutism in these social environments associated with social, occupational or academic impairment, further child psychiatric evaluation is recommended. Whereas children will probably remain silent in the clinical encounter with the phoniatrician, they may hesitantly communicate nonverbally, for example, by nodding or shaking their head. Receptive language tests may be performed by having the child point to responses. Expressive language may be evaluated on the basis of audiotaped speech in familiar social settings (Manassis 2009). While it is not appropriate to urge children with SM to speak, social interaction with them should not be missed, in order to challenge social avoidance behaviour and to create new opportunities for them to gain social experiences in a safe setting.

References

American Psychiatric Association (2013) Attention-deficit/hyperactivity disorder. In: Diagnostic and statistical manual of mental disorders, 5th edition (DSM-5™). American Psychiatric Publishing, Washington, DC, pp 59–65

Baldwin EJ, Gibberd FB, Harley C et al (2010) The effectiveness of long-term dietary therapy in the treatment of adult Refsum disease. J Neurol Neurosurg Psychiatry 81(9):954–957

Beutel M, Schulz H (2011) Epidemiologie psychisch komorbider Störungen bei chronisch körperlichen Erkrankungen. Bundesgesundheitsblatt Gesundheitsförderung Gesundheitsschutz 54(1):15–21

Billard C, Fluss J, Pinton F (2009) Specific language impairment versus Landau Kleffner syndrome. Epilepsia 50(Suppl 7):21–24

Biyani S, Morgan PS, Hotchkiss K et al (2015) Autism spectrum disorder 101: a primer for pediatric otolaryngologists. Int J Pediatr Otorhinolaryngol 79(12):798–802

Boucher J (2012) Putting theory of mind in its place: psychological explanations of the socio-emotional-communicative impairments in autistic spectrum disorder. Autism 16(3):226–246

Brandao-Almeida IL, Hage SR, Oliveira EP et al (2008) Congenital bilateral perisylvian syndrome: familial occurrence, clinical and psycholinguistic aspects correlated with MRI. Neuropediatrics 39(3):139–145

Buschmann A, Jooss B, Rupp A et al (2009) Parent based language intervention for 2-year-old children with specific expressive language delay: a randomised controlled trial. Arch Dis Child 94(2):110–116. https://doi.org/10.1136/adc.2008.141572

Cable AL, Domsch C (2011) Systematic review of the literature on the treatment of children with late language emergence. Int J Lang Commun Disord 46(2):138–154. https://doi.org/10.3109/13682822.2010.487883

Centers for Disease Control and Prevention (2014) Prevalence of autism spectrum disorder among children aged 8 years—autism and developmental disabilities monitoring network, 11 sites, United States, 2010. Morb Mortal Wkly Rep 63(37)

Chonchaiya W, Pruksananonda C (2008) Television viewing associates with delayed language development. Acta Paediatr 97(7):977–982

Christen HJ, Hanefeld F, Kruse E et al (2000) Foix-Chavany-Marie (anterior operculum) syndrome in childhood: a reappraisal of Worster-Drought syndrome. Dev Med Child Neurol 42(2):122–132

Cleary MA, Wraith JE (1993) Management of mucopolysaccharidosis type III. Arch Dis Child 69(3):403–406

Constantino JN, Charman T (2015) Diagnosis of autism spectrum disorder: reconciling the syndrome, its diverse origins, and variation in expression. Lancet Neurol 15(3):279–291. https://doi.org/10.1016/S1474-4422(15)00151-9

Cortese S, Holtmann M, Banaschewski T et al (2013) Practitioner review: current best practice in the management of adverse events during treatment with ADHD medications in children and adolescents. J Child Psychol Psychiatry 54(3):227–246

Deonna T, Roulet-Perez E (2010) Early-onset acquired epileptic aphasia (Landau-Kleffner syndrome, LKS) and regressive autistic disorders with epileptic EEG abnormalities: the continuing debate. Brain Dev 32(9):746–752

Deonna TW, Roulet E, Fontan D et al (1993) Speech and oromotor deficits of epileptic origin in benign partial epilepsy of childhood with rolandic spikes (BPERS). Relationship to the acquired aphasia-epilepsy syndrome. Neuropediatrics 24(2):83–87

Deutsche Angestellten-Krankenkasse (DAK) (2011) Gesundheitsreport 2011. Available via http://www.dak.de/dak/download/Gesundheitsreport_2011-1117028.pdf. Accessed 8 Oct 2015

Eckhardt-Henn A, Heuft G, Hochapfel G et al (2009) Neurotische Störungen und Psychosomatische Medizin, 8th edn. Schattauer, Stuttgart

Eisenberger T, Neuhaus C, Khan AO et al (2013) Increasing the yield in targeted next-generation sequencing by implicating CNV analysis, non-coding exons and the overall variant load: the example of retinal dystrophies. PLoS One 8(11):e78496

Fakhoury M (2015) Autistic spectrum disorders: a review of clinical features, theories and diagnosis. Int J Dev Neurosci 43:70–77

Faraone SV, Biederman J, Mick E (2006) The age dependent decline of attention-deficit/hyperactivity disorder: a meta-analysis of follow-up studies. Psychol Med 36(2):159–165

Faraone SV, Asherson P, Banaschewski T et al (2015) Attention-deficit/hyperactivity disorder. Nat Rev Dis Primers 1:1–23

Fernandez Filho JA, Shapiro BE (2004) Tay-Sachs disease. Arch Neurol 61(9):1466–1468

Fletcher JC, Berg K, Tranøy KE (1985) Ethical aspects of medical genetics. A proposal for guidelines in genetic counseling, prenatal diagnosis and screening. Clin Genet 27(2):199–205

Frankenburg WK, Dodds J, Archer P et al (1992) The Denver II: a major revision and restandardization of the Denver Developmental Screening Test. Pediatrics 89(1):91–97

Fuhrmann W, Vogel F (1983) Genetic counselling, 3rd edn. Springer, Berlin

Goorhuis-Brouwer SM, Dikkers FG, Robinson PH et al (2003) Specific language impairment in children with velocardiofacial syndrome: four case studies. Cleft Palate Craniofac J 40(2):190–196

Grimm T, Zerres K (2010) Genetic counseling and prenatal diagnosis. In: Speicher MR et al (eds) Human genetics. Problems and approaches, 4th edn. Springer, Berlin, pp 845–866

Guerreiro MM, Hage SR, Guimaraes CA et al (2002) Developmental language disorder associated with polymicrogyria. Neurology 59(2):245–250

Harper PS (2010) Practical genetic counselling, 7th edn. Arnold, London

Hautzinger M, Bailer M, Woral H et al (1994) Beck-Depressions-Inventar (BDI). Huber, Bern

Hilgert N, Smith RJ, Van Camp G (2009) Forty-six genes causing nonsyndromic hearing impairment: which ones should be analyzed in DNA diagnostics? Mutat Res 681(2–3):189–196

Hochlehnert A, Niehoff D, Herzog W et al (2007) Höhere Kosten bei internistischen Krankenhauspatienten mit psychischer Komorbidität: Fehlende Abbildung im DRG-System. Psychother Psychosom Med Psychol 57(2):70–75

Hua A, Major N (2016) Selective mutism. Curr Opin Pediatr 28(1):114–120

Keeton CP, Crosby Budinger M (2012) Social phobia and selective mutism. Child Adolesc Psychiatr Clin N Am 21(3):621–641

Kohlschütter A, Santer R, Lukacs Z et al (2012) A child with night blindness: preventing serious symptoms of Refsum disease. J Child Neurol 27(5):654–656

Landau WM, Kleffner FR (1957) Syndrome of acquired aphasia with convulsive disorder in children. Neurology 7(8):523–530

Larsson H, Chang Z, D'Onofrio BM et al (2014) The heritability of clinically diagnosed attention-deficit/hyperactivity disorder across the lifespan. Psychol Med 44(10):2223–2229

Lillywhite L, Saling M, Harvey S et al (2009) Neuropsychological and functional MRI studies provide converging evidence of anterior language dysfunction in BECTS. Epilepsia 50(10):2276–2284

Limbrock GJ, Castillo-Morales R, Hoyer H et al (1993) The Castillo-Morales approach to orofacial pathology in Down syndrome. Int J Orofacial Myology 19:30–37

Liukkonen E, Kantola-Sorsa E, Paetau R et al (2010) Long-term outcome of 32 children with encephalopathy with status epilepticus during sleep, or ESES syndrome. Epilepsia 51(10):2023–2032

Lord C, Bishop SL (2015) Recent advances in autism research as reflected in DSM-5 criteria for autism spectrum disorder. Annu Rev Clin Psychol 28(11):53–70

Lord C, Jones RM (2012) Annual research review: rethinking the classification of autism spectrum disorders. J Child Psychol Psychiatry 53(5):490–509

Lord C, Rutter M, Le Couteur A (1994) Autism diagnostic interview-revised: a revised version of a diagnostic interview for caregivers of individuals with possible pervasive developmental disorders. J Autism Dev Disord 24(5):659–685

Manassis K (2009) Silent suffering: understanding and treating children with selective mutism. Expert Rev Neurother 9(2):235–243

Mandy W, Lai MC (2016) Annual research review: the role of the environment in the developmental psychopathology of autism spectrum condition. J Child Psychol Psychiatry 57(3):271–292

Muris PEHM, Ollendick TH (2015) Children who are anxious in silence: a review on selective mutism, the new anxiety disorder in DSM-5. Clin Child Fam Psychol Rev 18(2):151–169

Nass R, Trauner DA (2012) Developmental language disorders. In: Swaiman KF et al (eds) Pediatric neurology: principles and practice, 5th edn. Elsevier Saunders, Philadelphia

Nevo Y, Segev Y, Gelman Y et al (2001) Worster-Drought and congenital perisylvian syndromes—a continuum. Pediatr Neurol 24(2):153–155

Online Mendelian Inheritance in Man (OMIM®) McKusick-Nathans Institute of Genetic Medicine, Johns Hopkins University (2016) An Online Catalog of Human Genes and Genetic Disorders. Available via http://omim.org/. Accessed 8 Dec 2016

Oono IP, Honey EJ, McConachie H (2013) Parent-mediated early intervention for young children with autism spectrum disorders (ASD). Cochrane Database Syst Rev 30(4):CD009774

Overvliet GM, Besseling RM, Vles JS et al (2010) Nocturnal epileptiform discharges, nocturnal epileptiform seizures and language impairment in children: review of the literature. Epilepsy Behav 19(4):550–558

Parker M, Bitner-Glindzicz M (2015) Genetic investigations in childhood deafness. Arch Dis Child 100(3):271–278. https://doi.org/10.1136/archdischild-2014-306099. Epub 2014 Oct 16. Review

Pina-Garza JE (2013) Psychomotor retardation and regression. In: Pina-Garza JE (ed) Fenichel's clinical pediatric neurology. Elsevier Saunders, Philadelphia

Polanczyk G, de Lima MS, Horta BL et al (2007) The worldwide prevalence of ADHD: a systematic review and metaregression analysis. Am J Psychiatry 164(6):942–948

Polanczyk GV, Willcutt EG, Salum GA et al (2014) ADHD prevalence estimates across three decades: an updated systematic review and meta-regression analysis. Int J Epidemiol 43(2):434–442

Rehm HL (2013) Disease-targeted sequencing: a cornerstone in the clinic. Nat Rev Genet 14(4):295–300

Rescorla L, Roberts J, Dahlsgaard K (1997) Late talkers at 2: Outcome at age 3. J Speech Hear Res 40(3):556–566

Resta RG (2006) Defining and redefining the scope and goals of genetic counselling. Am J Med Genet C Semin Med Genet 142C(4):269–275

Roberts MY, Kaiser AP (2011) The effectiveness of parent-implemented language interventions: a meta-analysis. Am J Speech Lang Pathol 20(3):180–199. https://doi.org/10.1044/1058-0360(2011/10-0055

Roberts MY, Kaiser AP (2015) Early intervention for toddlers with language delays: a randomized controlled trial. Pediatrics 135(4):686–694. https://doi.org/10.1542/peds.2014-2134

Robertson SB, Weismer SE (1999) Effects of treatment on linguistic and social skills in toddlers with delayed language development. J Speech Lang Hear Res 42(5):1234–1248. https://doi.org/10.1044/jslhr.4205.1234

Robins D, Fine D, Barton M (2016) Modified Checklist for Autism in Toddlers, Revised (M-CHAT-R™). Available via https://www.autismspeaks.org/what-autism/diagnosis/mchat. Accessed 23 Feb 2016

Rozanski A, Blumenthal JA, Davidson KW et al (2005) The epidemiology, pathophysiology, and management of psychosocial risk factors in cardiac practice. J Am Coll Cardiol 45(5):637–651

Ruether K, Baldwin E, Casteels M et al (2010) Adult Refsum disease: a form of tapetoretinal dystrophy accessible to therapy. Surv Ophthalmol 55(6):531–538

Scott S, Beidel DC (2011) Selective mutism: an update and suggestions for future research. Curr Psychiatry Rep 13(4):251–257

Shepard TH, Lemire RI (2010) Catalog of teratogenic agents, 13th edn. John Hopkins University Press, Baltimore

Shevell M, Ashwal S, Donley D et al (2003) Practice parameter: evaluation of the child with global developmental delay. Report of the Quality Standards Committee of the American Academy of Neurology and the Practice Committee of the Child Neurology Society. Neurology 60(3):367–380

Simon V, Czobor P, Balint S et al (2009) Prevalence and correlates of adult attention-deficit/hyperactivity disorder: meta-analysis. Br J Psychiatry 194(3):204–211

Sonuga-Barke EJ, Brandeis D, Cortese S et al (2013) Nonpharmacological interventions for ADHD: systematic review and meta-analyses of randomized controlled trials of dietary and psychological treatments. Am J Psychiatry 170(3):275–289

Speicher MR, Antonorakis SE, Motulsky AG (eds) (2010) Human genetics. Problems and approaches, 4th edn. Springer, Berlin

Steinhausen HC, Nøvik TS, Baldursson G et al (2006) Co-existing psychiatric problems in ADHD in the ADORE cohort. Eur Child Adolesc Psychiatry 15(Suppl 1):125–129

Suresh PA, Deepa C (2004) Congenital suprabulbar palsy: a distinct clinical syndrome of heterogeneous aetiology. Dev Med Child Neurol 46(9):617–625

Tellegen PJ, Winkel M, Wijnberg-Williams BJ et al (1998) Snijders-Oomen Nonverbal intelligence test. SON-R 2 ½-7 manual and research report. Swets & Zeitlicher BV, Lisse

Van Camp G, Smith RJH (2015) Hereditary hearing loss homepage. Available via http://hereditaryhearingloss.org. Accessed 19 Apr 2016

van Dijk EL, Auger H, Jaszczyszyn Y et al (2014) Ten years of next-generation sequencing technology. Trends Genet 30(9):418–426

Viana AG, Beidel DC, Rabian B (2009) Selective mutism: a review and integration of the last 15 years. Clin Psychol Rev 29(1):57–67

Vodopiutz J, Item CB, Hausler M et al (2007) Severe speech delay as the presenting symptom of guanidinoacetate methyltransferase deficiency. J Child Neurol 22(6):773–774

Wittchen HU, Jacobi F, Rehm J et al (2011) The size and burden of mental disorders and other disorders of the brain in Europe 2010. Eur Neuropsychopharmacol 21(9):655–679

Wong P (2010) Selective mutism: a review of etiology, comorbidities and treatment. Psychiatry 7(3):23–31

World Health Organization (2016a) ICD-11 beta draft. International classification of diseases 11th revision. Available via http://apps.who.int/classifications/icd11/browse/f/en. Accessed 29 Feb 2016

World Health Organization (2016b) ICD-11 beta draft. International classification of diseases 11th revision. Available via https://icd.who.int/dev11/l-m/en. Accessed 3 Mar 2016

Worster-Drought C (1974) Suprabulbar paresis. Congenital suprabulbar paresis and its differential diagnosis, with special reference to acquired suprabulbar paresis. Dev Med Child Neurol 30(Suppl 30):1–33

Zaki MS, Heller R, Thoenes M et al (2016) PEX6 is expressed in photoreceptor cilia and mutated in deaf-blindness with enamel dysplasia and microcephaly. Hum Mutat 37(2):170–174

Zipfel S, Schneider A, Wild B et al (2002) Effect of depressive symptoms on survival after heart transplantation. Psychosom Med 64(5):740–747

Part II

Voice Disorders Including Rehabilitation of Tumour Patients

Editors: Bożena Wiskirska-Woźnica,
Jürgen Wendler,
Antoinette am Zehnhoff-Dinnesen

Lectors: Jürgen Wendler, Tadeus Nawka,
John Rubin, Philippe Dejonckere

Basics of Voice Disorders

4

Sevtap Akbulut, Antoinette am Zehnhoff-Dinnesen,
Felix de Jong, Matthias Echternach, Ulrich Eysholdt,
Michael Fuchs, Tamás Hacki, Krzysztof Izdebski,
Annerose Keilmann, Peter Kummer,
Sanila Mahmood, Willy Mattheus, Dirk Mürbe,
Tadeus Nawka, Haldun Oguz, Ekaterina Osipenko,
Friedemann Pabst, Mette Pedersen,
Rainer Schönweiler, Amélie Elisabeth Tillmanns,
and Erkki Vilkman

Electronic Supplementary Material The online version
of this chapter (https://doi.org/10.1007/978-3-662-46780-
0_4) contains supplementary material, which is available
to authorized users.

S. Akbulut
Department of Otolaryngology, Yeditepe University,
Istanbul, Turkey

A. am Zehnhoff-Dinnesen · A. E. Tillmanns
Clinic of Phoniatrics and Pedaudiology,
University Hospital Münster, Münster,
Germany
e-mail: am.zehnhoff@uni-muenster.de;
AmelieElisabeth.Tillmanns@ukmuenster.de

F. de Jong
Research Group ExpORL, University Hospitals, KU
Leuven, Leuven, Belgium
e-mail: Felix.DeJong@med.kuleuven.be

M. Echternach
Department of Otorhinolaryngology, Division of
Phoniatrics and Pediatric Audiology, Munich University
Hospital (LMU), Campus Großhadern, Munich, Germany
e-mail: Matthias.Echternach@med.uni-muenchen.de

U. Eysholdt
Department of Medical Physics and Acoustics/
Medical Physics and Cluster of Excellence
Hearing4all, Carl von Ossietzky-Universität
Oldenburg, Oldenburg, Germany
e-mail: ulrich.eysholdt@uni-oldenburg.de

M. Fuchs
Section of Phoniatrics and Audiology,
University of Leipzig, Leipzig, Germany
e-mail: Michael.Fuchs@medizin.uni-leipzig.de

T. Hacki
Department of Otorhinolaryngology, Head and Neck
Surgery, Semmelweis University Budapest, Budapest,
Hungary

K. Izdebski
Department of Otolaryngology, Head and Neck
Surgery, David Geffen School of Medicine, UCLA,
Los Angeles, CA, USA
e-mail: kizdebski@pvsf.org

A. Keilmann
Voice Care Center Bad Rappenau, Bad Rappenau,
Germany
e-mail: Keilmann@kommunikation.klinik.uni-mainz.de

P. Kummer
Phoniatrics and Pediatric Audiology,
University Hospital Regensburg, Regensburg,
Germany,
e-mail: peter.kummer@ukr.de

S. Mahmood · M. Pedersen
Voice Unit, The Medical Center,
Copenhagen, Denmark
e-mail: dcn175@alumni.ku.dk; m.f.pedersen@dadlnet.dk

W. Mattheus
Division of Phoniatrics and Audiology and Saxonian
Cochlear Implant Center, University Hospital Carl Gustav
Carus, Technische Universität Dresden,
Dresden, Germany
e-mail: Willy.Mattheus@uniklinikum-dresden.de

D. Mürbe · T. Nawka
Department of Audiology and Phoniatrics,
Charité—University Medicine Berlin,
Berlin, Germany
e-mail: dirk.muerbe@charite.de;
tadeus.nawka@charite.de

H. Oguz
Fonomer, Ankara, Turkey

E. Osipenko
Phoniatrics Department, Federal Research Clinical
Centre of Otorhinolaryngology, Moscow, Russia

F. Pabst
ENT Department, Municipal Hospital Dresden,
Dresden, Germany
e-mail: Pabst-Fr@khdf.de

R. Schönweiler
Department of Phoniatrics and Pediatric Audiology,
University Clinic of Schleswig-Holstein, Campus
Lübeck, Lübeck, Germany
e-mail: rainer.schoenweiler@phoniatrie.uni-luebeck.de

E. Vilkman
Department of Otolaryngology and Phoniatrics –
Head and Neck Surgery, Helsinki University
Hospital, Helsinki, Finland
e-mail: Erkki.Vilkman@hus.fi

4.1   Definition of Voice Disorders

Dirk Mürbe

Voice disorders are mainly characterised by a persistent disturbance in the sound of the voice. Commonly, hoarseness is the disturbed sound of the voice. However, voice disorders are also defined by limited laryngeal efficiency or vocal endurance and sensations of laryngeal discomfort. The latter might include, e.g. globus sensation and dryness. Voice disorders restrict vocal communication skills and accordingly social interactions.

The definition of voice disorders should be consistent with the WHO's International Classification of Functioning, Disability and Health (ICF) with health as a multidimensional concept. Health is a state of physical, mental and social well-being and not merely the absence of disease or infirmity. Thus, voice problems are not always identified as impairment but are at least partly captured by activity and participation, the 'life-area domains' in the ICF scheme (Titze and Verdolini Abbott 2012).

Traditionally, systematic classification of voice disorders distinguishes two major classes: organic disorders and functional disorders. Organic voice disorders are those with a specific lesion in some part of the sound production system. Functional disorders are those without any structural or neurological laryngeal pathology.

However, relationships and boundaries between the organic and functional are not always clear. For example, organic voice problems are often associated with secondary functional voice disorders and vice versa, and functional voice disorders can lead to secondary organic lesions. The definition and sub-classification of functional voice disorders in particular have been discussed for a long time (see Sect. 5.1). Several problems are encountered with the traditional scheme, in particular with regard to the role of the central nervous system in phonation. Functional voice disorders have often been assumed to be (partly) psychogenic. However, psychogenic causes also require proven clinical evidence, not just the absence of physical findings. Other clinicians view functional disorders as those that are brought about by the individual's improper use of the voice (Titze and Verdolini Abbott 2012).

Because of these limitations, several attempts have been made to establish alternative classifications of voice disorders. Titze (1994) suggests classifying voice disorders as responses of the biomechanical laryngeal oscillator to environmental, systemic or traumatic conditions. Hacki (2014) proposes an aetiologically based classification with the implementation of malregulative dysphonia instead of functional dysphonia (see Sect. 4.2).

Further, it should be emphasised that the boundaries between normal and distorted voices are not fixed and that they also depend on the given cultural environment. Especially for professional voice users, harsh voices can either be a desirable effect or represent a devastating voice disorder. Thus, by reflection of the mentioned WHO concept of health, when hoarse professional voice users experience well-being, we cannot necessarily talk about disease. Apart from the deficit in well-being, disease is additionally determined by neediness and deficits in efficiency and performance. If these aspects become dominant, we are entering the clinically relevant area, and therapeutic consequences have to be considered. The limit of deviant voice production should be the auto-destruction of the voice apparatus, meaning here phono-traumatic lesions, simply because these will impose a permanent functional restriction. But there is, obviously, a trend to a more tolerant attitude towards an acceptance of distorted voices in the public. Without ignoring these tendencies, clinicians have to keep in mind that reliable functionality is more likely for clear than harsh voices (Wendler et al. 2014).

4.2 Considerations Regarding the Aetiological Definition of Phonation Disorders: 'Malregulative Dysphonia' Instead of 'Functional Dysphonia'

Tamás Hacki, Tadeus Nawka, Dirk Mürbe, Michael Fuchs, Peter Kummer, Friedemann Pabst, Rainer Schönweiler, Annerose Keilmann, and Felix de Jong

4.2.1 Background

Phonation is an essential component of communication and is therefore an essential component of human functioning, activity and participation (WHO 2001). It is an expression of the individual's bodily state, emotions and personality. The complex function of phonation is embedded within biological and psychosocial contexts. Biologically, phonation is based on the vocal structures (collectively, the vocal tract: trachea, larynx, pharynx, oral and nasal cavity) and their neural and hormonal regulation.

In terms of their aetiology, phonatory disorders (dysphonia) are traditionally divided into 'organic' and 'functional' categories. Vocal dysfunctions having psychosocial causes (psychogenesis, maladaptation to personal and occupational demands, voice overload, habits, etc.) are frequently described imprecisely as 'functional dysphonia'.

Despite many criticisms, the phrase 'functional dysphonia' has been used for years. The word 'functional' is problematical because it refers to (1) aetiology as well as (2) symptomatology (signs and symptoms) and therefore lacks precision (Pahn and Friemert 1988):

- Regarding (1), 'functional' is used to mean 'non-organic in origin'. Here, the term is used in its aetiological sense (see detailed explanation in the 'Definitions' subsection).
- Regarding (2), 'functional disorder' is used instead of 'dysfunction'.

If someone asks what dysphonia looks like 'functionally', they may also ask what function can be identified, or indeed can a dysfunction be identified?

The term 'functional disorder' here stands for signs, especially dysfunctions (or sub-dysfunctions; see below), that are revealed during investigation.

Certain functions of the three functional levels of the phonatory system (breathing, voice generation and articulation) can be referred to as subfunctions: ab- and adduction of the vocal folds, contraction and relaxation of the muscles, vibratory behaviour of the vocal folds, the course of phonatory breathing, movement of the articulators, etc.

Thus the term 'functional dysphonia' only indicates that a sign, a dysfunction, can be detected.

4.2.2 Definitions

Phoniatricians have been working on definitions of non-organic phonatory disorders (dysphonia, phonatory disorders, voice disorders[1]) since the early twentieth century. The term 'functional' has been criticised because of its lack of precision (Barth 1911; Stern 1924; Weiss 1934; Gundermann 1970) when paired with the phrases 'non-organic' and 'not identifiable', which carry negative connotations.

> The aetiological possibilities are constricted but not substantially differentiated by the use of these negating-phrases,
> warned Pahn and Friemert (1988).

In contrast, Hartlieb (1968) and Schultz-Coulon (1980) defined what can be understood by the term 'functional': the incorrect control and regulation of phonation. Böhme's formulation (Böhme 2004) also lies in this direction:

> Functional dysphonias are the result of uncoordinated movement of the phonatory apparatus.

More recent clarifications of the terminology of dysphonia follow various principles:

- Titze's (Titze 1994) aetiologically grounded characterisation of phonation disorders places the voice generator in the centre and allows for an interesting physical-physiological view of the patho-mechanism of vibratory disorders of the vocal folds and, with it, the origin of 'hoarseness'.
- The nomenclature of Morrison and Rammage (1993) comes from the level of symptomatology (signs and symptoms). The terms 'muscle misuse voice disorder' and 'muscular tension dysphonia' merely indicate incorrect muscular tension.
- In Mathieson's aetiological system (Mathieson 2001), two major components are positioned in opposition to each other: the 'behavioural' and the 'organic'. The behavioural component includes 'psychogenic' and 'hyperfunctional'

disorders (hyperfunction, overly strained voice, incorrect use of the voice and excessive muscle tension). All other clinical presentations are part of the organic dysphonia category: structural, congenital changes and trauma; neurogenic, endocrine disorders; and acquired laryngeal disorders.

- Roy (2003) summarises the imprecise views of functional dysphonia based mainly on the Anglo-American literature:

> Functional dysphonia - a voice disturbance in the absence of structural or neurologic laryngeal pathology - is an enigmatic and controversial voice disorder... Poorly regulated activity of the ...laryngeal muscles is cited as the proximal cause... (functional dysphonia) is frequently transient, and varies in its response to treatment. Some confusion surrounds the diagnostic category of functional dysphonia because it includes an assortment of medically unexplained voice disorders: psychogenic, conversion, hysterical, tension-fatigue syndrome, hyperfunctional, muscle misuse, or muscle tension dysphonia.

Aetiological criteria should be the fundamental part of any new definition of dysphonia, avoiding symptom-based components and replacing the imprecise term 'functional'.

4.2.3 Newly Proposed Definition

The aetiological basis for Hacki's new definition of dysphonia (Hacki 2013, 2014) is that the complex functionality of our organism depends on the organs/structures and their regulation:

> 'Dysphonia' is a complex phonatory disorder that is based on pathological structural changes and/or impaired neural/hormonal regulation of the vocal structures (collectively, the vocal tract: trachea, larynx, pharynx, oral and nasal cavity).

Hence a taxonomy is proposed on the basis of the structural and regulatory integrity of the vocal structures (Table 4.1).

Structural Dysphonia A phonatory disorder that is caused by a structural change in the vocal structures is denoted structural dysphonia. We reject the oft-used aetiological term 'organic dysphonia' in favour of 'structural dysphonia', to denote dys-

---

[1] 'Dysphonia' or 'phonatory disorder' is the more precise phrase because 'voice disorder' merely indicates the product 'voice' rather than the complex phonatory function.

Table 4.1 Aetiological system of dysphonia, following the principle of 'alteration to the structure and/or disrupted regulation'

Structural dysphonia
Regulatory dysphonia
   Hormonal dysphonia
   Neurogenic (central, peripheral) dysphonia
   Malregulative dysphonia
Structural-regulatory dysphonia

phonia that is based on structural lesions of the vocal structures, i.e. the larynx itself, or that arises from the organs involved in voice production.

Regulatory Dysphonia A dysphonia that is caused by anomalies of hormonal or neural regulation including both the central and peripheral (upper and lower) and the afferent and efferent neural systems[2] is denoted regulatory dysphonia. All 'non-organic' and nonstructural disorders fall within this classification.

Regulatory dysphonia is classified accordingly:

- *Hormonal dysphonia* (e.g. some types of mutational voice disorder) arises from a hormonal disorder.
- *Central or peripheral neurogenic dysphonia* arises through change in the central or peripheral parts of the nervous system (stroke, trauma, extrapyramidal diseases, central and peripheral paralysis, etc.).
- *Malregulative dysphonia* arises through a 'lapse' or 'derailment', an often temporary dysregulation that occurs for reasons other than the above-mentioned structural nervous system changes. This category classifies dysphonias that arise from disorders of the psychomotor or sensorimotor regulation without structural changes: psychogenic, behavioural (voice misuse, muscle tension, etc.) or sensory dysphonia[3] (stemming from disrupted auditory or somatosensory feedback). Use of the phrase 'malregulative dysphonia' rather than 'functional dysphonia' is advised.

---

[2] In order that clarity be preserved, this classification does not include the level of cell regulation.
[3] Suggested by Pahn and Friemert (1988).

Combined Structural-Regulatory Dysphonia When structural changes are accompanied by regulatory aetiologies (e.g. particular hormonal phonatory disorders such as acromegaly or psychosomatic dysphonias such as contact granuloma (Table 4.1)), combined structural-regulatory dysphonias arise.

The terms 'structural' and 'regulatory' allude only to aetiology, and all symptomatic connotations such as 'hyper-', 'hypo-' or 'muscle tension' are avoided (e.g. hyperfunctional dysphonia). It is better not to burden aetiology with superfluous symptomatologies.

4.2.4 Conclusion

The reduction of nonstructural phonatory disorders to the phrase 'functional dysphonia' does not convey information that sufficiently describes the aetiology. Instead, it merely defines what something is not, narrowing it to a description of a 'non-organic' disorder. In contrast, 'regulatory' concretely describes disrupted regulation, be it neurogenic or hormonal. The term 'malregulative' is a way of describing faulty regulation or 'lapses' of the nervous system in the absence of central or peripheral changes. We therefore propose replacing the aetiologically imprecise and ambiguous term 'functional dysphonia' with the term 'malregulative dysphonia'.

4.3 Parameters of Voice Production Relevant for Clinical Investigation

Ulrich Eysholdt

Describing the functional ability of an organ according to the extremes of its capability is very common within medicine, for example, describing the maximal and minimal angles of stretch/bend of the knee. This extremum principle is also used in voice diagnostics; it does not apply, however, to all diagnostic categories. A healthy voice must be able successfully to perform the communication tasks that are placed upon it. It must therefore be possible to vary the pitch and intensity of the voice sufficiently, the voice must sound acceptable and these tasks must be performed reliably over time.

4.3.1 Fundamental Frequency, Mean Fundamental Frequency of the Speaking Voice and Vocal Frequency Range

A voiced sound consists of a fundamental frequency and a series of harmonics (or overtones) the frequencies of which are integer multiples of the fundamental. Frequency is a physical quantity (dimension: Hz = 1 cycle/s) which corresponds to the psychoacoustic perception of pitch. The concept of a voice being 'high' or 'low' is widely used, even colloquially.

The fundamental frequency of a voice can be perceived and auditorily determined in spoken language in the same way as from a sung or sustained tone. When a patient is allowed to speak freely, he automatically uses the pitch that is most comfortable for him. With only little experience, the investigator can easily identify the fundamental frequency to within a semitone by comparing the pitch to that produced by a tone-generator. The more strongly a patient is affected by the emotional content of what they say, the more tension there is in their entire body, including in their voice. The mean fundamental frequency of the speaking voice correspondingly increases.

Determining the mean fundamental frequency of the speaking voice with technology is complex and vulnerable to technical error. Because of this, we restrict ourselves to estimating the pitch perceptually, which in general is equal to the mean fundamental frequency of the speaking voice. The mean fundamental frequency of spoken language can only be measured with considerable software expenditure; thus the patient is only allowed to sustain a tone that most closely corresponds to his natural speaking voice.

Errors in numerical pitch calculation may result from the evaluation of the fundamental frequency of a voice signal, which, if they go unnoticed, can lead to inconsistencies within the findings, such as certifying that a man has a female voice. While calculating the power spectrum is unproblematic when using the rapid algorithm of fast Fourier transform (FFT), the identification of the harmonic series sometimes may be erroneous owing to an octave error (usually upwards, which can be explained by simple algorithms incorrectly identifying a prominent first harmonic as the fundamental, whereas subharmonics almost never exist). Plausibility checks by the investigator are therefore essential.

The fundamental frequency is particularly dependent on the physical dimensions of the vibrating structures and resonance cavities and is correlated with body size, age and sex. Babies' voices have a fundamental frequency of approximately 400 Hz, whereas the voices of children and juveniles are 280–350 Hz. Differences according to sex are apparent following the hormone-dependent voice change during puberty (the mutation). The voice of an adult woman is approximately 200–250 Hz and that of a man 100–140 Hz. Women's voices tend to sink in pitch following menopause and older men's voices increase slightly. As a physiological reference, the so-called indifference level can be used. This is a pitch that is generated by a well-balanced action of all muscles involved with an optimal relation of muscular effort and vocal output. It is located at the transition area from the lower to the middle third of the pitch range. To avoid overloading of the speaker's voice apparatus by permanent upward deviation, this pitch should be kept during speaking at the average or mean speaking pitch or, at least, to which it should be brought back regularly.

The term *vocal frequency range* or *pitch range* denotes the interval between the fundamentals of the highest and lowest frequencies (f_{max}, f_{min}) that a person can sing. The range is usually described with musical terminology and covers just less than two octaves in men and women. An octave encompasses 12 semitones and corresponds in physical terms to a doubling of frequency. The conversion between these units can be performed by means of any pocket calculator, using the following formulae:

$$\text{Interval in Octaves} = \log_2\left(\frac{f_{max}}{f_{min}}\right) = \frac{\log_{10}\left(\frac{f_{max}}{f_{min}}\right)}{\log_{10} 2} = 3.322 \times \log_{10}\left(\frac{f_{max}}{f_{min}}\right) \tag{4.1}$$

$$\text{Interval in Semitones} = 39.864 \times \log_{10}\left(\frac{f_{max}}{f_{min}}\right) \tag{4.2}$$

4.3.2 Dynamic Range and Voice Range Profile

The average rate at which acoustic energy contained in the radiating sound of the voice passes through a unit area is called *intensity*, measured in watts per square centimetre. For practical reasons in terms of comparing intensities, the *intensity level* preferred for measurement is the logarithmic dB(A) scale (see Sect. 1.3). Such measurement enables analysis of the extremely wide range of intensity in relation to the normal threshold of hearing. A calibrated measuring station featuring a sound-level meter (commercially available) and following the manufacturer's standardised measurement conditions are required. The type of microphone used and the distance between the microphone and the patient's mouth are of critical importance. The patient must be clearly instructed and well-motivated in order to produce sounds at the limits of their vocal ability.

A minimal amount of energy is required in order to evoke vibration in the vocal folds. A lower amount of energy does not result in vocal sound. This minimal energy level is known as the *phonation threshold* (L_{min}) and corresponds to an intensity level of 35–40 dB(A) for the normal voice, though this varies individually.

At the other end of the intensity scale, the upper limit of phonation (L_{max}) of the untrained voice is 95–100 dB(A). Both limits $L_{max}(f)$ and $L_{min}(f)$ are frequency-dependent and increase with higher frequency. The difference between these limits

$$R(f) = L_{max}(f) - L_{min}(f) \tag{4.3}$$

is the frequency-dependent *dynamic range*.

A diagram of intensity level against frequency shows the upper and lower limits of phonation, inside which is the area known as the *voice range profile*. A normal voice range profile looks like a diagonal ellipse. A large vocal field is suggestive of a powerful voice and a small vocal field suggests a weak voice. Generating and evaluating a vocal field is highly dependent on experience, and the patient must have a very clear understanding of their task.

The limits of a normal vocal range profile can be taken as:

- Frequency range ≥1.5 octaves
- Dynamic range ≥30 dB(A)
- Smooth edges without significant distortion
- Mean fundamental frequency of the speaking voice is approximately at the transition between the lowest frequency and the middle third of the frequency range (on the frequency axis)

The terminology in this field is somewhat unclear and redundant, so for the avoidance of error, the following must be emphasised: the vocal frequency range is the interval between the highest and lowest frequencies of the voice, not the extent of the voice range profile.

A voice range profile cannot successfully be evaluated quantitatively, despite many attempts to achieve this. Measuring the area of the voice range profile is not necessarily sensible because (a) both axes of the voice range profile are logarithmic and (b) the edges of the voice range profile are indicated only by discrete points between which interpolation must be used. The specific type of interpolation used (linear or spline interpolation) influences the results as much as does the density of the data points. Measuring the extent of the voice range profile is undermined by fractal geometry, wherein the range of a real area is dependent upon the particular scale being used. Approximating the shape by using model calculations is possible in individual cases but has no clinical value. Instead of quantitative evaluation, the main value of the voice range profile is providing useful information on basic features of a voice at a glance.

4.3.3 Acoustic Parameters

The computational power of a small mobile phone processor is enough to extract an entire series of features from a speech signal almost in real time. A method of digital signal analysis that has been substantially adapted to voice investigations is used. The most-developed software, 'Praat' (a Dutch expression meaning 'talk'), comes from the Netherlands and is a free-to-download open-source product (http://praat.en.softonic.com/). Commercial alternatives are expensive but have practical advantages in clinical use because of their simplified user interfaces.

The patient should sing a sustained tone lasting at least 3 s into a microphone ('sustained phonation'). From the microphone signal the stable vibratory part is cut out ('windowing') and presented as an almost-periodic signal, which can be analysed with respect to two groups of parameters: perturbation and breathiness.

4.3.3.1 Perturbation Parameters

Perturbation parameters quantitatively describe how periodic the signal is. If N is the number of cycles contained in the signal and T_i is the duration of the ith cycle, then the average period is

$$\bar{T} = \frac{1}{N}\sum_{i=1}^{N} T_i \quad [\text{s}] \qquad (4.4)$$

The magnitude of the difference between an individual cycle and the mean

$$\Delta_i = |T_i - \bar{T}| \quad [\text{s}] \qquad (4.5)$$

is averaged ($\bar{\Delta} \geq 0$). The *jitter* (J) is defined as

$$J = 100\frac{\bar{\Delta}}{\bar{T}} \quad [\%] \qquad (4.6)$$

(Hollien et al. 1971)

Jitter expresses the mean deviation of the periods from the mean period as a percentage.

There are many other similar formulae expressing jitter besides that of Hollien et al. (1971), and each provides different normal values. The appropriate norms can be found in the software manuals.

A perfectly periodic voice signal has a constant cycle duration $T_1 = T_2 = \ldots = T_{N-1} = T_N = \bar{T}$: consequently $\bar{\Delta} = 0$ and Jitter = 0%. But such an ideal voice signal never occurs. Real voice signals are only almost periodic and have jitter values greater than 0%.

Analogously, the reproducibility of individual volume peaks is termed *shimmer*. The overall amplitude is averaged, and the deviation of individual amplitudes from the average is calculated and then itself averaged and expressed as a percentage.

Normal and pathological values are:

	Normal (%)	Neither-nor (%)	Pathological (%)	Not evaluable (%)
Jitter	<0.6	0.6–1.0	>1.0	≥5
Shimmer	<2.5	2.5–4.0	>4.0	≥25

There are a great number of roughness parameters besides jitter and shimmer, all of which are based on these two parameters. They all have specific uses but cannot be considered in this overview.

4.3.3.2 Breathiness Parameters (Noise Measurements)

Calculating the parameters of breathiness is more complex than calculating those of perturbation. After transforming the time signal into a power spectrum via FFT, it is split into two components, one harmonic and the other nonharmonic. Typical parameters include:

- Harmonics-to-noise ratio (HNR)
- Normalised noise energy (NNE)
- Glottal-to-noise excitation ratio (GNE)

There is no standardised calculation algorithm for these parameters. The related normal values therefore depend strongly upon the measurement software used. Clinical evaluation of these measures makes sense only when:

- The individual laboratory follows a standardised approach
- The results can be compared with standard values that have been generated with the same procedure

4.3.4 Maximum Phonation Time

The maximum phonation time (MPT) is the most important clinical parameter of the aerodynamics of the voice. As suggested by its name, MPT is the maximum time for which a patient can sing and hold a tone. As this procedure requires cooperation of the patient, compliance with standardised conditions is necessary in order to obtain a reliable measurement: the patient must practise once before the actual measurement, so that the investigator is certain that the patient has understood the instructions. For the measurement itself, the patient must breathe three times 'normally' and then inhale once to their maximum limit before they begin

singing. A target tone is unnecessary; it is best if the patient uses a comfortable pitch. Usually it corresponds to the mean fundamental frequency of their speaking voice.

Real measured MPT values can be divided into two categories and one less reliable interim area:

	Normal	Neither-nor	Abnormal
MPT (s)	>15	10–15	<10

The diagnostic selectivity of MPT is therefore not especially good.

MPT is closely correlated with the vital capacity (VC) of the lungs. Although the VC is sex-dependent (VC is almost 800 mL lower in women than in men), both sexes have a similar MPT. Because women have smaller larynxes than men and correspondingly small flow diameters, they require less air for phonation. This lower air consumption compensates the lower female VC, meaning that MPT is ultimately similar between the sexes.

The glottal flow rate (GFR) is the volume flow of air expired through the glottis during phonation. Its average can be calculated from the parameters MPT and VC from the formula:

$$GFR = \frac{VC}{MPT} \quad \left[\frac{mL}{s} \right] \qquad (4.7)$$

Because the VC is sex-dependent but MPT is not, the GFR is differentiated by sex. Values for women are 170–220 mL/s and values for men are 250–300 mL/s.

4.4 Types of Phonation

Ulrich Eysholdt

4.4.1 Definition

Phonation is the process of voluntary sound generation by an airstream through the larynx (from Greek φωνή = voice). Involuntary laryngeal sound is not under consideration here. Phonation is possible in both directions of the respiratory airstream, inspiratory and expiratory. The scope of this article is restricted to the expiratory airstream only. In physical terms, the larynx is a tube with a rigid outer wall and soft tissue cover inside. In earlier stages of evolution, the larynx worked as a valve in order to separate respiration from swallowing. Later on, as an acquirement of evolution, the voice function was added and arrived at its highest level in human beings. Phonation makes use of the soft tissue of the endolarynx, which consists mainly of muscles. They are able to change their position, shape and viscoelasticity (stiffness) very rapidly. In that way the muscles vary the cross-sectional area of the larynx as well as the wall impedance and influence the expiratory airstream. Each constriction of this tube is a possible source of sound generation. The narrowest opening, even in its most opened state, is the glottis, the area between the vocal folds (Greek γλῶττα = tongue, as in ancient times people suspected the tongue to be the source of voice and speech). However, sound production may even take place more cranially (supraglottal). Subglottal sound production is possible in pathological constriction of the trachea-laryngeal section (stenosis) but does not contribute to the normal or disordered voice and is not considered here. As a rough classification, the produced sound can be categorised as 'voiced' or 'unvoiced' (Titze 1994). A phonatory sound is called 'voiced' when the harmonic components are predominant and form a series of overtones. 'Unvoiced' sound production shows no harmonic components; the power spectrum is continuous and corresponds to a noise, sometimes without any frequency dependence.

Voiced articulation refers to vowels and some consonants, while unvoiced articulation is related only to certain consonants. There is no sharp border between 'voiced' and 'unvoiced', neither perceptually nor analytically.

4.4.2 Sound Sources within the Larynx

An expiratory airstream passing the glottis produces sound from three different sources:

- Volume-induced
- Eddy-induced
- Tissue-induced

The *volume-induced sound* is generated by the vibrating vocal folds: in the glottal plane, they regularly interrupt the continuous airstream, thus forming a sequence of air pulses in the supraglottal space. This is the most dominant sound component during normal phonation. The equidistant pulses have a fundamental frequency and a series of harmonic frequencies.

The *eddy-induced sound* results from turbulence near the mucosal surface. Between the superficial mucus and the mainstream, there is a boundary layer of turbulent air, which varies in structure and thickness and leads to a noise component. In normal phonation, eddy-induced sound contributes only little to the voice. By means of digital signal analysis and synthesis, it is possible to eliminate the eddy-induced voice component completely. However, a human listener perceives such computerised clean voice as unnatural and too clear. Obviously, a minimum noise component is necessary for a voice to be accepted as natural. When, on the other hand, the eddy-induced sound is increased, it may even dominate the volume-induced components. In this case the voice sounds altered, rough or breathy. Human auditory perception is very sensitive to such voice alterations.

Any vibrating mechanical structure produces a sound of itself, like a vibrating string or a vibrating wall. The vibrating structures within the larynx are the vocal folds, which generate *tissue-induced sound* components. Depending on the vibration, the tissue-induced components may be harmonic or not. In general they contribute low energy only, but compared with the noise components, they seem to be necessary for a voice to be perceived as natural. Under pathological conditions, i.e. when tissue may not vibrate, as when being stiffened by a scar, tissue-induced sound vanishes completely (Eysholdt 2014).

4.4.3 Glottal Phonation

Variables that change the phonation in the glottal plane are:

- The glottal opening
- The muscular tension of the endolaryngeal soft tissue
- The subglottal air pressure

The vocal folds form the glottis and receive their shape mainly by the M. vocalis. While the vocal muscle at its ventral end is fixed to the thyroid cartilage, it can be moved and positioned by the arytenoid cartilage at the dorsal end. During respiration, the vocal folds are abducted, and during phonation, they are adducted. The ad- and ab-duction movement is symmetrically performed by the tilting and rotating arytenoid cartilages. These movements are called *respiratory mobility*.

The opening width is the most important variable for regulating the glottal airstream. There is a continuous transition between maximum opening and closure:

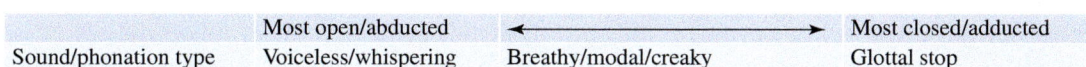

	Most open/abducted	← —————————————————— →	Most closed/adducted
Sound/phonation type	Voiceless/whispering	Breathy/modal/creaky	Glottal stop

Although there are audible differences, there is no clear perceptual boundary between the neighbouring phonation types. The overlap from one type to the next prevents the phonation type from being used as a sharp diagnostic criterion. Different phonation types make use of the same or similar laryngeal mechanisms. Additionally, in European languages the different phonation types transfer emotions, not meaning. For the European voice clinician, that and how these differences are used by different languages in the world to articulate meaningful speech sounds is of only minor importance (Laver 1980).

The *voiceless* condition with open glottis and relaxed vocal muscles corresponds to breathing: no vibrations are excited. When the glottis remains open and the muscles are stiffened, the resulting sound production is called whispering. The eddy-induced components increase, while the volume-induced sound is low. They can be used as primary signal for articulation; the whispering phonation type is used to express secrecy or confidentiality (Laver 1980).

In general, economic sound production needs adduction of the vocal folds and tension of the vocal muscles (or either of them). The transition from *whispering* to the *normal* speaking voice is a *breathy* phonation, which is the result of a (too) low muscular tonus or a (too) large glottal gap. The volume-induced sound components increase, while the eddy-induced components slightly decrease. The downregulation of the muscular tonus leads to a lower tissue stiffness, thus increasing the vibrating mass and consequently decreasing the fundamental frequency.

Breathy voice differs from a whisper because of the weaker medial compression, less muscular tension and the smaller degree of voicing effort.

Case Study 4.1

A pensioner (72 years old) has suffered from a hoarse and weak voice for several years. His voice is worse in the evening. Voice therapy was not successful. Except for high blood pressure, he has no other diseases. The video shows bowing of the vocal folds due to atrophy of the vocalis muscle. The closed phase pattern is characterised by an oval gap. The voice sound during the examination is breathy and partially aphonic, and only at higher frequencies in falsetto register do the vocal folds vibrate. Closure at higher volume is better but still not complete. The habitual pitch of the speaking voice is at about G4 (200 Hz), which is too high for a male voice. The voice sound is mildly breathy (R0 B1 H1).

For *normal* speech the modal phonation type is used, which means a neutral mode, economical in the sense that it requires least vocal effort. During modal phonation, subglottal pressure and muscular tension build up a dynamic equilibrium, each at moderate values, thus exciting the vocal folds to a sustained vibration. The vibration is a rotational motion in three dimensions, which can roughly be compared to that of a skipping rope with its maximum amplitude in the middle third. During a regular vibration pattern, the glottal gap is completely closed (except for a dorsal chink in women). The glottal vibration interrupts the expiratory airstream and leads to a predominantly volume-induced sound. Modal voice requires an anatomically normal larynx and a normal innervation. The reverse argument is not true: a larynx that is normally configured and has normal innervation is definitely able to produce nonmodal phonation.

Case Study 4.2
A 26-year-old man with a normal male voice wants to apply for singing studies. He has no complaints and strives to develop his bass baritone voice.

Case Study 4.3
A 26-year-old woman with a normal female voice wants to become a music teacher. The organic and functional findings do not give rise to any reservations.

Case Study 4.4
A 48-year-old owner of a record store complains about pain when speaking, a lump in the throat, hoarseness after slight vocal load, dry mouth, a salty taste and the feeling as if having drunk a hot liquid. Speaking is strenuous. It causes pain in the chest and the bronchi, sometimes only the next day. Otherwise the patient has no complaints. There is an obvious impossibility to phonate with a clear voice during stroboscopic examination. The vocal folds are pressed against each other which leads to a creaky phonation. Additionally, the video reveals a very slight atrophy of the right vocal fold and, for compensation, a hardly noticeable crossing of the vocal processes, the real so-called arytaenoid crossing (between 9 and 15 s of the video). When recording the voice range profile, he refused to produce loud tones. His speaking voice is almost normal (R1 B0 H1).

Creaky phonation is also called vocal fry. Characterised by a very low frequency at high subglottal pressure, it is the result of low stiffness in the vocal muscle and high adduction forces that close the glottis completely. Creaky phonation shows irregular periods (i.e. has no fundamental frequency) and has a comparatively low intensity. The voice production is 'uneconomic'. This voice sound in general is not used for communication but for performing art purposes (Titze 1994). Sometimes the falsetto (from Ital. falso = 'false') is considered as a phonation type. The larynx is antero-ventrally tilted and the vibrating mass reduced by stretching the vocal folds. The fundamental frequency is usually remarkably higher than in modal voice. As the falsetto mechanism makes use of the whole vocal tract instead of the laryngeal soft tissues, it is considered here as a vocal register (see Sect. 4.5) rather than phonation type.

4.4.4 Supraglottal Phonation

As sound can be generated at any constriction of the vocal tract, the same mechanisms described for the glottis apply to supraglottal structures, where the most important sound source are the ventricular folds. Although they contain muscular structures, their control is quite imprecise. The result is usually an irregular, very rough voice without audible fundamental frequency that sounds deep and strange. While some artists make use of this special sound (most famous: Louis Armstrong), this type of phonation is of importance for patients after a laryngeal operation (cordectomy). In this situation, a scarred vocal pseudo-fold is formed, which, owing to its stiffness, cannot take part in sound production. Then supraglottal phonation can replace the glottal and enable the patient to articulate speech sounds without any external device (Eysholdt 2014).

Case Study 4.5
A 40-year-old woman had an idiopathic subglottal stenosis that started 8 years ago. She underwent altogether eight interventions with glottal

and subglottal enlargement. The vocal folds lost their function in the course of this treatment. She developed a voice that is produced by her ventricular folds. The vocal range is markedly reduced. The voice is soft and severely hoarse with typical pauses of audible inspiration when breathing in between the phrases.

Case Study 4.6

A 46-year-old singer and professor of pop vocals demonstrates the distortion of vocal fold vibration by adducting the ventricular folds (video clip). In the case the ventricular folds contact and start to vibrate (not demonstrated here), the characteristic supraglottal phonation results, which has become the distinctive vocal sound of Louis Armstrong as mentioned in the text (audio clip).

4.5   Vocal Registers

Matthias Echternach

4.5.1   Introduction

The frequency ranges of voices are not consistent entities. At different locations in the frequency spectrum, the voice may change its perceptible character rapidly. An obvious example can be observed in male voices which imitate the female voice, where the voice not only changes the fundamental frequency but also changes its perceptual character. In untrained voices in particular, a rise of fundamental frequency is often associated with sudden uncontrolled pitch jumps to higher frequency regions (Fig. 4.1).

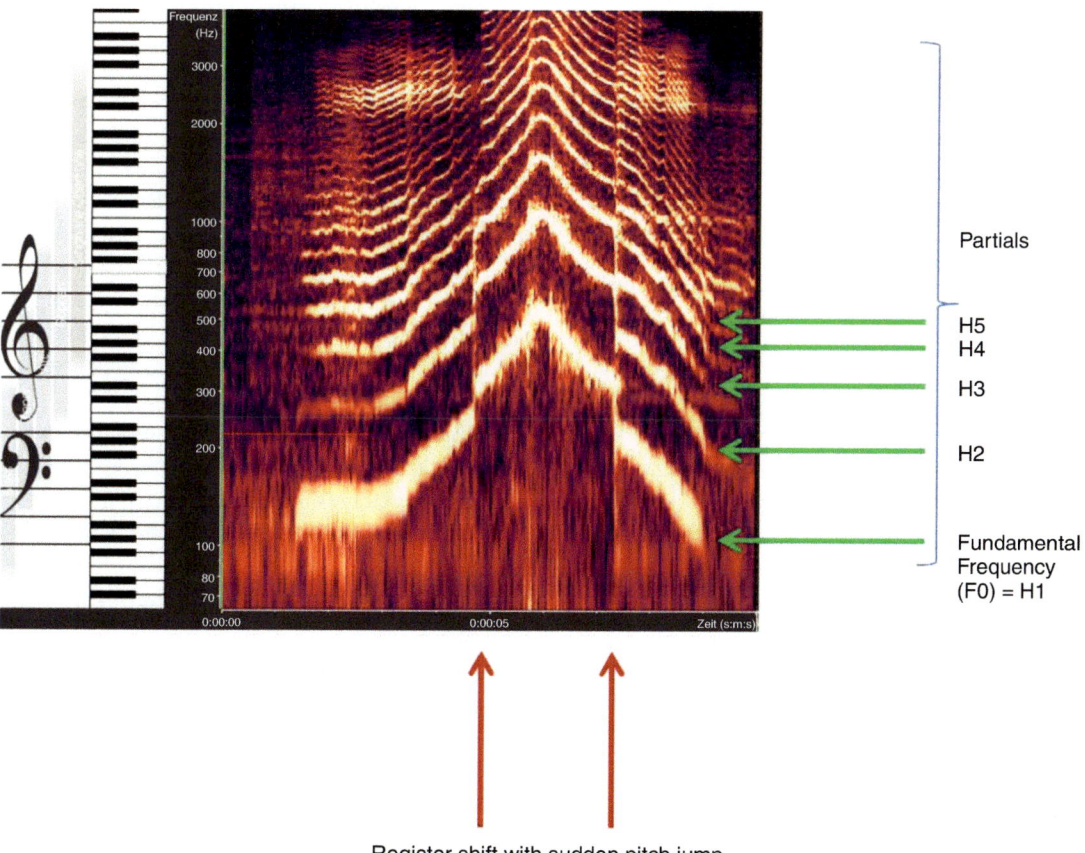

Register shift with sudden pitch jump

Fig. 4.1 Acoustic spectrum with a sudden pitch jump reflecting a register shift from modal to falsetto and back to modal register in a male subject. H1–H5 refer to partial of the radiated sound spectrum at the mouth

Regions with similar sound characteristics are, in analogy to organ registers, commonly denoted as vocal registers. The region where register transitions would usually occur is often described as the passaggio region.

The description of the mechanisms underlying vocal registers has been one of the more discussed issues of voice physiology. However, there is as yet no agreement on the underlying mechanisms or the number of registers. Furthermore, there is no agreement on the definition and the related terminology of the term register.

Manuel Garcia II in the 1840s provided one of the early definitions of registers:

> Par le mot registre, nous entendons une série de sons consécutifs et homogènes allant du grave à l'aigu, produits par le développement du même principe mécanique, et dont la nature diffère essentiellement d'une autre série de sons également consécutifs et homogènes, produits par une autre principe mécanique.
>
> Garcia (1847)

Translation as published by Henrich (2006) in accordance with Miller (2000):

> By the word register we mean a series of consecutive and homogeneous tones going from low to high, produced by the same mechanical principle, and whose nature differs essentially from another series of tones equally consecutive and homogeneous produced by another mechanical principle. All the tones belonging to the same register are consequently of the same nature, whatever may be the modifications of timbre or of the force to which one subjects them.

This definition is based on the concept of a uniform mechanical (laryngeal) principle of vocal registers. Indeed, for some registers, i.e. modal and falsetto, it has been shown that there are strong differences in oscillation patterns, tensions and laryngeal muscle activities.

However, many scientists expect that the perceptual differences between registers are not just related to the voice source but suppose that there could be interactions of neighbouring systems, such as the subglottal and vocal tract cavities, to the airflow or the vocal fold oscillations. Therefore an isolated definition of laryngeal mechanisms which neglects the rest of the voice production system seems inappropriate to many scientists who prefer a more perceptual definition of registers.

> The term register has been used to describe perceptually distinct regions of vocal quality that can be maintained over some ranges of pitch and loudness.
>
> Titze (1994)

In addition to these definitions, many more complex definitions have been published, which include breathing patterns, acoustic properties, etc.

As a result of the number of different definitions and varying expectations about the underlying mechanisms, there is still no uniform terminology for the different registers. In particular there is no agreement on the question of how many registers actually exist. Terms associated with registers are related to different outcome criteria. For example, the register in which most humans' speaking voice is located could be called 'M1' if the reader follows a laryngeal oscillatory description, where M stands for the mechanical principle. Also in the same way, the term 'lower thick' could be used, which is related to the morphology of the vocal folds. The same register could be called 'chest', 'Brust' or 'poitrine', which would relate the term to the awareness that the vibrations felt during the sound production are often experienced in the chest region. Lastly, the register could be denoted as modal register which refers to physical properties of the oscillatory system.

More confusion is caused by the fact that different professions prefer different terms. Different languages also contribute to the lack of a uniform terminology. Furthermore, sometimes the same term is used to describe different registers. In this respect the term *head register* is sometimes used to describe a stage voice above passaggio for male singers, while the same term is sometimes used synonymously with the male falsetto register. For female voices the term is often associated with pitch, being the first register occurring above the modal register. However, some people also use 'head' for the second register to occur above modal register (above a middle register), a register denoted by others as the upper register.

As a consequence of these ambiguities in terminology, as early as 1963, Mörner et al. (1963) found more than 100 terms for registers. Attempts to unify terminology have so far failed. The author explicitly emphasises that the terminology used in this section is not definitive and is used only to provide, for the reader, the possibility of comparing data.

The following description of the characterisation of registers is organised in order of the frequency range of the registers (low to high). Since many studies have focused on differences between different registers, in some cases characterisations of upper registers are referred to during the discussion of a lower register. However, a detailed description of such registers is offered later in the section.

4.5.2   Pulse Register

The term pulse register (related terms: vocal fry, creak, M0, #1, Strohbassregister, Kehlbassregister) describes the register in the very lowest part of the frequency spectrum of the human voice. This register is used only rarely in humans, and even then it is mostly related to speech but not singing. Nearly all descriptions and characterisations in literature are related to male voices. In this register it is thought that many different mechanisms such as double or triple impulses can occur. The voice signal can be periodic or aperiodic. It has also been shown that there can be an increase of perturbation measures, such as jitter and shimmer.

However, apart from the physical processes involved in voicing at these low fundamental frequencies, the perceptual pulse-like nature of this register might have another cause. In this respect Titze (1994) noted that for complex tones below a fundamental frequency of 70–80 Hz, single sound waves can be perceived by the human auditory system as a series of pulses. Therefore, from the perceptual aspect of register concepts, the underlying reason for the pulse register is not related to the sound producer but more to the listener.

4.5.3   Modal Register

The modal register (related terms: chest, heavy, #2, M1, Brustregister, poitrine) is the register where the speaking voice is usually located. It has been shown that the vocal folds oscillate along the whole length of the membranous portion. There are strong oscillatory amplitudes and mucosal waves. The closed phase is much longer than that within the next higher register. This is also reflected in a greater electro-glottographic contact quotient for the modal register. From electromyographic studies, it is thought that vocalis muscle activity dominates, whereas for the next higher register, the cricothyroid muscle dominates. As a consequence there is a greater mass in action for the modal register. The medial surface of the vocal folds is much greater than that in the higher registers.

The voice source spectrum is characterised by the strong intensities of overtones. In this respect the difference in level between the first partial (f_o or H1, with H standing for the harmonic) and the second partial ($2f_o$ or H2) is smaller than that for the higher register. Subglottal pressure is also higher in the modal register than in the pulse register.

The transition from the modal register to the next higher register—falsetto for male and middle for female voices—is frequently called the first passaggio.

4.5.4   Male Falsetto

The male falsetto (derived from *falsus, false*, as to the auditory impression, male voice sounding like female) is the register above the modal register. It has been shown that the oscillatory amplitudes and mucosal waves are smaller, and the open quotient greater, than in the modal register. Cadaver and electromyographic experiments suggest that, in contrast to the modal register, the cricothyroid muscle dominates the vocalis muscle in this register. The resulting sound and subglottal pressures are lower, and the intensities of overtones weaker, for falsetto than those of the modal register.

As a consequence of these acoustic characteristics, falsetto is only rarely used for singing on stage. However, in the case of a counter-tenor's singing, it is thought that a greater closed phase is achieved through the greater degree of vocal fold adduction for stage falsetto. Furthermore, vocal tract shapes differ between a naïve falsetto and stage falsetto (Wendler et al. 1985).

4.5.5 Side Note Concerning Higher Female Registers

In the literature the concepts of female vocal registers above the modal register are very contradictory. There are some scientists who suggest that there is a second register shift about one octave above the transition from modal to the middle register, whereas other scientists deny the existence of such a passaggio. Nevertheless a second passaggio of this kind is often confirmed by many female professional singers in clinical practice. If such a passaggio is assumed to exist, then the lower register could be denoted as middle and the upper as upper register. Miller (2000) postulated that a register shift around 500 Hz occurs because at that point, the fundamental frequency reaches the frequency of the first formant. Titze (1994) also found some evidence for a register transition in this frequency range. He hypothesised that subglottal resonances would amplify frequencies around 500 Hz, which would lead to vocal fold instabilities.

It should be noted that some authors refer to the upper register as being the register for the very highest fundamental frequencies; in this section this is referred to as the whistle register.

4.5.6 Middle Register

The middle register (related terms: head, Mittelregister, #2a) is the register above the modal register and below the upper register. Usually the frequency range for this register is between 300–500 and 500–800 Hz. In contrast to the modal register, the longitudinal tension of the vocal folds is increased, and the oscillatory amplitudes and mucosal waves are decreased. There is also a greater open phase during the glottal cycle. Using laryngostroboscopy, Svec and co-workers (Svec et al. 2008) described less adduction of the arytenoid cartilages, resulting in a small persistent gap in the posterior part of the vocal folds.

In comparison with the modal register, the middle register is associated with weak overtone intensities, a consequence of which is that the fundamental frequency intensity is relatively strong.

4.5.7 First Passaggio

The first passaggio is the region in the frequency spectrum where the transition from modal register to falsetto or middle register usually occurs, at around 300–500 Hz. In this area the modal and middle registers overlap, and therefore any particular fundamental frequency in this region could be produced in both registers (amphoteric sounds). The frequency range of the female passaggio is only very slightly higher than that of the male passaggio. Many scientists believe that this transition is primarily a laryngeal event. Indeed, when vocal tract shapes were analysed by means of dynamic real-time MRI, a recent study failed to show major differences between the modal and falsetto or middle registers (Echternach et al. 2010). Equalisation of registers, therefore, should be related to a gradual change in oscillatory patterns (Fig. 4.2).

4.5.8 Upper Register

Depending on which of the different classifications of registers is used, the frequency range for the upper register (related terms: light, #3) differs greatly. Nevertheless, some authors describe this register at a range of 700 to 1000–1100 Hz.

The reason for the existence of this register is not understood in detail. However, some authors have observed changes in vocal fold oscillation patterns, meaning that the oscillatory amplitudes and mucosal waves are small in relation to the

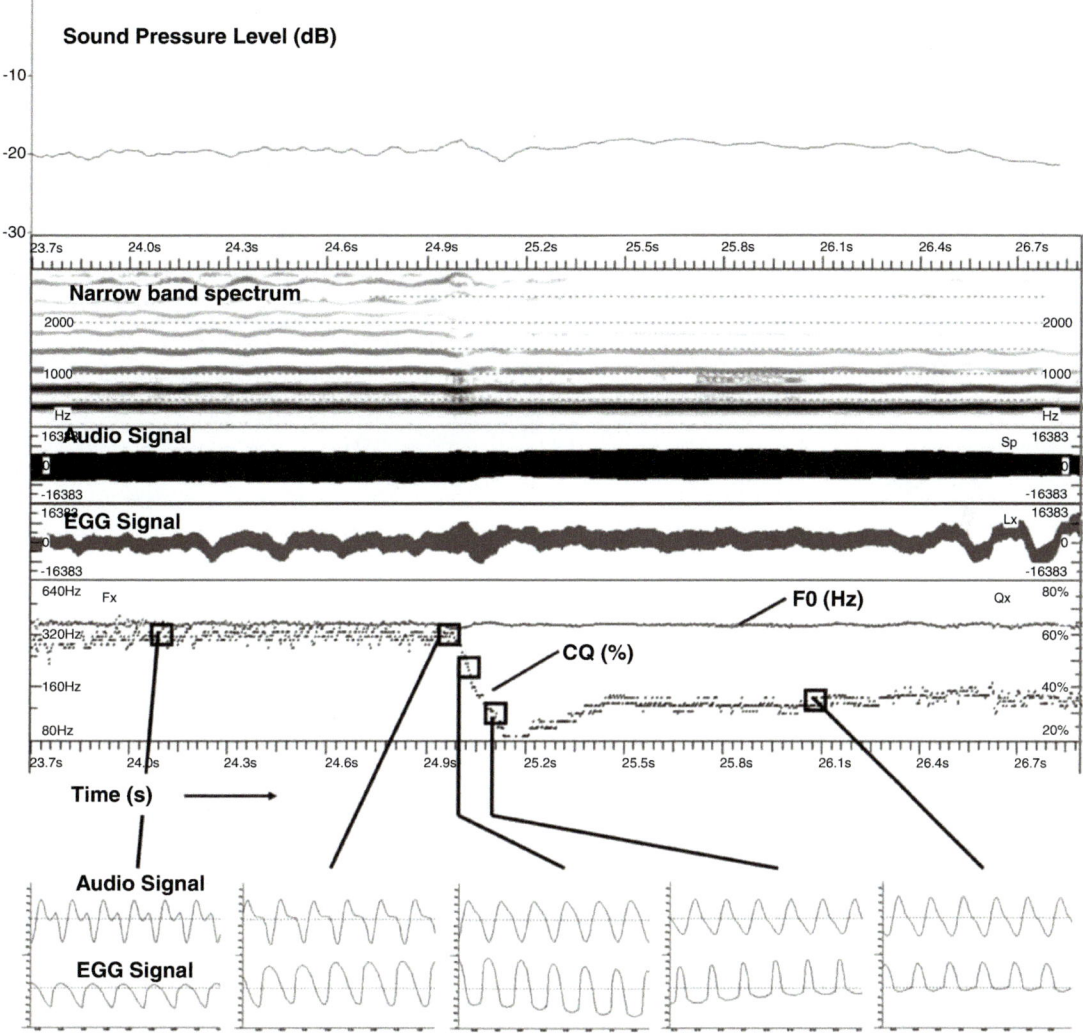

Fig. 4.2 Example of a register transition from modal to falsetto register in a professional singer without a clear sudden register transition event in the audio or electro-glottographic (EGG) signals. Here the voice is starting in modal register. At 24.9 s the subject starts to change registration to the falsetto register, as demonstrated by the change of the electro-glottographic contact quotient (CQ). The change takes about 300 ms and therefore about 100 glottal cycles. At the same time, no major changes of fundamental frequency (F0) or changes in the radiated spectrum at the mouth were present. Taken from Echternach et al. (2012). Copyright with kind permission from Elsevier

middle registers. In videokymographic studies, Svec and co-workers (Svec et al. 2008) observed persistent gaps during glottal closure. Furthermore they showed shorter opening and closing phases.

From an acoustic standpoint, the fundamental frequency is relatively strong in the upper register compared with that of the middle register. It has also been shown that strong vocal tract shape modifications occur in this register. Furthermore,

at least for professional voices, a formant tuning strategy (Sundberg 1975) is often observed in the upper register.

4.5.9 Second Passaggio

As indicated in the side note above, the passaggio between the middle and upper registers is still a matter of discussion. On the one hand, some

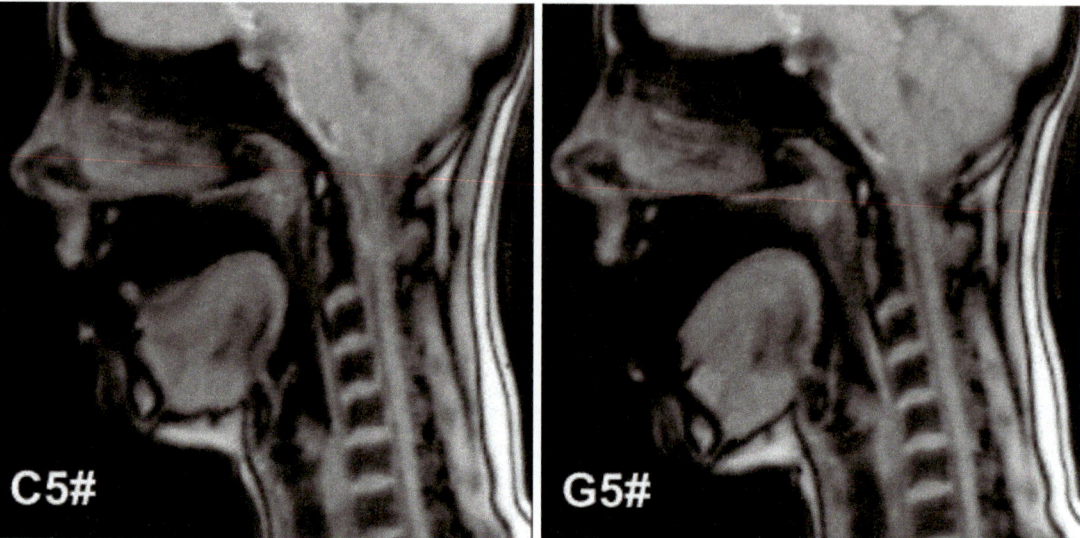

Fig. 4.3 Mid-sagittal vocal tract shapes from real-time MRI data for the pitches C5# and G5#. As can be seen, the tongue position differs markedly. Furthermore, the larynx is elevated and the lips are opened for G5#

authors do not believe in such a passaggio at all. For those who do consider it to exist, its cause remains unclear. It has been shown in some studies that, even when the vowel condition remains the same, the vocal tract shape is modified for fundamental frequencies higher than 750 Hz (Echternach et al. 2010) (Fig. 4.3).

If associated with a register transition, as expected by Miller (2000), who suggests that the transition is caused because the fundamental frequency reaches the first formant (F1), it could be argued that the register transition should occur at different frequency regions for the different vowel conditions, e.g. lower for vowels with low F1, such as /u/ or /i/. To the best of the author's knowledge, however, this register transition is thought to be at a nearly stable frequency. However, there are also studies suggesting a laryngeal event as cause of the second passaggio. Svec et al. (2008) observed two qualitatively different transitions above the first passaggio: one around 670 Hz associated with sudden pitch jumps and another at 1000 Hz where the sound pressure amplitudes and intensities of overtones decreased (Svec et al. 2008). Many singing pedagogues and some scientists think that the change of vowel quality might be a means to achieve register equalisation.

4.5.10 Whistle Register

Many singers and scientists commonly notice an additional register transition in the frequency range of 1000–1200 Hz. Voice production above these fundamental frequencies has been the subject of much scientific debate for many decades. Competing hypotheses have been postulated, including sound production in analogy to whistles, turbulence formed from vocal tract/voice source interactions, and a flageolet-like mechanism and modification of the airflow by oscillating vocal folds. In a recent study with transnasal high-speed endoscopy at a frame rate of 20,000 fps, it was shown for a single professional singer subject that at fundamental frequencies up to 1568 Hz, the vocal folds oscillated and closed completely during the glottal cycle (Echternach et al. 2013) (Fig. 4.4).

Endoscopic and MRI data for the register shift from upper to whistle register showed, in a single subject, no major changes in vocal tract shape and consequently no change in formants (Echternach et al. 2015). However, tuning strategies might differ between individuals at these high fundamental frequencies (Garnier et al. 2010). There is a need for further research, which may be provided by using the newest high-speed imaging techniques.

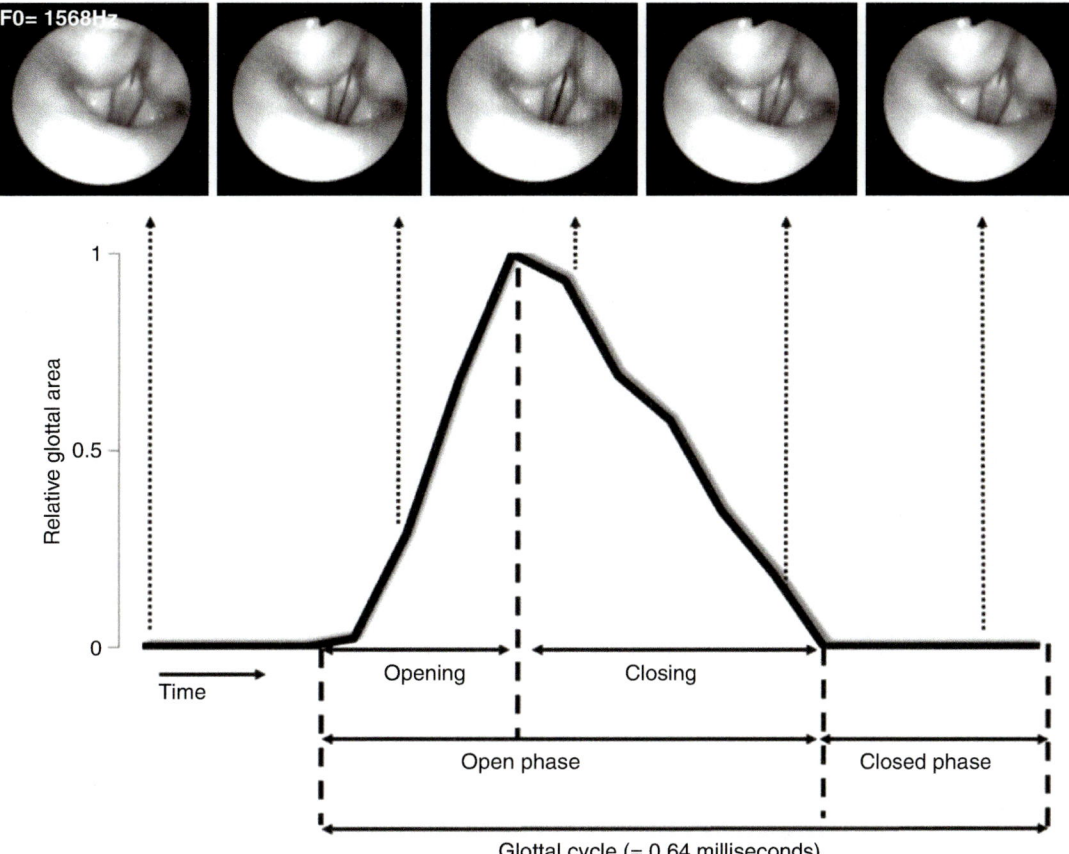

Fig. 4.4 Representative images from laryngoscopic high-speed material representing one glottal cycle in relation to a glottal area waveform. The pictures refer to voice production at a fundamental frequency of G6 (1568 Hz). Therefore one glottal cycle is related to the time of 0.64 ms. Taken from Echternach et al. (2013). Copyright with kind permission from the Acoustic Society of America

4.5.11 Belting as Register Function

In musical theatre a singing technique called belting is often used (Sundberg et al. 2012). It has been shown that belting exhibits differences in all aspects of voice production. It is often assumed that belting is associated with a loud voice and high subglottal pressure, but it has been found that the voice source fundamental is stronger (i.e. that the intensity for H1 is greater than that of H2) for the female classical voice than a heavy belt. The closed quotient and the electro-glottographic contact quotient are also greater in belting.

Many scientists believe that this vocal technique is related to a register function. In this respect, it is assumed that belting is considered an extension of the modal register to higher fundamental frequencies across the first passaggio. However, it should be mentioned that belting implies not only registration but also concerns aesthetic characteristics. Furthermore, it should be noted that there are many substyles of belting that might also contribute to different hypotheses and conclusions (Sundberg et al. 2012).

4.5.12 Yodelling

Yodelling is a special kind of phonation that is common in many cultures across the world. In addition to special vocalisation of syllables and ornaments, yodelling is characterised by sudden pitch changes, and it is often assumed that these pitch changes are accompanied by register changes. Pitch jumps occur very suddenly in yodelling, but in contrast to untrained voices, professional yodelling subjects show very precise placements of fundamental frequencies and well-defined changes in vocal tract shapes. Therefore, these pitch changes seem very coordinated. Additionally, perturbation measures such as jitter and shimmer are lower for professional yodelling subjects. Interestingly, for female voices yodelling only involves the change from modal to middle register and vice versa but not transitions to higher registers.

4.6 External Laryngeal Muscles and Their Role in Voice Production

Erkki Vilkman

4.6.1 External Laryngeal Frame in Voice Production

The hyoid and laryngeal structures are connected to each other and to other adjacent structures with spring-like attachments (ligaments, muscles) within which a state of equilibrium appears to exist. From a biomechanical point of view, the external mechanisms include not only a great number of muscles but also the often overlooked tracheal pull. Tracheal pull, i.e. the inferior force produced by the mass and tension of the trachea, is transmitted to the larynx through the cricoid cartilage and adjacent soft tissues. This complex interactive system is called the external frame of the larynx (Sonninen 1968).

The external muscles considered to be capable of contributing to voice production include the strap muscles, i.e. the sternothyroid (ST), the hyothyroid (HT) and the sternohyoid (SH) muscles, of which the ST and HT, together with the inferior pharyngeal muscles, i.e. the cricopharyngeal (CP) and the thyropharyngeal (TP) muscles, are directly connected to the larynx. The

suprahyoid muscles, i.e. the digastric, the mylohyoid, the geniohyoid (GH), the hyoglossus and the genioglossus muscles, as well as the infrahyoid muscles (SH, omohyoid), have an indirect effect on the larynx. Other indirect muscular forces include those produced by the palatal, oesophageal and nuchal musculature, of which the palatopharyngeal muscle also has a partially direct connection to the larynx. As regards vocal fold biomechanics, it is important to note that with the exception of the CP muscle, the forces produced by the extrinsic laryngeal muscles act directly on the thyroid cartilage (see Vilkman et al. 1996 for a review). A detailed description of the anatomy of the laryngeal region as well as vocal tract acoustics is not within the scope of this article (but see the scheme in Fig. 4.5 and Sects. 1.2 and 1.11).

4.6.2 Folding and Unfolding of the Laryngeal Structures

The deformation of the laryngeal tract associated with, e.g. pitch lowering, swallowing and effort closure of the larynx, should be considered a result of the folding of the laryngeal walls due to vertical changes in the structures, especially the approximation of the thyroid and hyoid cartilages, rather than a true sphincter action (Fink and Demarest 1978). In cadaver larynges the changes in the laryngeal structures caused by an increased hyoid-to-thyroid distance can be summarised as follows: the epiglottis rises, the vestibule of the larynx expands and the ventricular folds and the vocal folds abduct owing to a reduction in the folding of these structures with increasing vertical tension. This phenomenon is accompanied by a slight increase in F0 (Vilkman and Karma 1989). An example of 'unfolding' from everyday clinical practice is the examination technique for indirect laryngoscopy. In order to improve the view of the larynx, the relatively high-pitched vowels /i/ and /e/ and tongue pull are used. Vowel articulation modifies the laryngeal structures considerably. Non-phonatory laryngeal functions are, to a great extent, based on reflex interplay between relevant structures.

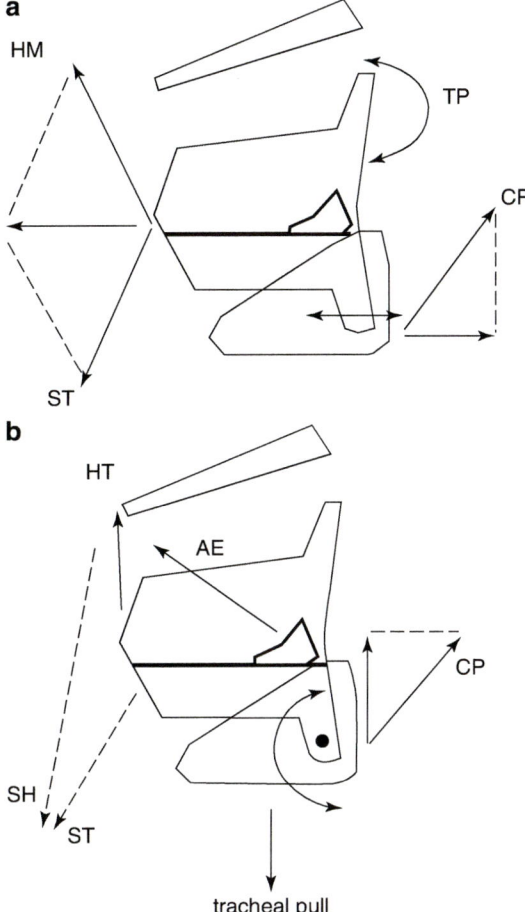

Fig. 4.5 Schematic representation of external laryngeal forces. (**a**) Forces lengthening the vocal folds and raising F0. (**b**) Forces shortening the vocal folds and lowering F0. *CP* cricopharyngeal muscle; *ST* sternothyroid muscle; *TP* thyropharyngeal muscle; *AE* aryepiglottic muscle; *HM* hyomandibular muscles; *HT* hyothyroid muscle; *SH* sternohyoid muscle. Taken from Vilkman et al. (1996). Copyright with kind permission from Elsevier

It is obvious that in some voice disorders, the phylogenetically young phonatory mechanism is more or less replaced by the archaic mechanism. In hyperfunctional dysphonia, for instance, the position of the larynx is high and the space of the laryngeal vestibule is small (e.g. Wendler and Seidner 1987). This change can be explained as occurring because of an approximation of the thyroid cartilage to the hyoid bone and increased folding, as observed during swallowing and effort closure.

External forces together with the cricothyroid system may contribute to the cross-sectional shape of the vocal folds. This is important, for instance, from the point of view of controlling registers and modes of phonation. Vertical changes in the laryngeal column may, in addition to slight fundamental frequency (F0) changes and abductory-adductory influence, also affect the register control of phonation (Wendler and Seidner 1987).

4.6.3   Length Adjustment of the Vocal Folds

For untrained singers especially, the correlation between pitch and laryngeal height is very strong. This is probably why the contribution of external laryngeal muscles has traditionally been suspected to play a major role in pitch control. During recent decades, however, research has revealed that in trained singers, the laryngeal height is not positively correlated with pitch, and the correlation can even be negative (Shipp and Izdebski 1975). The most important means of pitch control is connected with adjusting the length of the vocal folds, in which intrinsic muscles, notably the cricothyroid (CT) muscles, have an important role. As far as vocal fold elongation is concerned, the CT does not necessarily need assistance from the external laryngeal muscles. As to shortening of the vocal folds, it is plausible that tracheal pull (Zenker and Glaninger 1959) with controlled CT muscle relaxation is the main control mechanism (see Vilkman et al. 1996 for a review). A model based on an extensive literature review (Vilkman et al. 1996) of how external mechanisms might influence the pitch is presented in Fig. 4.5. Pitch may be raised (Fig. 4.5a) by a forward movement of the thyroid cartilage that is caused by the activity of the strap muscles and the musculature of the bottom of the mouth; in this case, the CP muscle pulls the cricoid cartilage posteriorly. The cricothyroid joint generally permits gliding in an anteroposterior direction to some extent. Figure 4.5a also illustrates that the TP may contribute to the lengthening of the vocal folds by approximating the thyroid laminae

(Zenker and Zenker 1960). Owing to changes concomitant with ageing, this mechanism is probably possible in young persons only. The option for pitch lowering can be summarised as follows (Fig. 4.5b). The lowering of the thyroid cartilage caused by ST and SH activity creates circumstances in which the contraction of the CP muscle, by opposing the cranial displacement of the larynx, rotates the cricoid cartilage around the axis of the CT joint, and thus the vocal folds are shortened (Fig. 4.5). Simultaneous CT relaxation, or at least CT deactivation, is also necessary. In addition, tracheal pull, although diminished because of a lowered larynx position, may contribute to the opening of the CT visor. Assisted by contractions of the SH and TH muscles, these events pull the hyoid bone towards the thyroid cartilage, which leads to changes in the laryngeal column, to increased folding in particular, as often seen in laryngoscopic examinations. In addition to the effects brought about by the hyoid-to-thyroid approximation, the function of the aryepiglottic muscles may also contribute to F0 change by pulling the arytenoids forward (lowering the epiglottis) or by rotating the cricoid cartilage.

4.6.4   Laryngeal Height in Voice Pedagogy and Therapy

In both speech therapy and singing pedagogy, maintaining a low position of the larynx has traditionally been considered favourable for good quality voice production. Clinical and pedagogical experience suggests that the physiological basis of this concept is related not only to resonatory and muscular tension aspects in general, but probably also to an intentional avoidance of excessive vocal fold folding, such as observed in an effort type of glottal closure in connection with a TH approximation. Considering the external factors and changes in the laryngeal column, there seem to be some grounds for a tentative formulation of a basic principle probably underlying the laryngeal control of voice production as follows: in good quality voice production, the intrinsic laryngeal muscles have to be allowed maximum independence in the delicate control of the stiffness and cross-sectional shape of the vocal folds. In this framework, increased folding, due to either articular rotation in the cricothyroid joint or hyoid-thyroid cartilage approximation, would be a violation of an important laryngeal setting. The high larynx position in high-pitched singing probably makes delicate adjustments, such as the so-called covering of the voice (e.g. Sonninen et al. 1999) with rising pitch in classical singing, difficult or even impossible, because of the circumstances created in the vocal fold tissues.

4.6.5   Conclusion

To summarise, the 'physiological larynx' has to be considered a complex interactive system, which is not restricted to the anatomical structures of the larynx. Some of the significant factors in this interactive system include tracheal pull and its interaction with CT activity, the gross vertical movements of the larynx, the interplay between thyroid cartilage biomechanics and CP muscle function and finally the sparse muscular connections to the cricoid cartilage.

4.7   Epidemiology of Dysphonia

Ekaterina Osipenko, Krzysztof Izdebski, and Amélie Elisabeth Tillmanns

4.7.1   Introduction

In a modern society, voice is an important tool for work and for social communication. Serious social and economical consequences occur when voice is injured. Identification of possible causations, risk factors and prevention of voice injury, clinically referred to as dysphonia, are of a paramount importance to the society at large (Duff et al. 2004; Bhattacharyya 2014). Treatment of dysphonia can be complicated, lengthy and costly and interrupt social and professional life. Hence knowledge of the epidemiological factors is of significant value in understanding the risk factors and improving prevention and treatments of dysphonia (Morabia 2004; Mayou and Farmer 2002; Hill 1965). However, epidemiological data about voice disorders are still rare and studies are just beginning to emerge. Additionally, nonstandardised definitions about the different forms of dysphonia make data collection and analyses even more challenging.

Traditionally, voice disorders are divided into organic/structural dysphonia and functional/malregulative dysphonia (see Sects. 4.1 and 4.2). However, the relationships and boundaries between organic and functional are not always clear. For example, an organic voice problem may be associated with secondary functional voice disorders or vice versa, and functional voice disorders may lead to organic lesions. The definition and sub-classification of functional voice disorders have been discussed for a long time. Correlating specific dysphonias to specific epidemiological factors is often complicated (Duff et al. 2004; Verdolini and Ramig 2001; Roy et al. 2004; Mayou and Farmer 2002). Another confusing factor is revision of the initial diagnosis, which occurs in up to 3% of all cases (Cohen et al. 2012).

In this section, we present literature about global findings on dysphonias with regard to age, sex, professional subgroups, risks and environmental and geographical/linguistic factors. Because providing epidemiological evidence on all types of dysphonia is beyond the scope of this section, discussion is limited to selected dysphonias. The many different forms of dysphonia are listed and explained elsewhere (see Sects. 5.1–5.16).

According to new large-scale epidemiological studies, up to almost half of the general population experiences voice disorders at least once in the lifetime (Roy et al. 2004, 2005, 2007; Behlau et al. 2012; Bhattacharyya 2014; Cohen et al. 2012). While the epidemiological characteristics of dysphonic cohorts appear to be universal, meaning that the epidemiological factors are non-specific for geography, race, language or social status, a higher risk for certain professions is, however, observed (Behlau et al. 2012;

Villanueva-Reyes 2011; Roy et al. 2004, 2005; Koufman and Blalock 1982; Izdebski et al. 2000; Duff et al. 2004; Verdolini and Ramig 2001; Carding et al. 2006). A sizable number of these voice disorders comprise acute, short-lasting voice problems, but between 20 and 60% of dysphonias that last longer than 4 weeks are also reported (Roy et al. 2005, 2007). Various reports also list a higher prevalence of dysphonias in women than in men (Roy et al. 2005; Garcia Martins et al. 2015; Behlau et al. 2012; Cohen et al. 2012; Bhattacharyya 2014).

Voice disorders occur at all ages. In childhood, the incidence is estimated between 0.12 and 38% with a higher prevalence in boys (Carding et al. 2006; Verduyckt et al. 2011; Cohen et al. 2012). Newer studies list vocal cord nodules, cysts and acute laryngitis as the main reasons for acquired juvenile dysphonias (Garcia Martins et al. 2015). In adults, functional dysphonia, acid laryngitis and vocal polyps are reported most frequently (Garcia Martins et al. 2015). Around 20% of the geriatric population suffers from voice disorders, often co-occurring with hearing loss, and increasing age is considered to be a risk factor for dysphonia (Cohen and Turley 2009; Cohen et al. 2012; Roy et al. 2007). Besides presbyphonia, functional dysphonia and Reinke's oedema occur often in the elderly (Garcia Martins et al. 2015).

Among professional voice users such as teachers, singers, radio and TV announcers, voice-over artists, military personnel, call-centre workers, voice or sports coaches, the lifetime prevalence of voice disorders is even higher. Different studies show that teachers have almost twice the risk of voice problems in their life as non-teachers (Behlau et al. 2012; Roy et al. 2004; Garcia Martins et al. 2014b). Voice disorders in the speaking professions also adversely affect work performance, work attendance and work loyalty (Roy et al. 2004, 2005; Bhattacharyya 2014). One report has stated that 16% of teachers considered changing their occupation because of recurring voice problems (Behlau et al. 2012). Costs of lost productivity due to untreated voice disorders in occupations like teaching are estimated to almost $3 billion annually in the USA.

Other important risk factors for voice disorders include smoking history and alcohol consumption, while gastro-oesophageal reflux association is questionable (Roy et al. 2004).

4.7.2 Organic/Structural Dysphonia

In various adult populations, organic dysphonia is described as being less frequent than functional dysphonia (Garcia Martins et al. 2015; Preciado et al. 2005; Van Houtte et al. 2010). From childhood to adulthood, the most frequent organic causations include acute laryngitis, accounting for about 40% of cases (Cohen et al. 2012; Bhattacharyya 2014), with benign vocal cord lesions such as nodules, polyps or cysts (Garcia Martins et al. 2015; ASHA 2015; Kılıç et al. 2004; Preciado et al. 2005). Chronic laryngitis was detected in 3.47 per 1000 people in a primary care cohort, with a mean age of 52.9 years (Stein and Nordzij 2013). With a reported incidence in dysphonic patients of about 17% in the age group between 7 and 12 years of age, vocal cord nodules occur predominantly in boys, while in the age group from 12 years of age to adulthood, nodules are more frequent in the female population (Garcia Martins et al. 2015). The literature is seemingly clear that voice overuse is a significant risk factor in vocal cord nodule formation in youngsters and adults and also that mucous retention cysts may have a functional cofactor, but congenital epidermoid cysts are important as well (Altman 2007; Duff et al. 2004; Behlau et al. 2012; Villanueva-Reyes 2011; Johns 2003; Garcia Martins et al. 2015). Voice overuse is probably the reason nodules are the most frequent organic cause of dysphonia in teachers (Preciado et al. 2005; Garcia Martins et al. 2014b).

In the population over 40 years old, acid laryngitis and smoking-related changes, such as Reinke's oedema, become more frequent (Garcia Martins et al. 2015). The incidence of dysphonia further increases in the group of patients over 60 years old (Garcia Martins et al. 2015). On one hand, various organic causes appear more frequently, partly due to the rising frequency of systemic diseases and decreased respiratory function, and on the other, presbyphonia occurs, as senescence profoundly affects the phonatory system through loss of elastic fibres, atrophy of the vocal folds, prominence of vocal apophysis and vocal tremor (Garcia Martins et al. 2014a, 2015; Marino and Johns 2014; Vaca et al. 2015) (see Sect. 5.15). The prevalence of voice disorders in seniors is shown to be around 19–29%, often co-occurring with hearing loss and severely affecting quality of life (Roy et al. 2007; Cohen and Turley 2009).

Another organic cause of dysphonia is carcinoma, with dysphonia often being the first presenting symptom (Schultz 2011). Cancer prevalence in patients seeking treatment because of dysphonia is reported to be 2.2% and greatest among males over 70 years of age (Cohen et al. 2012).

4.7.3 Functional/Malregulative Dysphonia

Functional or malregulative dysphonia (Hacki 2014) describes all types of dysphonia that are not due to structural or pathologically defined 'visible' causes (see Sects. 4.1 and 4.2) (Izdebski 2019; Koufman and Blalock 1982; Garcia Martins et al. 2015; Preciado et al. 2005). The incidence in a treatment-seeking population is 30%, predominating in young adults, adult women and elderly patients (Izdebski 2019; Cohen et al. 2012; Van Houtte et al. 2010).

Functional dysphonia can be due to constitutional differences, speaking habits, misuse or abuse of the voice, changing voice in puberty or aspects of personality (see Sects. 4.1 and 4.2). Teachers and other professional voice users are at a much higher risk of developing functional dysphonia. In one study, hyperfunctional dysphonia was found in 17.4% of teachers compared with 7.2% of controls, and incomplete glottal closure was reported in 13.9% of teachers compared with 1.2% in controls (Sliwinska-Kowalska et al. 2006). Another study showed that 50% of patients with functional dysphonia were professional voice users (Deary and Miller 2011).

Functional dysphonia has been shown to be associated with psychosocial factors such as anxiety or depression in about 30% of cases (Deary and Miller 2011; Misono et al. 2014), but epidemiological data on the frequency of psychogenic voice disorders are rare, mainly because of difficulties in differential diagnosis, as these often include multifactorial conditions (see Sect. 5.9). Psychogenic aphonia is rare (0.4%) but with a predominant occurrence in women (Kollbrunner et al. 2010).

4.8 Aetiology and Pathogenesis of Dysphonia: An Overview with Focus on Malformations, Inflammatory/Systemic Diseases, Malignancies and Traumata Affecting the Larynx, Resonance Disorders and Presbyphonia

Sevtap Akbulut and Haldun Oguz

4.8.1 Malformations
(see Figs. 1.16–1.18 in Sect. 1.2)

4.8.1.1 Laryngomalacia
Laryngomalacia is the most common laryngeal anomaly and cause of stridor in infancy. It is characterised by a collapse of the supraglottal larynx during inspiration. The stridor is typically only heard during inspiration and it is worse with feeding, crying and the supine position.

It is diagnosed by flexible laryngoscopy. Typical findings include an omega-shaped epiglottis, foreshortening of the aryepiglottic folds and forward prolapsing arytenoid cartilages and supra-arytenoid tissue obstructing airflow, with poor visualisation of the vocal folds. Flexible laryngoscopy may also provide a chance to exclude other supraglottal or subglottal pathologies that may contribute to stridor.

Laryngomalacia is usually a self-limiting disease that rarely requires surgical intervention.

Although it often worsens over the first few months, it usually resolves between 18 and 24 months of age (Solomons and Prescott 1987). It rarely persists in late childhood.

Most often, observation is the treatment of choice. During periods of acute laryngitis, special attention is required owing to worsening by swelling of the mucosa. Rarely, children may present with more severe problems such as feeding difficulties, cyanosis or failure to thrive. At that time, different techniques of supraglottoplasty, such as supraglottic trimming, resection of the aryepiglottic folds or dividing the aryepiglottic fold and excision of the cuneiform cartilage, may become the treatment choices (Roger et al. 1995; Solomons and Prescott 1987).

4.8.1.2 Congenital Vocal Fold Paralysis
Congenital vocal fold paralysis or paresis is one of the more common causes of neonatal stridor. Most of the children who present with paralysis have no demonstrable aetiology. There may be associated cardiac or neurological disorders based on, e.g. the Arnold-Chiari malformation, infection, neoplasm or birth trauma. Workup must include a thorough neurological and cardiac evaluation (Cohen et al. 1982).

Vocal fold paralysis may present as unilateral or bilateral. Unilateral paralysis is usually associated with breathy vocalisation, choking or aspiration. Stridor is less common. Usually observation is the only treatment that is needed for unilateral paralysis. Return of function is possible in about 6 months.

There is a high-pitched cry and inspiratory stridor in bilateral vocal fold paralysis. The vocal folds are passively moved apart on exhalation, so there is no expiratory stridor. Airway obstruction is frequently severe enough to require tracheotomy. Bilateral vocal fold paralysis is often associated with Arnold-Chiari malformation (Boey et al. 1995). Decompression can reverse the paralysis.

4.8.1.3 Laryngeal Atresia and Webs
The embryological origin of these rare conditions is a failure of recanalisation of the larynx during prenatal development. Laryngeal webs are most

commonly seen at the glottal level. The web may be thin with minimal fibrous tissue or thick and long involving supra- or subglottal areas. A thin web may be ruptured by intubation. The thicker the web, the harder it is to treat. Thick webs can present at birth as aphonia and rapid asphyxia if not immediately addressed. Surgical management of thick webs may require tracheotomy until the larynx is larger and more amenable to surgical correction (Milczuk et al. 2000).

Congenital laryngeal atresia can be associated with a tracheo-oesophageal fistula or many other congenital anomalies. The neonate with a laryngeal atresia has nearly no pathway for the air and needs immediate tracheotomy. Often the severity of associated anomalies does not let the child live long, even with a tracheotomy.

Thin and moderate anterior webs are usually not diagnosed at birth, as they may not produce airway obstruction symptoms. The treatment of choice is placement of a laryngeal keel with laryngofissure.

4.8.1.4 Laryngocele

A dilated laryngeal saccule that communicates with the laryngeal lumen is called a laryngocoele. It may be internal and confined to the larynx. This causes bulging of the ventricular or aryepiglottic fold. When a laryngocele extends beyond these confines into the neck, it is called an external laryngocele. If intra- and extra-laryngeal components occur together, it is named a combined laryngocele. The cyst is typically air-filled and occasionally contains some mucus. If there is no connection with the laryngeal lumen, the dilation is called a saccular cyst, which is filled with mucus. Complete excision by a microlaryngeal endoscopic approach and marsupialisation are usually successful; open laryngeal excision is rarely needed (Mysiorek and Persky 1989).

4.8.1.5 Subglottal Stenosis

Subglottal stenoses may be congenital or acquired. Congenital subglottal stenosis may present with airway obstruction in the neonatal period or with recurrent 'croup' (see Sect. 4.8.2) at a later period. The stenoses are less severe than acquired subglottal stenosis, which most commonly occurs secondarily to prolonged intubation. Diagnosis is made by direct laryngoscopy and bronchoscopy. Congenital deformity of the cricoid ring is usually the main problem for the congenital subglottic stenosis. Sizing of a subglottal stenosis with an endotracheal tube allows a more accurate understanding of the severity. Most subglottal stenoses that require surgical management are acquired in origin (Thompson and Kershner 2007).

4.8.1.6 Hemangioma

Subglottal and tracheal hemangiomas are benign, congenital vascular malformations derived from mesodermal remnants. They are relatively uncommon. Patients are usually asymptomatic at birth but present with stridor within the first few months of life. Asymmetric subglottal narrowing is the classic finding on soft tissue neck radiographs. Asymmetric submucosal mass with a bluish, reddish discolouration, which is most often found in the posterolateral subglottis, is diagnostic on endoscopic examination. They usually resolve spontaneously. Fifty percent regression is expected by 5 years of age. The treatment of choice is laser excision (Sie et al. 1994). Treatment of hemangioma with steroids or interferon may also be helpful in extensive or massive lesions (Ezekowitz et al. 1992).

4.8.2 Localised Inflammatory Diseases Affecting the Larynx

4.8.2.1 Acute Viral Infections

Infectious laryngitis is most commonly due to viral upper respiratory tract infections. Symptoms include dysphonia, cough, fever, generalised malaise and symptoms of rhinitis. Laryngoscopic findings are erythema and oedema of the vocal folds and supraglottis. The posterior larynx is usually irritated by coughing and throat clearing. Treatment includes hydration and voice rest. It is usually self-limited and resolves in about 5–7 days.

Pseudo-Croup Pseudo-croup (to differentiate it from diphtheria-caused croup) is a viral infection characterised by inspiratory stridor, a barking cough and hoarseness. It is mostly seen in pre-school children, usually in spring and autumn. The common viruses that cause pseudo-croup are *parainfluenza* and *influenza viruses* (Stroud and Friedman 2001). It starts with a clinical picture similar to that of upper respiratory tract infection, and then gradually increased inspiratory stridor and coughs develop. The severity of symptoms is related to the extent of subglottal oedema. Lateral neck filming may be helpful to make a diagnosis of pseudo-croup as it reveals subglottal narrowing and a normal epiglottis. An anteroposterior film shows the classic steeple sign in 50% of patients.

Treatment for pseudo-croup is supportive. Oral hydration and mist therapy can be helpful to decrease the subglottal inflammation and for thinning the secretions. Patients with stridor at rest may need to be sent to hospital. Nebulised racemic epinephrine has been shown to relieve airway obstruction. Patients benefit from the use of corticosteroids orally or parenterally ('intravenous tracheotomy'). A mixture of helium and oxygen can be used for respiratory distress (Stroud and Friedman 2001).

4.8.2.2 Acute Bacterial Infections

Acute Epiglottitis and Supraglottitis Acute epiglottitis is almost always caused by *Haemophilus influenzae* type B. A resultant inflammation and swelling of the supraglottal structures can develop rapidly and lead to life-threatening upper airway obstruction in children. Although it is thought of as a disease of childhood, because of efficient *Haemophilus influenzae* type B immunisation in children, it has become relatively more common in adults (Shah et al. 2004).

Patients present with symptoms that range from fever and dysphagia to drooling, muffled voice, stridor and cyanosis. Diagnosis in children is based on clinical suspicion. Lateral neck films show the 'thumbprint sign' of epiglottal oedema. Definitive diagnosis is made by direct inspection of the epiglottis, a procedure that should usually be done in the operating room by an experienced clinician. The main aim of the management is to secure the airway. In children this involves an intubation in the operating room, while in adults observation in the intensive care unit, intubation or even a tracheotomy may be necessary. Appropriate intravenous antibiotherapy for *H. Influenzae*, or for streptococcus and staphylococcus, especially in patients who are vaccinated for *H. Influenzae* type B, should be started (Gorelick and Baker 1994).

Bacterial Tracheitis Bacterial tracheitis (pseudomembranous 'croup') is a severe form of laryngotracheobronchitis. Most often the isolated agent is *Staphylococcus aureus*, although *Streptococcus pyogenes* and *Haemophilus influenzae* have also been reported. Presenting symptoms are high fever, dyspnoea progressing to stridor, dysphonia and cough. The diagnosis is made on the basis of thick purulent discharge and crusts in the airway, erythema and laryngeal oedema. The condition can be particularly dangerous in children owing to the small size of the airways. Intubation is almost always necessary in children (Donaldson and Maltby 1989).

Diphtheria Diphtheria is caused by *Corynebacterium diphtheriae*. It is a rare disease because of the widespread use of diphtheria-pertussis immunisation. The typical clinical picture is two- to three-day febrile illness with hoarseness, followed by dyspnoea and stridor. Characteristic signs include an odour that smells of a 'wet mouse' (or apple) and a grey laryngeal membrane seen on laryngeal examination. Diagnosis is based on Gram's stain and culture of the membrane. Differential diagnosis should include infectious mononucleosis, streptococcal pharyngitis and ulcerative pharyngitis. Treatment includes airway management, antitoxin and antibiotics (Adler et al. 2013).

4.8.2.3 Laryngeal Candidiasis

Laryngeal candidiasis is a commonly seen fungal infection by *Candida albicans*. It can occur in both immunocompromised patients and healthy individuals with predisposing factors such as use of corticosteroids, especially inhaled steroids, broad-spectrum antibiotics, diabetes mellitus, endotracheal intubation and recent laryngitis. Laryngoscopic examination reveals diffuse laryngeal erythema with an irregular, white exudate usually involving the true vocal folds. Invasive laryngeal candidiasis can be seen in the immunocompromised patients who present with mucosal oedema, ulceration and possibly tissue necrosis. Treatment consists of topical antifungal gargles with or without systemic antifungal agents. For invasive candidiasis intravenous amphotericin-B is recommended (Sulica 2005).

4.8.2.4 Chronic Laryngitis

Continuous irritation of the larynx by causes such as allergy, excessive smoking and alcohol use, postnasal drip from chronic rhinosinusitis, laryngopharyngeal reflux and vocal abuse or vocal overuse leads to chronic non-specific laryngitis (Fig. 4.6). Laryngeal examination reveals oedema and erythema of the vocal folds with increased vascular dilation (Woodson 2003).

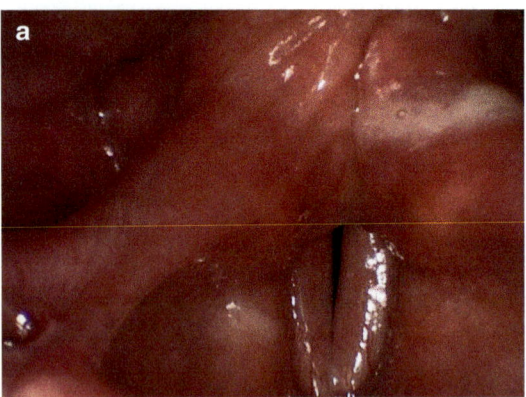

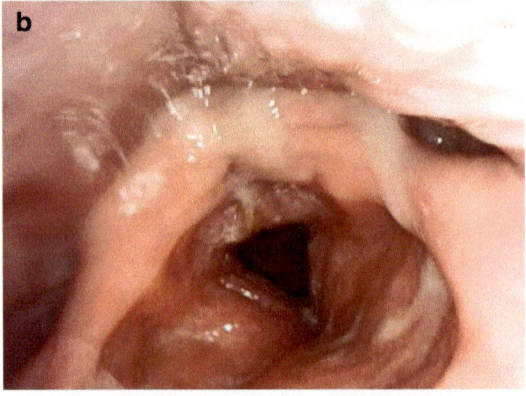

Fig. 4.6 (**a** and **b**) Examples of chronic laryngitis

Prolonged voice use, talking over loud noise and irritants should be avoided. Throat clearing should be strongly discouraged, and irritative cough should be treated with medication. Causative factors, such as chronic rhinosinusitis, allergy and reflux should be taken under control. Smoking should be discouraged.

When laryngitis does not resolve despite adequate medical therapy, other causes of hoarseness should be considered. Chronic vocal misuse is the most common cause of persisting laryngitis. Voice therapy would be very helpful in these subjects.

Patients with chronic laryngitis may develop dysplasias in terms of precancerous manifestations and therefore require close follow-up.

4.8.2.5 Laryngopharyngeal Reflux

Laryngopharyngeal reflux (LPR) is defined as the passage of gastric contents above the upper oesophageal sphincter, causing symptoms and tissue damage in the upper airway. It is estimated that more than half of patients with hoarseness have LPR. The most common symptoms associated with LPR are hoarseness, cough, throat clearing, globus sensation, excessive throat mucus, choking and sore throat (Oğuz et al. 2007).

There is no specific laryngeal finding pathognomonic for LPR. Oedema or hypertrophy and sometimes erythema of the posterior glottis are the more frequent laryngeal findings.

The treatment alternatives for LPR include lifestyle modifications, medical treatment and surgical therapy. Lifestyle modifications include decreased intake of fat, citrus fruits, tomato, caffeine, chocolate and alcohol; elevation of the head of the bed; cessation of smoking; and avoiding lying down and sleeping for 3 h after meals. Pharmacological acid suppression, including antacids, histamine receptor antagonists (H2 blockers) and gastric proton pump inhibitors, is the most important treatment method of LPR (for details see Sect. 5.5).

Nissen fundoplication may be an alternative option for patients who obtain partial relief from medications or for those who prefer surgical treatment to the possibility of long-term PPI treatment (Lindstrom et al. 2002).

4.8.2.6 Laryngitis Secondary to Irritation with Chemicals

Inhalation of toxic vapours can acutely irritate the larynx and lead to laryngitis (Pospiech et al. 1996). The symptoms of inhalation trauma include swelling, inflammation, stridor, wheezing and hoarseness, depending on the severity of the trauma and the type of gases or fumes inhaled. Intubation or tracheotomy may be required to manage the airway obstruction. Any patient who presents with laryngitis of obscure origin should be questioned about possible environmental or occupational exposure to inhaled substances (Woodson 2003). Long-term toxic exposure can lead to metaplasia (Pospiech et al. 1996).

4.8.3 Systemic Inflammatory Diseases Affecting the Larynx (see Figs. 5.27–5.32 in Sect. 5.13)

4.8.3.1 Tuberculosis

Laryngeal tuberculosis is a chronic bacterial infection caused by *Mycobacterium tuberculosis*. Patients present with hoarseness, odynophagia, dysphagia, cough, as well as the typical constitutional symptoms of tuberculosis with fatigue, weight loss and night sweats. The entire larynx including the true vocal folds, the arytenoids and the epiglottis can be involved, with tubercular lesions varying from mucosal oedema with local ulceration to granular nodular areas with exophytic fungating lesions. Chronic inflammatory changes restricted to one vocal fold are often associated with tuberculosis. It can mimic carcinoma of the larynx. The standard treatment of laryngeal tuberculosis is long-term administration of multiple antituberculous medications (Shin et al. 2000).

4.8.3.2 Histoplasmosis

Histoplasmosis is caused by *Histoplasma capsulatum*. Oropharyngeal and laryngeal involvement is frequent when a disseminated disease is present. It is characterised by oropharyngeal or laryngeal ulcers. The examination of the larynx may reveal a variety of lesions ranging from pearly white plaques to nodular granulomas.

Biopsy demonstrates granulomatous tissue changes containing necrosis with giant cells, lymphocytes and large numbers of macrophages with intracellular yeast forms observed on PAS or Gomori methenamine silver staining. Intravenous amphotericin-B is the treatment of choice (Sataloff et al. 1993).

4.8.3.3 Blastomycosis

Blastomycosis is a chronic pulmonary infection caused by the fungus *Blastomyces dermatitidis*. Laryngeal involvement occurs in 2–5% of all cases. Patients present with severe hoarseness, dysphagia, coughing and dyspnoea. The true vocal folds are the most commonly involved site. Laryngeal lesions usually appear as erythematous, granulomatous masses with irregular borders. Advanced disease may present with vocal cord fixation. Biopsies will show caseation necrosis with acute inflammatory infiltration and micro-abscesses. It is treated with intravenous amphotericin-B with good response (Reder and Neel 1993).

4.8.3.4 Sarcoidosis

Sarcoidosis is a chronic idiopathic systemic granulomatous disease. Laryngeal involvement is typically diffuse enlargement of the supraglottis, including the epiglottis, the aryepiglottic folds, arytenoids and false vocal folds. It spares the true vocal folds but the subglottis can be involved. Diagnosis is made on the basis of clinical features such as fever, hilar lymphadenopathy, cough and dyspnoea. Biopsy reveals non-caseating granulomas. Patients with laryngeal sarcoidosis may be treated by observation. Systemic and intra-lesional steroids demonstrate efficacy (Gallivan and Landis 1991).

4.8.3.5 Wegener Granulomatosis (Granulomatosis with Polyangiitis)

Wegener granulomatosis is a rare idiopathic disease. It involves mainly three regions: the renal system, lower respiratory tract and the head and neck region. Laryngeal involvement results in non-specific signs including wheezing or stridor, dyspnoea and dysphonia. Subglottal stenosis is the main problem while vocal folds are usually not involved. It is described by three pathological findings: necrosis, granulomatous inflammation and vasculitis. Diagnosis is based on identification of anti-neutrophil cytoplasmic antibody (ANCA) and more specifically the cytoplasmic c-ANCA in blood. Systemic treatment includes use of corticosteroids and other immunosuppressive drugs, especially cyclophosphamide. Endoscopic or open surgical procedures are treatment alternatives for severe airway stenosis. Good medical control before surgery is mandatory to have a successful airway outcome (Devaney et al. 1998; Herridge et al. 1996).

4.8.3.6 Amyloidosis

Laryngeal amyloidosis accounts for less than 1% of benign laryngeal pathologies. It is a benign idiopathic disease characterised by the extracellular accumulation of normally soluble proteins in an abnormal fibrillar form leading to tissue damage and disease. Amyloidosis comprises a family of disorders. Deposition of amyloid may be either localised or systemic and either primary or secondary (Akst and Thompson 2003). It can be associated with multiple myeloma, medullary thyroid carcinoma and small-cell carcinoma when it presents in a secondary form. Tumour-like, organ-limited amyloidosis is a relatively rare but well-recognised condition. It is usually not accompanied with plasma cell dycrasia and not followed by systemic disease. The common sites of involvement include the respiratory tract, skin and urinary bladder (Oğuz et al. 2007). Localised amyloidosis in the larynx results in slowly progressive dysphonia and dyspnoea. Amyloid lesions are described typically as 'firm, non-ulcerating, epithelial nodules'. It is definitely diagnosed with the histopathological presence of amyloid fibrils in a twisted β-pleated sheet pattern with affinity for Congo red dye. The underlying condition in the secondary form needs treatment, but systemic treatment usually does not eliminate the amyloid deposits. Surgical treatment is necessary for the lesions when the airway or voice is compromised (Akst and Thompson 2003; Bartels et al. 2004).

4.8.3.7 Other Systemic Inflammatory Diseases

Systemic Lupus Erythematosus Systemic lupus erythematosus is an autoimmune collagen vascular disease. It may present with laryngeal manifestations. Typical symptoms include hoarseness, odynophagia and dysphagia. Generalised vocal fold oedema or ulcerations are typical laryngeal findings. Vocal fold paralysis can also be seen. The usual treatment of this disease includes corticosteroids (Teitel et al. 1992).

Rheumatoid Arthritis Rheumatoid arthritis is an autoimmune disorder resulting in polyarthropathy. Laryngeal involvement is not uncommon. Rheumatoid lesions on vocal folds or cricoarytenoid arthritis can be responsible for dysphonia. Rheumatoid lesions can respond to systemic medical treatment; if they persist or cause a functional voice problem, surgery is warranted (Woo et al. 1995). Vocal cord hypomobility or immobility associated with cricoarytenoid arthritis may resolve with systemic treatment or with steroid injection into the cricoarytenoid joint (Nanke et al. 2001).

Relapsing Polychondritis Relapsing polychondritis is an idiopathic autoimmune disorder characterised by recurrent cartilage inflammation. Laryngeal symptoms include dyspnoea, hoarseness, cough, stridor and pain. There are no pathognomonic signs. Treatment consists of surgical airway management and medical therapies including steroids or dapsone (Estes 1983).

4.8.4 Malignancies of the Larynx

4.8.4.1 Squamous Cell Carcinoma

Squamous cell carcinoma makes up over 95% of malignant laryngeal neoplasms. The greatest incidence of laryngeal cancer occurs in the fifth to seventh decades. The male-to-female ratio varies from 5 to 20:1. The risk factors for laryngeal cancer are smoking, alcohol intake, HPV infection and laryngopharyngeal reflux disease (Falk et al. 1989; Kiyabu et al. 1989).

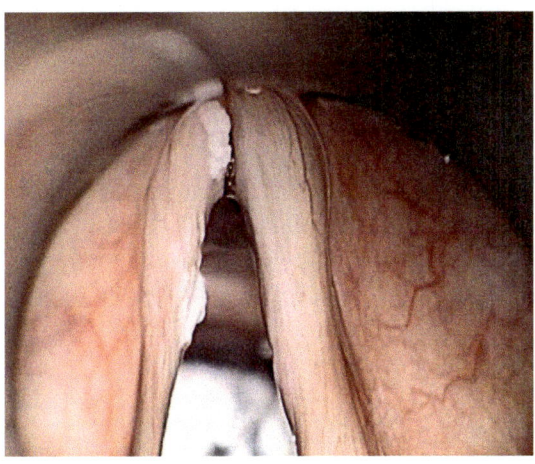

Fig. 4.7 Leukoplakia. With kind permission from the German Voice Clinic, Hamburg

The larynx is lined with stratified squamous epithelium down to the level of the true vocal folds; this transitions to a pseudostratified respiratory epithelium. Normally the epithelium matures from the basement membrane to the surface. Redundancy of the epithelial layers results in abnormal epithelial hypertrophy which is called as *keratosis*. When the normal epithelium is replaced by cells with malignant characteristics from the basement membrane to the surface, it is termed as *dysplasia*. It is graded mild to severe. Figure 4.7 shows changes appearing as so-called leukoplakia.

Carcinoma in situ is defined as dysplasia which fills the entire epithelium but does not extend below the basal membrane. Once abnormal epithelial cells invade beneath the basement membrane, the condition is then defined as a *carcinoma* or *microinvasive carcinoma*.

Keratosis is often associated with carcinoma in situ and invasive carcinoma, but the incidence of isolated keratosis becoming invasive cancer appears to be low (3%). Keratosis usually involves the true vocal folds and is related to smoking, vocal fold phonotrauma and laryngopharyngeal reflux. Even though the majority of patients with keratosis will not develop a malignancy, they should require close follow-up. Carcinoma in situ is indistinguishable grossly from keratosis or carcinoma. Complete excision of dysplasia or carcinoma in situ is crucial, as, if left untreated, carcinoma in situ will progress to invasive carcinoma.

The common symptoms of laryngeal cancer are dysphonia, dyspnoea, stridor, pain, dysphagia, odynophagia and cough, depending on the site and stage of the lesion. Hemoptysis, weight loss, halitosis and swelling in the neck may be seen in the late stages of the disease. Supraglottal tumours usually present late with associated symptoms, glottal tumours usually present early with voice change, and subglottal tumours present late with airway obstruction.

Complete endoscopic evaluation for staging requires a plan for airway management and examination of all at-risk mucosal surfaces. The neck must be examined and second primaries must be ruled out. Direct laryngoscopy under general anaesthesia is performed both to obtain specimens and to define the exact distribution of the lesion accurately.

Radiographic imaging allows evaluation of deep laryngeal spaces, involvement of cartilage and extrinsic muscles of the neck. Both computed tomography and magnetic resonance imaging are useful radiographic modalities for radiographic evaluation.

Lymphatic spread of the tumour occurs in a predictable fashion (Akmansu et al. 2004). This allows surgeons to limit neck dissections to include only the lymph nodes at risk. Glottal cancer has a lower incidence of lymphatic spread than supraglottal cancer. The rich lymphatic network of the supraglottis predisposes it to bilateral lymph node metastasis.

The tumour, node and metastasis (TNM) staging system of the American Joint Committee on Cancer is helpful for treatment planning. It is based on characteristics of the primary tumour, cervical lymph node status and distant metastases (Greene et al. 2002).

Early-stage cancers are usually treated with a single modality (surgery or radiotherapy) in most cases. Survival rates are similar with surgical therapy or radiation therapy in early-stage cancers, and both therapy methods have advantages and potential disadvantages. Treatment decisions should be based on many imprecise factors such as assessment of the tumour, the patient's medical state and goals, toxicities and, most important, the surgeon's personal experience and judgement. Surgical procedure involves some form of conservation technique or a total laryngectomy.

Advanced-staged lesions often require multimodality treatment with surgery followed by radiation or radiation with the addition of chemotherapy. There is a need for a multidisciplinary approach and consideration of each case on an individual basis (Castellanos et al. 1996; Hunt and McWhorter 2007; Sinard et al. 2003).

4.8.4.2 Verrucous Carcinoma

This is a low-grade squamous cell carcinoma that does not metastasise. The lesion is usually amenable to conservative surgery; radiation therapy is ineffective. Its anaplastic conversion after radiotherapy is controversial (Kumar 2004).

4.8.4.3 Sarcomas

Multiple sarcomas have been described in the larynx: chondrosarcoma, osteosarcoma, fibrosarcoma, liposarcoma and angiosarcoma.

Chondrosarcoma is the most prevalent of this tumour class. The majority of these tumours arise from the cricoid cartilage and present with airway obstruction symptoms. The prognosis is good.

4.8.4.4 Neuroendocrine Tumours

These are composed of atypical carcinoids, paragangliomas, large-cell tumours and small-cell tumours. This similar group of tumours behaves very differently, and correct diagnosis through immunohistochemistry is essential. Atypical carcinoids are the most common neuroendocrine tumour and are usually found in the supraglottis. They are aggressive tumours and surgical excision is needed. These carry a poor prognosis. Paragangliomas are relatively indolent tumours found usually in the supraglottis. Surgical excision is the main treatment for them. Small-cell tumours are the most aggressive of the neuroendocrine tumours and are treated with chemo-radiation therapy.

4.8.4.5 Minor Salivary Gland Tumours

There is a variety of minor salivary malignancies that occur in the larynx, including adenoid cystic carcinoma, mucoepidermoid carcinoma, acinic cell carcinoma, adenocarcinoma and malignant mixed carcinoma. They are typically found in the supraglottis. They behave like typical minor salivary gland neoplasms in other head and neck sites. Adenocarcinomas have the least favourable prognosis. Adenoid cystic carcinomas have a tendency to neural invasion with high local recurrence rates. Mucoepidermoid carcinomas are graded on their degree of differentiation, with high-grade tumours being more aggressive.

4.8.5 Traumata

4.8.5.1 Vocal Trauma and Traumatic Laryngitis

Overuse of the voice at a specific event, such as a football game or a party, can lead to functional laryngitis or traumatic laryngitis. As a result of excessive and strained vocalisation, mucosal oedema or even submucosal bleeding can occur in the vocal folds. Eliminating the abuse permits the vocal mechanism to return to its natural state. Complete voice rest is usually enough for irritated vocal folds to return to normal. The history of the patient is very important for being able to define the events that cause traumatic laryngitis. If such hyperfunctional behaviour continues over time, organic changes as vocal nodules, vocal polyps and polypoid chorditis may occur (Boone and McFarlane 2000).

4.8.5.2 Direct Blunt/Sharp Injury to Larynx

Different traumatic injuries may affect the larynx. These may include a penetrating neck wound, blunt trauma from a blow to the neck or attempted strangulation. The structures of the larynx may be severely damaged or fractured leading to airway problems. In most cases of trauma, medical or surgical treatment is needed.

4.8.6 Resonance Disorders

Resonance disorders may be classified as either functional or organic. Functional resonance problems may be habitual or may result from anatomical changes occurring after nasopharyngeal surgery, e.g. adenoidectomy, or from extreme emotional reactions such as in conversion behavioural problems. Organic resonation disorders include cleft palate, submucous cleft palate and velopharyngeal insufficiency caused by neurological disorders affecting the peripheral cranial nerves V, IX, X and XI. Medical or surgical therapy and speech therapy are treatment alternatives for organic causes of resonance problems (Stemple 1993).

Hypernasality occurs when vowels and voice consonants receive excessive nasal resonance owing to failure of the velopharyngeal sphincter to close adequately. It may be accompanied by excessive nasal airflow during the production of pressure consonants.

Hyponasality is the absence of normal resonation on nasal consonants caused by overclosure of velopharyngeal sphincter or blockage of the nasal cavity.

4.8.7 Presbyphonia

Presbyphonia is the condition caused by age-related changes in the larynx. It generally presents in the fifth decade of life or later. It is a process that involves not only loss of muscle bulk but also loss or degeneration of the layers of the lamina propria, as well as cricoarytenoid joint changes. The symptoms of patients are dysphonia, lack of volume/projection and vocal fatigue. Laryngoscopic examination reveals bilateral vocal fold bowing and incomplete glottal closure.

Parkinson disease often has an identical presentation to that of presbyphonia; however patients with Parkinson disease are more likely to have vocal tremor and monotone pitch. Voice therapy and surgical treatment alternatives such as bilateral medialisation laryngoplasty or injection augmentation are effective for presbyphonia (Oğuz and Akbulut 2013). For details see Sect. 5.15.

- *Functional voice disorders* (see Sect. 5.1)
- *Benign lesions of the larynx* (see Sect. 5.4)
- *Neurogenic disorders of the larynx* (see Sects. 5.6, 5.7 and 5.8)

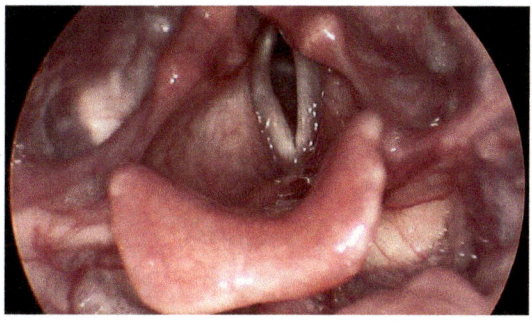

Fig. 4.8 Bilateral vocal fold paralysis after suture lateralisation and cordotomy

Figure 4.8 shows an example of a bilateral vocal fold paralysis after suture lateralisation and cordotomy.

- *Psychogenic dysphonia* (see Sect. 5.9)
- *Endocrinological causes of larynx diseases* (see Sect. 5.10)

4.9 Genetic Background of Voice Disorders and Genetic Perspectives in Voice Treatment

Mette Pedersen, Antoinette am Zehnhoff-Dinnesen, and Sanila Mahmood

4.9.1 Introduction

Knowledge about genetic predisposition and its consequence for health maintenance, disease development and individual treatment is a great challenge in the area of voice disorders. Genetic background and diagnostic and therapeutic options, as well as some aspects of personalised medicine/genomic medicine, are introduced.

4.9.2 Genetic Background of Voice Disorders

Some examples are presented in Table 4.2.

Table 4.2 Genetic background of voice disorders

Gene/chromosome/locus	Genetic details/pathophysiology	Illness/syndrome	Voice pathology	Theory
Vocal fold microstructure				
Gene for elastin *ELN* 7q11.23	Protein is tropoelastin, requires two functioning alleles for normal structural development of the vocal fold lamina propria (Watts et al. 2011)	Lack of one normal ELN allele in supravalvular aortic stenosis (SVAS) and Williams syndrome (WS)	Voice abnormal in individuals with SVAS/WS	Heterozygous *ELN* abnormalities possibly influence vocal fold biomechanics negatively (Watts et al. 2008)
Mucin genes, about 20 on different chromosomes	Encode gel-forming proteins, role of mucin gene profile for the mucosal barrier (Samuels et al. 2008)	Reflux-attributed laryngeal injury or disease	Reflux laryngitis	Genetic differences in the mucin gene profiles of the normal laryngeal epithelium compared with the epithelium of patients with reflux laryngitis (Samuels et al. 2008)
Vocal fold bowing				
DNA polymorphisms in twins	DNA polymorphisms in male twins concordant for 10 out of 10 short tandem repeats DNA markers, indicating monozygosity with a greater than 99% probability (Tanner et al. 2010)	Vocal fold bowing in twins	Hoarseness, breathiness	Genetic factor of voice pathology
Vocal fold inflammation				
Inflammatory mRNA	In an animal model by raised intensity phonation significant increase in vocal fold inflammatory mRNA expression (Rousseau et al. 2009)		Vocal disorder after vocal load	Relation between vocal load and inflammatory mRNA (Rousseau et al. 2009)
Laryngeal carcinoma				
Inhibitory interfering RNA segment	Copies of a small interfering RNA segment directed against the *HuR* gene were transfected into Hep-2 cells (*HuR* regulates expression of stress-sensitive genes, mediates inflammatory response in human endothelial cells) (Hep-2 cells: cell line from cancer patient) (Shen et al. 2010)	Cancer disease	Laryngeal carcinoma	Inhibitory effect of *HuR* gene small interfering RNA segment on laryngeal carcinoma Hep-2 cell growth (Shen et al. 2010)
Examples of voice disorders in syndromes/genetic disorders				
299 syndromes known with voice and resonance disorders according to Van Borsel (2004)				
Overview given in Sataloff (1995)				

Turner syndrome (TS)	Missing X-chromosome	45,X/45,XO	Higher frequency of pitched voice than in non-TS women	Growth factor normalises speech frequency in Turner syndrome (Andersson-Wallgren et al. 2008)
DiGeorge syndrome	Deletion of chromosome 22	22q11.2 deletion	Recurrent infections of the larynx, laryngeal atresia occasionally reported (Fokstuen et al. 1997)	Immune disorder causes infections (Cichocki et al. 2008)
Hyalinosis cutis et mucosae (Vago et al. 2007) or lipoid proteinosis, autosomal recessive (Dertlioğlu et al. 2014), early onset	Mutations of *ECM-1* 1q21	Mutations of extracellular matrix protein gene (*ECM-1*), deposits of hyaline material around the basement membrane of the skin and mucosa	Hoarseness, yellow deposits in the surface of the vocal folds (Xu et al. 2010), papular verrucae skin changes	Mutations are underlying defect of hoarseness, successful treatment attempt with acitretin (Dertlioğlu et al. 2014)
Hereditary systemic apolipoprotein A-1-derived amyloidosis	Mutations in several genes causing protein variants	Extracellular deposition of amyloid fibrils, protein variants in these 2 cases → apoA-1 Leu174Ser and apoA-1 Leu178Pro (Hazenberg et al. 2009)	2 cases with laryngeal amyloid (Hazenberg et al. 2009)	In patients with laryngeal amyloidosis, apoA-1 genotyping should be performed (Hazenberg et al. 2009)
Androgen insensitivity syndrome (Gottlieb et al. 2007), male individuals affected, degree from spermatogenic effect to female habitus	Mutation of androgen receptor gene, locus Xq11-Xq12	X-linked recessive or de novo mutation, possibly post-zygotic with somatic mosaicism	High-pitched voice	Mutational disorder by genetic defect
Examples of voice disorders in genetic neurological diseases				
TOR1A(DYT1) 9q34	Oppenheim dystonia in Ashkenazi Jewish population	Codes for the protein torsin A, an ATPase functioning in restoring damaged proteins in membranes, mutated TOR1A gene results in reduced ATPase activity (Lisak et al. 2007)	Focal dystonia in the larynx	Dystonia by mutated *TOR1A* gene
TUBB4 (DYT4) 19p13.3-p13.2	*DYT4* dystonia, autosomal dominant mode, craniocervical dystonia with prominent spasmodic dysphonia, thin face and body habitus (Lohmann et al. 2013)	c.4C>G mutation	Whispering dysphonia	*TUBB4* is neurally expressed tubulin, possibly abnormal microtubule function (Lohmann et al. 2013)

(continued)

Table 4.2 (continued)

Gene/chromosome/locus	Genetic details/pathophysiology	Illness/syndrome	Voice pathology	Theory
THAP1 (DYT6) 8p11.21	*DYT6* autosomal dominant mode	*DYT6* dystonia with prominent laryngeal and oromandibular involvement (Groen et al. 2011)	Spasmodic dysphonia	*THAP1* mutations causal for up to 25% of familial cases with generalised dystonia and prominent laryngeal involvement (Bressman et al. 2009)
THAP1 c.71+9C>A within intron 1 of *THAP1*				Risk factor for adult-onset primary dystonia with laryngeal dystonia (Vemula et al. 2014) Genetic screening by *DYT1/4/6* with low diagnostic yield in patients with spasmodic dysphonia (de Gusmão et al. 2016), clinical subtyping seems to be necessary
MATR3 5q31	Expressed in skeletal muscle, codes for nuclear matrix protein matrin 3 (Senderek et al. 2009)	Adult-onset, progressive autosomal dominant distal myopathy	Frequently associated with dysphonia (and dysphagia)	Genetic myopathy involves vocal muscles
ATXN7 3p12–21.1	Expanded cytosine-adenine-guanine (CAG) trinucleotide repeat	Spinocerebellar ataxia type 7 (SCA7)	Dysarthrophonia	Voice impairment possibly a result of extra-cerebellar manifestations of the disease with perturbation of the central nervous system leading to changes in laryngeal muscle tone (Gómez-Coello et al. 2017)
No specific genetic associations confirmed in tremor	Several areas (loci) on particular chromosomes were studied, in most families autosomal dominant pattern	Essential tremor, head tremor (Louis and Michalec 2014)	Voice tremor	Increased sensitivity in patients with head tremor and voice tremor (Louis and Michalec 2014)

4.9.3 Genetic Perspectives in Diagnostics and Treatment of Voice Disorders

Some examples are presented in Table 4.3.

4.9.4 Interindividual Tolerance of Drugs and Personalised Medicine/Genomic Medicine

Interindividual tolerance of drugs, including the likelihood of toxicity, may have a genetic background (Sattler et al. 2008; Abuzeid et al. 2011). In personalised medicine genetic information allows an adaptation of treatment (e.g. kind of drug, dose) to the individual preconditions of the patient's body (Pedersen and Eeg 2012). Genomic medicine offers a variety of options in diagnosis, prognosis, risk factor management and treatment.

Modern sequencing platforms, microarrays, high-throughput detection technologies, gene transcript profiling, quantitative multiplexed proteomics (indexing all proteins of the human organism and decoding their function), computational

Table 4.3 Genetic perspectives in diagnostics and treatment of voice disorders

Illness	Method	Approach
Defective tissue/scar/atrophy		
Oral mucosa	Tissue engineering	Biomaterial composed of chitosan (a polysaccharide) and fish scale collagen was developed that allows cell attachment and cell growth from underlying host tissue (Terada et al. 2012)
Vocal fold mucosa	Tissue engineering *Implantation of a regeneration scaffold*	Cells and necessary regulators come from surrounding tissue (Hirano 2011)
	Tissue engineering *Extracellular matrix preparations*	Stem cells implanted in atelocollagen sheets produce fibronectin (Hirano 2011)
	Tissue engineering *Cell transplantation* (carcinogenic risk concerning stem cells, Gugatschka et al. 2012)	Autologous bone marrow-derived mesenchymal (stromal) stem cells (BM-MSC)/adipose tissue-derived mesenchymal (stromal) stem cells (AT-MSC) (Hirano 2011) Wound healing profile of vocal fold fibroblasts more similar to BM-MSC, osteogenic capacity low in vibrated and scaffold condition (Bartlett et al. 2015)
	Tissue engineering *Growth factor treatment*	Hepatocyte growth factor in scars (HGF)/basic fibroblast growth factor (bFGF) in atrophy (Hirano 2011)
	Tissue engineering *Vibratory stimulation*	Vibratory stimulation of fibroblasts produces gene expression and synthesis of extracellular matrix reducing scar formation (Kutty and Webb 2010) By vibration secretion of profibrotic cytokine, TGFβ1 is induced which increases extracellular matrix proteins fibronectin and collagen type 1; stiffness is enhanced (Wolchok et al. 2009)
	Tissue engineering *Small interfering RNA*	Smad3 (protein interfering wound healing) siRNA decreases the fibrotic fibroblast phenotype in vitro (Paul et al. 2014)
Cartilage	Polypropylene mesh coated with collagen sponge alone or with embedded BM-derived stromal cells (Yamashita et al. 2007a, b)	Promising results in tracheal defects, not in larynx (Yamashita et al. 2007a, b)
Benign lesions	Fine-needle aspiration (FNA) biopsy for molecular testing of benign vocal fold lesions	FNA samples provide sufficient RNA material to generate transcript data (Li et al. 2013)
Cancer	*Cytoreductive therapy*	Inducing death of cancer cell
	Corrective therapy	Repairing genetic defects underlying malignancy
	Immune modulation	Promoting immune response against cancer (Sattler et al. 2008; Abuzeid et al. 2011)

simulations, gene knockouts, animal studies on drug effects, virtual patient models and establishing databases may be useful tools in developing strategies in personalised treatment of voice disorders (Auffray et al. 2010; Akama et al. 2011; Vodovotz et al. 2010).

Individual metabolism of food products should also be taken into account.

An example for the need of immunogenetics is the growing number of diseases associated with human leukocyte antigen (HLA) (Charron 2011).

4.9.5 Outlook

There is a need for enhanced genetic understanding of voice. This understanding must be documented with randomised controlled trials. A great challenge for evidence-based research lies ahead.

Acknowledgements Bilal Hussain Akram, Mohammad Shezad Mahmood and Manuel Pais Clemente are thanked for the idea for this overview of genetic knowledge related to phoniatrics.

4.10 Symptomatic Profile: Pathophysiology of Phonation

Dirk Mürbe and Willy Mattheus

4.10.1 Introduction

Voice disorders are defined by a disturbance in the sound of the voice, vocal fatigue from increased effort required during voice production or sensations of laryngeal discomfort. In most cases, there is no clear relationship between a specific voice disorder and one specific symptom. Further, almost every voice disorder is associated with more than one symptom.

It is not possible to assess the complex pathophysiology of phonation by technical devices. Thus, it is necessary to investigate the parameters that determine this process individually and evaluate their impact on the sound of the voice. This assessment needs to be referred to healthy voices and the underlying basic principle that air from the lungs is used to generate sound by means of aerodynamic forces that induce vibration of the two human vocal folds. The entire process of sound generation in human phonation is influenced by a complex anatomical system, which is permanently modified and adjusted. From these insights into the function of this combined 'string-wind-instrument' (Titze 2009), many parameters of the complete system of voice production have been analysed and evaluated for their influence on adequate assessment of the voice (see Sect. 4.3).

Hoarseness is a major aspect of disturbance to the sound of the voice, characterised by noticeable noise components. Commonly, the terms roughness and breathiness are used to describe the two main categories contributing to the assessment of hoarseness. In principle, irregularities of vocal fold vibration patterns cause roughness in the voice source signal, originating directly from the compression and rarefaction of air at the air-tissue border of the vocal folds' surface. In contrast, noisy voice sounds that are perceived as breathy are caused by a higher degree of vortical airflow or turbulence, e.g. due to glottal closure insufficiency, supraglottal or pharyngeal constrictions. It is obvious that the causes of roughness and breathiness in the voice signal cannot be clearly separated into independent issues because they influence each other. Therefore, in the following, some of the major parameters that drive the process of flow-induced vibration of the vocal folds are analysed with regard to distorted voices.

4.10.2 Subglottal Pressure

A minimum subglottal pressure and a time-varying component of physical interaction forces between airflow and vocal folds are required to start 'resonant' oscillation of the vocal folds. The higher the subglottal pressure the louder the source signal. This is appropriate for a 'resonant' oscillation of the vocal folds. As the subglottal pressure represents the energy potential that can be used to drive the oscillation process, it is plausible that more of it generates stronger oscillations and therewith sound waves of higher amplitude. An upper threshold of the subglottal pressure for 'resonant oscillation' is given by the effect of 'overblowing' of the vocal folds. In this case the amplitudes of oscillation get weaker, owing to high subglottal pressure, and the vocal folds are no longer able to close completely within one oscillation period. The flowrate of the air passing the glottal gap increases and flow-induced noisy components are added to the source signal (Sundberg et al. 2013). On the other hand, the lowest subglottal pressure needed for obtaining and sustaining vocal fold oscillation (the phonation threshold pressure) has been found to be useful in the assessment of disturbed voices, since it increases in cases of vocal fatigue or vocal fold swelling, e.g. following extensive vocal load (Enflo et al. 2013; Halpern et al. 2009).

The influence of a subglottal stenosis on the phonation process plays only a minor role or is indirect (Oren et al. 2009). Since the air flowrate in the trachea during phonation is much smaller than that during breathing, the aerodynamic resistance of the stenosis during phonation is very low compared with the resistance of the vocal folds. During breathing this relation is reversed and so the limited breathing function may have an impact on the ability to phonate.

4.10.3 Asymmetries of Distribution of Mass, Shape and Tension of the Vocal Folds

The excitation of the vibration of the vocal folds is sensitive to the transglottal airflow that exerts pressure forces onto the vocal folds. These forces would be the same for both vocal folds if the flow field in the glottal gap were uniformly distributed

and the two vocal folds were identical. This is not the case because vocal folds differ in distribution of mass, shape and tension. Consequently, the transglottal airflow is non-uniform, exerting non-uniform pressure onto the vocal folds. However, this non-uniformity does not necessarily mean that the generated sound and the resulting voice signal are disordered. As mentioned above a time dependence is necessary to start the process of oscillation and sound generation. The effect of any asymmetries on the voice signal and the differentiation between normal and disturbed sound is not yet clearly understood and is the object of ongoing research (Howe and McGowan 2013; Mittal et al. 2013; Erath et al. 2013). Basically, the ability of the sound generation system to produce a 'healthy' voice signal is dependent on the combination and interaction of all parameters, and there is not one parameter that has to fit into a certain range. This also implies that there are limitations to measuring or quantifying one parameter isolated from others.

Asymmetries of distribution of mass, shape and tension of the vocal folds are frequent causes of many voice disorders, both for organic and functional reasons. Thus, structural or functional larynx asymmetry leads to characteristic conditions of vocal pathophysiology:

- The asymmetrical shape of the vocal folds causes asymmetrical pressure forces of the flow field acting onto the vocal folds' surfaces. This results in asymmetrical counteracting forces of the vocal folds. All in all it is crucial that this coupled system is able to sustain oscillations.
- The excitation is also sensitive to the physical (material) parameters of the vocal folds because tension, elasticity and distribution of mass are responsible for the back-reaction forces of the vocal folds onto the airflow. The vibratory system of each vocal fold is often abstracted to a multi-mass-spring-damper model, so that its behaviour can be predicted by a computer model (Yang et al. 2012). Asymmetrical distribution of mass influences the inertia of the vocal folds.

Further, the spatio-temporal pattern of the oscillation has an impact on the supraglottal flow field. The pulsating airflow produces small puffs of air every period of oscillation. The airflow can be subdivided into acoustic fluid motion, which is often modelled as an alternating current (AC) component, and non-acoustic (aerodynamic) fluid motion, often modelled as a direct current (DC) component.

The acoustic flow propagates with the speed of sound through the vocal tract towards the mouth opening. The aerodynamic flow exits the glottal gap as a small jet that is disintegrated within the epilarynx. This disintegration is the source of an aero-acoustically generated sound that is broadband and that contributes to the noisy component of voice. For a system of oscillating vocal folds that are closing completely, this noisy component is relatively small and vanishes in the strong tonal component generated by the oscillating vocal folds. But for incomplete closure of the glottal gap during oscillation, as well as for whispery voice, this noisy component is more dominant.

4.10.4 Supraglottal Shape of the Vocal Tract

The supraglottal part of the vocal tract with ventricular folds, epilarynx tube and the hypopharyngeal area is the most sensitive region to flow-induced noisy sound sources. The airflow that exits the vibrating glottal gap in the form of a pulsating jet contains vortices that are referred to as turbulence, which can cause noisy sound components that are perceived as breathiness (Lighthill 1962; Howe and McGowan 2007). The amount of this noisy sound depends on the amount of airflow that passes the glottal gap as a DC component, e.g. owing to glottal closure insufficiency. Furthermore, it depends to a great extent on the degree of turbulence of this airflow. For instance, a narrow supraglottal passage and an incomplete glottal closure increase the amount of noisy components in the voice signal and thus the perceived breathiness. These noisy components exist in every voice signal, no matter if

healthy or pathological, because transglottal airflow is necessary to generate the vibration of the vocal folds and supraglottal vortical airflow is always present. It is the ratio of the harmonic components of the vibrating vocal folds and the noisy components of the supraglottal airflow that determines the degree of breathiness of the voice signal.

The dominant mechanism of sound generation for a very breathy voice is the same as for a whispery voice, but with differences in the adjustment of the vocal folds. A patient with a pathological breathy voice tries to adjust the vocal folds to achieve a phonation onset, but the airflow passes the glottal gap, and no oscillation or a very weak oscillation is induced. Accordingly, the dominant sound sources are the supraglottal vortical flow structures that interact with the pharyngeal wall.

In case of severe malfunction of vocal fold vibration, complete absence of the vocal folds, e.g. after cordectomy, but also in artistically intended cases, the ventricular folds can act as an oscillator. It seems much more difficult for these anatomical structures to be precisely adjusted for vibration in comparison with the vocal folds. Usually, incomplete closure during vibration is observed and often a very breathy sound is generated. Simultaneously the lung volume is consumed more rapidly and phonation time is decreased.

In summary, the basic pathophysiology of roughness and breathiness in the sound of the voice is schematically illustrated in Fig. 4.9. However, it has to be emphasised that, apart from hoarseness, voice disorders may be characterised by increased vocal effort, vocal fatigue and subsequent limitations in pitch and loudness. Further, commonly raised vocal effort leads to increased strain in speaking, which may be associated with tension in neck muscles and sensations of laryngeal discomfort. Often, the imbalance between vocal demands and individual vocal efficiency results in such secondary neuromuscular symptoms, associated with voice production, which may include the perilaryngeal area and further musculature of the neck, as well as the laryngeal

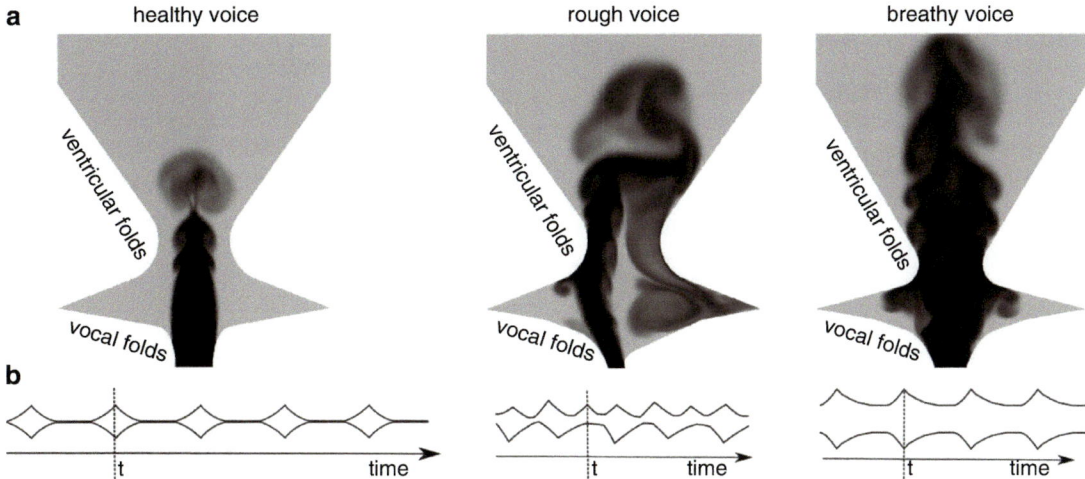

a healthy voice   rough voice   breathy voice

ventricular folds

vocal folds

b

Fig. 4.9 Schematic representation of healthy, rough and breathy voices with characteristic (**a**) supraglottal airflow visualised in a computational model (Mattheus and Brücker 2011) at instant of time *t* and (**b**) contours of the glottal gap visualised by videokymography (VKG) (see Sect. 6.5)

muscles. This underlines once more that our view on the pathophysiology of phonation must not be limited to the glottal area.

References

Abuzeid WM, Li D, O'Malley BW Jr (2011) Gene therapy for head and neck cancer. In: Alford RL, Sutton VR (eds) Medical genetics in the clinical practice of ORL. Karger, Basel, pp 141–151

Adler NR, Mahony A, Friedman ND (2013) Diphtheria: forgotten, but not gone. Intern Med J 43(2):206–210

Akama K, Horikoshi T, Nakayama T et al (2011) Proteomic identification of differentially expressed genes in neural stem cells and neurons differentiated from embryonic stem cells of cynomolgus monkey (*Macaca fascicularis*) in vitro. Biochim Biophys Acta 1814(2):265–276

Akmansu H, Oğuz H, Atasever T et al (2004) Evaluation of sentinel nodes in the assessment of cervical metastases from head and neck squamous cell carcinomas. Tumori 90(6):596–599

Akst LM, Thompson LDR (2003) Larynx amyloidosis. Ear Nose Throat J 82(11):844–845

Altman KW (2007) Vocal fold masses. Otolaryngol Clin North Am 40(5):1091–1108

Andersson-Wallgren G, Ohlsson AC, Albertsson-Wikland K et al (2008) Growth promoting treatment normalizes speech frequency in Turner syndrome. Laryngoscope 118(6):1125–1130

Auffray C, Charron D, Hood L (2010) Predictive, preventive, personalized and participatory medicine: back to the future. Genome Med 2(8):57

Bartels H, Dikkers FG, Lokhorst HM et al (2004) Laryngeal amyloidosis: localized versus systemic disease and update on diagnosis and therapy. Ann Otol Rhinol Laryngol 113(9):741–748

Barth E (1911) Einführung in die Physiologie, Pathologie und Hygiene der menschlichen Stimme. Thieme, Leipzig, p 411

Bartlett RS, Gaston JD, Yen TY et al (2015) Biomechanical screening of cell therapies for vocal fold scar. Tissue Eng Part A 21(17–18):2437–2447. https://doi.org/10.1089/ten.TEA.2015.0168

Behlau M, Zambon F, Guerrieri AC et al (2012) Epidemiology of voice disorders in teachers and non-teachers in Brazil: prevalence and adverse effects. J Voice 26(5):665.e9–665.18

Bhattacharyya N (2014) The prevalence of voice problems among adults in the United States. Laryngoscope 124(10):2359–2362

Boey HP, Cunningham MJ, Weber AL (1995) Central nervous system imaging in the evaluation of children with true vocal cord paralysis. Ann Otol Rhinol Laryngol 104(1):76–77

Böhme G (2004) Sprach-, Sprech-, Stimm- und Schluckstörungen. Urban & Fischer, München, Jena

Boone DR, McFarlane SC (2000) The voice and voice therapy, 6th edn. Pearson Education, Needham Heights, MA

Bressman SB, Raymond D, Fuchs T et al (2009) Mutations in THAP1 (DYT6) in early-onset dystonia: a genetic screening study. Lancet Neurol 8(5):441–446

Carding PN, Roulstone S, Northstone K et al (2006) The prevalence of childhood dysphonia: a cross-sectional study. J Voice 20(4):623–630

Castellanos PF, Spector JG, Kaiser TH (1996) Tumors of the larynx and laryngopharynx. In: Ballenger JC et al (eds) Otorhinolaryngology, 15th edn. Williams & Wilkins, Media, PA

Charron D (2011) HLA, immunogenetics, pharmacogenetics and personalized medicine. Vox Sang 100(1):163–166

Cichocki M, Singer G, Beyerlein S et al (2008) A case of necrotizing enterocolitis associated with adenovirus infection in a term infant with 22q11 deletion syndrome. J Pediatr Surg 43(4):e5–e8

Cohen SM, Turley R (2009) Coprevalence and impact of dysphonia and hearing loss in the elderly. Laryngoscope 119(9):1870–1873

Cohen SR, Geller KA, Birns JW et al (1982) Laryngeal paralysis in children: a long-term retrospective study. Ann Otol Rhinol Laryngol 91(4. Pt 1):417–424

Cohen SM, Kim J, Roy N et al (2012) Prevalence and causes of dysphonia in a large treatment-seeking population. Laryngoscope 122(2):343–348

de Gusmão CM, Fuchs T, Moses A et al (2016) Dystonia-causing mutations as a contribution to the etiology of spasmodic dysphonia. Otolaryngol Head Neck Surg 155(4):624–628

Deary V, Miller T (2011) Reconsidering the role of psychosocial factors in functional dysphonia. Curr Opin Otolaryngol Head Neck Surg 19(3):150–154

Dertlioğlu SB, Çalık M, Çiçek D (2014) Demographic, clinical, and radiologic signs and treatment responses of lipoid proteinosis patients: a 10-case series from Şanlıurfa. Int J Dermatol 53(4):516–523. https://doi.org/10.1111/ijd.12254

Devaney K, Ferlito A, Devaney SL et al (1998) Clinicopathological consultation: Wegener's granulamatosis of the head and neck. Ann Otol Rhinol Laryngol 107(5):439–445

Donaldson JD, Maltby CC (1989) Bacterial tracheitis in children. J Otolaryngol 18(3):101–104

Duff MC, Proctor A, Yairi E et al (2004) Prevalence of voice disorders in African American and European American preschoolers. J Voice 18(3):348–353

Echternach M, Sundberg J, Arndt S et al (2010) Vocal tract in female registers—a dynamic real-time MRI study. J Voice 24(2):133–139

Echternach M, Traser L, Richter B (2012) Perturbation of voice signals in register transitions on sustained frequency in professional tenors. J Voice 26(5):674.e9–674.e15

Echternach M, Dollinger M, Sundberg J et al (2013) Vocal fold vibrations at high soprano fundamental frequencies. J Acoust Soc Am 133(2):EL82–EL87

Echternach M, Birkholz P, Traser L et al (2015) Articulation and vocal tract acoustics at soprano subject's high fundamental frequencies. J Acoust Soc Am 137(5):2586–2595

Enflo L, Sundberg J, McAllister A (2013) Collision and phonation threshold pressures before and after loud, prolonged vocalization in trained and untrained voices. J Voice 27(5):527–530

Erath BD, Zañartu M, Stewart KC et al (2013) A review of lumped-element models of voiced speech. Speech Commun 55(5):667–690

Estes SA (1983) Relapsing polychondritis. A case report and literature review. Cutis 32(5):471–474

Eysholdt U (2014) Heiserkeit—Biomechanik und quantitative Laryngoskopie. HNO 62(7):541–552. https://doi.org/10.1007/s00106-014-2868-7

Ezekowitz RA, Mulliken JB, Folkman J (1992) Interferon alpha-2a therapy for life-threatening hemangiomas of infancy. N Engl J Med 326(22):1456–1463

Falk RT, Pickle LW, Brown LM et al (1989) Effect of smoking and alcohol consumption on laryngeal cancer risk in coastal Texas. Cancer Res 49(14):4024–4029

Fink B, Demarest R (1978) Laryngeal biomechanics. Harvard University Press, Cambridge

Fokstuen S, Bottani A, Medeiros PF et al (1997) Laryngeal atresia type III (glottic web) with 22q11.2 microdeletion: report of three patients. Am J Med Genet 70(2):130–133

Gallivan GJ, Landis JN (1991) Sarcoidosis of the larynx: presenting and restoring airway and professional voice. J Voice 47(1):81–94

Garcia M (1847) Mémoire sur la voix humaine présenté à l'Académie des Sciences en 1840, 2nd edn. Imprimerie d'E Duverger, Paris

Garcia Martins RH, Gonçalvez AM, Benito Pessin AB et al (2014a) Aging voice: presbyphonia. Aging Clin Exp Res 26(1):1–5

Garcia Martins RH, Bóia Neves Pereira ER, Hidalgo CB et al (2014b) Voice disorders in teachers. A review. J Voice 28(6):716–724

Garcia Martins RH, do Amaral HA, Tavares EL et al (2015) Voice disorders: etiology and diagnosis. J Voice 26(1):1–5

Garnier M, Henrich N, Smith J et al (2010) Vocal tract adjustments in the high soprano range. J Acoust Soc Am 127(6):3771–3780

Gómez-Coello A, Valadez-Jiménez VM, Cisneros B et al (2017) Voice alterations in patients with spinocerebellar ataxia type 7 (SCA7): clinical-genetic correlations. J Voice 31(1):123.e1–123.e5. https://doi.org/10.1016/j.jvoice.2016.01.010

Gorelick MH, Baker MD (1994) Epiglottitis in children, 1979 through 1992. Effects of haemophilus influenzae type b immunization. Arch Pediatr Adolesc Med 148(1):47–50

Gottlieb B, Beitel LK, Trifiro MA (2007) Androgen insensitivity syndrome [androgen resistance syndrome, testicular feminization. Includes: complete androgen insensitivity syndrome (CAIS), partial androgen insensitivity syndrome (PAIS), mild androgen insensitivity syndrome (MAIS)]. GeneReviews. https://www.researchgate.net/publication/221964322_Androgen_Insensitivity_Syndrome. Accessed 20 Aug 2016

Greene FL, Page DL, Fleming ID et al (2002) American joint committee on cancer: AJCC cancer staging manual, 6th edn. Springer Verlag, Berlin, pp 47–57

Groen JL, Yildirim E, Ritz K et al (2011) THAP1 mutations are infrequent in spasmodic dysphonia. Mov Disord 26(10):1952–1954. https://doi.org/10.1002/mds.23682. Epub 2011 Apr 29

Gugatschka M, Ohno S, Saxena A et al (2012) Regenerative medicine of the larynx. Where are we today? A review. J Voice 26(5):670.e7–670.13. https://doi.org/10.1016/j.jvoice.2012.03.009

Gundermann H (1970) Die Berufsdysphonie. In: VEB. Thieme, Leipzig

Hacki T (2013) Stimmphysiologie, -pathologie und -therapie. In: Hirschberg J et al (eds) Foniátria és társtudományok. Eötvös Kiadó, Budapest

Hacki T (2014) Eine Überlegung zur ätiologischen Strukturierung von Stimmstörungen: "dysregulative Dysphonie" statt "funktioneller Dysphonie". In: Gross M, Schönweiler R (eds) Aktuelle phoniatrische Aspekte. Medical Science GMS Publishing House, Düsseldorf. ISBN 978-3-00-047098-1

Halpern M, Hurd JL, Zuckerman JD (2009) Occupational shoulder disorders. In: Matsen F et al (eds) Rockwood and Matsen's the shoulder. Saunders Elsevier, Philadelphia, pp 1489–1508

Hartlieb K (1968) Stimm- und Sprachheilkunde aus biokybernetischer Sicht Teil III. Die Korrektur der funktionell gestörten Stimme und Sprache. Folia Phoniatr 20:43–56

Hazenberg AJ, Dikkers FG, Hawkins PN et al (2009) Laryngeal presentation of systemic apolipoprotein A-I-derived amyloidosis. Laryngoscope 119(3):608–615. https://doi.org/10.1002/lary.20106

Henrich N (2006) Mirroring the voice from Garcia to the present day: some insights into singing voice registers. Logoped Phoniatr Vocol 31(1):3–14

Herridge MS, Pearson FG, Downey GP (1996) Subglottic stenosis complicating Wegener's granulamatosis: surgical repair as a viable treatment option. J Thorac Cardiovasc Surg 111(5):961–966

Hill AB (1965) The environment and disease: association or causation? Proc R Soc Med 58(5):295–300

Hirano S (2011) Tissue engineering for voice disorder. JMAJ 54(4):254–257

Hollien H, Dew D, Philips P (1971) Phonational frequency ranges of adults. J Speech Hear Res 14(4):755–760

Howe MS, McGowan RS (2007) Sound generated by aerodynamic sources near a deformable body, with application to voiced speech. J Fluid Mech 592:367–392

Howe MS, McGowan RS (2013) Aerodynamic sound of a body in arbitrary, deformable motion, with application to phonation. J Sound Vib 332(17):3909–3923

Hunt JP, McWhorter AJ (2007) Malignant neoplasms of the larynx. In: Merati AL, Bielamowicz SA (eds) Textbook of laryngology. Plural Publishing, San Diego, CA

Izdebski K (2019) Voice assessment. In: Lalwani A (ed) Current diagnosis & treatment in otolaryngology, head and neck surgery, 4th edn. Lange Publications, New York, NY, pp 416–429

Izdebski K, Manace ED, Skiljo Haris J (2000) The challenge of determining work related voice/speech disabilities in California. In: Dejonckere P (ed) Occupational voice: care and cure. Kugler, The Hague, pp 149–154

Johns MM (2003) Update on the etiology, diagnosis, and treatment of vocal fold nodules, polyps, and cysts. Curr Opin Otolaryngol Head Neck Surg 11(6):456–461

Kılıç MA, Okur E, Yıldırım I et al (2004) The prevalence of vocal fold nodules in school age children. Int J Pediatr Otorhinolaryngol 68(4):409–412

Kiyabu MT, Shibata D, Arnheim N et al (1989) Detection of human papilloma virus in formalin-fixed, invasive squamous cell carcinoma using polymerase chain reaction. Am J Surg Pathol 13(3):221–224

Kollbrunner J, Menet AD, Seifert E (2010) Psychogenic aphonia: no fixation even after a lengthy period of aphonia. Swiss Med Wkly 140(1–2):12–17

Koufman J, Blalock PD (1982) Classification and approach to patients with functional voice disorders. Ann Otol Rhinol Laryngol 91(4 Pt 1):372–377

Kumar P (2004) Radiation therapy in larynx and hypopharynx. In: Cummings CW et al (eds) Otolaryngology head and neck surgery. Elsevier Mosby, pp 2401–2409

Kutty JK, Webb K (2010) Vibration stimulates vocal mucosa-like matrix expression by hydrogel-encapsulated fibroblasts. J Tissue Eng Regen Med 4(1):62–72

Laver J (1980) Phonetic description of voice quality. Cambridge University Press, Cambridge

Li NY, Dailey S, Thibeault SL (2013) Assessment of fine needle aspiration feasibility and specimen adequacy for molecular diagnostics of benign vocal fold lesions. Laryngoscope 123(4):960–965. https://doi.org/10.1002/lary.23703. Epub 2013 Feb 12

Lighthill MJ (1962) Sound generated aerodynamically. Proc R Soc Lond Ser A 267(1329):147–182

Lindstrom DR, Wallace J, Loehrl TA et al (2002) Nissen fundoplication surgery for extraesophageal reflux (EER). Laryngoscope 112(10):1762–1765

Lisak RP, Truong DD, Carroll WM et al (2007) International neurology. A clinical approach. Wiley-Blackwell, Hoboken, NJ, p 168

Lohmann K, Wilcox RA, Winkler S et al (2013) Whispering dysphonia (DYT4 dystonia) is caused by a mutation in the TUBB4 gene. Ann Neurol 73(4):537–545. https://doi.org/10.1002/ana.23829. Epub 2013 Apr 17

Louis ED, Michalec M (2014) Validity of a screening question for head tremor: an analysis of four essential tremor case samples. Neuroepidemiology 43(1):65–70. https://doi.org/10.1159/000365991. Epub 2014 Oct 16

Marino J, Johns M III (2014) The epidemiology of dysphonia in the aging population. Curr Opin Otolaryngol Head Neck Surg 22(6):455–459

Mathieson L (2001) The Voice & Its Disorders, 6th edn. Whurr Publishers, London

Mattheus W, Brücker C (2011) Asymmetric glottal jet deflection: differences of two- and three-dimensional models. J Acoust Soc Am 130(6):EL373–EL379

Mayou R, Farmer A (2002) ABC of psychological medicine: functional somatic symptoms and syndromes. BMJ 325(7358):265–268

Milczuk HA, Smith JD, Everts EC (2000) Congenital laryngeal webs: surgical management and clinical embryology. Int J Pediatr Otorhinolaryngol 52(1):1–9

Miller DG (2000) Registers in singing: empirical and systematic studies in the theory of the singing voice. Ponsen & Looijen BV, Wageningen

Misono S, Peterson CB, Meredith L et al (2014) Psychosocial distress in patients presenting with voice concerns. J Voice 28(6):753–761

Mittal R, Erath BD, Plesniak MW (2013) Fluid dynamics of human phonation and speech. Annu Rev Fluid Mech 45(1):437–467

Morabia A (2004) A history of epidemiologic methods and concepts. Part I. Birkhauser Verlag, Basel

Mörner M, Fransson F, Fant G (1963) Voice register terminology and standard pitch. STL-QPSR 4(4):17–23

Morrison MD, Rammage LA (1993) Muscle misuse disorders: description and classification. Acta Otolaryngol 113(3):428–434

Mysiorek D, Persky M (1989) Laser endoscopic treatment of laryngocele and laryngeal cysts. Otolaryngol Head Neck Surg 100(6):538–541

Nanke Y, Kotake S, Yonemoto K et al (2001) Cricoarytenoid arthritis with rheumatoid arthritis and systemic lupus erythematosus. J Rheumatol 28(3):624–626

Oğuz H, Akbulut S (2013) Ses Bozukluklarında Tedavi Seçimi Türkiye Klinikleri. J ENT Spec Topics 6(2):1–9

Oğuz H, Tarhan E, Korkmaz M et al (2007) Acoustic analysis findings in objective laryngopharyngeal reflux patients. J Voice 21(2):203–210

Oren L, Khosla S, Murugappan S et al (2009) Role of subglottal shape in turbulence reduction. Ann Otol Rhinol Laryngol 118(3):232–240

Pahn J, Friemert K (1988) Differentialdiagnostische und terminologische Erwägungen bei sogenannten funktionellen Störungen im neuropsychiatrischen und phoniatrischen Fachgebiet. 2. Phoniatrischer Aspekt. Folia Phoniatr 40:168–174

Paul BC, Rafii BY, Gandonu S et al (2014) Smad3: an emerging target for vocal fold fibrosis. Laryngoscope 124(10):2327–2331. https://doi.org/10.1002/lary.24723. Epub 2014 May 27

Pedersen M, Eeg M (2012) Does treatment of the laryngeal mucosa reduce dystonic symptoms? A prospective clinical cohort study of mannose binding lectin and other immunological parameters with diagnostic use of phonatory function studies. Eur Arch Otorhinolaryngol 269(5):1477–1482

Pospiech L, Kuzniar J, Roskowka-Nadolska B et al (1996) Influence of vapours of paint and toxic dusts on mucous membranes of the upper airways in paint and varnish factory workers. Med Pr 47(5):445–453

Preciado J, Pérez C, Calzada M et al (2005) Incidencia y prevalencia de los trastornos de la voz en el personal docente de La Rioja Estudio clínico: cuestionario, examen de la función vocal, análisis acústico y vídeo-olaringoestroboscopia. (Prevalence and incidence studies of voice disorders among teaching staff of La Rioja, Spain. Clinical study: questionnaire, function vocal examination, acoustic analysis and videolaryngostroboscopy). Acta Otorrinolaringol Esp 56(5):202–210

Reder PA, Neel HB (1993) Blastomycosis in otolaryngology: review of a large series. Laryngoscope 103(1 Pt 1):53–58

Roger G, Denoyelle F, Triglia JM et al (1995) Severe laryngomalacia: surgical indications and results in 115 patients. Laryngoscope 105(10):1111–1117

Rousseau B, Abdollahian D, Ohno T et al (2009) Effects of raised phonation on vocal fold gene expression. Otolaryngol Head Neck Surg 141(3):P64–P64

Roy N (2003) Functional dysphonia. Curr Opin Otolaryngol Head Neck Surg 11(3):144–148

Roy N, Merrill RM, Thibeault S et al (2004) Voice disorders in teachers and the general population: effects on work performance, attendance and future career choices. J Speech Lang Hear Res 47(3):542–551

Roy N, Merrill RM, Gray SD et al (2005) Voice disorders in the general population: prevalence, risk factors, and occupational impact. Laryngoscope 115(11):1988–1995

Roy N, Stemple J, Merrill RM et al (2007) Epidemiology of voice disorders in the elderly: preliminary findings. Laryngoscope 117(4):628–633

Samuels TL, Handler E, Syring ML et al (2008) Mucin gene expression in human laryngeal epithelia: effect of laryngopharyngeal reflux. Ann Otol Rhinol Laryngol 117(9):688–695

Sataloff RT (1995) Genetics of the voice. J Voice 9(1):16–19

Sataloff RT, Willborn A, Prestipino A et al (1993) Histoplasmosis of the larynx. Am J Otolaryngol 14(3):199–205

Sattler M, Abidoye O, Salgia R (2008) EGFR-targeted therapeutics: focus on SCCHN and NSCLC. ScientificWorldJournal 8:909–919

Schultz P (2011) Vocal fold cancer. Eur Ann Otorhinolaryngol Head Neck Dis 128(6):301–308

Schultz-Coulon HJ (1980) Die Diagnostik der gestörten Stimmfunktion. Arch Otorhinolaryngol 227:1–169

Senderek J, Garvey SM, Krieger M et al (2009) Autosomal-dominant distal myopathy associated with a recurrent missense mutation in the gene encoding the nuclear matrix protein, matrin 3. Am J Hum Genet 84(4):511–518

Shah RK, Roberson DW, Jones DT (2004) Epiglottitis in the *Hemophilus influenza type B* vaccine era: changing trends. Laryngoscope 114(3):557–560

Shen Z, Ye D, Zhang X et al (2010) Inhibitory effect of HuR gene small interfering RNA segment on laryngeal carcinoma Hep-2 cell growth. J Laryngol Otol 124(11):1183–1189

Shin JE, Nam SY, Yoo SY et al (2000) Changing trends in clinical manifestations of laryngeal tuberculosis. Laryngoscope 110(11):1950–1953

Shipp T, Izdebski K (1975) Vocal frequency and vertical larynx positioning in singers and non-singers. J Acoust Soc Am 58(5):1104–1106

Sie KC, McGill T, Healy GB (1994) Subglottic hemangioma: ten years' experience with the carbon dioxide laser. Ann Otol Rhinol Laryngol 103(3): 167–172

Sinard RJ, Netterville JL, Ossoff RH (2003) Squamous cell cancer of the larynx. In: Ossoff RH et al (eds) The larynx. Lippincott Williams & Wilkins, Philadelphia, PA

Sliwinska-Kowalska M, Niebudek-Bogusz E, Fiszer M et al (2006) The prevalence and risk factors for occupational voice disorders in teachers. Folia Phoniatr Logop 58(2):85–101

Solomons NB, Prescott CA (1987) Laryngomalacia. A review and the surgical management. Int J Pediatr Otorhinolaryngol 13(1):31–39

Sonninen A (1968) The external frame function in the control of pitch in the human voice. In: Bouhuys A (ed) Sound production in man. Ann N Y Acad Sci 155(1):68–90

Sonninen A, Hurme P, Laukkanen AM (1999) The external frame function in the control of pitch, register and singing mode: radiographic observations of a female singer. J Voice 13(3):319–340

Stein DJ, Nordzij JP (2013) Incidence of chronic laryngitis. Ann Otol Rhinol Laryngol 122(12):771–774

Stemple JC (1993) Voice therapy clinical studies. Mosby, St. Louis, MO

Stern H (1924) Klinik und Therapie der Krankheiten der Stimme. Mschr Ohrenheilk 58:1–53

Stroud RH, Friedman NR (2001) An update on inflammatory disorders of the pediatric airway: epiglottis, croup, and tracheitis. Am J Otolaryngol 22(4):268–275

Sulica L (2005) Laryngeal thrush. Ann Otol Rhinol Laryngol 114(5):369–375

Sundberg J (1975) Formant technique in a professional female singer. Acust 32(2):89–96

Sundberg J, Thalen M, Popeil L (2012) Substyles of belting: phonatory and resonatory characteristics. J Voice 26(1):44–50

Sundberg J, Scherer R, Hess M et al (2013) Subglottal pressure oscillations accompanying phonation. J Voice 27(4):411–421

Svec JG, Sundberg J, Hertegard S (2008) Three registers in an untrained female singer analyzed by videokymography, strobolaryngoscopy and sound spectrography. J Acoust Soc Am 123(1):347–353

Tanner K, Sauder C, Thibeault SL et al (2010) Vocal fold bowing in elderly male monozygotic twins: a case study. J Voice 24(4):470–476

Teitel AD, MacKenzie CR, Stern R et al (1992) Laryngeal involvement in systemic lupus erythematosus. Semin Arthritis Rheum 22(3):203–214

Terada M, Izumi K, Ohnuki H et al (2012) Construction and characterization of a tissue-engineered oral mucosa equivalent based on a chitosan-fish scale collagen composite. J Biomed Mater Res B Appl Biomater 100(7):1792–1802

The ASHA Leader Blog (2015) The problem of limited health care coverage voice disorder treatment. Podcast: Episode 33. https://blog.asha.org/2015/11/04/limited-health-care-coverage-for-treatment-of-voice-disorders/ Accessed 29 Jan 2018

Thompson DM, Kershner JE (2007) Pediatric laryngology. In: Merati AL, Bielamowicz SA (eds) Textbook of laryngology. Plural Publishing, San Diego, CA

Titze IR (1994) Principles of voice production. Prentice-Hall, Englewood Cliffs, NJ

Titze IR (2009) Das Saitenblasinstrument Spektrum der Wissenschaft, vol 2, pp 54–60

Titze IR, Verdolini Abbott K (2012) Vocology—the science and practice of voice habilitation. National Center for Voice and Speech, Salt Lake City

Vaca M, Mora E, Cobeta I (2015) The aging voice: influence of respiratory and laryngeal changes. Otolaryngol Head Neck Surg 153(3):409–413

Vago B, Hausser I, Hennies HC et al (2007) Hyalinosis cutis et mucosae. J Dtsch Dermatol Ges 5(5):401–405

Van Borsel J (2004) Voice and resonance disorders in genetic syndromes: a meta-analysis. Folia Phoniatr Logop 56(2):83–92

Van Houtte E, Van Lierde K, D'Haeseleer E et al (2010) The prevalence of laryngeal pathology in a treatment-seeking population with dysphonia. Laryngoscope 120(2):306–312

Vemula SR, Xiao J, Zhao Y et al (2014) A rare sequence variant in intron 1 of THAP1 is associated with primary dystonia. Mol Genet Genomic Med 2(3):261–272. https://doi.org/10.1002/mgg3.67. Epub 2014 Feb 11

Verdolini K, Ramig LO (2001) Review: occupational risks for voice problems. Logoped Phoniatr Vocol 26(1):37–46

Verduyckt I, Remacle M, Jamart J et al (2011) Voice-related complaints in the pediatric population. J Voice 25(3):373–380

Vilkman E, Karma P (1989) Vertical hyoid bone displacement and fundamental frequency of phonation. Acta Otolaryngol 108(1–2):142–151

Vilkman E, Sonninen A, Hurme P et al (1996) External laryngeal frame function in voice production revisited: a review. J Voice 10(1):78–92

Villanueva-Reyes A (2011) Voice disorders in the metropolitan area of San Juan, Puerto Rico: profiles of occupational groups. J Voice 25(1):83–87

Vodovotz Y, Constantine G, Faeder J et al (2010) Translational systems approaches to the biology of inflammation and healing. Immunopharmacol Immunotoxicol 32(2):181–195

Watts CR, Awan SN, Marler JA (2008) An investigation of voice quality in individuals with inherited elastin gene abnormalities. Clin Linguist Phon 22(3):199–213

Watts CR, Knutsen RH, Ciliberto C et al (2011) Evidence for heterozygous abnormalities of the elastin gene (ELN) affecting the quantity of vocal fold elastic fibers: a pilot study. J Voice 25(2):e85–e90

Weiss DA (1934) Der Begriff des Funktionellen mit besonderer Berücksichtigung der Sprach- und Stimmheilkunde. Mschr Ohrenheilk 68:830–832

Wendler J, Seidner W (1987) Lehrbuch der Phoniatrie, 2nd edn. VEB Georg Thieme, Leipzig

Wendler J, Fischer S, Seidner W et al (1985) *Stroboglottometric* and acoustic measures of natural vocal registers. In: Askenfelt A et al (eds) Proceedings of the Stockholm Music Acoustics Conference 1983 (SMAC 83) 46(1): 261–268. Royal Swedish Academy of Music, Stockholm

Wendler J, Dejonckere PH, Wienhausen S et al (2014) Therapeutic consequences from changing voice ideals (clear to harsh, pleasant to jarring): summarizing report on a round-table discussion at the 5th World Voice Congress, Luxor, Egypt, 27-31 October 2012. Logoped Phoniatr Vocol 39(4):188–190

Wolchok JC, Brokopp C, Underwood CJ et al (2009) The effect of bioreactor induced vibrational stimulation on extracellular matrix production from human derived fibroblasts. Biomaterials 30(3):327–335

Woo P, Mendelsohn J, Humphrey D (1995) Rheumatoid nodules of the larynx. Ear Nose Throat J 113(1):147–150

Woodson GE (2003) Laryngitis. In: Ossoff RH et al (eds) The larynx. Lippincott Williams & Wilkins, Philadelphia, PA

World Health Organization (2001) International classification of functioning, disability and health (ICF). WHO, Geneva

Xu W, Wang L, Zhang L et al (2010) Otolaryngological manifestations and genetic characteristics of lipoid proteinosis. Ann Otol Rhinol Laryngol 119(11): 767–771

Yamashita M, Omori K, Kanemaru S et al (2007a) Experimental regeneration of canine larynx: a trial with tissue engineering techniques. Acta Otolaryngol 127(Suppl 557):66–72

Yamashita M, Kanemaru S, Hirano S et al (2007b) Tracheal regeneration after partial resection: a tissue engineering approach. Laryngoscope 117(3): 497–502

Yang A, Berry DA, Kaltenbacher M et al (2012) Three-dimensional biomechanical properties of human vocal folds: parameter optimization of a numerical model to match in vitro dynamics. J Acoust Soc Am 131(2):1378–1390

Zenker W, Glaninger J (1959) Die Stärke des Trachealzuges beim lebenden Menschen und seine Bedeutung für die Kehlkopfmechanik. Ztschr Biol 111: 155–164

Zenker W, Zenker A (1960) Über die Regelung der Stimmlippenspannung durch von außen eingreifende Mechanismen. Folia Phoniatr (Basel) 12(1): 1–36

Special Kinds and Clinical Manifestation of Voice Disorders

5

Antoinette am Zehnhoff-Dinnesen,
Sevtap Akbulut, Eugenia Chávez Calderón,
Muhittin Demir, Dirk Deuster, Michael Fuchs,
Ahmed Geneid, Thomas Murry,
Tadeus Nawka, Christiane Neuschaefer-Rube,
Ewa Niebudek-Bogusz, Andrzej Obrębowski,
Haldun Oguz, Arno Olthoff,
Anders Overgård Jønsson,
Mette Pedersen, Bernhard Richter,
John Rubin, Berit Schneider-Stickler,
Kevin Shields, Mariola Śliwińska-Kowalska,
Bożena Wiskirska-Woźnica, Virginie Woisard,
and Waldemar Wojnowski

Electronic Supplementary Material The online version
of this chapter (https://doi.org/10.1007/978-3-662-46780-
0_5) contains supplementary material, which is available
to authorized users.

A. am Zehnhoff-Dinnesen · D. Deuster
Clinic of Phoniatrics and Pedaudiology,
University Hospital Münster, Münster, Germany
e-mail: am.zehnhoff@uni-muenster.de;
deusted@uni-muenster.de

S. Akbulut
Department of Otolaryngology, Yeditepe University,
Istanbul, Turkey

E. Chávez Calderón
Centro de Foniatría y Audiología,
Mexico City, Mexico

M. Demir
Section of Phoniatrics and Audiology,
ENT Clinic, University Hospital Essen,
Essen, Germany
e-mail: Muhittin.Demir@uk-essen.de

M. Fuchs
Section of Phoniatrics and Audiology,
University of Leipzig, Leipzig, Germany
e-mail: Michael.Fuchs@medizin.uni-leipzig.de

A. Geneid
Department of Otolaryngology and Phoniatrics –
Head and Neck Surgery, Helsinki University Central
Hospital, Helsinki, Finland
e-mail: Ahmed.Geneid@hus.fi

T. Murry
Department of Otolaryngology-Head and Neck
Surgery, Loma Linda Voice and Swallowing Center,
Loma Linda Medical University,
Loma Linda, CA, USA
e-mail: tmurry@llu.edu

T. Nawka
Department of Audiology and Phoniatrics,
Charité—University Medicine Berlin, Berlin, Germany
e-mail: tadeus.nawka@charite.de

C. Neuschaefer-Rube
Clinic of Phoniatrics, Pedaudiology and
Communication Disorders, School of Medicine of the
RWTH Aachen University, University Hospital
Aachen, Aachen, Germany
e-mail: cneuschaefer@ukaachen.de

E. Niebudek-Bogusz · M. Śliwińska-Kowalska
Department of Audiology and Phoniatrics,
Nofer Institute of Occupational Medicine,
Łódź, Poland
e-mail: Ewa.Bogusz@imp.lodz.pl; marsliw@imp.lodz.pl

A. Obrębowski · B. Wiskirska-Woznica
W. Wojnowski
Department of Phoniatrics and Audiology, Poznan
University of Medical Sciences, Poznan, Poland
e-mail: aobrebow@ump.edu.pl

H. Oguz
Fonomer, Ankara, Turkey

A. Olthoff
Department of Otorhinolaryngology, Phoniatrics and
Pedaudiology, University Medical Center Göttingen,
Göttingen, Germany
e-mail: olthoff@med.uni-goettingen.de

A. Overgård Jønsson
University of Copenhagen, Copenhagen, Denmark
e-mail: hbk777@alumni.ku.dk

M. Pedersen
Voice Unit, The Medical Center,
Copenhagen, Denmark
e-mail: m.f.pedersen@dadlnet.dk

B. Richter
Freiburger Institut für Musikermedizin,
Hochschule für Musik und Universitätsklinikum
Freiburg, Freiburg, Germany
e-mail: Bernhard.Richter@uniklinik-freiburg.de

J. Rubin
University College London, London, UK
e-mail: mail@johnrubin.co.uk

B. Schneider-Stickler
Division of Phoniatrics-Logopedics, Department of
Otorhinolaryngology, Medical University Vienna,
Wien, Austria
e-mail: berit.schneider-stickler@meduniwien.ac.at

K. Shields
National Hospital for Neurology and Neurosurgery,
London, UK
e-mail: kevin.shields@uclh.nhs.uk

V. Woisard
Voice and Deglutition Unit, ENT Department,
Toulouse University Hospital, Toulouse, France
e-mail: Woisard.v@chu-toulouse.fr

5.1 Functional Voice Disorders

Berit Schneider-Stickler

5.1.1 Definition

Functional dysphonia is by definition characterised as disturbance of the voice sound (mostly hoarseness), a limited vocal endurance of the voice and several abnormal sensations (i.e. globus sensation, dryness, feelings of laryngeal discomfort). In contrast to organic dysphonia, functional dysphonia is a voice disorder without any structural or neurological laryngeal pathology and with no organic alterations being detectable (Wendler et al. 1973; Roy 2003). The term 'functional' implies a voice problem due to pathophysiological malfunction rather than morphological alteration of the laryngeal structures.

The terms 'organic' and 'functional' define opposite diagnoses; nevertheless, organic lesions of laryngeal structures can lead to secondary functional voice problems and functional voice disorders to secondary organic lesions.

Functional voice disorders usually occur in voice users. People who do not have any verbal communication requirements usually do not complain about voice malfunction. Vocal abuse and overuse are the most important factors for phonotrauma and the development of first functional voice disorders, and subsequent phonation-associated ('secondary organic') vocal fold alterations.

5.1.2 Terminology

For a long time, the term 'functional dysphonia' has been used for psychogenic voice problems. Even patients still associate 'functional problem' with psychogenic impairment. The number of patients with functional voice disorders seems to be increasing, owing to societal changes, increase of verbal communication tasks and the increased level of stress. Negative stress impact and insufficient stress-coping strategies seem to be high risk factors in developing psychosomatic symptoms and non-organic disorders; these symptoms can also affect voice use. Stress, negative emotions and psychological conflicts might influence the mechanism of phonation with inappropriate subglottal pressure, loudness and fundamental frequency.

The literature shows a quite confusing variety of synonymous expressions for functional dysphonia (Roy 2003; Morrison et al. 1983; Morrison and Rammage 1993; Koufman and Blalock 1982, 1988) (see Sects. 4.1 and 4.2): psychogenic, conversion, hysterical, tension-fatigue syndrome, hyperfunctional, muscle misuse, malregulative and muscle tension dysphonia.

5.1.3 Aetiology of Functional Dysphonia

The main categories of the aetiology of functional voice disorders are according to Wendler et al. (1973):

- Constitutional
- Habitual
- Ponogenic
- Symptomatic
- Psychogenic

The term *constitution* describes the basic nature of a person. Each individual has an innate, natural physical and mental disposition. Voice can be trained to a certain degree (voice condition) as can any other muscle system. Each individual has physical limits. Concerning voice use, all people have different vocal power and endurance limits. It was shown by Schneider et al. (2006) that people with weak vocal constitution (constitutional vocal hypofunction) are at risk of developing occupational voice disorders if vocal demands exceed the vocal capacities.

A constitutionally weak voice (vocal hypofunction) can be defined as a voice with reduced ability to increase vocal intensity; in voice range profile measurements, the maximum sound pressure for shouting and loud singing does not reach values higher than 90 dB(A).

Habitual voice use means behaving in a regular manner (habit). Vocally healthy habits will seldom lead to functional voice problems, but habitual overuse (i.e. too much) and misuse (i.e. too loud, too fast, pressed) of voice might have an impact on developing a functional dysphonia. In voice diagnostics, the voice use in the family, in the workplace environment as well as in leisure time has to be critically examined. Poor vocal habits are at high risk of developing into voice problems.

Occupational voice use (*ponogenic* factors) with high vocal demands is without doubt of increasing interest in laryngology and phoniatrics (Gundermann 1970). Szabo Portela et al. (2013) showed, by using a voice accumulator, that most test subjects have higher phonation time during work than in leisure time. Interestingly the fundamental frequency was used at higher levels during work time.

Voice disorders affect professional voice users considerably more than non-professional users. The classification of voice use, based on profession by Koufman and Isaacson (1991), has become legendary.

- Level I refers to an 'elite vocal performer' such as singers and actors
- Level II describes a 'professional voice user' such as pedagogists, lecturers and clergy
- Level III patients are 'nonvocal professionals', such as lawyers, doctors
- Level IV users are 'nonvocal non-professionals' without any need for professional voice use

Although this classification is useful as a general categorisation, there is a trend to higher communication requirements in almost all professions. With increasing vocal demands and increasing costs for occupational health and safety, occupational voice users will be increasingly in the focus of voice care programmes.

Symptomatic cofactors describe functional voice problems within the scope of a basic general debilitating illness. Patients in general poor health with physical weakness will also tend to have a poor voice quality.

Psychogenic factors can be related to any negative stress-coping strategies and depressive mood situations. They do not include psychiatric disorders, although voice problems can also be a symptom of a psychiatric disease.

5.1.4 Hyperfunctional and Hypofunctional Dysphonia

'Muscle tension dysphonia' has become the preferred diagnostic label to describe functional voice problems, presumably related to dysregulated or imbalanced laryngeal and para-laryngeal muscle activity (Morrison et al. 1983; Morrison and Rammage 1993; Roy et al. 1996).

Glottal and supraglottal contraction patterns are responsible for muscle tension dysphonia/ functional dysphonia. In clinical practice it is common to distinguish between hyper- and hypo-functional dysphonias, depending on whether these functional disorders are based on 'too much' (hyperfunctional) or 'too little' (hypofunctional) muscular tension. Primarily respiratory activity, vocal fold tension, the adjustment of the muscles of the vocal tract and the entire body are affected, and thus, disturbances of balance between subglottal pressure, the myoelastic forces of the glottis and the resonatory features of the vocal tract are usually predominant in the complex of phonatory symptoms.

Several classification systems have been suggested, especially to describe laryngoscopic features (Morrison and Rammage 1994; Morrison 1997; Van Lawrence 1987). Often-cited laryngeal manifestations of dysregulated laryngeal muscle tension include the following: tight mediolateral glottal or supraglottal contraction, anteroposterior glottal or supraglottal compression, incomplete glottal closure, posterior glottal gap and bowing.

However, stroboscopic research has not shown evidence of subtypes of hyperfunctional or hypofunctional dysphonia (Schneider et al. 2002).

5.1.5 Dysodia

Within the group of functional voice disorders, dysodia is the exclusive dysfunction of the singing voice without impairment of the speaking voice. The subtle voice performance is limited, especially when singing high and piano notes. The unexpected or gradual loss of a singing voice, which had functioned well before a certain point, belongs to one of the more frightening and unpleasant experiences singers can confront in the course of their career. Accordingly, any impairment of the singing voice should be diagnosed as early as possible. When confronted with a dysphonia, talented musicians often suffer a crisis of self-confidence, which may propel them towards maladaptive compensations; these may destabilise their usual techniques, already disrupted by the changes in their vocal acoustics (Faure et al. 2010).

5.1.6 Clinical Diagnostics

The clinical diagnosis of a functional voice disorder is commonly made after exclusion of any organic laryngeal pathology. A comprehensive anamnesis might give first directions to functional voice problems being present. The examination of any patient with functional voice complaints should include the examinations recommended by the European Laryngological Society (Dejonckere et al. 2001).

Table 5.1 summarises the more important clinical impressions and diagnostic approaches.

The currently used subclassification into hyper- and hypo-functional dysphonias is often made on the basis of stroboscopy. Stroboscopic parameters of clinical interest are usually maximum amplitude, relative mucosal wave, closed phase, phase differences and symmetry of vibrations.

Arndt and Schäfer (1994) introduced the width-length relationship as a quotient between maximum amplitude and total vocal fold length. They could successfully differentiate healthy voices from functional dysphonias by using this parameter, whereas the comparison of hyper- and

Table 5.1 Comparison of hyper- and hypo-functional dysphonia in clinical diagnostics

	Hyperfunctional dysphonia	Hypofunctional dysphonia
Pathological mechanism	Irregularities of vocal fold vibration due to increased glottal resistance	Glottal closure insufficiency due to decreased glottal resistance
Subjective complaints	Vocal discomfort and voice sound alteration with longer voice use	Rapid vocal exhaustion, loss of voice brilliance
Auditory perceptual voice sound evaluation (GRBAS)	Rough, strained	Breathy, asthenic
General appearance	General muscle hypertension, thoracic breathing pattern, tight articulation pattern, cervical tension	General muscle hypotension, tendency towards shallow breathing
Laryngostroboscopy	Supraglottal hypertension, reduced open phase, reduced maximum amplitudes, long closure phase	Insufficient glottal closure even in loud phonation, enlarged maximum amplitude, long open phase, short closure phase
Voice range profile measurement	Loss of piano function	Loss of forte function

hypo-functional dysphonias by using strobo-scopic parameters revealed no difference (Schneider et al. 2002). Schneider et al. failed to find stroboscopic evidence (correlates) of subtypes of functional dysphonia, and for the diagnostics of functional dysphonias, stroboscopy did not provide high expectations.

Voice range profile measurements can easily differentiate subtypes of functional dysphonias. A hypofunctional dysphonia is usually characterised by a limitation of loud phonation (see Case Study 5.1). These patients can produce very low sound pressure levels in soft speaking and soft singing, but the increase in vocal intensity is reduced, and they mostly reach maximum sound pressure levels of less than 90 dB.

Case Study 5.1

A 46-year-old kindergarten teacher had undergone a viral infection of the upper respiratory tract 1 month before. She took antibiotics and cortisone. Now she has still a weak voice. In her history, there is a period of anorexia that is stable now and symptom-free. During leisure time, she sings in a choir. Video-laryngostroboscopy shows incomplete closure. The vocal range is mildly restricted, voice quality mildly breathy (R0 B1 H1).

In contrast, a hyperfunctional dysphonic patient usually reaches quite loud intensities while loud singing and shouting. With loud phonation, maximum values of sound pressure of more than 90 dB can easily be produced, whereas the ability of soft voice production is disturbed (see Case Study 5.2). Patients can hardly phonate at sound pressure level values lower than 55 dB.

Case Study 5.2

A 27-year-old actor occasionally has problems with his voice after having acted on stage the day before. He is sensitive to cold. His voice range profile shows an elevated curve of the softest tones. He is well able to project his voice. The voice sounds rough (R1 B0 H1).

5.1.7 Management

In general, for therapy of a voice disorder, a clinician usually has to choose between conservative therapy, application of drugs and surgical approaches/phonosurgery. In functional dysphonia phonosurgery is not indicated. The only clinical exception is a severe hyperfunctional dysphonia without response to conservative voice therapy. In this case an indirect laryngeal application of botulinum toxin might be indicated. In extreme muscular hypertension, the application of muscle relaxants or so-called neuromuscular blocking agents can also be discussed. In cases of cervical problems, a pain analgesic medication, orthopaedic therapy or physiotherapy might also be helpful before entering voice therapy.

Functional voice dysphonias are first of all a domain of conservative voice treatment despite the considerable controversial discussion about causal aetiological mechanisms. The literature is replete with evidence that symptomatic voice therapy for functional voice disorders can often result in rapid and dramatic voice improvement (Roy 2003; Roy and Leeper 1993; Ziegler et al. 2014; Moore 2012; Van Houtte et al. 2011; Hazlett et al. 2011; Marszałek et al. 2012; Van Lierde et al. 2010).

Many voice therapies include yawn-sigh, resonant voice therapy, visual and electromyographic biofeedback, progressive muscle relaxation and perilaryngeal massage to reduce or rebalance muscular tension. Manual/digital techniques have been described to determine the presence and degree of laryngeal musculoskeletal tension, as have methods to relieve such tension during the diagnostic assessment and management session.

5.2 Occupational Voice Disorders

Ewa Niebudek-Bogusz and
Mariola Śliwińska-Kowalska

5.2.1 Introduction

In recent decades, voice has assumed an important role in occupational activities. According to some studies, about one-third of the workforce relies on the voice to perform the job (Carding 2007). The increasing role of verbal communication in developing society and the heavy vocal demands associated with particular professions induce the growing risk of occupational voice disorders having a serious impact on working ability (Dejonckere 2001; Vilkman 2004; Niebudek-Bogusz and Sliwinska-Kowalska 2013).

5.2.2 Definition

Occupational voice disorders are work-related self-reported symptoms and clinical signs of dysphonia occurring in subjects whose job demands voice use as a critical aspect of the work.

A job can be classified as vocally demanding with regard to the vocal effort or vocal load needed in specific job activities. According to the Union of the European Phoniatricians recommendation (cited after Obrębowski 2008), the professions should be classified as follows:

- Group I—professions demanding high quality of voice, e.g. singers, actors and other vocal performers
- Group II—professions demanding permanent vocal load, e.g. teachers, interpreters, speakers
- Group III—professions demanding more than average endurance of vocal apparatus because of some voice tasks performed in noisy environment, e.g. lawyers, physicians, clergy, military men

5.2.3 Epidemiology

Data from the United Kingdom show that more than five million workers are routinely affected by voice impairments at an annual cost of approximately £200 million (Carding 2007). It has been suggested that some professional groups, such as teachers, performers and telemarketing staff, are more at risk of developing voice disorders than other voice-demanding professions. Several randomised studies proved that the prevalence of dysphonia is around two to three times higher in teachers than in controls (Roy et al. 2005; Sliwinska-Kowalska et al. 2006). Data from various countries confirm that teaching is an occupation with the greatest risk (de Jong 2010). They indicate that from about 11–38% of the investigated teachers experience current voice problems, but more than 57% of them report at least one occurrence of voice disorders during their life. Additionally, at least one in three teachers claims that teaching has a detrimental effect on his or her voice and they are sometimes even forced to change profession (Roy et al. 2005).

Another emerging group of employees with a high risk of voice disorders is that of call centre industry workers. This group has dramatically grown over the past decade. Approximately 5%

of the workforce in the United States works in call centres, compared with an estimated 2% in the EU. The incidence of voice disorders is expected to grow, owing to the highly demanding vocal load in this professional group and work-related stress factors in call centres (Schneider-Stickler et al. 2012). Raising the retirement age of voice professionals is an additional factor that can contribute to the increasing number of cases of occupation-related dysphonia in some EU countries.

Thus occupational dysphonia can not only affect the quality of life and social well-being of employees but also the economic efficiency of companies.

5.2.4 Aetiology and Risk Factors for Occupational Dysphonia

Occupational voice disorders have a multifactorial aetiology. Conditions at work may affect voice, whereas individual-specific factors may influence the employees' susceptibility to dysphonia.

The factors that can cause occupational voice disorders include the following (see Table 5.2):

- Voice loading: a crucial factor in the development of professional voice problems (see also Sect. 6.8). The load-related changes in the vocal tract are caused by prolonged speaking: at high intensity (more than 70 dB (A)), at a pitch outside the normal range, with improper intonation and abnormal resonance (Niebudek-Bogusz et al. 2006). The study of Remacle et al. (2012) indicated that 2 h of continuous oral reading with intensity 70–75 dB(A) could

be phonotraumatic for normophonic females. It should be stressed that research to establish safety standards concerning the duration and intensity level of loading factors is still in progress (Echternach et al. 2014)
- Environmental factors: dust, pollution, poor humidity and exposure to fluctuations of temperature may affect the condition of the mucosa of the upper respiratory tract. Other important ergonomic factors are background noise and improper acoustic conditions with poor reverberation time, which decrease the Speech Transmission Index (STI). STI expresses speech transmission in space. Poor room acoustics frequently lead to an increase in vocal effort. In order to be heard in deficient acoustic conditions, a speaker involuntarily tries to increase voice intensity; estimated subglottal pressure (ESP) and sound pressure level (SPL) have shown it is kept about 10–15 dB above the environmental noise (the Lombard effect)
- Psycho-emotional factors, which play an important role in handling the demands of a professional voice: voicing with an adverse psycho-emotional attitude increases the prevalence of voice disorders. Many voice professionals with dysphonia have entered a vicious circle: the psychological factors exacerbate voice pathology, and voice disabilities interfere with job satisfaction, performance and attendance, affecting psychological well-being (de Jong 2010)
- Lack of vocal hygiene and incorrect voice production techniques, which may cause pathological compensation of heavy vocal load and in consequence induce muscle tension in the area of the pharynx, larynx and neck, affecting

Table 5.2 Risk factors of occupational voice disorders

Ergonomic factors	Health factors	Personal characteristics
Voice loading	Respiratory tract diseases	Gender (female)
Background noise	Allergy	Family history of voice disorders
Poor acoustics	LPR (Laryngopharyngeal reflux)	Incorrect phonation technique
Indoor air quality:	Mucosal problems	Posture
Humidity	Hormonal disturbances	Smoking
Temperature	Musculoskeletal abnormalities	Personality features
Irritants	Deterioration of general	Physical and mental activity
Work-related stress	physical/mental condition	Ability to cope with stress

body posture and the breathing pathway. Moreover, the lack of coping strategies in occupational stress enhances muscle strain (Koufman 2003; Marszałek et al. 2012)

According to some cross-sectional studies, lifetime vocal load, incorrect techniques of voice production and psychological predispositions constitute the major risk factors for developing occupation-related voice disorders (Sliwinska-Kowalska et al. 2006; Bermudez de Alvear et al. 2010) (see Table 5.2). The individual-specific factors that can contribute to voice disorders are multiple, including frequent infections of the upper respiratory tract, allergies, laryngopharyngeal reflux and hormonal disturbances. Moreover, some studies report a gender predisposition to occupational dysphonia. The glottal cycle dose is much higher in females than in men owing to the nearly doubled fundamental frequency F0. Moreover, the female larynx seems to be more vulnerable (Dejonckere 2001) because of the following physiological differences: (1) being subjected to lifelong hormone-mediated effects, (2) the curving shape of the vocal folds contributing to insufficient glottal closure and to the hourglass-shaped oscillation pattern (characteristic of vocal nodules) and (3) reduced lubrication of the female laryngeal mucosa causing lower levels of hyaluronic acid in mucus secretions, which interferes with vocal fold vibration and decreases resistance to vocal loading. The relation between the above-mentioned factors is complex, and the relative influence of each factor varies among individuals.

5.2.5 Diagnostic Procedures

Adequate management of occupational dysphonia requires (1) proving the relationship between pathologies of the glottis and occupational vocal load; (2) assessing the efficiency of the vocal function—'voice fitness for duty'; (3) determining the prognosis; and (4) monitoring of changes after a recovery period or voice therapy (Calcinoni and Niebudek-Bogusz 2014). Consequently, considering the multidimensional nature of occupational dysphonia, diagnostics of voice should be,

in voice professionals as well as in all patients with impairment of vocal function, multidimensional and include the following:

- The patient's history
- ENT/phoniatric examination
- Perceptual assessment of voice quality (e.g. GRBAS)
- Self-assessment of voice (e.g. Voice Handicap Index)
- Video-laryngostroboscopy—standard in diagnosing voice disorders and imaging of the larynx function
- Objective evaluation of the vocal function via acoustic and aerodynamic measurements, in an attempt to quantify the severity of voice pathology

At this point, the following issues should be emphasised:

- *Occupational History* (see Table 5.3) should be specific and concern the following: the subject's current job, duration of employment (for teachers—the type of school and class, the number of class hours per day and per week as well as the number of students per class) and environmental work conditions (ambient temperature, humidity, dust, pollution, etc.). A more detailed enquiry should concern subjective vocal symptoms appearing over the entire working life, including recurrent or permanent hoarseness, vocal fatigue, loss of voice or aphonia, chronic dryness and the sensation of a 'lump' in the throat or persistent dry cough. Odynophonia—pain caused by using the voice can be a disturbing symptom. The history should also refer to current and past laryngological or phoniatric care (including voice training) and sick leave due to voice disorders. Further questions should be asked about non-occupational risk factors, e.g. smoking or other habits, previous or concomitant ENT and other diseases (including sinusitis, pharyngitis and allergies, bronchitis, reflux disease, thyroid diseases, sexual hormonal imbalances, anaemia, cervical spine problems). Careful questioning as to current medications including antihistamines, diuretic, birth control pills

Table 5.3 Occupational history

Job-related factors	Vocal symptoms	Nonoccupational risk factors
Kind of job, work load	Chronic/recurrent hoarseness	Smoking, alcohol consumption, drugs
Hours of vocal effort per day/week	Vocal fatigue	Improper diet or daily fluid intake
Work environment	Loss of voice/aphonia	ENT diseases (e.g. sinusitis, pharyngitis)
Access to sound amplifier	Difficulty in being heard	Other diseases (e.g. reflux, allergies,
Psychosocial conditions	Throat clearing	hearing loss)
Frequent business trips	Chronic dryness in the throat	Extra-occupational voice loading
Jet-lag risk	'Lump' in the throat	Voice demanding hobby
	Sore throat	Current medication (e.g. antihistamines,
	Odynophonia	diuretics, oral contraceptives)
	Persistent dry cough	Previous operations, anaesthesia

and vitamins is needed. A history of previous surgery, particularly performed under anaesthesia, is also important. Laryngeal surgery is a matter of great concern

During the conversation the physician is able to supplement historical information, fitting the questions individually to the patient's complaints. Moreover, during the conversation it is possible to evaluate voice production perceptually.

- *Self-Assessment of Voice* is a valuable tool of comprehensive voice diagnosis, particularly important among professional voice users, because it enables evaluation of the level of handicap that the subject experiences as a result of voice disorders. In reference to the WHO multidimensional concept of health, the patient's subjective opinion should not be ignored in assessing the health consequence of disability, for example, the extent of impairment. One of the more common instruments of voice self-assessment is the Voice Handicap Index (VHI)—a 30-item questionnaire evaluating complaints and signs of disability due to voice disorders. This scale has been shown to have validity and reliability in various countries, and thus it can be used as a valuable screening tool (Cheng and Woo 2010; Herbst et al. 2015). The assessment of voice handicap ought to be taken into account, particularly in voice professionals, for whom voice disorders may not only have an impact on their general health condition but also bring about employment-related problems. Other common methods of voice self-assessment include V-RQOL (Voice-Related Quality of Life),

VOS (Voice Outcome Survey), VoiSS (Voice Symptom Scale) and VTDS (Vocal Tract Discomfort Scale) (Bermudez de Alvear et al. 2010; Woznicka et al. 2012)

5.2.6 The Assessment of Vocal Load Effects

A crucial issue in diagnosing occupational dysphonia is the evaluation of the influence of vocal load on the voice apparatus (Hunter and Titze 2009). The evaluation of vocal load effects may be performed by means of the following.

Laboratory Tests Including Vocal Loading Tasks The most popular vocal loading task (see also Sect. 6.8) consists of reading aloud a text for 30 min at the level of background (white) noise of 85 dB SPL (decibels sound pressure level).

The following pre- and post-vocal loading voice parameters are compared:

- Subjective self-ratings: specific surveys including questions concerning symptoms that accompany vocal effort have been developed by using a visual analogue scale (VAS) (Laukkanen et al. 2004). However, the common VHI questionnaire also covers complaints indicating vocal fatigue
- Acoustic analysis:
  - Comparison of the pre- and post-test acoustic parameter values obtained by using the Multidimensional Voice Program. The most frequent changes are observed in the average fundamental frequency and in

the parameters of jitter and shimmer groups (Niebudek-Bogusz et al. 2008; Remacle et al. 2012)

- Comparison of the pre- and post-test voice range profile (VRP): a decrease in the maximum post-vocal loading VRP is considered to be a voice reduction test (cited after Obrębowski 2008)
- Aerodynamic parameters: pre- and post-test values of maximum phonation time (MPT), estimated subglottal pressure (ESP) and sound pressure level (SPL) have been shown to be relevant for the assessment of vocal efficiency (Chang and Karnell 2004; Remacle et al. 2012; Echternach et al. 2014)

The changes of objective measurements may be accompanied by laryngo-videostroboscopic signs after the vocal loading test. The effects of poorly compensated vocal effort may affect dimensions of phonatory functions, including deterioration of the quality of the mucosal wave or incompleteness of phonatory glottal closure. A negative vocal loading test without deterioration after vocal effort has been noted in subjects with a well-functioning voice apparatus and sufficient voice capacity.

Individual Dosimeters Dosimeters used in the workplace are portable devices worn by subject in order to extract and collect important parameters of vocal behaviour over an entire daily working time. Evaluation by means of dosimeters is particularly useful in assessing individual vocal load in specific job conditions and recovery time in various options of multimodal communications.

The most frequently used dosimeters are the following (Echternach et al. 2014):

- Ambulatory Phonation Monitor, which extracts the following data: the voicing percentage (%), the average fundamental frequency (Hz) and amplitude (dBSPL), glottal cycle dose and also distance dose—the length 'covered' by the vocal fold mucosa in the whole cycle of daily working activities (m)

- Voxlog—a voice accumulator that registers phonation time, the fundamental frequency, voice sound pressure level, the background noise level, cycle and distance dose and energy dissipation and radiated energy dose (www.sonvox.com/voxlog/)

Individual dosimeters or vocal loading tasks seem to be valuable tools for the assessment of 'voice fitness for duty' in professional voice users and may enable clinicians to detect even early stages of occupational dysphonia. They can be used not only for predicting dysphonic severity but also for biofeedback and for the monitoring of the results of vocal training (Calcinoni and Niebudek-Bogusz 2014).

5.2.7 Clinical Aspects of Occupational Voice Disorders

Negative voice adaptation under conditions of chronic vocal load may result in the development of vocal fatigue and, as a consequence, reduced vocal endurance, leading to occupational voice disorders.

Occupational dysphonia may produce multiple voice symptoms, including recurrent or chronic hoarseness, sensation of dry throat or a lump in the pharynx, even pain, dry cough, loss of the singing range, voice tiredness or voicelessness (aphonia).

Types of occupationally determined voice disorder may take the form of:

- *Functional (Non-organic) Dysphonia*—the most frequent form of hyperfunctional origin (see also Sect. 5.1); phonation with excessive muscular forces leads to chronic abuse syndrome, inducing vocal fatigue and reduced voice capacity. Phoniatric examination may reveal incorrect type of breathing, excessive neck muscle tension, incorrect resonator activation and 'hard' phonation with rough voice, accompanied by abnormal vibration parameters observed by means of videostroboscopy (e.g. diminished amplitude of vocal fold vibration, reduced mucosal wave or glottal sphinc-ter closure with vestibular phonation). Long-lasting functional dysphonia often leads to irreversible laryngeal lesions, frequently of organic type

• *Organic Dysphonia*—the most common organic outcomes of vocal hyperfunction include vocal nodules, hypertrophy of the vocal folds margin, vascular lesions of the glottis, contact ulcers and asthenia of the internal larynx muscles contributing to glottal insufficiency. Vocal nodules are con-sidered to be the most frequent occupation-related pathology. Vocal nodules are the effect of chronic phono-trauma and occur mostly in females (in adult age), which can be explained by the sex differences described above. These organic lesions are frequently preceded by prenodules—reversible sym-metric slight oedema of vocal fold edges, which accompanies functional dysphonia, with muscular tension imbalance and an hourglass-shaped vibration pattern. In cases of the chronic vocal injuries, these oedemas may change into permanent hyalinised fibrous nodules or into epithelial calluses occurring around the free edge of the vocal folds, at the anteroposterior midpoint of the membranous folds. The vocal nodules, typi-cally, are whitish, small, generally bilateral and symmetrical (Fig. 5.1)

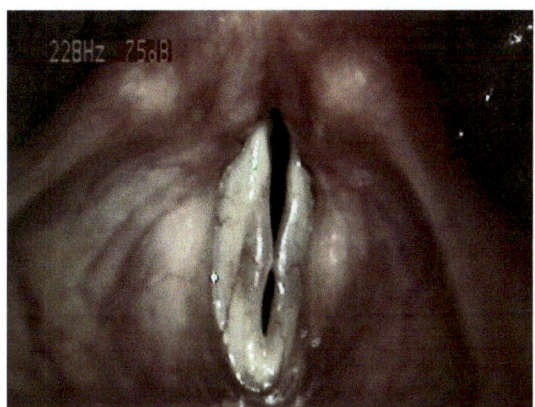

Fig. 5.2 Polypoid degeneration of vocal nodules in an older female teacher—image of the larynx during phonation

Females of older age, particularly teachers suffering from vocal nodules for a long time, par-ticularly with coexisting inflammatory factor can develop polypoid hypertrophy of those lesions (like those presented in Fig. 5.2). Many other vocal fold injuries may occur in connection with chronic phono-trauma. Hypertrophy of the vocal folds secondary to vocal effort often takes the form of benign vocal fold masses, mainly polyp-oid or fibrovascular changes localised on the edges of the vocal folds. Signs of laryngeal impairment in voice professionals may be associ-ated with other nonoccupational risk factors: e.g. acute laryngitis, LPR (laryngopharyngeal reflux), Reinke's oedema, sulcus vocalis and leukoplakia. Sometimes in such cases differential diagnosis and the assessment of the main risk factors are not simple.

Case Study 5.3

A 40-year-old teacher of music and sports at a high school had voice problems for the last 3 years. When singing high notes, she feels that there is no closure of the vocal folds. She had studied singing and conducts five choirs besides her teaching activities. At the age of 34, she suf-fered two heart attacks and was fitted with a bypass. She takes beta-blockers and clopidogrel and additionally thyroxine because of Hashimoto's struma.

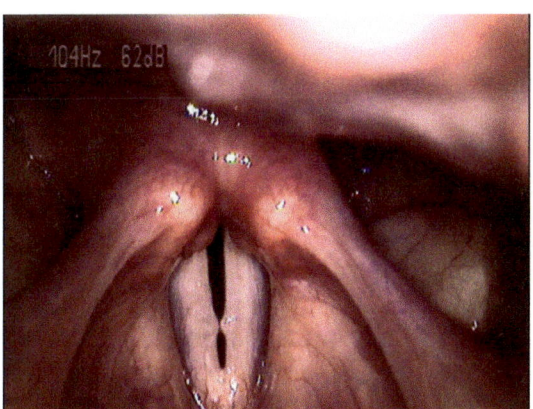

Fig. 5.1 Vocal nodules—image of the larynx during phonation

There is characteristic marginal oedema on both vocal folds in the middle of the membranous part. Closure is complete in the chest register but hourglass-shaped at soft phonation. The voice range profile shows that high notes cannot be sung softly; otherwise, it is inconspicuous. The voice at connected speech is normal (R0 B0 H0) as is the singing voice in the low register.

Case Study 5.4

A 26-year-old event manager providing much professional talking had voice problems for years. After vocal load the voice is hoarse up to aphonic and regularly worse in the evening. There are no diseases in her history.

The video shows vocal fold nodules in the characteristic location and an hourglass-shaped closure. Vocal range is restricted. The speaking voice is mildly hoarse (R1 B1 H1) and has a tendency to pressed phonation.

5.2.8 Differential Diagnosis

The main role is played by videostroboscopic imaging, which enables physicians to detect pathological alterations of the vocal folds that are a consequence of repeated movements and collisions of the vocal folds during chronic vocal overload (Rubin et al. 2014). Different types of benign vocal fold masses (BVFM) located at the vocal fold edge (e.g. nodules, chronic oedema and polypoid hypertrophy) seem especially to be secondary to vocal effort (Fig. 5.3). These pathologies are sometimes unilateral at first but, with the progress of the disease the contralateral fold, can also be affected. Occupation-related vocal fold hypertrophy should be differentiated from Reinke's oedema, which includes major polypoid corditis changes that are causally associated with cigarette smoking.

Furthermore, the following parameters of the phonatory function should be taken into consideration: (1) the quality of the mucosal wave; (2) the regularity of vocal fold vibrations; (3) the amplitude of the vocal fold movement; and (4)

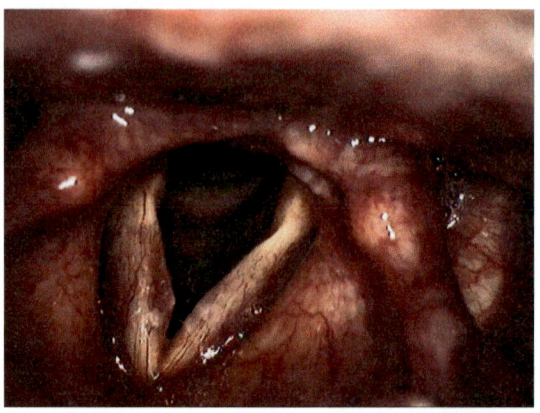

Fig. 5.3 Hypertrophy of the vocal folds (secondary to vocal effort)—image of the larynx during breathing

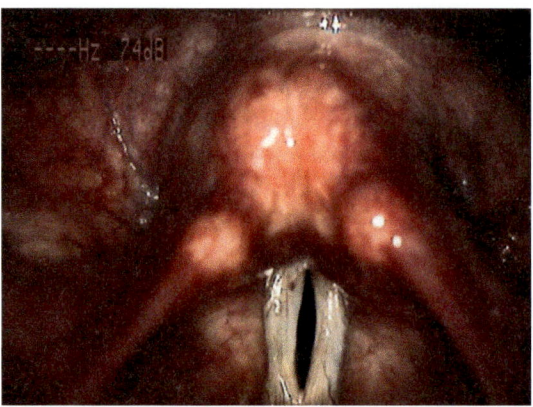

Fig. 5.4 Asthenia of the internal larynx muscles, which contributes to irreversible glottal insufficiency (spindle-shaped glottal closure) and to permanent dysphonia—image of the larynx during phonation

the configuration of glottal closure. It is assumed that slightly insufficient posterior glottal closure should be regarded as normal, particularly in women, while other types of glottal incompleteness are considered pathological. For example, vocal nodules are characterised by hourglass-shaped glottal closure, whereas overload asthenia of the internal larynx muscles displays spindle-shaped glottal closure (Fig. 5.4). This latter voice disorder seems to be related to long-lasting vocal fatigue, which can indicate occupational hazard as a risk factor (European Economic Community Brussels 2003).

5.2.9 Management in Occupational Voice Disorders

Occupation-related voice disorders are becoming a global multifocal health problem, involving social, economic and public health aspects. The prevention and treatment of occupational dysphonia call for improving occupational safety regulations and introducing better health arrangements for professional voice users.

5.2.9.1 Treatment

It should be stressed that phoniatricians or laryngologists who treat professional voice users should be aware of the fact that voice is crucial to their professional career (Nawka 2008). In view of the multifactorial aetiology of occupational dysphonia, the multidimensional model of therapy should be recommended. The therapy should be fitted to individual needs. The battery of frequently applied therapeutic methods is large and includes the following: pharmacological treatments, phonosurgery, psychotherapy, manual therapy, osteopathic therapy and forms of voice rehabilitation, such as vocal training and teaching skills of target behaviour eliminating vocal abuse. The methods of voice treatment are described in Sects. 8.2 and 8.3 of this book. At this point, it needs to be stressed that the treatment of occupational dysphonia ought to focus on the following elements:

- Education on voice hygiene: stressing that the vocal effort should be followed by an appropriate period of voice rest
- Vocal training: an important method of voice therapy that can improve vocal capacity and the ability to compensate for vocal load. It can significantly increase "voice fitness for duty" in professional voice users and may enable them to continue working
- Coping strategies for dealing with occupational stress and burn-out symptoms: this is a particularly important module in the treatment of functional occupational dysphonia, since psycho-emotional factors constitute a considerable risk of persisting voice problems in some individuals

Management of occupational dysphonia should be holistic and should rely on a close collaboration of phoniatricians, otolaryngologists, speech therapists, psychologists and physiotherapists or osteopaths or other clinicians if needed (Marszałek et al. 2012). Extensive treatment of occupational voice disorders performed in a health spa frequently produces better results than those from treatment in an outpatient clinic.

5.2.9.2 Certification

In many EU countries, the problem of occupational voice disorders is undervalued, perhaps because of the lack of this disease entity in the basic list of occupational diseases specified in the EU Commission Recommendation 2003/670/EC. Only in some countries, for example, in Poland, are occupational voice disorders included in the list of occupational diseases and regarded as a medicolegal issue (Calcinoni and Niebudek-Bogusz 2014). For example, according to Polish law, a certified occupational voice disorder entitles the person to financial compensation in the form of a single financial indemnity (calculated proportionally to the percentage of the loss of health, ranging between 10 and 40%). If partial permanent work disability due to occupational disease is proven, a pension may be provided. The pension is granted frequently for 1–2 years only, and the person is expected to retrain in order to get another job.

High-quality documentation of voice examination from the whole employment period plays a crucial role in the certification procedure. The phoniatric evaluation, including videostroboscopic imaging and the instrumental assessment of work-related vocal load, should be documented and archived as relevant evidence in the diagnostic procedure of occupational voice disorders and in the monitoring of the voice improvement in the course of treatment.

5.2.9.3 Prophylaxis

The important role of the prevention of occupational voice disorders has already been recognised in some studies, but only a few countries have been introducing better health arrangements for voice professionals in the last few decades.

For example, in Poland, teachers employed in public schools are examined by laryngologists before they start work, and then the examination is repeated at obligatorily set periods. One of the Polish preventive programmes has resulted in the introduction of an optional new subject into the syllabus of pedagogical colleges: education on vocal hygiene and proper vocal behaviour (Niebudek-Bogusz and Sliwinska-Kowalska 2013). Several other countries, e.g. Scandinavian countries and Austria, have introduced many preventive programmes for professional voice users (Vilkman 2004; Schneider-Stickler et al. 2012).

Prevention should also concern other vocally demanding professions, including the still-growing staff of the call centre companies. Therefore, new technologies of instrumental voice evaluation, including the assessment of vocal loading effects, ought to be developed and implemented. They can facilitate the diagnostics of the risk of occupation-related dysphonia and the detection of changes in its early stages. They can also support therapy (biofeedback). The prophylactic programmes should be developed on the basis of multidisciplinary treatment of occupational dysphonia and by the collaboration of laryngologists, phoniatricians and speech therapists, as well as occupational medicine doctors.

To sum up, in view of the increasing impact of voice disorders on people's ability to work, more relevant prevention strategies are needed.

5.3 Singing Voice Disorders

Bernhard Richter

5.3.1 Introduction

Human voice production is accomplished through the perfect coordination of breathing, laryngeal movement and articulation. The movement patterns employed in this process are some of the more complex movements of which the human body is capable.

In general, any dysfunction of the human voice is called dysphonia. According to the underlying complex mechanisms of voice production, there are multiple causes of dysphonia. The cardinal symptom of dysphonia is hoarseness, irrespective of its aetiology. In daily clinical work, a rough classification of organ-related and organ-unrelated dysphonias has proved useful.

Organic voice dysfunctions may have an inflammatory or a traumatic origin. Other causes may be benign or malignant lesions of the vocal cords.

In singers, this classification can be applied as well; but additional criteria—more adapted to the singers' special needs and skills—should be included. Therefore, for singers, other distinctions can be made:

- Dysphonia-causing dysfunctions of the voice-producing organ itself
- Dysfunctions accompanying general diseases (e.g. influenza), in which a more or less severe impairment of the body or vocal capability is intrinsic

In the latter case, the vocal dysfunction is not a disease of the vocal organ but a symptom of the general disease (Wendler and Seidner 2005).

5.3.2 Special Issues in the Evaluation of Singers' Voices

For the evaluation of a singer's voice, it is mandatory for the examiner to be aware that a singer's larynx may show visible abnormalities or deviations that do not cause any voice impairment.

Structural modifications such as asymmetries, unilateral vocal cord swelling, oedema, polyps, varices, etc. are not unusual in a professional singer's larynx. Systematic studies in professional singers have shown that these 'anatomical lesions' do not necessarily affect tone production or the vocal sound; moreover, no impairment of vocal sound production and sound stability may be perceived either by the singers themselves or by the person listening to them (Traser et al. 2012). For the appropriate classification of stroboscopic images with regard to functional aspects of voice production, the sound quality of the voice, as well as the vocal capacity and singing skills, has to be considered before any decision is made about whether a treatment should be initiated and, especially for singers, what the specific treatment procedures should be.

With the purpose of systematic classification of singing voice disorders, the following distinctions can be made:

- Dysfunctions that have their cause primarily in the singing voice (singing-related disorders)
- Dysfunctions that have other causes but that also hamper singing

5.3.3 Singing-Related Disorders

5.3.3.1 Acute Symptoms of Vocal 'Overuse'

The onset of respiratory infections is often associated with acute symptoms of vocal 'overuse'. These mostly start with a rhinitic medical condition of viral origin as an ordinary 'cold'. Young singers in particular lose control of their singing voice when they are affected by a rhinitis. They do not only perceive a change in the sound of vocal consonants, but they also sense a kinaesthetic change.

This kinaesthetic perception is one of the essential feedback systems employed during professional singing (Mürbe et al. 2002, 2004). In the case that this control mechanism is constrained, singers often try to compensate by 'pressing' or 'pushing' the voice which, in turn, may cause an increase of the subglottal pressure as well as the mechanical strain of the vocal cords (Sundberg 1987; Jiang et al. 2000). This may result in either a swelling at the free edge of the vocal fold, oedema or even bleeding into the vocal folds (see Figs. 5.5 and 5.6).

Such haematomas require special care if acetylsalicylic acid had been taken during the infection, since acetylsalicylic acid, as well as diclofenac, enhances the disposition for bleeding.

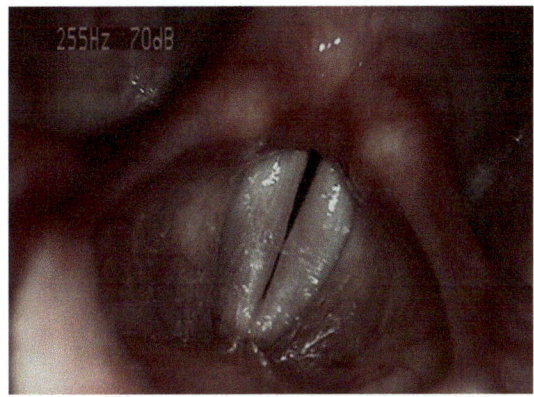

Fig. 5.5 Swelling at the free edge of the vocal fold

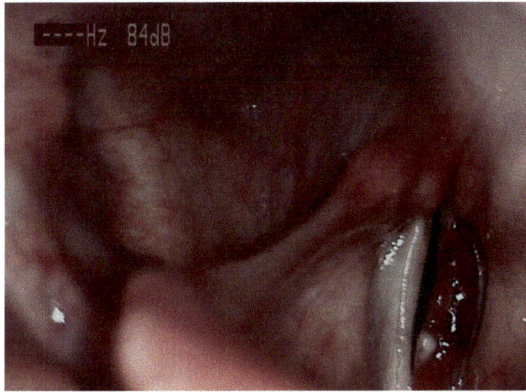

Fig. 5.6 Vocal fold haematoma

When affected by a respiratory infection, those with a high occupational use of the voice—singers and actors—are confronted with the decision whether to sing or speak despite the infection. The answer to this depends on the individual conditions and on the expected vocal strain.

In general, three crucial questions are to be considered for the evaluation of vocal strain:

- Is the patient hoarse?
- Does the patient show any laryngitic symptoms?
- How good are the patient's vocal skills?

Singers, irrespective of their experience, should not put any strain on the voice in the case of hoarseness or any signs of inflammation in the laryngeal area. The voice must not be strained under any circumstances when the acute disease comes with hoarseness. If signs and symptoms of laryngitis are proven by an ENT or phoniatrician during careful strobo-scopic examination, singers and actors should not perform at all.

A hoarse voice must also not be used for singing in a choir because the auditory sound control is hampered when singing in an ensemble. This so-called Lombard-effect is an impair-ment of the auditory feedback system during voice production and is due to the increased sur-rounding noise volume (Lombard 1911). Individuals without special vocal training or experience automatically increase their speak-ing or singing volume when speaking or singing in surroundings with a noise volume over 70 decibels, as is often the case in a choir. Moreover, when the singing takes place in a choir, onset of hoarseness is not immediately perceived, and, since the affected singer does not want to lose face in front of his choral associates, the singing is often continued despite increasing voice problems.

Highly experienced singers with fully devel-oped singing skills are able to sing even when suffering from an infection—as long as there is no hoarseness or laryngitis. In general, singers have learned to use their voice without increased strain even in the case of altered auditory or kin-aesthetic feedback.

5.3.3.2 Chronic Overuse (Misuse)

As a rule, overuse results from a disproportion of vocal strain to vocal capacity. This diagnosis especially applies to continuous (chronic) vocal overuse.

From the beginning of the nineteenth century, a paradigm change regarding the vocal exigen-cies can be observed: from lyrical to dramatic singing. Along with the alteration to more dra-matic demands in opera, reports of vocal crises and on chronic overuse in opera singers have been increasing. Accordingly, vocal overuse is not a new phenomenon in professional singers; it is also not at all rare. The world-famous Swedish singer Jenny Lind (1820–1887), who had her debut at the age of 17 singing the role of Agathe

in *Freischütz*, is known to have suffered an existential vocal crisis at the age of 21. Another example is Enrico Caruso (1873–1921) who needed two vocal cord surgeries in the course of his career (Springer 2002). Unrelated to these operations, Caruso again paused from perfor-mance for 7 months in 1911. His biographer, Springer (2002), attributed this break to Caruso's general exhaustion. In the middle of her career, Christa Ludwig repeatedly suffered from vocal haematoma resulting from voice overuse (Ludwig 1999).

Some of the composers who were responsible for the growing dramatisation of operas, e.g. Richard Wagner and Giuseppe Verdi, were quite aware of the high—and increased—vocal exigen-cies inherent to their scores. In 1875, Wagner complained in correspondence with Julius Hey (1832–1909):

> […] since the quite suggesting and commonly used term 'Sprechgesang (chant)' only referred to a strongly enhanced speaking of texts that had to combat the unequal battle with the orchestra. No wonder that this senseless proceeding ruined num-berless beautiful voices. I am to blame for all this.
> Hey (1911)

On the occasion of the planned representation of his innovative 'dramatic' opera MACBETH in Naples in 1848, Verdi wrote about the singer Eugenia Tadolini (1809–1851) who was planning to sing the Lady Macbeth part:

> Tadolini's qualities are far too good for that role! This may seem absurd to you!! … […] Tadolini has a stupendous voice, clear, limpid, powerful; and I would like the Lady to have a harsh, stifled, and hol-low voice. Tadolini's voice has an angelic quality; I would like the Lady's voice to be diabolical. […].
> Gossett (2007)

One should not derive from Verdi's expression that he preferred 'ugly' voices; but it becomes obvious that also for him the dramatisation of the singing technique became increasingly important in the course of his creative career.

As a reaction to this growing dramatisation of operas, the writer and music critic George Bernard Shaw (1856–1950) expressed his opin-ion on Verdi's compositional style and its health consequences for singers:

The whole secret of a healthy voice writing lies in keeping the normal plane of music, and therefore the bulk of the singers' work, in the middle of the voice. Unfortunately, the middle of the voice is not the prettiest part of it; and in immature or badly and insufficiently trained voices it is often the weakest part. There is, therefore, a constant temptation for composers to use the upper fifth of the voice almost exclusively; and this is exactly what Verdi did without remorse. He practically treated that upper fifth as the whole voice, and pitched his melodies in the middle of it instead of the middle of the entire compass, the result being a frightful strain on the singer.

In order to avoid vocal overuse, the roles of the singing teacher as well as of the physician are crucial. The singing teacher is, together with the student, responsible for the teaching content and for choosing the appropriate exercises and scores. The singing teacher has a very high responsibility for the prophylactic avoidance of vocal overuse. Here, essential support comes from the phoniatrician who may be addressed whenever the singing teacher or the student have open questions or need help.

It is essential and important that any phoniatrician in charge of professional voice users be very experienced (see Sect. 1.10). The phoniatrician should also have profound knowledge of psychological issues (see Sect. 5.9). Ideally, the phoniatrician should have professional voice training.

With the phoniatrician's and the singing teacher's help, young singers should develop awareness that singing should only take place within one's own voice category (*Fach*). A prerequisite for this is the teaching of knowledge about voice categories. Furthermore, active advice based on comprehensive experience is required (see Sect. 1.10).

It is very wise for a singer to avoid any voice overuse. A singer has to be aware that the more the voice is strained by difficult scores, the more agility and stretching of the relevant muscles are needed for it to recover. Therefore, the messa di voce (see Sect. 1.8) for the coloratura and others should under no circumstances be removed from the training programme but, on the contrary, be further practised. Dramatic and highly dramatic singing—including some subgroups of jazz and pop-rock singing, as well as belting in general—

represent an especially complex challenge in terms of voice physiology and treatment by any voice specialist. In phoniatric practice, the question of the right time for singers to turn to dramatic scores often arises only when signs of overuse become apparent.

Here, three major mistakes—the 'magic 3 t's'—can be observed: (1) Singers start too early in their career to sing dramatic scores; (2) the scores chosen are too difficult; (3) the practising of the scores is too long and loud. Consequently, voice specialists should generally recommend a slow and careful start to singing development. Young singers who in particular do not have the pressure of time constraints should not rush to change towards the dramatic *Fach*: it is observed that this development is usually adopted too early.

Vocal overuse can be treated through competent phoniatric care and adequate involvement of the singer in the treatment procedure. Chronic overuse may lead to a functional voice disorder and, especially in singers, to dysodia (see Sect. 5.2). Various other voice problems may also arise from chronic or acute overuse. These are called benign organic voice disorders and are explained in detail in Sect. 5.4.

5.3.4 Dysfunctions and Diseases Hampering Singing

Organic Voice Disorders Organic voice disorders may—besides original alterations—result either from functional disorders, which cause a purely mechanical impairment of the vocal fold mobility, or from functional disorders of the muscles and corresponding nerves that are responsible for the tension and mobility of the vocal cords.

Acute Inflammation Acute respiratory infections are often accompanied by signs of laryngitis of viral or bacterial origin. Regardless of the underlying pathological cause, this laryngitis leads to swelling of the vocal cords and to hoarseness. In these cases singing and speaking should be strictly limited to avoid acute or chronic overuse of the voice.

Chronic Inflammation There are various causes of chronic inflammation. Inhaled noxious agents such as cigarette smoke, dust and vapours may lead to chronic inflammation (Richter et al. 2002). In this context, of particular note are the chronic inflammatory changes associated with inhalatory steroid therapy used in the treatment of asthma. These changes are often accompanied by fungal colonisation of the larynx. However, continuous overuse of the voice may also lead to chronic inflammatory laryngeal changes. Furthermore, more general medical conditions such as rheumatic diseases may be a cause of chronic inflammatory changes in the larynx (see Sect. 5.13).

Hormonal Influences Hormone-related voice disorders are explained in detail in Sect. 5.10.

Significant Changes in the Vocal Tract Singing voice disorders are not only restricted to problems of laryngeal origin. Modifications of the vocal tract might lead to or promote dysphonia. Diseases that involve disorders of the functioning of the vocal tract, such as movement disorders of the soft palate, or impairments of the velopharyngeal closure after tonsillectomy, possibly influence the acoustic properties of the vocal tract: impairment of formant clustering and formant tuning as well as influences on the voice source by means of non-linear relationships may be involved (Titze 2008). These variables might explain dysphonia in conditions without impairment of vocal fold function. Therefore, the diagnostics of dysphonia should not be reduced to functional analysis of vocal fold oscillations (Echternach et al. 2011).

Indoor Air Climate The climatic conditions of an opera stage—especially the air's humidity—may deviate considerably from those recommended for singers (Richter et al. 2000). This is particularly so when there is no effective air conditioning. From considering these conditions, along with the fact that singers may suffer a substantial dryness of the mouth because of the adrenergic stress reaction of stage fright, the importance of the optimisation of the indoor air climate becomes quite clear and unquestionable.

Reflux Reflux-related posterior laryngitis is a disease that is not specific to singers, but singers who suffer from reflux (GERD, gastrooesophageal reflux disease) often develop a posterior laryngitis (Cammarota et al. 2007). In all cases, singers suffering from GERD should undergo thorough medical examination (see Sect. 5.5).

Tumours To date, there is no literature that provides descriptions of malignant vocal cord tumours related to or caused by vocal strain. Accordingly, these lesions are no more common in singers than in people with no vocal profession. There may even be a lower rate of malignant tumours in singers since they, for the reason of voice hygiene, usually consume less noxious agents (alcohol and nicotine) than average members of the population. Nevertheless, any hoarseness of unknown origin lasting longer than 3 weeks should be examined by an ENT physician or a phoniatrician. Since there are various diseases with hoarseness as a symptom, a thorough diagnosis is required in order to exclude any malign lesions.

Vocal Fold Movement Disorders So far there have been no descriptions of strain-related vocal cord movement disorders. Accordingly, vocal fold movement disorders are no more common in singers than in non-professional voice users (see Sects. 5.6–5.8). Where a singer requires surgery in the region of the nervus laryngeus recurrens and the nervus laryngeus superior (e.g. thyroid gland operation), a very careful medical procedure in the context of voice hygiene is required, including neuro-monitoring. Given the surgeons' awareness of this risk, dysfunctions that arise from such surgery (e.g. nerve paralysis) may even be rarer in singers than in the average population.

Case Study 5.5
A 40-year-old pop and soul singer had voice problems with her singing voice. She had no other diseases and takes no medication. The examination with video-laryngostroboscopy revealed vocal fold nodules. The voice range

profile shows loss of high notes especially for soft tones. The speaking voice is normal. When singing, she fails to hit the passaggio note C5 (523 Hz), whereas the next one, D5 (587 Hz), is possible. This does not happen regularly. Usually singers avoid such accidents by pushing their voice.

Case Study 5.6
A 39-year-old musical singer and actor had some problems with his high voice. He had a phonosurgical intervention years ago, but it is not known which vocal fold was operated on. During video-laryngostroboscopy, there is a hardly noticeable swelling of the left vocal fold. He is a high baritone, and his voice range profile is adequate to the requirements of a musical singer. The speaking voice is normal as is the singing voice. However, he feels insecure about the performance and does not always trust his voice.

Case Study 5.7
A 43-year-old opera singer (soprano) had trouble with her high notes and needed a long time (more than 48 h) for recovery after performances. Video-laryngostroboscopy shows marginal oedema on both vocal folds in the middle of the membranous part where amplitudes are largest and collision and shearing forces strongest. When singing, she loses control over the high notes that tend to slide up. The speaking voice sounds mildly rough (R1 B0 H0).

Case Study 5.8
This 40-year-old baritone sings dramatic opera roles but wants to be a lyric singer. His voice is a bit heavy after he had sung performances with a cold. The video-laryngostroboscopy shows mucus/phlegm on the vocal folds. The margins are macerated, and on the right side, there is a small swelling. These are typical signs of an inflammation after vocal load. The vocal range is not affected. He has a very strong singer's formant. His speaking voice sounds a little rough (R1 B0 H0). When singing, he tends to push his voice. After a few days of voice rest he will recover.

5.4 Benign Organic Voice Disorders

Mette Pedersen, Anders Overgård Jønsson, Sevtap Akbulut, Haldun Oguz, and Tadeus Nawka

5.4.1 Lesions of the Lamina Propria of the Vocal Folds

5.4.1.1 Vocal Fold Nodules
Vocal fold nodules are the most common benign lesions of the vocal folds in both children and adults. The prevalence of nodules in the general population is not known but has been reported as being the cause of hoarseness in up to 23.4% of children, 0.5–1.3% of ENT clinic attendances and 6% of phoniatric clinic attendances. The prevalence of nodules in female teachers was found to be 43% of 218 cases with dysphonia, in a population of 1046 female teachers in a study in Spain. Teachers speak for an average of 102 min per 8 h. Nodules were found in 25% of hoarse singers (Pedersen and McGlashan 2012).

Definition Vocal fold nodules are mostly symmetrical thickenings of the vocal fold margin due to oedematous swelling of the lamina propria and distension of the overlying epithelium.

Causes Vocal fold nodules usually result from continuous vocal abuse, misuse or overload. This rather simplistic view should be extended because they may appear on the one hand as localised oedemas and on the other as epithelial thickenings. The main cause is certainly vocal stress, but there are other contributing factors that are not known. In recent years, attention has been focused on another aspect of aetiology, namely, epithelial tissue deviations in the region of the nodules. The development of nodules does not seem to be related to age but rather to functional load when speaking and singing (Martins et al. 2010).

Signs and Symptoms Nodules are generally bilateral lesions located at the mid-membranous vocal fold. There are two types of nodule that may not necessarily have the same aetiology or prognosis. The first type consists in the beginning of fairly soft and pliable diffuse swellings. The histological abnormality seems to be more concentrated in the superficial lamina propria. They may increase over time owing to chronic vocal load up to the size of Reinke's oedema. The other kind of nodule is characterised by focal hard and fibrotic epithelial thickenings.

Laryngostroboscopic examination demonstrates an hourglass-closure pattern and normal or minimally reduced mucosal wave vibratory activity.

Treatment The standard treatment is voice therapy. Many people try to avoid surgical intervention. In terms of lasting improvement, phonosurgery is the better choice when combined with voice therapy.

Prognosis These lesions may respond to a combination of voice rest or voice ergonomics and voice therapy when the patient is compliant, and the therapy is done in an appropriate fashion. However, they will not cease completely and may recur after renewed vocal load such as vocal recitals. After phonosurgery, the prerequisites for voice therapy and adjustments of singing technique are better. Even then, vocal fold nodules may recur.

5.4.1.2 Vocal Fold Polyps

Definition Vocal polyps, more often unilateral than bilateral, are typically exophytic or pedunculated lesions of the middle part of the membranous vocal folds.

Causes Polyps result from vocal hyperfunction, as do vocal nodules. However, unlike vocal nodules, polyps are often precipitated by a single vocal event, such as screaming. Once a small polyp begins, any continued vocal abuse or misuse will irritate the area and lead to its continued growth.

Signs and Symptoms There are two types of polyp: hyaline or glassy ones of pale colour and haemorrhagic ones that are red. Polyps have a sharply delimited margin to the surrounding epithelium. Stroboscopic evaluation reveals a variable closure pattern according to size and localisation of the polyp. Pedunculated polyps are pressed below the vocal fold level into the inframarginal region, or they topple over during phonation and sit on the superior plane of the vocal fold. Polyps originating from the medial vocal fold edge may lead to an hourglass-closure pattern. The mucosal wave is inhibited at the site of the polyp, whereas other parts of the vocal folds may vibrate in a normal fashion.

Treatment Voice therapy may help the symptoms of polyps, but generally surgical excision of the lesion is the treatment of choice. The distended epithelium covering the polyp should be resected as a whole, leaving the surrounding strong epithelium intact. Lamina propria material should not be removed below the epithelial level, to provide a matrix for epithelial regeneration. The microflap technique is not advisable.

Prognosis There is a good prognosis for voice function after polyp excision, provided the intervention is limited to the pathological structures. Polyps usually do not recur.

Case Study 5.9
A 39-year-old construction engineer had suffered from hoarseness for 6 months. The vocal fold polyp may have developed when she used her loud voice on construction sites. She had no other health-related problems. She has lost her head voice and is unable to sing. The speaking voice sounds moderately rough (R2 B1 H2), and it feels as if she needs to clear her throat from phlegm in order to speak normally.

5.4.1.3 Polypoid Corditis (Reinke's Oedema)

Definition Reinke's oedema is a pathological condition of the vocal folds, which involves accumulation of a gelatinous type of fluid under the vocal fold cover in Reinke's space.

Causes The most common aetiological factors of Reinke's oedema involve tobacco use, LPR (laryngopharyngeal reflux) and chronic vocal abuse. Upper airway infection can often be present in patients with Reinke's oedema, but there is no clinical evidence that supports infection as an aetiological factor.

Signs and Symptoms Reinke's oedema can considerably increase the mass and volume of the vocal folds. That typically lowers the pitch of the voice and causes increased vocal effort and instability. The aetiological factors should be addressed before surgical treatment.

Treatment Phono-microsurgery is indicated once Reinke's oedemas have reached a significant size. It is not likely that they will reform after cessation of smoking or after treating laryngopharyngeal reflux. The operation may be carried out on both vocal folds at the same time when done properly (see Sect. 8.10). Vocal effort may increase after removal of the oedema when a gap arises between the vocal folds. That is why the thin and fragile epithelium covering the gelatinous masses should never be resected completely. A so-called stripping is definitely malpractice and leads inevitably to scarring and irreparable vocal damage. Such side effects of the operation cause more discomfort than the oedema itself. Voice therapy before surgery is helpful in eliminating the vocal abuse and obtaining a better result after the surgery.

Prognosis After surgical removal, Reinke's oedema usually does not recur. In case of removal in an exact fashion, voice can improve significantly. Otherwise, it is nearly impossible to correct resulting scar formation when too much of the epithelium has been removed.

Case Study 5.10
A 54-year-old woman, a smoker with 45 pack-years, has been hoarse for many years. The video shows giant Reinke's oedema on both vocal folds. The pitch of the speaking voice is in the region of male voices, but the timbre is still female. She is unable to speak up or sing.

5.4.2 Secondary Pathological Changes of the Vocal Folds and the Larynx

5.4.2.1 Vocal Fold Cysts

Definition Vocal fold cysts are swellings below the epithelium of the vocal fold. They contain mucus or a caseous mass.

Causes Epidermoid cysts may be secondary to vocal abuse or to remaining epithelium trapped inside the lamina propria. They have a lining of stratified squamous and keratinised epithelium and a duct that ends blindly on the inferior margin of the vocal fold.

Mucous-retention cysts develop from the obstruction of the glandular ducts caused by different conditions, such as voice overuse, laryngitis secondary to gastro-oesophageal reflux or upper-airway infections. The cavity is covered by a ciliated cylindrical epithelium. The cysts are more common in adults but can also be diagnosed in children (Martins et al. 2011).

Signs and Symptoms Patients complain about increasing hoarseness of the voice. Dynamic and pitch range are restricted. Intra-cordal cysts appear as small spheres on the margins of the vocal folds and sometimes on the superior surface. They are predominantly unilateral. Epidermoid cysts are white, while mucus retention cysts are often yellowish. On stroboscopic evaluation, mucosal wave vibratory activity may be normal to disrupted, depending on the size of the cyst, with an hour-glass-closure pattern.

Treatment Phonosurgery is generally required for symptomatic cysts. The epithelium does not have to be resected but just divided to dissect the subepithelial cyst, and remove it completely.

Prognosis Epidermoid cysts fill with mucus and grow with time. Sometimes the duct opens and the mucus drains off. The small duct may close and the cyst may fill up again. Ruptured cysts may generate sulcus vocalis or mucosal bridges (Bouchayer et al. 1985). When removed properly, the vocal ligament heals without sequelae. Cysts may recur when parts of the epithelium stay inside the vocal fold.

Case Study 5.11

A 42-year-old lawyer had hoarseness for 4 years. A cyst of the left vocal fold had been operated on 2 years ago but had now recurred. Therapy should be aimed at a complete removal of the encapsulated epithelium within the lamina propria. The voice sounds mildly rough and breathy (R1 B1 H1). Dynamic vocal range is slightly restricted, which is noticed by the patient only after an above-average vocal load.

5.4.2.2 Sulcus Vocalis

Definition Sulcus vocalis is a narrow, linear depression in the surface of the vocal fold running longitudinally along the vocal folds. It is a deficiency of the lamina propria of the vocal fold and the covering epithelium, which is thin and not pliable.

Causes The aetiology of sulcus vocalis is uncertain (Ford et al. 1996). Possible aetiological factors are congenital, developmental or traumatic. In the elderly a sulcus vocalis may develop after inflammation such as laryngitis or myositis.

Signs and Symptoms The longitudinal extent of the furrow is variable, as is its depth (type I superficial, type IIa vergeture involving deeper layers of the lamina propria, type IIb similar to an open cyst (Giovanni et al. 2007)). It frequently disrupts normal vibration of the vocal folds. It is seen as a deepening or a line between the upper and lower edge of the vocal folds on laryngostroboscopic examination.

Treatment It is extremely difficult to treat a sulcus vocalis successfully, especially after myositis. Several surgical methods have been described. In principle scarred tissue is mobilised, or the thin epithelium is separated from the ligament. Augmentation is used in some cases. As the original structure of the sulcus is not changed by augmentation, this procedure seems to be the least invasive and best function-preserving one.

Prognosis Surgical results are often unsatisfactory owing to the lack of lamina propria substance, the attachment of epithelium to the vocal ligament and the frequently associated scar (Ford et al. 1996; Pontes and Behlau 1993).

Case Study 5.12

A 33-year-old student of theology had voice problems for more than 10 years. She is allergic to animals, moulds and some foods. Moreover, she has bronchial asthma and takes ciclesonide as an inhaled steroid. A cyst of the left vocal fold had been removed 2 years ago. The video shows scars on both vocal folds in the middle of the membranous part. The left vocal fold is thicker than the right one. There is a phase shift of about 45°, i.e. the left vocal fold moves later to the midline, with an incomplete closure. The voice range profile indicates that her vocal capacity is sufficient for a voice professional. The voice is normal (R0 B0 H0). Note a mild dyslalia in the form of a lisp, an interdental sigmatism.

5.4.2.3 Laryngocele

Definition A laryngocele is an air containing dilation of Morgagni's ventricle. It communicates with the ventricle via a narrow stalk. In cases of obliteration, the cavity fills with mucus. It expands either internally or externally or both.

Causes Congenital laryngoceles are lined with respiratory epithelium and filled with serous liquid. They are located in the paraglottal space lateral to the vocal folds or in the epiglottic vallecula. Acquired laryngoceles develop after closure of the laryngeal ventricle by inflammation, trauma or dispersed epithelium in the ventricular folds. The cystic dilation of the laryngeal saccule is filled by secretion from the encapsulated epithelium.

Signs and Symptoms Congenital laryngoceles lead to stridor and dyspnea. Acquired epithelial laryngoceles remain symptom-free over decades. The first sign of increase is hoarseness and only rarely dysphagia or dyspnoea. The contents may become infected and accumulate pus (laryngopyocele). This leads quickly to these symptoms, which are accompanied by pain.

The full clinical shape of laryngoceles mostly appears in adults. The ventricular fold, aryepiglottic fold or vocal fold is swollen. Even the epiglottic vallecula or piriform recess may be filled. The ventricular fold may cover the vocal fold and narrow the laryngeal entrance. In cases of expansion from the larynx through the thyrohyoid membrane, the external laryngocele may form a swelling of the neck. Internal laryngoceles are within the larynx itself and do not cross the thyrohyoid membrane. External laryngoceles penetrate the thyrohyoid membrane at the neurovascular bundle. The segment confined by the membrane is of normal size and connects normally with the laryngeal ventricle, whereas the portion outside the membrane is dilated. Mixed laryngoceles are dilated in both segments.

The secretion is serous in the beginning and thickens over time. It acquires a yellowish hue and resembles pus although bacteria are rarely detected. Laryngoceles are diagnosed by videolaryngostroboscopy. In cases of an external laryngocele, a CT scan may support the planning of surgery.

Treatment Laryngoceles are resected via microlaryngoscopy with a CO_2 laser. During surgery care has to be taken not to injure the vocal folds. External laryngoceles can be pulled into the inner larynx during micro-laryngoscopy and then excised. Open surgery from the neck can be avoided in most cases (Rosen and Simpson 2008).

Prognosis There is hardly a recurrence of laryngoceles when the lining epithelium is completely resected. Voice and respiration usually normalise and swallowing difficulties disappear.

Case Study 5.13

A 59-year-old pensioner noticed deterioration of her voice half a year ago without remarkable cause. Breathing and swallowing were not impaired. She has slipped discs between C5 and C7, suffers from an anxiety disorder treated by psychotherapy and has problems with her meniscus and nodes of the thyroid gland. None of these problems had anything to do with the laryngocele that inhibits the vibration of the right vocal fold,

restricts the voice range and leads to a moderately hoarse voice dominated by roughness (R2 B1 H2). After laser surgery voice function was restored.

5.4.2.4 Contact Ulcer/Contact Granuloma

Definition A contact ulcer or granuloma is primitive granulomatous tissue at the vocal process of the arytenoid cartilage arising from a defect in the mucosal lining.

Causes The literature suggests that these two clinical problems are probably the same disorder and seem to result from one of three causes or a combination of these. The first cause is intubation trauma during surgery (intubation granuloma); the second is glottal trauma from abuse-misuse, and the third aetiology, possibly the largest group, is laryngopharyngeal reflux (LPR). The risk of having intubation trauma leading to contact ulcer/granuloma is particularly high in children and women, as they have smaller airways and are thus more often traumatised by large tubes (Whited 1979). Excessive slamming of the arytenoids during production of low-pitched phonation coupled with excessively hard glottal attack and possibly increased loudness with frequent throat clearing and coughing may result in contact injury of the vocal folds (Boone and McFarlane 2000). A far larger group of patients with contact injury seems to be in the class of LPR. Stomach acid is forced up the oesophagus and irritates the area between the arytenoids in reflux patients (Koufman 1991).

Other causes that are not evident in the literature may be conscious or unconscious mental stress and insufficient glottal closure due to atrophy of the vocalis muscle. The latter may cause involuntary increase of adduction forces between the arytenoid cartilages or crossing of the vocal processes of the arytenoids thereby fostering the formation of contact granuloma.

Signs and Symptoms Patients with contact ulcer or contact granuloma may present with vocal fatigue accompanied with pain in the laryngeal area, severe dysphonia and frequent throat clearing.

Contact ulcers and contact granulomas generally arise from the vocal process of the arytenoid cartilage. They may also be above the glottal level when arytenoid apices contact during phonation. They may be on one side or appear on both and be complementary in shape, such as a hammer and anvil. The size may range from a shallow bowl-shaped area to a large exophytic ball lying on the vocal fold and thereby impeding vocal fold vibrations.

Treatment In case the diagnosis has not been confirmed by histological examination, the tissue should be removed. This is best performed via micro-laryngoscopy with jet ventilation and the use of a CO_2 laser. Voice therapy is helpful in case of habitually pressed voice to regain a normal voice.

Prognosis Contact granulomas often recur shortly after excision. In this case repeated interventions should be made only when the voice is affected. Once the aetiological trauma and irritants that initiated the contact granuloma/ulcer are removed, they will spontaneously resolve within months.

5.4.2.5 Papilloma

Definition Papillomas are wartlike growths originating from the epithelium of the vocal folds and the mucosa of the larynx after infection with human papilloma virus (HPV).

Causes Recurrent respiratory papillomatosis is most commonly caused by and associated with HPV-6 and HPV-11 subtypes. It may be transferred during vaginal birth from mother to child. There is no evidence that it is transmitted through oral sex, and it is not considered a sexually transmitted disease.

Signs and Symptoms Papillomas involving the larynx frequently occur in young children. They are the most common laryngeal tumour in children. Clinical presentation of laryngeal papilloma is progressive airway obstruction and dysphonia that may even progress to aphonia.

Treatment Surgical treatment in most cases is laser surgery. In order to protect deeper layers of the lamina propria, papilloma should be vaporised only down to the epithelial level, not below it. In order not to implant epithelial cells into the vocal fold, subepithelial infusion should be applied before laser vaporisation. Some surgeons prefer conventional excision surgery in order to prevent scattering viable papillomatous cells into deeper layers of the vocal folds. The use of a micro-debrider is also possible but it should be handled with great care. Scars can easily form when the epithelium has been removed completely. Repeated surgery can lead to postsurgical webbing of the vocal folds and to vocal fold scar formation. Hence papillomas should only be removed when they interfere with the airway (Boone and McFarlane 2000; Wetmore et al. 1985) or cause loss of voice. Radiation therapy is obsolete.

Adjuvant medical therapies, such as interferon therapy, retinoic acid, indol-3-carbinol and cidofovir (Lundquist et al. 1984; Thompson and Kershner 2007) have been tried, but all failed to cure the disease.

In adult men, laryngeal secretions tend to become negative, and serum antibody titres tend to increase after vaccination with Gardasil. However, there was no significant difference between serum level of antibodies, negative laryngeal secretions and the presence of papillomatosis 1 year later (Hirai et al. 2018; Makiyama et al. 2017).

A promising line of therapy based on successful case reports includes systemic application of bevacizumab as well as cidofovir and epidermal growth factor receptor (EGFR) inhibitors such as gefitinib and erlotinib for emergency treatment when the airway is severely compromised and other therapeutic measures fail (Best et al. 2012; Fernandez-Bussy et al. 2018; Kalanjeri et al. 2017; Mohr et al. 2014; Nagel et al. 2009; Rogers et al. 2013).

Prognosis Papilloma of the airway in children is serious, because of its recurrent and persistent threat to compromise the small airway. There is no proof that papillomatosis stops recurring about the time of puberty. There is no cure for this benign disease.

Case Study 5.14

A 66-year-old woman had been suffering from hoarseness for 6 months. In her history she had undergone surgery for a meningioma of the falx cerebri 3 years ago and has underactivity of the thyroid gland. The laryngeal examination revealed a papilloma of both vocal folds. Her voice has nearly disappeared. Vocal range is restricted to a mere whisper. After careful removal of the flat papilloma spread along the vocal fold margins, her voice improved towards near normal function.

5.4.2.6 Benign Neoplasia

Definition Benign neoplasia is an uncontrolled propagation of vascular or neural cells. One may also find extracellular deposition of substances leading to vocal fold bulging and dysphonia.

Causes The causes of benign neoplasia often cannot be determined.

Signs and Symptoms Neurofibromas are the most common benign laryngeal tumours. They appear very similar to inclusion cysts and rarely cause symptoms. They are much firmer than inclusion cysts (Anderson 2007). Adult haemangiomas may arise from the glottis or the supraglottis. They tend to form uniform submucosal masses.

Treatment Biopsy is needed for diagnosis, and they can generally be treated with complete surgical excision. Treatment is determined by the severity of dysphonia or airway obstruction (Hoffman et al. 2003). Asymptomatic laryngeal masses with a benign appearance can be observed without a biopsy in most cases.

Prognosis Benign laryngeal neoplasms are rare and the course of disease cannot be predicted. Usually there is no recurrence after surgical treatment.

Case Study 5.15

A 46-year-old pastry cook who worked formerly as a kindergarten teacher had been suffering from voice impairment for 1.5 year. She is otherwise healthy and takes no medication. The video shows a markedly bulging left vocal fold. Surgery was planned under the suspicion of a laryngocele. However, it turned out to be a solid mass that was histologically diagnosed as a neurofibroma. The speaking voice is a bit higher than normal, the vocal range restricted. The voice sound is moderately hoarse (R2 B2H2).

Case Study 5.16

A 45-year-old pharmaceutical representative had been suffering from reduced vocal capacity and recurring hoarseness for several years. Laryngeal examination revealed a swelling of the right ventricular fold and a small oedema of the right vocal fold margin. Surgery was planned on the suspicion of a laryngeal cyst. However, during the intervention a solid mass was discovered under the surface which turned out to be bulging cartilage. Vocal range is restricted; the voice is mildly hoarse (R1 B1 H1).

Examples of benign lesions of the larynx are shown in Fig. 5.7.

5.5 Gastro-oesopharyngeal Reflux Influences on Larynx and Voice

Virginie Woisard

5.5.1 What Is Gastro-oesophageal Reflux?

Gastro-oesophageal reflux (GER) occurs when stomach contents flow back up into the oesophagus. This reflux is a physiological phenomenon with an average of 50 episodes per day, mainly after meals. Gastro-oesophageal reflux disease (GERD) is a more serious, chronic—or long-lasting—form of GER. The backward flow of stomach acid into the oesophagus causes symptoms or oesophageal mucosal lesions. The diagnosis is based on pH monitoring studies. GERD is defined (Richter 2003) by up to 50 reflux episodes below pH 4.0 per day into the oesophagus or a time below pH 4.0 up to 1.5% of the whole time of the monitoring (24 h). Classical symptoms are heartburn (uncomfortable,

Vocal fold nodules often seen in singers

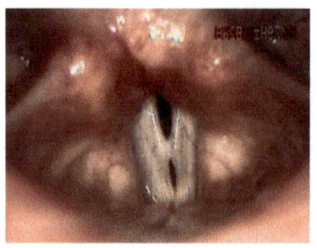

Vocal fold papilloma

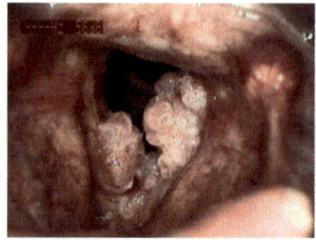

Oedema and phlebectasia secondary to reflux, allergy and infection

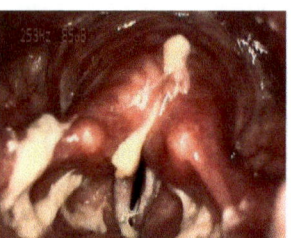

Reinke's oedema

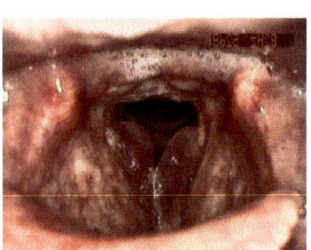

Laryngocele ventriculus laryngis

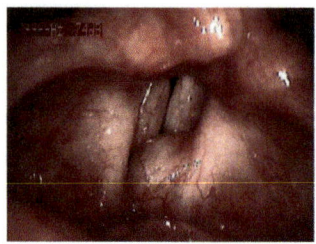

Fig. 5.7 Benign lesions of the larynx with tabular characterisation

upward burning feeling in the mid-chest, behind the breastbone), acid regurgitation and foul-smelling eructations. They may be absent in more than half the patients presenting with extra-digestive manifestations (Jaspersen et al. 2003). Other non-typical manifestations may involve the upper aero-digestive tract (hoarseness, cough, throat clearing, globus pharyngeus, laryngeal hyperirritability, laryngospasm, pharyngitis, otitis media, laryngitis, laryngeal pyogenic granuloma, glottal and subglottal stenosis, laryngeal carcinoma) or lungs (asthma, bronchitis, bronchiectasis, aspiration pneumonia, idiopathic fibrosis) (Galli et al. 2006; Balkissoon and Kenn 2012).

Digestive symptoms, endoscopic findings and pH measurement allow the establishment of guidelines for the follow-up of patients with GERD by gastroenterologists, with the aim of decreasing the symptoms and prevent oesophageal complications (mainly oesophagitis with haemorrhagic or cancer risks). Thus three types of reflux are usually described:

- Physiological reflux occurring just after a meal. This is regurgitation of some of the stomach's digestive juices and food without pain symptoms
- Symptomatic reflux giving discrete signs of digestive dysfunction, such as heartburn and dyspepsia, the sensations of more or less acid reflux into the pharynx, which are perfectly tolerated. This is not a real disease because there is no complication
- Pathological reflux, meaning that the patient suffers signs of hurting with the GER. These signs can be digestive or not, related to GERD or to laryngopharyngeal reflux (LPR). Proton pump inhibitor (PPI) therapy remains the cornerstone of treatment (Koufman 2002; Richter 2003)

Furthermore, heavy reflux may occur with aspiration of much material (mostly during sleep) leading to laryngospasm and threatening and frightening apnoea.

5.5.2 What Is Laryngopharyngeal Reflux?

Laryngopharyngeal reflux (LPR) refers to the backflow of stomach contents into the laryngopharynx. There are numerous synonyms for LPR in the medical literature; the most accepted of these terms is extra-oesophageal reflux.

Koufman (1991, 2002) demonstrated the existence of pharyngeal reflux by a double-probe pH monitoring (oesophageal and pharyngeal) performed on an ambulatory basis over 24 h. Of the 206 otolaryngology patients with GERD undergoing diagnostic pH monitoring, 62% had abnormal oesophageal pH, and 30% demonstrated reflux into the pharynx. Pharyngeal reflux was present in 58% of patients presenting laryngeal symptoms. Its duration was shorter and it arose more frequently in a vertical position. Lower oesophageal sphincter dysfunction and oesophageal motility disorders were frequently suspected. Other studies also support a role for LPR. For example, in patients with resected benign true vocal fold lesions, the prevalence of laryngopharyngeal reflux is higher than that of pathological gastro-oesophageal reflux (Beltsis et al. 2011). The diagnosis of LPR is often missed because symptoms associated classically with reflux, such as dyspepsia and pyrosis, are frequently absent because patients with LPR either do not develop *oesophagitis* or do not respond to acid reflux with typical symptoms such as heartburn (Ford 2005).

Despite these arguments, controversy exists because of difficulties in making the diagnosis. An LPR event is evident when pH in the proximal sensor abruptly drops to less than 4 during or immediately after distal acid exposure (exposure near the lower oesophageal sphincter). LPR is confirmed when total acid exposure time (percentage of time during 24-h monitoring when the sensor detects pH levels <4) is more than 1% (Kawamura et al. 2004). However, there are no standardised and normative data to consider pathological versus physiological reflux. That is why the most frequently used tools are the reflux find-ing score (RFS) and the reflux symptom index (RSI) developed by Belafsky et al. (2001b, 2002b). Currently, the two main diagnostic tools are laryngoscopy and reflux monitoring of LPR. On laryngoscopy, the signs most commonly used to diagnose LPR are erythema and oedema of the larynx; however, these signs are not specific for LPR, may be associated with other causes and may even be found in healthy individuals. In addition, pH testing has low sensitivity in diagnosing gastro-oesophageal reflux disease-related laryngeal findings (Abou-Ismail and Vaezi 2011).

RSI and RFS are easy to administer in the routine care of patients suspected of having laryngopharyngeal reflux. These scales are described in Table 5.4.

By implementation in daily use, most patients may not need examination in the first-line assessment of LPR. These examinations can be reserved for nonresponders, restricting uncontrolled prescription of PPIs (Habermann et al. 2012).

However, disagreement persists regarding optimum diagnostic techniques, criteria of normality and treatment efficacy. Because of a paucity of convincing evidence regarding techniques for establishing a definitive diagnosis and causation in individual patients, and because of a plethora of imperfect studies that have produced conflicting conclusions, LPR diagnosis and management remain controversial (Sataloff et al. 2010; Hawkshaw et al. 2013). For this reason, new approaches are being explored, such as pepsin immunohistochemical staining of the laryngeal mucosal epithelia (Jiang et al. 2011).

5.5.3 Reflux and Larynx

Traditionally, laryngeal abnormalities may be caused by direct injury or by a secondary mechanism. Direct injury is due to contact of acid and pepsin with the laryngeal mucosa, resulting in mucosal damage (Koufman 1991; Delahunty and Cherry 1968; Cherry and Margulies 1968; Lillemoe

Table 5.4 Description of the reflux symptom index and the reflux finding score developed from Belafsky et al. (2001b, 2002b)

	The reflux symptom index (RSI)	The reflux finding score (RFS)
Instructions	Within the past month, how did the following problems affect you? Ordinal scale: 0–5 (0, no problem; 5, severe problem)	Assign a grade of intensity to the different laryngoscopic signs Ordinal scale, specific for each item
Items	Hoarseness or other voice problems	Infraglottic oedema (pseudosulcus). Scale: 0–2 0, absent; 2, present
	Clearing throat	Ventricular obliteration. Scale: 0–4 0, none; 2, partial; 4, complete
	Excess throat mucus or postnasal drip	Erythema/hyperaemia. Scale 0–4 0, none; 2, arytenoids only; 4, diffuse
	Difficulty swallowing food, liquid or pills	Vocal fold oedema. Scale 0–4 0, none; 1, mild; 2, moderate; 3, severe; 4, polypoid
	Coughing after eating or after lying down	Diffuse laryngeal oedema. Scale 0–4 0, none; 1, mild; 2, moderate; 3, severe; 4, obstructing
	Breathing difficulties or choking episodes	Posterior commissure hypertrophy. Scale 0–4 0, none; 1, mild; 2, moderate; 3, severe; 4, obstructing
	Troublesome or annoying cough	Granuloma/granulation. Scale 0–2 0, absent; 2, present
	Sensations of something sticking in the throat or lump in throat	Thick endolaryngeal mucus. Scale 0–2 0, absent; 2, present
	Heartburn, chest pain, indigestion or stomach acid coming up	
Interpretation of the scores	An RSI >9 indicates patients symptomatic for LPR	An RFS >7 predicts a 95% certainty of patients with LPR

et al. 1982). Alternatively, irritation of the distal oesophagus by acid may cause a reflex mediated by the *vagus nerve*, resulting in chronic cough and throat clearing, which may produce traumatic injury to the laryngeal mucosa (Ramet 1994; Sacre and Vandenplas 1989). Recently, some authors have been focusing on the specific molecular aetiopathology of LPR. Researchers have considered that the failure of intrinsic defences in the larynx may cause changes in laryngeal epithelium, such as alterations in carbonic anhydrases and E-cadherin (Wood et al. 2011). Mucin expression also varies according to the severity of reflux. Moreover, they have discovered the presence of H^+/K^+-ATPase pumps around the submucosal glands of the human larynx. The lack of carbonic anhydrase in the epithelium of the vocal folds in cases of LPR supports the hypothesis that reflux-related damage mainly affects the glottal area. Finally, pepsin is often found on laryngeal epithelial biopsy and in sputum of patients with pH test-proven GERD and symptoms of LPR. Pepsin, at pH 7, in non-acidic refluxes causes damage by becoming reactivated inside the cell. Inhibitors of peptic activity hold promise as a new therapy for reflux (Wassenaar et al. 2011; Johnston et al. 2010). Further research is required to identify a definitive mechanism for mucosal injury.

For laryngeal disorders, the most recent evidence indicates that LPR represents a complex spectrum of abnormalities. LPR appears to be associated strongly with, or be a significant aetiological cofactor in, about half of these patients (Garrigues et al. 2003). Typical laryngoscopic findings described as diagnostic of reflux in the literature are:

- Posterior laryngitis (Kamel et al. 1994; Garrigues et al. 2003; Ulualp et al. 1999; Ylitalo et al. 2001)
- Subglottal stenosis (Little et al. 1985)
- Pseudosulcus (see Fig. 5.8a and in comparison sulcus in Fig. 5.8b) and partial effacement or obliteration of the laryngeal ventricle (Belafsky et al. 2002a; Belafsky 2003; Hickson et al. 2001)

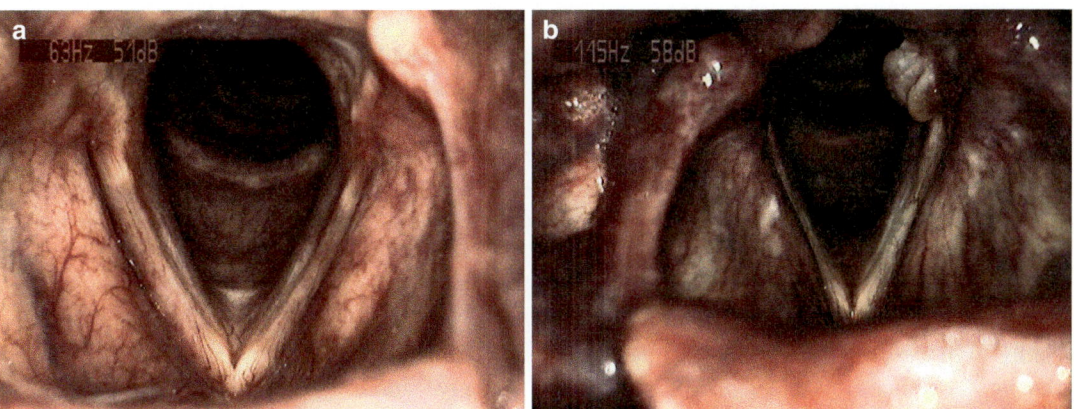

Fig. 5.8 (**a**) Pseudosulcus. With kind permission from Prof. Tadeus Nawka, Berlin. (**b**) Granuloma and sulcus for comparison with pseudosulcus in (**a**). With kind permission from Prof. Tadeus Nawka, Berlin

Table 5.5 Suggestive laryngeal aspects

TYPE of LESION		LOCALISATION
Erythema		Posterior margins
Oedema		
Pachydermia		Posterior third of the vocal folds
Granulation tissue		
Ulceration		The whole vocal fold
Granuloma		
Leucoplasia		The whole larynx

The arrow describes the decreasing frequency

These diagnostic criteria combine the type and the localisation of the lesion. They are reported in Table 5.5 by decreasing frequency (Woisard et al. 1996).

On the other hand, oedema of the interarytenoid mucosa seen on endoscopy is related to endoscopic-positive oesophagitis (EE) and is an independent predictor of EE.

Unfortunately, laryngoscopy cannot be considered as a tool determining the diagnosis of reflux because of the poor intra- and inter-assessor agreements of the scores developed to establish the clinical laryngoscopic diagnosis (Sataloff et al. 2010; Branski et al. 2002; Welby-Gieusse et al. 2008). The diagnosis reflux laryngeal disease remains too examiner-dependent.

Moreover, the association of several factors may lead to the apparition of specific laryngeal lesion. For example, mechanical laryngeal trauma and reflux are factors provoking granuloma; reflux and inhaled corticosteroids can promote fungal laryngitis.

According to recent advances, it is assumed that the gastro-oesophageal reflux (GER) is a possible co-promoting factor for squamous cell carcinoma development in the upper parts of the gastrointestinal and respiratory systems, considering the higher frequency of acid-dependent lesions in the population suffering GER. Laryngopharyngeal reflux appears to be an important risk factor in the development of laryngeal carcinoma. Some authors have demonstrated that gastric reflux is an independent risk factor for laryngopharyngeal carcinoma (Ozlugedik et al. 2006; Mercante et al. 2003; Langevin et al. 2013; Coca-Pelaz et al. 2013), while the prevalence of *Helicobacter pylori* is lower than the prevalence of LPR and is not correlated with the risk of cancer (Cekin et al. 2012).

Finally, reflux dysphonia is possible without posterior laryngitis in laryngoscopy.

5.5.4 Reflux and Voice

GER is a vocal risk factor often entangled with other factors such as stress, poisoning from smoking and vocal overload. It is systematically sought in vocal disorders, but the multifactorial aspect of dysphonia makes difficult the precise determination of the role of each factor. Therefore, if the reality of a causal relationship between the GER and laryngeal symptoms is no longer discussed, highlighting it in clinical practice remains difficult.

The problems of voice affect more than 30% of the population at some period of life. The GER is also a very frequent phenomenon. Its prevalence in adults is from 30 to 40% for one episode at least monthly and from 5 to 10% for a daily episode. Prevalence of the extra-digestive symptoms is estimated at 30% (Jaspersen et al. 2003). Recently, Randhawa et al. (2009) highlighted the risk of masking of GER by other factors, such as allergy and food intolerance, that lead to overestimation of the role of the reflux. Allergy, more specifically allergic rhinitis, affects approximately 24% of the population. These authors note the very high frequency of this effect and the difficulties it presents to highlight causal relations between these various other entities.

Therefore GER and LPR cannot be considered as a disease per se within the framework of ENT manifestations. They act as cofactors and must be integrated into a multifactorial causation with regard to the symptom from which the patient suffers. Richter illustrated this construct (Fig. 5.9) by a pyramid with a decreasing prevalence of the GER in the extra-digestive manifestations. He also suggested that the need for therapeutic tests with omeprazole decreases with the decreasing specificity of the disease for GER.

Thus, in the presence of an ENT manifestation of reflux, the physician has to adopt a holistic approach, analysing the various factors contributing to the emergence of the symptom.

This situation leads to an overdiagnosis of laryngopharyngeal reflux as the cause of hoarseness (Thomas and Zubiaur 2013).

Regarding the treatment, one proposal is to plan empirical anti-reflux treatment according to the reflux index system (RSI) and reflux finding score (RFS). There is no agreement about the modalities of the therapeutic test, but some authors recommend the use of a double dose of a proton pump inhibitor for 3 months.

Proton pump inhibitors (PPIs) are medications that are ubiquitous in a gastroenterologist's practice.

Their safety among pharmacological agents has been recognised despite the reports of

Fig. 5.9 GER prevalence and digestive and extra-digestive manifestations (with kind permission from Elsevier, adapted from Richter (2003), in the top triangle Misc replaced by Infections)

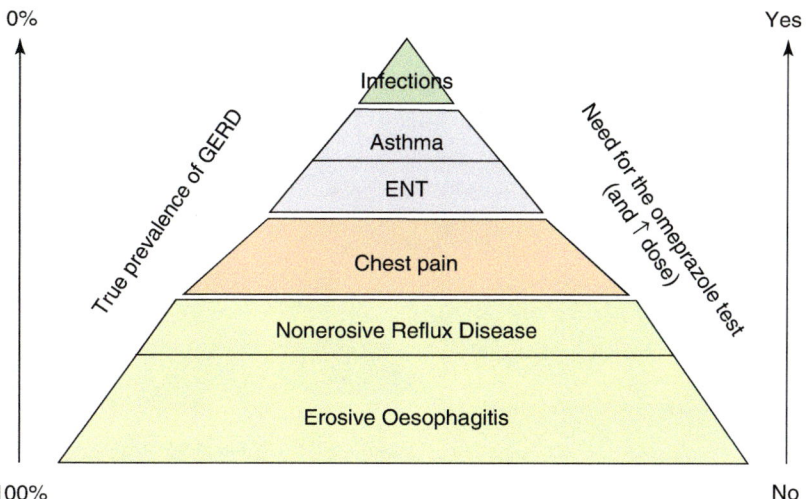

potential adverse effects associated with their use. These potential interactions have ranged from alteration of the absorption of vitamins and minerals, metabolic effects on bone density, alteration of pharmacokinetics/pharmacodynamics and related drug interactions and alterations of intended effect, infection risk to hypersensitivity responses with consequent organ damage (de la Coba et al. 2016).

In the study of Naiboglu et al. (2011), antireflux treatment led to significantly reduced laryngopharyngeal symptoms and signs. Longer times of treatment may be needed for complete resolution of symptoms. This method seems to be effective, but the level of proof remains low because of the lack of placebo controls. Therefore, many physicians empirically prescribe reflux medication as a primary therapy, even when symptoms of gastro-oesophageal reflux disease are not present (Ruiz et al. 2014). The current management recommendation for this group of patients is empirical therapy with twice-daily PPIs for 1–3 months. In the majority of those who are unresponsive to such therapy, other causes of laryngeal irritation should be considered. Surgical fundoplication is most effective in those who are responsive to acid-suppressive therapy.

In broad outline, three situations can be met in phoniatric practice with a therapeutic proposal, as communicated here.

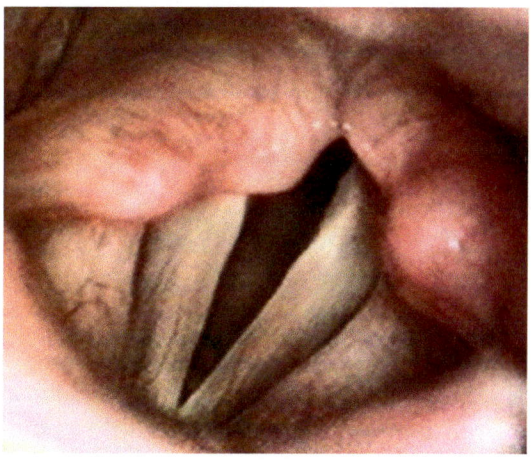

Fig. 5.10 Oedema of the posterior margin

First Situation Dysphonia is associated with suggestive signs of GER, but the reflux is not in the foreground. The medical history may or may not highlight a pyrosis or other digestive symptoms. The laryngeal lesions due to the reflux are limited to an erythema or oedema of the posterior margin (Fig. 5.10) more or less associated with a thickening of the interarytenoid area (Fig. 5.13).

The GER is only retained as an associated risk factor. The main factor may be dysfunctional, psychological or anatomical. The treatment is based on the hygiene and dietary measures associated with a medical treatment according to the degree of posterior inflammation of the larynx.

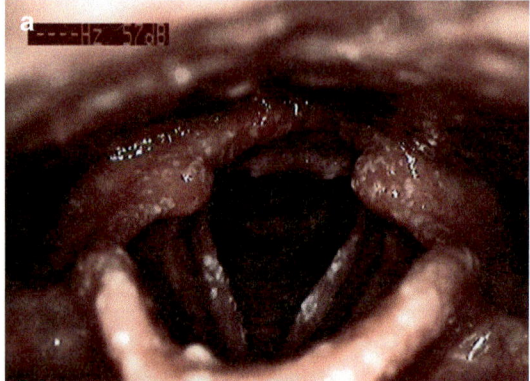

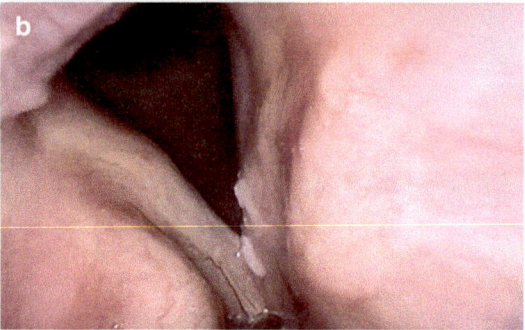

Fig. 5.11 (**a**) Fungal laryngitis. With kind permission from Prof. Tadeus Nawka, Berlin. (**b**) Leukokeratosis. With kind permission from the German Voice Clinic, Hamburg

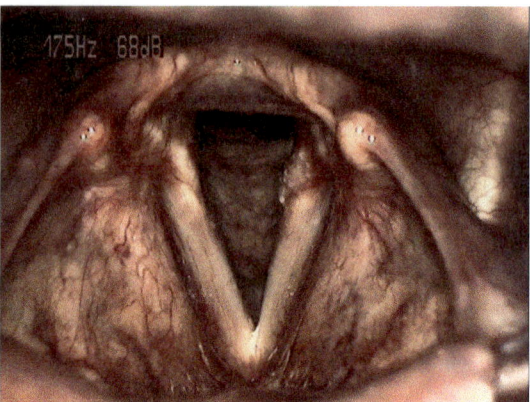

Fig. 5.12 Contact ulcerations on the left side and thickening of the interarytenoid area. With kind permission from Prof. Tadeus Nawka, Berlin

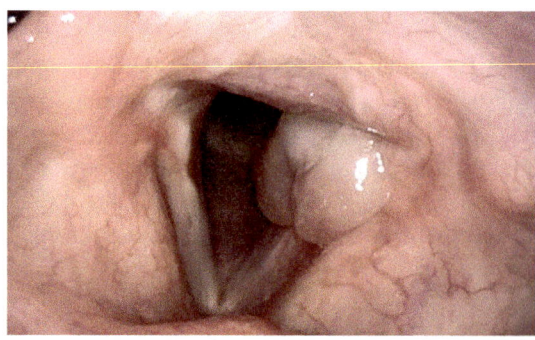

Fig. 5.13 Erythema of the posterior margin, thickening of the interarytenoid area and granuloma. With kind permission from the German Voice Clinic, Hamburg

Taking into consideration the GER in case of laryngeal surgery is important and may lead to a preventive treatment before and after the surgery.

Second Situation GER may be the main aetiological factor of the vocal disorder. It leads to more 'specific' lesions. In the absence of other associated irritating factors, chronic laryngitis is observed. It is necessary to look for fungal infection in the presence of an aspect of white lesions such as leukokeratosis laryngitis (Fig. 5.11a, b).

Associated with vocal overload or with closed glottis efforts, the GER promotes contact ulcerations (Fig. 5.12), which cannot heal completely, giving a granuloma (Fig. 5.13). The concomitant association of episodes of pyrosis and closed glottis efforts can provoke painful posterior laryngitis.

Finally, in a context of intubation, reflux favours complications such as granuloma and laryngeal synechia.

Medical treatment is necessary by inhibiting the proton pump. A tri-therapy can be proposed: antacids, prokinetic and antisecretory. It is always associated with the hygiene and dietary measures and with the management of the various associated vocal risk factors, to avoid relapse upon stopping the treatment.

Third Situation This is very rare and corresponds to an atypical laryngeal lesion in a GER context resistant to the medical treatment and may be an indication for surgery. This is an anterior granuloma or a granulomatous laryngitis (Fig. 5.14). This latter lesion involves the whole larynx and corresponds to an unspecific inflammation seen in the histology. Despite the GER treatment, the treatment remains problematic with questions about its evolution.

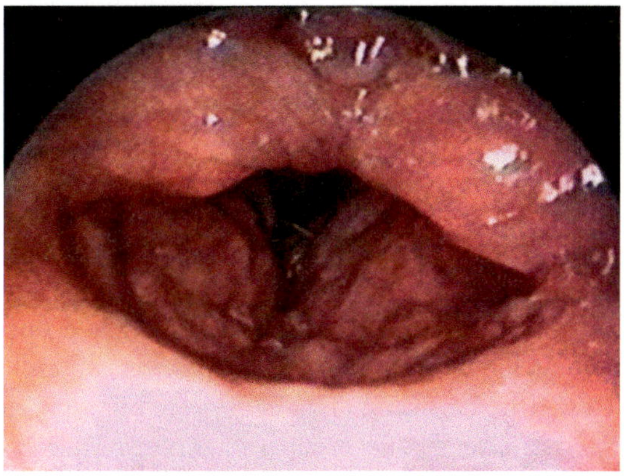

Fig. 5.14 Anterior granuloma or a granulomatous laryngitis

Another aspect of the question is the physiological interaction of speech or singing with reflux. Vocal load without singing is probably not an important aetiological factor for laryngopharyngeal reflux. However, the increase of intra-abdominal pressure and stress appears to increase GER in singers (Cammarota et al. 2007), and some authors have described that laryngopharyngeal reflux affects choristers more often than teachers or control subjects without vocal load at work (Hočevar-Boltežar et al. 2012). These results suggest that singing as the main professional activity can notably contribute to the development of the reflux.

Case Study 5.17
A 42-year-old driver at an embassy had an operation on the larynx 6 years ago. For about 2 years, he had noticed a 'flap', a foreign body, during breathing. A biopsy taken 2 weeks ago revealed an unspecific granulation polyp. The patient has type 2 diabetes and takes metformin. Contact granuloma may be associated with reflux, but not necessarily. The video shows a typical contact granuloma on the left that during adduction extends above and below the right vocal process on the opposite side and inhibits complete closure. Note that there is also a small inframarginal cyst on the right side. Vocal range is markedly reduced; the voice is mildly hoarse (R1 B1 H1).

Case Study 5.18
A 62-year-old housewife has always had a dark voice. After an infection of the upper airways her voice had become worse. She suffers from reflux. Her medication is pantoprazole because of reflux, thyroxine because of a thyroidectomy and clopidogrel because of heart attacks. She stopped smoking a year ago. The video shows chronic laryngitis. The epithelium and the inter-arytenoid region are swollen and keratotic. The vocal range is reduced; the voice quality mildly hoarse (R1 B1 H1).

5.5.5 Conclusion

It can be assumed that reflux that reaches the larynx can damage it. Because the symptoms possibly related to LPR can be linked to other causes, a careful consideration of the patient's medical history is of utmost importance, followed by mandatory laryngoscopy. Several laryngeal and vocal risk factors are often present in voice disorders, highlighting a frequent multifactorial context. This level of complexity explains the poor level of scientific proof and why the role of GER remains a 'myth' fed by practical clinical observations. The search for the different factors involved and their organisation into a hierarchy allow the determination of a strategy of care, by ranking the various therapeutic options.

Diagnostic procedures, such as the trial administration of proton pump inhibitors or long-term pH measurement, should be used selectively. Depending on the individual symptoms, lifestyle changes, breathing or voice therapy or PPI therapy might be useful.

5.6 Central Neurogenic Voice Disorders

John Rubin and Kevin Shields

5.6.1 Introduction

This section focuses on central neurological issues. For further information on the peripheral neurological system, please see Sects. 1.2 and 5.7.

In the twenty-first century, voice remains the primary means of human communication, in spite of the massive increase in the use of electronic devices. With the advent of Skype and telemedicine communications, it is the authors' opinion that an increasing number of currently non-verbal teletextual types of electronic communication will incorporate the human voice owing to the richness of the signal that it includes.

Sound signals are used to communicate intellectual content, linguistic and paralinguistic content and emotional content. There is little doubt that the voice and the vocal tract are interlinked to emotions and feelings. It is a common experience that the phone will ring, the listener will hear a sound (that is frequently frequency-limited) and within a matter of moments, even if the speaker has not been heard from in many months or years, the listener will be able to both recognise the listener, the paralinguistic as well as the linguistic message, and respond. This response may well be influenced by a sudden change in the listener's autonomic system as well as central nervous system. How can this occur?

In an attempt to respond to the question posed above, we need to go back to basics. The brain has approximately 100 billion neurons. These include nerve cells and glial (support) cells. The neurons, in essence, act as 'on-off' switches. When 'on' they transmit nerve signals-electrical signals/current. Neurons are made up of a cell body (soma), nucleus, dendrites (that can branch multiple times and communicate with other cells) and axons (that can be very long (metres)). Synapses connect the neurons; they are found between somas and dendrites of nerve fibres or axonal terminals. Each neuron has between 1000 and 10,000 synapses. When an action potential reaches a synapse, it triggers the release of tiny amounts (quanta) of neurotransmitter causing depolarisation of the postsynaptic region. There are hundreds of neurotransmitters, both excitatory and inhibitory. Well-known ones include dopamine, serotonin, acetylcholine, noradrenaline and gamma aminobutyric acid (GABA). Whether or not an action potential is generated in the target neuron will depend on a variety of factors, including the integration and summation of inhibitory and excitatory synaptic inputs to that cell. Thus the heart of neural function is part electrical part chemical.

Information tends to reach the brain via neural networks. A typical, rather simple, but powerful neural network is that of the laryngeal adductor reflex. As an example, imagine that the readers were eating crisps at the time they were reading this section and a crisp accidently irritated one side of the epiglottis or lateral pharyngeal wall. This irritation would elicit neurons to fire, via the internal branch of the superior laryngeal nerve, and neural activity will go up to the nodose ganglion and then to the ipsilateral nucleus tractus solitarius. At this point there would be interneural connections to both nucleus ambiguus. This would effect a bilateral motor response to the internal laryngeal muscles with a resultant glottal closure reflex. This reflex arc is very fast, the conduction velocity in the extracranial nerves being approximately 60 m/s, leading to a glottal closure response in less than 60 ms from the stimulating event. Had the stimulating event been at the glottis or subglottal level, the effector would have been via the recurrent rather than the superior laryngeal nerve.

The surface of the brain is grey-brown, the colour of the neuronal cell bodies (grey matter) and the neuropil (dendrites and unmyelinated axons). Grey matter regions are typically involved in muscle control and sensory perception. They can be thought of as the Chief Executive Officers and Trustees, performing executive functions of the brain, processing information. Deep to this lie the axon layers with white sheath (myelinated). This is the white matter and can perhaps be thought of as the personal administrators and middle managers—white matter tends to carry information.

Historically the brain was anatomically divided into separate lobes that were functionally distinct, whereby the frontal lobe is involved in speech planning and reason and contains the primary and supplementary motor cortices; the parietal lobe in sensory perception and praxis, with sensory feedback from the body; the temporal lobe with speech perception, some memory and hearing; the occipital lobe with the visual cortex;

the cerebellum with movement and balance; and the brainstem with breathing and swallowing. The brain also has two hemispheres connected by the corpus callosum. In general the right hemisphere is said to deal with visual activities. It is more 'intuitive' than the left hemisphere and can be thought of as putting information together, grouping it. For example, if a car is viewed, the right hemisphere activity might be to note 'I recognise that, it is a car'. The left hemisphere is said to be dominant in 95% of the population. It is more analytical than the right hemisphere, analysing the information collected by the right hemisphere. It also tends to deal more with language, understanding and expression.

5.6.2   Language

In terms of language, the left temporal and frontal areas are dominant in 95% of individuals for language. Please see Figs. 1.47 and 1.48 in Sect. 1.2, demonstrating areas active in language on the brain surface (Fig. 1.47) and functional anatomy of language processing (Fig. 1.48). The right side is somewhat equivalent for environmental noise, spatial skills and prosody (Nasreddine et al. 1999). Wernicke's area is one of the two parts of the cerebral cortex that have been linked to speech since the nineteenth century. It is located in the posterior section of the superior temporal gyrus in the left (or dominant) cerebral hemisphere and encircles the auditory cortex on the Sylvian fissure. It is neuroanatomically described as being in the posterior part of Brodmann's area (BA 22). Wernicke's area is the site that on functional MRI studies is most consistently implicated in understanding of written and spoken language/word recognition (DeWitt and Rauschecker 2012). Broca's area is the other classically recognised speech-related area. It is a region of the frontal lobe of the left hemisphere usually identified as the pars opercularis and pars triangularis of the inferior frontal gyrus, neuroanatomically as Brodmann's area 44 and 45 (BA 44, 45). It abuts on and instructs the motor cortex regarding articulation and speech.

Previously it was believed that information passed from Wernicke's to Broca's area through the arcuate fasciculus, a band of white matter deep to the supramarginal gyrus connecting both language areas, but this is in dispute. Broca's area initiates a motor plan that is transmitted to the primary motor cortex (Brodmann's area 4) to pronounce the words. The motor cortex, in coordination with the supplementary motor area, basal ganglia and cerebellum, sends corticobulbar fibres to implement speech sounds (Nasreddine et al. 1999). More recent functional imaging has supported a larger range of processing areas for speech reception and language processing, and the last word has certainly not been written on this subject (Newman et al. 2010).

According to Jürgens and colleagues, in many mammals there is a visceromotor subcortical network of brain regions dedicated to phonatory species-specific calls. In a sense the periacqueductal grey can be considered at the core, regulating neurons of the lower brainstem via the reticular formation from the lateral pontomedullary- and limbic-related regions. There are cortical laryngeal projections from the anterior cingulate gyrus (Jürgens 2002a, b, 2009). In humans, some aspects of emotive voicing exploit this older pathway. However, for linguistic and paralinguistic speech, there are more direct corticobulbar projections to the reticular formation in effect bypassing the limbic system. Temporal lobe activity is critical for auditory self-regulation. The time from a thought to sound is approximately 130 ms.

In the mammalian brainstem the nucleus ambiguus and retroambiguus are of particular importance from an effector standpoint for laryngeal and expiratory muscle control. The midbrain and cerebellum are substantially involved in feedback and timing (Benninger et al. 2006; Jürgens 2002a, b, 2009; Kuypers 1958).

5.6.3   Neurolaryngology History-Taking

History taking in neurological voice disorders is of paramount importance (Woodson 2008).

Temporal development of the disorder, symptom description, associated features, handedness, associated intercurrent or past medical disease, past psychiatric history and family history have all been highlighted as integral to the neurological history (Nasreddine et al. 1999). We also feel that emphasis should be placed on aspects relating to the psychosocial history, as this is often the key to successful management and rehabilitation.

Vocal fatigue, vocal weakness, pain when speaking, increased effort relating to speech, glottal tightness, pitch breaks and tremor all point towards a neurological cause of the disorder (Woodson 2008). Changes in normal vocal quality (strain/strangle, harshness), vocal effort (range, breathiness, fatigue), vocal pitch (monopitch, loss of stability of pitch with yodelling or pitch breaks, etc.) and vocal tremor should all be ascertained and may point to problems at the level of the vocal folds. Speech-related problems such as articulatory issues, slurred or unintelligible speech, velopharyngeal insufficiency with hypernasality point towards bulbar or suprabulbar pathology. Woodson (2008) notes that hoarseness in isolation is far less likely to point to a neurological cause than when associated with dysphagia. Again the history is crucial.

5.6.4 The Clinical Examination: General

When evaluating a patient with a suspected neurological voice (or swallow) disorder, the patient will often come in with the diagnosis already substantiated. None the less, the first assessment by the ENT surgeon/phoniatrician should be global rather than ENT-specific; otherwise it is easy to miss a critical clue to diagnosis and management. In particular affect, gait, posture and coordination, movement (spontaneous, tremor, etc.), reflexes and tone all need reviewing, before the more-focused ENT/phoniatric examination. Let us review these.

Affect Flattening of the intonation could be indicative of depression. It can also be seen in neurological disorders affecting the frontal lobes and subcortical white matter. Parkinsonian movement disorders cause hypomimia with a paucity of facial expression. Hypothyroidism should be considered. A labile affect could be seen in a bipolar disorder, and potentially also in thyrotoxicosis. It can also be seen in a variety of neurological disorders, but it should be remembered that certain psychoactive medications (e.g. dopaminergic agonists) can cause behavioural abnormalities.

Gait, Posture and Coordination Gait and posture in Parkinsonism are characterised by small steps (marche a petit pas) with successively more rapid steps (festination). Posture is not uncommonly forward-held with the spine bent forward, head down, immobile (akinesia) and rigid. Gait and posture in individuals with cerebellar disease can be broad-based, with a coarse trunk tremor (titubation). Gait is often ataxic with lurching from side to side or staggering. Patients with Huntington's chorea will have continuous twisting movements of the trunk and limbs that may be worsened by walking. Sufferers with muscular dystrophy often have weak trunk and lower limb muscles. As they rise up from a chair, a characteristic posture is to flex at the hip and push upwards with help from the hands on the upper thighs (Gower's sign). Owing to pelvic weakness, they often 'waddle' when walking forwards with legs spread and shoulders sloping down (Gilman 1998).

Coordination abnormalities are common in individuals with cerebellar pathology, whereby finger-to-nose testing is problematic, sloppy and dysmetric with a side-to-side tremor coming from the shoulder. In Parkinsonism coordination may be slow and hypometric. In corticospinal tract disorders, it may be slow and clumsy (Nutt 1999).

Movement Spontaneous movement can be seen in individuals with basal ganglia disease (e.g. chorea, dystonia, rest tremor). Patients with Huntington's chorea may have spontaneous grimacing of the facial muscles. Patients with Tourette's may have spontaneous facial movements as well as spontaneous vocal tics. Craniocervical dystonia patients may have involuntary movements of the facial or neck musculature. On the other hand, patients with Parkinson's typically have akinesia, with difficulty in initiating movement.

Tremor Tremor at rest is consistent with Parkinsonism or extrapyramidal disease (Nasreddine et al. 1999); intention tremor is suggestive of cerebellar disease.

Reflexes and Tone Hyper-reflexia and spasticity are upper motor neuron signs, consistent with corticospinal tract disorders. Spastic paralysis involving one side of the body in association with spastic type speech points to a lesion of the subcortical white matter and internal capsule. Hyporeflexia is commonly seen in association with peripheral nerve diseases causing weakness or proprioceptive sensory loss.

As part of the ENT/phoniatric examination all of the cranial nerves should be tested. The ears should be examined to make certain that cerumen impaction or middle ear pathology is not impacting upon the patient's ability to hear. 'Glue' ear may also be indicative of pathology of the Eustachian tube, post nasal space, nose or the soft palate. The mouth and oropharynx are of particular importance as many patients with neurological disorders present with dysarthrophonia. The lips should be evaluated for adequate ability to seal the tongue for fasciculations (often a sign of neurodegenerative pathology such as motor neuron disease) and for fullness of movement. Skull base lesions could lead to hypoglossal nerve (XII cranial nerve) dysfunction. Subtle tongue dysfunction, particularly after repeated movement could 'unmask' a neuromuscular junction pathology such as myasthenia gravis. Tongue dysfunction is a not infrequent sequela of stroke. The soft palate should be looked at for evidence of clonus (such as seen in myoclonus). Assessment of voluntary function is also necessary. Loss of such function is not uncommon in stroke or severe head injury and can be associated with velopharyngeal dysfunction as well as speech issues. Soft palate, tongue and facial muscle problems can lead to dysphagia as well as speech disorders.

The key ENT/phoniatric examination in anyone suspected of neurological voice, speech or swallow disturbance is flexible nasendoscopy, preferably in combination with stroboscopy (Woodson et al. 1991). En route to the larynx the nose, post nasal space and soft palate can be comprehensively studied for altered anatomical and physiological function. The degree of closure of the soft palate against Passavant's ridge can be assessed and the integrity of the velum confirmed.

The larynx should be observed at rest as well as in function. At rest, clonic or other spontaneous activity can be looked for. In function, gentle adduction, sphincteric closure, cough, quiet breathing and vigorous abduction are all reviewed. The larynx is 'stressed' by repeated counting and repeated 'e-sniff' manoeuvres. This permits the examiner to look for laryngeal muscular fatigue or incompetence or both related to work, a sign of neuromuscular junction pathology. Asymmetry of abduction or adduction over time may be a subtle sign for vocal fold paralysis or paresis. General laryngeal incoordination may be a sign of suprabulbar pathology. The use of stroboscopy allows routine qualitative assessment. Of particular importance from the standpoint of management is identification of bowing or incompetent valving/closure of the glottis. This can be addressed with speech therapy intervention or surgical augmentation.

Laryngeal EMG is of great importance. It can help determine if functional recovery is feasible or if there is ongoing neuronal degeneration. It can also assist in determining which nerves have been injured. In certain forms of myopathy and motor neuron disorders, it can be diagnostic. If botulinum toxin is being considered for a spastic or spasmodic condition, EMG will assist the surgeon in locating the tip of the injecting needle (Sulica et al. 2006; Blitzer et al. 1985; Brin et al. 1992).

5.6.5 Neurological Speech and Voice Disorder Terms

As we begin to discuss specific disorders, certain terms are helpful. Dysphasia or aphasia is a partial or complete impairment of the ability to communicate, resulting from brain injury, usually brought on by damage to the cortex. Aphasia types include, amongst others, expressive aphasia, receptive aphasia, conduction aphasia, anomic aphasia, global aphasia and primary progressive aphasias. In essence expressive (Broca's) aphasia is associated with the expressive difficulty in word finding and putting words together. Patients with expressive aphasia have lesions to the medial insular cortex (Dronkers et al. 2007; Masdeu 2000). Receptive (Wernicke's/sensory) aphasia is associated with the inability to comprehend meanings. It is associated with damage to the medial temporal lobe and underlying white matter (Kolb et al. 2003).

Verbal apraxia or dyspraxia is an oro-motor speech disorder characterised by the inability to speak correctly and consistently. It is not due to weakness or paralysis of the speech musculature individually; conversely, it affects the purposeful control of the movements necessary for speech. Verbal dyspraxia may occur in children, and thus it is also known as developmental articulatory dyspraxia.

Ataxia is loss of muscular coordination. Ataxia-phasia is the inability to form connected sentences—only single intelligible words. Dysarthria signifies a disturbance of articulation generally due to paralysis, incoordination or spasticity of the muscles used for creating spoken language. Dysarthrophonia is a speech dysfunction that affects respiration, phonation, articulation and prosody of speech.

Case Study 5.19

This is a case of dysarthrophonia in a 72-year-old woman who had noticed a fading voice for the last 5–6 years. The larynx shows a tremor that cannot be suppressed at will. The voice is shaking during examination with the rigid endoscope. The voice range profile reveals that she is neither able to produce soft sounds nor loud tones.

5.6.6 Clinical Approach

In our Neurological Voice Clinic at the National Hospital for Neurology and Neurosurgery, we find it helpful to consider voice disorders from the standpoint of their effects at the level of the larynx (and speech disorders from the standpoint of their effects on the vocal tract especially the articulators). To that end we use a modified version of the Ramig classification (Smith and Ramig 2006). From a laryngeal standpoint, we look at vocal fold adduction/abduction. In this portion of the section, we shall focus on certain disorders with hypo-adduction, hyper-adduction and mal-adduction.

5.6.6.1 Hypo-adduction

This section is aimed primarily at central causes of neurological voice disorders. Consequently, peripheral disorders of the muscle, neuromuscular junction, peripheral nerve and nucleus, all relatively common causes of hypo-adduction will not be reviewed here; peripheral neurogenic voice disorders can be found in Sect. 5.7.

Parkinsonism

Parkinsonism is a constellation of disorders that have hypo-adduction as a typical laryngeal finding. More than 80% of these cases are caused by Parkinson's disease, which will be the focus of this discussion. Parkinson's disease is a disorder of the nigrostriatal region characterised by dopamine deficiency (Hornykiewicz 1966). Typical findings include bradykinesia, rigidity, postural instability and resting tremor of 4–7 Hz (Jankovic and Stacy 1999). Prevalence is 1 per 1000, but in the elderly it is closer to 1 per 100 population. Approximately 1.5 million individuals are known to suffer from Parkinson's disease in the United States and ten million worldwide, and approximately 90% are said to have voice problems (Logemann et al. 1978; Hartelius and Svensson 1994; Ho et al. 1998, 2008; Sapir et al. 2001). That said, a study in Boston identified some Parkinsonian features in 34% of the elderly (Bennet et al. 1996). Voice symptoms appear early in the disorder and are often progressive (Harel et al. 2004; Rusz et al. 2011; Holmes et al. 2000). From a vocal perspective, the voice is often soft, breathy and lacking in projection. It also lacks pitch variation, sounding monotonous. The laryngeal exam often shows bowing of the vocal folds with incomplete apposition. Articulation is also often poor, as is intelligibility (Smith and Ramig 2006). Rate of speech is high. EMG studies have shown reduction in activation and increase in variability of firing of thyroarytenoid muscles (Baker et al. 1998; Luschei et al. 1991); this is believed to be due to reduced central drive. Management with levodopa treatment has not proven consistently beneficial to voice and speech production; neither has deep brain stimulation (Ho et al. 2008; Skodda 2012). Augmentation of the vocal folds has been tested. Temporary improvement with collagen injection was found. Sewall et al. (2006) and Berke et al. (1999a, b) found similar benefits.

Although traditional speech therapy has proven to be of little benefit, the Lee Silverman technique has now been used for over 20 years with proven efficacy in patients with Parkinson's disease. Benefits have been demonstrated in sound pressure level and subglottal pressure (Ramig et al. 2002).

Parkinson-plus syndromes are multisystem neurodegenerative disorders that incorporate Parkinsonian features with other neurological symptoms. These syndromes include progressive supranuclear palsy (PSP), multiple systems atrophy (MSA) and corticobasal degeneration (CBGD) and are due to abnormalities in tau- and alpha-synuclein function (Sjoström et al. 2002; Williams and Lees 2009). In PSP, dopaminergic, cholinergic and adrenergic neurotransmitter systems are involved; in MSA the Parkinsonism is poorly responsive to levodopa therapy together with varying degrees of autonomic, cerebellar and pyramidal dysfunction.

CBGD is distinctive owing to the Parkinsonism plus certain specific cortical signs as well as limb apraxia which at times is so dysfunctional as to be called 'alien limb' (Doody and Jankovic 1992). Voice and speech symptoms are common and early features, particularly in MSA, consisting of mixed type dysarthria with hypokinetic as well as spastic components (Skodda et al. 2010). Blumin and Berke (2002) found five of seven patients presenting with neurological disorders and with bilateral abductor vocal cord paresis to have MSA.

Case Study 5.20

A patient received deep brain stimulation because of Parkinson disease at the age of 70. His voice became weak in the course of the disease during the last years. In his history there is a myocardial infarction years ago and diabetes type 2. His medication comprises L-DOPA, insulin, acetylsalicylic acid and a beta-blocker. The vocal folds are bowed with atrophy of the vocalis muscle and lamina propria. The closure pattern shows a complete glottal gap. The mucosal wave is reduced. The voice sounds monotonous, breathy and faint. The vocal range is severely restricted.

Case Study 5.21

A 62-year-old former shop assistant had been suffering from hoarseness, articulation disorder, dyspnoea on exertion and swallowing difficulty for 1 year. She reports mild reflux without heartburn, has bronchial hyperreactivity and had overcome an episode of depression. By the time of examination, restricted mobility of the orofacial musculature, the soft palate and the larynx were present. No other neurologic symptoms were found. Examination of pharyngeal and laryngeal structures reveals reduced constriction of the nasopharynx, incomplete velar closure, bowed vocal folds and attenuated abduction of the left vocal fold. These findings are typical for multiple system atrophy of central origin. During phonation, the vocal folds vibrate and the closure pattern shows complete closure. Speech is dominated by slow, slurred articulation and voice quality by roughness (R2 B1 H2). The vocal range is severely restricted.

Closed Head Trauma (Traumatic Brain Injury)

Among a constellation of other signs and symptoms, closed head trauma is a cause of speech disorders. It is a major cause of death and disability, particularly among both children and young adults. The most common areas to have focal lesions in non-penetrating traumatic brain injury are the orbitofrontal cortex and the anterior temporal lobes. Aphasia or dysarthrophonia can occur when somewhat less commonly affected areas such as motor or language areas are, respectively, damaged. In one study of closed head-injured patients requiring admission to a rehabilitation unit, 87% had speech-related issues. Thirty percent were aphasic, 25% had motor speech disorders, and 32% had mixed speech deficits (Menon et al. 1993). In another study, McHenry et al. (1994) found reduction in laryngeal airway resistance and concomitant increase in glottal airflow, likely consistent with hypo-adduction and breathiness.

Motor Neuron Disorders (MND)

Motor neuron disorders are a group of neurodegenerative disorders (motor neuronopathies) that include amyotrophic lateral sclerosis (ALS), progressive muscular atrophy, primary lateral sclerosis and progressive bulbar palsy. These disorders all affect the motor neurons and have generalised and usually progressive voluntary motor disorders, including swallowing, speech and voice. The muscles supporting expiration are also generally very weak. Voluntary muscle atrophy and fasciculations are common. Dysarthria, dysphagia and dyspnoea are frequent. From a voice perspective, patients suffering from MND often have weak breathy voices, particularly in bulbar onset, but they can also present with spasticity and hyperfunction. Once the respiratory muscles become involved, the voice is likely to become progressively breathy. Articulation also becomes more problematic owing to denervation of the muscles. ALS is the most common of the disorders. Other ENT/Phoniatric manifestations often include velopharyngeal insufficiency as well as swallowing problems and difficulty with managing secretions. Roughly one quarter of cases present with bulbar onset ALS. In this group ENT/phoniatric symptoms may predate limb symptoms. A smaller group will present with respiratory onset ALS whereby the intercostal muscles weaken first, leading to breathing issues. There is both upper and lower motor neuronal degeneration. At times tracheotomy is required along with management of secretions. Management is generally supportive (Smith and Ramig 2006; Rowland 2000).

5.6.6.2 Hyper-adduction Disorders

Hyper-adduction disorders can be reviewed from the standpoint of constancy of strain and lack of constancy (Brin et al. 1992). This includes the 'pseudobulbar' or supranuclear palsies, the choreas and the dystonias.

'Pseudobulbar' or Supranuclear Palsies

Pseudobulbar palsy typically refers to injuries (usually bilateral) of the corticobulbar tracts. It is characterised by spastic dysarthria (also called upper motor neuron dysarthria) (Nasreddine et al. 1999). Speech and swallowing disorders are due to bilateral injury of these pathways. The interruption may occur at any point from the cortex to the brain stem, but most commonly the interruption is due to ischaemic injury. Clinical findings indicative of cerebral lesions producing these pseudobulbar symptoms may include aphasia, sensory changes and corticospinal tract findings such as limb spasticity, increased tendon and jaw jerk reflexes and an extensor plantar response. Patients with pseudobulbar palsy also may have impaired emotional control, with pathological laughter or crying, and emergence of primitive reflexes such as suck and snout (Hermanowicz and Truong 1999).

Choreas

Huntington's chorea is the example of chorea that we shall use. It is an autosomal dominant disease, caused by an unstable trinucleotide repeat mutation on chromosome 4. Incidence is approximately 5–10 per 100,000 (Huntington's Disease Collaboration Research Group 1993). Pathological findings in the brain include generalised atrophy with cortical neuronal degeneration. Marked caudate atrophy is the pathological hallmark of the disease (Penney and Young 1998). Almost any part of the body can be involved with jerky involuntary sudden movements and motor impermanence. This can also affect the laryngeal muscles leading to sudden pitch and loudness changes that generally have a strained quality to them. General medical management includes use of dopaminergic depleters such as tetrabenazine. Laryngeal botulinum toxin injections have also been tested in trials with some success.

Other genetic causes of chorea are rare, including some of the spinocerebellar ataxias,

Friedrich's ataxia, brain iron accumulation disorders, etc. Acquired causes include some HIV infections in association with cryptococcal disease, Sydenham's chorea and a group of other disorders.

Spasmodic Dysphonia

Although relatively uncommon (approximate incidence 1:60,000 to 1:100,000), there is a substantial body of ENT-related information on spasmodic dysphonia (SD), most likely due to our ability to treat symptoms with botulinum toxin injections. Spasmodic dysphonia is a dystonia that affects the laryngeal muscles. Dystonias are a family of movement disorders characterised by abnormal involuntary movements of voluntary muscle groups. Classification depends on age of onset and distribution of the dystonic activity. In some cases these involuntary contractions only occur during certain task-specific activities. In the larynx this tends to manifest as speech-related pitch breaks. Mutations have been identified for several familial forms of dystonias (e.g. *DYT1*, *DYT4*, *DYT6*). These tend to have clinical manifestations in childhood. Cases of focal adult onset SD are rare, and a genetic locus for SD has yet to be found (Blumin and Ludlow 2014; Xiao et al. 2010).

Spasmodic dysphonia (SD) has been subdivided into adductor and abductor types. The pure adductor type is commonest (approximately 85–90%), and a pure abductor type is very unusual, only representing about 2–3%. There is also a mixed adductor/abductor type. In this subsection we will focus on the more common adductor type. Typical pitch breaks with adductor SD occur in association with vowel sounds, particularly the \a\ and \e\ vowels. It is particularly apparent when one word ends with a vowel followed by a word beginning with a vowel such as occurs in the phrase 'I eat apples every day' or in words with concurrent or consequential vowel sounds such as 'eighty'. The voice is said to sound strangled/strained. EMG demonstrates bursts of muscular activity overlying a normal interference pattern (Ludlow 2006; Blitzer et al. 1985).

As far as management is concerned, many approaches have been tested. There is no curative management protocol yet available. Speech ther-

apy may be helpful as an adjunct but is not the primary treatment. Surgical management has included nerve section (Dedo 1976), thyroplasty or laryngeal nerve section with reinnervation (Berke et al. 1999a, b). To date no peripheral surgical manipulation has regularly proven curative. To the authors' knowledge there are no controlled neuropharmacological studies demonstrating significant symptom relief, and the role of medications in SD is only adjunctive (Blumin and Ludlow 2014). Most commonly, low-dose botulinum toxin is used in peripheral laryngeal muscles, usually the thyroarytenoid (Truong et al. 1991; Lees et al. 1992). Our experience is that low-dose unilateral injections appear as efficacious as bilateral (Upile et al. 2009). Thus as of the time of press, botulinum toxin injection is still the generally preferred treatment (Blumin and Ludlow 2014). That said, the risk of development of antibodies though rare, does exist.

Case Study 5.22

A 69-year-old woman had been suffering from pressed voice for more than 20 years. She underwent multiple injections of botulinum toxin which was applied trans-orally directly into the vocal folds. On a nearly regular basis, she is treated every 3–4 months when speaking becomes strenuous. The voice sound is rough, breathy and groaning. The video shows inconspicuous vocal folds. Dynamic range and pitch range are reduced. The second video of this case shows the trans-oral injection of botulinum toxin under local anaesthesia.

Case Study 5.23

This 47-year-old woman had been hoarse for 2 years. The thyroid gland, allegedly pressed against the larynx, had been removed 2 months ago. The voice did not improve afterwards. Voice therapy was ineffective, too. This case is an example of abductor spasmodic dysphonia. In the video one observes the difficulty in adducting the vocal folds. But this phenomenon is not as characteristic as the voice sound. During speaking the voice is interrupted by aphonic passages at the onset of words as well as in the middle of phonation. The vocal range is markedly reduced.

5.6.6.3 Tremor

Long-term tremor is seen in essential tremor, Parkinson's disease and cerebellar/dystonic tremor. It is also present in many instances of spasmodic dysphonia. We will use essential tremor as the example of this discussion. Without doubt, essential tremor is the commonest of the hyperkinetic movement disorders. Incidence has been reported to be between 4 and 60 per thousand individuals and increases with increasing age; prevalence is 2–5%. Although the hands and head are more commonly affected, the voice can be affected in up to 20% of individuals (Elble and Koller 1990). An autosomal dominance pattern has been established in approximately 50% (Murray 1981); thus, the term familial tremor is often used. Typical tremor varies from 3 to 7 Hertz. Abnormalities in the olivocerebellar tracts have been identified on PET scanning (Jenkins et al. 1993), and it is likely that peripheral somatosensory feedback loops are involved, leading to disturbances in rhythmicity (Deuschl and Elble 2000). Unlike resting tremors such as are found in Parkinson's disease, essential tremor is a postural tremor (Jankovic and Stacy 1999). Women are affected more often than men, the tremor generally appearing in middle age.

Management of essential tremor should include a beta-blocker unless contraindicated. That said, beta-blockers have only limited benefit for vocal tremor. At the time of publication, no pharmacologic trials have demonstrated evidence of significant vocal benefit in patients with essential tremor. Deep brain stimulation in the thalamus has been noted to have benefited a few patients with vocal tremor (Yoon et al. 1999), but these are still just case reports. Botulinum toxin has been injected into the thyroarytenoid muscles with some benefit. However, the more widespread the tremor, the less likely the efficacy of the laryngeal botulinum (Blumin and Ludlow 2014). We have substantial experience of botulinum injection in tremor. Our experience is that prolonged breathiness following injection is more likely than in cases of SD. Thus we tend to limit our injections to very low-dose unilateral injections, with some benefit (JR personal observation).

5.6.7 Summary

This section has reviewed central neurological disorders. It introduced the subject by reviewing some basic aspects of brain function and of language. It then presented the neuro-laryngological history and physical examination, emphasising ENT/phoniatric manifestations.

Specific central neurological disorders were then described, using the context of the effect at a voice (laryngeal) level and speech (articulatory) level. Parkinson's disease, closed head trauma, motor neuron disease, spasmodic dysphonia and tremor were reviewed in some detail.

5.7 Peripheral Neurogenic Voice Disorders

Arno Olthoff

5.7.1 Introduction

Physiological positions of vocal folds are 'median' during phonation and 'lateral' during respiration. In cases of vocal fold paralysis, the impaired adduction and abduction of vocal folds lead to different positions between 'median' and 'lateral'.

For the majority of textbooks, vocal fold mobility impairments are classified by their 'paramedian' or 'intermediate' position. Additionally 'cadaveric' positions are described with a bowed vocal fold in a most lateral position.

This common classification does not consider further variables (e.g. time course, functional deficits) and does not entirely meet the high variability of laryngoscopic and videostroboscopic findings.

Paralyses have to be identified and characterised in order to indicate necessary diagnostics and to arrange obligatory or facultative therapies. Therefore the knowledge of laryngeal innervation, possible reasons for their dysfunction and options for recreation or rehabilitation are essential.

This section will give the anatomical and physiological background and intends to be a useful guide for clinical tasks.

5.7.2   Brief Historical Review

Because a historical review is not common in textbooks, I would like to offer this to interested readers. There is an ongoing discussion about laryngeal innervation, and the readers' own clinical experience can be compared with current theories and classifications.

Since the first studies of vocal fold paralyses (Gerhardt 1863), the aim was to conclude the site of nerve lesion from the position of paralysed vocal folds. 'Semon's law' (Clerf and Baltzell 1953) and the 'Wagner-Grossmann-Theory' (Grossmann 1897) have to be mentioned first in this context. Early contradictory publications came from Lemére (1933), Clerf and Baltzell (1953) and Tschiassny (1957) who suspected that different affected nerve branches were responsible for vocal fold position. More recent publications from Crumley (1989), Sanders et al. (1994), Sanudo et al. (1999) and Olthoff et al. (2007) have illustrated an ongoing discussion about the laryngeal motoric system.

Trying to incorporate all different kinds of vocal fold impairment under the generic term 'paralysis of the recurrent nerve' implies an indissoluble problem: in our human motoric system, competing abductors and adductors (e.g. flexors and tensors in our extremities) are innervated by different nerves. Transferring this fact to the laryngeal motoric system, the only opener of the larynx (the posterior cricoarytenoid muscle) should have an exclusive innervation. Hence, the recurrent laryngeal nerve must be 'more than one' and needs further analysis to reveal whether at least separated fibres allow the innervation of antagonistic muscles. The different theories that were intended to show separate innervation of laryngeal adductors and the sole abductor will be briefly highlighted.

The main intent of all authors has been to interpret the cause of 'paramedian' positions of paralysed vocal folds. Semon (Clerf and Baltzell 1953) found a separation of the recurrent laryngeal nerve into abductor and adductor fibres and stated that a higher vulnerability of abductor fibres led to 'paramedian' vocal fold positions. In case of recurrent laryngeal nerve lesion, Wagner-Grossmann (Grossmann 1897) defined the external branch of the superior laryngeal nerve as the only competing nerve that enables a 'paramedian' vocal fold position resulting from the exclusive innervation of the adductory cricothyroid muscle. Even though this theory was rejected by other authors (Woodson 1993; Koufman et al. 1995), it became consensus in the European literature. Lemére (1933) supported Semon's aspect of fibre separation, and later Miehlke et al. (1973) used this aspect for reinnervation procedures. Lemére (1933) additionally suspected that the only unpaired muscle of the larynx, the interarytenoid muscle, was responsible for 'paramedian' findings owing to its adductor competence and bilateral innervation. The unaffected opposite nerve could cause the adduction and paramedian position. To explain bilateral 'paramedian' paralyses, Clerf and Baltzell (1953) and Tschiassny (1957) implicated motoric fibres in the internal branch of the superior laryngeal nerve that run to the interarytenoid muscle. In case of recurrent laryngeal nerve lesion, the preserved adductory fibres from the superior laryngeal nerve would lead to bilateral 'paramedian' vocal fold positions. This theory was supported later from Sanders et al. (1994) who visualised these fibres with a special staining technique. The existence of motoric fibres in internal branches that run into the interarytenoid muscle could not be proved by histochemical analyses (Olthoff and Ehrlich 2010). Lemére (1933) and Rueger (1972) demonstrated these fibres running through the interarytenoid muscle without motoric but with sensory endings in the laryngeal mucosa. Other studies with retrograde tracers also proved that fibres from the internal branch of the superior laryngeal nerve run to the posterior cricoarytenoid muscle with motoric projection to the rostral ambiguous nucleus. A collateral reinnervation and neuromuscular sprouting of these fibres in the case of recurrent laryngeal nerve lesions were interpreted as evidence for motoric reinnervation (Hydman and Mattsson 2008).

Apart from vagal innervation and all mentioned laryngeal muscles, Réthi (1952) described a 'stylopharyngeal muscle system' in order to interpret ventricular phonation and dystonic voice disorders. The involved stylopharyngeal muscle is innervated from the glossopharyngeal nerve, and its insertion into the supraglottal area might enable some supraglottal adduction in the case of vagal nerve paralyses.

In later studies the aspect of spontaneous or surgical reinnervation was emphasised as the main reason for 'paramedian' vocal fold positions caused by increased adductor muscle tension (Crumley 1989). The fixation of vocal folds was interpreted by concurrent innervation of antagonistic muscles ('synkinesis') that causes an 'autoparalysis' that was first described for facial innervation (Stennert 1982). But as the regeneration of nerve fibres needs time (several months), the idea of 'reinnervation' could not explain immediate bilateral paramedian vocal fold paralysis after thyroid surgery.

More recent macroscopic studies have revealed new findings of very vulnerable recurrent laryngeal nerve fibres running to the posterior cricoarytenoid muscle. These fibres are highly endangered in, for example, thyroid surgery, and their injury is potentially responsible for 'paramedian' paralyses (Olthoff et al. 2007). Additionally, a branch that runs from the external branch of the superior laryngeal nerve into the endolarynx might support a 'paramedian' vocal fold position and may redirect the discussion of the 'Wagner-Grossmann-Theory' (Wu et al. 1994; Olthoff et al. 2007).

As an 'up-to-date hypothesis', we could state that synkinesis will be crucial for paramedian vocal fold positions in paralyses older than 3–6 months.

Paramedian vocal fold positions in earlier stages will be caused by injuries of abductor fibres owing to incomplete lesions of the recurrent trunk fibres. In incomplete lesions the superior number of adductor fibres will cause paramedian positions.

Thus, a paramedian vocal fold position is based on an imbalance between adductor and abductor muscle activities for the reasons above. A more lateral ('intermediate') position will consequently indicate an additional lesion of adductor fibres or refer to a more complete lesion of the recurrent trunk.

This knowledge was the basis for the current advantage in laryngeal pacing. The first target of stimulation was the laryngeal abductor muscle (posterior cricoarytenoid muscle) to free patients with bilateral paramedian vocal fold paralysis from dyspnoea (Li et al. 2013). Because the bilateral paramedian vocal folds' position implies imbalanced adductor muscle activity, the stimulation of the laryngeal opener tends to restore the muscular balance.

5.7.3 Anatomy and Physiology

The efferent laryngeal vagal nerve fibres (cranial nerve X) derive from the nucleus ambiguus and run together with fibres from the spinal nuclei of the accessory nerve (cranial nerve XI) through the jugular foramen. Afferent laryngeal fibres run back to the nuclei of the solitary tract (Sasaki et al. 2001). Because muscle spindles are proven to be in laryngeal muscles (Baken and Noback 1971; Malannino 1974; Tellis et al. 2004), a reflex motoric system can be stated following the general principles of our human motoric system. Afferent proprioceptive fibres will run with the internal branch of the superior laryngeal nerve (Lemére 1933; Sanudo et al. 1999; Sasaki et al. 2001).

Owing to the cortical representation of laryngeal muscles, functional magnetic resonance imaging techniques have given new insights and revealed a more medial area than traditionally known from Penfield's 'homunculus' (Olthoff et al. 2008; Brown et al. 2008). The site is located adjacent to the lateral hand area. Transcranial magnetic stimulations were optimal in the same site and confirmed these findings (Rödel et al. 2004) (Fig. 5.15).

Fig. 5.15 The red area represents the sensorimotor area of the hand and the lateral adjacent blue area the sensorimotor area of the larynx (arrow). Parts of Penfield's 'homunculus' are pictured for orientation

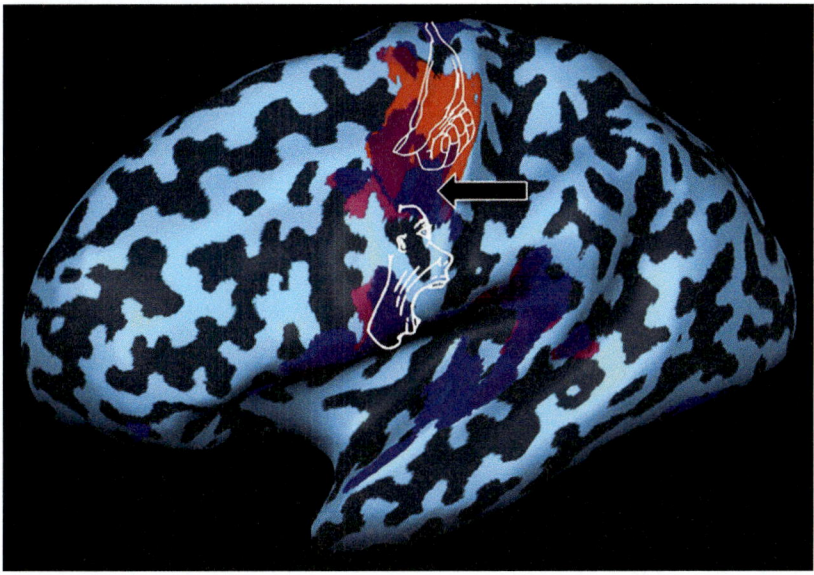

5.7.4   Laryngeal Innervation

After passage of the jugular foramen the *superior laryngeal nerve* separates from the vagus nerve and sends one internal sensoric branch through the hyothyroid membrane into the larynx and one *external motoric branch* to the cricothyroid muscle. Deriving from the external nerve, a branch runs into the larynx that was first called 'communicating nerve' and later 'ventricular branch' owing to its course into the ventricular muscle (Wu et al. 1994, Olthoff et al. 2007).

After parting from the vagal nerve, the right recurrent nerve curves around the brachiocephalic trunk, and the left recurrent nerve around the aortic arch, before running upwards to the larynx. The recurrent laryngeal nerves pass close to the trachea and reach the larynx from the rear laterally. Before entering the larynx, the ansa galeni leaves the recurrent nerve and joins the internal branch of the superior laryngeal nerve. Directly before the dorsal entrance into the larynx, very thin and vulnerable fibres leave the recurrent nerve and enter the posterior cricoarytenoid muscle, which is the only opener of the larynx (posticus). These extralaryngeal fibres (Rr. postici) are

highly endangered in surgical treatment, such as thyroid surgery, even by just moving the recurrent nerve.

After the laryngeal entrance, and covered by the posterior cricoarytenoid muscle, the *posterior ramus* runs to the interarytenoid muscle. The *anterior ramus* supplies the medial and lateral thyroarytenoid and the lateral cricoarytenoid muscle, which are synergistic adductors of the vocal fold (Fig. 5.16). Over the course of more than 100 years, the anatomical nomenclature of the posterior ramus changed in anatomical textbooks. In contrast to our classification that was based on fundamental studies from Lang et al. (1986), the posterior branch is sometimes seen as the branch that turns to the ansa galeni (Mattsson et al. 2015). This fact is mentioned to prevent misunderstandings.

Apart from their vagal innervation, the stylopharyngeal muscles insert bilaterally into the supraglottis and are also innervated from the glossopharyngeal nerve. They are still discussed as supporting the elevation of the larynx during swallowing. Owing to their supraglottal insertion, they might be able to induce some supraglottal adductions.

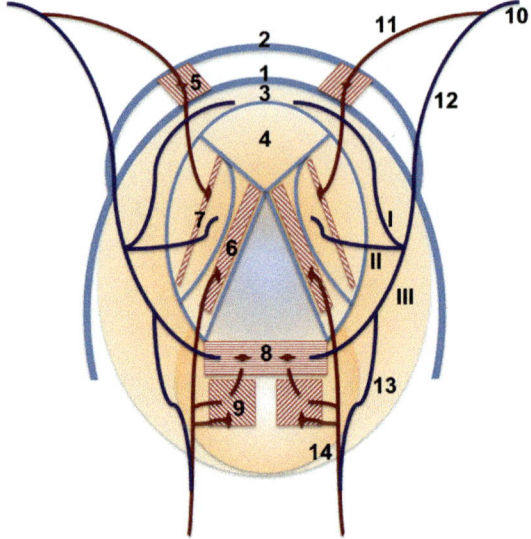

Fig. 5.16 A schematic view of the larynx and its innervation. (1) Thyroid cartilage, (2) cricoid cartilage, (3) lingual epiglottis, (4) laryngeal epiglottis, (5) cricothyroid muscle, (6) 'vocalis' muscle, (7) ventricular muscle, (8) interarytenoid muscle, (9) 'posticus' muscle, (10) superior laryngeal nerve (SLN), (11) external branch of the SLN, (12) internal branch of the SLN, (13) 'ansa galeni', (14) recurrent laryngeal nerve; (I) anterior, (II) middle, (III) posterior branches of 12. Red lines represent motoric and blue lines sensoric or proprioceptive nerves

5.7.5 Laryngeal Motoric System

Except for the posterior cricoarytenoid muscle, every laryngeal muscle tends to narrow the laryngeal lumen. The exclusive opener of the larynx enables an abduction of vocal folds exceeding the cadaveric position that is caused by the elastic laryngeal tissues.

The adduction of vocal and ventricular folds, combined with the approach of the arytenoids against the caudal part of the epiglottis, leads to a complete sphincteric closure of the larynx that is essential for airway protection during swallowing. More differentiated adduction is present in throat clearing, coughing and phonation.

This might explain the presence of various adductors that in concert are able to perform the different adductor tasks. Laryngeal opening is a comparatively simple but essential function. Therefore only one abductor muscle, namely, the posterior cricoarytenoid muscle, proves to be sufficient.

In detail the adductors are the *lateral cricoarytenoid muscle*, the strongest adductor of the ligaments of the vocal folds, owing to its insertion to the anterior part of the muscular process of the arytenoid cartilage (opposite and antagonistic to the posterior cricoarytenoid muscle, which inserts on the posterior surface). The *interarytenoid muscle* is responsible for the closure of the cartilaginous part of the glottis by narrowing the arytenoid bodies to the midline. Transverse and oblique fibres work in a synergistic manner (Schiel et al. 2004). The internal and external *thyroarytenoid muscles* are responsible for the fine-tuning of vocal fold tension. An increased vocal fold tension tends to support adduction. The *cricothyroid muscles* narrow the cricoid against the thyroid cartilage anteriorly. Owing to the dorsal articulation between both cartilages, this approximation leads to a tension and consequently adductory support of the vocal folds. This effect depends on a sufficient tension of the thyroarytenoid muscles.

The origins and insertions are shown in a figure that serves as a crib using hands and fingers ('rule of thumb') (Fig. 5.17).

The above-mentioned 'stylopharyngeal muscle system' (Réthi 1952) might enable some supraglottal (ventricular) adductions owing to its insertion, away from all mentioned laryngeal muscles, into the supraglottis.

5.7.6 Laryngeal Tasks and Function

The distinctive feature of the aerodigestive tract is the common use of one anatomical area (the larynx) for two essential but incompatible functions: breathing and swallowing. Even if textbooks, anatomical atlases and clinical diagnostics, such as videofluoroscopies, show sagittal views as the most common aspect of our aerodigestive tract, they give the wrong impression of a digestive hose behind a ventilation tube. For the correct impression, we have to look at the axial view: the airway is combined with and surrounded by our digestive tract. Irrespective of the separation of mouth and nose, the division of our aerodigestive tract starts with the larynx. In newborns we can clearly see the anatomical position of the larynx in the centre of the digestive tract: a high-riding epiglottis, the aryepiglottic folds and the

posterior commissure form a protecting 'tube' against aspiration. In adults this aspect becomes less explicit, and the protection of our airway depends essentially on an adequate sphincteric closure of glottal and supraglottal structures (described above) (Fig. 5.18).

5.7.7 Laryngeal Competence and Incompetence

Airway opening during respiration and the protection of the airway during swallowing are the two primary and essential functions of our larynx. In humans the evolution of voice production is a secondary function: speech is evolutionarily younger than nutrition (Negus 1929). Just as the secondary use of the masticatory organs is for articulation, the larynx is used secondarily for vocalisation to allow speech production.

Each of the three functions mentioned can be impaired after lesions of laryngeal innervation. The lesion sites might be central (e.g. after stroke) or peripheral (e.g. bulbar or nerve lesions). Because the laryngeal cortical representation is bilateral, unilateral paralyses are only evident after peripheral injuries (not after central lesions). Possible clinical impairments of central or peripheral lesions are dyspnoea, dysphagia and dysphonia. In central or bulbar lesions, additionally affected adjacent structures (glossopharyngeal, hypoglossal) often influence clinical findings.

For more details see Sect. 5.6.

Fig. 5.17 The backs of both hands are shown schematically after crossing forearms. Hands act as arytenoid bodies. Arrows represent laryngeal muscles and their function can be simulated: (1) thyroarytenoid 'vocalis' muscle (tension, closure), (2) lateral cricoarytenoid muscle (strong closure of the ligament part), (3) posterior cricoarytenoid 'posticus' muscle (only opener), (4) interarytenoid muscle (closure of the cartilage part)

Fig. 5.18 Digestive tract (D) and airway (A) are shown schematically. The axial (endoscopic) view reveals: the digestive (oral, oropharyngeal and hypopharyngeal) tract is not behind the airway but surrounds the airway. This schematic view illustrates the importance of the laryngeal protective morphology and function

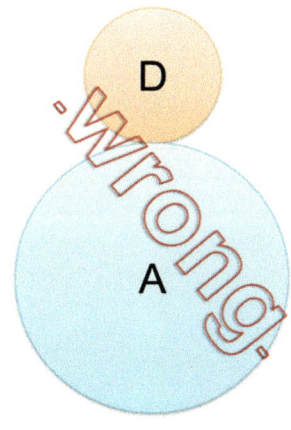

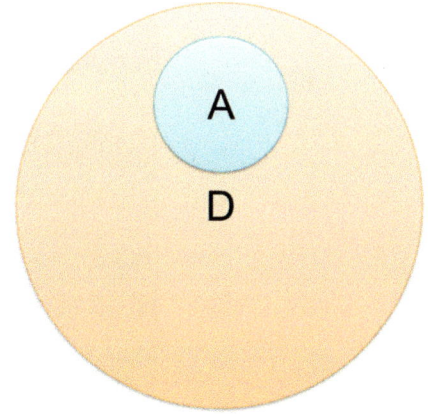

5.7.8 Diagnostics

5.7.8.1 Causes of Peripheral Lesions and Laryngeal Paralyses

More than 80% of laryngeal nerve lesions are iatrogenic and mainly caused by thyroid surgery; followed by carotid, cervical spine, thoracic or cardiac surgery and neck surgery done for different purposes. The remaining cases are caused by primary or secondary tumours and metastases or induced by neurotropic viruses (varicella zoster, Epstein-Barr, herpes simplex, *Cytomegalovirus*, Coxsackie, *adenovirus*, diphasic meningoencephalitis) or bacteria (*Borrelia*). Many of these acquired infections cannot be proved by serological tests, and paralyses are often classified as 'idiopathic'. Some cases are post-traumatic but often not clearly separable from side effects of salvage surgery. Bulbar lesions impose similar peripheral lesions. These are rare cases in tumours, vascular insults or neuromuscular diseases.

In the case of a bilateral *intermediate position* of vocal folds after intubation, a high-riding cuff from a ventilation tube that compresses the internal branch (anterior ramus) against the inner surface of the thyroid cartilage has to be discussed as a possible cause (Olthoff and Kruse 2004). In these rare cases, an isolated lesion of adductor fibres is stated as a cause of imbalanced abductor muscle activity (Fig. 5.19).

5.7.8.2 Diagnostic Tasks and Schedules

The classification of laryngeal paralyses is driven from endoscopic findings. Hence, diagnostics start with *endoscopic laryngoscopy* that shows vocal fold mobility impairment. The endoscopic impressions are focused on reduced or absent abductions or adductions of the paralysed vocal fold with different degrees of muscle tension. Various findings of straight and bowed vocal folds in several positions to the glottal midline can be observed. A separation is limited to paramedian and intermediate vocal fold position (see below).

The endoscopy is enhanced by *videostroboscopy* that gives information about the tone of the vocalis muscle and the quality of glottal competence during phonation.

Fig. 5.19 Examples of two different (paramedian, intermediate) bilateral paralyses are shown in a typical trans-oral endoscopic view

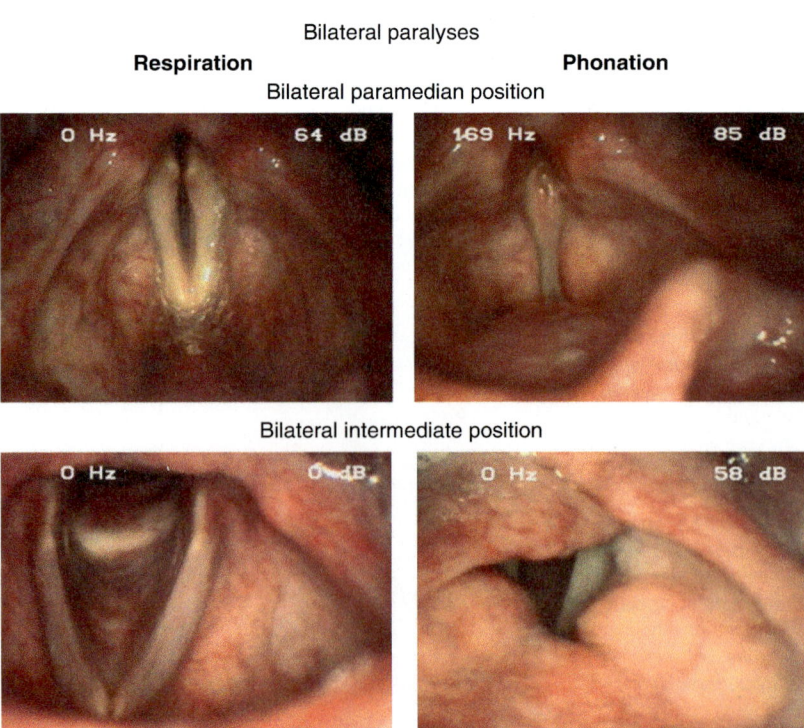

Bilateral paralyses

Respiration   Phonation

Bilateral paramedian position

Bilateral intermediate position

Voice disorders can be perceptively described by using the roughness-breathiness-hoarseness-scale ('RBH'-*scale*) and quantified by computerised analysis of voice quality (e.g. Göttingen Hoarseness Diagram). To assess the impact of dysphonia on the quality of life, a standardised questionnaire for self-assessment of quality of voice should be used. For this, functional scales such as the 'Voice Handicap Index' (VHI) (Nawka et al. 2003) and the 'Voice-Related Quality of Life' (V-RQOL) (Hogikyan and Sethuraman 1999) are suitable.

For more information on voice analyses, see Chap. 6.

Respiratory distress should be quantified by body plethysmographic examination. The central airway resistance (R_{AW}) is independent of effort and gives an ideal reference for glottal obstruction (Olthoff et al. 2005). Others consider the peak flow the best reference value. It depends on sex, age and body height and is available in norm tables. It is effort-dependent and ranges from some 6–10 L/s. The risk range is at 40–50%, and values <40% are considered a strong indication of glottal dilation.

In case of iatrogenic lesions most paralyses are temporary. The extent of nerve lesions can be classified as 'neurapraxia', 'axonotmesis' and 'neurotmesis' (Seddon 1942). 'Neurapraxia' describes the mildest nerve injury with an intact axon and intact endo-, peri- and epineurium. It implies the best prognosis. 'Axonotmesis' names a nerve lesion with an affected axon but intact endo-, peri- and epineurium. In case of 'neurotmesis', the continuity of the entire nerve is lost, which implies the worst prognosis. A classification can be obtained by laryngeal electromyographic (EMG) diagnostics, but a precise prospective and treatment-relevant result cannot be concluded from EMG findings (Laskawi et al. 1994; Sataloff et al. 2003). However, an EMG diagnostic is essential in the verification of paralyses of the cricothyroid muscle because endoscopic findings are not specific. A spontaneous recovery cannot be excluded even if EMG shows findings fitting to a 'neurotmesis'. The nerve's ability to heal spontaneously averages 1 mm per day. Presuming a mean length of 300 mm (measured from nucleus ambiguus to the laryngeal muscle), spontaneous recoveries last up to 10 months. Within this period of time, no irreversible surgical treatments should be performed to restore laryngeal functions. In case of an unclear onset time of paralyses, or in case of partial cure, this period could be extended to 12 months. An early intervention, such as a tracheostomy, is intended to be temporary and focused on the management of serious complaints.

If the anamnesis suggests an 'idiopathic lesion', this term should be avoided until the exclusion of neurogenic viral infections, neuromuscular diseases and tumours as possible causes, for which serum analyses, computed tomographic (CT) scans and interdisciplinary (neurological) diagnostics are mandatory (Table 5.6).

5.7.8.3 Clinical Findings and Classification of Laryngeal Paralyses

The first step of classification starts by distinguishing unilateral from bilateral paralysis.

In unilateral paralysis the position of the impaired vocal folds may have two classical positions: paramedian and intermediate. Our clinical experience shows more than the mentioned classical positions. Owing to the remaining or recovered nerve function, we additionally see vocal fold positions 'in between' and also lateral positions with atonic and excavated vocal folds and additionally atonic supraglottal structures. Paralysis might be incomplete and partial adductions or abductions can remain or be recovered. The time period between onset of paralysis and clinical examination has an enormous impact on the interpretation of clinical findings.

In *unilateral paralysis* the main symptoms are dysphonia of different degrees and duration. In rare cases a normal phonation may persist or recover in spite of unilateral mobility impairment. The absence of an impact on voice quality does not exclude a paralysis, e.g. after thyroid surgery, which shows the importance of endoscopic evaluations. The quality of voice is not correlated perforce with the respiratory position of the paralysed vocal fold (paramedian or

Table 5.6 Recommended treatments in unclear origin or degree of lesion

	Until 3 months	Until 6 months	Until 9 months	Until 12 months
Unilateral pareses (paramedian, intermediate)	**D**: Laryngoscopy, videostroboscopy, voice analyses, serum analyses, CT scan, MRI (brainstem, neck incl. thyroid gland, thorax), optional EMG	**D**: Laryngoscopy, videostroboscopy, voice analyses	**D**: Laryngoscopy, videostroboscopy, voice analyses	**D**: Laryngoscopy, videostroboscopy, voice analyses, CT scan, MRI (brainstem, neck incl. thyroid gland, thorax)
	Th: Voice therapy, optional temporal augmentation	**Th**: Optional temporal augmentation	**Th**: Optional temporal augmentation	**Th**: Permanent augmentation, medialisation (thyroplasty type I)
Bilateral paramedian pareses	**D**: Laryngoscopy, videostroboscopy, voice analyses, body plethysmography, serum analyses, CT scan, MRI (brainstem, neck incl. thyroid gland, thorax), optional EMG	**D**: Laryngoscopy, videostroboscopy, voice analyses, body plethysmography	**D**: Laryngoscopy, videostroboscopy, voice analyses, body plethysmography	**D**: Laryngoscopy, videostroboscopy, voice analyses, body plethysmography, CT scan, MRI (brainstem, neck incl. thyroid gland, thorax)
	Th: Depends on degree of dyspnoea: tracheotomy or 'wait and see' possibly botulinum toxin injection[a]	**Th**: Depends on degree of dyspnoea: tracheotomy or 'wait and see'	**Th**: Depends on degree of dyspnoea: tracheotomy or 'wait and see'	**Th**: Dorsal glottectomy Optional: Laryngeal pacer
Bilateral intermediate pareses	**D**: Laryngoscopy, videostroboscopy, voice analyses, serum analyses, CT scan, MRI (brainstem, neck incl. thyroid gland, thorax), optional EMG	**D**: Laryngoscopy, videostroboscopy, voice analyses	**D**: Laryngoscopy, videostroboscopy, voice analyses	**D**: Laryngoscopy, videostroboscopy, voice analyses, CT-scan, MRI (brainstem, neck incl. thyroid gland, thorax)
	Th: Voice therapy	**Th**: None	**Th**: None	**Th**: Optional: augmentation, medialisation (CAVE: respiration)
CT-pareses	**D**: Laryngoscopy, videostroboscopy, voice analyses, EMG, optional serum analyses, optional CT scan, MRI (brainstem, neck, thorax)	**D**: Laryngoscopy, videostroboscopy, voice analyses	**D**: Laryngoscopy, videostroboscopy, voice analyses	**D**: Laryngoscopy, videostroboscopy, voice analyses
	Th: Voice therapy	**Th**: Voice therapy	**Th**: None	**Th**: None

CT cricothyroid muscle; *D* diagnostics; *Th* therapies; *EMG* electromyography

[a]Botulinum toxin injections can be administered trans-orally to the lateral cricoarytenoid and interarytenoid muscle or on trial from outside to the cricothyroid muscle

intermediate) but with the remaining adductory power during phonation (Fig. 5.20).

Dysphagia often appears for a short period at the onset of paralysis and is rarely associated with aspiration. Paroxysmal dyspnoea might occur because of 'vocal fold dysfunction' (VFD) or the synonymous 'inducible laryngeal obstruction' (ILO) that frequently indicates an incomplete or reconvalescent palsy. Any treatment that exceeds clarifying, advising and reassuring of patients should be avoided.

In *bilateral paralysis* the classical finding after peripheral nerve lesions (Rr. postici) is a bilateral paramedian position of the vocal folds. Depending on the remaining opening of the glottis, patients suffer from dyspnoea of different degrees.

Rare lesions of the internal adductor branch (mainly caused by a high-riding cuff of a

Fig. 5.20 Examples of two different (paramedian, intermediate) unilateral paralyses are shown in a typical trans-oral endoscopic view

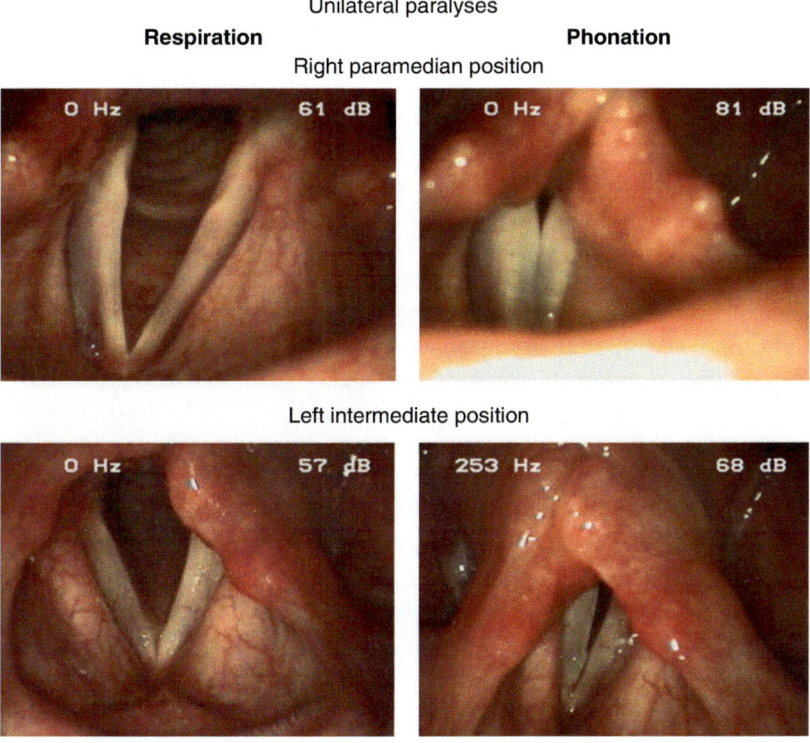

Unilateral paralyses

Respiration   **Phonation**

Right paramedian position

Left intermediate position

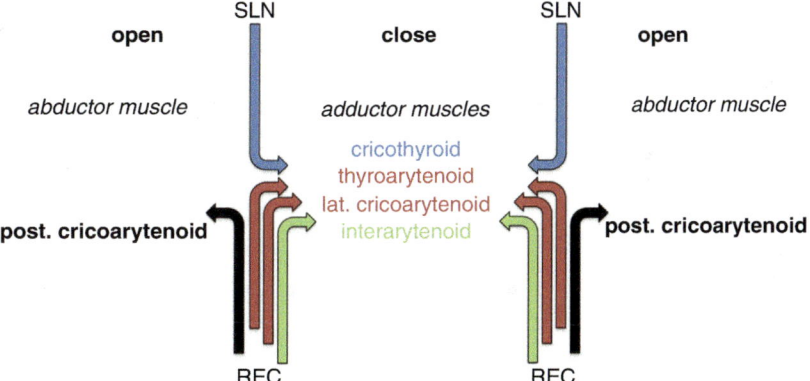

Fig. 5.21 A schematic model of the laryngeal innervation is given. The external branch of the superior laryngeal nerve (SLN) is blue. The recurrent laryngeal nerve (REC) is subdivided into the Rr. postici (black), the anterior ramus (red) and the posterior ramus (green)

ventilation tube that compresses the internal branch against the inner surface of the thyroid cartilage) lead to a bilateral intermediate position of the vocal folds.

Following the anatomical model of this section, the explanation of the early diagnosed (within 3 months after onset) post-traumatic paramedian position is an exclusive lesion of the very vulnerable Rr. postici. A normal function of the remaining adductory fibres that run with the dorsal and anterior branch would cause a paramedian position. Another reason for early observed paramedian mobility impairments can be an incomplete lesion of the recurrent trunk and major surviving adductory fibres (Fig. 5.21). An intermediate position of the vocal folds is explained by affected intra-laryngeal fibres that run with the anterior branch to the main adductor muscles. Another explanation is the complete lesion of the recurrent trunk affecting every adductor (and of course abductor) nerve fibre. Both assumptions also explain atonic and excavated vocal folds that cause aphonia.

In case of later diagnoses (more than 3 months after onset), reinnervation and synkinesis will determine the position of vocal folds and impede conclusions regarding the lesion's site.

Because adductor and abductor fibres derive from one recurrent nerve trunk, various clinical findings may result from different kinds, degrees and periods of recurrent laryngeal nerve injuries.

An affected external ramus of the superior laryngeal nerve would cause paralysis of the cricothyroid muscle and of the ventricular muscle, owing to its intra-laryngeal branch.

Hence, mobility of vocal folds is unaffected but their tension is reduced. This leads, in cases of bilateral lesions, to restrictions of the upper pitch range. These patients are unable to shout. Unilateral lesions may appear more or less symptomless.

Lesions of the internal ramus of the superior laryngeal nerve are not certainly accessible in clinical diagnostics. Various clinical symptoms, such as hypaesthesia or dysaesthesia with slight dysphageal manifestations or laryngeal movement disorder due to affected proprioceptive fibres, could be assumed. Actual findings like these are difficult to verify and rarely presented to clinicians.

5.7.9 Therapy

5.7.9.1 Therapeutic Options and Aims

The choice of treatment depends on the kind, duration and degree of impairment.

If adjacent nervous areas are not involved, an associated dysphagia normally occurs temporarily and rarely causes aspiration. In most cases an intervention is not necessary. A swallowing therapy can be prescribed in extraordinary cases.

Owing to the possible recovery of nerve fibres, the time course has a high impact on the interpretation of clinical findings and the choice of treatments. In the *early period* of paralysis and depending on the vocal fold position and degree of dysphonia due to *unilateral paralyses*, voice therapy is the first choice. Temporal phonosurgical interventions (augmentation) are often recommendable simultaneously to improve glottal closure right away. If no operation is required, voice therapy aims to improve voice and to avoid strain. It may be combined with electrical stimulation of the vocal muscle to minimise atrophy, but the effect is highly questionable. During the period of possible nerve recovery, no permanent surgical treatment should be carried out. In this period for temporary augmentations of paralysed vocal folds, resorbing materials such as hyaluronic acid are suited.

After *10–12 months*, materials such as autologous fat or cartilage (thyroplasty type I), but also foreign materials (such as titanium or Goretex®), can be used for medialisation of impaired vocal folds. A medialisation can also be combined with surgical rotation of the arytenoid body to medialise the cartilage part (dorsal third) of the vocal folds. From the mentioned timings, the choice between different phonosurgical options depends on the videostroboscopic findings, the surgeon's expertise and the patient's preference. For details see Sect. 8.10.

Depending on the degree of dyspnoea in *bilateral paramedian* positions after a period of 10–12 months, a permanent widening of the glottis is recommended. During this period of about 1 year, a temporary tracheostomy might become necessary. As an alternative, repeated botulinum toxin injections may be tried to achieve a change of positions from paramedian to intermediate by lowering of the vocal fold tension. For most effective injections, the lateral cricoarytenoid and interarytenoid muscles can be treated. Less effective but easier to treat, the cricothyroid muscles can be injected. Several methods of vocal fold lateralisation are described in the literature. The aim of these methods is to ensure respiration and to avoid dysphagia but to accept aphonia. Nowadays the aim is to improve respiration and avoid aphonia. The laser surgical dorsal widening of the glottis (partial arytenoidectomy) is carried out as the optimal compromise between sufficient respiration without tracheostomy and voice quality (Olthoff et al. 2005). Dysphagia only rarely appears temporarily in the post-operative period.

In a bilateral intermediate vocal fold position, a 'wait and see' policy is recommended. Owing to the pathomechanism of a compressed nerve, a neurapraxia can be expected. Fortunately, most of them recover after 6–12 months. In permanent cases phonosurgical options are limited and have to be decided on individually. Voice therapies can establish a ventricular phonation.

In the case of an affected external branch of the superior laryngeal nerve (paralysis of the cricothyroid muscle), voice therapy can be carried out including 'glissando' exercises to improve the pitch range of voice, but the results are barely satisfying owing to the lack of compensatory possibilities.

5.7.9.2 Therapeutic Outlook

Nerve anastomoses or neuromuscular flaps are beginning to show encouraging results, but they are not yet standard surgical procedures. The main effects are seen with healing defects (synkinesis, autoparalysis) that are also mentioned as 'successful regeneration' in the literature (Crumley 1990).

Encouraging results are also seen with regard to the implantation of laryngeal electrodes into the larynx (Med-El) that stimulate the posterior cricoarytenoid muscle, as an option to treat bilateral paramedian paralyses. If laryngeal adduction is sufficient to ensure phonation and laryngeal closure for deglutition, an electric pacer is suited to provide the counterpart (Li et al. 2013).

Case Study 5.24
A 32-year-old attorney underwent surgery of a stenosis of the aortic isthmus 13 months ago. After surgery the left vocal fold was paralysed. She had 30 sessions of voice therapy without sufficient effect. The paralysed vocal fold is bowed and has no respiratory mobility. It is in the paramedian position. The closure pattern is characterised by a complete gap. The sound of the speaking voice is pressed, moderately rough (R2 B1 H2). The voice range profile is markedly restricted. The patient is not able to speak up.

Case Study 5.25
A 52-year-old lecturer and business coach had an aortic dissection 18 months ago. After the vascular reconstruction, during recovery he developed paranoid schizophrenia. His voice is not sufficient to meet the requirements of his profession. The left vocal fold is paralysed in the lateral position. During phonation there is a large gap, and the vocal folds have no contact. Phonation time is extremely short (1.2 s). When reading he runs out of air after a few syllables. The voice sounds severely rough and moderately breathy (R3 B2 H3). Note that in spite of the large glottal gap, the prevailing quality is not breathiness but roughness, which is due to the decoupled vibrations of the vocal folds.

Case Study 5.26
This 74-year-old woman had lung cancer and was operated on. During surgery the left recurrent nerve was severed. One month later neither vocal fold could abduct. Nothing was reported about the right recurrent nerve. She has breathing difficulties especially under exertion but was not tracheotomised. Her voice is impaired as well. During inspiration the vocal folds are driven medially because of the Bernoulli effect. Voice is moderately hoarse (R2 B1 H2). During pauses one can hear how she breathes heavily. The voice range profile is narrow with little dynamic range and no projection of voice.

5.8 Laryngeal Sensory Neuropathy

Thomas Murry

5.8.1 Introduction

The sensory system of the larynx has been shown to affect phonation, swallowing, breathing and reaction to noxious stimuli resulting in cough (Henriquez et al. 2007). In addition, laryngeal sensory neuropathy has been identified in patients with chronic cough, rhinosinusitis and gastro-oesophageal reflux disease (GERD) (Harding

Table 5.7 Diagnoses that may have a sensory component

Vocal fold paralysis
Vocal fold paresis
Chronic cough
Laryngospasm
Spasmodic dysphonia
Bronchitis
Autosomal diseases
Paradoxical vocal fold motion (vocal cord dysfunction)
Irritable larynx syndrome
Pertussis
Exercise induced asthma
Gastro-oesophageal reflux
Laryngo-oesophageal reflux
Idiopathic cough
Unexplained hoarseness (functional dysphonia)

These may be primary or secondary diagnoses

and Richter 1997; Lee and Woo 2005). Sensory integrity of the laryngopharynx is crucial in maintaining upper airway protection to prevent choking and to maintain normal swallowing. Laryngeal sensation is also involved in the control of the cough reflex. Disorders of laryngeal sensitivity are the common denominator in many disorders of the larynx and vocal folds (Wani and Woodson 1999). Chronic cough, paradoxical vocal fold motion and laryngospasm are common disorders that all have a component of abnormal laryngeal sensitivity (Murry and Sapienza 2010). Table 5.7 is a comprehensive list of diagnoses that may have a sensory component. With the proper diagnosis and follow-up treatments, disorders of laryngeal sensory neuropathy improve in the majority of cases. Treatments may include medication, surgery or behavioural rehabilitation. This section describes recent findings of sensory laryngeal neuropathy and its relation to cough and other laryngeal disorders.

5.8.2 Evidence for Laryngeal Sensory Neuropathy

The lamina propria (LP) mucosa develops hyper- or hypo-responsive sensitivity when irritated, inflamed or injured, and no longer transmits information to the vocal folds accurately. This may result in paradoxical vocal fold motion (PVFM) primarily upon inspiration (although it may occur on expiration), following cough or choking. The finding of abnormal vocal fold movement has been shown to result in coughing or shortness of breath (Mazzone 2005).

Another theory is that decreased lamina propria sensation leads to reduced chemosensitivity and results in increased collection of particulate matter in the laryngopharynx and the cough reflex is simply an adaptive mechanism that has evolved to clear the larynx (Cukier-Blaj et al. 2008). Paradoxical adduction of the vocal cords during inspiration in this context can be protective in preventing further inhalation of particulate matter if LP sensation is not intact.

Laryngeal sensory neuropathy that manifests itself as a chronic, intractable cough is associated with sensory changes in the vagus nerve. Whether it is hypo- or hypersensitivity of the LP mucosa, numerous investigations have found a relationship between cough and sensory changes. It remains controversial what type of sensory changes trigger the cough events (Murry et al. 2004; Phua et al. 2005; Zargi et al. 2013). Morrison et al. (1999) described the irritable larynx syndrome (ILS), an entity in which there are central nervous system changes resulting in sensorimotor pathways being left in a hyperexcitable state and an alteration in the way that the central neurons react to incoming stimuli. They suggest that the sensitivity threshold for the cough behaviour is thought to be remapped in the brain.

Paradoxical vocal fold movement (PVFM), a syndrome whereby the vocal folds adduct involuntarily usually during inspiration, has been linked to chronic cough in ILS. Symptoms of PVFM include cough, dysphonia, dyspnoea and choking sensations (Murry and Sapienza 2010). Vertigan et al. (2006) describe some sensory postulates to link chronic cough and PVFM. Cough can be a symptom of PVFM, or a more causal relationship is defined, such as coughing as an adaptive mechanism to help open the vocal folds during an attack of PVFM, as suggested by Cukier-Blaj et al. (2008). Other authors also describe an association among reflux disease, chronic cough and PVFM (Altman and Irwin 2010). Chronic cough has been noted in up to 40% of patients with laryngopharyngeal reflux (LPR) and 80% of patients with PVFM (Newman et al. 1995; Harding and Richter 1997; Sifrim et al. 2005).

Sensitivity of afferent laryngeal nerves can be affected by the presence of inflammatory mediators in the airway and is an important pathophysiological mechanism in the development of chronic cough (Murry et al. 2004). One such inflammatory mediator is recurrent irritation of the laryngopharyngeal (LP) region by stomach acid. In a study by Phua et al. (2005), a calibrated air pulse technique (FEESST method) was used to test for the lowest air pressure (most sensitive) required to elicit the laryngeal adductor reflex (LAR) in 2 groups: 15 patients with chronic cough and GERD and 10 healthy subjects without GERD. The method of using air pulse stimulation to assess laryngopharyngeal sensitivity (LPS) was first described by Aviv et al. (1993), where air pulses of varying calibrated pressures are delivered to the aryepiglottic folds to elicit an involuntary transient adduction of the vocal folds, also known as the LAR. In the study by Phua et al. (2005), the mean baseline LAR threshold of the patient group with chronic cough and GERD was significantly higher (9.5 mm Hg) than that in the normal subjects (3.68 mm Hg), which suggested that the patient group with GERD had significantly impaired LPS.

A condition known as autosomal dominant hereditary sensory neuropathy (HSN I) demonstrates another link between cough and sensory neuropathy. Symptoms of paroxysmal cough, GERD and distal sensory loss are commonly described among those with HSN 1. Neurophysiological and pathological studies demonstrate a sensory axonal neuropathy. Cough in these patients is most likely due to a combination of denervation and hypersensitivity of the upper airways and oesophagus (Spring et al. 2005).

Chronic cough remains with a multifactorial presentation and offers a challenge to the clinician. In addition, it causes social and functional disruption in the patient's quality of life. Despite short-term treatments—some with temporary success—the problem rarely has a long-term solution when treated with a single therapy. It is known that chronic cough can be a manifestation of laryngeal neuropathy (Henriquez et al. 2007) and that chronic cough is seen in patients with PVFM (Murry et al. 2004). Furthermore, patients with LPR have decreased LP sensitivity (Harding and Richter 1997; Phua et al. 2005), and LP sensitivity and cough severity improve in these patients with PPI treatment (Harding and Richter 1997; Murry et al. 2004).

Sensory neuropathy, regardless of measures of hyper- or hyposensitivity, should be considered when patients present with long-term chronic cough. While many patients with chronic cough do have allergies, rhinosinusitis or reflux, medications should resolve those conditions and thus decrease or eliminate the cough. When symptoms persist, sensory neuropathy should be considered as the underlying basis for the disease.

In the case of chronic cough, the presence of symptoms despite various treatments may be due to repeated or extensive exposure to noxious stimuli such as acid reflux, chemicals and environmental pollution or to pneumonia or viral illnesses such as a cold, influenza or upper respiratory infection. Even continued traumatic misuse of the vocal muscles in speaking or repeated throat clearing may lead to long-term cough, as is the case with contact vocal process granuloma. These repetitive events lead to remodelling the normal response in the central nervous system, causing the larynx to respond inappropriately with either a hypo- or hyperactive response, specifically with cough.

Murry et al. (2004) proposed that PVFM and chronic cough were associated with sensory neuropathy of the larynx caused by LPR and could be improved with PPI treatment and with behavioural management, such as that first described by Christopher and colleagues (Rogers and Stell 1978; Christopher et al. 1983). In that study, air pulse stimulation of the aryepiglottic area delivered via a channelled flexible endoscope (Aviv et al. 1999, 2000) was used to elicit the presence of a normal or abnormal response. The study by Phua et al. (2005) also used the calibrated air pulse technique developed by Aviv et al. (1993) to compare LP sensation between patients with GERD and healthy subjects. They concluded that patients with GERD had impaired LP mechanosensitivity and that normal subjects also developed decreased LP mechanosensitivity after infusion of hydrochloric acid. However, the patients with GERD were never treated with medication, and there was no post-treatment evaluation or testing done. Their study also examined patients with isolated GERD, who did not have additional symptoms of cough, hoarseness, laryngospasm or a diagnosis of PVFM.

Lee and Woo (2005) found that gabapentin, an anticonvulsive medication, was helpful in improvement of symptoms in over 65% of the patients with observable laryngeal motor neuropathy. They identified patients with partial paralysis of the vocal folds and the presence of cough and treated them with gabapentin. They interpreted the results as an indication that sensory neuropathy was a contributor to the chronic cough.

5.8.3 Summary

Numerous disorders of the upper airway may have a sensory component. Development of protocols to exclude other diseases has been the primary method for detecting sensory neuropathology. Improved patient assessment often leads to a sensory basis for chronic cough. Improved assessment of sensation, or the lack of it, often leads to satisfactory resolution of the primary problem. For many patients with chronic cough, a combination of factors is often identified as controlling the underlying disease. Chronic cough, when refractory to treatment with typical medications for allergy, reflux disease or sinus conditions, should be considered to be neuropathic in nature. While single treatments of anticonvulsive medications may be helpful, long-term chronic cough is rarely managed successfully with a single treatment regimen. Combined modality treatment of medication plus behavioural management has been shown to offer improvement or resolution for cough when sensory factors are considered as part of the under-

lying cause (Murry et al. 2004; Lee and Woo 2005; Vertigan et al. 2006; Mishriki 2007). Assessment of long-term chronic cough may be extensive, to rule out other conditions, such as asthma, pulmonary disease or rhinosinusitis, or to include them in the treatment regimen.

5.9 Psychosomatic Voice Dysfunction

Dirk Deuster

5.9.1 The Role of Voice in Communication

The voice is the basis of oral communication. To understand why the voice especially can be affected in mental health problems, the nature of different aspects of communication has to be regarded first.

In their communication model, Paul Watzlawick and colleagues formulated 'some tentative axioms of communication', which are very useful for understanding different aspects of communication, as well as the role the voice plays in this process (Watzlawick et al. 2011). Before pointing out three of these axioms with regard to voice, it must be recognised that communication is not only oral speech but also vocal (e.g. prosodic elements including melody and fluency), nonvocal and even nonlinguistic (e.g. facial expression and body movement) behaviour. Therefore, voice is not only the tone generator of oral speech but sends autonomous information comprising non-verbal behaviour, too (Pittam 1994). To realise this, just imagine key voice differences between a friendly discussion and a vehement dispute and the possibility of recognising such differences solely on the basis of voice sound.

In the first axiom 'the content and relationship levels of communication', Watzlawick et al. (2011) describe that communication always includes both the content and relationship level and the authors emphasise that the relationship aspect becomes more important when relationships are 'sick' because of a 'constant struggle about the nature of the relationship' and vice versa. The axiom 'digital and analogue communication' means that communication uses analogue and digital (e.g. words) signals, whereby analogue communication is almost always all non-verbal communication. It should be noted that 'non-verbal' does not mean 'mute' but includes vocal and nonvocal behaviour. When considered together, both axioms acquire special significance: communication is not only oral speech but any kind of behaviour and consists of content and a relationship level. It might be reasonably assumed that the relationship level is conveyed mainly by analogue means and acquires more impact when relationships are disturbed. By supposing that the voice or prosody is a part of analogue communication, it becomes clear why the voice expresses emotional states and is vulnerable to mental and behavioural disorders.

Last, 'the impossibility of noncommunication' has far-reaching consequences: because it is not possible 'not to behave', it is consequently not possible not to communicate either, and thus the voice sends information continuously, even—or in particular—if the voice is aphonic.

5.9.2   Mental Illness in Phoniatric Practice

In general, phoniatricians encounter patients with directly relevant psychological disorders (see Fig. 5.22) or without a direct connection to a phoniatric disease or condition. The first group comprises certain patients with a 'phoniatric manifestation' of a mental illness such as a dissociative motor disorder (F44.4), an acute stress reaction (F43.0) or adjustment disorders (F43.2) as a result of a phoniatric disease, psychological factors affecting a phoniatric disease or condition (F54) or a phoniatric disease as one symptom of a mental illness (e.g. voice changes within a mood disorder, sore throat as part of a somatoform pain disorder). The second group includes patients with mental and behavioural disorders clearly perceived by the phoniatrician but without a causal link to the phoniatric disease or condition, which occur especially in patients with personality disorders (F60).

Thus, different psychological disorders may affect a voice disorder. Conversely, a voice disorder is neither pathognomonic for a specific

Fig. 5.22 Examples of psychological disorders (diagnoses with ICD-10) directly relevant to voice disorders

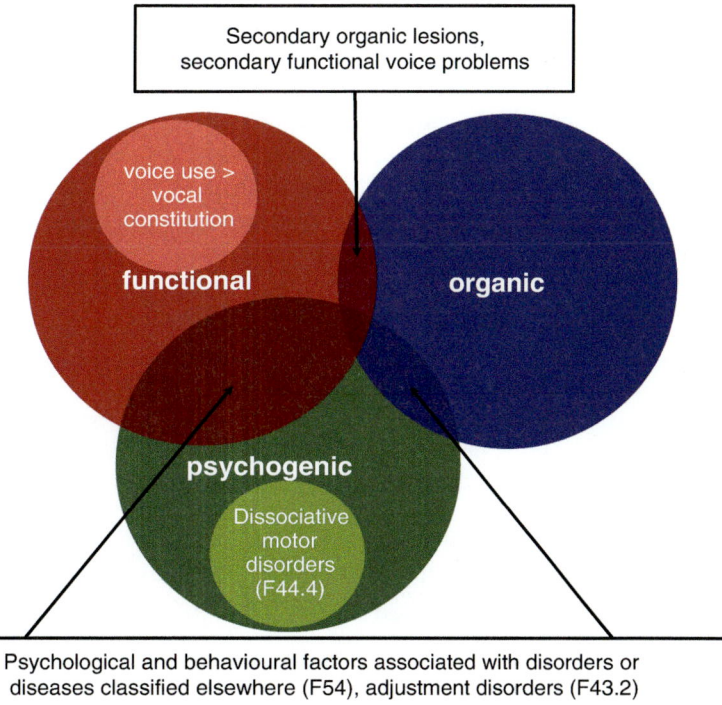

mental illness nor for a specific intrapsychic or interpersonal process. Therefore, if a mental illness is suspected, specific examination methods are needed and diagnostic criteria have to be fulfilled to make a definite diagnosis.

5.9.3 Psychogenic Aphonia

Psychogenic aphonia is a very impressive disorder condition. In ICD10 (World Health Organization 2014), it belongs to the dissociative disorders (F44), specifically to the dissociative motor disorders (F44.4). ICD10 describes dissociative disorders as

> […] a partial or complete loss of the normal integration between […] control of bodily movements,

whereas

> medical examination and investigation do not reveal the presence of any known physical or neurological disorder.
>
> WHO (2014)

This means in case of psychogenic aphonia that volitional movements to close the vocal folds for phonation are not possible without an apparent (organic) cause. Figure 5.23 shows typical laryngostroboscopic findings of a patient with a psychogenic aphonia. In addition, a 'hyperfunctional' type of aphonia exists with a floating transition to psychogenic dysphonia. This form is more rare and is in some cases an attempt of hyperfunctional compensation for the lack of glottis closure in 'hypofunctional' aphonia. But whether the vocal folds cannot vibrate because of a lack of glottal closure or an excessive tension, either way the result is a more or less voiceless communication. However, the differentiation between a hypo- and hyperfunctional form is important for differential diagnosis (e.g. spasmodic dysphonia) and voice therapy.

According to the literature, psychogenic aphonia is a rare disease with a point prevalence of 0.4%, and women are hugely over-represented (Kollbrunner et al. 2010). However, the fact that dissociative disorders tend to recede after days to weeks with or without therapeutic interventions makes it difficult to obtain exact data. In particular, it may be assumed that patients with short-term aphonia were either not referred to phoniatricians regularly or lost the typical aphonic symptomatology until phoniatric investigation, so that the diagnosis or suspected diagnosis is based only on medical history. The following symptoms and history information are landmark information for psychogenic aphonia:

- Sudden-onset beginning (and end) of aphonia
- Voiced throat-clearing or coughing, voiced laughing and crying
- No explanatory physical/neurological disorder
- Close association in time with 'traumatic events, insoluble and intolerable problems, or disturbed relationships' (ICD10 criteria). Although, this association cannot be always verified in a first interview
- Because of the recurring character of psychogenic aphonia, most patients report periods with an aphonic voice in the past

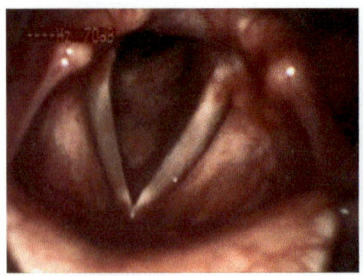 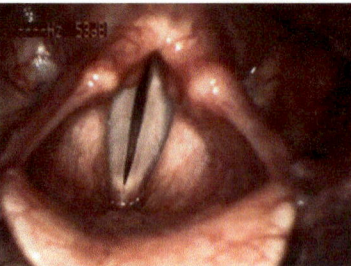 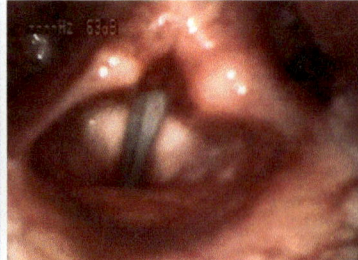

Fig. 5.23 Patient (female, 24 years of age) with a psychogenic aphonia while breathing, trying to vocalise, and coughing (from left to right)

It may be confusing when a patient with an aphonic voice shows a complete glottal closure within the laryngoscopic investigation. Because the examination situation is not comparable with that of free conversation, this phenomenon occasionally occurs and should not prevent the diagnosis of a psychogenic aphonia.

In addition, the following information in the medical history should be requested:

- The beginning and course of aphonia provide information about possible traumatic events. In this respect it is important to understand that aphonia does not have to be a catastrophic event but must be interpreted with regard to the biographical background of the patient
- The assumed cause of aphonia gives information about the patient's disease concept and is useful for patient counselling
- Limitations in everyday life due to aphonia may provide information about a morbid gain
- Previous diagnostics and treatment can point to somatisation factors and is also necessary for patient counselling

Patients are usually not conscious of the psychogenic origin. Quite to the contrary, most patients have a somatic disease concept, and this concept will be reinforced with the beginning or logical assignment of the aphonia with a real or supposed upper respiratory infection and a corresponding somatic treatment by physicians. Because psychogenic aphonia disorders tend to recede, the somatic treatment will be perceived as successful (known as somatisation). However, it occasionally happens that an upper respiratory infection occurs before the first appearance of an aphonia. Unfortunately, the phoniatrician is often referred to only when aphonic periods become more frequent or sustained, and it is more difficult at this stage to discuss a psychogenic origin than at the onset of symptoms. It is very important to note that organic changes in the larynx do not exclude a dissociative motor disorder. What is relevant is whether an organic change adequately explains the extent and progress of (sudden) aphonia.

Case Study 5.27
A 24-year-old woman works as a dentist's assistant. She underwent surgery of the vocal folds because of alleged Reinke's oedema 2 years ago. The voice was recorded 1 day and 3 months after the intervention. No injuries were seen on the vocal folds during video-laryngostroboscopy. She was able to speak with a normal voice but felt that it did not improve. On the contrary the voice gradually vanished. At the moment there is no voice at all. Voice therapy did not lead to a restitution of the voice. She received psychotherapy but lost the motivation to continue. The video shows incomplete adduction of the vocal folds as if there was a blockage. She has spoken in a whisper for more than 1 year.

5.9.4 Psychogenic Dysphonia and Psychogenic Aspects of Functional Dysphonia

In comparison with psychogenic aphonia with its typical symptoms, a definition and diagnosis of psychogenic dysphonia are much more difficult. Studies have shown that dysphonic patients have high levels of mental/psychosocial distress irrespective of the cause of dysphonia (Millar et al. 1999; Misono et al. 2014) so that psychological factors can be a cause as well as an effect of a dysphonia. However, not only the cause but the severity of mental illness is crucial for the need of adequate therapeutic interventions.

As described in the Sect. 5.1, psychogenic aspects are one aetiological factor for functional voice disorders so that a differentiation between 'functional' and 'psychogenic' is not always possible but rather a matter of degree. Normally, a multifactorial condition with more (e.g. dissociative dysphonia) or fewer (e.g. occupational voice disorder with concomitant occupational distress) psychological factors exists.

From a diagnostic point of view, some information in the medical history and clinical investigation point to underlying psychological factors:

- The voice symptoms are more situation-related than dependent on voice use and may change several times per day

- Long courses of voice therapy without a sustained improvement of voice function
- Drawing attention to the voice during the history interview or clinical investigation exacerbates the dysphonia, so that examination results are unexpectedly bad
- The voice quality may change when the patient talks about triggering psychosocial factors, e.g. the partner, the illness or death of a family member or the professional situation (Bauer 1990)

The last point is a main factor in clinical examination since, in contrast to psychogenic aphonia, a typical finding in laryngostroboscopic examination is lacking. The laryngostroboscopic findings are very different. Often patients present a pronounced glottal and supraglottal hypertension with a sound like a hyperfunctional or spasmodic dysphonia, but also more hypofunctional forms with breathy or pulse register-like sounds or tremolando and dysarthria-like sounds are possible. Hence, apart from the psychosocial medical history (distress, personal or professional conflicts, etc.), differential diagnostics plays an important role in the diagnosis of a psychogenic dysphonia.

Case Study 5.28

Three months ago, this 32-year-old kindergarten teacher had an acute respiratory infection and lost her voice. After recovery the voice remained impaired. She was not able to go to work because of the reduced vocal loading capacity. The video demonstrates incomplete closure during phonation in an otherwise normal larynx. The voice range profile is shifted to higher frequencies; the maximal volume is too low for professional purposes. The voice sound is soft and breathy. It has many aphonic insets and no 'core' (R1 B2 H2).

5.9.5 Psychogenic Aspects of Mutational Falsetto

Different forms of disorders of the voice with regard to mutation are known (see Sect. 5.10).

From a psychosomatic viewpoint, the persistent fistular voice or mutational falsetto in men is particularly interesting. Subject to an absence of a hormonal and organic cause, a 'child voice' persists owing to an excessive tension of the cricothyroid muscle.

To understand a possibly psychogenic aetiology of this phenomenon, a view of the psychosocial development in the constituting phase of mutational falsetto, puberty, is helpful. It is the stage of transition from childhood to adulthood and substantial body changes, particularly the altering of the voice, reflect this transition. But this transition and finding one's role in the adult world is a complex development for young men. Erikson described the 'Who am I and what can I be?' as the existential question and 'identity versus role confusion' as the psychosocial crisis at this stage (Erikson 1959).

It is therefore obvious that the retention of the high 'child voice' can be an (unconscious) expression of problems of accepting or fulfilling the new role. Another factor cited in this context is a strong emotional bond with the mother. There is however a lack of systematic investigations of these links, probably owing to the small number of patients with mutational falsetto.

Case Study 5.29

A 25-year-old man did not have voice change. He had androgen therapy when he was 14. The testosterone level is normal now. At present he takes a tricyclic antidepressant. His height is 156 cm and his weight 48 kg. The thyroid cartilage has grown. The Adam's apple is clearly visible. Beard growth is sparse. He is the only child and still lives with his parents. He speaks in his falsetto voice, and sometimes growling low sounds intermingle. When looking at this shy and timid person, one may well imagine that he might be frightened by his own masculine voice that would be in sharp contrast to his delicate body. He only uses his child voice as recorded in the voice range profile. The larynx has a normal adult size. The vocal folds are tense and do not contact during phonation.

5.9.6 Therapeutic Strategies for Psychosomatic Voice Dysfunctions

The key task for the phoniatrician is to recognise a patient's mental illness. In the case of psychogenic aphonia, the symptoms themselves lead to the diagnosis; in other cases the medical history as well as a possible discrepancy between phoniatric findings and the patient's condition hint at psychological factors. The phonatrician's thoughts should be discussed with the patient, and in this respect it is particularly important to be sensitive and empathic, because patients mostly perceive their problems as somatic and psychogenic origins are potentially unconscious. Thus, confronted with the diagnosis of a psychogenic origin, patients often do not really feel they are being taken seriously. It can be helpful to use the term 'distress' for a start, because it is readily understandable and does not normally have a negative connotation as does 'mental illness'. In this regard, apart from basic psychosomatic competence, a special qualification in communication skills and a Balint group is helpful and recommended for phoniatricians.

A psychotherapy or psychopharmacological drug treatment is not required for all patients, but if a mental illness is suspected, the diagnosis and the need for treatment must be determined. Normally this requires a psychosomatic or psychiatric examination in addition; experience shows that it is beneficial for the patient when the phoniatrician, as a specialist for voice disorders, acts as advisor and guide for the patient.

Because we have to pick up the patients where they are, a symptomatic voice therapy, which should include exercises for voice and body perception, is most often helpful for the patient and sufficient with regard to their current voice function. However, the 'causative therapy' has to be kept in mind, too, so that—especially in recurring psychogenic aphonia—close medical supervision from the phoniatrician in cooperation with a psychosomatic or psychotherapeutic colleague is needed, in order not to overlook underlying intrapsychic or interpersonal processes after voice restitution.

5.10 Hormone-Related Dysphonia

Andrzej Obrębowski and Dirk Deuster

5.10.1 Introduction

The endocrine system controls the inner environment by secreting hormones affecting metabolism, homeostasis and reproductive processes. Specificity of hormone actions depends on their receptors, located in target organs.

The human voice organ is sensitive to the action of hormones and sex hormones in particular (Abitbol et al. 1999), although the underlying mechanisms are not clear in detail. Even though investigations of the expression of sexual hormone receptors have shown conflicting results (Newman et al. 2000; Schneider et al. 2007; Cohen et al. 2009; Nacci et al. 2011; Voelter et al. 2008), it is undisputed that changes in the level of sexual hormones lead to voice changes (Raj et al. 2010; D'haeseleer et al. 2009; Harries et al. 1997; Damste 1964). Therefore, the larynx is considered to represent a secondary sex characteristic.

Pruszewicz and Obrębowski (1992) found that hormonally conditioned voice disturbances comprise around 15% of all disturbances of voice in women.

5.10.2 Influence of Sex Hormones

With puberty, sex differences in the development of the larynx are observable, resulting from a larger larynx and longer vocal folds in men. The larger growth in men is a result of an increasing testosterone production (Fuchs et al. 1999; Harries et al. 1997). After puberty, the laryngeal cartilage begins to ossify, and from then on endogenous or exogenous testosterone leads to a voice deepening, but no longer to a growth of the cartilage. Studies suggest that androgens influence the expression of alkaline phosphatase and mineralisation in the male thyroid cartilage (Claassen et al. 2006). In women, different levels of oestrogen and progesterone may effect vocal fold and voice changes within the menstrual cycle, pregnancy and menopause (e.g. Barillari et al. 2016; Chernobelsky 2002; Chae et al. 2001; Davis and Davis 1993; Moses et al. 1997; D'haeseleer et al. 2012; Raj et al. 2010; Abitbol et al. 1999).

5.10.2.1 Mutation and Its Disturbances

In European children, the first signs of pubertal development ((in boys testicular growth, Tanner stage G2, and in girls breast development, Tanner stage B2 (Tanner 1962)) can be identified at the age at about 11.5 years in boys and 11 years in girls (Parent et al. 2003). Voice change, also known as mutation, manifests later during the subsequent course of puberty, approximately at the age of 12. Relating to testicular growth, mutation will start in less than a year if testicular volume reaches 20 mL (Tanner stage G5) (Fuchs et al. 1999). At mutation, the voice of boys becomes lowered on the average by one octave, in girls by three to four semitones with a parallel change of vocal range (Fuchs 2008; Hollien et al. 1994).

Three stages of mutation course are distinguished (e.g. Seeman 1959):

- Pre-mutation period: the voice becomes flat, occasionally hoarse
- Proper mutational period: a hoarse voice with sudden alterations in its pitch, uncertain intonation
- Post-mutation period: gradual maturation of voice to a quality appropriate for a given individual

Most frequently the mutational alterations last 8–12 weeks, however, the post-mutation period may extend to 2–3 years. Laryngological alterations sometimes suggest an inflammatory condition of the larynx. The alterations may involve phonatory insufficiency of the posterior glottis, in the form of the so-called mutational triangle.

According to Seeman (1959), the most frequent disturbances of mutation include:

- Persistent fistular voice (vox fistularis persistens): excessive tension of the cricothyroid muscle leads to a high pitch of voice. Frontal compression of thyroid cartilage (Bresgen's manoeuvre) and overcoming of the tension may result in an immediate effect of lowering the voice pitch to an individually appropriate one
- Prolonged mutation (mutatio prolongata): the alterations typical for mutation persist occasionally for several months
- Premature mutation (mutatio precox): a decrease in pitch of voice at the age of 8–10 years, it requires endocrinological diagnosis (tumours of adrenal cortex)
- Perverse mutation (mutatio perversa): a significant decrease in pitch of voice during mutation in girls, frequently linked to an excessive growth of the larynx, which requires endocrinological diagnosis

In very rare cases, disorders of sexual development (DSD) are the underlying reasons for a lacking or unexpected voice change in puberty (e.g. Klinefelter syndrome, androgen insensitivity syndrome, congenital adrenal hyperplasia). In these cases, in addition to the voice development, other physical aspects of sexual development are affected such as the growth of height, pubic hair, beard, testis or breast and the menarche. In cases of doubt, gynaecological, urological and endocrinological examinations should be performed (Hiort et al. 2014).

5.10.2.2 Voice Disturbances in the Menstrual Cycle and in Menopausal Women

Fluctuations in hormone levels - in the follicular phase an increase of oestrogens with a low level of progesterone, in the luteal phase a gradual increase in progesterone with a decrease in oestrogen - may have an effect on women's voice. Therefore, in the premenstrual and menstrual phases, vocal folds and voice changes are described, whereby the current data are heterogeneous (e.g. Barillari et al. 2016; Chernobelsky 2002; Chae et al. 2001; Davis and Davis 1993). These voice changes are discrete and affect in

...g voice (Nawka and Wirth

...omparing different phases of the menstruation cycle, Raj et al. (2010) found the 'best voice quality' in the phase with the highest oestrogen level, the ovulatory phase (days 13–15) and the 'worst voice quality' in the premenstrual phase (days 24–28). But these differences are discrete and group effects, so that it is not possible to specify the phase of menstruation on the basis of voice parameter.

The relative increase of testosterone in postmenopausal women might lead to a voice deepening (D'haeseleer et al. 2012, Raj et al. 2010, Abitbol et al. 1999).

5.10.2.3 Voice Disturbances in the Course of Pregnancy

In the course of pregnancy, changes of the laryngeal mucosa such as oedema, dry mucosa and occasional crusting may impair voice functions (Moses et al. 1997). These changes are known as laryngopathia gravidarum and occur in a more oedematous form and a more dry form (Laryngitis sicca gravidarum) (Nawka and Wirth 2008; Höing and Seitzer 1988). Some case reports have described severe stenotic laryngeal oedema associated with pre-eclampsia (Höing and Seitzer 1988). In addition, in the course of pregnancy, gastro-oesophageal reflux frequently causes vocal function to become worse.

5.10.3 Dysfunction of the Pituitary Gland

Of the many hormones produced by the frontal lobe of the pituitary gland, disturbances in growth hormone (GH) secretion especially influence voice. Untreated hypopituitary children, with a lack of GH, show higher mean speaking fundamental frequencies than healthy children of the same age (Hoffman et al. 1984). Conversely, adults with active acromegaly (excessive GH secretion), most frequently as a result of an adenoma of the pituitary gland, have lower mean speaking fundamental frequencies and higher perturbation parameters than healthy adults,

whereas the mean speaking fundamental frequencies are, with only a few exceptions, in the normal reference range (Bogazzi et al. 2010; Williams et al. 1994). Aydin et al. (2013) found no significant differences in the mean speaking fundamental frequencies but also different perturbation parameter values.

5.10.4 Dysfunction of the Thyroid and Parathyroid Glands

Thyroid hormones (thyroxine, tri-iodothyronine) represent iodine-containing amino acids. They are formed under the effect of pituitary and hypothalamic hormones. Thyroid hormones regulate energy expenditure and biological development.

Despite the neighbourhood of the larynx and the thyroid gland, voice dysfunction in thyroidal disease is caused by the general impact of a hypothyroid or hyperthyroid metabolic status. In hyperthyroidism, analogous to the typical symptoms of neuromuscular tremor, nervousness, hyperactivity and dyspnoea (De Leo et al. 2016), voice symptoms similar to those of functional dysphonia, a vocal tremor or a shortness of breath may occur.

Infants with congenital hypothyroidism (cretinism) show crying abnormalities such as greater vibrato contour and lower crying frequencies (Boero et al. 2000). In adults with non-congenital hypothyroidism, hoarseness, lowered pitch, vocal fatigue and reduced range of voice have been described as possible voice symptoms (Birkent et al. 2008). In the author's (OA) observation, an increased mass of the vocal folds is observed with parallel muscular atrophy. In hypothyroid patients, most often in long-standing or severe hypothyroidism, myxedema, an accumulation of glycosaminoglycans in subcutaneous and other interstitial tissues, may occur, but it is rare today (Braverman and Utiger 2005). In addition, hypothyroidism may cause respiratory problems with influence on voice function, for example, by actions on the ventilatory control system, diaphragmatic muscle function or a goitre-caused upper airway obstruction (Sorensen et al. 2016).

Regardless of hormonal status, diseases of the thyroid gland with goitre can cause symptoms such as globus sensation, the feeling of a foreign body and dysphagia, by a mechanical effect.

Similar to those in thyroid gland diseases, voice dysfunctions in parathyroid gland diseases are results of a general effect, which is either a hypocalcaemia in hypoparathyroidism or hypercalcaemia in hyperparathyroidism. Therefore, in hyperparathyroidism muscle weakness and easy fatigability, and in hypoparathyroidism various symptoms of neuromuscular irritability including laryngospasm, can occur (Silverberg and Bilezikian 2001; Jan De Beur et al. 2001).

5.10.5 Dysfunction of the Suprarenal Glands

The abnormal secretion of cortisol or other adrenocortical steroids shows clinical manifestations in many organ systems (Cushing syndrome) (Schteingart 2001). Cushing-specific voice disorders are not described in detail. In adrenal insufficiency (Addison disease), general weakness and fatigue can similarly alter voice.

5.10.6 Voice Disturbances in Diabetes Mellitus

In the pancreas, the endocrine function is fulfilled by the pancreatic islands, which secrete the anabolic polypeptide insulin. Its deficit results in diabetes mellitus. Apart from the typical symptoms, voice disturbances termed xerophonia or dry voice may develop (Sataloff et al. 1997). In addition, diabetic neuropathy seems to be relevant in the larynx with positive sensory symptoms such as limb numbness and burning pain or reduced sensibility (Hamdan et al. 2014).

5.10.7 Virilisation of the Female Voice Organ

Endogenous virilisation of the voice organ can be induced by tumours of the ovary or adrenal cortex, polycystic ovaries, functional disturbances in the ovarian stroma cellular system or within DSD (congenital adrenal hyperplasia); see Sect. 5.10.2.1. Exogenous virilisation results from administration of drugs that contain androgens, anabolic steroids or progestogens.

As described in Sect. 5.12, androgens influence the larynx with the result of a voice deepening and, depending on ossification status, a laryngeal growth. Laryngostroboscopic findings in adults show different results: Obrębowski (1983) found that the virilising lesions are significantly promoted by morphological-functional asymmetries within the larynx and professional loading of voice, whereas Deuster (2017) detected no significant visible changes of the larynx of women treated with testosterone because of a female-to-male transsexualism (see Sect. 5.12). However, it is well known that androgenic or anabolic steroids promote muscle mass, so that one can assume that an increasing mass of vocal muscle is at least partly responsible for voice deepening.

The prodromal signs of virilisation are important, including lustreless voice with progressive alteration in its timbre, intonational insecurity. The range of the voice gradually becomes reduced from the top frequencies, the duration of phonation becomes shortened, and the mean timbre of voice becomes changed.

In anabolic dysphonia, analysis of basic frequency, apart from disturbances in periodicity and intonational alterations, demonstrates an initial lowering (Pruszewicz et al. 1973). The lowering of the mean frequency of voice remains irreversible.

5.11 A Survey on Gender Vocology Focused on the Demands of Male-to-Female Transsexuals

Christiane Neuschaefer-Rube

5.11.1 Introduction

Gender vocology, apart from the historical and cultural topic of the castrate's voice, and the medical problems in the context of the mutational voice, has its origin in the rising number of individuals who feel a very deep attraction to live in the sex opposite to that they were born in. Unlike hermaphrodites, the chromosomal and genital appearance of these transsexuals is in accordance, and their sex organs are complete. It was Benjamin who described as early as 1953 that the transsexual is firmly convinced that his or her psychological gender is the opposite of his or her anatomical gender (Benjamin 1953, 1966). In everyday life, these individuals have a strong desire to belong to this opposite sex in respect of their body, their outfit, and their communicational skills and habits with special emphasis of their voice. Since a hormonal treatment of female-to-male (FM) transsexuals has the desired side effect in lowering their voice, the phoniatric patients asking for gender-related voice fitting are mainly male-to-female (MF) transsexuals. The present section is focused on the demands of this patient group, introduced by summaries of physiological voice perception and production in male and female adults.

5.11.2 Terminology

In diagnostic terms, the so-called *gender dysphoria* is categorised as a *gender identity disorder* encoding transsexualism as F64.0 within the International Classification of Diseases (WHO 2010). Further criteria of gender identity disorders are summarised in different versions of the *Diagnostic and Statistical Manual of Mental Disorders* (DSM) (Cohen-Kettenis and Pfäfflin 2010). It is of importance that the label *GID*, being the abbreviation of gender identity disorder, is often used in a less-specific meaning than the terms transsexualism and trans-identity (Cohen-Kettenis and Pfäfflin 2010). In respect of the latter, the term *transsexual* is mainly focused on the biological qualities such as one's chromosomal, gonadal, morphological and hormonal characteristics, whereas the terms *transgender* and *transident* mainly pronounce their social context and gender identity (Migeon and Wisniewski 1998).

5.11.3 What Do We Know About the Epidemiology and Aetiology of Transsexualism?

The prevalence of transsexualism in Europe is high and seems to have been increasing since the 1960s of the last century (for an overview see Michel et al. 2001, Olyslager and Conway 2007). However, the epidemiological data in the past were typically estimated by indirect statistics and by questionnaires given to divergent patient groups (cf. Gómez-Gil et al. 2009), since formal epidemiological studies had not been conducted by then (Zucker and Lawrence 2009). Having these restrictions in mind, the following statistics are often quoted: for Germany a prevalence of 1:94,000–1:104,000 for female-to-male (FM) transsexuals has been reported in contrast to that of 1:36,000–1:42,000 for male-to-female (MF) transsexuals (Weitze and Osburg 1996). The prevalence in the Netherlands shows a ratio of 1:30,400 for FMs and one of 1:11,900 for MFs. For the population in Belgium, the data were quite similar when estimated some years ago (de Cuypere et al. 2007). Data from Spain revealed a prevalence of 1:48,096 (FMs) and 1:21,031 (MFs) for the population of Catalonia (Gómez-Gil et al. 2006). Probably the number of transident individuals in all countries is considerably higher, since not all patients undertake all steps of the medical and legal gender fitting process, so that an unknown number of them remain uncounted. For most European countries, the ratio of transsexuals changing from male to female is two or more times higher than that of transsexuals in the opposite manner (Garrels et al. 2000; Gómez-Gil et al. 2009; Michel et al. 2001; Olyslager and Conway 2007).

However, the aetiology of transsexualism and transidentity is not established as yet. While there are some investigators who define these groups mainly as a problem of cultural education and role (e.g. Butler 1990; Hirschauer 1999), there are a growing number of researchers who have reported biological evidence of transsexualism. The main areas of evidence deal with the alterations in hormonal interactions in these individuals and with alterations in brain function and morphology (Michel et al. 2001). For example, the data of Kranz et al. (2014) support the hypothesis of a lateralised serotonergic system that seems to be absent from the mid-cingulum, indicating a circumscribed absence of brain masculinisation in that region in MFs, and Kruijver et al. (2000) report MFs having female neuron numbers in a limbic nucleus. Our own group has investigated cerebral correlates of voice gender perception in response to natural and opposite-gender morphed voices in healthy men and women (Junger et al. 2013) and in MFs (Junger et al. 2014). In these studies, the fMRI data of the transsexuals compared with the two healthy groups showed differences in a widespread neural network.

5.11.4 Gender-Specific Voice Perception

Voice is of evolutionary significance in respect of mating and belongs to the secondary sex characteristics. In a recent study we could show that healthy men and women perceive male and female voices differently. For men and women, it is true that they identify voice samples of the opposite sex faster and more accurately than those of their own sex. The neural correlates of this opposite gender-related voice perception could be identified and localised mainly in the right medial prefrontal cortex, the left orbitofrontal cortex and the left middle temporal gyrus (Junger et al. 2013). Interestingly, this improved perception of voices belonging to the opposite sex has been proven not to be true for MFs. MFs showed different fMRI patterns in the neural network when listening to male vs. female voices from those of healthy men and women. These differences were even true for opposite-sex morphed voices. In respect of the latter, the cerebral reaction pattern of MFs was more similar to those of women than to those of men (Junger et al. 2014).

Influences of special gender-related voice characteristics were investigated by Van Borsel et al. (2009). They could show that vowels spoken by healthy women using a breathy voice were rated as more feminine than those spoken in a natural voice by male listeners. In studies reporting that men prefer women with high pitched voices, it could be shown that they prefer raised pitch in females at all levels of starting pitch (Feinberg et al. 2008).

5.11.5 Gender-Specific Voice Production

The voice production during life starts with a uniform cry at birth of 450–520 Hz (Michelsson et al. 2002). Following a developmental voice dimorphism, the performance of mean fundamental frequencies, formants, prosody, semantic and gestural habits are quite different in adult males and females. Although different hormone receptors have been localised within the vocal folds (Newman et al. 2000), in contrast to primary females, a cross-hormone therapy in biological males does not change their glottal function and voice. For healthy adults, the rule of thumb is that the speaking voice of females is twice the mean fundamental frequency (F0) of that of males, whose voice is an octave lower. In detail, according to Oates and Dacakis (1997), the mean F0 for males is reported as 107–132 Hz (range: 80–165 Hz) and the mean F0 for females as 196–224 Hz (range: 145–275 Hz), whereas the pitch range between 145 and 165 Hz represents the gender-ambiguous range. The same authors quoted that transsexuals with an F0 ≥160 Hz are likely to be perceived as females, in contrast to those with F0 <160 Hz who are perceived as males (Oates and Dacakis 1997). These data are similar to those of Wolfe et al. (1990) who observed 155 Hz as the lowest F0 identified as female. However, not only vocal artists such as voice imitators cross their borders. Therefore, Oates and Dacakis (1997) pointed out that these data should be considered as sex-preferential rather than sex-exclusive. In addition to the sex-related differences of the mean fundamental frequencies, there are sex-related varieties of formants as well. A large study was performed by Gunnar Fant in the 1970s who examined vowels in six different languages. Some of the reported differences between adult males and females were positive shifts of F1 for the vowel /a/ resulting from the smaller size of the pharynx in females. Differences in respect of the F2 for /i/ were explained by the fact that this formant forms the λ/2-resonance of the pharynx, and differences of the F3 for /u/ result from the sex difference between the pharynx-to-oral cavity length (Fant 1975).

5.11.6   General Treatment of Male-to-Female Transgenders

It is obvious that the rules of medical and legal approval of transsexualism vary in different European countries. In some countries there are no rules; in others there are very specific regulations (for overview, see Steinmetzer and Groß 2008). However, in this section the author will focus on principles representing some sort of current consensus. It is usual in most of the countries that individuals assigning themselves as transsexuals have to visit a psychiatrist to have the diagnosis verified. In different stages of treatment, a so-called real-life test is carried out. This means that the MF has lived in the role of the opposite gender for a defined period. Since this test is mostly performed before cross-sexual hormone therapy, breast and genital assignment surgery and before voice therapy, it is difficult to put into practice. The sense of this activity is to explore sociocultural changes in living the target role, to confirm the purposes of the predominantly irreversible treatments. In respect of legal identity, there is an important difference between an official change of name adjusted to the target sex and a change of legal sex attribution. In countries in which same-sex unions are unusual, a change of legal sex attribution may initiate divorce. This is very difficult for many transsexuals, since their families and partners are often important assistants during their gender and body transition. In addition, those relatives need some time to orientate themselves for further life as well. Thus, in the author's experience, there is a considerable number of MFs who delay their legal female attribution to prolong their social relationships.

5.11.7   Gender-Specific Voice Fitting in Male-to-Female Transgenders

What are the aims of a gender-specific voice fitting in male-to-female transgenders?

- To define an individual therapeutic target voice that matches the voice ideals with the transgender's body, age, peer group and private and professional demands
- To achieve gender conformity in self-perception of voice in respect of the speaker's self-identity with her target sex
- A very important goal is to achieve a perceptual voice gender conformity for listeners, which means learning to avoid a mismatch between sex and voice in private and occupational situations

Following these demands to develop a female voice production, there are further therapeutic goals and strategies to consider. It is important to compound a sustainment or improvement of voice quality, endurance and resilience according to individual demands, avoiding hyperfunctional dysphonia resulting from inadequate voice training. In this context, it is important to note that in the author's experience, a great number of transgenders are professional speakers. Since the mean fundamental frequency does not fit for all male-to-female transgenders, it is necessary to use complementary strategies. They underline the social role performance of the persons. Examples are to fit prosodic habits, diction, gestures, facial expression based on female outfit, standing and walking. Although only some of the MF individuals need phonosurgical voice adjustment, the specific techniques will be presented first.

5.11.7.1   Phonosurgical Approaches
The main concepts of phonosurgical treatments in male-to-female transgenders to feminise the voice are laryngeal framework surgery and endolaryngeal glottal surgery. It is usual to combine this phonosurgery, often as a sandwich strategy with conservative voice training. In addition,

epilation, thyroid chondroplasty to reduce the silhouette of the male thyroid cartilage, genioplasty, rhinoplasty and other facial adjustments (Becking et al. 1996) are sometimes added as strategies to fulfil a feminisation of the facio-cervical appearance of the former males.

The framework surgery was invented by Isshiki who described a cricothyroid approximation (Isshiki et al. 1974) often cited as Isshiki's type IV thyroplasty (e.g. Brown et al. 2000). The functional principle of this surgery is an increase in vocal cord tension to raise the speaking fundamental frequencies. In experiments on excised human larynxes, Kitajima et al. (1979) found a linear relation between cricothyroid distance and fundamental frequency of approximately 0.15–0.90 semitones per mm of approximation, up to a plateau found by force application of 30–50 gm. Kanagalingam et al. (2005) extended the approximation technique by an additional anterior subluxation of the thyroid cartilage. Further modifications are the cricothyroidopexy with use of titanium mini-plates as a common strategy (Neumann et al. 2003; Neumann and Welzel 2004). Other techniques such as anterior commissure advancement (LeJeune et al. 1983) or the modification of Tucker (1985), as well as the A-P expansion of the thyroid ala by vertical strip insertion (Isshiki 1989) performed through a cartilage window from the external approach, are to the author's knowledge not frequently carried out any more. It is important to recognise that in contrast to the glottal surgery, and to framework surgery combined with excisions of the anterior vocal cords (Kunachak et al. 2000), the cricothyroid approximation is to some extent reversible.

Reports on the outcome following cricothyroid approximation 6 months and later after surgery present data of an overall fundamental frequency gain for the speaking voice of 56.9 Hz, estimated by EGG, representing a mean raise of approximately five semitones (Kanagalingam et al. 2005). Other authors found an acoustically estimated F0-rise of 3–5 semitones in 32% and of more than 6 semitones in 42% of 59 patients following cricothyroidopexy, including 7% who achieved a rise of more than eight semitones (Neumann et al. 2003). However, 26% of the patients did not achieve even a rise of three semitones. One third of the group remained in the category of male f0 (A1-C#3), another third rose to the gender-ambiguous range (D3-E3), and only the last third achieved that of a female f0 (>F3) (Neumann et al. 2003). In a long-term survey over an 8-year period of 45 MF responders, the satisfaction rate of long-lasting voice improvements reached 70%. It is noticeable in this context that only 55% of the individuals estimated this result as a surgical effect whereas 21% thought that voice therapy was more effective (Matai et al. 2003). In a perceptual rating of femaleness of the voice of MFs compared with those of natural men and women in an auditory only, and in an audiovisual setting, the rating scores of the MFs lay between those of the natural groups in both settings (Van Borsel et al. 2008).

Glottal surgery presented as a technique following a laryngofissure with denudation and approximation of the anterior third of the vocal cords (Donald 1982) has been substituted by endolaryngeal glottal surgery carried out during microlaryngoscopy by Wendler (1994). The endolaryngeal glottal surgery is sometimes performed as a vocal fold stripping and more often as a glottoplasty, whereby the anterior part of the vocal folds is sutured after precise rim deep epithelisation by laser (Wendler 1994). The main intention of the stripping is to increase vocal fold stiffness by mass reduction and scarification (Gross 1999, 2008). The goal of the glottoplasty is a reduction of the vibrating mass (Gross 2008).

While the glottoplasty is irreversible, the outcome seems to be better than that of the frame surgery. Thus, Gross (1999) presented a group of 10 MFs in a follow-up of 3–4 years after their glottoplasty showing a pitch elevation of 7–13 semitones with a mean of 9.2 semitones. Eight out of ten MFs performed habitual fundamental frequencies within the normative female range (>165 Hz), and only two were situated in the gender-ambiguous frequency range.

Case Study 5.30

A 53-year-old former policeman is a CEO of an IT company now. He is married and has two grown-up children. Only half a year ago, he started hormone therapy, taking oestradiol and cyproterone acetate, the usual therapy for transgender women. He had a warm and sonorous baritone voice with a normal male larynx.

After glottoplasty the voice shifted upwards and lost the tell-tale masculine tones. One year later, her voice harmonised with her outer appearance. She is well accepted at work and in her personal life.

However, regarding phonosurgical voice adjustments as such, all of the framework and endolaryngeal interventions focus on the glottis being the sound generator, while sex differences in vocal tract configuration and formant behaviour are ignored. This may be one reason for unsatisfying auditory gender identification despite properly raised pitch. Thus it takes some time and vocal practice to coordinate the phonatory components after surgery. Therefore, phonosurgery is usually embedded in an initial and postsurgical voice training.

5.11.7.2 Voice Fitting by Training

Before starting the voice training, it is necessary to evaluate the current voice characteristics and function by voice assessment. Depending on the available equipment, the diagnostics are merely perceptual ratings (GRBAS, RBH index, mean pitch, etc.) or objective acoustical measurements (HNR, jitter, shimmer, fundamental frequency and formant measurements, etc.). Laryngoscopy, stroboscopy and high-speed glottal imaging are performed to describe the laryngeal size, the glottal closure and the oscillatory function of the vocal cords. Phonetography is an important tool as well, since it is useful for determining the prognosis of a conservative voice fitting. It is the experience of the author that individuals having a voice range that covers the extent of both sexes, combined with physiological voice dynamics, are better in outcome than those showing a typical male phonetogram. Other parameters belonging to tonus, phonatory respiration, voice quality, articulation, loading capacity, etc. are estimated to exclude or to confirm a hyperfunctional pathology of the patients. The basic therapeutic demands in the latter are similar to those of non-transsexual voice patients. Before raising the pitch of the MFs, techniques to soften their

phonation, i.e. to diminish the hyperfunctional habits, have to be practised.

In order to define an individual therapeutic target voice, there are two main strategies. The first is to listen to voice samples of female relatives of the MFs and samples of popular personalities such as female actors and politicians. The second strategy is the use of voice morphing. Thereby a voice record of the MF reading a standard text (e.g. Rainbow Passage) will be stepwise transformed to the female gender by combined F0 and formant adaption. We use PRAAT software from Boersma and Weenink (Link: www.praat.org) to produce an ascending pitch sequence by 2-semitone steps (up to 12 semitones) combined with a vocal tract (formant) adaptation of 3% per 2 semitones. Together with the phoniatrician and the voice therapist, the MF patient can discuss her voice ideal in regard of body size, age, peer group and everyday demands. In most of the cases, a pitch rise morphed for more than 6–8 semitones sounds artificial, and a habitual rise of 6–8 semitones combined with female prosodics is sufficient for the patients.

A literature research for studies of non-surgical gender fitting of voice disclosed different imponderabilities. Thus, most of the studies are casuistic (e.g. Kaye et al. 1993) or studies of fewer than five cases (e.g. Chaloner 1991; Mészáros et al. 2005). Long-term studies including sufficient follow-up data are very rare. Often, the therapeutic settings and training items are not specified in detail or represent concepts that were designed for other purposes. Last, but not least, the therapeutic goal in most of the studies resembles a terminological black box called 'naturalness of voice' (cf. De Bruin et al. 2000).

What do we know about the essential (voice) characteristics of gender fitting in male-to-female transsexuals? In reports on voice fitting, the rise of the fundamental frequency is most often described (Gelfer 1999), although its percentage contribution to the perception of femaleness is further under discussion (see overview of Dacakis et al. 2012). In comparison with F0, the necessity of formant adaption has been less regarded so far. It is recognised by Carew et al. (2007), who report exercises to increase the vowel formants F1, F2, F3 and the oral resonance by lip spreading and forward placing of the tongue. In addition, there is evidence from a perception study conducted with synthetic voice samples that increasing F0 and formant frequencies simultaneously is more effective in gaining a female rating than modifying only one component (Hillenbrand and Clark 2009). In respect of intonation, a more lively prosodic pattern of increased use of upward inflection, rather than avoidance of downward inflection and an increased use of rise and fall inflections, is reported. An increase of the used pitch range during running speech is recommended (Dacakis 2002). This implies that the mean pitch should be targeted not too high to preserve some prosodic dynamics (Gelfer 1999). During voice fitting, a reduction of chest resonance substituted by increased head resonance seems to be of importance (De Bruin et al. 2000; Dacakis 2002). In respect of voice quality, some breathiness will contribute to the gender fitting (Gorham-Rowan and Morris 2006; Van Borsel et al. 2009). Whether a reduced vocal loudness contributes to the female gender fitting, as Dacakis et al. (2012) recommend, may be decided by the social habits within the peer groups of the MFs. The social role contributes elementarily to the voice performance. It is experienced by linguistic adaption, training of facial expression and body language and changing the individual outfit. On a much more intimate level, sexual experiences in the target gender role can initiate an important advance in respect of the gender and voice fitting process. The change process has been fully successful if voice reflexes are performed according to the desired gender.

5.12 Special Aspects in Female-to-Male Transsexuals

Dirk Deuster

5.12.1 Testosterone-Induced Voice Alteration in Female-to-Male Transsexual Persons

Testosterone treatment in female-to-male (FM) transsexual persons leads to a significant voice lowering. As a consequence, FMs only rarely request medical services because of voice problems so our knowledge about these persons is much lower than for male-to-female (MF) transsexuals. Studies have shown that voice lowering starts a few weeks after, and reaches a steady state at the end of the first year of treatment (Van Borsel et al. 2000; Damrose 2009; Nygren et al. 2015; Deuster et al. 2016), and compared with a group of biological men, there are no significant differences of pitch, intonation and perturbation parameters after long-term androgen treatment (Cosyns et al. 2014; Deuster et al. 2016).

5.12.2 Tasks of Phoniatricians in Female-to-Male Transsexuals

Owing to the low number of FM patients, no exact information about the prevalence of voice disorders is available. From a large investigation, voice lowering difficulties can be expected in about 10% of cases (Cosyns et al. 2014). Various causes may explain insufficiencies in voice lowering: a reduced androgen sensitivity (see Sect. 5.10), an insufficient testosterone dose, other organic/constitutional causes or functional causes comparable to a prolonged mutation or mutational falsetto in biological men.

From a diagnostic view, the laryngoscopic examination is of little help because testosterone treatment does not cause any significant visible changes of the larynx in each case (see Fig. 5.24): testosterone application in adults does not result in a growth of the laryngeal framework with a lengthening of the vocal folds but just in an increase of their muscular mass not appearing in the laryngoscopic view. A voice range profile, in particular the lowest possible frequency, may indicate if there is a problem in the testosterone-induced changes of the larynx or with the adaptation to it.

Therapeutic options should be determined in cooperation with the attending endocrinologist, and testosterone treatment should be optimised with regard to the voice, if necessary. Voice therapy is useful when functional causes for insufficiency of voice lowering exist, characterised by an

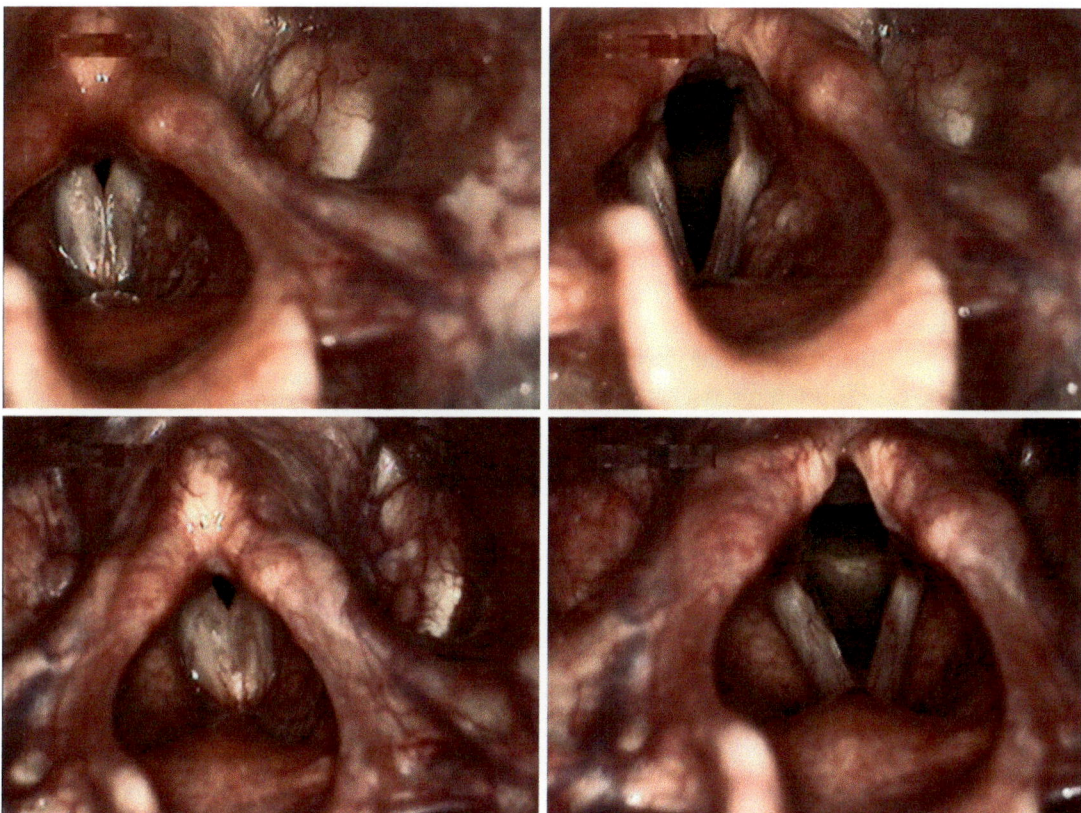

Fig. 5.24 Largely unchanged laryngostroboscopic findings in a 24-year-old female-to-male transsexual before (above) and 36 weeks after (below) beginning of testosterone treatment. Speaking fundamental frequency was 177 Hz and 96 Hz, respectively

unphysiologically large distance between speaking fundamental frequency and the lowest possible frequency or a pitch instability. But before beginning voice therapy, it is necessary to exchange mutual therapeutic expectations, because self- and external-assessment of the voice may be different, which is true for FM as well as MF clients (Adler et al. 2006; Sandmann et al. 2014). If an adequate voice lowering does not occur after testosterone treatment and voice therapy, there should be a surgical shortening of the anteroposterior thyroid ala (thyroplasty III), as described by Isshiki (Adler et al. 2006; Isshiki et al. 1983).

Apart from voice lowering difficulties, other voice disorders such as hoarseness and limited vocal endurance may occur, possibly triggered by the hormonal treatment. In these cases, the therapeutic options correspond largely to those of non-transsexual individuals. However, in voice therapy it should be taken into account

that, in contrast to non-transsexual individuals in particular, organic changes of the larynx and voice instabilities should be expected in the first year after beginning the testosterone treatment.

5.13 Dysphonia in Systemic Diseases

Waldemar Wojnowski and
Bożena Wiskirska-Woźnica

5.13.1 Laryngeal Granuloma in Reflux Disease

Gastro-oesophageal reflux disease (GERD) is the most common cause of laryngeal inflammation; 10–50% of patients with laryngeal complaints have a GERD-related underlying cause. The highest incidence of reflux is found in patients with laryngeal neoplasms (88%) and muscle tension dysphonias (70%) (Bain et al. 1983; Castell et al. 1985; Little et al. 1985; Littlejohn et al. 1998; Ulualp and Toohill 2000).

Laryngopharyngeal reflux (LPR) affects both children and adults and may be associated with an acute, chronic or intermittent pattern of laryngitis, with or without granuloma formation. The symptoms of LPR are quite different from those of classic GERD as seen in the gastroenterology patient, who characteristically has heartburn, regurgitation and oesophagitis. Patients with 'reflux laryngitis' (LPR) present with hoarseness but almost two-thirds deny ever having heartburn. Other throat symptoms, such as globus pharyngeus (a sensation of a lump in the throat), dysphagia, chronic throat clearing and coughing, are often associated with LPR (Burton et al. 1992; Koufman et al. 2000; Koufman 1991, 1994; Ossakow et al. 1987). Physical findings of LPR can range from mild, isolated oedema or erythema of the area of the arytenoid cartilages to diffuse laryngeal oedema and hyperaemia with granuloma formation and airway obstruction (Belafsky et al. 2001a; Jindal et al. 1994).

Pseudosulcus vocalis refers to a pattern of subglottal oedema that extends from the anterior commissure to the posterior part of the larynx; it appears like a groove or sulcus. It can easily be differentiated from a true sulcus (sulcus vergeture), which is the adherence of the vocal fold epithelium to the vocal ligament secondary to the absence of the superficial layer of lamina propria. True sulcus is related to scarring of the vocal fold(s) in the phonatory striking zone. Whereas true sulcus stops at the vocal process and is in the midportion of the striking zone, pseudosulcus vocalis (see Sect. 5.5) extends all the way to the back of the larynx. Some disorders associated with supra-oesophageal complications of reflux disease include laryngeal contact ulcer and granuloma (Koufman et al. 2000, Koufman 1994) (Figs. 5.25 and 5.26).

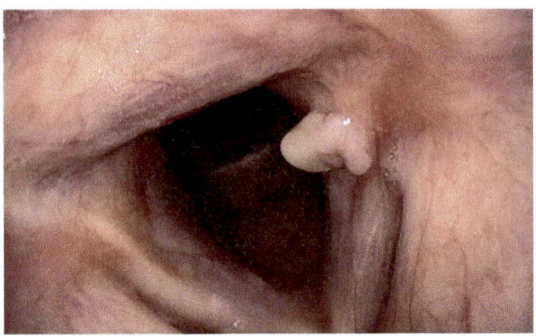

Fig. 5.25 Laryngeal granuloma in reflux disease. With kind permission from the German Voice Clinic, Hamburg

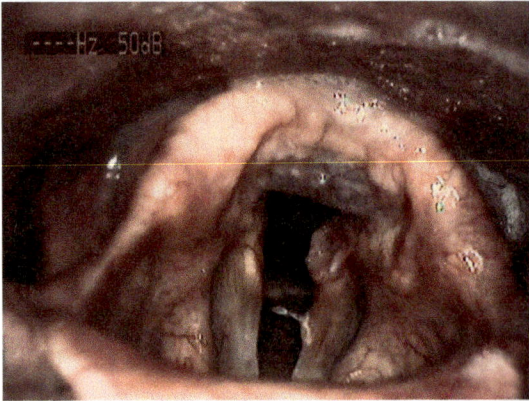

Fig. 5.26 Laryngeal contact granuloma (ulcer) in reflux disease. With kind permission from Prof. Tadeus Nawka, Berlin

5.13.2 Sarcoidosis

Sarcoidosis is a slowly progressive, rarely fatal, systemic granulomatous disease of unknown cause. The lungs and skin are most commonly involved, and laryngeal sarcoidosis occurs in 1–5% of cases usually in the supraglottal region (Gallivan and Landis 1993; Neel and McDonald 1982). When the skin of the nasal rim is affected, upper respiratory sarcoidosis involvement is seen in approximately 75% of cases (Jorizzo et al. 1990). The larynx is rarely involved without clinical or radiographic evidence of lung involvement. Dyspnoea and dry cough are common symptoms. The true vocal folds are rarely involved. Patients may present hoarseness owing to nodules on the vocal folds. Sarcoidosis is

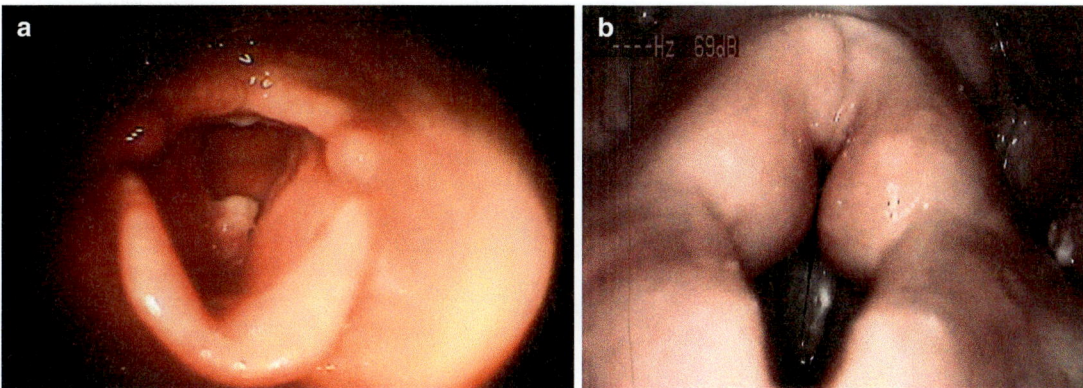

Fig. 5.27 (**a**) Sarcoidosis of the right vocal fold. (**b**) Laryngeal sarcoidosis. With kind permission from Prof. Tadeus Nawka, Berlin

rarely painful and may present with symptoms of airway obstruction (Gallivan and Landis 1993). Characteristically the entire supraglottis appears pale pink and massively oedematous, sometimes obscuring visualisation of the vocal folds. Less commonly, some laryngeal sarcoidosis patients present with a few discrete, sometimes haemorrhagic, nodules (up to 1 cm in diameter) on the epiglottis or other supraglottal structures (Bower et al. 1980; Loehrl and Smith 2001; Neel and McDonald 1982).

The diagnosis of sarcoidosis requires the following three components: involvement of at least two organ systems, non-caseating granulomas and exclusion of other granulomatous diseases (Fig. 5.27a, b). Physical examination often reveals enlarged and tender lymph nodes, dry cough and skin and eye manifestations (McCaffrey and McDonald 1983). Systemic high-dose steroids are recommended as primary treatment for laryngeal sarcoidosis. In the cases of large masses of sarcoid and dyspnoea or the failure to respond to conservative treatment, surgery is recommended—endoscopic laser—to reduce masses.

5.13.3 Tuberculous Laryngitis

With the discovery of effective anti-tuberculosis drugs, the incidence of both pulmonary and laryngeal tuberculosis rapidly declined. Nevertheless, tuberculous laryngitis remains one of the more common granulomatous diseases of the larynx, but today is frequently not associated with advanced active pulmonary disease (Harney et al. 2000; Loehrl and Smith 2001). In the nodular, ulcerative (later) stages, tuberculosis may easily be confused with laryngeal carcinoma (Delap et al. 1997; Flanagan and McIlwain 1993). Patients with laryngeal tuberculosis commonly present in their third to fourth decade of life with varying symptoms, including hoarseness, odynophagia and otalgia. Symptoms may include hoarseness, cough, pain (and referred otalgia), dyspnoea and stridor. Additionally, tuberculous laryngitis may result in perichondritis and cartilage necrosis with resultant airway compromise. Respiratory obstruction may develop in later stages of the disease. Laryngeal examination may reveal diffuse oedema and a hyperaemic, hypertrophic mucosa involving the posterior third of the larynx, or the process may be diffuse, nodular and ulcerative (Fig. 5.28) (Harney et al. 2000; Levenson et al. 1984; Ramadan et al. 1993; Soda et al. 1989). It is a misconception that interarytenoid (posterior commissure) involvement alone is the most commonly observed pattern. In the modern era, the true vocal folds appear to be the most commonly involved site (Harney et al. 2000).

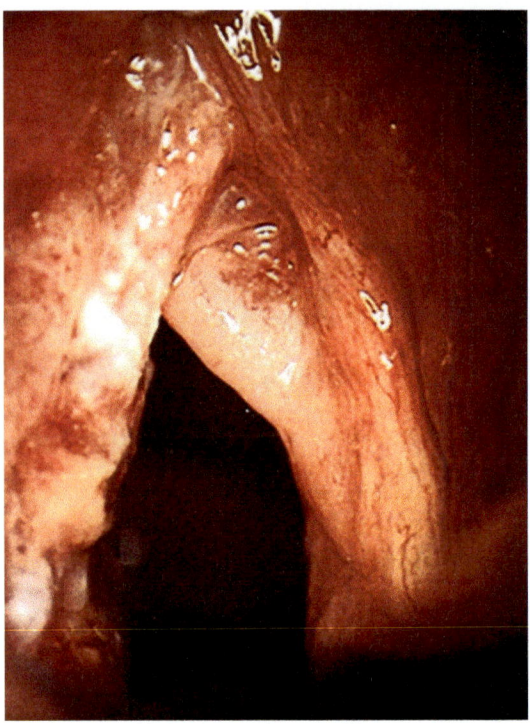

Fig. 5.28 Laryngeal tuberculosis. With kind permission from Prof. Tadeus Nawka, Berlin

5.13.4 Rheumatoid Arthritis

Rheumatoid arthritis (RA) is a systemic autoimmune disorder of unknown cause that can affect any organ in the body. Its most common manifestation is symmetric polyarthritis, but it also can cause inflammation of non-joint structures, vasculitis and pulmonary changes. Rheumatoid arthritis may affect the larynx both directly and indirectly (Arnett et al. 1988). Rheumatoid involvement of the cricoarytenoid joints may cause hoarseness or airway obstruction. At postmortem examination, up to 87% of patients with rheumatoid arthritis have cricoarytenoid joint changes, but from laryngoscopy only 17–33% of patients have clinical signs of laryngeal involvement, namely, posterior laryngeal inflammation and decreased arytenoid cartilage mobility (Jurik et al. 1985; Lofgren and Montgomery 1962). Woo et al. (1995) described rheumatic nodules within the submucosal spaces of the vocal folds,

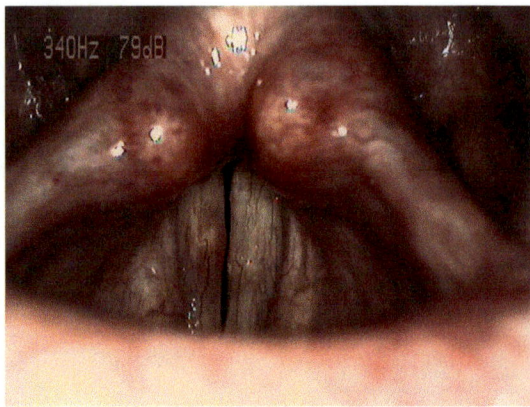

Fig. 5.29 Rheumatic white submucosal nodules, smaller on the left side. With kind permission from Prof. Tadeus Nawka, Berlin

which were similar to rheumatic nodules found elsewhere. Rheumatoid nodules may occur anywhere in the larynx or within the substance of the vocal folds itself, leading to hoarseness. The gross appearance of rheumatoid laryngeal nodules is variable. They may appear as white submucosal nodules (Fig. 5.29), or nodules in the form of bamboo shoots (bamboo nodes), as ulcerated friable polypoid lesions or as ill-defined masses deep within the substance of the vocal folds (Friedman and Rice 1975; Ossakow et al. 1987; Osipenko et al. 2016; Woo et al. 1995) (Fig. 5.30a, b). Bamboo node lesion should be treated by local laryngeal injections (1–3 times) with steroids as the first line of therapy; in some cases surgery can be a useful treatment to improve voice quality (Ossakow et al. 1987). Voice disorders in the course of RA are usually manifested by hoarseness of various intensity, a feeling of a 'lump' in the throat, problems with swallowing, sometimes also dyspnoea and sore throat with larynx ache radiating to the ears. These symptoms are often connected with inflammation of the cricoarytenoid joints. Acute inflammation of the synovia of the cricoarytenoid joints can lead to limiting their mobility. In a severe case, limited mobility of the joints can result in dyspnoea when tracheotomy can appear to be necessary. The inflammation of laryngeal arteries can lead to

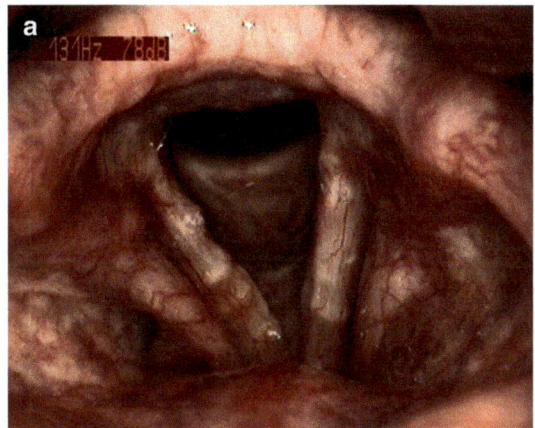

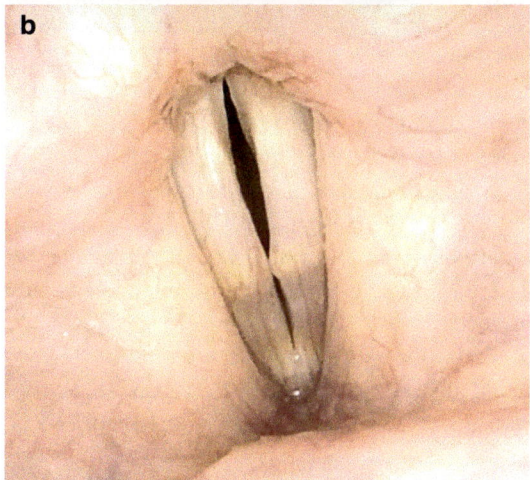

Fig. 5.30 (**a**) Rheumatic nodules like 'bamboo shoots'. (**b**) Rheumatic nodules like 'bamboo shoots'. With kind permission from the German Voice Clinic, Hamburg

laryngeal nerve ischemia, neuron degeneration and eventually to laryngeal muscle atrophy (Loehrl and Smith 2001; McCaffrey and McDonald 1983).

Case Study 5.31
A native English-speaking woman (51 years old) working as costumer and communicating with artists, as well as working freelance as a speaker, noticed increasing hoarseness a year ago. She had had autoimmune processes for 3 years expressing as colitis ulcerosa, giant cell arteritis and rheumatoid arthritis. The vocal folds show bamboo nodes, one on the left and two on the right.

The dynamic range of the voice is diminished. Voice quality is moderately impaired owing to permanent roughness (R2 B1 H2).

5.13.5 Amyloidosis

Amyloidosis is a dysproteinaemia in which a characteristic, amorphous, eosinophilic substance is deposited in the tissues of various organs. Amyloidosis is classified as being either 'systemic' or 'localised' (Lewis et al. 1992). Cohen has provided a detailed classification:

• Primary amyloidosis in which there is no coexisting disease (50–60%)
• Amyloidosis associated with multiple myeloma (20–30%)
• Secondary amyloidosis of chronic disease (10%)
• Hereditary amyloidosis (1%)
• Amyloidosis associated with ageing (10–20%)
• Local amyloidosis, tumour-like deposits without systemic disease (10%) (Clevens et al. 1994)

The 'localised' type of amyloidosis is almost never fatal and is the type that most commonly involves the larynx. On laryngoscopy, amyloidosis appears as diffuse mucosal thickening or subepithelial nodules, localised mainly to the anterior part of the subglottis. Patients are usually asymptomatic until the deposits involve the vocal folds or critically narrow the airway (Figs. 5.31a, b and 5.32). Laryngeal amyloidosis usually has a benign course (Clevens et al. 1994; Gertz and Kyle 1989).

Case Study 5.32
A 34-year-old office worker perceived increasing strain when speaking during the last year. Gradually breathing became exhausting during recent months. The video shows typical protrusions of the subglottal region beginning right at the lower edge of both vocal folds. Histological examination of these masses yielded a localised form of light chain amyloidosis.

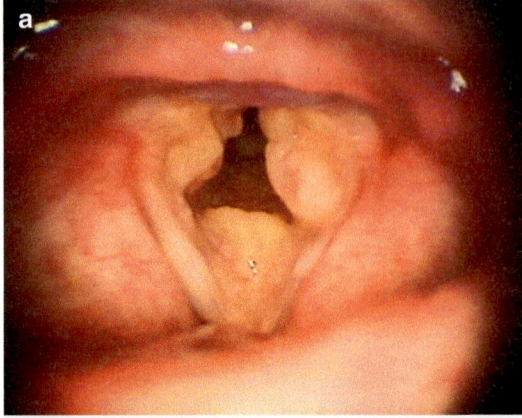

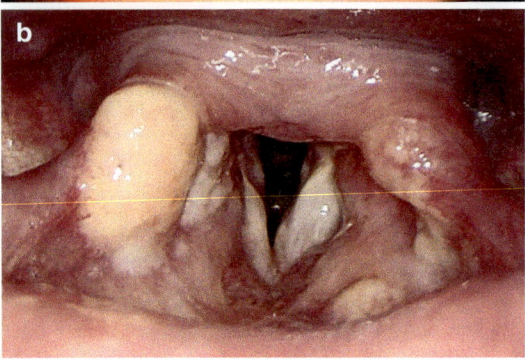

Fig. 5.31 (**a**) larynx amyloidosis—masses narrowing the subglottal region. (**b**) Larynx amyloidosis. With kind permission from the German Voice Clinic, Hamburg

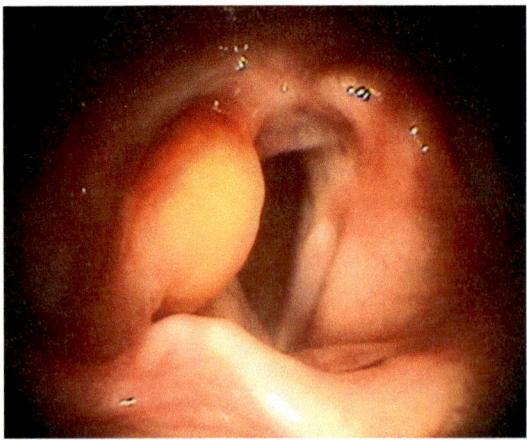

Fig. 5.32 Subepithelial cyst-like amyloid in the epiglottal region

5.13.6 Systemic Lupus Erythematosus

Lupus is a systemic, autoimmune disease of unknown aetiology. It affects women (primarily those of child-bearing age) more commonly than men and usually presents in the second and third decades of life. Circulating immune complexes cause damage to blood vessels, connective tissue and mucosal surfaces (Campbell et al. 1983; Gallivan and Landis 1993; Loehrl and Smith 2001). The lesions may be variable, for example, petechiae, ulcerations or raised non-ulcerated lesions with erythematous borders. Laryngeal involvement is reported to occur in 0.3–13% of patients. Laryngeal symptoms rarely present as isolated findings. Hoarseness, throat pain or dyspnoea all may be presenting symptoms depending on the site of involvement. The larynx may also be involved by these mucosal lesions or, on occasion, by cricoarytenoid arthritis. The glottis and cricoarytenoid joints seem to be the most commonly involved sites. Laryngeal involvement usually occurs at times of acute exacerbation of the systemic disease (Smith and Ferguson 1989; Tan et al. 1982; Teitel et al. 1992; Toomey et al. 1974).

5.13.7 Granulomatosis with Polyangiitis of the Larynx (Wegener's Granulomatosis)

Wegener's granulomatosis is a systemic disease of unknown aetiology characterised by necrotising granuloma with vasculitis involving the upper respiratory tract, lungs and kidneys. Clinically, Wegener's granulomatosis is manifested by bilateral pneumonitis (95%), rhinosinusitis (90%), renal disease (80%) and laryngeal ulceration and oedema (25%). It most commonly occurs in the fourth and fifth decades of life, and there is a 2:1 male predominance (Allen 1996; Littlejohn et al. 1998; Loehrl and Smith 2001). The more common head and neck manifestations involve the sinonasal region. Laryngeal involvement may resemble acute laryngitis, but the eventual development of granulomatous ulcers throughout the larynx may lead the clinician to suspect the diagnosis. Subglottal stenosis, which eventually develops in 8.5% of patients, usually presents with a smooth, submucosal mass that is a poor prognostic sign, occurs in approximately 20% of cases and can lead to significant airway obstruction, requiring tracheostomy and surgical correction of the stenosis (Waxman and Bose 1986). Diagnosis is based on typical histological findings of necrotising granulomas and vasculitis. The anti-cytoplasmic autoantibody test (C-ANCA) is highly specific for Wegener's granulomatosis. Recommended treatment includes cyclophosphamide with corticosteroids (Allen 1996, Littlejohn et al. 1998, Loehrl and Smith 2001).

Case Study 5.33

A 28-year-old woman with Wegener's granulomatosis. She has suffered from subglottal stenosis which was operated on a year ago. The video shows erosions and thick mucus on the nasal mucosa. The vocal folds are slightly atrophic, otherwise without pathological findings. During phonation the ventricular folds adduct for compensation. The subglottis is narrowed by granulomatous tissue and scars. Granuloma indicate a still active disease.

The voice is mildly hoarse (R1 B1 H1); the vocal range is clearly restricted.

5.14 Voice, Environment and Allergy

Eugenia Chávez Calderòn (original scientific work), Muhittin Demir, and Antoinette am Zehnhoff-Dinnesen (derivative scientific work)

5.14.1 Principles of Allergic Reactions

Allergic diseases are a global health problem with increasing prevalence (Chávez 2018). According to a Finnish study in 2012, physician-diagnosed bronchial asthma was reported in 9.5% of men and 10.8% of women, hay fever in 28.1% of men and 36.1% of women (Jousilahti et al. 2016). Allergic diseases of the upper and lower respiratory tract can affect vocal quality.

Allergy describes all forms of hypersensitivity of the human immune system against foreign substances with detrimental consequences for the host and comprises type I, IgE-mediated or cell-mediated reactions. Gell and Coombs (1975) first classified four types of hypersensitivity reactions (Table 5.8).

Although the pathogenesis of allergic diseases is not completely understood today, some studies indicate a contribution of genetics and environment, especially at the stage of allergen sensitisation (Wang 2005). Respiratory allergic reactions are increased by environmental factors (Chávez 2006, 2007, 2009, 2010a, b, 2012); the following are possible causes of allergic diseases: increased air pollution, reduced contact with environmental microbiota (Jousilahti et al. 2016) and changed lifestyle (hygiene standards, food, vaccination, stress and ownership of pets). Depending on the allergen, allergic reactions typically of the skin, the gastrointestinal and respiratory tracts are observed.

The immunological response of the respiratory system to an allergen is inflammation of the respiratory mucosa. For adequate immune protection of mucosal surfaces in the respiratory tract, there are two main systems in the human body, termed innate and adaptive immunity.

Innate Immunity Three systems belong to innate immunity:

- Epithelium: mucosal barriers, limits entrance of foreign particles into the airway system
- Phagocytotic system: employing monocytes and macrophages, supported by the destructive effects of neutrophils and natural killer cells
- Complement system: inactivates the foreign body by assembling a membrane attack complex (Dempsey et al. 2003), which has effects on regulation of inflammation and attracts lymphocytes

Table 5.8 Classification of hypersensitivity (modified according to Gell and Coombs 1975)

Classification	Mechanism	Typical clinical manifestation	Timing of reaction
Type I (IgE-mediated)	IgE	Anaphylaxis, angio-oedema, urticaria	Immediate, minutes to hours
Type II (cytotoxic)	IgM, IgG, complement, phagocytosis	Cytopenia, nephritis, haemolytic anaemia	Variable
Type III (immune complex)	IgM, IgG, complement, precipitins	Serum sickness, vasculitis, glomerulonephritis	1–3 weeks' post-exposure
Type IV (delayed cell-mediated)	T-lymphocytosis	Contact dermatitis	48–72 h

Adaptive Immunity By adaptive immunity the body learns to detect the unique antigens of a pathogen and creates an antigen-specific response to eliminate it (Dempsey et al. 2003). There are two types of adaptive immune responses: humoral immunity, mediated by antibodies produced by B-lymphocytes, and cell-mediated immunity, activating antigen-specific cytotoxic T lymphocytes. Cytokines, proteins important in cell signalling, play a role in both mechanisms.

5.14.2 Allergens and Irritants

Allergens mostly belong to the family of proteins and cause an allergic reaction via triggering the production of IgE antibodies. They can be classified in four groups:

- Indoor allergens (mites, animal allergens, cockroaches and moulds): proteolytic enzymes (serine and cysteine proteases), lipocalins or ligand-binding proteins, tropomyosins, albumins, calcium-binding proteins
- Outdoor allergens (grass, tree and weed pollens and mould spores): plant pathogenesis-related (e.g. PR-10) proteins, calcium-binding proteins, pectate lyases, β-expansins, trypsin inhibitors
- Plant and animal food allergens (fruits, vegetables, nuts, milk, eggs, shellfish and certain types of fish): lipid-transfer proteins, profilins, seed storage proteins, tropomyosins (Chapman et al. 2007)
- Injected allergens (insect venoms and some therapeutic proteins): phospholipases, hyaluronidases

Allergens that are dispersed in the air are known as aeroallergens (tree, grass and weed pollens, yeasts und dust), which are the most frequent allergens. Meteorological changes can have an impact on the production, distribution and dispersion of these aeroallergens.

Irritants are substances that cause non-IgE-mediated inflammation of mucosal membranes of the respiratory tract. There is often a synergistic process of allergens and irritants, which leads to hoarseness of voice, shortness of breath, wheezing, coughing and difficulty in breathing in.

An allergic reaction to food (vegetables or meats: tomato, chocolate, milk products, nuts, corn, wheat, chicken, beef, turkey or pork) can affect the respiratory tract and change the quality of the pitch of the voice.

Even drugs can cause allergic and pseudo-allergic reactions (PAR, without immunological specificity), which are mainly induced by the immunogenicity of drugs, drug metabolic products or drug additives. The most common drugs that cause adverse drug reactions (ADR) are penicillin, sulphonamides, tetracycline antibiotics and cephalosporins, non-steroidal anti-inflammatory drugs and acetylsalicylic acid, general or local anaesthetics, chemotherapy drugs and radio-contrast media (Warrington and Silviu-Dan 2011). They can produce immediate or delayed allergic reactions.

5.14.3 The Environment

The environment influences our respiratory system (Chávez 2006, 2007, 2009, 2010a, b, 2012). Inhaled air and its pollutants especially affect the respiratory tract including the larynx and the bronchial and alveolar system, which is responsible for the process of gas exchange between the external environment and the human organism. The allergic reaction to these pollutants is an important factor in the aetiopathogenesis of laryngeal mucosal lesions. The pollutants accumulate on mucus, and their absorption in the respiratory mucosa leads to irritation, inflammation, oedema, swelling in the nose, pharynx, larynx and bronchia as well as to obstruction of the ostia of the sinuses (Trevino 1996). If the allergic patient has respiratory hyperactivity (possibly in the form of bronchial hyper-responsiveness with easily triggered bronchospasm) and presents allergic reactions to different environmental substances, the harm to the larynx by cough and oedema increases the voice pathology.

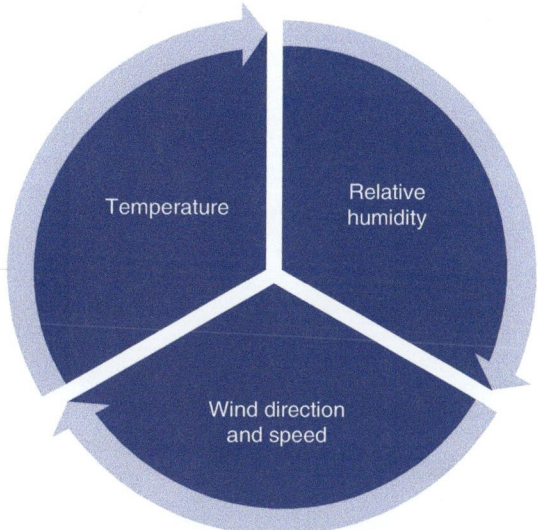

Fig. 5.33 Meteorological factors affecting allergic reactions

5.14.4 Air Pollution

Air pollutants can be classified by their source, chemical composition, size and mode of release into indoor or outdoor environments (Bernstein 2004). They can also be subdivided into primary (emitted directly) versus secondary (result of chemical reactions with other pollutants or gases), indoor (e.g. building materials, smoking) versus outdoor (e.g. industrial, agricultural) and gaseous (e.g. ozone) versus particulate pollutants. There are meteorological factors (Fig. 5.33) that can affect the different environments of each town or city, and this situation can worsen an allergic reaction.

Primary and secondary pollutants, volatile organic compounds (e.g. from certain trees), UV-radiation and heat are the basis of photochemical reactions leading to photochemical smog (Miller and Spoolman 2014). The main outdoor pollutants are ozone, sulphur dioxide, nitrogen dioxide, carbon monoxide and particles smaller than 10 μm (Fig. 5.34).

Voice production needs a healthy mucosa in the vocal folds and in the resonating chambers, permitting a normal mucosal waveform and a proper vocal resonance. There are two mechanisms that maintain a healthy mucosa:

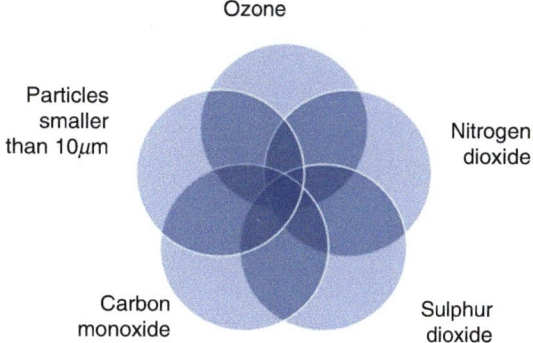

Fig. 5.34 Pollutants affecting allergic reactions

- Lubrication: mucous elasticity and viscosity with a balanced chemical composition
- Transportation: ciliary movement with beating at 12–15 Hz in waves of metachronal motion

The mucus is propelled cephalad at 4–20 mm/min through the vocal cords into the pharynx. About 30 ml of respiratory mucus are expectorated or swallowed daily (Tilley et al. 2015; Fahy and Dickey 2010).

The exact pathogenesis by which air pollutants cause harmful health effects is complex. Studies have shown, for example, that

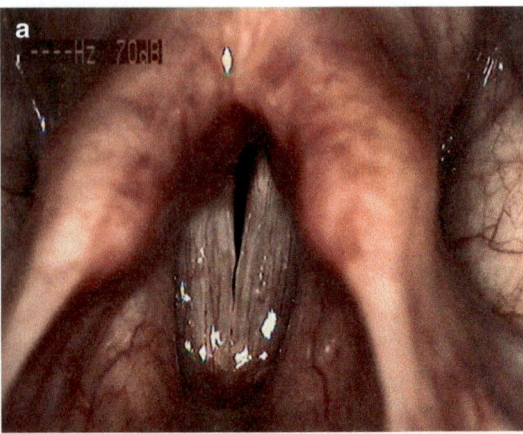

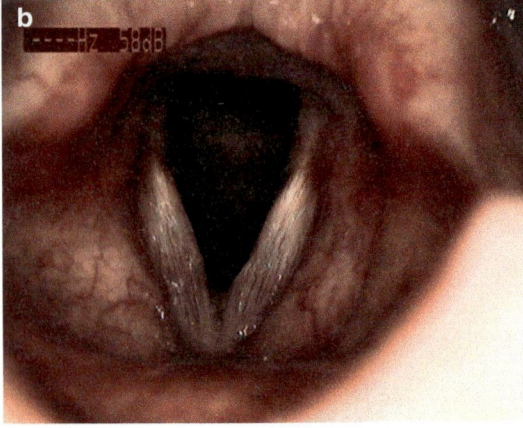

Fig. 5.35 (**a**, **b**) Signs due to air pollution. With kind permission from Prof. Tadeus Nawka, Berlin

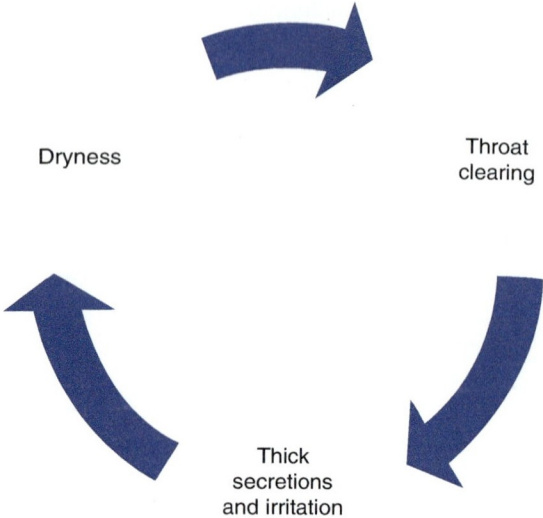

Fig. 5.36 Air pollution symptoms influencing voice

5.14.5 Signs and Symptoms

The immune system of all individuals recognises the triggering antigens as foreign. Upon exposure to an allergen, atopic individuals develop pathological immune responses. In allergic respiratory pathologies, allergens trigger the production of IgE by allergen-specific B lymphocytes controlled by interleukin 4, which is produced by allergen-specific CD4 T lymphocytes. Persistent airway inflammation and oedema depend on these control mechanisms (Fig. 5.36) (Lambrecht and Hammad 2014).

The most frequent signs due to respiratory allergies are dryness, itching, burning, foreign body sensation, oedema and erythema of the respiratory tract, including the larynx with the vocal folds (Fig. 5.37). The inflammation and oedema accompanied with tenacious mucus, can be originated from the upper or lower respiratory tract (Jackson-Menaldi et al. 1999), cause dysphonia, lack of vocal flexibility, lack of brilliance and an increased need for throat clearing and coughing (Chávez 2006; Stemple et al. 2000).

Moreover, singers especially will suffer from diminished auditory perception, lack of brilliance in high tones and changes in vocal flexibility and pitch accuracy. If the nose is congested by oedema in the inferior and intermediate turbinates

particulate matter (PM) can provoke pulmonary inflammation, immunotoxic effects, oxidative stress, stimulation of nociceptors and the autonomic nervous system (Gerlofs-Nijland et al. 2005) and affects the cardiopulmonary system and the voice production.

The clinical respiratory tract signs can be nasal and pharyngeal mucosal dryness, inflammation of the throat and vocal folds, thickness of mucus or slight oedema in the vocal folds (Fig. 5.35a, b). Throat clearing may become necessary because of mucosal dryness and thick tenacious secretions. A constant irritation of the vocal folds may also be observed (Fig. 5.36). A well-functioning lubrication of the nose, pharynx and larynx helps to avoid voice problems.

Fig. 5.37 Symptoms of allergy affecting voice

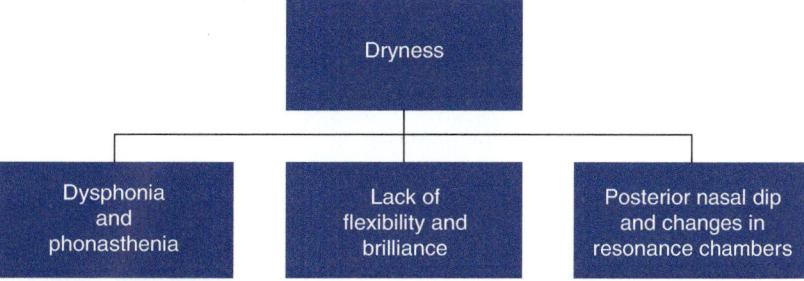

and secretions, the patient may complain about oral breathing, sore throat, pharyngeal itching or inflammation and obstruction sensations when speaking or singing (Fig. 5.38).

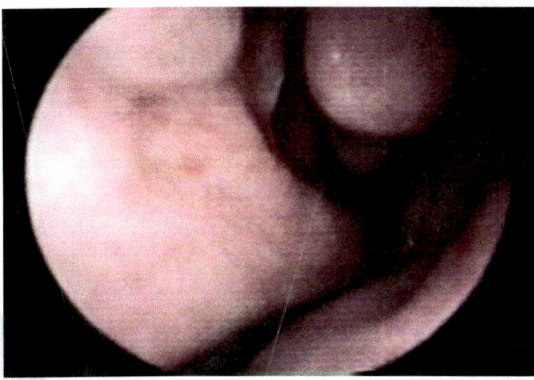

Fig. 5.38 Oedema, paleness and hypertrophy of the inferior turbinates. (Revista de la Facultad de Medicina—with kind permission of the Universidad Nacional de Colombia) (Zabala-Parra et al. 2017)

5.14.6 Diagnostics

History and Physical Examinations Diagnosis of allergic disorders begins with a detailed personal and family history (because of a possible genetic background), preferably on the basis of a well-designed questionnaire (Gill and Dhingra 2016).

Complaints such as seasonality; triggered by exposures at home, at workplace or at school; on the streets; and medicaments should be considered (Gill and Dhingra 2016). The physical examination should comprise the inspection of the eyes, ears, nose, oro-nasopharynx and larynx and the assessment of sinuses, the respiratory system (Gill and Dhingra 2016) and hearing.

Allergen Testing The history of symptoms, typical physical findings and association of symptoms with allergen exposure indicate allergen testing.

Since the 1940s several diagnostic methods (in vivo and in vitro) have been practised to identify which allergens cause pathologies. The diagnosis of allergic disease requires a careful and critical evaluation of laboratory test results, e.g. the serum total IgE level is increased not only in allergic diseases but also in cases of parasite infestation or haematological diseases. Allergen-specific IgE can nowadays be detected by radioallergosorbent tests (RAST), fluorescence-enzyme-immunoassays (FEIA) and enzyme-linked immunosorbent assays (ELISA) belonging to enzyme immunoassays (EAI); see below.

In Vivo Immunoallergic Tests Skin-prick tests, intradermal tests (Skin and Titration Set), patch tests and provocation tests are in vivo immunoallergic tests. Currently, the skin-prick test (SPT) (Niederberger et al. 2014) and the Set are the more widely used in vivo diagnostic tools for immediate-type allergic reactions. Set and SPT are easy to perform, inexpensive and safe and allow a visualisation of sensitization.

In Vitro Immunoallergic Tests The measurement of total serum IgE, radioallergosorbent tests (RAST) and enzyme-linked immunoassays (EIA with ELISA, FEIA) belong to in vitro immunoallergic tests. In general total IgE measures the overall quantity of immunoglobulin E in the blood and it is used as a screening test. Quantitative RAST is a reliable test and as ELISA allows the detection of allergen-specific IgE antibodies in nanograms per millilitre of serum (Gill and Dhingra 2016). But quantitative measurements of allergen antibodies provide sometimes limited information about the severity of the allergic disease. It is necessary to have the clinical picture. A screening for a specific IgE can be performed by multi-parameter testing, which provides the investigation of a wide spectrum of allergens (Gosink 2015).

In vitro tests offer the advantages of safety (no danger of anaphylaxis) and good reproducibility. No unknown or adverse reactions are to be expected.

RAST is the most reliable allergen test in phoniatric patients (respiratory and food allergens).

Provocation Tests Such tests comprise nasal, bronchial and conjunctival provocation. The possibility to use them in special cases in spite of the risk of a severe reaction has to be considered carefully. Resuscitation equipment and emergency medication must be available; close medical supervision is necessary in all cases. Usually such tests are not necessary in phoniatric patients.

Pulmonary Investigations/Pulmonary Function Testing These investigations/testing consist of, for example, chest X-ray examinations, arterial blood gas analysis, diffusing capacity of carbon monoxide, oxygen desaturation during exercise and plethysmography (Cantani 2008). They concern a variety of lung disorders, including airflow obstruction, restrictive disorders, bronchial hyperactivity and exercise limitations (Wanger 2011).

The phoniatrician will indicate a consultation with a pulmonologist if necessary.

5.14.7 Examination of the Upper Respiratory Tract

The resonating chambers (nose, sinuses, oral cavity, pharynx, supraglottal area) are responsible for vocal quality and perceived characteristics of speech sounds (Simberg et al. 2009).

The following diagnostic methods can be used to evaluate allergic effects on the larynx and the supraglottal vocal tract:

- Endoscopy of nose and sinuses
- Endolaryngoscopy with stroboscopy for detecting and assessing pathology of the laryngeal mucosa, vocal fold motion biomechanics and mucosal vibration (Rosen 2005)
- Acoustic analysis of voice

Laryngoscopy may show allergic signs such as vocal fold erythema, subglottal oedema and polypoid degeneration (Figs. 5.39 and 5.40). Stroboscopy shows failure in glottal closure and vertical wave irregularities may be demonstrated by stroboscopy (Fig. 5.39).

5.14.8 Therapeutic Approaches

The management of allergic diseases consists of the following categories of treatment:

Fig. 5.39 Allergy signs in vocal folds

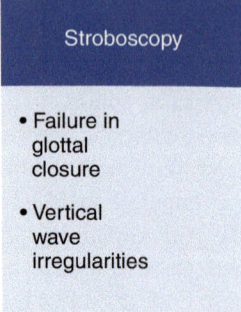

Vocal fold body	Vocal fold edge	Stroboscopy
• Oedema • Erythema	• Subglottal oedema • Polypoid degeneration	• Failure in glottal closure • Vertical wave irregularities

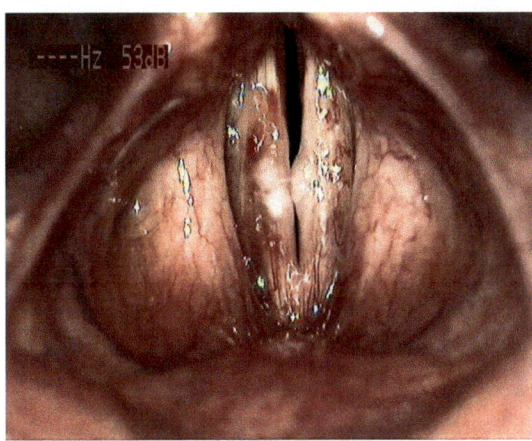

Fig. 5.40 Erythema and polypoid degeneration due to allergy. With kind permission from Prof. Tadeus Nawka, Berlin

- Non-pharmacological management (e.g. allergen avoidance) (US Department of Health and Human Services 2007)
- Pharmacological therapy, immunotherapy

5.14.8.1 Non-pharmacological Approaches and Prevention

In the therapy of allergic diseases, it is imperative to identify and avoid factors that may worsen the course of the disease. Studies have shown that a low level of environmental allergens reduces some respiratory symptoms in the first year of life in high-risk infants (Custovic et al. 2001; Green et al. 2003).

Environmental protection is necessary in all environments, especially in urban areas. Various protective methods are necessary, including air measurements, the use of catalytic convertors and start-stop systems in cars, car-pooling programmes and improvements in public transportation, as well as programmes to retain or plant trees.

The protection of urban woodland, especially old, tall trees, has a positive effect on air quality, and the management of particles and contaminants lowers temperatures and increases wind movement.

Individuals should avoid sport and exercise during periods of high pollutant concentration and, if possible, avoid traffic during rush hours.

The speed of climate change could be reduced if cities were to change their policies on energy use and the production of CO_2, for example, capturing CO_2 by trees, protecting rural woodland and avoiding fires for agricultural purposes or waste management.

In order to maintain healthy immune system regulation, it is advisable to avoid frequent respiratory diseases, keep well hydrated and reduce allergenic overload (e.g. by reducing exposure to chemicals for personal or environmental use). Sufficient cardiovascular and respiratory training in patients diminishes the hypersensitivity of the airway. It is necessary to avoid active or passive smoking. The use of HEPA (High-Efficiency Particulate Air) purifiers helps to maintain a healthy environment during sleep. The environmental conditions of the bedroom, office or television areas should be as free from dust as possible. It is important to maintain the humidity of the airway as much as possible owing to damage caused by different air pollutants.

Airway dryness and voice misuse should be avoided.

5.14.8.2 Pharmacological Treatment

The symptomatic treatment addresses inflammation, production of secretions and the immune response of airways system. There are different pharmacological options for controlling the allergic response to environmental allergens:

- Antihistamines
- Mast cell stabilisers
- Anti-inflammatory agents
- Corticosteroids
- Anti-leukotriene agents
- Transfer factor (TF)
- Mucolytics

Antihistamines Probably the best known type of allergy medication are antihistamines. They improve early-phase H1-receptor-mediated symptoms such as sneezing, itching, rhinorrhoea and, to a lesser degree, nasal congestion. A side effect of antihistamines is dryness of the mucosa with reduced lubrication of the vocal folds and diminished voice quality. Further side effects of modern antihistamines may be headache and gastrointestinal symptoms, whereas sleepiness is less common in contrast to drugs of the first generation. Fexofenadine, desloratadine and levocetirizine have less side effects on the voice.

Mast Cell Stabilisers These are cromone medications that hinder the release of histamine by blocking a calcium channel important for mast cell degranulation. They can be inhaled or applied in the form of nasal sprays and eye drops. Full effect is reached after 1 or 2 weeks. Drug tolerability is good.

Non-steroidal Anti-inflammatory Drugs (NSAIDs) Some common examples of NSAIDs are aspirin, ibuprofen and naproxen; similar drugs are ketoprofen, meloxicam, serratio peptidasa and wobenzym (different enzymes). A variety of side effects (e.g. gastric erosions and kidney damage) has to be considered.

Corticosteroids Intranasal application of corticosteroids can be considered for treating not only the acute phase symptoms but also the late phase reaction (Petersen and Agertoft 2016).

Nasal steroids may be administered for long periods. But local side effects such as nasal mucosal dryness, nasopharyngitis, stinging sensations and nasal ulcerations with epistaxis must be considered (Ratner et al. 2009).

Inhaled steroids are an essential therapy option in asthma. Possible side effects are dysphonia, throat irritation, coughing and mycosis. To avoid voice problems, the use of ciclesonide, for example, is advantageous, a prodrug that is converted only in the lung to an active metabolite.

Sometimes the use of a short-term cortisone, such as betamethasone in one intramuscular application, or prednisone for 1–2 weeks, in decreasing dosage, is indicated. Side effects of cortisone medicaments have to be considered.

Anti-leukotrienes As highly potent inflammatory mediators leukotrienes stimulate broncho-constriction, inflammation and mucus secretion in asthma. Anti-leukotrienes oppose leukotrienes by inhibiting related enzyme or receptor function (Singh et al. 2013). They alleviate the symptoms of asthma, allergic rhinitis and related diseases. Side effects may be a feeling of nervousness, headache, nausea and nasal congestion (Riccioni et al. 2007).

Transfer Factor (TF) Cell-mediated immunity can be transferred from immune healthy donors to immune-deficient recipients by transfer factor (TF). The application of TF improves immune regulatory mechanisms in allergic patients and provides a better resolution of allergic reactions (Gómez et al. 2010).

Mucolytic Agents The gel structure of mucus is broken down by mucolytic agents, and its elasticity and viscosity is decreased (Henke and Ratjen 2007). The use of mucolytics, such as carbocisteine, ambroxol, and nebulisation with dexpanthenol, may be helpful in improving mucosal lubrication.

Allergen-Specific Immunotherapy This immunotherapy represents the potentially curative treatment of several allergic diseases (Akdis and Akdis 2011) and comprises subcutaneous immunotherapy (SCIT) and sublingual immunotherapy (SLIT). SCIT involves weekly subcutaneous injections of increasing amounts of allergen, beginning with very small doses and gradually increasing to higher doses. SLIT involves placement of allergen in the form of dissolvable tablets or drops or extracts in the sublingual region. To handle the continuous increasing desensitisation with personal vaccines is relatively simple; the risks from SLIT are very low. The time of desensitisation can last for 2–3 years depending on the extent of the allergy. Sometimes reinforcement is necessary.

5.14.9 Conclusion

Allergies can harm the mucosa of the nose, sinuses, pharynx, larynx and lungs and diminish voice function. Respiratory and food allergies have to be specified and the modern repertoire of therapeutic options should be considered as early as possible. The following recommendations may be helpful:

- Diminish allergenic overload (respiratory, digestive and chemical); the reduction of environmental pollutants helps to reduce inflammatory reactions of the larynx
- Desensitisation should be considered as an important therapeutic tool
- Gastro-oesophageal reflux as another factor needs to be consequently investigated and treated
- Treatment measures to stabilise voice pathologies should be applied
- Allergic symptoms and signs have to be regularly controlled, new allergic reactions may appear

5.15   Voice in the Elderly

Ahmed Geneid

5.15.1 Definition

Ageing is a complicated process in which calendrical age differs from the biological one. Calendrical age is linear without much individual variability. However, biological ageing is nonlinear; its rate can be slowed and can speed up, causing wide individual variability in the course of ageing process and its effects. Voice in the elderly has a number of characteristics that make it a rather different entity from the normal voice of the younger population. However, this entity also entails wide individual variability and represents itself a continuum on which normal voice and vocal folds are at one end, and marked physiological ageing changes in the vocal folds and presbyphonia stand at the other. Presbyphonia means ageing voice. Such ageing voice entails a special challenge to the phoniatrician in terms of the functional impact it has on the ageing person and his need for socially related interactions. The population pyramid of Europe has already turned into a cylinder. The population pyramid is a graphical illustration showing the distribution of various age groups in a population and forms the shape of a pyramid with its base representing the percentage of the young in the population in comparison with the aged at the top of the pyramid. Such a change imposes an increasing magnitude of presbyphonic voice problems and their increasing presentation in phoniatric clinics around Europe. This change in the population pyramid is also taking place in developing countries.

Nearly one fourth of the aged population reports dysphonia with one fourth of these being linked to ageing (Roy et al. 2007; Turley and Cohen 2009). However, it should be noted that only 19% of patients older than 65 years and with voice problems have bowing of the vocal folds. In other words, many other laryngeal findings can occur in old age, other than bowing of the vocal folds, that are attributed to senile changes of the larynx (Lundy et al. 1998). Nevertheless, in terminology presbyphonia and presbydysphonia are different terms. Presbyphonia by definition means an ageing voice, whereas presbydysphonia means hoarseness in an ageing voice. However, the latter term does not take into account the functionality of the voice. Presbyphonia is the term commonly used and will be used in this section, being the one best known and mostly used. As with other voice conditions, presbyphonia needs treatment when the patient is not able to cope with it functionally. Thus, a presbyphonic voice that does not limit the functionality of the patient is normal.

5.15.2 Aetiology

The larynx, as other parts and organs of the body, undergoes a number of senile changes that affect the functionality of the organ. The ageing process is also evident in the larynx. The effects of the ageing process in the larynx tend to appear around the end of the fifth decade of life and increase with age. The ageing process with senile changes happening includes changes in the voice source, the vocal folds as well as the frame of the larynx itself.

Changes in the Skeletal and Muscular System of the Larynx These include calcification of the cartilage, mild erosion of articular surfaces and atrophy of the muscles. In addition, it is postulated that tremors of voice seen among the elderly may result from a reduction in neuromuscular control (Martins et al. 2014; Paulsen et al. 2000).

Changes in the Vocal Folds The quantity of elastic fibres tends to reduce with age. This results in decreased elasticity of the intermediate layer of the lamina propria (Martins et al. 2014). Accordingly, this transitional layer over the deep collagen-rich layer is no longer able to maintain the same elasticity as in young populations. The collagen fibres, on the other hand, show an increase in number through the lamina propria, especially in its deep and intermediate layers. The superficial layer also shows morphological changes, such as forming high-intensity bundles, with spaces between them and interstitial spaces for extracellular matrices decreasing. In addition, twisting of the collagen fibrils occurs (Sato et al. 2002). These changes lead to increased stiffness and reduction of elasticity of the vocal folds. Such changes are attributed to genetic factors (Ximenes Filho et al. 2003). In addition, mucus production tends to decrease with age, decreasing the smoothness of vibration owing to dryness of surface of the vocal folds.

In addition, the lamina propria is decreased in thickness among the elderly in comparison with the younger population. Much atrophy is also evident in the thyroarytenoid muscle leading to reduction in the mass of the vocal folds. Atrophy of the muscle along with the reduction of the mass of lamina propria leads to the commonly found bowing of the vocal folds. Ageing-related changes other than in the larynx can also lead to effects on voice production and its quality. Ageing effects on the respiratory system are also similar to those in other organs. Respiratory functions decrease with age with reduction of the driving power of phonation.

5.15.3 Diagnosis

Presbyphonia is a diagnosis of exclusion and is best done by a good medical history as well as laryngeal imaging. Acoustic analysis of voice is complementary and is best used for follow-up treatment.

Medical History Patients usually present with symptoms of weak, breathy voice, with reduced projection and unsteadiness, in addition to pitch changes (Baken 2005). Pulmonary function may be reduced owing to comorbidities and age, resulting in low subglottal pressure leading to reduced vocal loudness. Tremor may be associated with the previous findings. Auditory perceptual assessment is mandatory, as with other voice disorders.

Findings on Laryngeal Imaging Senile changes in the vocal folds cause bowing of the vocal folds and irregularity of the vibration. Vocal folds usually appear narrower with reduced thickness (Sulter et al. 1996). Such changes result in the spindle- and oval-shaped glottis associated with atrophy of the vocal folds and prominence of vocal processes among patients with presbyphonia (Honjo and Isshiki 1980; Pontes et al. 2005) (Fig. 5.41).

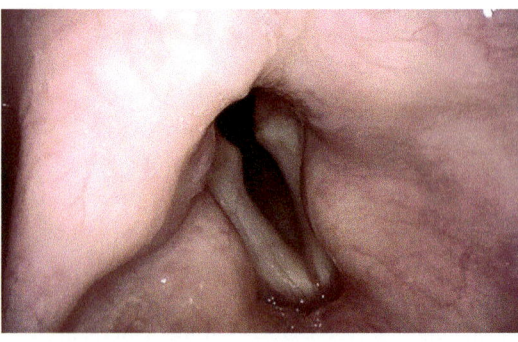

Fig. 5.41 Presbylarynx. With kind permission from the German Voice Clinic, Hamburg

Findings on the Acoustic Analysis of Voice Samples F0 tends to be higher for elderly males and lower for elderly females with greater jitter and shimmer than in the young and middle-aged. In addition, the harmonics-to-noise ratio is also lower among the elderly (Dehqan et al. 2013).

5.15.4 Treatment

The ageing voice does not need treatment in the absence of functional impairment. Patients differ in their needs and how they regard the functional impairment resulting from presbyphonia. It is not uncommon to encounter elderly with mild presbyphonia who do not complain of their voice and regard it as a normal process that they are able to cope with. Accordingly, treatment options are to be offered according to the patient needs and the findings in his larynx.

Treatment options available are either voice therapy or surgical intervention such as injection laryngoplasty or thyroplasty (laryngeal framework surgery). Surgical treatment of presbyphonia aims to correct the gap of the glottis. When the gap is smaller, the wasted air escaping from the glottis is saved. This results in less air escaping from the glottis and subsequently less breathiness of the voice.

Voice Therapy Voice therapy comes to be the first option in the treatment of the ageing voice. It includes respiratory and phonatory exercises in addition to vocal educational advice. Vocal educational advice should always include taking enough water to avoid dehydration and improve humidity within the larynx. This results in subjective improvement of the voice as well as quality of life (Berg et al. 2008). However, severe cases of vocal fold atrophy hardly benefit from voice therapy.

Injection Laryngoplasty The most common is injection laryngoplasty in which the vocal folds are injected with a filler (fat, fascia, hydroxyapatite or others) under general or local anaesthesia. This method has been commonly used for vocal fold paralysis but is effective as well in the treatment of vocal fold atrophy (Postma et al. 1998).

Laryngeal Framework Surgery/Thyroplasty Thyroplasty is often reserved for patients with severe atrophy of the vocal folds and large gaps of the glottis. In this procedure, the vocal fold is medialised statically by inserting an implant in the paraglottal space. This is done bilaterally for patients and atrophy of the vocal folds (Netterville et al. 1993).

This procedure, as well as injection laryngoplasty, reduces the glottal gap; however, it neither improves the vocal fold atrophy nor the senile changes of the lamina propria.

5.15.5 Prognosis

Senile changes of the larynx progress; this is a normal process that develops among all elderly but at different rates. Accordingly, these changes and presbyphonia are expected to be more evident with increase in age. However, the pace of such changes and their effects on the patient are quite hard to predict. This is due to the effects of comorbidities as well as the functionality of patient himself.

Case Study 5.34
A 64-year-old pensioner with asthma and hypertension had gradually lost his voice during the last few years. Four years ago an augmentation of the vocal folds improved his voice but did not last for long. The larynx shows an age-related atrophy of the vocalis muscle and scarring of the epithelium on both vocal folds. The vocal folds hardly vibrate, and there is a large glottal gap during attempted phonation. This leads to an aphonic voice (Rx B3 H3). No sustained tones are registered. The speaking voice profile is not interpretable.

5.16 Voice in Childhood and Adolescence: Special Challenges

Michael Fuchs

5.16.1 Introduction

This section specifically addresses the special issues of age- and development-related voice diagnostics in children and adolescents for three reasons:

- Dysphonia can frequently be found in these age groups. The international literature rates its prevalence as 6–24%, in some cases even well above that (Connor et al. 2008)
- Dysphonia has a direct relevance for young patients. It affects their communicative behaviour and their psychological well-being and leads to a more negative assessment by adults as well as other children and adolescents
- The voice diagnostic conditions and experiences gained during adulthood cannot be immediately and directly applied to children and adolescents. It is particularly important to take into account the dynamics of development and the resulting normative value ranges

It is also important to take into account the wide range of symptoms and lack of knowledge of these symptoms by the parents, carers and colleagues: often parents or other persons of reference do not adequately perceive the hoarseness of a child or adolescent as a cardinal symptom of a dysphonia, so that much time passes before a visit is paid to a physician. In a current and representative British study of 7389 8-year-olds, 6% were diagnosed with an atypical voice tone, which only 22% of the parents involved had noticed (Carding et al. 2006).

In addition, even when hoarseness is found within the framework of a more general medical examination, the cases are not always forwarded to corresponding specialists of phoniatrics and pedaudiology or otorhinolaryngology.

Apart from the possible organic causes that often require treatment, dysphonia has additional consequences for the affected child: children with a pathological voice are assessed more negatively by peers and adults than children with a healthy voice. Furthermore, changes in vocal sound have emotional effects (sadness, anger, frustration) in 40–80% of children and impair social contacts (reduced vocal contribution during classes and recreational activities) (Eckel et al. 2000).

In the international literature there is a knowledge gap in normative data of vocal development and of sociocultural and educational influences on voice in childhood and adolescence. These data are needed for both the diagnostics and therapy of dysphonia and dysodia and the care of increased vocal activities in individual voice training or in membership of choirs.

5.16.2 Landmarks of Voice Development and Normative Values

Anatomical and histopathological knowledge has a direct clinical relevance and should be considered in a much more decisive manner than hitherto. At the time of birth, the length of the vocal folds is approximately 2.5–3.0 mm. In adult females it is between 11 and 15 mm and in adult males between 17 and 21 mm. With increasing age the vocal folds also become thinner and differ in their histological structure with the typical three-layered lamina propria. Plastinated infantile larynxes have been used to provide a detailed anatomical description of the development of the glottis and subglottis during the first 5 years of life (Eckel et al. 2000).

For this reason surgical interventions, particularly for vocal fold nodules, are out of the question until the larynx has completed growth, and the vocal folds have differentiated, since scarring of the vulnerable tissue bears the risk of permanent vocal limitations. In contrast to this, with juvenile larynx papillomatosis or rare suspected tumorous changes, surgical interventions to the vocal folds often cannot be avoided even in childhood.

When assessing an individual's voice development, it must be remembered that the vocal apparatus does not grow at a constant speed. Phases with more rapid growth can be differentiated from phases in which there is a relatively slow, continuous development. During the first 2 years of life and during voice breaking (mutation), the voice organ changes within a short period.

5.16.3 Development of Vocal Performance and Quality

The first vocal performance is the cry of a newborn. It usually has a frequency of approximately 440 Hz, which corresponds to the musical concert pitch a1 (A4) and apparently represents a purely vocal expression that is not superimposed upon by the articulators of speech. It requires an active breathing function for generating the subglottal pressure. Even when the voice tone while crying is characterised by elements of hoarseness (throatiness and breathiness) as well as pressed vocalisation during the first days of life, these can be reliably differentiated from pathological inspiratory or expiratory breathing sounds. Within the first few weeks and months of life, melodic and rhythmic elements develop. They are initially an expression of the infant's momentary emotions and needs but progress increasingly to preliminary stages of speaking and singing (Wermke 2007). Before mutation, the average pitch of unstressed speaking develops equally for girls and boys. The average pitch frequencies range from 220 Hz (a) to 262 Hz (c1) for boys and from 211 Hz (gis) to 281 Hz (cis1) for girls, whereby there are no statistically significant differences between the sexes. Following mutational growth of the larynx and lengthening of the vocal folds, men reach an average pitch ranging from 87 Hz (F) to 147 Hz (d), and women from 175 Hz (f) to 293 Hz (d1).

The increase in pitch range and dynamics with age depends very much on sociocultural and (singing) educational influences. In our own studies, we were able to show that both regular voice activity and phonation lead to a significant broadening of both parameter values (Frank and Sparber 1970;

Fuchs et al. 2009). Table 5.9 shows the parameters' pitch and sound pressure level, as well as maximum phonation time, that have been compiled from normative value ranges obtained from the literature. The measurement of these parameters is most widely spread in clinical practice.

Numerous publications on vocal pitch range employ so-called normative voice range profiles, which are practicable for diagnostics, although less suitable for the representation of age development chosen here. Representative data and our own results were thus selected by means of example. However, this overview also clearly shows the lack of knowledge about normative values, particularly with respect to small children.

5.16.4 Medical History: Typical Symptoms of Dysphonia in Childhood and Adolescence

As is the case with adults, children and adolescents with dysphonia typically complain about symptoms that can be subdivided into three groups: changes in voice tone, limitation of vocal ability and physical discomfort in the head and throat area. At an early age, instabilities (involuntary changes between the vocal registers and diplophonia) as well as open and closed nasalisation appear frequently as a change in sound.

In clinical routine, combined voice and speech disorders predominate and are characterised as rhinophonia. Up to about the age of 4, children do not become aware of the change in sound by themselves, but the changes are partly noticed by parents and other persons of reference (Eckel et al. 2000). Thereafter children are increasingly able to assess the sound of their own voice and its effect on other persons but also the peculiarities of the voices of other children and adults (Fuchs et al. 2009).

Vocal limitations can relate to the pitch range, the dynamic range and also the duration for which the child's voice can be stressed without complaint or harm. For example, children may not be able to speak and sing loudly or very loudly, so that they have problems in very noisy situations and cannot vocally communicate their

Table 5.9 Mean values of vocal pitch range boundaries (musical notation), dynamic boundaries (dB(A)) and maximum phonation time (seconds) for untrained and trained voices

Age	Voice education	3 years	4 years	5 years	6 years	7 years	8 years	9 years	10 years	11 years	12 years	13 years	14 years	15 years	16 years
Mean values of vocal pitch range boundaries (musical notation)	Untrained							Boys: fis - d² Girls: f - e² [3]				Boys: Gis - e¹ Girls: f - fis² [3]			
		Boys: h - h¹ Girls: h - h¹ [2]				Boys: g - c³ Girls g - c³ [1]									
			Boys: b - c² Girls: h - c² [2]	Boys: b - c² Girls: h - c² [2]	Boys: a - e2 Girls: h - f² [2]	Boys: Pre-mutation: f - g² Mutation: c - e¹ Post-mutation: G - e¹ [2]									
			Boys: ais - d² Girls: ais - d² [4]	Boys: a - f² Girls: ais - fis² [4]	Boys: a - a² Girls: ais - gis² [4]	Boys: a - gis² Girls: a - gis² [4]	Boys: g - g² Girls: a - g² [4]	Boys: f - gis² Girls: g - ais² [4]	Boys: g - a² Girls: g - h² [4]	Boys: fis - ais² Girls: ais - fis² [4]	Boys: fis - a² Girls: g - c³ [4]				
	Trained							Boys: f - gis² Girls: f< gis² [3]				Boys: Ais - c² Girls: e - gis² [3]			
Mean values of dynamic boundaries (dB(A))	Untrained					Boys: 63.8-83.8 Girls: 62.3-82.1 [1]		Boys: 54.5-75.8 Girls: 52.6-76.3 [3]				Boys: 52.8-76.0 Girls: 52.3-77.6 [3]			

	3 years	4 years	5 years	6 years	7 years	8 years	9 years	10 years	11 years	12 years	13 years	14 years	15 years	16 years
Trained		Boys: 53–80 Girls: 53–79 [4]	Boys: 52–80 Girls: 53–82 [4]	Boys: 52–85 Girls: 52–82 [4]	Boys: 52–85 Girls: 52–83 [4]	Boys: 56–86 Girls: 53–82 [4]	Boys: 51–83 Girls: 51–82 [4] Boys: 48.2–92.5 Girls: 48.8–49.6 [3]	Boys: 51–83 Girls: 51–80 [4]	Boys: 50–83 Girls: 51–83 [4]	Boys: 50–86 Girls: 51–80 [4]	Boys: 48.8–89.6 Girls: 50.0–88.1 [3]			
Mean values of maximum phonation time (seconds) — Untrained				Boys: 10.4 Girls: 10.6 [3]			Boys: 16.8 Girls: 14.4 [3]				Boys: 14.8 Girls: 18.0 [3]			
Mean values of maximum phonation time (seconds) — Trained							Boys: 13.7 Girls: 11.8 [3]				Boys: 14.3 Girls: 13.7 [3]			
Age	3 years	4 years	5 years	6 years	7 years	8 years	9 years	10 years	11 years	12 years	13 years	14 years	15 years	16 years
Voice education														

[1] Böhme G, Stuchlik G (1995) Voice profiles and standard voice profile of untrained children. J Voice 9(3):304–307. [2] Frank F, Sparber M (1970) Stimmumfänge bei Kindern aus neuer Sicht. Folia Phoniatr 22:397–402. [3] Fuchs M, Heide S, Hentschel B et al. (2006) Stimmleistungsparameter bei Kindern und Jugendlichen: Einfluss der körperlichen Entwicklung und der sängerischen Aktivität. HNO 54(12):971–980. [4] Hacki T, Heitmüller S (1999) Development of the child's voice: permutation and mutation. Int J Pediatr Otorhinolaryngol 49(Suppl 1):141–144

needs and their personality within a group. Frequently, however, there are also limitations at minimal intensity: the affected children are less successful at speaking and singing softly than vocally healthy children.

A further aspect is quick vocal fatigue: a significant deterioration of vocal quality after just a short strain of the voice (loud speaking, vocally intensive recreational activities, singing) and an extended recovery phase, when the complaints do not regress completely overnight. All of the named limitations ultimately lead to a deprivation in vocal and emotional options for expression.

The discomfort felt by children and youths mainly include (burning) sore throat, feelings of exertion, compulsion to clear the throat, tickling of the throat and the feeling of being out of breath, while the typical feeling of a lump in the throat (globus pharyngis) is the most frequent symptom complained of in adulthood. These voice-related complaints are made by 45–65% of affected children aged 4 and above and by 25–40% of cases with youths (Eckel et al. 2000).

5.16.5 Organic Diagnostics of the Vocal Apparatus

With newborns as well as infants, indirect video laryngoscopy is performed with a flexible scope (diameter: 2.8–3.4 mm). Stroboscopic assessments by flexible chip-tip pharyngo-laryngoscopes can be successfully performed even on newborns. However, good clinical experience has also been made with rigid scopes, whereby the tongue is not protruded but only pressed down lightly. From about age 3 onwards, rigid optics are mainly used.

With small children, the use of special optics with a shortened distance between the handpiece and the tip of the endoscope (diameter: 7 mm) has been used extensively (Fig. 5.42). On the other hand, optics with an even smaller diameter (4 mm) and with considerably greater image detail than with flexible optics bring a greater risk of injury due to warding off movements by the child because of the narrow endoscopic tip.

The optics with the largest diameter (12 mm) are, owing to their heat-protective attachment, currently the camera systems used in high-speed glottography. Clinical experience has shown, because of the anatomical conditions in the oro-pharynx, that these cannot be tolerated before the age of 12. An analysis of vocal fold oscillations can be performed on children by means of stro-boscopy from the age of birth and by means of high-speed video from the ages of 12–14.

Direct laryngoscopy under anaesthesia is possible from the age of birth and even with prema-ture infants. The younger the child, the more

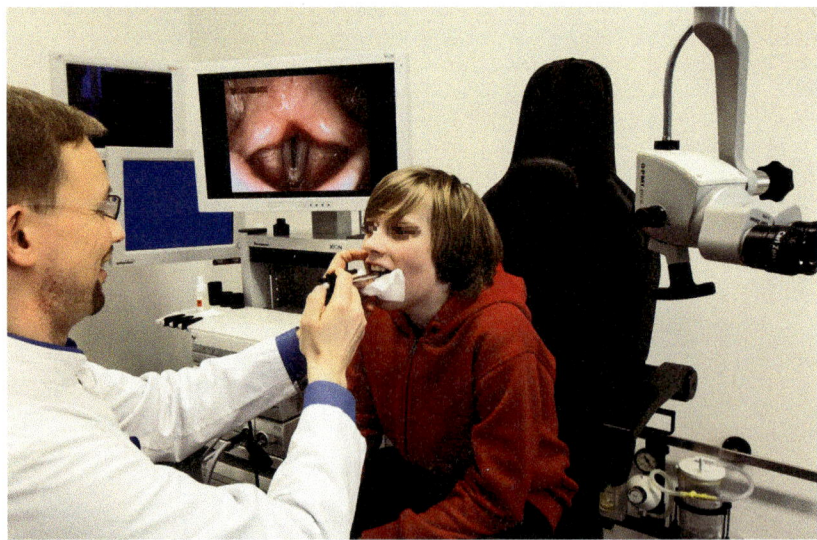

Fig. 5.42 Examination conditions with videolaryngoscope and digital image processing

important it is to conduct intensive preoperative preparations and to have close collaboration between the surgeon and the anaesthetist and paediatricians (neonatologists, paediatric intensivists). Even though malignant tumours are exceptionally rare as the cause for dysphonia in childhood and adolescence, the more frequent other organic causes (particularly papillomas) are reason enough to clarify endoscopically the cause of any hoarseness that lasts longer than 3 weeks.

Case Study 5.35
Vocal fold nodules of a 10-year-old boy. He has always been hoarse and after extreme vocal abuse the voice became completely aphonic. The video shows in very short sequences bilateral vocal fold protrusions in the middle of the membranous vocal fold. The voice range is clearly restricted. The sound of the speaking voice is mildly rough and breathy (R1 B1 H1).

Case Study 5.36
Vocal fold cyst of an 11-year-old boy. He sings a leading role in a musical. His voice gradually lost the high tones even though mutation had not begun yet. The dynamic range is still good. The speaking voice is strained and reveals a mild roughness and breathiness (R1 B1 H1).

Case Study 5.37
Papillomatosis in a 5-year-old girl. Her voice varies between severely hoarse and aphonic (R3 B3 H3). Usually she has to make great effort to produce voice. She becomes short of breath on exertion.

5.16.6 Functional Diagnostics

In the diagnosis of vocal performance and quality, auditory perceptual analysis of the voice is the main method used during the early years of life. Initially, parameters of throatiness, breathiness and hoarseness, the average speaking pitch and vocalisation can be assessed on the basis of spontaneous vocal and linguistic expressions. From preschool age onwards, additional parameters (exertion, tiredness, instability) as well as

the pitch range are assessed. Standardised, phonetically balanced texts should be used as soon as the child has a firm command of reading.

When measuring the profile of spoken pitch, besides minimal voice intensity, two or three further levels up to maximum intensity are required. Experience has shown this can be accomplished from school age onwards. For measuring the profile of the singing voice, the child must be able to repeat a given tone as softly and loudly as possible (Figs. 5.43 and 5.44). Children actively engaged in singing accomplish this at preschool age. Furthermore, the new generation of software available for acquiring voice range profiles also records held tones that deviate from the demanded pitch. The advantages of the voice range profile lie in the frequency-related representation of the dynamic width of the singing voice and the simultaneous presentation of findings of the speaking-voice profile in the form of a diagram that makes it possible to grasp more quickly the vocal performance capability. State-of-the-art software also records each individual voice tone produced while measuring the singing voice profile, so that more detailed acoustic analyses of the vocal performance can be added to explain the findings.

A tool for qualitative evaluation of the singing voice profile in children is the Voice Range Profile Index for Children (Heylen et al. 1998). Furthermore, individual voice quality assessments can be made with numerous applicable acoustic analysis methods that can even work with vocal expressions lasting just a few seconds (Fuchs et al. 2007).

In assessing vocal performance and quality in children and adolescents, auditory voice findings, as well as the speaking and singing voice range profile including acoustic analyses, are of particular diagnostic value.

5.16.7 Supplementary Diagnostic Methods

Currently there is only limited experience with questionnaires that examine children's own vocal limitations and their effects on well-being and

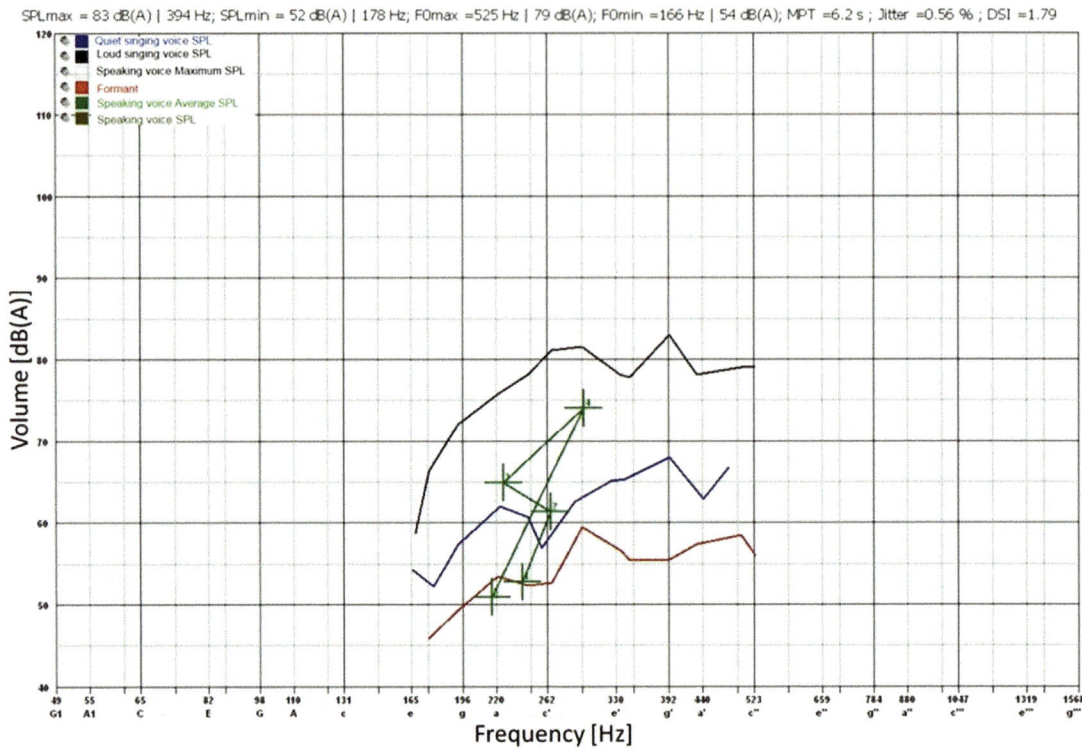

SPLmax = 83 dB(A) | 394 Hz; SPLmin = 52 dB(A) | 178 Hz; F0max =525 Hz | 79 dB(A); F0min =166 Hz | 54 dB(A); MPT =6.2 s ; Jitter =0.56 % ; DSI =1.79

Fig. 5.43 A singing and speaking voice range profile

Fig. 5.44 Singing and speaking voice range profile of a 14-year-old boy at the beginning of mutation, with conspicuous limitations in the vocal pitch range and dynamic width while singing, as well as a reduced ability to raise the speaking voice. The fundamental speaking frequency is still in the range of that of a small boy

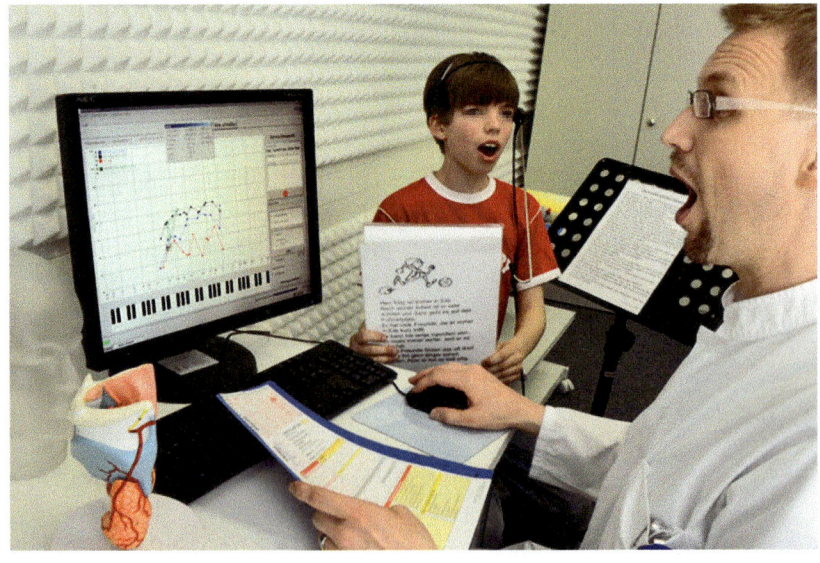

quality of life. Directed interviews that take into account the physical, functional, social and emotional factors have been well tried in this respect (Eckel et al. 2000). There are comprehensive concepts (Kollbrunner 2006; Nienkerke-Springer et al. 2005) available for psychosomatic diagnostics. However, their application requires that the diagnostician who is generally first confronted with a child's dysphonia, i.e. the specialist for phoniatrics and pedaudiology or ENT medicine, is aware of these aetiological relationships and the corresponding method (including consultation and therapy) and that such cooperation is possible on-site. Besides anamnestic dialogues, diagnostic methods are special instruments for parent interviews, such as questionnaires about the subject of voice and family sociograms (Kollbrunner 2006).

Within the framework of clinical voice diagnostics for children and adolescents, it should be determined whether the occurrence of dysphonia could also be due to an unfavourable, dynamic family situation. In this case it would be recommended to consult a specialist in child and adult psychology.

In practice, a representation of the vocal apparatus from image-generating processes (particularly CT and MRT) is almost always considered only in conjunction with organic causes for dysphonia, and even then it is reserved for special questions.

5.16.8 Relevance for the Clinical Assessment of Suitability for Increased Vocal Activities

When it is to be assessed whether a child's vocal apparatus is suitable for increased vocal stress—for example, as encountered by a member of a children's and adolescents' choir or for solo tasks in the music room and opera—the diagnostic methods above, taking into account the normative values, can provide an initial assessment. Where organic or functional limitations in vocal performance and quality can be excluded, an in-depth anamnestic dialogue should be performed to assess whether the child can meet the musical and psychosocial requirements necessary for the respective vocal delivery. Very often the assessing person is faced with the problem that so far there has been no vocal training and vocal stress, so that even the effects cannot as of yet be estimated. Repeated examinations at intervals of 3–6 months are well proven to account for the dynamic development. Thus, given educational training in singing, an initially constitutionally 'small voice' can experience a significant increase

in vocal performance and quality so that it is in a better position to meet the increased vocal challenges. On the other hand, high vocal stress without accompanying phonation can lead to dysphonia because the vocal requirements are being chronically overtaxed.

As a tool for estimating vocal activity in daily clinical routine and for scientific examinations, the Leipzig Workgroup has developed a classification system that facilitates a reliably reproducible classification that is independent of the professional group (physicians, phonation educators, choir masters, music teachers, lay people) performing the assessment. The normative value ranges presented help to detect and treat deviations from regular physiological development (Fuchs et al. 2008).

Dysphonia before adulthood is often left untreated, particularly when it is not very pronounced and not deteriorating significantly. This is despite the fact that the negative consequences of untreated dysphonia not only have a direct effect on childhood and adolescence but also extend into adulthood. Diagnostic and therapeutic measures should be specific to the respective age and development of the child; new technical devices also facilitate precise outpatient diagnostics at an early age in childhood. Besides endoscopic methods, there are also acoustic methods that facilitate a precise documentation of findings and easy comparability. Not only organic but also functional dysphonia requires increased attention.

References

Abitbol J, Abitbol P, Abitbol B (1999) Sex hormones and the female voice. J Voice 13(3):424–446

Abou-Ismail A, Vaezi MF (2011) Evaluation of patients with suspected laryngopharyngeal reflux: a practical approach. Curr Gastroenterol Rep 13(3):213–218

Adler RK, Hirsch S, Mordaunt M (eds) (2006) Voice and communication therapy for the transgender/transsexual client. A comprehensive clinical guide. Plural Publishing, San Diego, CA

Akdis CA, Akdis M (2011) Mechanisms of allergen-specific immunotherapy. J Allergy Clin Immunol 127(1):18–27

Allen NB (1996) Wegener's granulomatosis. In: Bennett JC, Plum F (eds) Cecil's essentials of medicine. WB Saunders, Philadelphia, pp 1494–1498

Altman KW, Irwin RS (2010) Cough specialists collaborate for an interdisciplinary problem. Otolaryngol Clin N Am 43(1):xv–xix

Anderson TD (2007) Benign lesions of the larynx. In: Merati AL, Bielamowicz SA (eds) Textbook of laryngology. Plural Publishing, San Diego, CA

Arndt HJ, Schäfer A (1994) Der Weiten-Längen-Quotient der Glottis als Mass für die Amplitudengrösse. (The width-length quotient of the glottis as a measure of amplitude values). Folia Phoniatr Logop 46(6):265–270

Arnett FC, Edworthy SM, Block DA et al (1988) The American Rheumatism Association 1987 revised criteria for the classification of rheumatoid arthritis. Arthritis Rheumatol 31(3):315–324

Aviv JE, Martin JH, Keen MS et al (1993) Air pulse quantification of supraglottic and pharyngeal sensation: a new technique. Ann Otol Rhinol Laryngol 102(10):777–780

Aviv JE, Martin JH, Kim T et al (1999) Laryngopharyngeal sensory discrimination testing and the laryngeal adductor reflex. Ann Otol Rhinol Laryngol 108(8):725–730

Aviv JE, Liu H, Parides M et al (2000) Laryngopharyngeal sensory deficits in patients with laryngopharyngeal reflux and dysphagia. Ann Otol Rhinol Laryngol 109(11):1000–1006

Aydin K, Turkyilmaz D, Ozturk B et al (2013) Voice characteristics of acromegaly. Eur Arch Otorhinolaryngol 270(4):1391–1396

Bain WM, Harrington JW, Thomas LE et al (1983) Head and neck manifestations of gastroesophageal reflux. Laryngoscope 93(2):175–179

Baken RJ, Noback CR (1971) Neuromuscular spindles in intrinsic muscles of a human larynx. J Speech Hear Res 14(3):513–518

Baken RJ (2005) The aged voice: a new hypothesis. J Voice 19(3):317–325

Baker K, Ramig L, Luschei E et al (1998) Thyroarytenoid muscle activity associated with hypophonia in Parkinson disease and aging. Neurology 51(6):1592–1598

Balkissoon R, Kenn K (2012) Asthma: vocal cord dysfunction (VCD) and other dysfunctional breathing disorders. Semin Respir Crit Care Med 33(6):595–605

Barillari MR, Volpe U, Innaro N et al (2016) Is menstrual dysphonia associated with greater disability and lower quality of life? J Voice 30(1):88–92

Bauer H (1990) Störungen der stimme. In: Uexküll T (ed) Psychosomatische medizin. Urban und Schwarzenberg, Munich

Becking AG, Tuinzing DB, Hage JJ et al (1996) Facial corrections in male to female transsexuals: a preliminary report on 16 patients. J Oral Maxillofac Surg 54(4):413–418

Belafsky P, Postma G, Koufman J (2001a) Laryngopharyngeal reflux symptoms improve before changes in physical findings. Laryngoscope 111(6):979–981

Belafsky PC, Postma GN, Koufman JA (2001b) The validity and reliability of the reflux finding score (RFS). Laryngoscope 111(8):1313–1317

Belafsky PC, Postma GN, Koufman JA (2002a) The association between laryngeal pseudosulcus and laryngopharyngeal reflux. Otolaryngol Head Neck Surg 126(6):649–652

Belafsky PC, Postma GN, Koufman JA (2002b) Validity and reliability of the reflux symptom score (RSI). J Voice 16(2):274–277

Belafsky PC (2003) Abnormal endoscopic pharyngeal and laryngeal findings attributable to reflux. Am J Med 115(Suppl 3A):90S–96S

Beltsis A, Katsinelos P, Kountouras J et al (2011) Double probe pH-monitoring findings in patients with benign lesions of the true vocal folds: comparison with typical GERD and the effect of smoking. Eur Arch Otorhinolaryngol 268(8):1169–1174

Benjamin H (1953) Transvestism and transsexualism. Int J Sexol 7:12–14

Benjamin H (1966) The transsexual phenomenon. Julian Press, New York

Bennet DA, Beckett CA, Murray AM et al (1996) Prevalence of parkinsonian signs and associated mortality in a community population of older people. N Engl J Med 334(2):71–76

Benninger MS, Gardner GM, Schwimmer C et al (2006) Laryngeal neurophysiology. In: Rubin JS et al (eds) Diagnosis and treatment of voice disorders, 3rd edn. Plural Publishing, San Diego, CA, pp 109–114

Berg EE, Hapner E, Klein A et al (2008) Voice therapy improves quality of life in age-related dysphonia: a case-control study. J Voice 22(1):70–74

Berke GS, Blackwell KE, Gerratt BR et al (1999a) Selective laryngeal adductor denervation-reinnervation: a new surgical treatment for adductor spasmodic dysphonia. Ann Otol Rhinol Laryngol 108(3):227–231

Berke GS, Gerratt B, Kreiman J et al (1999b) Treatment of Parkinson Hypophonia with autologous collagen augmentation. Laryngoscope 109(8):1295–1299

Bermudez de Alvear R, Martinez-Arquero G, Barón FJ et al (2010) An interdisciplinary approach to teachers' voice disorders and psychosocial working conditions. Folia Phoniatr Logop 62(1–2):24–34

Bernstein JA (2004) Health effects of air pollution. J Allergy Clin Immunol 114(5):1116–1123

Best SR, Friedman AD, Landau-Zemer T et al (2012) Safety and dosing of bevacizumab (Avastin) for the treatment of recurrent respiratory papillomatosis. Ann Otol Rhinol Laryngol 121:587–593

Birkent H, Karacalioglu O, Merati AL et al (2008) Prospective study of the impact of thyroid hormone replacement on objective voice parameters. Ann Otol Rhinol Laryngol 117(7):523–527

Blitzer A, Lovelace RE, Brin MF et al (1985) Electromyographic findings in focal laryngeal dystonia. Ann Otol Rhinol Laryngol 94(6 Pt 1):591–594

Blumin JH, Berke GS (2002) Bilateral vocal fold paresis and multiple system atrophy. Arch Otolaryngol Head Neck Surg 128(12):1404–1407

Blumin JH, Ludlow CL (2014) Management of the spasmodic dysphonias. In: Rubin JS, Sataloff RT, Korovin GK (eds) Diagnosis and treatment of voice disorders, 4th edn. Plural Publishers, San Diego

Boero DL, Weber G, Vigone MC et al (2000) Crying abnormalities in congenital hypothyroidism: preliminary spectrographic study. J Child Neurol 15(9):603–608

Bogazzi F, Nacci A, Campomori A et al (2010) Analysis of voice in patients with untreated active acromegaly. J Endocrinol Investig 33(3):178–185

Boone DR, McFarlane SC (2000) The voice and voice therapy, 6th edn. A Pearson Education Company, Needham Heights, MA

Bouchayer M, Cornut G, Witzig E et al (1985) Epidermoid cyst, sulci, and mucosal bridges of the true vocal cord: a report of 157 cases. Laryngoscope 95(9):1081–1094

Bower JS, Belen JE, Weg JG et al (1980) Manifestations and treatment of laryngeal sarcoidosis. Am Rev Respir Dis 122(2):325–332

Branski RC, Bhattacharyya N, Shapiro J (2002) The reliability of the assessment of endoscopic laryngeal findings associated with laryngopharyngeal reflux disease. Laryngoscope 112(6):1019–1024

Braverman LE, Utiger RD (2005) Introduction to hypothyroidism. In: Braverman LE, Utiger RD (eds) Werner & Ingbar's the thyroid: a fundamental and clinical text, 9th edn. Lippincott Williams & Wilkins, Philadelphia

Brin MF, Fahn S, Blitzer A et al (1992) Movement disorders of the larynx. In: Blitzer A et al (eds) Neurologic disorders of the larynx. Thieme Medical Publishers, New York, pp 248–278

Brown M, Perry A, Cheesman AD et al (2000) Pitch change in male-to-female transsexuals. Has phonosurgery a role to play? Int J Lang Commun Disord 35(1):129–136

Brown S, Ngan E, Liotti M (2008) A larynx area in the human motor cortex. Cereb Cortex 18(4):837–845

Burton DM, Pransky SM, Katz RM et al (1992) Pediatric airway manifestations of gastroesophageal reflux. Ann Otol Rhinol Laryngol 101(9):742–749

Butler J (1990) Gender trouble. Feminism and the subversion of identity. Routledge, New York

Calcinoni O, Niebudek-Bogusz E (2014) Occupational voice. In: Rubin J et al (eds) Diagnosis and treatment of voice disorders, 4th edn. Plural Publishing, San Diego, pp 735–762

Cammarota G, Masala G, Cianci R et al (2007) Reflux symptoms in professional opera choristers. Gastroenterology 132(3):890–898

Campbell SM, Montanaro A, Bardana EJ (1983) Head and neck manifestations of autoimmune disease. Am J Otolaryngol 4(3):187–216

Cantani A (2008) Pediatric allergy, asthma and immunology. Springer, Berlin, Heidelberg

Carding PN, Roulstone S, Northstone K et al (2006) The prevalence of childhood dysphonia: a cross-sectional study. J Voice 20(4):623–630

Carding P (2007) Occupational voice disorders: is there a firm case for industrial injuries disablement benefit? Logoped Phoniatr Vocol 32(1):47–48

Carew L, Dacakis G, Oates J (2007) The effectiveness of oral resonance therapy on the perception of femininity of voice in male-to-female transsexuals. J Voice 21(5):591–603

Castell DO, Wu WC, Ott DJ (eds) (1985) Gastroesophageal reflux disease, pathogenesis, diagnosis, therapy. Futura Pub Co, Mt. Kisko, New York

Cekin E, Ozyurt M, Erkul E et al (2012) The association between Helicobacter pylori and laryngopharyngeal reflux in laryngeal pathologies. Ear Nose Throat J 91(3):E6–E9

Chae SW, Choi G, Kang HJ et al (2001) Clinical analysis of voice change as a parameter of premenstrual syndrome. J Voice 15(2):278–283

Chaloner J (1991) The voice of the transsexual. In: Fawcus M (ed) Voice disorders and their management, 2nd edn. Chapman & Hall, London, New York, Tokio, pp 245–267

Chang A, Karnell MP (2004) Perceived phonatory effort and phonation threshold pressure across a prolonged voice loading task: a study of vocal fatigue. J Voice 18(4):454–466

Chapman MD, Pomés A, Breiteneder H et al (2007) Nomenclature and structural biology of allergens. J Allergy Clin Immunol 119(2):414–420

Chávez RE (2006) The effect of environmental conditions on voice. Paper presented at the 3rd World Voice Congress, Istanbul, 19–22 June, 2006

Chávez RE (2007) Environmental and respiratory allergies effects on the voice. Paper presented at the 36th Symposium of the Voice Foundation, Philadelphia, USA, 31 May 2007

Chávez RE (2009) Alteraciones de la voz por patología alérgica, La influencia del ambiente en el Canto. Paper presented at the VII. Congreso Internacional de Alergia y Medicina Ambiental, Mexico, 2009

Chávez RE (2010a) Environment, smoking and voice. Paper presented at the 4th Congress of the World Voice Consortium, Seoul, Korea, 6–9 September 2010

Chávez RE (2010b) Vocal pathology in singers and actors due to respiratory allergies and harmful environment. Paper presented at the 4th Congress of the World Voice Consortium, Seoul, Korea, 6–9 September 2010

Chávez RE (2012) Ambiente, alergia y voz. Paper presented at the Congreso 52 SMORL y CCC, CanCun, Mexico, 30 April 2012

Chávez RE (2018) Voice patients with respiratory allergies. New results. (in preparation for publication)

Cheng J, Woo P (2010) Correlation between the Voice Handicap Index and voice laboratory measurements after phonosurgery. Ear Nose Throat J 89(4):183–188

Chernobelsky SI (2002) A study of menses-related changes to the larynx in singers with voice abuse. Folia Phoniatr Logop 54(1):2–7

Cherry J, Margulies SI (1968) Contact ulcer of the larynx. Laryngoscope 78(11):1937–1940

Christopher KL, Wood RP 2nd, Eckert RC et al (1983) Vocal-cord dysfunction presenting as asthma. N Engl J Med 308(26):1566–1570

Claassen H, Monig H, Sel S et al (2006) Androgen receptors and gender-specific distribution of alkaline phosphatase in human thyroid cartilage. Histochem Cell Biol 126(3):381–388

Clerf LH, Baltzell WH (1953) Re-evaluation of Semon's hypothesis. Laryngoscope 63(8):693–699

Clevens RA, Eslamado RM, DelGaudio JM et al (1994) Amyloidoma of the neck: case report and review of the literature. Head Neck 16(2):191–195

Coca-Pelaz A, Rodrigo JP, Takes RP et al (2013) Relationship between reflux and laryngeal cancer. Head Neck 35(12):1814–1818

Cohen E, Kolbus A, van Trotsenburg M et al (2009) Immunohistochemical examinations of sex hormone receptors in benign vocal fold lesions. Folia Phoniatr Logop 61(5):259–262

Cohen-Kettenis PT, Pfäfflin F (2010) The DSM diagnostic criteria for gender identity disorder in adolescents and adults. Arch Sex Behav 39(2):499–513

Connor NP, Cohen SB, Theis SM et al (2008) Attitudes of children with dysphonia. J Voice 22(2):197–209

Cosyns M, Van Borsel J, Wierckx K et al (2014) Voice in female-to-male transsexual persons after long-term androgen therapy. Laryngoscope 124(6):1409–1414

Crumley RL (1989) Laryngeal synkinesis: its significance to the laryngologist. Ann Otol Rhinol Laryngol 98(2):87–92

Crumley RL (1990) Repair of the recurrent laryngeal nerve. Otolaryngol Clin N Am 23(3):553–563

Cukier-Blaj S, Bewley A, Aviv JE et al (2008) Paradoxical vocal fold motion: a sensory-motor laryngeal disorder. Laryngoscope 118(2):367–370

Custovic A, Simpson BM, Simpson A et al (2001) Effect of environmental manipulation in pregnancy and early life on respiratory symptoms and atopy during first year of life: a randomised trial. Lancet 358(9277):188–193

Dacakis G (2002) The role of voice therapy in male-to-female transsexuals. Curr Opinion Otolaryngol Head Neck Surg 10(3):173–177

Dacakis G, Oates J, Douglas J (2012) Beyond voice: perceptions of gender in male-to-female transsexuals. Curr Opin Otolaryngol Head Neck Surg 20(3):165–170

Damrose EJ (2009) Quantifying the impact of androgen therapy on the female larynx. Auris Nasus Larynx 36(1):110–112

Damste PH (1964) Virilization of the voice due to anabolic steroids. Folia Phoniatr (Basel) 16:10–18

Davis CB, Davis ML (1993) The effects of premenstrual syndrome (PMS) on the female singer. J Voice 7(4):337–353

De Bruin MD, Coerts MJ, Greven AJ (2000) Speech therapy in the management of male-to-female transsexuals. Folia Phoniatr Logop 52(5):220–227

De Cuypere G, Van Hemelrijck M, Michel A et al (2007) Prevalence and demography of transsexualism in Belgium. Eur Psychiatry 22(3):137–141

Dedo HH (1976) Recurrent laryngeal nerve section for spastic dysphonia. Ann Otol Rhinol Laryngol 85(4):451–459

Dehqan A, Scherer RC, Dashti G et al (2013) The effects of aging on acoustic parameters of voice. Folia Phoniatr Logop 64(6):265–270

Dejonckere PH (2001) Occupational voice—care and cure. Kugler Publications, The Hague, The Netherlands

Dejonckere PH, Bradley P, Clemente P et al (2001) A basic protocol for functional assessment of voice pathology, especially for investigating the efficacy of (phonosurgical) treatments and evaluating new assessment techniques. Guideline elaborated by the Committee on Phoniatrics of the European Laryngological Society (ELS). Eur Arch Otorhinolaryngol 258(2):77–82

de Jong F (2010) An introduction to the teacher's voice in a biopsychosocial perspective. Folia Phoniatr Logop 62(1–2):5–8

de la Coba OC, Arias A, de Argila de Prados M et al (2016) Proton-pump inhibitors adverse effects: a review of the evidence and position statement by the Sociedad Española de Patología Digestiva. Rev Esp Enferm Dig 108(4):207–224. https://doi.org/10.17235/reed.2016.4232/2016

Delahunty JE, Cherry J (1968) Experimentally produced vocal cord granulomas. Laryngoscope 78(11):1941–1947

Delap TG, Lavy JA, Alusi G et al (1997) Tuberculosis presenting as a laryngeal tumor. J Infect 34(2):139–141

De Leo S, Lee SY, Braverman LE (2016) Hyperthyroidism. Lancet 388(10047):906–918

Dempsey PW, Vaidya SA, Cheng G (2003) The art of war: innate and adaptive immune responses. Cell Mol Life Sci 60(12):2604–2621

Deuschl G, Elble RJ (2000) The pathophysiology of essential tremor. Neurology 54(Suppl 4):S14–S20

Deuster D, Matulat P, Knief A et al (2016) Voice deepening under testosterone treatment in female-to-male gender dysphoric individuals. Eur Arch Otorhinolaryngol 273(4):959–965

Deuster D (2017) Testosteron-induzierte Stimm- und Kehlkopfveränderungen bei Frau-zu-Mann-Transsexualismus. In: Caffier PP, Deuster D (eds) Aktuelle phoniatrisch-pädaudiologische Aspekte. Frick Kreativbüro und Onlinedruckerei e. K, Krumbach

DeWitt I, Rauschecker JP (2012) Phoneme and word recognition in the auditory ventral stream. Proc Natl Acad Sci U S A 109(8):E505–E514. https://doi.org/10.1073/pnas.1113427109

D'haeseleer E, Depypere H, Claeys S et al (2009) The menopause and the female larynx, clinical aspects and therapeutic options: a literature review. Maturitas 64(1):27–32

D'haeseleer E, Depypere H, Claeys S et al (2012) The impact of hormone therapy on vocal quality in postmenopausal women. J Voice 26(5):671.e1–671.e7

Donald PJ (1982) Voice change surgery in the transsexual. Head & Neck Surg 4:433–437

Doody RS, Jankovic J (1992) The alien hand and related signs. J Neurol Neurosurg Psychiatry 55(9):806–810

Dronkers NF, Plaisant O, Iba-Zizen MT et al (2007) Paul Broca's historic cases: high resolution MR imaging of the brains of Leborgne and Lelong. Brain 130(Pt 5):1432–1441

Echternach M, Traser L, Richter B (2011) Pathophysiologische Betrachtungen zur Dysphonie durch Erkrankung im Bereich des Vokaltraktes bei reizlosen Stimmlippen. Sprache Stimme Gehör 35(04):139–143

Echternach M, Nusseck M, Dippold S et al (2014) Fundamental frequency, sound pressure level and vocal dose of a vocal loading test in comparison to real teaching situation. Eur Arch Otorhinolaryngol 271(12):3263–3268

Eckel HE, Sprinzl GM, Sittel C et al (2000) Zur Anatomie von Glottis und Subglottis beim kindlichen Kehlkopf. HNO 48(7):501–507

Elble RK, Koller WC (1990) Tremor. Johns Hopkins University Press, Baltimore

Erikson EH (1959) Identity and the life cycle. International University Press, New York

European Economic Community Brussels (2003) Council Directive 2003/670/CE, Brussels. http://eur-lex. europa.eu. Accessed 7 Oct 2014

Fahy JV, Dickey BF (2010) Airway mucus function and dysfunction. N Engl J Med 363(23):2233–2247

Fant G (1975) Nonuniform vowel normalization. STL-QPSR 16(2–3):1–19

Faure MA, Perouse AR, Coulombeau B (2010) Therapeutic choices for curing dysodia?... three clinical cases. Rev Laryngol Otol Rhinol (Bord) 131(1):59–60

Feinberg DR, DeBruine LM, Jones BC et al (2008) The role of femininity and averageness of voice pitch in aesthetic judgements of women's voices. Perception 37(4):615–623

Fernandez-Bussy S, Labarca G, Vial MR et al (2018) Recurrent respiratory papillomatosis and bevacizumab treatment. Am J Respir Crit Care Med 197(4):539–541

Flanagan PM, McIlwain JC (1993) Tuberculosis of the larynx in a lepromatous patient. J Laryngol Otol 107(9):845–847

Ford CN, Inagi K, Khidr A et al (1996) Sulcus vocalis: a rational analytical approach to diagnosis and management. Ann Otol Rhinol Laryngol 105(3):189–200

Ford CN (2005) Evaluation and management of laryngopharyngeal reflux. JAMA 294(12):1534–1540

Frank F, Sparber M (1970) Stimmumfänge bei Kindern aus neuer Sicht. Folia Phoniatr 22(6):397–402

Friedman BA, Rice DH (1975) Rheumatoid nodules of the larynx. Arch Otolaryngol 101(6):361–363

Fuchs M, Behrendt W, Keller E et al (1999) Prediction of the onset of voice mutation in singers of professional Boys' choirs: investigation of members of the Thomaner choir, Leipzig. Folia Phoniatr Logop 51(6):261–271

Fuchs M, Fröhlich M, Hentschel B et al (2007) Predicting mutational change in the speaking voice of boys. J Voice 21(2):169–178

Fuchs M (2008) Landmarken der physiologischen Entwicklung der Stimme bei Kindern und Jugendlichen (Teil 1). ((Landmarks of physiological development of the voice in childhood and adolescence (Part 1)). Laryngorhinootologie 87(1):10–16

Fuchs M, Meuret S, Geister D et al (2008) Empirical criteria for establishing a classification of singing activity in children and adolescents. J Voice 22(6):649–657

Fuchs M, Meuret S, Thiel S et al (2009) Influence of singing activity, age and sex on voice performance parameters, on subjects' perception and use of their voice in childhood and adolescence. J Voice 23(2):182–189

Galli J, Cammarota G, Volante M et al (2006) Laryngeal carcinoma and laryngo-pharyngeal reflux disease. Acta Otorhinolaryngol 26(5):260–263

Gallivan GJ, Landis JN (1993) Sarcoidosis of the larynx: preserving and restoring airway and professional voice. J Voice 7(1):81–94

Garrels L, Köckott G, Michael N et al (2000) Sex ratio of transsexuals in Germany: the development over three decades. Acta Psychiatr Scand 102(6):445–448

Garrigues V, Gisbert L, Bastida G et al (2003) Manifestations of gastroesophageal reflux and response to omeprazole therapy in patients with chronic posterior laryngitis: an evaluation based on clinical practice. Dig Dis Sci 48(11):2117–2123

Gelfer MP (1999) Voice treatment for the male-to-female transgendered client. Am J Speech Lang Pathol 8(3):201–208

Gell PGH, Coombs RRA (1975) Classification of allergic reactions responsible for hypersensitivity and disease. In: Gell PGH et al (eds) Clinical aspects of immunology. Blackwell, Oxford, pp 761–781

Gerhardt C (1863) Studien und Beobachtungen über Stimmbandlähmung. Virchows Arch Pathol Anat 27:68–98, 296–321

Gerlofs-Nijland ME, Boere AJF, Leseman DLAC et al (2005) Effects of particulate matter on the pulmonary and vascular system: time course in spontaneously hypertensive rats. Part Fibre Toxicol 2(1):2–2

Gertz MA, Kyle RA (1989) Primary systemic amyloidosis-a diagnostic primer. Mayo Clin Proc 64(12):1505–1519

Gill NK, Dhingra S (2016) Diagnosis of Allergy. Indian J L Sci 5(2):123–134

Gilman S (1998) Cerebellar disorders. In: Rosenberg R, Pleasure DE (eds) Comprehensive neurology, 2nd edn. Wiley, New York, pp 415–433

Giovanni A, Chanteret C, Lagier A (2007) Sulcus vocalis: a review. Eur Arch Otorhinolaryngol 264(4):337–344

Gómez VJ, Chávez Sánchez R, Flores Sandoval G (2010) Transfer factor and allergy. Rev Alerg Mex 57(6):208–214

Gómez-Gil E, Trilla García A, Godás Sieso T et al (2006) Estimación d la prevalencia, incidenia y razón de sexos del transexualismo en Cataluña según la demanda asistencial. Actas Esp Pysiquiatr 34(0):295–301

Gómez-Gil E, Trilla A, Salamero M et al (2009) Sociodemographic, clinical and psychiatric characteristics of transsexuals from Spain. Arch Sex Behav 38(3):378–392

Gorham-Rowan M, Morris R (2006) Aerodynamic analysis of male-to-female transgender voice. J Voice 20(2):251–262

Gosink J (2015) Precise diagnosis of allergies by multiplex profiling. https://www.euroimmun.com/fileadmin/ euroimmun/pdf/news/article/HP_3000_L_UK_C.pdf. Accessed 22 Apr 2016

Gossett P (2007) Censorship and the Definition of a National Idiom. http://glimmerglass.org/files/1513/8126/5939/Gossett_ShowTalk.pdf. Accessed 12 Jan 2018

Green RH, Brightling CE, Pavord ID et al (2003) Management of asthma in adults: current therapy and future directions. Postgrad Med 79:259–267

Gross M (1999) Pitch-raising surgery in male-to-female transsexuals. J Voice 13(2):246–250

Gross M (2008) Phonochirurgie bei Transsexuellen—Nutzen und Risiken. In: Groß D et al (eds) Transsexualität und Intersexualität. Medizinische, ethische, soziale und juristische Aspekte. Medizinisch Wissenschaftliche Verlagsgesellschaft, Berlin, pp 201–206

Grossmann M (1897) Experimentelle Beiträge zur Lehre von der Posticuslähmung. Arch Laryngol 6:282–360

Gundermann H (1970) Die Berufsdysphonie. VEB Georg Thieme, Leipzig

Habermann W, Schmid C, Neumann K et al (2012) Reflux symptom index and reflux finding score in otolaryngologic practice. J Voice 26(3):e123–e127

Hamdan AL, Dowli A, Barazi R et al (2014) Laryngeal sensory neuropathy in patients with diabetes mellitus. J Laryngol Otol 128(8):725–729

Harding SM, Richter JE (1997) The role of gastroesophageal reflux in chronic cough and asthma. Chest 111(5):1389–1402

Harel B, Cannizzaro M, Snyder P (2004) Variability in fundamental frequency during speech in prodromal and incipient Parkinson's disease: a longitudinal case study. Brain Cogn 56(1):24–29

Harney M, Hone S, Timon C et al (2000) Laryngeal tuberculosis: an important diagnosis. J Laryngol Otol 114(11):878–880

Harries ML, Walker JM, Williams DM et al (1997) Changes in the male voice at puberty. Arch Dis Child 77(5):445–447

Hartelius L, Svensson P (1994) Speech and swallowing symptoms associated with Parkinson's disease and multiple sclerosis: a survey. Folia Phoniatr Logo 46(1):9–17

Hawkshaw MJ, Pebdani P, Sataloff RT (2013) Reflux laryngitis: an update, 2009–2012. J Voice 27(4):486–494

Hazlett DE, Duffy OM, Moorhead SA (2011) Review of the impact of voice training on the vocal quality of professional voice users: implications for vocal health and recommendations for further research. J Voice 25(2):181–191. https://doi.org/10.1016/j.jvoice.2009.08.005. Epub 2010 Feb 4

Henke MO, Ratjen F (2007) Mucolytics in cystic fibrosis. Paediatr Resp Rev 8(1):24–29

Henriquez VM, Schulz GM, Bielamowicz S et al (2007) Laryngeal reflex responses are not modulated during human voice and respiratory tasks. J Physiol 585(Pt 3):779–789

Herbst CT, Oh J, Vydrová J et al (2015) Digital VHI-a freeware open-source software application to capture the Voice Handicap Index and other questionnaire data in various languages. Logop Phoniatr Vocol 40(2):72–76

Hermanowicz N, Truong DD (1999) Cranial Nerves IX (Glossopharyngeal) and X (Vagus). In: Goetz CG, Pappert EJ (eds) Textbook of clinical neurology. WB Saunders, Philadelphia

Hey J (1911) Richard Wagner als Vortragsmeister. In: Hey H (ed) Breitkopf & Härtels Musikbücher. Breitkopf & Härtel, Leipzig, pp 1864–1876

Heylen L, Wuyts FL, Mertens F et al (1998) Evaluation of the vocal performance of children using a voice range profile index. J Speech Lang Hear Res 41(2):232–238

Hickson C, Simpson CB, Falcon R (2001) Laryngeal pseudosulcus as a predictor of laryngopharyngeal reflux. Laryngoscope 111(10):1742–1745

Hillenbrand JM, Clark MJ (2009) The role of F0 and formant frequencies in distinguishing the voices of men and women. Atten Percept Psychophys 71(5):1150–1166

Hiort O, Birnbaum W, Marshall L et al (2014) Management of disorders of sex development. Nat Rev Endocrinol 10(9):520–529

Hirai R, Makiyama K, Matsuzaki H et al (2018) Gardasil vaccination for recurrent laryngeal papillomatosis in adult men second report: negative conversion of HPV in laryngeal secretions. J Voice 32(4):488–491

Hirschauer S (1999) Die soziale Konstruktion der Transsexualität. Suhrkamp, Frankfurt a. M

Ho A, Iansek R, Marigliani C et al (1998) Speech impairment in a large sample of patients with Parkinson's disease. Behav Neurol 11(3):131–137

Ho AK, Bradshaw JL, Iansek R (2008) For better or worse: the effect of levodopa on speech in Parkinson's disease. Mov Disord 23(4):574–580

Hočevar-Boltežar I, Šereg-Bahar M, Kravos A et al (2012) Is an occupation with vocal load a risk factor for laryngopharyngeal reflux: a prospective, multicentre, multivariate comparative study. Clin Otolaryngol 37(5):362–368

Höing R, Seitzer D (1988) Zur Klinik der Laryngopathia gravidarum. Laryngol Rhinol Otol 67(11):564–566

Hoffman HT, Overholt EM, Karnell MP et al (2003) Granuloma contact ulcers and other posterior lesions. In: Ossoff RH et al (eds) The larynx. Lippincott Williams & Wilkins, Philadelphia

Hoffman WH, Supal C, Tosi O (1984) Computer analyses of acoustical parameters in hypopituitary children before and after growth hormone treatment. Int J Pediatr Otorhinolaryngol 7(1):1–9

Hogikyan ND, Sethuraman G (1999) Validation of an instrument to measure voice-related quality of life (V-RQOL). J Voice 13(4):557–569

Hollien H, Green R, Massey K (1994) Longitudinal research on adolescent voice change in males. J Acoust Soc Am 96(5 Pt 1):2646–2654

Holmes R, Oates JM, Phyland DJ et al (2000) Voice characteristics in the progression of Parkinson's disease. Int J Lang Commun Disord 35(3):407–418

Honjo I, Isshiki N (1980) Laryngoscopic and voice characteristics of aged persons. Arch Otolaryngol 106(3):149–150

Hornykiewicz O (1966) Metabolism of brain dopamine in human parkinsonism: neurochemical and clinical aspects. In: Costa E et al (eds) Biochemistry and Pharmacology of the Basal Ganglia: Proceedings of the Second Symposium of the Parkinson's Disease Information and Research Center, College of Physicians and Surgeons of Columbia University, November 29–30, 1965. Raven Press, New York

Hunter EJ, Titze IR (2009) Quantifying vocal fatigue recovery: dynamic vocal recovery trajectories after a vocal loading exercise. Ann Otol Rhinol Laryngol 118(6):449–460

Huntington's Disease Collaboration Research Group (1993) A novel gene containing a trinucleotide repeat that is expanded and unstable on Huntington's disease chromosomes. Cell 72(6):971–983

Hydman J, Mattsson P (2008) Collateral reinnervation by the superior laryngeal nerve after recurrent laryngeal nerve injury. Muscle Nerve 38(4):1280–1289

Isshiki N, Morita H, Okamura H et al (1974) Thyroplasty as a new phonosurgical technique. Acta Otolaryngol 78(5–6):451–457

Isshiki N, Taira T, Tanabe M (1983) Surgical alteration of the vocal pitch. J Otolaryngol 12(5):335–340

Isshiki N (1989) Surgery to elevate vocal pitch. In: Isshiki N (ed) Phonosurgery. Theory and Practice. Springer, Tokyo, Berlin, pp 141–156

Jackson-Menaldi CA, Dzul AI, Wayne SR (1999) Allergies and vocal fold edema: a preliminary report. J Voice 13(1):113–122

Jan De Beur SM, Elizabeth A, Streeten EA et al (2001) Hypoparathyroidism and other causes of hypocalcemia. In: Becker KL et al (eds) Principles and practice of endocrinology and metabolism, 3rd edn. Lippincott Williams & Wilkins, Philadelphia

Jankovic J, Stacy M (1999) Movement disorders. In: Goetz CG, Pappert SJ (eds) Textbook of clinical neurology. WB Saunders, Philadelphia, pp 639–661

Jaspersen D, Kulig M, Labenz J et al (2003) Prevalence of extra-oesophageal manifestations in gastro-oesophageal reflux disease: an analysis based on the ProGERD Study. Aliment Pharmacol Ther 17(12):1515–1520

Jenkins IH, Bain PG, Colebatch JG et al (1993) A positron emission tomography study of essential tremor: evidence for over activity of cerebellar connections. Ann Neurol 34(1):82–90

Jiang A, Liang M, Su Z et al (2011) Immunohistochemical detection of pepsin in laryngeal mucosa for diagnosing laryngopharyngeal reflux. Laryngoscope 121(7):1426–1430

Jiang J, Verdolini K, Aquino B et al (2000) Effects of dehydration on phonation in excised canine larynges. Ann Otol Rhinol Laryngol 109(6):568–575

Jindal JR, Milbrath MM, Shaker R et al (1994) Gastroesophageal reflux as a likely cause of "idiopathic" subglottic stenosis. Ann Otol Rhinol Laryngol 103(3):186–191

Johnston N, Wells CW, Samuels TL et al (2010) Rationale for targeting pepsin in the treatment of reflux disease. Ann Otol Rhinol Laryngol 119(8):547–558

Jorizzo JL, Koufman JA, Thompson JN et al (1990) Sarcoidosis of the upper respiratory tract in patients with nasal rim lesions: a pilot study. J Am Acad Dermatol 22(3):439–443

Jousilahti P, Haahtela T, Laatikainen T (2016) Asthma and respiratory allergy prevalence is still increasing among Finnish young adults. Eur Respir J 47(3):985–987

Jürgens U (2002a) Neural pathways underlying vocal control. Neurosci Biobehav Rev 26(2):235–258

Jürgens U (2002b) A study of the central control of vocalization using the squirrel monkey. Med Eng Phys 24(7–8):473–477

Jürgens U (2009) The neural control of vocalization in mammals: a review. J Voice 23(1):1–10

Junger J, Pauly K, Bröhr S et al (2013) Sex matters: neural correlates of voice gender perception. NeuroImage 79:275–287

Junger J, Habel U, Bröhr S et al (2014) More than just two sexes: the neural correlates of voice gender perception in gender dysphoria. PLoS One 9(11):e111672

Jurik AG, Pedersen U, Nrgård A (1985) Rheumatoid arthritis of the cricoarytenoid joints: a case of laryngeal obstruction due to acute and chronic joint changes. Laryngoscope 95(7 Pt 1):846–848

Kalanjeri S, Hoffman S, Farver C et al (2017) Diffuse tracheal papillomatosis. Am J Respir Crit Care Med 195:134–135

Kamel PL, Hanson D, Kahrilas PJ (1994) Omeprazole for the treatment of posterior laryngitis. Am J Med 96(4):321–326

Kanagalingam J, Georgalas C, Wood GR et al (2005) Cricothyroid approximation and subluxation in 21 male-to-female transsexuals. Laryngoscope 115(4):611–618

Kawamura O, Aslam M, Rittmann T et al (2004) Physical and pH properties of gastroesophagopharyngeal refluxate: a 24-hour simultaneous ambulatory impedance and pH monitoring study. Am J Gastroenterol 99(6):1000–1010

Kaye J, Bortz MA, Tuomi SK (1993) Evaluation of the effectiveness of voice therapy with a male-to-female transsexual subject. Scand J Log Phon 18(2–3):105–109

Kitajima K, Tanabe M, Isshiki N (1979) Cricothyroid distance and vocal pitch. Experimental surgical study to elevate the vocal pitch. Ann Otol 88(1 Pt 1): 52–55

Kolb SJ, Costello F, Lee AG et al (2003) Distinguishing ischemic stroke from the stroke-like lesions of MELAS using apparent diffusion coefficient mapping. J Neurol Sci 216(1):11–15

Kollbrunner J (2006) Funktionelle Dysphonien bei Kindern. Ein psycho- und familiendynamischer Therapieansatz, 1st edn. Schulz-Kirchner, Idastein

Kollbrunner J, Menet AD, Seifert E (2010) Psychogenic aphonia: no fixation even after a lengthy period of aphonia. Swiss Med Wkly 140(1–2):12–17

Koufman JA, Blalock PD (1982) Classification and approach to patients with functional voice disorders. Ann Otol Rhinol Laryngol 91(4 pt 1):372–377

Koufman JA, Blalock PD (1988) Vocal fatigue and dysphonia in the professional voice user: Bogart-Bacall syndrome. Laryngoscope 98(5):493-499

Koufman JA (1991) The otolaryngologic manifestations of gastroesophageal reflux disease (GERD): a clinical investigation of 225 patients using ambulatory 24 hour pH monitoring and an experimental investigation of the role of acid and pepsin in the development laryngeal injury. Laryngoscope 101(4 Pt 2 Suppl 53):1–78

Koufman JA, Isaacson G (1991) The spectrum of vocal dysfunction. Otolaryngol Clin N Am 24(5):985–988

Koufman JA (1994) Contact ulcer and granuloma of the larynx. In: Gates GA (ed) Current therapy in otolaryngology-head and neck surgery, 5th edn. Mosby, St. Louis, pp 456–459

Koufman A, Walker FO, Joharji GM (1995) The cricothyroid muscle does not influence vocal fold position in laryngeal paralysis. Laryngoscope 105(4 Pt 1):368–372

Koufman JA, Amin MR, Panetti M (2000) Prevalence of reflux in 113 consecutive patients with laryngeal and voice disorders. Otolaryngol Head Neck Surg 123(4):385–388

Koufman JA (2002) Laryngopharyngeal reflux 2002: a new paradigm of airway disease. Ear Nose Throat J 81(9 Supp 2):2–6

Koufman JA (2003) Laryngeal muscle tension patterns (MTPs). In: Rubin JS et al (eds) Diagnosis and treatment of voice disorders. Thomson Delmar Learning, New York, pp 175–182

Kranz GS, Hahn A, Kaufmann U et al (2014) White matter microstructure in transsexuals and controls investigated by diffusion tensor imaging. J Neurosci 34(46):15466–15475. https://doi.org/10.1523/JNEUROSCI.2488-14.2014

Kruijver FP, Zhou JN, Pool CW et al (2000) Male-to-female transsexuals have female neuron numbers in a limbic nucleus. J Clin Endocrinol Metab 85(5):2034–2041

Kunachak S, Prakunhungsit S, Sujjalak K (2000) Thyroid cartilage and vocal fold reduction: a new phonosurgical method for male-to-female transsexuals. Ann Otol 109(11):1082–1086

Kuypers HG (1958) Corticobulbar connexions to the pons and lower brain-stem in man: an anatomical study. Brain 81(3):364–388

Lambrecht BN, Hammad H (2014) Allergens and the airway epithelium response: gateway to allergic sensitization. J Allergy Clin Immunol 134(3):499–507

Lang J, Nachbaur S, Fischer K (1986) Nn. laryngei, Verzweigungen im Kehlkopfinneren. Gegenbaurs Morphol Jahrb 132:723–736

Langevin SM, Michaud DS, Marsit CJ et al (2013) Gastric reflux is an independent risk factor for laryngopharyngeal carcinoma. Cancer Epidemiol Biomark Prev 22(6):1061–1068

Laskawi R, Drobik C, Baaske C (1994) Prognostic value of electrodiagnosis of Bell's palsy. Laryngorhinootologie 73(6):338–341

Laukkanen AM, Järvinen K, Artkoski M et al (2004) Changes in voice and subjective sensations during a 45-min. vocal loading test in female subjects with vocal training. Folia Phoniatr Logop 56(6):335–346

Lee B, Woo P (2005) Chronic cough as a sign of laryngeal sensory neuropathy: diagnosis and treatment. Ann Otol Rhinol Laryngol 114(4):253–257

Lees AJ, Turjanski N, Rivest J et al (1992) Treatment of cervical dystonia, hand spasms and laryngeal dystonia with botulinum toxin. J Neurol 239(1):1–4

LeJeune FE, Guice CE, Samuels PM (1983) Early experiences with vocal ligament tightening. Ann Otol Rhinol Laryngol 92(5 Pt 1):475–477

Lemére F (1933) Innervation of the larynx (III) Experimental paralysis of the laryngeal nerve. Arch Otolaryngol 18(4):413–424

Levenson MJ, Ingerman M, Grimes C et al (1984) Laryngeal tuberculosis: review of twenty cases. Laryngoscope 94(8):1094–1097

Lewis JE, Olsen KD, Kurtin PJ et al (1992) Laryngeal amyloidosis: a clinicopathologic and immunohistochemical review. Otolaryngol Head Neck Surg 106(4):372–377

Li Y, Pearce EC, Mainthia R et al (2013) Comparison of ventilation and voice outcomes between unilateral laryngeal pacing and unilateral cordotomy for the treatment of bilateral vocal fold paralysis. ORL J Otorhinolaryngol Relat Spec 75(2):68–73

Lillemoe KD, Johnson LF, Harmon JW (1982) Role of the components of the gastroduodenal contents in experimental acid esophagitis. Surgery 92(2):276–284

Little FB, Koufman JA, Kohut RI et al (1985) Effect of gastric acid on the pathogenesis of subglottic stenosis. Ann Otol Rhinol Laryngol 94(5 Pt 1):516–519

Littlejohn MC, Bailey BJ, Yoo JK (1998) Granulomatous diseases of the head and neck. In: Bailey BJ et al (eds) Head and neck surgery-otolaryngology. Lippincott-Raven, Philadelphia, pp 205–218

Loehrl TA, Smith TL (2001) Inflammatory and granulomatous lesions of the larynx and pharynx. Am J Med 111(Suppl 8A):113–117

Lofgren RH, Montgomery WW (1962) Incidence of laryngeal involvement in rheumatoid arthritis. N Engl J Med 267:193–195

Logemann J, Fisher HB, Boshes B et al (1978) Frequency and cooccurrence of vocal tract dysfunctions in the speech of a large sample of Parkinson's patients. J Speech Hear Disord 43(1):47–57

Lombard É (1911) Le signe de l'élévation de la voix. Annales des Maladies de l'Oreille, du Larynx, du Nez et du Pharynx 37(2):101–119

Ludlow CL (2006) The Spasmodic dysphonias. In: Rubin JS et al (eds) Diagnosis and treatment of voice disorders, 3rd edn. Plural Publishers, San Diego

Ludwig C (1999) … und ich wäre so gern Primadonna gewesen. Henschel, Berlin

Lundquist PG, Haglund S, Carlson B et al (1984) Interferon therapy in juvenile laryngeal papillomatosis. Otolaryngol Head Neck Surg 92(4):386–391

Lundy DS, Silva C, Casiano RR et al (1998) Cause of hoarseness in elderly patients. Otolaryngol Head Neck Surg 118(4):481–485

Luschei E, Ramig L, Baker K et al (1991) Discharge characteristics of laryngeal single motor units during phonation in young and older adults and in persons with Parkinson disease. J Neurophysiol 81(5):2131–2139

Makiyama K, Hirai R, Matsuzaki H (2017) Gardasil vaccination for recurrent laryngeal papillomatosis in adult men: first report: changes in HPV antibody titer. J Voice 31(1):104–106

Malannino N (1974) Proceedings: laryngeal neuromuscular spindles and their possible function. Folia Phoniatr (Basel) 26(4):291–292

Marszałek S, Niebudek-Bogusz E, Woźnicka E et al (2012) Assessment of the influence of osteopathic myofascial techniques on normalization of the vocal tract functions in patients with occupational dysphonia. Int J Occup Med Environ Health 25(3):225–235. https://doi.org/10.2478/S13382-012-0041-7. Epub 2012 Jun 22

Martins RH, Defaveri J, Domingues MAC et al (2010) Vocal fold nodules: morphological and immunohistochemical investigations. J Voice 24(5):531–539

Martins RH, Santana MF, Mendes Tavares EL (2011) Vocal cysts: clinical, endoscopic, and surgical aspects. J Voice 25(1):107–110

Martins RHG, Gonçalvez TM, Pessin ABB et al (2014) Aging voice: presbyphonia. Aging Clin Exp Res 26(1):1–5

Masdeu JC (2000) Aphasia. Arch Neurol 57(6):892–895

Matai V, Cheesman AD, Clarke PM (2003) Cricothyroid approximation and thyroid chondroplasty: a patient survey. Otolaryngol Head Neck Surg 128(6):841–847

Mattsson P, Hydman J, Svensson M (2015) Recovery of laryngeal function after intraoperative injury to the recurrent laryngeal nerve. Gland Surg 4(1):27–35

Mazzone SB (2005) An overview of the sensory receptors regulating cough. Cough 1:2

McCaffrey TV, McDonald TJ (1983) Sarcoidosis of the nose and paranasal sinuses. Laryngoscope 93(10):1281–1284

McHenry J, Wilson RL, Minton JT (1994) Management of multiple physiologic system deficits following traumatic brain injury. J Med Speech Lang Path 2(1):59–74

Menon EB, Ravichandran S, Tan ES (1993) Speech disorders in closed head injury patients. Singap Med J 34(1):45–48

Mercante G, Bacciu A, Ferri T et al (2003) Gastroesophageal reflux as a possible co-promoting factor in the development of the squamous-cell carcinoma of the oral cavity, of the larynx and of the pharynx. Acta Otorhinolaryngol Belg 57(2):113–117

Mészáros K, Vitéz LC, Szabolcs I et al (2005) Efficacy of conservative voice treatment in male-to-female transsexuals. Folia Phoniatr Logop 57(2):111–118

Michel A, Mormont C, Legros JJ (2001) A psychoendocrinological overview of transsexualism. Eur J Endocrinol 145(4):365–376

Michelsson K, Eklund K, Leppänen P et al (2002) Cry characteristics of 172 healthy 1- to 7-day-old infants. Folia Phoniatr Logop 54(4):190–200

Miehlke A, Dal Ri H, Schätzle W et al (1973) Isolierte reinnervation der abduktionsmuskulatur des stimmbandes. (Isolated reinnervation of the abductor musculature of the vocal cord). Arch Klin Exp Ohren Nasen Kehlkopfheilkd 203(3):241–254

Migeon CJ, Wisniewski AB (1998) Sexual differentiation. From genes to gender. Horm Res 50(5):245–251

Millar A, Deary IJ, Wilson JA et al (1999) Is an organic/functional distinction psychologically meaningful in patients with dysphonia? J Psychosom Res 46(6):497–505

Miller TG, Spoolman S (2014) Sustaining the earth, 11th edn. Brooks Cole, Pacific Grove, CA

Mishriki YY (2007) Laryngeal neuropathy as a cause of chronic intractable cough. Am J Med 120(2):e5; author reply e7

Misono S, Peterson CB, Meredith L et al (2014) Psychosocial distress in patients presenting with voice concerns. J Voice 28(6):753–761

Mohr M, Schliemann C, Biermann C et al (2014) Rapid response to systemic bevacizumab therapy in recurrent respiratory papillomatosis. Oncol Lett 8:1912–1918

Moore C (2012) Reflections on clinical applications of yoga in voice therapy with MTD. Logoped Phoniatr Vocol 37(4):144–150. https://doi.org/10.3109/140154 39.2012.731080

Morrison MD, Rammage LA, Belisle GM et al (1983) Muscular tension dysphonia. J Otolaryngol 12(5):302–306

Morrison MD, Rammage L (1993) Muscle misuse voice disorders: description and classification. Acta Otolaryngol (Stockh) 113(3):428–434

Morrison MD, Rammage LA (1994) The management of voice disorders. Singular Publishing Group, San Diego

Morrison MD (1997) Pattern recognition in muscle misuse voice disorders: how I do it. J Voice 11(1):108–114

Morrison M, Rammage L, Emami AJ (1999) The irritable larynx syndrome. J Voice 13(3):447–455

Moses RL, Paige T, Cavalli G et al (1997) Laryngotracheobronchitis in pregnancy and its clinical implications. Otolaryngol Head Neck Surg 116(3):401–403

Mürbe D, Pabst F, Hofmann G et al (2002) Significance of auditory and kinesthetic feedback to singers' pitch control. J Voice 16(1):44–51

Mürbe D, Pabst F, Hofmann G et al (2004) Effects of a professional solo singer education on auditory and kinesthetic feedback—a longitudinal study of singers' pitch control. J Voice 18(2):236–241

Murray T (1981) Essential tremor. Can Med Assoc J 124(12):1559–1570

Murry T, Tabaee A, Aviv JE (2004) Respiratory retraining of refractory cough and laryngopharyngeal reflux in patients with paradoxical vocal fold movement disorder. Laryngoscope 114(8):1341–1345

Murry T, Sapienza C (2010) The role of voice therapy in the management of paradoxical vocal fold motion, chronic cough, and laryngospasm. Otolaryngol Clin N Am 43(1):73–83, viii–ix

Nacci A, Fattori B, Basolo F et al (2011) Sex hormone receptors in vocal fold tissue: a theory about the influence of sex hormones in the larynx. Folia Phoniatr Logop 63(2):77–82

Nagel S, Busch C, Blankenburg T et al (2009) Treatment of respiratory papillomatosis—a case report on systemic treatment with bevacizumab. Pneumologie 63:387–389

Naiboglu B, Durmus R, Tek A et al (2011) Do the laryngopharyngeal symptoms and signs ameliorate by empiric treatment in patients with suspected laryngopharyngeal reflux? Auris Nasus Larynx 38(5):622–627

Nasreddine ZS, Mendez MF, Cummings JL (1999) Speech and language. In: Goetz CG, Pappert EJ (eds) Textbook of clinical neurology. WB Saunders Company, Philadelphia

Nawka T, Wiesmann U, Gonnermann U et al (2003) Validierung des Voice Handicap Index (VHI) in der deutschen Fassung. (Validation of the German version of the Voice Handicap Index). HNO 51(11): 921–930

Nawka T (2008) Postoperative Betreuung in der operativen Laryngologie. (Postoperative care in operative laryngology). HNO 56(12):1183–1189

Nawka T, Wirth G (2008) Stimmstörungen, 5th edn. Deutscher Ärzte-Verlag GmbH, Köln

Neel HB, McDonald TJ (1982) Laryngeal sarcoidosis: report of 13 patients. Ann Otol Rhinol Laryngol 91(4 Pt 1):359–362

Negus VE (1929) The mechanism of the larynx. Chapter VI. Heinemann WM (Medical Books) Ltd, London, p 149

Netterville JL, Stone RE, Luken ES et al (1993) Silastic medialization and arytenoid adduction: the Vanderbilt experience. A review of 116 phonosurgical procedures. Ann Otol Rhinol Laryngol 102(6):413–424

Neumann K, Welzel C, Berghaus A (2003) Operative Stimmerhöhung bei Mann-zu-Frau-Transsexuellen. HNO 51(1):30–37

Neumann K, Welzel C (2004) The importance of the voice in male-to-female transsexualism. J Voice 18(1):153–167

Newman AJ, Supalla T, Hauser P et al (2010) Dissociating neural subsystems for grammar by contrasting word order and inflection. Proc Natl Acad Sci U S A 107(16):7539–7544

Newman KB, Mason UG 3rd, Schmaling KB (1995) Clinical features of vocal cord dysfunction. Am J Respir Crit Care Med 152(4 Pt 1):1382–1386

Newman SR, Butler J, Hammond EH et al (2000) Preliminary report on hormone receptors in the human vocal fold. J Voice 14(1):72–81

Niebudek-Bogusz E, Fiszer M, Kotyło P et al (2006) Diagnostic value of voice analysis in assessment of occupational voice pathologies in teachers. Logop Phoniatr Vocol 31(3):100–106

Niebudek-Bogusz E, Kotyło P, Politański P et al (2008) Acoustic analysis with vocal loading test in occupational voice disorders: outcomes before and after voice therapy. Int J Occup Med Environ Health 21(4):301–308

Niebudek-Bogusz E, Sliwinska-Kowalska M (2013) An overview of occupational voice disorders in Poland. Int J Occup Med Environ Health 26(5):659–669

Niederberger V, Eckl-Dorna J, Pauli G (2014) Recombinant allergen-based provocation testing. Methods (San Diego, Calif) 66(1):96–105. https://doi.org/10.1016/j.ymeth.2013.07.037

Nienkerke-Springer A, McAllister A, Sundberg J (2005) Effects of family therapy on children's voices. J Voice 19(1):103–113

Nutt JG (1999) Gait and balance. In: Goetz CG, Pappert EJ (eds) Clinical neurology. WB Saunders Company, Philadelphia

Nygren U, Nordenskjöld A, Arver S et al (2015) Effects on voice fundamental frequency and satisfaction with voice in Trans men during testosterone treatment—a longitudinal study. J Voice 30(6):766.e23–766.e34

Oates JM, Dacakis G (1997) Voice change in transsexuals. Venereology 10(3):178–187

Obrębowski A (1983) Badania kliniczne i elektroakustyczne nad egzogenną wirylizacją narządu głosu. (Clinical and electroacoustical examination in exogenic voice virilisation). Otolaryngol Pol 37:95–98

Obrębowski A (2008) Narząd głosu i jego znaczenie w komunikacji społecznej. Medical University of Poznań, Poznań

Olthoff A, Kruse E (2004) Peripher-motorische Innervation des Larynx. In: Gross M, Kruse E (eds) Aktuelle phoniatrisch-pädaudiologische Aspekte 12:52–59. Medicombooksde, Videel, Niebüll

Olthoff A, Zeiss D, Laskawi R et al (2005) Laser microsurgical bilateral posterior cordectomy for the treatment of bilateral vocal fold paralysis. Ann Otol Rhinol Laryngol 114(8):599–604

Olthoff A, Schiel R, Kruse E (2007) The supraglottic nerve supply: an anatomic study with clinical implications. Laryngoscope 117(11):1930–1933

Olthoff A, Baudewig J, Kruse E et al (2008) Cortical sensorimotor control in vocalization: a functional magnetic resonance imaging study. Laryngoscope 118(11):2091–2096

Olthoff A, Ehrlich T (2010) Enzymhistochemische Färbung von Nerven humaner und suiner Kehlköpfe. In: Gross M, am Zehnhoff-Dinnesen A (eds) Aktuelle phoniatrischpadaudiologische Aspekte 2010, 27. Wissenschaftliche Jahrestagung der Deutschen Gesellschaft fur Phoniatrie und Padaudiologie Aachen, Germany 17th–19th Sept. 2010, Vol 18,

Darpe Industriedruck GmbH & Co. KG, Münster, pp 121–124

Olyslager F, Conway L (2007) On the calculation of the prevalence of transsexualism. Paper presented at the WPATH 20th International Symposium, Chicago, IL, September 5–8. http://www.changelingaspects.com/PDF/Prevalence_of_Transsexualism.pdf. Accessed 5 Mar 2014

Osipenko EV, Izdebski K, Cruz RM et al (2016) Bamboo vocal folds (B-nodes) examination with white light and with NBI® illumination. A case for a non-traumatic etiology. In: Izdebski K et al (eds) Normal and abnormal vocal folds kinematics. High Speed Digital Phonoscopy (HSDP), Optical Coherence Tomography (OCT) and Narrow Band Imaging (NBI®), vol 2. Applications. Pacific Voice and Speech Foundation, San Francisco, CA, pp 398–396

Ossakow SJ, Elta G, Colturi T et al (1987) Esophageal reflux and dysmotility as the basis for persistent cervical symptoms. Ann Otol Rhinol Laryngol 96(4):387–392

Ozlugedik S, Yorulmaz I, Gokcan K (2006) Is laryngopharyngeal reflux an important risk factor in the development of laryngeal carcinoma? Eur Arch Otorhinolaryngol 263(4):339–343

Parent AS, Teilmann G, Juul A et al (2003) The timing of normal puberty and the age limits of sexual precocity: variations around the world, secular trends, and changes after migration. Endocr Rev 24(5):668–693

Paulsen F, Kimpel M, Lockemann U et al (2000) Effects of ageing on the insertion zones of the human vocal fold. J Anat 196(1):41–54

Pedersen M, McGlashan J (2012) Surgical versus non-surgical interventions for vocal cord nodules (Review). Cochrane Database Syst Rev 6:CD001934

Penney JB, Young AB (1998) Huntington's disease. In: Jankovic J, Tolosa E (eds) Parkinson's disease and other movement disorders, 3rd edn. Williams & Wilkins, Baltimore

Petersen TH, Agertoft L (2016) Corticosteroids for allergic rhinitis. Curr Treat Options Allergy 3(1):18–30

Phua SY, McGarvey LPA, Ngu MC et al (2005) Patients with gastro-oesophageal reflux disease and cough have impaired laryngopharyngeal mechanosensitivity. Thorax 60(6):488–491

Pittam J (1994) Voice in social interaction—an interdisciplinary approach. Sage Publications Inc, Thousand Oaks, CA

Pontes P, Behlau M (1993) Treatment of sulcus vocalis: auditory perceptual and acoustical analysis of the slicing mucosa surgical technique. J Voice 7(4):365–376

Pontes P, Brasolotto A, Behlau M (2005) Glottic characteristics and voice complaint in the elderly. J Voice 19(1):84–94

Postma GN, Blalock PD, Koufman JA (1998) Bilateral medialization laryngoplasty. Laryngoscope 108(10):1429–1434

Pruszewicz A, Obrębowski A, Jassem W et al (1973) Ausgeprägte akustische Merkmale virilisierter Mädchenstimmen. Folia Phoniatr Logop 25(5):331–341

Pruszewicz A, Obrębowski A (1992) Hormonalnie uwarunkowane zaburzenie głosu i mowy. (Hormonal conditioned voice and speech disorders). In: Pruszewicz A (ed) Foniatria Kliniczna. PZWL, Warszawa, pp 158–172

Raj A, Gupta B, Chowdhury A et al (2010) A study of voice changes in various phases of menstrual cycle and in postmenopausal women. J Voice 24(3):363–368

Ramadan HH, Tarazi AE, Baroudy FM (1993) Laryngeal tuberculosis: presentation of 16 cases and a review of the literature. J Otolaryngol 22(1):39–41

Ramet J (1994) Cardiac and respiratory reactivity to gastroesophageal reflux: experimental data in infants. Biol Neonate 65(3–4):240–246

Ramig LO, Fox C, Sapir S (2002) Parkinson's disease: speech and voice disorders and their treatment with the Lee Silverman Voice Treatment. Semin Speech Lang 25(2):169–180

Randhawa PS, Mansuri S, Rubin JS (2009) Is dysphonia due to allergic laryngitis being misdiagnosed as laryngopharyngeal reflux? Logoped Phoniatr Vocol 35:1):1–1):5

Ratner PH, Meltzer EO, Teper A (2009) Mometasone furoate nasal spray is safe and effective for 1-year treatment of children with perennial allergic rhinitis. Int J Pediatr Otorhinolaryngol 73(5):651–657

Remacle A, Finc C, Roche A et al (2012) Vocal impact of a prolonged reading task at two intensity levels: objective measurements and subjective self-ratings. J Voice 26(4):177–186

Réthi A (1952) Rolle des stylopharyngealen Muskelsystems im Krankheitsbild der Taschenbandstimme und der dysphonia spastica. Folia Phoniatr 4(4):201–216

Riccioni G, Bucciarelli T, Mancini B et al (2007) Antileukotriene drugs: clinical application, effectiveness and safety. Curr Med Chem 4(18):1966–1967

Richter B, Löhle E, Maier W et al (2000) Working conditions on stage: climatic considerations. Logoped Phoniatr Vocol 25(2):80–86

Richter B, Löhle E, Knapp B et al (2002) Harmful substances on the opera stage: possible negative effects on singers' respiratory tracts. J Voice 16(1):72–80

Richter JE (2003) Medical management of patients with esophageal or supraesophageal gastroesophageal reflux disease. Am J Med 115(Suppl 3A):179–187

Rödel RM, Olthoff A, Tergau F et al (2004) Human cortical motor representation of the larynx as assessed by transcranial magnetic stimulation (TMS). Laryngoscope 114(5):918–922

Rogers DJ, Ojha S, Maurer R et al (2013) Use of adjuvant intralesional bevacizumab for aggressive respiratory papillomatosis in children. JAMA Otolaryngol Head Neck Surg 139:496–501

Rogers JH, Stell PM (1978) Paradoxical movement of the vocal cords as a cause of stridor. J Laryngol Otol 92(2):157–158

Rosen CA (2005) Stroboscopy as a research instrument: development of a perceptual evaluation tool. Laryngoscope 115(3):423–428

Rosen CA, Simpson CB (2008) Operative techniques in laryngology. Springer, Berlin, Heidelberg

Rowland LP (2000) Signs and symptoms in neurologic diagnosis. In: Rowland LP et al (eds) Merritt's neurology, Textbook of neurology, 10th edn. Lippincott Williams & Wilkins, Philadelphia

Roy N, Leeper HA (1993) Effects of the manual laryngeal musculoskeletal tension reduction technique as a treatment for functional voice disorders: perceptual and acoustic measures. J Voice 7(3):242–249

Roy N, Ford CN, Bless DM (1996) Muscle tension dysphonia and spasmodic dysphonia: the role of manual laryngeal tension reduction in diagnosis and treatment. Ann Otol Rhinol Laryngol 105(11):851–856

Roy N (2003) Functional dysphonia. Curr Opin Otolaryngol Head Neck Surg 11(3):144–148

Roy N, Merril R, Gray S et al (2005) Voice disorders in the general population: prevalence, risk factors and occupational impact. Laryngoscope 115(11):1989–1995

Roy N, Stemple J, Merrill RM et al (2007) Epidemiology of voice disorders in the elderly: preliminary findings. Laryngoscope 117(4):628–633

Rubin JS, Sataloff RT, Korovin GS (eds) (2014) Diagnosis and treatment of voice disorder, 4th edn. Plural Publishing, San Diego

Rueger RS (1972) The superior laryngeal nerve and the interarytenoid muscle in humans: an anatomical study. Laryngoscope 82(11):2008–2203

Ruiz R, Jeswani S, Andrews K et al (2014) Hoarseness and laryngopharyngeal reflux: a survey of primary care physician practice patterns. JAMA Otolaryngol Head Neck Surg 140(3):192–196. https://doi.org/10.1001/jamaoto.2013.6533

Rusz J, Cmejla R, Ruzickova H et al (2011) Quantitative acoustic measurements for characterization of speech and voice disorders in early untreated Parkinson's disease. J Acoust Soc Am 129(1):350–367

Sacre L, Vandenplas Y (1989) Gastroesophageal reflux associated with respiratory abnormalities during sleep. J Pediatr Gastroenterol Nutr 9(1):28–33

Sanders I, Wu BL, Mu L et al (1994) The innervation of the human posterior cricoarytenoid muscle: evidence for at least two neuromuscular compartments. Laryngoscope 104(7):880–884

Sandmann K, am Zehnhoff-Dinnesen A, Schmidt CM et al (2014) Differences between self-assessment and external rating of voice with regard to sex characteristics, age, and attractiveness. J Voice 28(1):128. e11–128.e18

Sanudo JR, Maranillo E, Leon X et al (1999) An anatomical study of anastomoses between the laryngeal nerves. Laryngoscope 109(6):983–987

Sapir S, Pawlas AA, Ramig LO et al (2001) Voice and speech abnormalities in Parkinson disease: relation to severity of motor impairment, duration of disease, medication, depression, gender, and age. J Med Speech Lang Pathol 9(4):213–226

Sasaki CT, Ho S, Kim YH (2001) Critical role of central facilitation in the glottic closure reflex. Ann Otol Rhinol Laryngol 110(5 Pt 1):401–405

Sataloff RT, Emerich KA, Hoover CA (1997) Endocrine dysfunction. In: Sataloff RT (ed) Professional voice: the Science and Art of Clinical Care. Singular Publishing Group, San Diego, pp 291–297

Sataloff RT, Mandel S, Mann EA et al (2003) AAEM Laryngeal Task Force. Laryngeal electromyography: an evidence-based review. Muscle Nerve 28(6):767–772

Sataloff RT, Hawkshaw MJ, Gupta R (2010) Laryngopharyngeal reflux and voice disorders: an overview on disease mechanisms, treatments, and research advances. Discov Med 10(52):213–224

Sato K, Hirano M, Nakashima T (2002) Age-related changes of collagenous fibers in the human vocal fold mucosa. Ann Otol Rhinol Laryngol 111(1):15–20

Schiel R, Olthoff A, Kruse E (2004) Untersuchungen zur Anatomie des Ramus posterior des Nervus recurrens und seiner Beziehung zum Musculus interarytaenoideus. In: Gross M, Kruse E (eds) Aktuelle phoniatrisch-pädaudiologische Aspekte, vol 12. Medicom- books.de, Videel, Niebüll, pp 18–20

Schneider B, Wendler J, Seidner W (2002) The relevance of stroboscopy in functional dysphonias. Folia Phoniatr Logop 54(1):44–54

Schneider B, Enne R, Cecon M et al (2006) Effects of vocal constitution and autonomic stress-related reactivity on vocal endurance in female student teachers. J Voice 20(2):242–250. Epub 2005 Aug 10

Schneider B, Cohen E, Stani J et al (2007) Towards the expression of sex hormone receptors in the human vocal fold. J Voice 21(4):502–507

Schneider-Stickler B, Knell C, Aichstill B et al (2012) Biofeedback on voice use in call center agents in order to prevent occupational voice disorders. J Voice 26(1):51–62

Schteingart DE (2001) Cushing syndrome. In: Becker KL et al (eds) Principles and practice of endocrinology and metabolism, 3rd edn. Lippincott Williams & Wilkins, Philadelphia

Seddon HJ (1942) A classification of nerve injuries. Br Med J 2(4260):237–239

Seeman M (1959) Sprachstörungen bei Kindern. Carl Marhold Verlag, Halle, Germany

Sewall GK, Jiang J, Ford CN (2006) Clinical evaluation of Parkinson's-related dysphonia. Laryngoscope 116(10):1740–1744

Sifrim D, Dupont L, Blondeau K et al (2005) Weakly acidic reflux in patients with chronic unexplained cough during 24 hour pressure, pH, and impedance monitoring. Gut 54(4):449–454

Silverberg SJ, Bilezikian JP (2001) Primary hyperparathyroidism. In: Kenneth L et al (eds) Principles and practice of endocrinology and metabolism, 3rd edn. Lippincott Williams & Wilkins, Philadelphia

Simberg S, Sala E, Tuomainen J et al (2009) Vocal symptoms and allergy—a pilot study. J Voice 23(1):136–139

Singh RK, Tandon R, Dastidar SG et al (2013) A review on leukotrienes and their receptors with reference to asthma. J Asthma 50(9):922–931

Sjostrom AC, Holmberg B, Strang P (2002) Parkinson-plus patients-an unknown group with severe symptoms. J Neurosci Nurs 34(6):314–319

Skodda S, Visser W, Schlegel U (2010) Acoustical analysis of speech in progressive supranuclear palsy. J Voice 25(6):725–731. Epub 2010 May 8

Skodda S (2012) Effect of deep brain stimulation on speech performance in Parkinson's disease. Parkinsons Dis 2012:850596

Sliwinska-Kowalska M, Niebudek-Bogusz E, Fiszer M et al (2006) The prevalence and risk factors for occupational voice disorders in teachers. Folia Phoniatr Logop 58(2):85–101

Smith ME, Ramig LO (2006) Neurologic disorders and the voice. In: Rubin JS et al (eds) Diagnosis and treatment of voice disorders, 3rd edn. Plural Publishing, San Diego, pp 447–477

Smith RR, Ferguson GB (1989) Systemic lupus erythematosus causing subglottic stenosis. Laryngoscope 86(5):734–738

Soda A, Rubio H, Salazar M et al (1989) Tuberculosis of the larynx: clinical aspects in 19 patients. Laryngoscope 99(11):1147–1150

Springer C (2002) Enrico Caruso—Tenor der Moderne. Holzhausen. In: Wien

Stemple CJ, Glaze LE, Klaben BG (2000) Clinical voice pathology. Theory and management, 3rd edn. Singular Publishing Group, San Diego, CA

Stennert E (1982) The autoparalytic syndrome—a leading symptom of postparetic facial function. Arch Otorhinolaryngol 236(1):97–114

Sulica L, Blitzer A, Meyer T (2006) Laryngeal electromyography. In: Rubin JS et al (eds) Diagnosis and treatment of voice disorders, 3rd edn. Plural Publishers, San Diego, pp 249–260

Sulter AM, Schutte HK, Miller DG (1996) Standardized laryngeal videostroboscopic rating: differences between untrained and trained male and female subjects, and effects of varying sound intensity, fundamental frequency, and age. J Voice 10(2):175–189

Sundberg J (1987) The science of the singing voice. Northern Illinois University Press, DeKalb, IL

Sorensen JR, Winther KH, Bonnema SJ et al (2016) Respiratory manifestations of hypothyroidism: a systematic review. Thyroid 26(11):1519–1527

Spring PJ, Kok C, Nicholson GA et al (2005) Autosomal dominant hereditary sensory neuropathy with chronic cough and gastro-oesophageal reflux: clinical features in two families linked to chromosome 3p22-p24. Brain 128(Pt 12):2797–2810

Steinmetzer J, Groß D (2008) Der Umgang mit Transsexualität in der Europäischen Union unter besonderer Berücksichtigung von Belgien. In: Groß D et al (eds) Normal—anders—krank? Akzeptanz, Stigmatisierung und Pathologisierung im Kontext der Medizin. Medizinisch Wissenschaftliche Verlagsgesellschaft, Berlin, pp 153–169

Szabo Portela A, Hammarberg B, Södersten M (2013) Speaking fundamental frequency and phonation time during work and leisure time in vocally healthy preschool teachers measured with a voice accumulator. Folia Phoniatr Logop 65(2):84–90. Epub ahead of print

Tan EM, Cohen AS, Fries JF et al (1982) The 1982 revised criteria for the classification of systemic lupus erythematosus. Arthritis Rheumatol 25(11):1271–1277

Tanner JM (1962) Growth at adolescence, 2nd edn. Blackwell, Oxford

Teitel AD, MacKenzie CR, Stern R et al (1992) Laryngeal involvement in systemic lupus erythematosus. Semin Arthritis Rheumatol 22(3):203–214

Tellis CM, Rosen C, Thekdi A et al (2004) Anatomy and fiber type composition of human interarytenoid muscle. Ann Otol Rhinol Laryngol 113(2):97–107

Thomas JP, Zubiaur FM (2013) Over-diagnosis of laryngopharyngeal reflux as the cause of hoarseness. Eur Arch Otorhinolaryngol 270(3):995–999

Thompson DM, Kershner JE (2007) Pediatric laryngology. In: Merati AL, Bielamowicz SA (eds) Textbook of laryngology. Plural Publishing, San Diego, CA

Tilley AE, Walters MS, Shaykhiev R et al (2015) Crystal cilia dysfunction in lung disease. Annu Rev Physiol 77:379–406

Titze I (2008) Nonlinear source-filter coupling in phonation: theory. J Acoust Soc Am 123(5):2733–2749

Toomey JM, Snyder GG III, Maenza RM et al (1974) Acute epiglottitis due to systemic lupus erythematosus. Laryngoscope 84(4):522–527

Traser L, Richter B, Nusseck M et al (2012) Standardisierte Stimmdiagnostik bei professionellen Sopranistinnen in der musikermedizinischen Sängersprechstunde. Musikphysiologie und Musikermedizin 19(2):140–147

Trevino RJ (1996) Air pollution and its effect on the upper respiratory tract and on allergic rhinosinusitis. Otolaryngol Head Neck Surg 114:239–241

Truong DD, Rontal M, Rolnick M et al (1991) Double-blind controlled study of botulinum toxin in, prevalence adductor spasmodic dysphonia. Laryngoscope 101(6):630–634

Tschiassny K (1957) Therapeutically induced paralysis of the cricothyroid muscle or its removal in paralytic laryngeal stenosis. Arch Otolaryngol 65(2):133–142

Tucker HM (1985) Anterior laryngoplasty for adjustment of vocal fold tension. Ann Otol Rhinol Laryngol 94(6 Pt 1):547–549

Turley R, Cohen S (2009) Impact of voice and swallowing problems in the elderly. Otolaryngol Head Neck Surg 140(1):33–36

Ulualp SO, Toohill RJ, Hoffmann R et al (1999) Pharyngeal PH monitoring in patients with posterior laryngitis. Otolaryngol Head Neck Surg 120(5):672–677

Ulualp SO, Toohill RJ (2000) Laryngopharyngeal reflux: state of the art diagnosis and treatment. Otolaryngol Clin N Am 33(4):785–802

Upile T, Elmiyeh B, Jerjes W et al (2009) Unilateral versus bilateral thyroarytenoid Botulinum toxin injections in adductor spasmodic dysphonia: a prospective study. Head Face Med 5:20

US Department of Health and Human Services (2007) National Asthma Education and Prevention Program Expert Panel Report 3. Guidelines for the Diagnosis and Management of Asthma. https://www.nhlbi.nih.gov/files/docs/guidelines/asthsumm.pdf. Accessed 26 Jan 2018

Van Borsel J, De Cuypere G, Rubens R et al (2000) Voice problems in female-to-male transsexuals. Int J Lang Commun Disord 35(3):427–442

Van Borsel J, Van Eynde E, De Cuypere G et al (2008) Feminine after cricothyroid approximation? J Voice 22(3):379–384

Van Borsel J, Janssens J, De Bodt M (2009) Breathiness as a feminine voice characteristic: a perceptual approach. J Voice 23(3):291–294

Van Houtte E, Van Lierde K, Claeys S (2011) Pathophysiology and treatment of muscle tension dysphonia: a review of the current knowledge. J Voice 25(2):202–207. https://doi.org/10.1016/j.jvoice.2009.10.009. Epub 2010 Apr 18

Van Lawrence VL (1987) Suggested criteria for fibreoptic diagnosis of vocal hyperfunction. In: Care of the Professional Voice Symposium. The British Voice Association, London

Van Lierde KM, De Bodt M, Dhaeseleer E et al (2010) The treatment of muscle tension dysphonia: a comparison of two treatment techniques by means of an objective multiparameter approach. J Voice 24(3):294–301. https://doi.org/10.1016/j.jvoice.2008.09.003. Epub 2009 Jun 4

Vertigan AE, Theodoros DG, Gibson PG et al (2006) The relationship between chronic cough and paradoxical vocal fold movement: a review of the literature. J Voice 20(3):466–480

Vilkman E (2004) Occupational safety and health aspects of voice and speech professions. Folia Phoniatr Logop 56(4):220–253

Voelter C, Kleinsasser N, Joa P et al (2008) Detection of hormone receptors in the human vocal fold. Eur Arch Otorhinolaryngol 265(10):1239–1244

Wang DY (2005) Risk factors of allergic rhinitis: genetic or environmental? Ther Clin Risk Manag 1(2):115–123

Wanger J (2011) Pulmonary function testing. Jones & Bartlett Publishers, Burlington, MA

Wani MK, Woodson GE (1999) Paroxysmal laryngospasm after laryngeal nerve injury. Laryngoscope 109(5):694–697

Warrington R, Silviu-Dan F (2011) Drug allergy. Allergy Asthma Clin Immunol 7(Suppl 1):S10

Wassenaar E, Johnston N, Merati A et al (2011) Pepsin detection in patients with laryngopharyngeal reflux before and after fundoplication. Surg Endosc 25(12):3870–3876

Watzlawick P, Bavelas JB, Jackson DD (2011) Pragmatics of Human Communication: a study of interactional patterns, pathologies and paradoxes. WW Norton & Co, New York. (Reprint)

Waxman J, Bose WJ (1986) Laryngeal manifestations of Wegener's granulomatosis: case reports and review of the literature. J Rheumatol 13(2):408–411

Weitze C, Osburg S (1996) Transsexualism in Germany: empirical data on epidemiology and application of the German Transsexuals' Act during its first ten years. Arch Sex Behav 25(4):409–425

Welby-Gieusse M, Woisard V, Calas M et al (2008) Correlation between laryngoscopic examination and the gastroesophagial reflux in dysphonic patient. Rev Laryngol Otol Rhinol 129(2):107–114

Wendler J, Seidner W, Rose A et al (1973) Zur praktischen Nomenklatur der funktionellen Dysphonie. (Practical nomenclature of functional dysphonias). Folia Phoniatr (Basel) 25(1):30–38

Wendler J (1994) Glottoplasty for raising pitch. Abstract at the 3rd Intern. Symp. on Phonosurgery, pp 14, 63

Wendler J, Seidner W (2005) Klinik. In: Wendler J et al (eds) Lehrbuch der Phoniatrie und Pädaudiologie. Thieme, Stuttgart, pp 139–191

Wermke K (2007) Von einfachen zu komplexen Melodien: Über die frühesten Entwicklungsschritte auf dem Weg zur Sprache. In: Fuchs M (ed) Singen und Lernen. Logos, Berlin, pp 9–20

Wetmore SI, Key JM, Suen JY (1985) Complications of laser surgery for laryngeal papillomatosis. Laryngoscope 95(7 Pt 1):798–801

Whited RE (1979) Laryngeal dysfunction following prolonged intubation. Ann Otol Rhinol Laryngol 88(4 Pt 1):474–478

Williams DR, Lees AJ (2009) Progressive supranuclear palsy: clinicopathological concepts and diagnostic challenges. Lancet Neurol 8(3):270–279

Williams RG, Richards SH, Mills RG et al (1994) Voice changes in acromegaly. Laryngoscope 104(4):484–487

Woisard V, Percodani J, Serrano E et al (1996) Les manifestations laryngées du reflux gastrooesophagien. Bull Audiophonol 12(5–6):429–438

Wolfe VI, Ratusnik DL, Smith FH et al (1990) Intonation and fundamental frequency in male-to-female-transsexuals. J Speech Hear Disord 55(1):43–50

Woo P, Mendelsohn J, Humphrey D (1995) Rheumatoid nodules of the larynx. Otolaryngol Head Neck Surg 113(1):147–150

Wood JM, Hussey DJ, Woods CM et al (2011) Biomarkers and laryngopharyngeal reflux. J Laryngol Otol 125(12):1218–1224

Woodson GE, Zwirner P, Murry T et al (1991) Use of flexible fiberoptic laryngoscopy to assess patient with spasmodic dysphonia. J Voice 5(1):85–91

Woodson GE (1993) Configuration of the glottis in laryngeal paralysis. I: clinical study. II: animal experiments. Laryngoscope 103(11 Pt 1):1227–1241

Woodson G (2008) Management of neurologic disorders of the larynx. Ann Otol Rhinol Laryngol 117(5):317–326

World Health Organization (2010) International Classification of Diseases (ICD-10). http://apps. who.int/classifications/icd10/browse/2010/en#/F64. Accessed 5 Mar 2014

World Health Organization (2014) International Classification of Diseases (ICD) Version 2014. http:// www.who.int/classifications/icd/en/. Accessed 15 Nov 2016

Woznicka E, Niebudek-Bogusz E, Kwiecień J et al (2012) Applicability of the vocal tract discomfort (VTD) scale in evaluating the effects of voice therapy of occupational voice disorders. Med Pr 63(2):141–152

Wu BL, Sanders I, Mu L et al (1994) The human communicating nerve. An extension of the external superior laryngeal nerve that innervates the vocal cord. Arch Otolaryngol Head Neck Surg 120(12):1321–1328

Xiao J, Zhao Y, Bastian RW et al (2010) Novel THAP1 sequence variants in primary dystonia. Neurology 74(3):229–238

Ximenes Filho JA, Tsuji DH, Do Nascimento PH et al (2003) Histologic changes in human vocal folds correlated with aging: a histomorphometric study. Ann Otol Rhinol Laryngol 112(10):894–898

Ylitalo R, Lindestad PA, Ramel S (2001) Symptoms, laryngeal findings, and 24 hour pH monitoring in patients with suspected gastroesophagial reflux. Laryngoscope 111(10):1735–1741

Yoon MS, Munz M, Sataloff RT et al (1999) Vocal tremor reduction with deep brain stimulation. Stereotact Funct Neurosurg 72(2–4):241–244

Zabala-Parra SI, Amado-Galeano S, Gempeler-Rueda FE (2017) Fibronasolaringoscopia en el diagnóstico de síndrome de apnea-hipopnea obstructiva del sueño (SAHOS). Res Fac Med 65(Suppl 1):97–100

Zargi M, Hocevar-Boltezar I, Sereg-Bahar M et al (2013) Exercise induced laryngeal obstruction and laryngeal sensitivity. Poster presented at the European Academy of Otolaryngology—Head and Neck Surgery, Nice, France, 27–30 April 2013

Ziegler A, Dastolfo C, Hersan R et al (2014) Perceptions of voice therapy from patients diagnosed with primary muscle tension dysphonia and benign mid-membranous vocal fold lesions. J Voice 28(6):732–742. https://doi.org/10.1016/j. jvoice.2014.02.007. Epub ahead of print

Zucker KJ, Lawrence AA (2009) Epidemiology of gender identity disorder: recommendations for the Standards of care of the world professional association for transgender health. Intern J Transgenderism 11(1):8–18

Diagnosis and Differential Diagnosis of Voice Disorders

6

Wolfgang Angerstein, Giovanna Baracca,
Philippe Dejonckere, Matthias Echternach,
Ulrich Eysholdt, Franco Fussi, Ahmed Geneid,
Tamás Hacki, Katarzyna Karmelita-Katulska,
Renate Haubrich, František Šram, Jan G. švec,
Jitka Vydrová, and Bożena Wiskirska-Woźnica

Electronic Supplementary Material The online version
of this chapter (https://doi.org/10.1007/978-3-662-46780-
0_6) contains supplementary material, which is available
to authorized users.

W. Angerstein
Phoniatrie und Pädaudiologie,
Univ.-Klinikum Düsseldorf, Düsseldorf, Germany
e-mail: angerstein@med.uni-duesseldorf.de

G. Baracca
ENT Department, AO Niguarda Cà Granda,
Milan, Italy
e-mail: giovanna.baracca@gmail.com

P. Dejonckere
Federal Agency for Occupational Risks,
Brussels, Belgium
e-mail: Philippe.deJonckere@kuleuven.be

M. Echternach
Department of Otorhinolaryngology, Division of
Phoniatrics and Pediatric Audiology,
Munich University Hospital (LMU),
Campus Großhadern, Munich, Germany
e-mail: matthias.echternach@med.uni-muenchen.de

U. Eysholdt
Department of Medical Physics and Acoustics/
Medical Physics and Cluster of Excellence
Hearing4all, Carl von Ossietzky-Universität
Oldenburg, Oldenburg, Germany
e-mail: ulrich.eysholdt@uni-oldenburg.de

F. Fussi
AudioPhoniatric Centre, Azienda USL Romagna,
Ravenna, Italy
e-mail: ffussi@libero.it

A. Geneid
Department of Otolaryngology and Phoniatrics –
Head and Neck Surgery, Helsinki University Central
Hospital, Helsinki, Finland
e-mail: Ahmed.Geneid@hus.fi

T. Hacki
Department of Otorhinolaryngology, Head
and Neck Surgery, Semmelweis University Budapest,
Budapest, Hungary

K. Karmelita-Katulska
Department of Neuroradiology, University of Medical
Sciences in Poznan, Poznan, Poland
e-mail: katarzyna_katulska@op.pl

R. Haubrich
Evangelisches Klinikum Niederrhein
Duisburg-Nord, Zentrale Abteilung für
Diagnostische und Interventionelle Radiologie,
Duisburg, Germany
e-mail: R.Mauersberger@gmx.de

© Springer-Verlag GmbH Germany, part of Springer Nature 2020
A. am Zehnhoff-Dinnesen et al. (eds.), *Phoniatrics I*, European Manual of Medicine,
https://doi.org/10.1007/978-3-662-46780-0_6

F. Šram · J. Vydrová
Voice and Hearing Centre Prague, Prague 2,
Czech Republic
e-mail: sramfr@email.cz; vydrova@medico.cz

J. G. Švec
Department of Biophysics, Faculty of Science,
Palacky University, Olomouc, Czech Republic
e-mail: jan.svec@upol.cz

B. Wiskirska-Woźnica
Department of Phoniatrics and Audiology, Poznan
University of Medical Sciences, Poznan, Poland
e-mail: bozena.woznica@wp.pl

6.1 Methods of Non-instrumental Voice Examination and Voice Screening

Bożena Wiskirska-Woźnica

6.1.1 Introduction

The full non-instrumental assessment of the phonatory function of the larynx should include a medical history, adequately collected from the patient, as well as a physical examination (including respiration, hearing and velopharyngeal competence) and an auditory perceptual voice evaluation (Sataloff 2005a).

6.1.2 Diagnostic Interview

A medical history of voice disorders (Table 6.1) primarily consists of questions concerning the nature of the change in the timbre, the pitch, extent and loudness of voice, frequently reported hoarseness and its severity, any occurrence of episodes of voice loss and fatigability of voice. The history should be able to determine the onset and circumstances and effects of vocal problems, either sudden or prolonged, their appearance as an acute or chronic dysfunction, duration of the symptoms, any presence of a possible link to an excessive vocal effort, changes of voice quality during course of the day (e.g. in the morning voice problems in hypofunctional dysphonia, after voice load increasing voice problems in

Table 6.1 A medical history of voice disorders

Voice complaints	Timbre change
	Pitch
	Loudness
	Hoarseness
	Episodes of voice loss
Onset and nature of problems	Sudden/prolonged
	Acute/chronic
	Duration of symptoms
	Presence of fatigue voice
	Changes of voice quality during course of the day
Complaints accompanying phonation	Pharyngolaryngeal paraesthesia
	Dryness, irritation
	Sensation of having foreign body in the throat
Comorbidities	Respiratory tract infections
	Gastro-laryngeal reflux
	Neurological diseases, the use of medication
	Habits, e.g. smoking cigarettes
	Hormonal status (menstrual cycles, hormonal medications)
Occupational ailments	Onset and nature of voice complaints
	Daily loading of vocal organ
	Working conditions
	Number of working years

hyperfunctional dysphonia, alternating voice quality over the day in psychogenic dysphonia), infection or stress.

History taking should regard any complaints that may accompany phonation, such as pharyngolaryngeal paraesthesia, dryness, irritation or a sensation of having a foreign body in the pharynx and larynx. Moreover, questions in the medical interview should concern comorbidities, particularly respiratory tract infections, gastro-laryngeal reflux, neurological diseases, the use of medications, as well as any habits, especially cigarette smoking. In women, history taking should also involve the hormonal status: the regularity of menstrual cycles and the possible use of hormonal medications, including contraceptives or hormone replacement therapy. As far as professional voice users are concerned, it is necessary to establish the onset (after how many hours of using the voice) and the nature of voice complaints, the daily loading of the vocal organs, the working conditions and the number of years in the profession. In addition, information about systematic voice training during education and any former voice therapy may be useful (Aronson and Bless 2009).

6.1.3 Physical Examination Including Respiration and Velopharyngeal Competence

Any ENT examination should routinely pay special attention to the morphology of the vocal organ. Predominantly, palpation of the neck should be performed, with respect to the position of the larynx in relation to the other anatomical structures. The laryngeal skeleton and the surrounding structures should be palpated on respiration, phonation and swallowing. In particular, one should observe the formation of the thyroid cartilage and the laryngeal prominence, commonly known as the Adam's apple, more apparent in men. Furthermore, the *neck examination* includes observing any enlarged thyroid gland as well

as the laryngeal vertical mobility (e.g. upwards on swallowing). The Bresgen grip is a frontal pressure on the thyroid cartilage notch. In cases of mutational falsetto, as a result of compression of the flexible thyroid cartilage, the voice drops immediately about an octave down into the chest register owing to relaxation of the overtensed vocal folds. It does not occur when the cartilage is calcified, e.g. due to age or hormonal disorders.

The physical examination assessing vocal functions of the *larynx* should include a routine examination of the larynx (see Sect. 6.3); voice emission technique including breathing; body posture; voice projection strategies; coordination between respiration, phonation and articulation; the indication of aerodynamic parameters (in particular, the maximum phonation time); and voice self-assessment (see Sect. 6.2). The examination of the larynx with an endoscope or a laryngeal mirror as indirect laryngoscopy should be performed at the very beginning. For phoniatric purposes, attention should be focused on the oropharynx - the valleculae epiglotticae and the shape of the epiglottis; on the hypopharynx - its shape, the size and symmetry of piriform sinuses and the glossoepiglottic and aryepiglottic folds; and on the larynx - the arytenoids cartilage region, vestibular folds, ventricles, colour, length, width and movement of the vocal folds, the shape of the glottis during phonation and the subglottal area, as well as the colour, moisture of the mucosa and the presence of any abnormal tissue.

In the process of voice assessment, it is essential to examine not only the larynx but the whole *vocal tract*: the oral and nasal cavities and naso-, oro- and hypopharynx. These cavities significantly contribute to the timbre and the proper resonance of the voice. The closure of the nasopharynx due to muscle obstruction of the soft palate on articulation of oral consonants prevents pathological nasality. The evaluation requires the estimation of the size of these cavities, the condition of the mucosa and any possible morphological changes. One should observe the following criteria:·the shape, symmetry and mobility of the tongue; the symmetry and mobility of the lips; the arrangement of the teeth and occlusion; the mobility of jaws and the mandible; the condition and the relationship of the hard and soft palate; the presence of abnormal movements as myoclonus; the symmetrical mobility of the soft palate and the uvula; the size and symmetry of the palatine tonsils, hypertrophy and signs of possible inflammation; the size of the adenoids; the condition of the nasal cavity and nasal turbinates; possible nasal obstruction; the presence of allergic symptoms including swelling and bruising of the turbinates; colour and moisture of the mucosa; and any pathological contents in the nasal cavities or in the nasopharynx.

The evaluation of conditions by means of the phonation technique should first assess the *activity of extrinsic and intrinsic laryngeal muscles.* One should assess whether the voice is produced freely without any hypercontraction of muscles. In case of vocal hyperfunctionality, there is an excessive, pathological muscle tension and distension of the veins of the neck. In the opposite condition, i.e. vocal hypofunction, phonation is carried out with a weakening of the laryngeal muscle activity (Sataloff 2005b).

6.1.4 Examination of Types of Respiration

Proper breathing technique is an essential condition for the normal voice, in particular for professional voice users. Significant also is the use of the appropriate manner of respiration (inhalation/exhalation). There are three patterns of breath support: upper thoracic/clavicular, abdominal/diaphragmatic and mixed thoracic/abdominal.

The upper thoracic/clavicular breathing involves the expansion of mainly the upper part of the chest. Ribs and abdomen are at relative rest. This type of breathing allows only partial filling of the lungs with air and the breath is defective. Breathing with a predominance of costal track called mixed thoracic/abdominal breathing consists of the ribs moving apart on the outside and slightly upwards, while the chest expands in the lateral dimension. The most appropriate and the most efficient, optimal manner for phonation is abdominal/diaphragmatic breathing. This type of breathing with a predominance of abdominal track occurs when the duration of the inspiration movement of the lower ribs is minimal and the diaphragm contracts and moves downwards. It increases the size of the chest forwards and backwards (Pruszewicz 1992). In singing, the deepest and most appropriate breath is characterised by high amplitude movements of the diaphragm, allowing a deep breath, and ample work of the muscles of the ribs guarantees the correct support breathing (appogio) (Fig. 6.1).

A properly produced voice should manifest the ability to use the whole resonator of the vocal tract. On clinical examination it is possible to evaluate the function of head resonators on phonation of memoranda combined with a vowel phonation [mmae], [mmo], and [mmi].

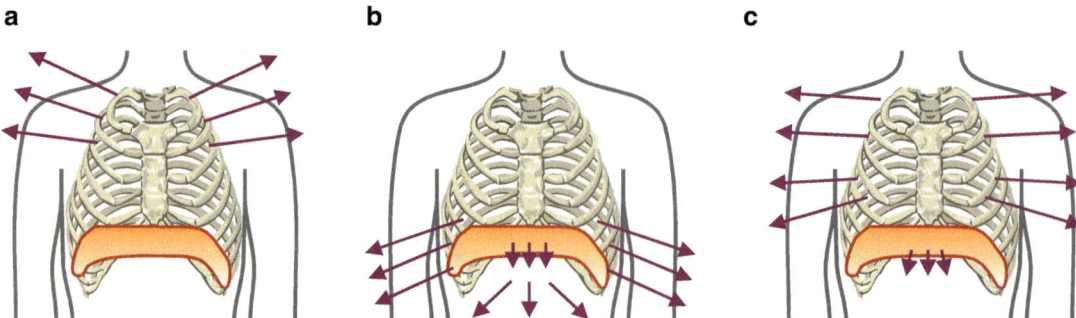

Fig. 6.1 Three patterns of breath support: (**a**) upper thoracic/clavicular, (**b**) abdominal/diaphragmatic and (**c**) mixed thoracic/abdominal

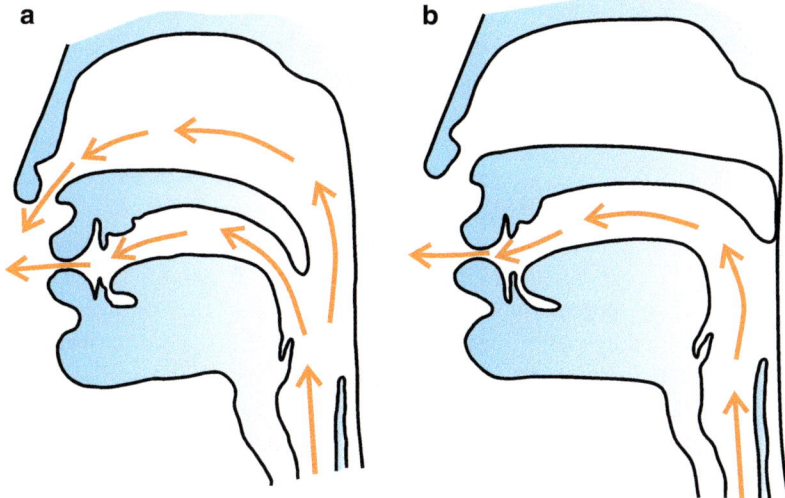

Fig. 6.2 The palatopharyngeal closure during production of (**a**) nasal and (**b**) oral sounds

6.1.5 Examination of Velopharyngeal Competence

The assessment includes velopharyngeal competence. This plays an important role in the presence of a normal nasal resonance in the voice. Normally, only on emission of nasal vowels (e.g. /m/, /n/) is the function of the velopharyngeal sphincter physiologically incomplete, and the airstream enters the nose (Fig. 6.2).

On phonation of oral sounds, when the velopharyngeal valving is not properly controlled and the airflows into the nose, the vowels and nonnasal consonants have an improper hypernasal resonance (open nasality). In hyponasality, the velopharyngeal valving is also improperly controlled, which results in the absence of a nasal resonance on nasal consonants. The closed nasality (rhinophonia clausa—hyponasality) arises as a consequence of a difficult passage of air through the nose. Most frequently, this happens as a consequence of mucosal oedema or polyps in the nose as well as adenoid hypertrophy. The nasal sounds /m/ and /n/ sound like /b/ and /d/, and the voice becomes muted. If there is both velopharyngeal insufficiency and nasal obstruction, the nasality can be mixed.

The diagnosis of open nasality (rhinophonia aperta—hypernasality) is primarily based on the results of three tests:

- The Gutzmann test, which consists of pronouncing the vowel /a/ several times on compression and release of the wings of the nose, which normally does not change the sound. In case of the open nasality, the vowel sound on compression varies and is clearly darker.
- The Czermak mirror test involves placing an unheated mirror in front of the nostrils, and the patient is asked to pronounce the syllables composed of vowels and explosive consonants such as /pa-pa, ba-ba/. If open nasality occurs, the air is released through the nose in the form of a mist cloud visible on the mirror.
- In the Seeman test, one olive of the otoscope is placed in the patient's nostrils, and the second one in the examiner's ear, while pronouncing vowels or consonants. If open nasality occurs, the murmur of the escaping through the nose can be heard (Pruszewicz 1992).

Otoscopy, performed as part of the ENT examination, may indicate possible changes in the middle ear, which as a possible cause of hearing loss may be the cause of abnormal phonation by means of its insufficient self-control. A pure tone *audiogram* should be performed in all cases of voice disorders owing to the feedback of hearing and voice.

6.1.6 Perceptual Evaluation of Voice Quality

The clinical evaluation of phonation (non-instrumental) should be started by identifying the timbre of spoken voice in the perceptual examination. *Voice quality* is a subjective concept from the auditory point of view. During the first contact with the patient, the assessment of voice disorders, as well as the evaluation of the efficacy of the treatment, is performed on the basis of the perceptual psychoacoustic evaluation of the voice (Bassich and Ludlow 1986). Hoarseness is the most common word that describes the quality of the voice characterised by noticeable noise components. It is a non-specific symptom caused mainly by irregularities of the normally almost periodic vibration of the vocal folds or lack of closure and most frequently accompanies organic diseases of the larynx (De Krom 1995). It can also be a symptom of innervation disorders of the larynx and occurs as a result of disturbed mechanisms of phonation in functional dysphonia. In addition, voice qualities are often described by the following words: harsh, breathy, rough, strained or squeezed.

It is important to mention that the same disease may lead to quite different manifestations in voice quality, and the same voice quality may have quite different causes of the underlying pathology (Kreiman et al. 1992, 1993). Thus, any deviant voice requires a complete physical examination (Bless and Baken 1992).

In order to standardise the terminology used to define dysphonia, a variety of *perceptual scales* have been developed to describe the quality of the voice (Dejonckere et al. 1993). Many phoneticians (Laver 1980), voice and speech physiologists and phoniatricians are convinced that it is necessary to create a universal scale for assessing perceptual voice. Currently, of many scales of subjective evaluation (de Bodt et al. 1996, 1997),

e.g. the Stockholm Voice Evaluation Approach (Hammarberg 2000), Buffalo Voice Profile System (Wilson 1987), Laver's Vocal Profile Analysis Scheme (Laver et al. 1992), Consensus Auditory-Perceptual Evaluation of Voice (CAPE-V) (Karnell et al. 2007) and Newcastle Audio Ranking (NeAR) (Gould et al. 2012), the best known and the most widely used is the scale of the Japan Society of Logopaedics and Phoniatrics, the GRBAS scale (Hirano 1989).

The GRBAS scale describes the voice disorder with the use of five well-defined parameters: G, the grade of hoarseness; R, roughness, an audible impression of irregularities of the vibration of the vocal folds; B, breathiness, an audible impression of the air leakage through the insufficient glottal closure; A, an asthenic voice; and S, a strained voice. This scale has four degrees of intensity of disturbances, where '0' indicates a normal voice, '1' mild disturbance, '2' moderate disturbance, and '3' severe disturbance, with respect to all the parameters. Thus, a normal voice is described as follows: G0R0B0A0S0, which means a sonorous voice, without rough elements, produced with a soft attitude, and with a complete glottis closure, produced freely without any excessive muscle tension. Dejonckere et al. (2000) proposed to expand this scale with another parameter: I—instability of the voice (i.e. variability over time)—and then the scale will have the GIRBAS form. The shortened modification of the GRBAS scale excluding A and S owing to the proven low inter- and intra-rater reliability is the RBH scale (Wendler et al. 1986), where /R/ is roughness, /B/ breathiness and /H/ hoarseness. In research the perceptual evaluation should be performed by at least three independent examiners/judges, and then all the results should be averaged (Gerratt et al. 1993; Fang-Ling and Matteson 2014).

Additionally, it should be noted (Bough et al. 1996) that the features of an individual voice depend on the number of certain properties, and therefore apart from the personality and emotional state, one should take into consideration the current body temperature, the degree of rest and rehydration of the body and even the time elapsed from the last meal.

Moreover, the phoniatrician should estimate perceptually whether the *pitch* of the spoken voice is appropriate for the patient's age and gender and whether it is stable. The speech tasks for perceptual voice assessment is generally limited to a 5-s sustained phonation of the vowel sounds /a/ and /i/, as well as a short reading of phonetically balanced texts, e.g. the Rainbow Passage for English language. The *mean speaking pitch* is different in male and female adults, and it changes with age. It is approximately 260 Hz (200–260 Hz, *g-c1*) and 130 Hz (100–130 Hz, *G-c*) in younger females and in males, respectively. The *vocal pitch range*, calculated as the difference between sung sounds at the lowest and highest pitch possible, should cover 1.5–2 octaves, and reaches, depending on the voice type, from d/c^1 to d^2/c^3 for females and D/c to d^1/c^2 for males. In running speech, an area of one octave is generally covered. Clinical observations are usually performed with respect to the patient's habitual pitch while speaking, in order to check whether it is too low or too high. Pitch is of striking importance for all kinds of professional speaking, especially for teachers, lecturers and public speakers. The physiological reference is the so-called indifference level, a pitch that is generated by a well-balanced action of all muscles involved with an optimal relation of muscular tension and vocal output. It is located at the transition area from the lower to the middle third of the pitch range.

This is the pitch that should be kept during speaking as the average or mean speaking pitch or at least to which it should be regularly brought back. Permanent upward deviation does not only mean an overloading of the speakers' voice apparatus but also that of the listener. As an effect of the so-called functional listening, listeners unconsciously mimic the speakers' muscular tension, get strained and tired and lose their attention.

For the purposes of complete voice evaluation, it is important to determine the *register of the voice*. The term 'register' means the type of voice, especially while singing, although the term may also refer to the mode of vibration (Niimi and Miyaji 2000). The laryngeal register reflects a specific mode of phonation. The phys-

iological register (modal), called the chest tone, occurs because of the normal vibrations of the vocal folds and is a record of the fundamental frequencies that appear mainly while speaking. The term 'falsetto' (head tone) occurs at very high frequencies and is often slightly breathy with an incomplete glottal closure and vibration of the only free edges of the vocal fold, with the tension of the posterior part. A creaky voice, or glottal fry, occurs at very low frequencies by means of the vibration of the frontal parts of the vocal folds and a tight closure of the glottis (see also Sect. 4.5).

A normal voice is produced with the appropriate *loudness*, not too loud and not too weak, and indicates the ability of the free and dynamic modulation of the volume.

The most important aerodynamic parameter of phonation is the measurement of the *maximum phonation time* (MPT) and the *s/z ratio* (Gelfer and Pazera 2006). MPT is the ability to pronounce the vowel /a/ freely at full exhaustion for as long as possible at a comfortable pitch and volume. According to Kent et al. (1987), for persons aged 17–41 years, on average it fluctuates between 15 s for women and 23 s for men and is reduced with age. Values depending on the age can range as low as 17.25–34.6 s for men and 12.10–26.5 s for women. The s/z ratio makes it possible to compare the ability to control airflow on phonation of the voiceless /s/ and voiced /z/, which is important for establishing the way in which the patient controls exhalation. In individuals with normal voices, the s/z ratio is near 1.0. Vital capacity (VC), measured parametrically by spirometry, is not a direct measurement of phonation but is used indirectly as a measure of lung function indicating the amount of air that can be used for phonation. Vital capacity is a combination of inspiratory reserve volume, expiratory reserve volume and tidal volume—this is total volume of air that can be inspired after total expiration (see Sect. 6.7). The average values of the normal vital capacity reach approximately 4800 mL for men and 3500 mL for women.

The *phonation quotient* (PQ) indicates the amount of air consumed on phonation and is obtained by division of the vital lung capacity by the maximum phonation time: PQ = VC/MPT. The normal values for this parameter vary from 145 to 269 mL/s for men and from 137 to 233 mL/s for women. Raes and Clement (1996) in their work presented the following results: for adult men at MPT 22.2 s and VC 4.800 mL, the PQ value was 269 mL/s; for women at MPT 18.4 s and VC 3.500 mL, the PQ was 233 mL/s.

The next issue to examine is *voice attacks*. There are three kinds of attack: the preferred soft mode—simultaneous, when the breath and the vibration occur at the same time; glottal, when vocal folds push against each other too strongly, making it difficult for them to vibrate; and breathy, when the breath occurs first and then the vocal folds begin to vibrate, but a gap in the incompletely closed glottis causes a portion of the air to be converted to the noise, rather than to the acoustic wave.

6.1.7 Articulation

Owing to the permanent interaction between vocal tract configuration and glottal function, proper articulation is also part of the specific technique of producing a normal voice. It should be characterised by a distinctive pronunciation of vowels and consonants, a moderate rate of speech and a mouth open wide with a suitable lowering of the mandible. What seems important is the ability of the correct movement of the lips, the palate (lifting and lowering) and the tongue.

6.1.8 Screening Methods

Screening is an investigation carried out in normal individuals to detect diseases in their early, subclinical stages. Screening of voice quality provides assessments to professional voice users, as well as candidates and students for occupations with special voice quality demands, or any lay person experiencing voice problems. Voice screening is also important for identification and early management of paediatric voice disorders, which can affect the child's education and psychosocial develop-

ment. A screening method as a first step is usually based on a review of voice history to identify any potential problems or on questionnaire concerning vocal symptoms. It can be administered by health-care personnel in order to select persons for further examination by a phoniatrician and should include the assessment of voice quality and visualisation of vocal fold function. There are screening tests that can be used to measure different aspects of voice rapidly. They are generally based on questionnaire data and voice analysis, i.e. the assessment of the quality of voice, pitch, loudness, maximum phonation time, respiration and resonance. Questionnaires usually contain typical questions concerning voice complaints, duration of intensive voice and speech use, smoking, subjective voice function assessment (e.g. GRBAS scale) and voice self-assessment (e.g. VHI). Both questionnaire and voice analysis are non-invasive multi-parameter monitoring tools for early detection of potential voice disorders and therefore very useful in preventive health care in phoniatrics.

Methods of screening presented by scientists are based on a questionnaire and voice analysis that concern various groups of adults and children, e.g. the Voice Assessment Protocol for Children and Adults (VAP) (Haynes et al. 2006), Boone Voice Program for Children (Boone 1993; Boone et al. 2005), Quick Screen for Voice (Lee et al. 2004) and Screening Index for Voice Disorders (SIVD) (Ghirardi et al. 2013). There are also other voice screening tests based on only one parameter, e.g. the Glottal to Noise Excitation Ratio presented by Spanish scientists (Godino-Llorente et al. 2010). They confirmed that this acoustic parameter is a good choice for screening purposes in discriminating normal and pathological voices. Johnson et al. (2014) presented a voice screening over the telephone; it can differentiate spasmodic dysphonia from other voice disorders. Ohlsson et al. (2012) performed screening in teacher students using questionnaire Screen6 (Simberg et al. 2001) and the Swedish Voice Handicap Index. They found an association between the number of potential vocal risk factors and the number of voice symptoms.

There is no doubt that laryngoscopy is the most important information source for screening voice disorders. Awan et al. (2016) presented voice screening with the Cepstral Spectral Index of Dysphonia (CSID), which contains three reference standards: auditory perceptual estimation, Voice Handicap Index and laryngoscopic description. They suggested that this CSID method with acoustic voice analysis could be used as a potential screening tool for voice disorder identification. Pernambuco et al. (2016a, b) presented in Portuguese (there is not yet an English translation) a new tool for epidemiological screening voice in older adults: the Rastreamento de Alteracoes Vocais em Idosos (RAVI), i.e. Screening for Voice Disorders in Older Adults. This test consists of 16 questions related to sensations and perceptions associated with the voice. The authors emphasise that RAVI is the first voice-related self-reported questionnaire for identifying voice disorders in older adults. Several other countries, e.g. Scandinavian countries and Austria, have introduced many preventive programmes for professional voice users (Vilkman 2004; Schneider-Stickler et al. 2012).

Some of these screening procedures are useful practically and can be recommended, for example, the Quick Screen for Voice (Lee et al. 2004). It is a rapid and widely administered (by SPL) screening test for children that contains many aspects of voice, respiration and resonance; it has been validated in a large group of kindergarten and preschool children and is used as part of a comprehensive speech, language and hearing screening. The Screening Index for Voice Disorders (SIVD) has been proved to be an efficient tool for screening occupational voice disorders and can be used as an instrument of epidemiologic vigilance (Ghirardi et al. 2013).

Voice screening procedures allow early detection of voice disorders in the subclinical stage and the administration of the treatment, rehabilitation and prevention; they can, if necessary, be used to dissuade people with voice dysfunction from the so-called voice professions.

6.2 Self-Administered Questionnaires for the Assessment of Voice Disorders in Normal and Professional Users

Franco Fussi and Giovanna Baracca

6.2.1 Introduction

Self-administered questionnaires are used to assess the impact of the health problems on the quality of life of the patients. The World Health Organization (1971) defines disability as:

> a restriction or lack of ability manifested in the performance of daily tasks

and handicap as

> a social, economic, or environmental disadvantage resulting from an impairment or disability.

Measuring the quality of life in case of a health problem, in addition to the physical examination, allows physicians to understand better the point of view of the patient related to his individual experience of a certain disease. An example of the different impacts produced by a voice problem follows: a vocal disability could increase when a patient is not able to speak at a certain pitch or loudness and a vocal handicap when a patient loses money because his voice becomes ineffective in communicating or performing. There is not necessarily a correlation between the results of the evaluation of dysphonia obtained by means of perceptive evaluation, video-laryngostroboscopy and acoustic/aerodynamic parameters and the severity of the subjective disturbance perceived by the patient in his daily life. Self-perceived impairment largely depends on how a person uses his voice. A professional speaker will be more strongly impaired by a breathy voice than a computer engineer; in the same way, a singer will face more serious consequences than a painter when his voice is hoarse. Self-assessment instruments, indeed, take into account the type of social activity, the environment where the voice is more utilised, the family habits, education, sex, gender, psychological traits and life style. The impact on the quality of life of a dysphonic problem is an important factor for clinicians not only to obtain a global evaluation but also to take the best therapeutic decision, in a field in which the prognosis is not with respect to life (quoad vitam) but with respect to health (quoad valetudinem). Moreover, questionnaires should be useful in providing a further element for measuring the outcomes of a voice treatment, be it surgical, pharmacological or rehabilitative.

6.2.2 List of Self-Assessment Questionnaires Utilised in Practice

In the literature, the administration of different types of questionnaire, all validated by means of statistical methodology, has demonstrated satisfactory psychometric qualities in terms of high internal consistency and test-retest reliability. Questionnaires are usually constituted by items individually scored on an ordinal scale from 0 to N, on the basis of how often each statement is experienced from the patient in daily life. The total score gives an indication of how the voice disorder creates annoyance in the life of the patient. The majority of questionnaires are also divided into subscales that score some specific aspects of the perception of the voice disturbance, such as the emotional, the physical or the social. The most well-known self-administration questionnaires include the Voice-Related Quality of Life (V-RQOL), the Voice Handicap Index (VHI), the Vocal Performance Questionnaire (VPQ), the Voice Activity and Participation Profile and the Voice Symptom Scale. There follows a brief description of each of these instruments.

The VPQ (Carding and Horsley 1992), developed in 1992, consists of 12 items concerning the physical and psychosocial impacts of a general voice disturbance on daily life. It has the advantage of being easily and briefly administered and demonstrates high internal consistency, but it does not investigate specific aspects of a voice problem. The VHI (Jacobson et al. 1997), validated in 1997, is the only self-assessment questionnaire that meets the criteria established by the Agency for Healthcare Research and Quality for

determining disability in speech-language disorders. The VHI (Table 6.2), translated into and validated in more than 20 languages, is a 30-item questionnaire, each one scored from 0 (never) to 4 (always), differentiated into 3 subscales about specific domains of the impact of voice problems (emotional, functional and physical). The functional subscale investigates the consequences of a voice disturbance on daily activities (disability); the physical subscale is related to the perception of the dysphonia in terms of physical symptoms (impairment); the emotional subscale measures the effects on the emotional life of a voice problem (handicap). The maximum score of the VHI is 120; a score from 0 to 14 corresponds to no disturbance, from 15 to 28 to a slight disturbance, from 29 to 50 to a moderate disturbance and over 51 to a severe disturbance.

Jacobson et al. (1997) found that VHI has good psychometric properties and a correlation with patient judgment of the voice-disorder severity. Furthermore, VHI demonstrates a high correlation with the Dysphonia Severity Index (Wuyts et al. 2000), and it is a good index of the self-perception of the voice modification after vocal fold surgery. Available online since 2013 (Herbst et al. 2015), the DigitalVHI, a free open-source software application for obtaining Voice Handicap Index (VHI) and other questionnaire data, can be used when filling in the information. The software makes the VHI scores directly available for analysis in a digital form. Reduced versions of the VHI have also been validated, such as the VHI-10 (Rosen et al. 2004) and the VHI-9i (Nawka et al. 2009), comprised, respectively, of 10 and 9 items extracted from the original version, that can be comfortably utilised for their brevity and ease of administration. Another questionnaire that obtained similar results to those of the VHI-10 in terms of psychometric properties is the Voice-Related Quality of Life (V-RQOL) (Hogikyan and Sethuraman 1999), developed and validated in 1999, comprising ten items, divided into socio-emotional and functional-physical subscales. The Voice Symptom Scale (VoiSS) (Wilson et al. 2004) is a 30-item questionnaire developed in 2004 and able to assess communication problems, psychological impact, perception of voice characteris-

Table 6.2 Voice Handicap Index (VHI)

		0	1	2	3	4
1	My voice makes it difficult for people to hear me					
2	I run out of air when I talk					
3	People have difficulty understanding me in a noisy room					
4	The sound of my voice varies throughout the day					
5	My family has difficulty hearing me when I call them throughout the house					
6	I use the phone less often than I would like					
7	I'm tense when talking with others because of my voice					
8	I tend to avoid groups of people because of my voice					
9	People seem irritated with my voice					
10	People ask, 'What's wrong with your voice?'					
11	I speak with friends, neighbours or relatives less often because of my voice					
12	People ask me to repeat myself when speaking face-to-face					
13	My voice sounds creaky and dry					
14	I feel as though I have to strain to produce voice					
15	I find other people do not understand my voice problem					
16	My voice difficulties restrict my personal and social life					
17	The clarity of my voice is unpredictable					
18	I try to change my voice to sound different					
19	I feel left out of conversations because of my voice					
20	I use a great deal of effort to speak					
21	My voice is worse in the evening					
22	My voice problem causes me to lose income					
23	My voice problem upsets me					
24	I am less outgoing because of my voice problem					
25	My voice makes me feel handicapped					
26	My voice 'gives out' on me in the middle of speaking					
27	I feel annoyed when people ask me to repeat					
28	I feel embarrassed when people ask me to repeat					
29	My voice makes me to feel incompetent					
30	I'm ashamed of my voice problem					

0 never; *1* almost never; *2* sometimes; *3* almost always; *4* always. Copyright with kind permission from the American Speech-Language-Hearing Association (ASHA)

tics and other respiratory symptoms. The Voice Activity and Participation Profile (VAPP) (Ma and Yiu 2001) is a 28-item questionnaire consisting of five subscales focused on the self-perception of the severity of voice disturbances, impact on job activity and daily communication and impact on social relationships and emotional life. The answers are provided by the patient on a visual analogue scale (VAS).

The self-assessment instruments can play an important role in creating, in a brief time, an empathic relationship between dysphonic patients and clinicians, helping the latter to understand the real effect of a voice problem on daily living and functioning. In addition, it has to be taken into account that questionnaire answers are affected by several individual variables, such as family and community support, cultural background and so on. It is necessary to include the self-assessment evaluation in a multistep evaluation of voice, as recommended by ELS Guidelines (Dejonckere et al. 2001). Self-administered questionnaire results must be considered as an aspect of the multidimensional evaluation of a voice disorder, also including perceptual, videostroboscopic, acoustic and aerodynamic assessments. The utilities of the self-administration questionnaires must be considered in the diagnostic phase, when the idea of how the patient perceives the voice disorder can improve the clinician's choice on the best treatment. Moreover, by analysing the results, the clinician can help the patient to become aware of his problem and manage it. Comparison of the answers pre- and post-treatment, rehabilitative or surgical, indicates the level of satisfaction of the patient with the results of therapy.

6.2.3 Questionnaires for Special Kinds of Voice Disorders

Self-assessment protocols must be specific for special categories of patients with voice disorders. This is the reason that some special instruments have been created and validated for particular groups of dysphonic people. It has already been reported that self-evaluation questionnaires are influenced by several factors such as age, sex, specific disease patterns, occupation and others. Considering the age factor, it cannot be neglected that children's voice disorders must be evaluated with specific self-assessment instruments able to take into account the impact of dysphonia on daily paediatric life. The Pediatric Voice Handicap Index (pVHI) (Zur et al. 2007), comparable to adult VHI, is characterised by high internal consistency and high test-retest reliability. It is able to measure the impact of child's voice quality on overall communication, development, education, social and family life. It is composed of 21 items divided into three subscales, functional, physical and emotional, concerning how much the parents perceive the impact of their child's voice disturbance on his or her daily life. In this case, indeed, the questionnaire must be filled in by the child's parents. Ricci-Maccarini et al. (2013) validated a self-assessment questionnaire in Italian specific for children from 8 to 14 years of age, in which each child fills in the interview autonomously. It demonstrated good clinical validity and responsiveness to treatment in case of paediatric dysphonia. In 2012 Verduyckt et al. (2012) created and validated a new self-assessment questionnaire for paediatric use, capable of measuring in parallel the impact of children's voice disorders by themselves and their parents, the Pediatric Voice Symptom Questionnaire (PVSQ). It is valid, reliable and easy to administer in children from 6 years of age, when they are conscious of their vocal symptoms (Verduyckt et al. 2011). Another category of people usually affected by voice dis-

orders in terms of low satisfaction with their voice parameters comprises transgenders, who often perceive their pitch too low and their voice disorder as a problematic factor in social life. In 2013 Dacakis et al. (2013) validated the Transgender Self-Evaluation Questionnaire able to provide a reliable self-report measure of vocal functioning in male-to-female transsexuals. It is structured as a self-administered interview composed of 30 items scored from 1 to 4 concerning voice problems in daily use experienced when living as a female. Another factor that must be taken in account is the awareness of the patient about his voice problem and his availability to modify his vocal strategies through a voice therapy. Some self-assessing instruments were created to be particularly useful in evaluating some variables important for the therapeutic choices. In particular, Epstein et al. (2009) created and validated the Voice Disability Coping Questionnaire (VDCQ), able to measure the coping processes in different patient groups. It is constituted by four coping subscales: 'social support', 'passive coping', 'avoidance' and 'information seeking' measured over 15 items. Coping in psychological medicine refers to the way in which people deal with the stress of illness. In case of voice disorders, this instrument helps people understand how to cope with voice problems. The questionnaire should be administered before voice therapy in order to address modification of coping and put it in relation to the outcomes.

6.2.4 Self-Administered Questionnaires for Professional Users

Singers constitute a specific population of professionals particularly at risk of voice problems. They are more likely to seek help and report problems related to their singing voice (Rosen and Murry 2000; Phyland et al. 1999). Singers represent 11.5% of all patients at voice consultations while constituting only 0.02% of the general population (Titze et al. 1997). Hoarseness frequently affects not only their speaking voice but also their singing voice and, consequently, their professional activity. This is partly due to the importance they give to their voice status, a critical social and occupational factor that can significantly affect their quality of life. The perception of a voice problem in singing is often related to specific symptoms, such as difficulty in the passaggio, vocal endurance and diminished range, aspects that are not assessed by the common self-assessment questionnaires. They are, indeed, more sensitive to vocal disabilities, which may have a higher impact on their quality of life than that of non-singers. Hence, to obtain a self-assessing instrument able to evaluate vocal disability in singers, in 2007, Cohen et al. (2007) created and validated a specific questionnaire, the Singing Voice Handicap Index (SVHI), aimed at measuring the physical, social, emotional and economic impacts of voice problems on the lives of the singers. The SVHI (Table 6.3) is a 36-item self-administered questionnaire that is used to

Table 6.3 Singing Voice Handicap Index (SVHI) (Reprinted with kind permission of Prof. Seth Cohen, Durham, North Carolina, USA)

		0	1	2	3	4
1	It takes a lot of effort to sing					
2	My voice cracks and breaks					
3	I am frustrated by my singing					
4	People ask 'What is wrong with your voice?' when I sing					
5	My ability to sing varies day to day					
6	My voice 'gives out' on me while I am singing					
7	My singing voice upsets me					
8	My singing problems make me not want to sing/perform					
9	I am embarrassed by my singing					
10	I am unable to use my 'high voice'					
11	I get nervous before I sing because of my singing problems					
12	My speaking voice is not normal					
13	My throat is dry when I sing					
14	I've had to eliminate certain songs from my singing/performances					
15	I have no confidence in my singing voice					
16	My singing voice is never normal					
17	I have trouble making my voice do what I want it to					
18	I have to 'push it' to produce my voice when singing					
19	I have trouble controlling the breathiness in my voice					
20	I have trouble controlling the raspiness in my voice					
21	I have trouble singing loudly					
22	I have difficulty staying on pitch when I sing					
23	I feel anxious about my singing					
24	My singing sounds forced					
25	My speaking voice is hoarse after I sing					
26	My voice quality is inconsistent					
27	My singing voice makes it difficult for the audience to hear me					
28	My singing makes me feel handicapped					
29	My singing voice tires easily					
30	I feel pain, tickling or choking when I sing					
31	I am unsure of what will come out when I sing					
32	I feel something is missing in my life because of my inability to sing					
33	I am worried my singing problems will cause me to lose money					
34	I feel left out of the music scene because of my voice					
35	My singing makes me feel incompetent					
36	I have to cancel performances, singing engagements, rehearsals or practices because of my singing					

0 never; *1* almost never; *2* sometimes; *3* almost always; *4* always

assess difficulties related to voice health status typical of the singing professional, as demonstrated by its psychometric properties of reliability and validity. The items address symptoms frequently reported to phoniatricians and speech pathologists by singers. Each item must be individually scored on a 5-point Likert scale (ordinal scale) ranging from never (score of 0) to always (score of 4) (Likert 1932).

The SVHI has demonstrated higher sensitivity to clinical changes than the VHI in singers, proving the validity of the SVHI in measuring outcomes in the singing population. In fact, VHI may underestimate the level of handicap related to voice problems in performers, especially for certain pathologies able to produce severe consequences for the professional activity, for example, reflux or allergies. These disturbances affect the singing voice more severely than the speaking voice, so it is necessary to have a specific tool able to measure the impact of any kind of voice problem peculiar to the singing activity. It is important for a self-assessment instrument to recognise changes in singing voice health status after surgical, pharmacological or rehabilitative treatments, and the SVHI demonstrates these properties in terms of clinical validity. The original English version of the SVHI has been translated into and validated in several languages, and it is utilised in different countries. Also developed and validated is an abbreviated version of the SVHI, the SVHI-10 (Cohen et al. 2009), composed of 10 items extracted from the 36 original, on the basis of the item-total correlation and better self-assessment of the voice disorders. SVHI-10 can be easily utilised to facilitate the assessment of the perceived handicap related to a singing voice problem, especially in the case of repeated administration or multidimensional assessment when the time for the evaluation is reduced.

Of course, singers constitute a peculiar population, but they are not so homogeneous: variables such as the singing styles performed, the amount of singing training and experience, the nature of singing demands and the performance environments can definitely affect the voice conditions of a singer and the perceived level of handicap. Voice disturbances, caused by vocal fold lesions, can in fact produce a different subjective disturbance depending on the number and duration of the performances, the amount of rehearsal needed and the characteristics of voice use during the performances. All these factors are influenced by the professional level and the singing style that a singer engages. Accordingly, singing style may be an important predictor of singing voice handicap requiring particular consideration. This evidence led Fussi (2005) and Moreti et al. (2012) to develop more specific self-assessment instruments, on the model of the SVHI, for the modern and classical singing voice. The two questionnaires, called the Classical Singing Voice Handicap Index (CSVHI) (Table 6.4) and the Modern Singing Voice Handicap Index (MSVHI) (Table 6.5), which are currently under validation on a large number of singers, are composed of 30 items grouped into 3 areas (impairment, disability, handicap). Each item is scored from 0 to 4 on the basis of how often it is experienced in the singing activity. The items are consistent with the peculiar use of the voice, depending on the singing style engaged. They investigate aspects of singing that can be perceived only in the case of a high level of self-confidence with their own voice. The two different instruments, for classical and modern singers, take into consideration the environments where singers perform; the theatre in the case of the classical style; open-spaces, restaurant or pubs in the case of modern style; the level of background noise that is minimum during the opera performance and could be very loud during parties; or other situations where modern singers often perform. Furthermore, the environments of classical concerts have similar acoustic characteristics, whereas modern music is performed in several different types of situations to which modern singers must adapt their voices each time. There are also some technical aspects in the use of voice that should be investigated differently for classical and modern singing: for the modern style, there is no definite vocal reg-

Table 6.4 Classical Singing Voice Handicap Index (CSVHI)

		0	1	2	3	4
1	I have difficulties during the performance in the theatre with modification of my vocal efficiency					
2	My vocal warm up has to be prolonged					
3	I am forced to modify my vocal technique because my voice problem influences my usual technical control					
4	My singing problem forces me to modify or limit my repertoire					
5	My singing problem forces me to limit my usual study time					
6	I have difficulties during my performance with modification of my vocal efficiency					
7	I have to prolong the vocal rest between two performance					
8	I have to avoid changes in the vocal intensity during the pianissimo execution to mask my voice problem					
9	To mask my singing problem, I am forced to undergo continuous medical therapy					
10	My singing problem forces me to limit the use of my voice in my social life					
11	I feel more anxious than usual before performances					
12	People around me do not recognise my singing voice problem					
13	I am subjected to justified criticism from people around me					
14	I get nervous and less sociable because of my singing problems					
15	I get worried when someone asks me to repeat a vocalism or a sung phrase					
16	I feel that my career is in danger because of my singing difficulties					
17	My colleagues, managers and critics have noticed my singing difficulties					
18	I have to cancel performances and other professional commitments					
19	I avoid planning my next professional commitments					
20	I avoid speaking to people					
21	I have trouble managing my breathing					
22	I feel my sung emission breathy and weak					
23	I feel my sung emission is rough, with noise					
24	I have difficulties in controlling the intensity of the sound (vocal breaks)					
25	My vocal range is reduced					
26	I have difficulties in balancing vocal registers and resonance					
27	I feel I have to force to produce my voice					
28	The voice quality goes down during the performance					
29	My speaking voice is tired and worse after the performance					
30	The vocal efficiency is reduced at certain times of the day					

0 never; *1* almost never; *2* sometimes; *3* almost always; *4* always. Copyright with kind permission from OMEGA EDIZIONI s.a.s. di Giacomo Soncini & C., Torino, Italia

ister as in classical, so the vocal texture is more adaptable to the repertoire. Singers in this case have the possibility of varying the timbre according to the songs, several times within the same performance, and to look for different vocal solutions. Classical style, conversely, needs homogeneous vocal emission and more rigour in the execution. It follows that performers can feel a different level of discomfort caused by a voice difficulty according to the singing style.

CSVHI and MSVHI are two specific instruments able to measure the level of handicap related to the singing voice differently for classical and modern styles and to evaluate peculiar aspects of the singing activity related to the singing style engaged.

In conclusion, the most utilised self-assessment questionnaires are the VHI for common dysphonic diseases, the PVHI for paediatric voice disorders and the SVHI for dysphonia in voice professional users.

Table 6.5 Modern Singing Voice Handicap Index (MSVHI)

		0	1	2	3	4
1	I feel vocal fatigue from the beginning of the performance					
2	My speaking voice is hoarse and tired during a performance					
3	I am forced to modify my vocal technique because my voice problem influences my usual technical control					
4	My singing problem forces me to eliminate or limit certain songs from my repertoire, also with transposition of tonality					
5	My singing problem forces me to limit my usual study time					
6	I have difficulties during my performance with modification of my vocal efficiency					
7	I cannot stand more than two consecutive performances					
8	I have to ask the sound engineer for help to hide the alterations of my voice					
9	To mask my singing problem, I am forced to undergo continuous medical therapy					
10	My singing problem forces me to limit the use of my voice in my social life					
11	I feel more anxious than usual before performances					
12	People around me do not recognise my singing voice problem					
13	I am subjected to justified criticism from people around me					
14	I get nervous and less sociable because of my singing problems					
15	I get worried when someone asks me to repeat a vocalism or a sung phrase					
16	I feel that my career is in danger because of my singing difficulties					
17	My colleagues, managers and critics have noticed my singing difficulties					
18	I have to cancel performances and other professional commitments					
19	I avoid planning my next professional commitments					
20	I avoid speaking to people					
21	I have trouble managing my breathing					
22	My vocal performance changes throughout the day					
23	I feel that my voice is breathy and weak					
24	I feel that my voice is rough					
25	I have to strain to produce my voice					
26	My vocal efficiency varies in an unpredictable manner during the performance					
27	I try to modify my voice to make it better					
28	It takes a lot of effort to sing					
29	My voice is worse in the evening					
30	My voice tires easily during a performance					

0 never; *1* almost never; *2* sometimes; *3* almost always; *4* always. Copyright with kind permission from OMEGA EDIZIONI s.a.s. di Giacomo Soncini & C., Torino, Italia

6.3 Laryngoscopy, Stroboscopy, High-Speed Video and Phonovibrogram

Ulrich Eysholdt

6.3.1 Light Sources

6.3.1.1 Cold Light

Light projectors for medical endoscopy have been built since the 1930s. All techniques of light production have a common problem: the brighter the light, the higher the temperature of the equipment from unwanted heat generated. A heat-absorbing glass is built into endoscopy light projectors for the protection of the patient. Because of this, this equipment is not quite as hot, and the promotionally euphemistic name 'cold light source' is now applied. Clinically available cold light sources use light generated by excited halogen (F, Cl, Br) or inert (Xe, Kr) gas molecules and have a typical power consumption of 250–300 W. Halogen light is 'warm white' and is therefore more comfortable for the doctor during an examination. When working with a Xe or Kr source, the doctor must, however, first accustom himself and his perception to the blueish 'cold white' light.

6.3.1.2 LED

Currently, cold light source technology is being superseded by LED (light-emitting diode) light. Coloured LEDs (green, red, etc.) have been on the market for decades, but white light LEDs of sufficient luminance have only recently become available. LEDs are very suitable for clinical use: they need less power and generate much less heat than cold light technology, meaning that the tip of the endoscope does not become hot over time. Current LEDs (in 2015) do not have quite the same degree of brightness as conventional xenon cold light sources. LED light sources have another advantage for laryngoscopy: in contrast to cold light sources, LEDs do not fluctuate with the 50 Hz mains voltage. LEDs are therefore ideal light sources for high-speed video recording (HSV).

6.3.1.3 Stroboscopic Light

Stroboscopy is based on a special flashing light source which—in a medical application—is solely used for examination of the vibratory movement of the vocal folds. Laryngostroboscopy can be performed just as well by using a simple laryngoscopy mirror or any type of endoscope. Stroboscopy (from the Greek στρόβος strobos, meaning whirl or rotation, from the first mechanical stroboscopes that used rotating perforated discs to interrupt the light beam) is a method of visualising rapid movements that are impossible to be seen by the eyes alone because the chemical regeneration of rhodopsin in the retina of human eyes allows a maximum frequency of movement perception of only 20 Hz. However, stroboscopy is only appropriate for the visualisation of periodic movements, which are movements that repeat their spatial position. The moving object is illuminated by a rapid series of light flashes, the frequency of which is designated by the repetition rate of the movement. If the frequency of the light flashes is identical to that of the movement, then every light flash illuminates the object in the same phase, meaning that the object appears to the observer to be static ('stroboscopy in standstill'). If the frequency of light flashes is faster than the movement, the flash will illuminate the object earlier and reveal another phase of the periodic movement. The object will seem to move slowly ('stroboscopy in slow motion', an optical illusion). In laryngostroboscopy the apparent vibration of the vocal folds is lowered to 1 Hz. The visual representation is so convincing that the methodical constraints are often forgotten:

A Stroboscopy only targets periodic (i.e. non-disturbed) vocal fold vibration during sustained phonation. The more irregular the vibration, the less effective the stroboscopy.

B The virtual slow-motion movement of stroboscopy is a visual illusion only. A quantitative evaluation is technically possible but physically meaningless.

In technical terms, stroboscopy violates the Nyquist condition of Shannon's sampling theorem. Nonetheless, stroboscopy has been an important element of the diagnostic investigation of the voice since 1960.

6.3.2 The Endoscope

An endoscope is defined as an optical instrument that can be used to view a cavity from the inside through a narrow opening. The superposition principle of geometrical optics is utilised, which states that two crossing beams of light do not influence each other. Illumination and observation occur simultaneously in the same optical system. The size of an endoscope is given in 'mm diameter' (D) and sometimes in the older Charrière (Ch) unit of measurement, which corresponds to 'mm circumference' (conversion: $D = Ch/\pi$, with $\pi = 3.14159 \ldots$ the circle constant). The length of the endoscope is unimportant for laryngeal endoscopy.

There are two main types of endoscope: rigid and flexible.

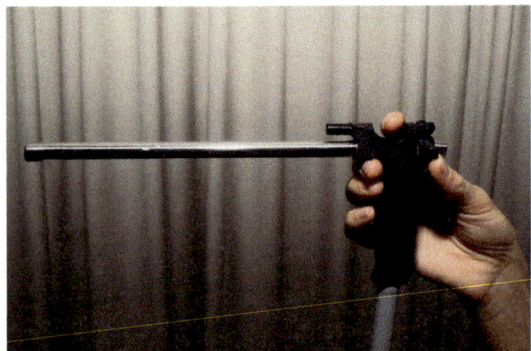

Fig. 6.3 Rigid endoscope 90°

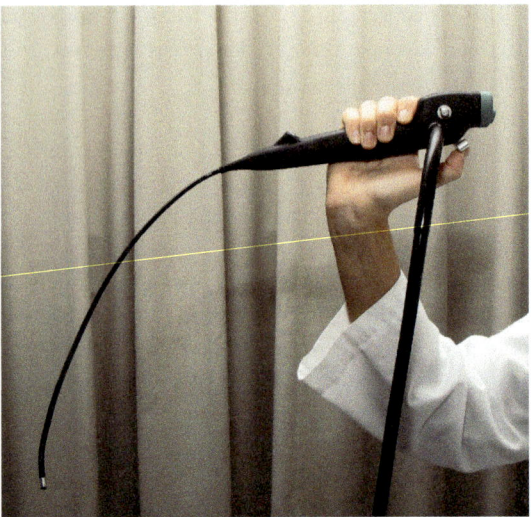

Fig. 6.4 Flexible endoscope

6.3.2.1 Rigid Endoscopy

Rigid endoscopes with a length of 3–50 cm are these days mainly used for examination of the upper respiratory tract. A typical rigid laryngoscope is a metal tube of 15–25 cm length that contains 'rod lenses' (glass cylinders with lens-shaped cavities that direct and focus light) as an imaging system. The light from the light source is directed laterally through a fibre-optic cable coupled to a semi-transparent beam splitter. At the tip of the endoscope, the light is reflected by a mirror and emitted. The reflection angle of this mirror defines the endoscope type (see Fig. 6.3). An angle of 70–90° is suitable for illuminating the larynx (90° is most common in Europe). Ninety degree or 70° laryngoscopes have today replaced the laryngoscopic mirror of the nineteenth century. The old term 'indirect' laryngoscopy is kept for this modern technique because the light is redirected at an angle. A 70° laryngoscope can be inserted a little deeper (and therefore be brought closer to the vocal folds), but a more subtle examination technique is required.

The image is observed through a magnifying eyepiece lens through which one can either directly look or to which a video camera can be attached. The eyepiece usually has fourfold magnification.

6.3.2.2 Flexible Endoscopy

In contrast to the rigid endoscope, a flexible endoscope can be directed around a curve. Conventional flexible endoscopes have the same design as rigid endoscopes, except that they have a bundle of flexible fibre-optic cables instead of a rod lens. Flexible laryngoscopes are approximately 40 cm long, and the tip can be directed by control knobs near the eyepiece (see Fig. 6.4). In contrast to a bronchoscope, flexible laryngoscopes do not have a suction tube or working tube next to the light channel, and it is therefore possible to manufacture very narrow flexible laryngoscopes (max. 5 mm, in contrast with the 6–8 mm of a bronchoscope). However, a not insignificant loss of light occurs with fibre optics; the longer the endoscope, the greater the amount of light lost. This loss of light must be compensated for during observation, either by performing observations in a darkened room or by using electronic light amplification within the video chain.

COTT ('Chip-on-the-Tip') Modern image sensors can be constructed so small that they can fit on the tip of a flexible laryngoscope. Image distortion must be corrected by an external computer, the camera processor. This 'chip-on-the-tip' technology produces very good images because it has almost no loss of light. It is, however, very expensive and is only used in combination with an HD standard high-quality video chain.

Transnasal Flexible Laryngoscopy The flexible laryngoscope is inserted through the nose (inferior nasal meatus), and the tip is usually positioned in the oropharynx. The insertion phase must be uninterrupted and is often performed with mucosal anaesthesia to avoid patient discomfort. If the endoscope is inserted and positioned correctly, the patient is able to tolerate it well and can speak and swallow during the examination. This technique is used for 'fibre-optic endoscopic examination of swallowing' (FEES) (see Vol. 2, Chap. 6).

The endoscope can be inserted beyond the oropharynx if required to investigate specific issues. The tip is then positioned in the endolarynx or in the trachea but is less well tolerated here because the mucous membranes are more sensitive.

6.3.2.3 Rigid or Flexible?

Rigid and flexible endoscopic techniques are both types of indirect laryngoscopy. The technique used depends upon the country and local customs. Flexible laryngoscopy is prevalent in Japan, but 90° rigid laryngoscopy is more often found in Europe and the west coast of the USA, while 70° rigid techniques are more common on the east coast of the USA. In general, the luminance of the rigid endoscope is higher than that of the flexible endoscope, but this difference has less relevance these days because both techniques are typically combined with video recording, which essentially nullifies the difference. Analogue video techniques following S-VHS or U-matic high band have long since been replaced by digital recordings and data storage on computer. With digital video signals, weaknesses in the primary signal can easily be improved before storage (in jargon, 'Photoshopping'). Other differences between endoscopes exist and are measureable but play no role within clinical practice. 'Rigid or flexible'—previously a matter of faith—is now not a question of quality but a question of habit.

6.3.3 Indirect Laryngoscopy

The patient should be sat upright in a chair, with his bottom firmly against the backrest and his upper body bent slightly forwards (approximately 15°). With a 70° endoscope, the patient's head should be flexed dorsally, and the investigator should stand during the investigation. With a 90° endoscope, the patient's head is held normally and the investigator should sit down. With a flexible transnasal endoscope, the patient should be seated as comfortably as possible; the investigator should also be seated in a relaxed position and not just on ergonomic grounds: he must be able to use the footswitch of the stroboscope without losing balance. The magnifying laryngoscope is inserted through the oral cavity with the tongue outstretched, despite the fact that the uvular veli palatini must be pushed to the side with the tip of the endoscope. The investigator needs to be skilful in order to avoid gag and swallowing reflexes.

The patients should be asked to produce a vocal tone that they can hold over time, such as [hæː]. Though this sound can hardly be produced with the endoscope in the throat, the intention alone makes the epiglottis rise, which permits a view into the larynx down to the glottis. When a patient is encouraged to produce this sound, the vocal folds, which are abducted for respiration, are then adducted. This transition of the larynx from respiratory to phonatory position can be visualised by laryngoscopy. A dynamic balance between the prephonatory tension of the vocal folds and the simultaneously raised subglottal pressure is generated within 80–150 ms, and the vocal folds begin to vibrate. This phase of prephonatory laryngeal alignment cannot be visualised by endoscopy, but once the vocal folds have established a steady oscillatory state (after 2–10 cycles of vibration), the voice level triggers the stroboscope, and the movement of the vocal folds can be observed in slow motion (Table 6.6).

Endoscopic imaging will continue to be improved by the advances in recording and analysis techniques afforded by video. The investigator should orientate himself on the monitor on which the 'moving image' is displayed. Despite the additional expenditure of time, it is common to record the video and assess it immediately after the actual investigation. It is important to concentrate on the management of the patient and the endoscope during the investigation itself in order to obtain good images.

Table 6.6 Transition from respiration to phonation

		Visible on laryngoscopy
Respiration	Vocal folds abducted, glottis open	Yes
Vocal insertion	Adductive movement of the vocal folds ('respiratory mobility')	Yes
	Prephonatory generation of • Vocal fold tension • Subglottal pressure	No
Phonation	Vocal fold adducted, glottis closed	Yes
	Vocal fold vibration ('phonatory mobility')	Only by using stroboscopic light or high-speed technology

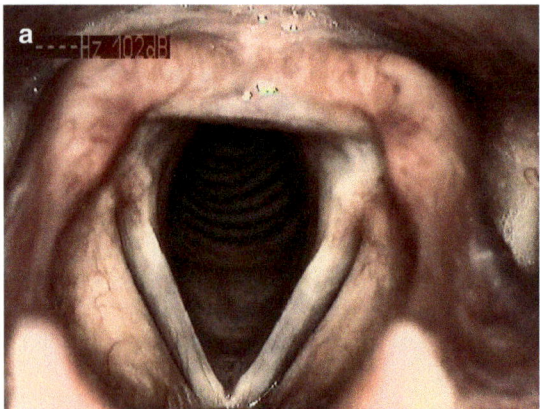 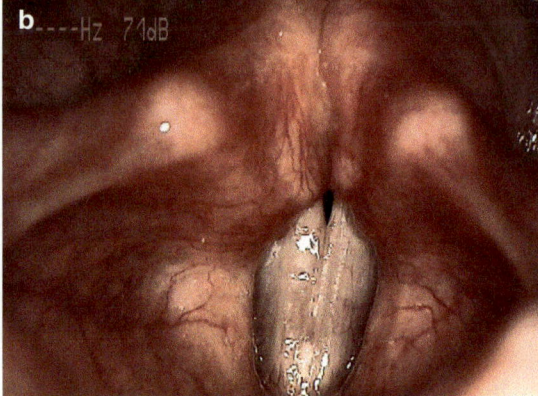

Fig. 6.5 Typical laryngoscopic images showing respiration in (**a**) and phonation in (**b**). With kind permission from Prof. Tadeus Nawka, Berlin

The monitor must be orientated according to (a) the redirection of light in the laryngoscope and (b) the patient's ability to interpret it. 'Up' on the monitor is the dorsal direction, 'down' is ventral, and the 'right' side of the monitor is the patient's left and vice versa. This sounds trivial but in fact cannot be emphasised strongly enough: the most severe treatment errors within hospitals occur because of wrong-side procedures.

Figure 6.5 shows typical laryngoscopic images, (a) in respiration and (b) in phonation mode. The criteria for assessment of the images are adjusted according to Virchow's disease classification (malformation, degeneration, trauma, inflammation and tumour). A laryngoscopic finding should describe:

- The morphology of the endolarynx
  - Vocal fold configuration (free edges and surface)
  - Inflammation
  - Trauma/haemorrhage
  - Neoplasia
  - Atrophy (degeneration)
  - Malformation
- Respiratory mobility
- Phonatory mobility

In order to orientate oneself rapidly, the triangular glottal opening, which is usually dark black, is bordered by the bright white vocal folds. The vocal folds, vestibular folds and arytenoids should be observed for the subsequent documentation of findings, and either the endoscope or the patient's head should be moved in order to look into the anterior commissure.

On phonation, the glottis closes and respiratory mobility is visible. Phonatory mobility (vibration of the vocal folds) cannot be visualised with a laryngoscope. This can be achieved by using stroboscopy (very widely used but methodically problematical; see Sect. 6.3.1.3 A and B) and recording techniques in real-time resolution such as 1D videokymography (VKG) (see Sect. 6.5) or 2D high-speed video recording (HSV).

6.3.4 Visualisation of Vocal Fold Vibration

Vocal fold vibration, which has a frequency ≥ 100 Hz, is so fast it cannot be seen with the eyes. Video recording and technical devices to assist with observation are necessary in order to transform the speed of the vocal folds into a form that can be perceived. Such technology includes:

- Stroboscopy. Dispenses with detailed movement and reflects only a split-second recording of each vibratory cycle in which the vibrating vocal folds are illuminated by a flashing light source.
- High-speed video endoscopy (HSV). Records video with a high frame rate (≥ 4000 frames per second (fps), equating to 15–40 images per cycle. Videokymography (VKG) is a simplified, inexpensive variant but has associated limitations.

Both techniques are similar in that they involve connecting a video recorder to a laryngoscope. We tend to avoid the inconvenient word 'video(laryngo)stroboscopy' in clinical jargon and instead just use the terms stroboscopy or HSV endoscopy.

6.3.4.1 Stroboscopy

Stroboscopy has been widely used for decades (Schönhärl 1960; Hirano 1981); the recording apparatus has been substantially simplified and regularly adapted to current technology. Despite its underlying limitations, stroboscopy sometimes is thought of as a kind of secret weapon in voice diagnosis, even by many ENT physicians. However, stroboscopy is very well suited to the analysis of vocal fold vibration as long as the voice is no more than slightly disturbed.

The light source is a flashing light, which is set to the frequency of the patient's voice. The trigger signal is the fundamental frequency of the

voice, which is continuously calculated by a microprocessor in the stroboscope. A very robust trigger signal for the stroboscope light source can be taken from EGG or from a contact microphone which the patient holds against the outside of his own larynx. Triggering by a microphone that is sensitive to airborne sound and is attached to the endoscope is simpler but gives a less robust signal: the airborne signal contains many harmonics, so it takes longer to identify the fundamental frequency (it may even be impossible within the appropriate time frame, by which time the stroboscope may have turned off).

Modern stroboscopic light sources can be triggered up to 600 Hz, at which frequency they can show an exact image for each vibratory cycle. Following the initial combination of all of the images from each vibratory cycle, a film of the moving image which appears to be slow motion can be shown on the monitor. Assessment criteria for video laryngoscopy are:

- Amplitude
- Mucosal wave
- Closure of the glottis
- Temporal and spatial symmetry of the vibration

All these parameters are highly dependent on pitch and loudness. Therefore, corresponding documentation is obligatory; otherwise the descriptions of any vibratory findings are definitely useless. The same is true for all methods used to assess vocal fold vibrations.

Consequently, a great deal of experience is required in order to evaluate and interpret results correctly. The complexity of voice function and its numerous mutual dependencies are difficult to interpret.

Amplitude denotes the distance of the vibrations of the vocal folds. Although the vocal folds vibrate in 3D rotatory movements, endoscopy only reveals a projection of the mediolateral component. This is interpreted as movement of the vocal muscle (musculus vocalis, thyroarytenoideus). The amplitude is smaller at higher frequencies (increased muscle tension resulting in lower vibratory mass) as well as at lower loudness. Amplitude is therefore best observed at a comfortable pitch and loudness for the patient (i.e. in the middle of his vocal range). It is categorised by using a four-step Likert scale: (1) enlarged, (2) normal, (3) small and (4) missing on both sides.

The phenomenon of the *mucosal wave* was first discovered by the use of stroboscopy. Mucosal waves are waves of the epithelium covering the vocal folds, which run laterally during the vibration of the medial edge of the vocal folds. They occur at the cranial and caudal surfaces of the vocal folds but are only observable at the cranial surfaces. Mucosal waves can only occur when the viscoelasticity of the lamina propria and Reinke's space is not impaired, when the epithelia of the vocal folds can be extended laterally within their own limits along the base. Mucosal waves are evaluated according to the following categories on stroboscopy:

1. Present
2. Restricted
3. Abolished
4. Extended/enhanced

where (1) corresponds to the normal condition and (2) and (3) indicate disruptions in viscoelasticity, which could have various causes (inflammation or tumour, or simply dysfunctional). Case (4) is essentially only found in Reinke's oedema, a specific type of chronic laryngitis featuring the pathological enlargement of Reinke's space and the build-up of gelatinous mucous.

The question of *glottal closure* (whether or not the glottis is closed completely) can only be answered by using stroboscopic or other visualisation techniques. As well as the binary decision:

- Glottis closed during phonation
- Glottis *not* closed during phonation

It is also important to describe the type of incomplete closure of the glottis. The following categories are distinguished:

- Ventral gap
- Dorsal gap

- Continuous chink-shaped gap
- Spindle-shaped gap
- Hour glass glottis
- Irregular gap

In principle, an incomplete glottal closure is considered to be pathological in most cases. One exception is the triangular dorsal gap in young women (the 'glottal chink'), which can also be observed during pubescent voice change in males (the 'mutation triangle').

The most complex stroboscopic evaluation category is *temporal and spatial vibration symmetry*. Human perception is very robust in the categories of shape, colour, size and texture but not very reliable for time-dependent processes. There are only two possible categories for evaluating the symmetry of vocal fold vibration with stroboscopy:

- Symmetrical
- (Clearly) asymmetrical

A European consensus paper proposed the use of quantitative values for stroboscopy, rather than the above categories. However, given the methodical restrictions and highly subjective nature of stroboscopy, this proposal is not sensible and suggests a level of accuracy that does not actually exist.

6.3.4.2 High-Speed Video (HSV)

High-speed video technology is well-established in sports coverage, where it is called slow-motion video. For laryngoscopy, it is not yet clinically established while being under evaluation. A high-quality HSV camera operating at 4000 fps (in comparison with the normal 25 fps) is required. This technology was first developed through military mass production and since then has become less expensive so that it can be used within medicine. To increase their recording rate, HSV cameras usually work in black-and-white mode. Indeed, HSV cameras exist that produce colour images with high temporal and spatial resolution. Using 4000 fps recording equipment, the camera takes 40 images during a single 100 Hz vibratory cycle and 16 images during a 250 Hz cycle. If the high-speed film is then played back at 25 fps, there is a time-stretch ratio of 1:160 which, in contrast to stroboscopy, is a true slow motion. HSV laryngoscopy is therefore always indicated in cases where the voice is so severely dysfunctional that stroboscopy cannot be reliably triggered.

An HSV camera can, in principle, be attached to any type of endoscope. However, at such a high recording rate, the video shutter is only open for approximately 10 μs, meaning that the intensity of the light is significantly reduced. To improve the luminance, HSV recordings are mostly created with 90° or 70° rigid laryngoscopes.

6.3.5   Data Compression: Phonovibrogram (PVG)

A 2-s video recording at a 1:160 time-stretch ratio takes 320 s (5 min 20 s) to watch: a clinically unacceptable duration. The only way to avoid this is by compressing the data, either by reducing the video image to a single line at the time of recording (videokymography, VKG) or by image processing after recording.

The phonovibrogram (PVG) is at present the only clinically evaluated data compression technique for HSV recordings. It uses post-recording image processing, in which the movement-relevant information is extracted from the whole HS video sequence and combined in a single image. The PVG is designed to visualise motion asymmetries between left and right vocal folds.

6.3.5.1 PVG Computation
The following calculation steps are performed for every individual image (step 0) of the HSV recording:

- Step 1: The glottis is segmented.
- Step 2: Anterior and posterior commissures are defined.
- Step 3: A connecting line is drawn from the anterior to the posterior commissure, called the main glottal axis. The main glottal axis is not a morphological structure; it simply indicates the line of symmetry.

- Step 4: Left and right vocal fold are distinguished, here indicated by colour.
- Step 5: The distance between the left or right vocal fold edge and the main glottal axis is now measured along the length of the axis, with the glottal opening either to the left or right. After this measurement, the remaining components of the image are completely removed.
- Step 6: Only the following image components are kept:
  – The left free edge of the vocal fold
  – The right free edge of the vocal fold
  – The anterior commissure
  – The posterior commissure
  – The main glottal axis
- Step 7: The image is then split up along the main glottal axis. The right vocal fold remains in position, and the left vocal fold (shown on the right side of the image) is rotated 180° around the posterior commissure. The length of the vocal folds (the main glottal axis) therefore appears to be doubled, as if the anterior commissure appears twice (as A_L at the top and A_R at the bottom).
- Step 8: In order to visualise them, the distance measurements from (Step 5), which define the glottal opening, are coded into red pixels. The wider the glottal opening, the brighter red of the corresponding pixel. The result is a column of red pixels of different brightness that is twice as long as the main glottal axis for each single video frame, showing the glottal opening left/right and ranging from the 'left' anterior commissure, over the posterior commissure, to the 'right' anterior commissure. By this procedure, each image of an HSV sequence is reduced to a column of coloured pixels, each of which represents the current glottal opening separated for left and right.
- Step 9: Steps 1–8 are applied to each single frame of the HSV sequence and produce as many pixel columns as there are video frames. Placed side by side, the columns form a 2D image showing the glottal opening over time, the phonovibrogram (PVG).

The ordinate is twice the main glottal axis, and the abscissa is time. The left side of the glottis is shown above the posterior commissure (point P), and the right side is shown below it. The parallel line that meets the abscissa at point P is the axis in relation to which the symmetry must be evaluated (Eysholdt and Lohscheller 2008).

Figures 6.6, 6.7, 6.8, 6.9, 6.10, 6.11, 6.12, 6.13, and 6.14 show PVG computation steps.

6.3.5.2 Evaluation of the PVG

A normal PVG of a clinical examination is shown in Fig. 6.15. Although it can be evaluated perceptually, a machine is usually used. The first step is to separate the oscillation cycles

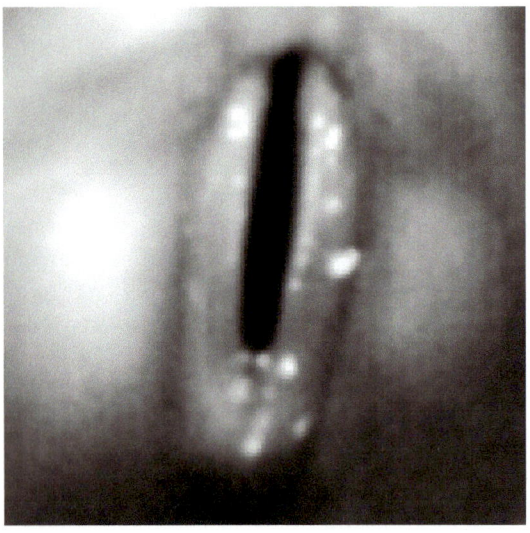

Fig. 6.6 PVG computation Step 0, the basis: Single image extracted out of a HS video sequence

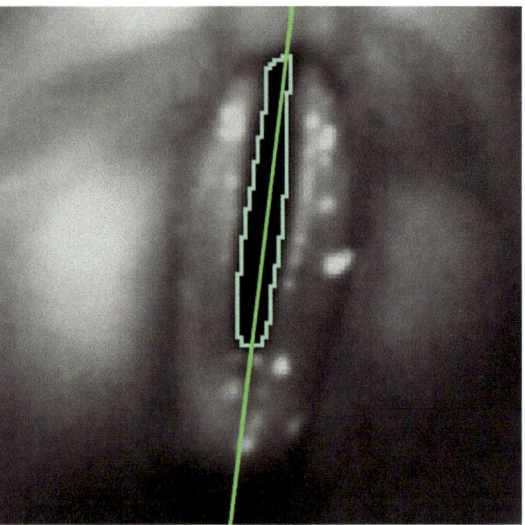

Fig. 6.8 PVG computation Step 3: Computation of the glottal midline (main axis)

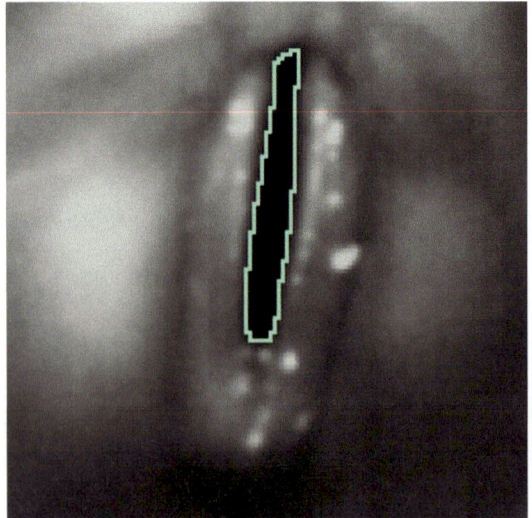

Fig. 6.7 PVG computation Steps 1 and 2: Segmentation of the glottis, i.e. detection of the vocal fold edges and anterior/posterior commissure

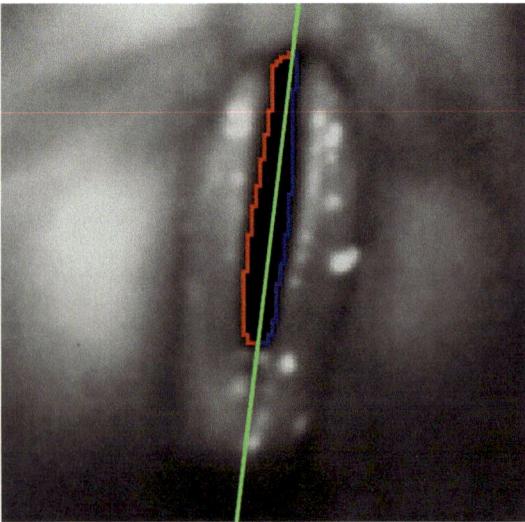

Fig. 6.9 PVG computation Step 4: Distinguishing between left and right vocal folds

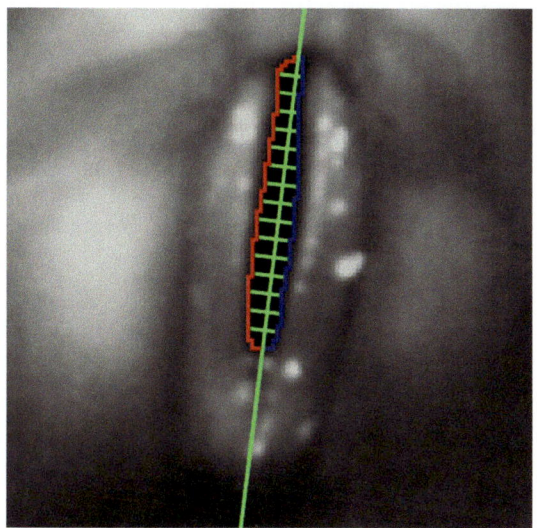

Fig. 6.10 PVG computation Step 5: Distance measurement between left/right vocal fold and glottal midline. After this, all image parts are suppressed except for the coloured structures

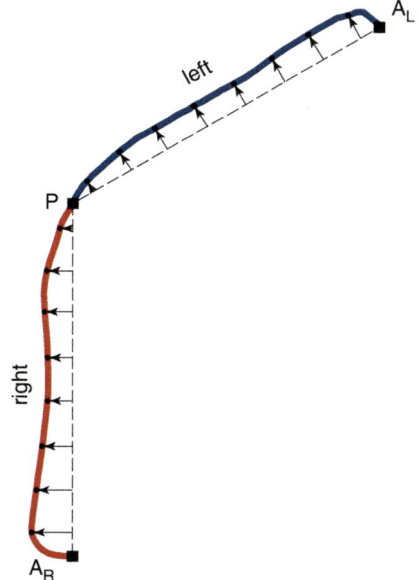

Fig. 6.12 PVG computation Step 7: the image is virtually split up along the dashed midline. The left vocal fold (blue) is rotated from the bottom up by 180° around P. Thus, the glottal length seems to be doubled, and the anterior commissure seems to appear twice (as A_L and A_R). The purpose of this visualisation procedure is to emphasise asymmetry between left and right

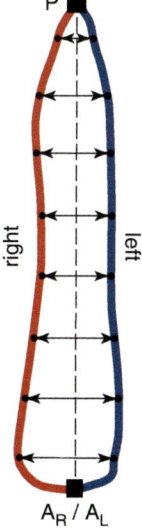

Fig. 6.11 PVG computation Step 6: Data-compressed laryngoscopic image after fading-off the non-moving parts. Components of the size-reduced image are: (1) Right vocal fold edge (red). (2) Left vocal fold edge (blue). (3) Anterior commissure A_L/A_R. (4) Posterior commissure P. (5) Glottal main axis (dashed), which is a reference line only

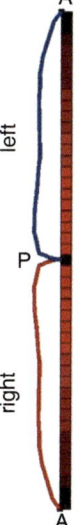

Fig. 6.13 PVG computation Step 8: the arrows from Step 7, which denote the side-dependent glottal widths, are replaced by red pixels. The wider the opening, the longer the arrow, the brighter the red pixel. All pixels together form a red vector containing the complete information about the glottal opening at the time T the image was taken

(Fig. 6.16). The regularity of the oscillation period is calculated; it corresponds to the acoustical jitter (Fig. 6.17). Within each cycle, the following measures are quantified and averaged over 40–200 cycles:

- Amplitude
- Right-left symmetry (Fig. 6.18)
- Glottal closure (Fig. 6.19)

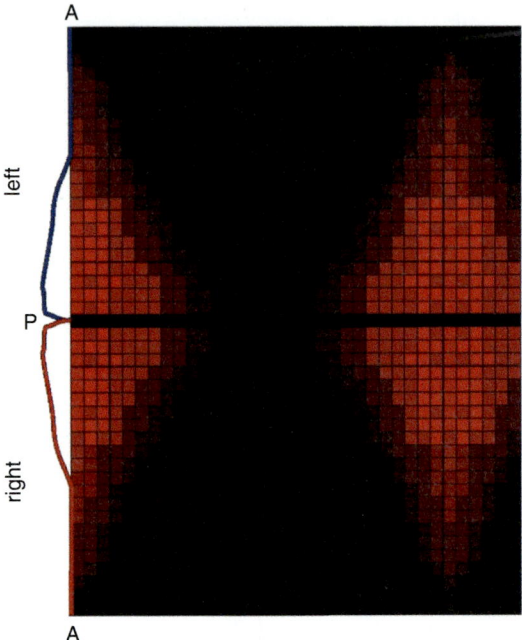
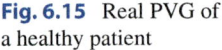

Fig. 6.14 PVG computation Step 9: Steps 1–8 are applied to each single image of the HS sequence. The resulting coloured columns are ordered side by side and form the PVG. This figure represents synthetic data, just for clarification of the image processing procedure

Apart from mucosal waves, PVGs are evaluated from the same criteria as in stroboscopy.

Many more details of the movement can be quantitatively extracted from this technique.

Advantages of PVG visualisation include:

- The possibility of evaluating the movement of left and right vocal folds independently.
- The speed and acceleration of each vocal fold can be measured at each position.
- The type of glottal opening and closure can be quantified.
- The symmetry of the movement can be quantified.
- The determination of irregular vibration modes (anterior-posterior).

These advantages of PVG over stroboscopy are not yet clinically used (Unger et al. 2016).

PVG is, at present, the only quantitative method of assessing vocal fold vibration. Because the technology is not very widespread, few people have clinical experience with PVG. The line between normal and abnormal/pathological patterns on PVG is still somewhat unclear, and it is not possible to predict the PVG pattern from the psychoacoustic impression from current models. Clinical observation so far indicates that a normal PVG is very variable and that many different PVG patterns could result from a healthy voice. Clearly defined criteria for pathology only exist for organic voice disorders (e.g. polyps, Reinke's oedema, uni- and bilateral paresis, carcinoma, etc.), but HSV techniques are not necessary in such cases.

Fig. 6.15 Real PVG of a healthy patient

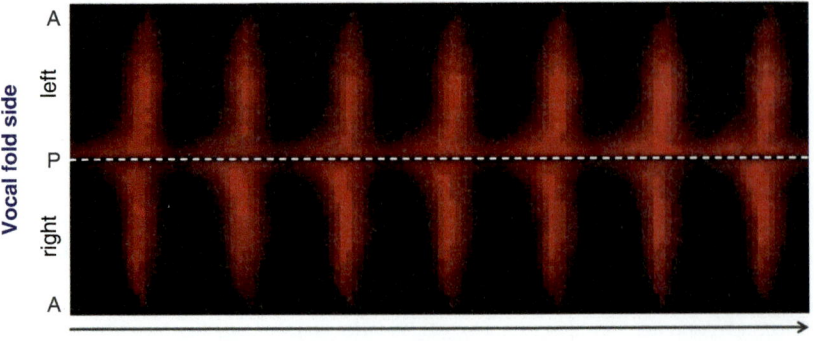

Fig. 6.16 PVG evaluation: identification of vibration cycles

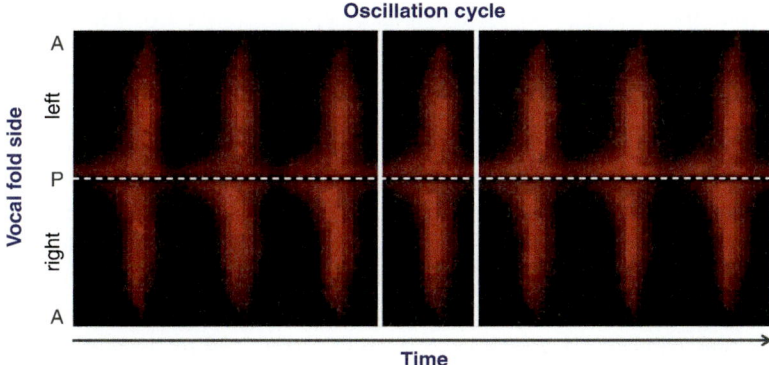

Fig. 6.17 PVG evaluation of regularity

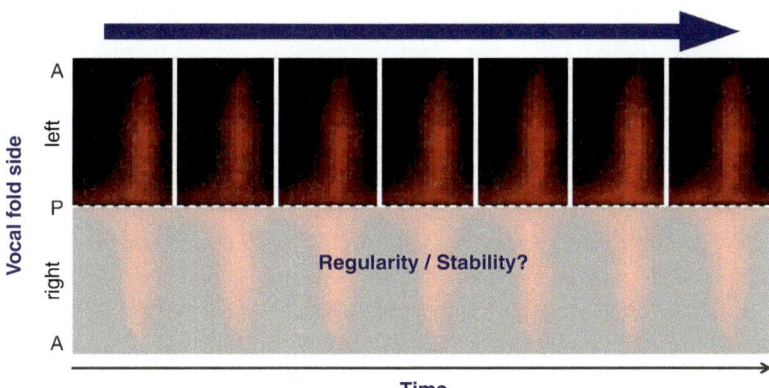

Fig. 6.18 PVG evaluation of symmetry

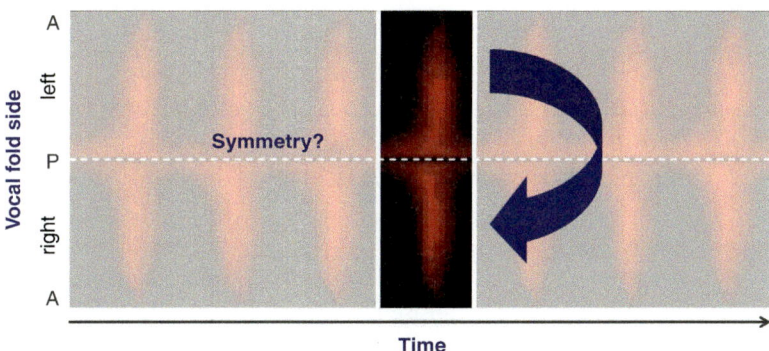

Fig. 6.19 PVG evaluation of glottal closure

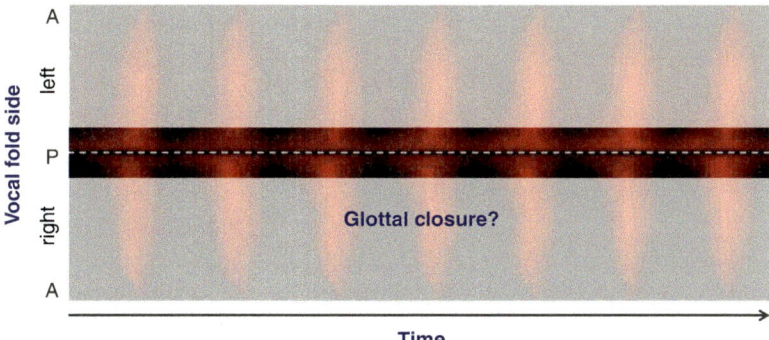

Asymmetrical modes of vibration are only visualisable by using PVG. These lateral differences can appear when phonatory contact at the midline between the vocal folds is too weak (right-left asymmetry, N cycles on one side over M on the other, $N \neq M$, usually with $N = M + 1$). Anterior-posterior asymmetry (in which right and left vocal folds vibrate evenly but dorsal and ventral vocal folds have different frequencies) appears much less often. Whereas right-left asymmetry can result from various disorders, such as post-operative condition, paresis in recovery and others, anterior-posterior asymmetry belongs under the general term functional dysphonia. However, the reverse does not hold: functional dysphonia is only occasionally anterior-posterior asymmetry (Eysholdt 2014).

PVG cannot show any morphological criteria of the endolarynx. Redness resulting from inflammation, change in shape due to swelling or a tumour and change in mucosal texture: none of these can be seen on PVG. This is a consequence of the great degree of data compression and reduction, which focus only on moving areas of the vocal folds. PVG exclusively shows movement.

6.4 Tips and Tricks for Laryngeal Examination: A Handy Guide

Ahmed Geneid

The contents of this section comprise four parts:

- Before the examination
- Carrying out the basic examination
- Having a better view
- Other tricks

6.4.1 Talking with the Patient Before the Examination

In psychology, priming is an effect in which exposure to a certain stimulus influences the response to another stimulus. The exposure stimulus can be perceptual or semantic. In other words, if you start talking to the patient about the gag reflex, repeat the word and explain it too much, then you may end up getting a more frightened patient with a more sensitive gag reflex than his norm. If you start talking about how easy it is to examine the larynx and give the necessary information, then you may expect more cooperation from the patient.

Shaky hands searching for the instruments give the impression of a less experienced clinician. The reason may be that you just had too much coffee in the morning or that the examination room changed and it is your first time in the new room. However, the patient is not aware of your reasons and is just interpreting unconsciously the perceptual impression received from you.

Give the needed information, and if, for one reason or another, you have much time before the examination, then feel free to talk about voice and how stroboscopy works and shape the discussion to the cultural and educational background of the patient.

6.4.2 Carrying Out the Basic Examination

6.4.2.1 Positioning of the Patient

Laryngeal examination can be rendered quite simple for both the phoniatrician and the patient when the patient is positioned the right way. Adhere to the following steps and watch the video of positioning the patient:

- Ask the patients to sit with hips to the back as far as possible, with a straight back. Then ask the patient to lean the back forward from the waist with the head extended. Usually this is called the 'sniffing the air' position. In Scandinavia, where I work, I would hint that the patient take the position of a ski jumper.
- Be sure that patient's shoulders are down and relaxed. The more the patient raises them, the less space you will have inside the throat.
- Patient's hands are best resting on knees. Legs uncrossed.

- Remember that a patient's retraction of the head will limit your vision of the vocal folds. Reposition the patient's head to have a better view.

6.4.2.2 Examination with a Rigid Laryngoscope

After the patient is positioned, I usually opt for what I call a 'dry training', in which I ask the patient to protrude his tongue; I support it gently and ask the patient to have a sustained /ee:/ (as in 'see'). This dry training is done first without the laryngoscope. The idea is to teach the right position to the patient and ease fears about the examination. After this dry training, I start with positioning the rigid laryngoscope. My aim is not to touch the structures from the base of the tongue and backwards. If the patient has a quite sensitive gag reflex, then I would introduce the rigid laryngoscope while the patient is phonating, and then I ask the patient to breathe while the endoscope is there. The sound /ee:/ (as in 'see') is best taught to before the examination. During the examination, it is common that the patient is not able to produce it, so instruct him to think about it while phonating; this will get you the area of vision needed. Spray anaesthesia should be used if the gag reflex hinders the examination. Especially for stroboscopy, it can prevent the muscular hypertension that may influence the vibratory pattern, but on the other hand, the tactile-kinaesthetic feedback may be influenced too.

6.4.2.3 Examination with a Flexible Endoscope

Many patients tolerate the flexible endoscope better than the rigid. However, some cannot stand the idea of something going through their nose. Positioning of the patient is important here as well but without the need for a full 'sniffing the air' position.

I usually tend to use anaesthesia coupled with decongestant on a cotton probe rather than spraying Xylocaine, which causes more irritation. Choose the nostril side that is better anatomically and apply the anaesthesia and decongestant in the middle meatus of the nasal cavity if you would also like to assess the velopharyngeal port, other-

wise you may find it enough to go through the lower meatus. Lidocaine jelly can also be used, taking care to apply it a few millimetres to the back from the scope lens to avoid disturbing the visualisation.

Hold the fibrescope in line with the nostril with your hands holding it below the level of the nose.

In functional endoscopic evaluation of swallowing, I prefer to carry it out without anaesthesia and also through the middle meatus. A decongestant can be applied. The idea is to avoid the anaesthetic leaking to the larynx and distorting the results of the examination. Another option is to apply a small amount of anaesthesia with a cotton probe to the front part of middle meatus.

Using the middle meatus enables the examination of the velum much better than if you have the fibrescope on the floor of the nasal cavity.

6.4.2.4 Positioning of Observers

In many cases there are people other than you and the patient in the examination room. They can be a nurse, spouse of the patient, students or other observers visiting your clinic. It is best if they are standing either behind the patient or in his blind spot. The patient may get quite distracted or even frightened by the reactions on the faces of the observers.

6.4.3   Having a Better View

6.4.3.1 Examining the Piriform Fossa

This can be done easily by blowing out the cheeks with the mouth closed. It is easier to perform with flexible nasofibrescopy. It also works well with the rigid laryngoscope and the patient rounding his lips around the laryngoscope and blowing his cheeks out.

6.4.3.2 Examining the Vocal Folds Closely Above and Below

Getting the endoscope quite close to the upper side of vocal folds during intermittent phonation can initiate the gag reflex, especially on touching the epiglottis or aryepiglottic folds. One way to avoid this is to move the endoscope down to the vocal fold level while the patient sustains phonation.

For certain patients, especially those with possible changes on the lower side of the vocal folds, you may want to get a closer look of the lower side of the vocal folds. Usually, it is quite tricky trying to get the scope down through the glottis without touching the vocal folds and starting a marked coughing episode. A nice trick for that deals with our innate reflex associated with inspiration, in other words the forced opening of the glottis during inspiration. Such forced opening is usually lengthened in duration with inspiration through only one nostril. Accordingly, with the flexible scope in one nostril, ask the patient to breathe in through the other while the mouth is closed. Apply a little pressure to close the nostril housing the flexible fibrescope. The result should be a long inspiration from the other nostril with sufficient opening of the glottis. This will give you the time to dip the tip of your fibrescope just below the vocal fold. Examine one vocal fold lower side at a time.

6.4.3.3 Visual Examination of the Valleculae and the Base of the Tongue

Visualising the valleculae and the base of the tongue with the rigid laryngoscope can be troublesome for a junior phoniatrician or laryngologist. It may give the feeling that the tongue base papillae and lingual tonsillar tissues are hypertrophied when they are not. palpation and the use of a laryngeal mirror should be performed when in doubt. It may add a few minutes to the examination time but will save unneeded consultations.

During flexible laryngoscopy, it is easy to get a better visualisation of this region by asking the patient to protrude the tongue.

6.4.3.4 Examining the Vertical Position of the Vocal Folds When Suspecting Superior Laryngeal Nerve Injury

A suspicion of superior laryngeal injury entails the need to examine the position of the vocal folds if they happen to be at different heights. Sometimes this can be easily detected if the difference is marked with one vocal fold hanging above the other. However, in many situations the difference in position may be quite small, and the monocular vision offered by the laryngoscope does not help in seeing it. In order to gain a binocular vision, you need to use both of your eyes. This can be done by using an otolaryngologic microscope and a laryngeal mirror. Focal distance should be changed to 35 cm from 20 cm, which is usually used for the ear.

6.4.4 Other Tricks

6.4.4.1 Stroboscope Is Not Available or Not Working

Stroboscopy or high-speed stroboscopy should always be used when carrying out laryngoscopic examination. However, if for one reason or another you do not have such possibility, then the vocal fold edge can be inspected while the vocal folds are abducted during respiration. This will enable you to assess with a sharp image the edge lesions that are usually blurred in phonation.

6.4.4.2 No Laryngoscope Available

Needless to say, you should really consider the administrative reason that left you, a phoniatrician, without your main tool. However, saving the day is possible. A nasal endoscope of 70° can be used for laryngeal examination; just remember to turn it upside down. The picture you get will be quite small in comparison with that from a laryngoscope. A laryngeal mirror combined with a microscope is also a good option and will enhance your experience in using such a demanding technique.

6.4.4.3 Working with Diplophonia and Triggering Problems

Stroboscopy is based on getting a stable audio signal from the patient. Irregularity of the signal will fail to trigger a regular series of light flashes, resulting in an inability to see to the vocal fold vibrations.

In cases of diplophonia, one good way of getting over this problem is to focus on one vocal fold at a time and search for the right frequency at which stroboscopy will work. This can be helped by asking the patient to phonate /ee:/ (as in 'see') at different frequencies following your examples. If this does not work, then one more trick that I use quite rarely is to have the stroboscope microphone attached to my neck rather than the patient's. By searching for the right frequency, you will get a better visualisation of the patient's vocal folds during vibration. You may end up seeing only one or two sustained phases of the vibration showing up a standstill pictures.

If the voice is relatively unstable, as it can be in cases of non-organic dysphonia, then ask the patient to phonate with closed lips. The result is elongation of the vocal tract by addition of the nasal cavities resulting in a more stabilised phonation.

6.4.4.4 Rigid Laryngoscopy and Fibrescopy for Children

Rigid laryngoscopy can work very well for children. The youngest I had was 3 years old. Refrain from using anaesthesia. Rigid laryngoscopy for children can be easier and more easily administered than nasofibrescopy, which requires more cooperation from the child.

Fibrescopy requires more preparation than rigid endoscopy. Use adrenaline or other constricting agents on a cotton bud to ensure more space for the fibrescope. I usually refrain from using Xylocaine spray owing to its irritating effect. The paediatric fibrescope has quite a small diameter that significantly limits the size of the obtained picture. However, it is better tolerated by small children. Requiring a paediatric fibrescope to drop from the middle to the lower meatus suggests that using an adult fibrescope is a better option. Adult fibrescopes can be used with children older than 5 years. Giving a lollipop to children is an excellent idea during fibrescopic examination. Its function in the examination is to make sure that the child is happily breathing through the nose resulting in opening of the velopharyngeal valve. Accordingly, the way will be open for the fibrescope from the nasal cavity downwards.

Acknowledgements Ideas mentioned in this article are the summation of what I have learned from colleagues or personally developed. The list of these colleagues is quite long. However, I am indebted to Nasser Kotby from Egypt, Per-Åke Lindestad from Sweden and Erkki Vilkman, Mari Markkanen-Leppänen, Teemu Kinnari and Maaria Ansaranta from Finland.

6.5 Videokymography

František Šram, Jan G. Švec, and Jitka Vydrová

6.5.1 Introduction: Videokymography (VKG) and Kymographic Techniques

The technique of videokymography (VKG) was developed as a low-cost, clinician-friendly version of laryngoscopic high-speed video (HSV) systems (Švec and Schutte 1996). It allows correct display of the patterns of vocal fold vibrations that cannot be properly visualised by stroboscopy (such as irregularities and instabilities, including severe hoarseness and register transitions). In contrast to the full HSV system, videokymography does not record the full images of the larynx but records only images from a single selected line at a high rate (currently 7200 line images per second). This reduces the amount of recorded data and makes the technique faster and less demanding on the recording and storage equipment than the full HSV. The VKG examination line can be placed at any location of the vocal folds. When captured, the line images are placed sequentially to form a new 'kymographic' image ('videokymogram', or in short 'kymogram') that displays the behaviour of the vocal folds at the specific selected location in real time.

The current generation videokymography (Qiu and Schutte 2006) utilises a special video camera (i.e. videokymographic camera) providing the kymographic images in real time, simultaneously and side by side with the standard laryngoscopic images of the vocal folds (Fig. 6.20). The immediate availability of the images makes the VKG method suitable for use in busy clinical practice, and it also distinguishes VKG from other HSV

Fig. 6.20 The standard laryngoscopic (left) and VKG (right) images, which are delivered simultaneously by the second-generation VKG camera. The VKG image shows the normal behaviour of the vocal folds in time (40 ms duration, time running from top to bottom) at the location marked by the line in the standard image. The examined subject was a 43-year-old male without voice problems. Symbols used: *rf/lf* right/left vocal fold; *rv/lv* right/left ventricular fold; *rm/lm* right/left laterally travelling mucosal wave

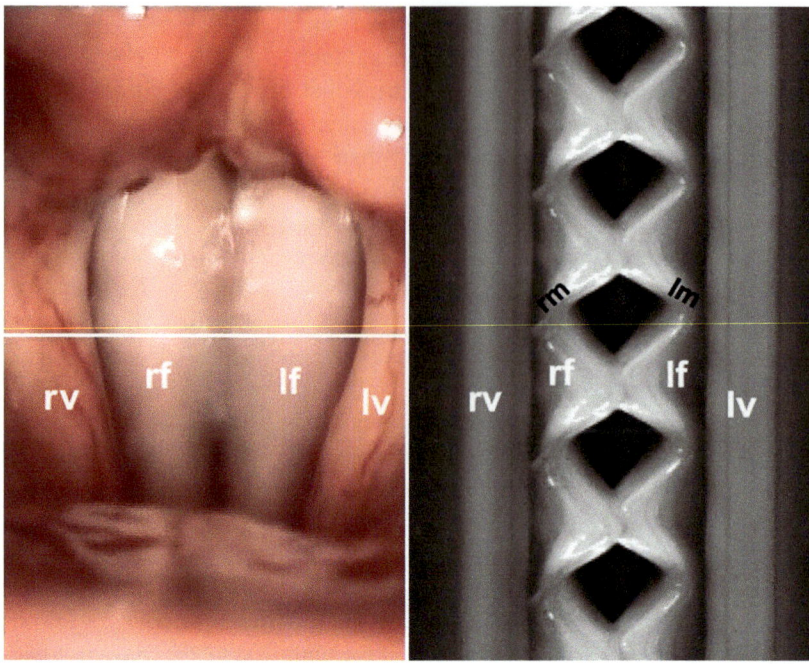

systems that can visualise or process the images only after the recording has taken place.

Apart from videokymography, which is based on a special video camera (hardware), the principle of kymographic imaging has also been applied to obtaining kymographic images from full high-speed videolaryngoscopic (*digital kymography*, DKG (Wittenberg et al. 2000)) and strobo-videoscopic recordings (*strobo-videokymography*, SVKG (Isogai 1994, Sung et al. 1999)). In contrast to VKG, which displays the kymographic images immediately during the examination, the two latter methods employ special software to construct the kymograms from previously obtained high-speed laryngoscopic or videostroboscopic recordings. The advantages and disadvantages of these three kymographic methods are discussed by Švec and Schutte (2012).

In contrast to classical laryngoscopy, which aims at observing and evaluating the *structural appearance* of the vocal folds and of the laryngeal structures, kymography aims at observing and evaluating the *vibratory function* of the vocal folds and of the surrounding tissues. In this sense, the method aims at diagnosing the vibrational, rather than the structural, problems of the laryn-geal tissues. Since voice is produced through vibration of laryngeal tissues, it provides a more detailed insight into the mechanism of voice disorders. *The method is especially useful for discovering vibrational problems in functional dysphonias where the vocal folds do not show any obvious structural abnormality, but the voice is impaired in some way.* The vibrational disorder problems reveal pathophysiological alterations of the vocal folds and surrounding tissues that are difficult to discover otherwise.

6.5.2 VKG Equipment and Examination Procedure

The basic equipment for videokymographic examination consists of (1) *a special videokymographic camera*, (2) *a laryngoscope*, (3) *a continuous light source of high intensity* (300 W xenon light is preferable), (4) *a standard video-capturing system* (computer or a video recorder), (5) *a video monitor* and (6) *a microphone* for capturing the voice signal (Fig. 6.21).

Generally, the examination procedure in videokymography is similar to the video-laryngostroboscopic procedure. The difference

Fig. 6.21 The equipment setup for videokymography

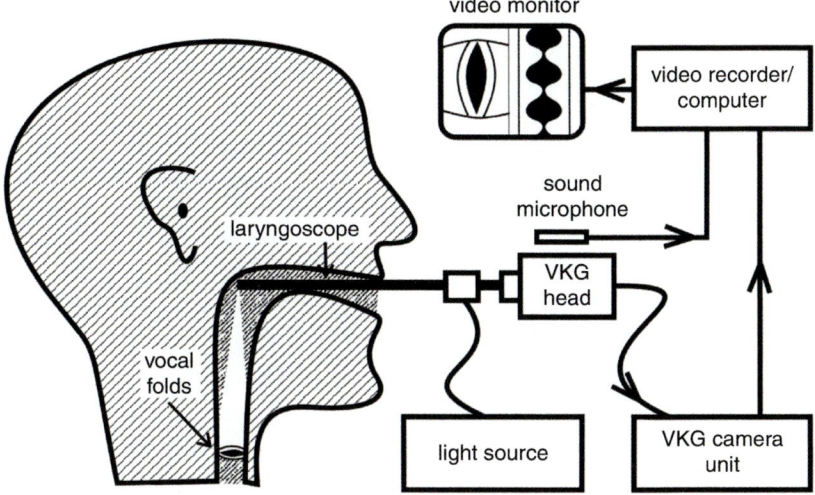

is that the clinician should make sure that during the examination procedure, the measurement line for VKG images is placed at the desirable location on the vocal folds, perpendicular to the glottal axis. Useful tips and tricks on the VKG examination procedure can be found in the publication of Švec and Šram (2011).

6.5.3 Normal VKG Findings

Sustained phonations at a comfortable pitch and loudness (measures to be documented for later comparisons) should ideally present the following properties, which are well visible in the videokymographic images of the vocal folds (recall Fig. 6.20):

- Both vocal folds are vibrating.
- Ventricular folds are not vibrating.
- Vibrational amplitudes of both vocal folds are approximately similar.
- Vibrational frequencies of both vocal folds are approximately the same.
- The vibrations are regular.
- The vibrations are free of aberrations.
- The vocal folds touch each other during vibration at the place of maximum vibration amplitude.

- The closed phase takes from ca. 5 to 65% of period duration at the place of maximum vibration amplitude.
- The shape of lateral peaks (i.e. the turn from opening to closing) is sharp.
- Mucosal waves propagate laterally on the upper vocal fold surface.
- No large left-right phase asymmetry is present.

The vocal fold vibrations vary when changing fundamental frequency (Fig. 6.22), loudness (Fig. 6.23) as well as vocal register (Fig. 6.24), so care should be taken to take these factors into account.

6.5.4 VKG Features in Voice Disorders

Alternations of vibratory features seen in VKG allow different types of vibrational disorders of the larynx to be distinguished (Fig. 6.25). The features and their possible causes are described in detail by Švec et al. (2007, 2009). Some of these are:

- *Completely Absent Vibration of the Vocal Fold* (Fig. 6.25a, rf)—a very serious finding, which can result from a tumour, scar or excessive vocal fold stiffness.

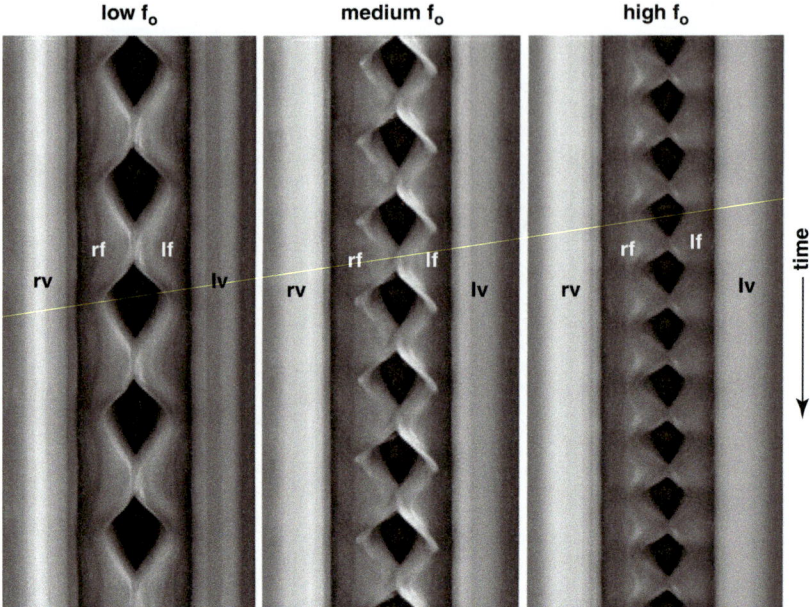

Fig. 6.22 The changes in vocal fold vibration due to increasing fundamental frequency (f_o) in a healthy male subject. Notice the increasing number of periods within the image (from left to right c. 5, 7¼ and 10 cycles, corresponding to the fundamental frequencies of c. 125, 181 and 250 Hz) and the decreasing amplitudes of vibration. The kymograms were obtained at the line perpendicular to glottal axis, in the middle of the membranous glottis. Total time displayed: 40 ms. For abbreviations see legend to Fig. 6.20

Fig. 6.23 The changes in vocal fold vibration due to increasing loudness in a healthy female subject. Notice particularly the enlargement of vibration amplitudes, prolongation of the closed phase and increasing vigour of the laterally travelling mucosal waves (rm, lm) with increasing loudness. The kymograms were obtained at the line perpendicular to glottal axis, in the middle of the membranous glottis. Total time displayed: 18.4 ms. For abbreviations see legend to Fig. 6.20

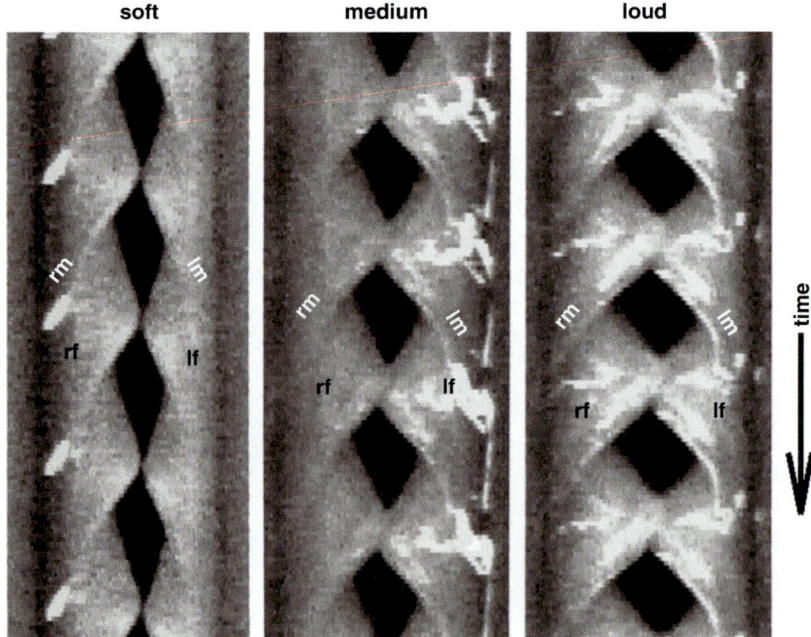

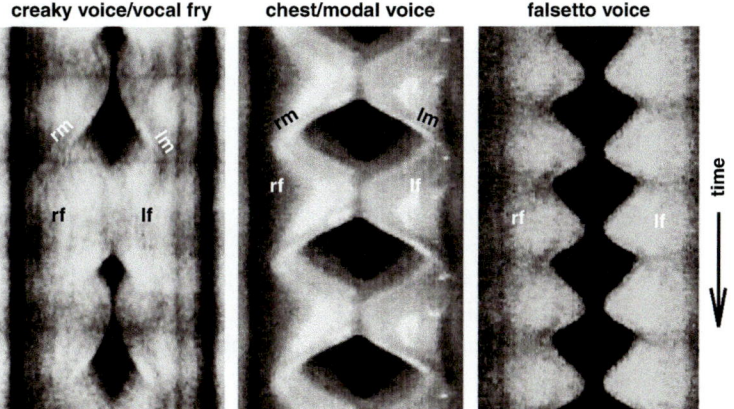

Fig. 6.24 The vocal fold vibration in different voice registers in a healthy male subject. Creaky voice/vocal fry register shows repetition of two different openings and smaller vibration amplitudes than in the typical pattern of the chest/modal register. The falsetto voice reveals no glottal closure, less sharp lateral peaks and reduced mucosal waves. In all the cases, the vibrations are left-right symmetric. The kymograms were obtained at the line perpendicular to glottal axis, in the middle of the membranous glottis. Total time displayed: 18.4 ms. For abbreviations see legend to Fig. 6.20

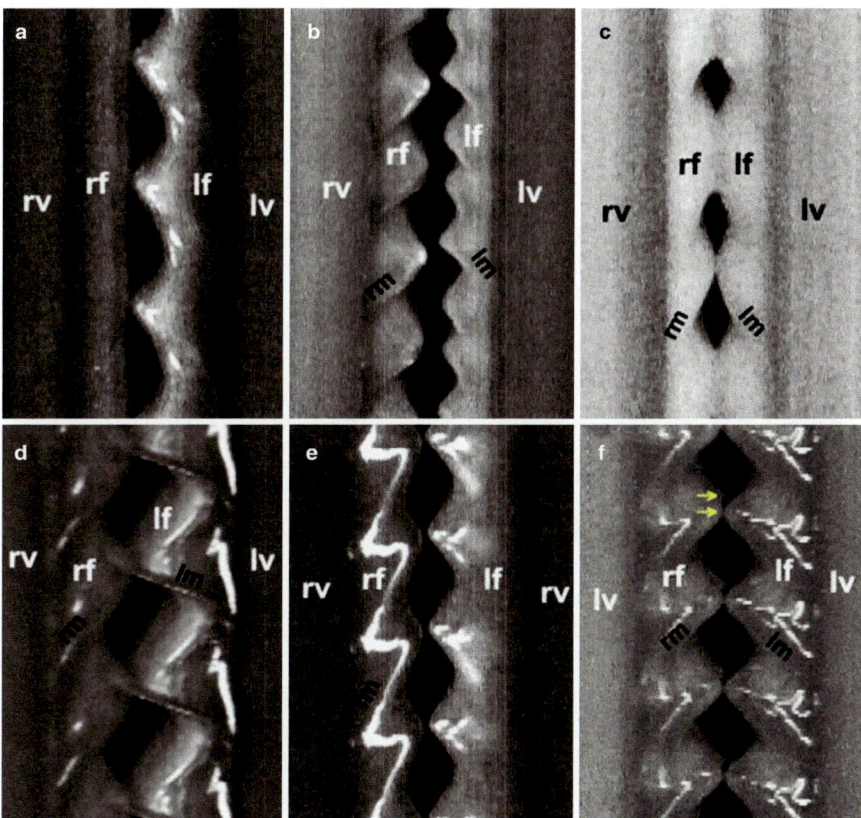

Fig. 6.25 Different types of vibration disorder of the vocal folds revealed in VKG images. Total time displayed in the VKG images: 18.4 ms (from top to bottom). (**a–f**) See the text. For abbreviations see legend to Fig. 6.20

- *Partly Absent Vibration of the Vocal Fold*—can be observed, e.g. when the body of the vocal fold is stiff or in case of a dislocated vocal fold implant.
- *Absence of Glottal Closure* (Fig. 6.25b)—when observed at the place of maximum vibration amplitude at comfortable pitch and loudness, this indicates serious problems with vocal fold adduction. It is typical of voices with strong breathiness. It is a physiological finding in high-pitched or in intentionally breathy voices.
- *Large Cycle-to-Cycle Variability* (Fig. 6.25b, c)—is typical of largely irregular voices and can result, e.g. from left-right vocal fold asymmetry, from anterior-posterior vocal fold asymmetry or from excessively low vocal fold tension.
- *Large Left-Right Amplitude Differences*—indicate large structural differences between the left and right vocal folds. These can result from unilateral laryngeal pathological conditions, such as from, e.g. unilateral vocal fold paralysis.
- *Left-Right Frequency Differences* (Fig. 6.25b)—are mainly observed in subjects with different tension of the left and right vocal folds and lack of glottal closure. They occur most often because of unilateral vocal fold paralysis. The finding usually relates to biphonia or diplophonia.
- *Large Left-Right Phase Differences* (Fig. 6.25d)—are a sign of left-right asymmetry in tension or mass of the vocal folds. This finding can often be observed, e.g. in subjects with unilateral vocal fold paralysis with good glottal closure (i.e. after medialisation surgery) but may also be found in singers complaining of voice problems. Perceptually the voice may sound rather normal, but the asymmetry may limit the usable frequency range.
- *Axis Shift During Closure* (Fig. 6.25d)—indicates left-right asymmetry in vocal fold tension or difference in level of the vocal folds.
- *Decreased Sharpness of Lateral Peaks* (Fig. 6.25a lf, Fig. 6.25e, rf)—indicates

reduced vertical phase differences of the vocal folds, which may result from an excessively stiff mucosa on its medial surface.
- *Absent or Reduced Mucosal Waves on the Upper Vocal Fold Surface* (Fig. 6.25a, lf, Fig. 6.25e, lf)—indicate that the mucosa is excessively stiff on the upper vocal fold surface.
- *Sharpened Medial Peaks* (Fig. 6.25e, lf)—indicate a thinned edge of the vocal fold. It is observable when glottal closure is absent.
- *Ripple (Aberration)*—this is frequently observed anteriorly to a localised lesion on the vocal fold (nodule, polyp, cyst) when the lesion interferes with the vibrations.
- *Double Medial Peak (Aberration)* (Fig. 6.25f, rf-double arrow)—most often indicates the presence of a sulcus or furrow on the medial vocal fold surface.
- *Lack of Smoothness of Medial Peaks (Aberration)*—indicates defective medial vocal fold shape.
- *Large Vibration of Surrounding Tissues (e.g. Ventricular Folds or Aryepiglottic Folds)*—may be found in larynges exhibiting hyperfunction or compensating for glottal insufficiency. Sometimes it can be used voluntarily for special voice effects, e.g. in rock singing (Borch et al. 2004; Lindestad et al. 2001).
- *Co-vibration of Fluids*—is a sign of too much fluid or mucus interfering with the vocal fold vibrations and causing slight irregularities of voice. This may be a result of laryngeal inflammation.

6.5.5 Clinical Examples

Case Study 6.1
A 63-year-old male suffering from dysphonia that arose after a cold and lasted for 4 months. He was a smoker (20 cigarettes daily).

VKG examination: Complete absence of vibration of the left vocal fold was revealed (Fig. 6.26, arrow).

Diagnosis: This raised a suspicion of tumorous infiltration of the left vocal fold. Laryngoscopy

Fig. 6.26 VKG examination images of a subject with left vocal fold carcinoma. The left vocal fold shows complete absence of vibrations (arrow), while the right vocal fold shows normal vibratory behaviour. Total time displayed in the VKG image: 40 ms (from top to bottom). For abbreviations see legend to Fig. 6.20

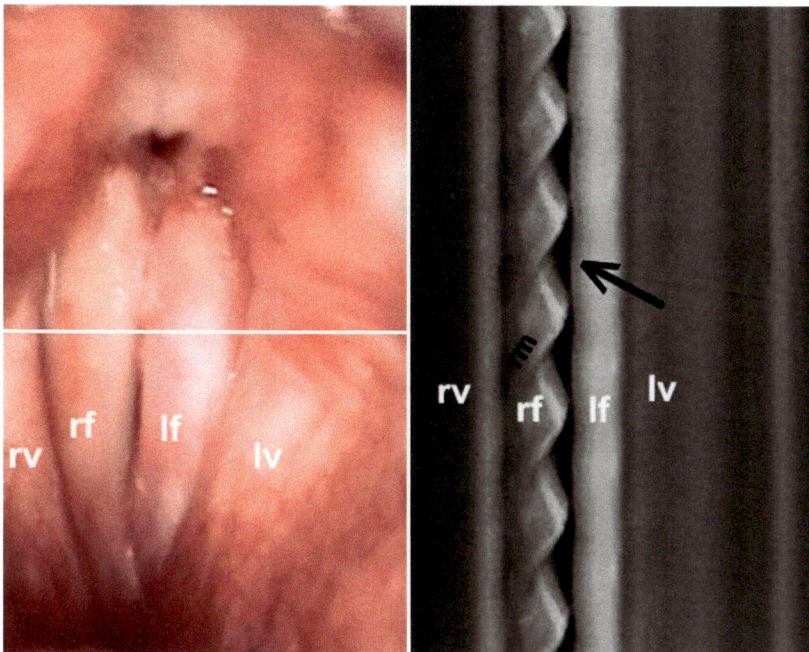

and histological exam revealed squamous cell carcinoma.

Therapy: Left-sided cordectomy.

Result: The patient comes for regular check-ups; currently he is in the fourth year without problems.

Case Study 6.2

A 52-year-old female, professional singer, member of the choir of the Prague Philharmonic Orchestra. Her original diagnosis was breast carcinoma for which she underwent complex therapy 2 years ago—breast ablation, radiotherapy and chemotherapy. Since then she had been on hormonal antioestrogenic medication (Arimidex). After the end of the therapy, she returned to the professional career of a choir singer. During the last 6 months, she experienced voice problems interfering seriously with her career—reduction of voice range, voice instabilities and hoarseness.

VKG examination (Fig. 6.27): Laryngoscopic view revealed slight structural unevenness of the posterior third of the right vocal fold. VKG view showed four abnormal vibrational characteristics revealing an impairment of vocal fold function-

ing: (1) large left-right phase asymmetry indicating different tensions of the two vocal folds; (2) axis shift during glottal closure, again indicating different tensions of the two vocal folds; (3) reduced sharpness of the right lateral peak indicating increased stiffness of the right vocal fold mucosa on the medial surface; and (4) reduced laterally travelling mucosal waves on the right vocal fold indicating increased stiffness of the mucosa of the right upper vocal fold surface.

Diagnosis: Chronic laryngitis with serious stiffening and potential scarification on the right vocal fold mucosa, most likely due to laryngopharyngeal reflux. Reflux episodes penetrating upper oesophageal sphincter were verified by using combined multichannel intraluminal impedance and pH monitoring (Mli-pH).

Therapy: PPI medications, reduced voice usage, work inability.

Result: Presently the patient requests a disability pension. It is probable that the voice problems are partly related to stress from the primary carcinoma diagnosis. There is also a likely relationship to the Arimidex antioestrogen therapy, which is, however, unavoidable in the case of breast carcinoma.

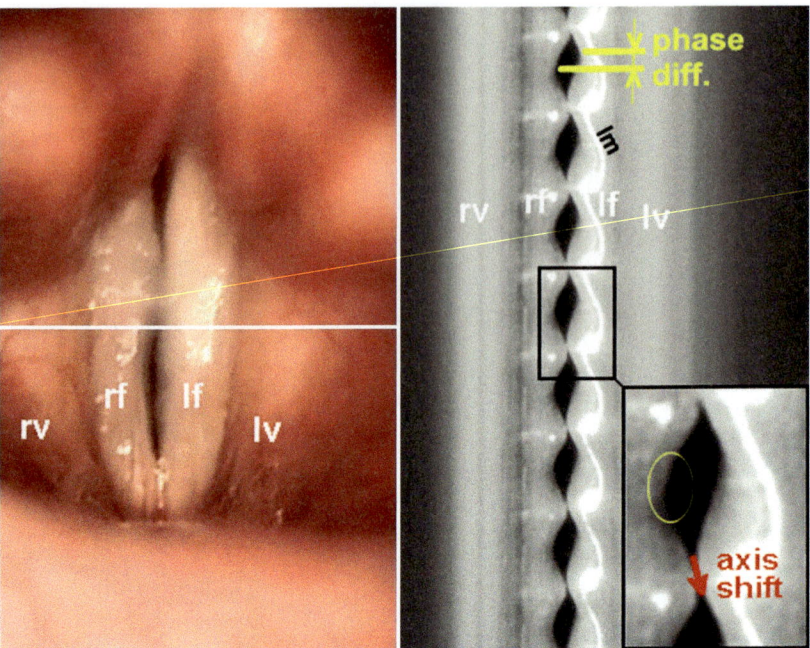

Fig. 6.27 VKG examination images of a female professional singer with decreased mucosal pliability of the right vocal fold. Notice (1) the left-right phase differences of the lateral peaks, (2) axis shift during glottal closure, (3) the markedly more rounded lateral peak on the right vocal fold (yellow ellipse) than on the left one and (4) hardly any presence of laterally travelling mucosal waves on the right vocal fold, whereas these are clearly present on the left one (lm). Total time displayed in the VKG image: 40 ms (from top to bottom). For abbreviations see legend to Fig. 6.20

Case Study 6.3

A 72-year-old male, retired accountant. The voice was husky, produced with an incorrect technique, usually pressed with breathiness, exhibiting poorly controlled changes in pitch and loudness.

VKG examination (Fig. 6.28): Laryngoscopic images showed rather normal-looking vocal folds with the vocal processes mostly pressed together during phonation. Intermittently, there was linear membranous glottal gap. VKG images revealed various vibratory patterns of the vocal folds, including regular, subharmonic and irregular patterns. The mucosal wave was present. Noticeably, all the patterns were left-right symmetric suggesting no problems with the left-right imbalance of the vocal folds.

Diagnosis: Aged voice, bilateral paresis m. interni, intermittent linear membranous glottal gap, laryngo-pharyngeal reflux.

Therapy: Voice hygiene, reflux treatment.

Result: The voice quality and the vibrational alterations correspond to the age of the patient.

6.5.6 Summary

Videokymography is an optical laryngoscopic examination method that is mainly aimed at diagnosing vibration disorders of the vocal folds. These are the basic cause of voice disorders. A special videokymographic camera is used to capture the standard laryngoscopic video images simultaneously with the high-speed kymographic images showing the vibratory pattern of the vocal folds at a selected location. This also allows diagnosis of small alterations of the vocal fold vibrations. These alterations could result from inflammatory as well as from tumorous infiltration of the vocal fold tissues. Furthermore, it

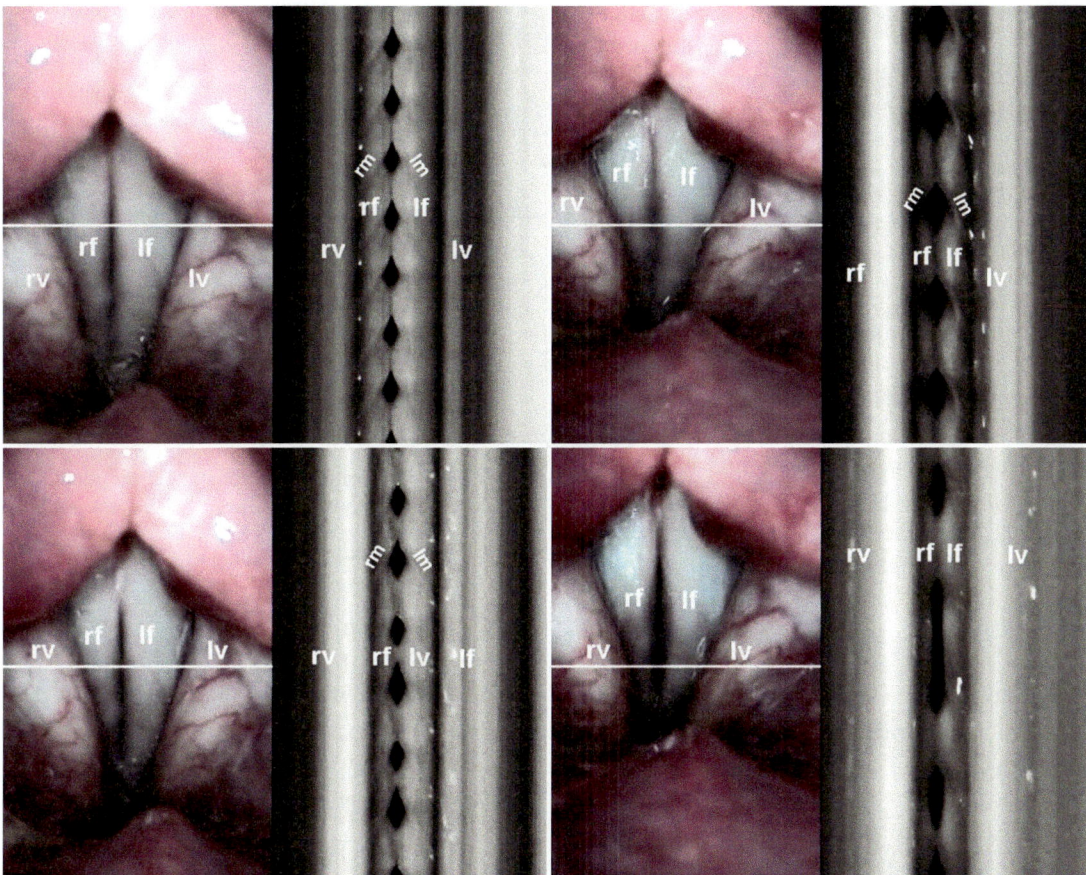

Fig. 6.28 Four VKG examination images of a male subject with an aged voice. Notice the variability of the vibration pattern of the vocal folds. Top: regular voice at higher (right) and lower (left) pitch. Bottom: dicrotic vocal fold vibration showing repetition of two glottal openings of different shapes at higher vocal fold tension (left) and irregular vocal fold vibration at lower vocal fold tension (right). Total time displayed in the VKG image: 40 ms (from top to bottom). For abbreviations see legend to Fig. 6.20

allows diagnosis of vocal fold mucosa impairments, small scars, submucosal blood vessel dilations and vocal fold oedema of allergic or hormonal origins. Visual clinical evaluation of the videokymographic pattern requires knowledge of the normal vocal fold vibratory pattern and of the correlation between the pattern alterations and the pathophysiology of the vocal fold tissue disorders. The method is very useful for early diagnosis of vocal fold cancer. It allows recognition of tissue pathology at the stages when the laryngoscopic or laryngostroboscopic images still look normal.

6.6 Stroboscopic and Kymographic Examinations of Lip Vibrations in Brass Musicians

Renate Haubrich and Wolfgang Angerstein

6.6.1 Introduction

Lip vibrations in brass musicians can be investigated and video-documented by stroboscopy and kymography. These non-invasive imaging techniques are relevant within the practice of musicians medicine for assessing the occupational (in)capacity of professional brass musicians. Helmholtz (1875) stated:

> Only two kinds of membranous tongues have to be considered as musical instruments: the human lips in brass instruments, and the human larynx in singing.

Sounds can be produced by vibration of the mucosal or muscular layers of the vocal folds. This is also true for the lips: the anatomical requirement for sound generation is the multilayered construction of both tone generators. In the larynx, the mucous membrane is connected to the vocal ligament and vocal muscle via a thin layer of connective tissue (Reinke's space). This multilayered construction of the vocal folds is also referred to as the 'body-cover model' (Hirano 1974; Story and Titze 1995). A similar multilayered construction also exists in the lips (internally to externally: the mucosa, submucosa with glands, orbicularis oris muscle, subcutis and epidermis) (Tillmann 1997; Paulsen 2010; Welsch 2006).

Phoniatricians have used imaging methods to examine high-frequency vibrations of the vocal folds for many decades (stroboscopy, Schönhärl 1960; Luchsinger 1949; Oertel 1878, 1895; Böhme and Gross 2001; kymography, Böhme and Gross 2001; Šram et al. 1998; Gall et al. 1971; Gross 1985). Therefore it is obviously justified to employ stroboscopy and kymography when lip vibrations of brass musicians are examined. Martin (1942) developed a method by which lip vibrations of a French horn player could be investigated stroboscopically. Damsté (1966) compared the vibrations of a singer's vocal folds to the vibrations of the lips of a trombonist. Kymographic studies of a trombonist's lip vibrations were described by Šram and Švec (2000).

6.6.2 Occupation-Specific Diseases

Embouchure is the word that wind instrumentalists use to describe the way the mouth is held during performance. It is derived from the French *bouche*, meaning mouth. The definition of embouchure normally refers to the lips and facial muscles, but the teeth and jaw are integral to its function and the embouchure could not function without them.

Campos (2005)

When this complex interaction of various muscle groups gets out of control, embouchure problems result: the physician Flesch (1925) reported on a trumpeter with

> convulsions in the orbicularis oris. The patient could not blow a tone.

Similar difficulties of the lower lip were described by the neurologist Singer (1926):

> The lower lip of a trumpeter slid off the mouthpiece 'as if paralysed'. Tones of a certain pitch could not be blown anymore (…). But there was no pain involved, only the feeling of a heavy 'chunk' in the mouth (cheek), the outblown airjet seemed to flee between the upper lip and the mouthpiece.

These painless disease patterns are nowadays called 'embouchure dystonia'. In early stages, the disease manifests as a:

> subtle deficiency of sound production, mainly in a certain register, a certain style or a clearly defined dynamic range.

Altenmüller and Jabusch (2008)

Later the disease expands to the whole ambitus and all dynamic ranges of the instrument. Then, control over the embouchure, articulation and breathing cannot be ensured for any kind of playing technique. Quite likely the sound will break off, and side tones will appear. Air leaks can occur besides the mouthpiece; brass players may have spasms or tremor of the involved musculature (Altenmüller and Jabusch 2008). Furthermore, tremor of the lips, involuntary closure of the lips ('liplock') and locking of the jaw can be experienced in embouchure dystonia (Frucht et al. 2001; Frucht 2009). The Meige syndrome in brass players is a combination of embouchure dystonia with blepharospasm (Frucht et al. 2001; Frucht 2009).

Even a rupture of the orbicularis oris muscle is possible when the lips are tensed excessively (especially when playing very high pitches) (Arcier and Vernay 1994; Papsin et al. 1996;

Donnet et al. 1996; Planas 1982, 1988; Maneiro 2014). A prominent patient who suffered from rupture of the lip musculature was Louis Armstrong. 'Satchmo's syndrome' (Planas 1982) is characterised by fatigability of the lip musculature and the inability to produce high pitches, often accompanied by pain (Papsin et al. 1996; Donnet et al. 1996; Maneiro 2014; Liu and Hayden 2002). An injury of the orbicularis oris muscle can force the brass musician to stop playing temporarily or may result in a permanent occupational incapacity, with serious economic consequences (Maneiro 2014). In the literature an operative reconstruction of the orbicularis oris muscle is highly recommended (Papsin et al. 1996; Planas 1982, 1988; Sullivan 1989).

Functional diseases (embouchure dystonia (Altenmüller and Jabusch 2006a)) as well as organic lesions of the lips (soft tissue wounds (Bumiller 1936), pressure-induced neuropathy (Zeller 1985; Loock and Lorenz 1981; Schuppert and Altenmüller 2000) and Satchmo's syndrome (Arcier and Vernay 1994; Planas 1982, 1988; Maneiro 2014)) can lead to an incapacity for work in brass players. Landeck (1974) reported that in the vast majority of brass players with chronic lesions of the lip, an early retirement or an occupational retraining is inevitable.

Thirteen per cent of German orchestra musicians have to give up their profession for health reasons (Böckelmann and Schneyer 2009), about 1% of professional musicians suffer from occupation-specific dystonia (musicians dystonia) (Altenmüller and Jabusch 2006b; Rozanski et al. 2015). Damage of the lip nerves due to pressure exerted by the mouthpiece is recognised as a pathogenetic agent for an occupational disease in brass players (BK-Nr. 2106, Ärztl. Sachverständigenrat beim Bundesministerium für Arbeit u. Sozialordnung (BMA) 2002). Thus, musicians dystonia as an 'occupation-specific and occupational disease' should be included in the schedule of occupational diseases (Rozanski et al. 2015). Assessment of the embouchure function in brass players is therefore relevant for entitlements from institutions for statutory accident insurance and prevention.

6.6.3   Methodology

Brass musicians lips are observed while playing by using a rigid endoscope inserted into a bore hole of the mouthpiece.

The optimal position for the bore hole can be determined separately for each individual mouthpiece. This is done by positioning the 70° endoscope above the cup of the mouthpiece so that the outer rim of the mouthpiece is completely visible through the endoscope. The distance between endoscope tip and outer rim is measured and mirrored on a horizontal axis along the outer rim. This measurement defines the optimal position for the bore hole. The bore hole is drilled at a 70° angle into the cup of the mouthpiece, and a thread is tapped into it.

A guiding sleeve with a knurled screw is subsequently screwed into the hole (cf. Fig. 6.29, lower image). The 70° endoscope (cf. Fig. 6.29, upper image) is inserted into the guiding sleeve and fixed with a coupler.

Fine adjustments may be done by turning the knurled screw of the guiding sleeve slightly upwards or downwards, depending on the configuration of the mouthpiece (semi-spherical or conical cups). Lighting is provided by a fibre optic cable, screwed onto the endoscope. The mouthpiece is connected to the instrument, and a stroboscopy or kymography camera is clipped onto the endoscope (cf. Fig. 6.30).

An airborne-sound microphone mounted on a stand approximately 1 m from the bell of the

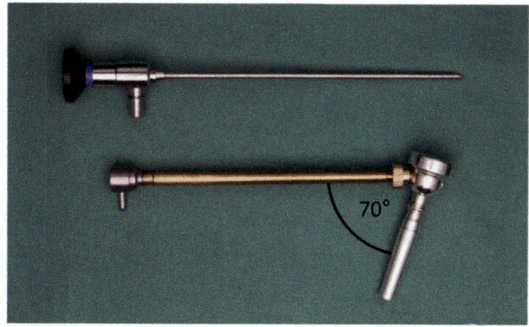

Fig. 6.29 Trumpet mouthpiece with fixed guiding sleeve and a separate 70° endoscope (© Mauersberger 2016)

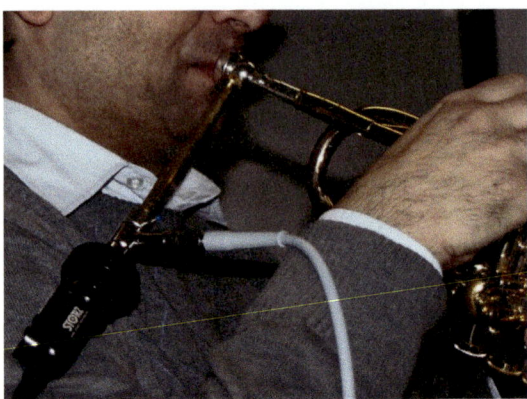

Fig. 6.30 Trumpeter's examination by a mouthpiece with lateral bore hole, guiding sleeve, attached endoscope and camera (© Mauersberger 2016)

instrument triggers the stroboscope. Alternatively, a contact microphone can be placed on one cheek, near the corner of the mouth.

For the observation of lip vibrations, this standardised device with fixed coupling between endoscope and camera on the one hand and mouthpiece with instrument on the other hand is suitable. Thus, motion artefacts (e.g. generated when using freehand endoscopy) are avoided. In contrast to the depiction of the vibrating lips via fenestrated mouthpieces, this technique allows the instrument to be played without loss of air. Near-real playing conditions are created by using the musician's own instrument with a modified commercial quality mouthpiece.

6.6.4 Examination

Before the examination, the musicians should be asked to play 'dry' (i.e. without moistening the lips with saliva), and the mouthpiece should be slightly warmed (e.g. through submerging it in warm water) in order to reduce misting of the optics from the player's breath.

Examination of lip vibrations begins after an individual warm-up period. The exercises that are to be played should be passages consisting of various dynamics (pianissimo to fortissimo), articulations (staccato and legato) and pitches. They should cover the entire technical spectrum

of the instrument in order to imitate the player's 'natural strain' (such as in a concert or opera) as closely as possible.

6.6.5 Evaluation

6.6.5.1 Stroboscopy

Vibration Phases Opening, closing, open and closed phases of the lip vibration cycle can be distinguished by stroboscopy, analogously to those of the vocal folds (Böhme and Gross 2001; Nawka 2012).

During the opening phase (see Fig. 6.31; 45–180°), the distance between the lips increases. In the closing phase (see Fig. 6.31; 180–315°), the upper and lower lips come closer to each other. The complete time period during which the lips are open (see Fig. 6.31; 45–315°) is known as the open phase. The open phase is therefore the sum of the opening and closing phases. In the closed phase (see Fig. 6.31; 0° und 360°), the oral fissure is completely shut.

Embouchure Types Various embouchure types of brass players were described by Leno (1971, 1974, 1995, 2009) through stroboscopic visualisation and were more precisely distinguished by Reinhardt (1973): by mouthpiece position and direction of exhaled airstream, upstream or downstream types can be classified (Leno 1971, 1974, 1995, 2009). The downstream type (see Fig. 6.32) is characterised by a prominent upper lip, which directs the airstream downwards into the mouthpiece. The mouthpiece is positioned high (Leno 1971, 1974, 1995, 2009; Wilken 2009). The upstream type (see Fig. 6.33) is characterised by a prominent lower lip, which directs the airstream upwards into the mouthpiece. The mouthpiece is positioned low. This embouchure type is much less common than the downstream type (Leno 1971, 1974, 1995, 2009; Wilken 2009).

The embouchure type depends on the individual anatomy (including positioning of the teeth, distance between oral fissure and columella base

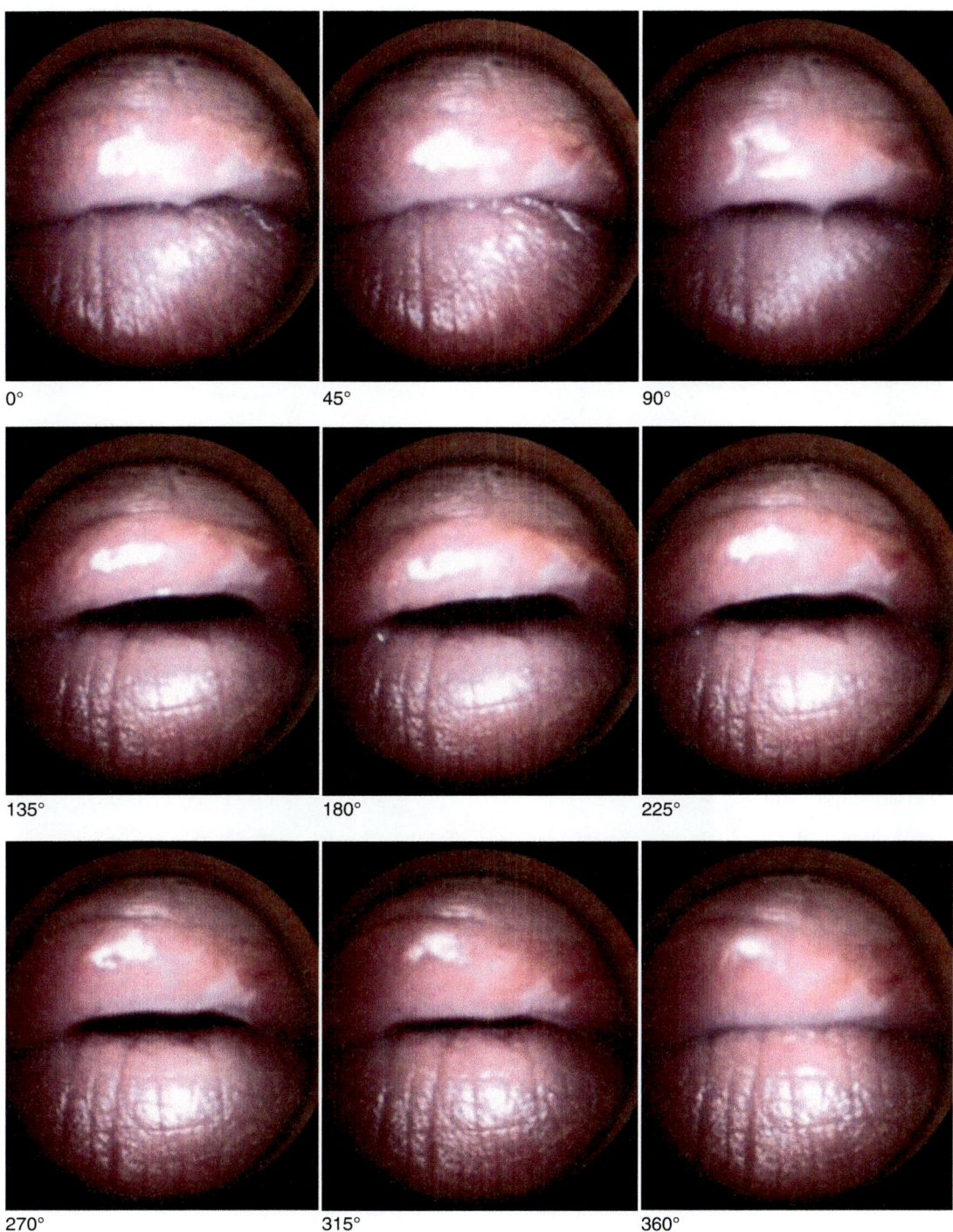

Fig. 6.31   Stroboscopic vibration cycle of a trumpeter's lips (266 Hz, C4, mezzo forte) (© Mauersberger 2016)

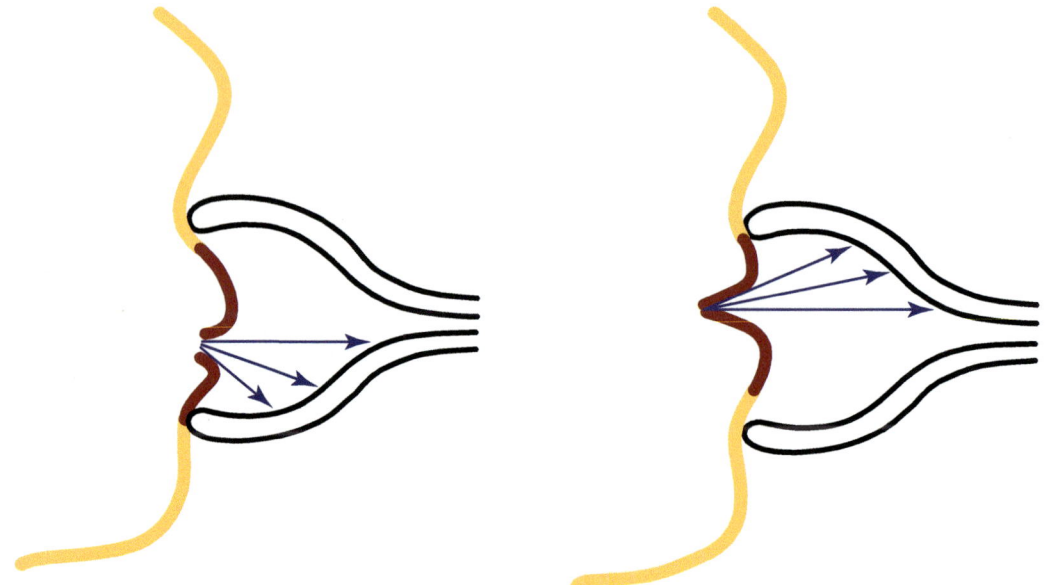

Fig. 6.32 Downstream type (© Mauersberger 2016)

Fig. 6.33 Upstream type (© Mauersberger 2016)

Fig. 6.34 Horizontal mucosal waves (**a**) on the upper lip of a trombonist (downstream type) and (**b**) on the lower lip of a trombonist (upstream type), (© Mauersberger 2016)

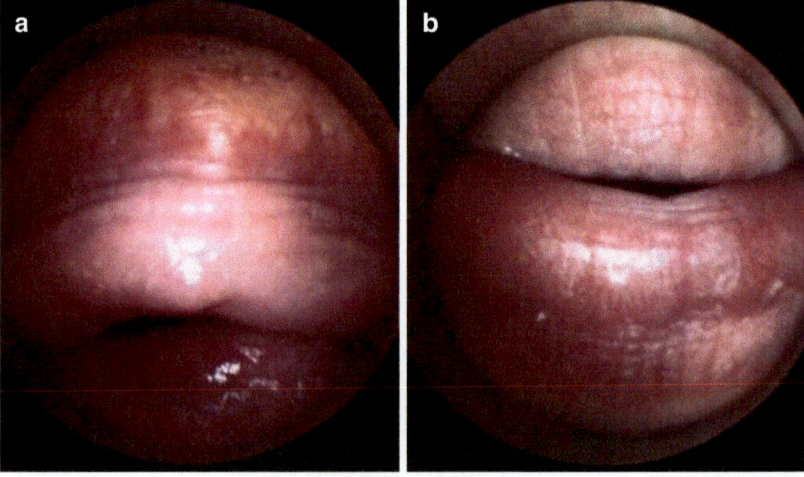

and lip morphology) and cannot be trained (Wilken 2009). Upstream and downstream types are possible with both high embouchure (mouthpiece closer to the nose) and low embouchure (mouthpiece closer to the chin) (Wilken 2009).

Functional Analyses As for the vocal folds, the vibrating lips of a brass player should be initially assessed for the sufficiency of lip closure and phase synchronicity (comparison of upper and lower lip vibrations). In addition, mucosal waves can often be observed on the vibrating lips, analogously to the displacement of the marginal edge of the vocal folds (see Fig. 6.34).

Seidner and Eysholdt (2005) identify the displacements of the marginal edge of the vocal folds as

> movements of the superficial mucosa sliding on a gliding layer […] over the muscle.

Fig. 6.35 Functional mucosal distensions of the upper lip (**a**) in the middle, swinging towards the examiner in the sagittal plane, and (**b**) right paramedian, swinging downwards into the oral fissure in the frontal plane (© Mauersberger 2016)

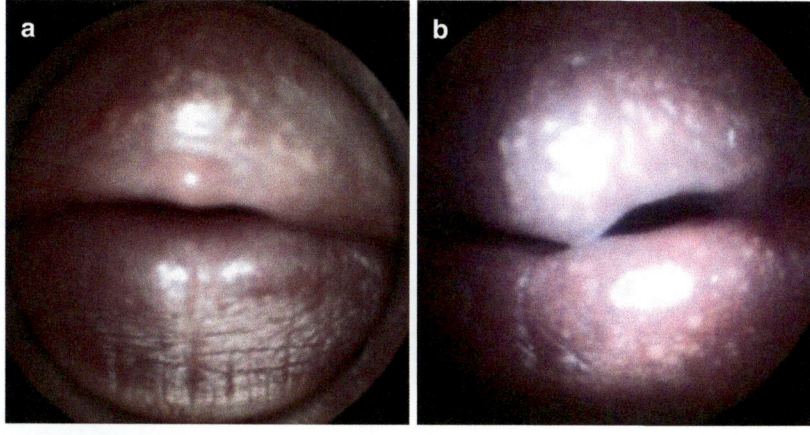

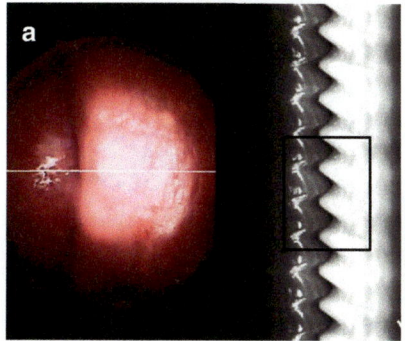

Fig. 6.36 (**a**) Opening, closing, open and closed phases of the lip vibration cycle, observed in a trumpeter (247 Hz, H3, mezzo forte); (**b**) detailed image enlargement rotated 90° to the left: red arrow, opening phase; blue arrow, closing phase; purple arrow, open phase; green arrow, closed phase (© Mauersberger 2016)

Similar

movements of the superficial mucosa […] over the muscle

also exist on the lips.

Functional mucosal distensions are occasionally seen, which presumably arise through the Bernoulli suction and should not necessarily be evaluated as pathological (see Fig. 6.35).

6.6.5.2 Kymography

In kymographic images (Figs. 6.36, 6.37, 6.38, 6.39, 6.40, and 6.41), the upper lip is displayed on the right and the lower lip on the left side.

Vibration Phases Analogous to stroboscopic observations, opening, closing, open and closed phases can also be distinguished by kymographic examinations (see Fig. 6.36). This phase classification of lip vibration cycles is based on the

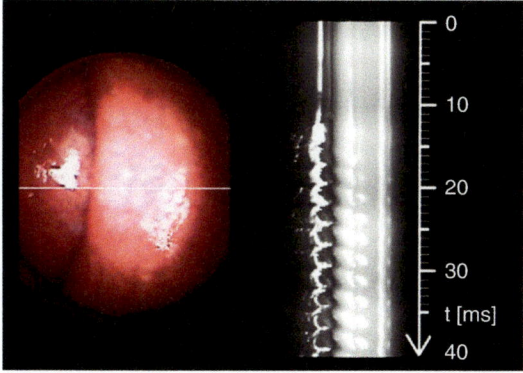

Fig. 6.37 Onset phase of a trumpeter (© Mauersberger 2016)

kymographic analysis of vocal fold vibrations by Gall and Hanson (1973) and by Švec's research group (Böhme and Gross 2001; Švec et al. 1999; Švec and Šram 2002).

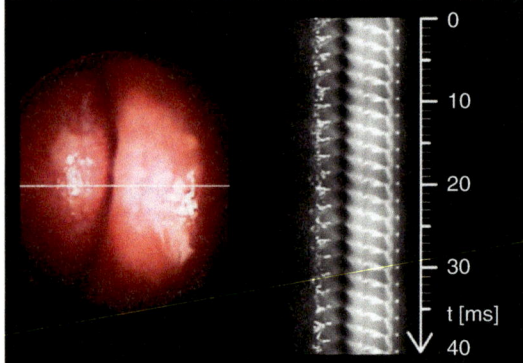

Fig. 6.38 Steady-state phase with low amplitudes (494 Hz, H4, mezzo forte) of a trumpeter (© Mauersberger 2016)

Additionally, onset, steady-state and offset phases may be distinguished, since each individual lip vibration is captured separately by this high-speed line scanning technique. During tone onset (see Fig. 6.37), lip vibration amplitudes increase. A constant amplitude during the blown tone characterises the steady-state phase (see Figs. 6.38 and 6.39). The amplitude varies due to the frequency (see Figs. 6.38 and 6.39). During the offset phase (see Fig. 6.40), the blown tone ends as a result of the decreasing lip vibration amplitudes.

Amplitude Measurements Single lip vibration amplitudes can be measured by a multistep

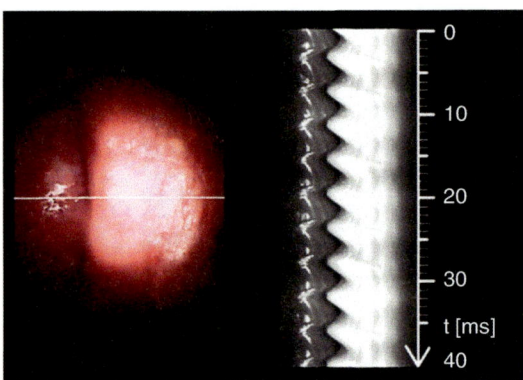

Fig. 6.39 Steady-state phase with large amplitudes (247 Hz, H3, mezzo forte) of a trumpeter (© Mauersberger 2016)

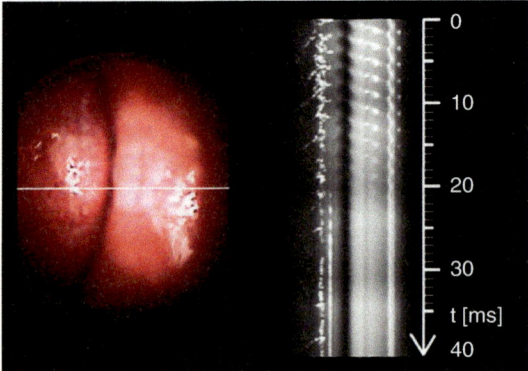

Fig. 6.40 Offset phase of a trumpeter (© Mauersberger 2016)

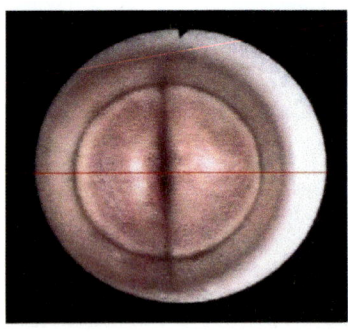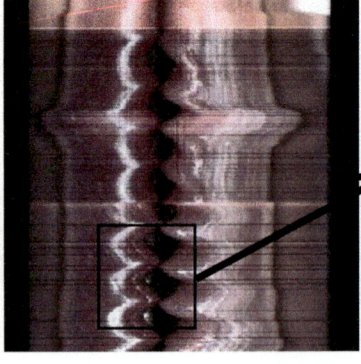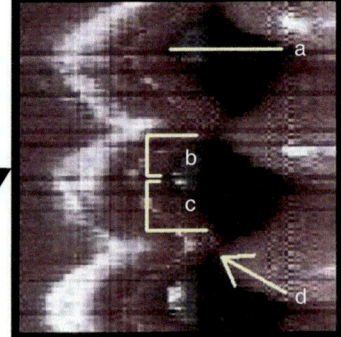

Fig. 6.41 Colour strobe kymography of a trombonist's lips. Left image, photograph of lips with recording line; middle image, reconstructed colour strobe kymography; right image, detailed enlargement of middle image; *a* maximal lip opening; *b* opening phase; *c* closing phase; *b + c* open phase; *d* closed phase (© Mauersberger 2016)

evaluation algorithm with rpSzene® software (rpSzene® version 8.0 (2006–2010)/Rehder/Partner GmbH/Hamburg) (Mauersberger 2016). Vibrations of the lower lip are partially overlaid by vibrations of the upper lip in most brass players (downstream type; see e.g. Figs. 6.36, 6.37, 6.38, 6.39, and 6.40). Therefore, lower lip vibrations of downstream-type players are only partly visible and mostly not measurable.

As with the singer's vocal folds (Schutte and Seidner 2005), there is a negative correlation between pitch and amplitude of the upper lip in brass players: the higher the frequency played, the smaller the amplitudes of the upper lip and vice versa. In addition, the amplitudes vary with intensity: the louder the tone played, the larger the amplitudes of the upper lip and vice versa (Mauersberger 2016).

Methodological limitations may be found in cases of significant overlapping of the lower lip by the upper lip (extreme downstream type) or of the upper lip by the lower lip (extreme upstream type). High-frequency tones that are played in pianissimo may have very small amplitudes (<0.1 mm), which are not measurable (Mauersberger 2016).

6.6.6 Conclusions

Kymography and stroboscopy are non-invasive imaging techniques for detailed real-time functional analyses of lip vibrations. They allow the brass musician to play his or her own instrument. By using a mouthpiece with lateral bore hole, fixed guiding sleeve, attached endoscope and camera, image artefacts and loss of air can be avoided so that the lips are examined in near-real brass instrument playing conditions.

One advantage of kymography over stroboscopy is that each individual lip vibration can be examined along a predetermined line (kymography, high-speed line scanning). In contrast to high-speed recordings of lip vibrations (e.g.

Bromage et al. 2005, 2010; Bromage 2007; Chick et al. 2005; Stevenson et al. 2009; Newton et al. 2008; Boutin et al. 2015), the volume of accumulated data is considerably lower in kymography. The sampling rates of lip vibrations are similar (7.200 lines per second in kymography (Mauersberger 2016), compared with 2000 (Newton et al. 2008)–11,025 (Boutin et al. 2015) frames per second in high-speed recordings of lip vibrations).

Stroboscopic examinations are more suitable for pictorial, descriptive representations than for measurements and statistical analyses of lip vibrations. Stroboscopic cameras are much less expensive than kymographic cameras and are therefore used more often in clinical practice. With special software, a colour strobe kymographic image can be derived and reconstructed from a stroboscopic video sequence of the lips (see Fig. 6.41) in the same way as for the vocal folds (see Nawka 2012). For this purpose, a previously defined recording line is extracted from consecutive single images of the stroboscopic video sequence (see left image of Fig. 6.41). The single images are then placed one below the other in chronological order (see middle image of Fig. 6.41).

This is an inexpensive alternative to real-time kymography (where a separate kymographic camera is needed), because only one camera is necessary for both stroboscopy and kymography.

Ideally, kymography and stroboscopy should be complemented by further diagnostic methods to evaluate the brass player's embouchure: a non-invasive morphological lip examination is carried out clinically and sonographically (mainly for evaluation of the orbicularis oris muscle). The lower end of the vocal tract with the larynx can be studied by common phoniatric techniques (e.g. laryngoscopy, stroboscopy, kymography, acoustic signal analyses, rating scales).

In clinical practice and outpatient departments for musicians medicine, embouchure investigations of brass players are closely related to insurance, legal and economic aspects relevant to professional liability: for accident and illness coverage and for professional liability insurances, the question of (in)capacity to work largely depends on these embouchure evaluations. In the context of rehabilitation programmes and litigation, those examinations can provide valuable information to judge brass musicians (in)capacity to perform (e.g. assessment of post-traumatic (Satchmo's syndrome), post-operative or strain-induced (embouchure dystonia) alterations of the lips). Therefore, stroboscopic and kymographic studies of lip vibrations are recommended for routine use in musicians medicine consultations.

Case Study 6.4: Stroboscopy of the Lips

Three herniated discs cause cervical myelocompression and a discrete right hemisyndrome. The lip vibrations are mostly uncoordinated. One can see irregular high-frequency fluttering and trembling of the upper lip with markedly reduced amplitudes. Normal cycles are rare. Additionally, an insufficient lip closure with uncontrollable salivation can be observed.

6.7 Instrumental Methods for Assessment of Laryngeal Phonatory Function

Philippe Dejonckere

6.7.1 Introduction

The voice laboratory can be considered an essential tool for the assessment and treatment evaluation of voice patients and for clinical research on voice disorders.

Several specific questions may be answered from the information obtained in the voice laboratory:

- Is a given voice or voice function measurement to be considered as normal (within normal limits) or pathological?
- If the voice or voice function is to be considered pathological, how severe is the alteration?

- Which aspects or mechanisms of voice production are concerned with the voice disorder? How does the primary (medical) aetiology or lesion explain the components of voice production that are perceived or analysed as deviant (e.g. by limiting vocal fold closure or by eliciting irregular vibrations related to vocal fold asymmetry), and how do they account for the patient's complaints (e.g. voice fatigue or compensation mechanisms)? Is a measure specific for a certain nosologic entity (diagnostics in a narrower sense)? However, as a rule, no acoustic parameter may be considered as pathognomonic for a specific medical aetiological diagnosis.
- What is the result of a comparison of voice production at two or more times (e.g. before and after therapy) or in two or several situations or voicing conditions (spontaneously vs. louder, or during an Isshiki manoeuvre or when applying a defined therapeutic technique)? Have the changes returned the voice to normal function as indicated by voice measurement (Dejonckere 2000)?

6.7.2 A Prerequisite: Recording a Voice Sample

Audio recording is the most important basic requisite for voice quality assessment. Once a high-quality recording has been made, it can be stored and remains available—as a document—for performing additional investigations at a later time, as, e.g. blind perceptual evaluation by a panel or sophisticated acoustic analyses (Titze 1995). A sampling frequency of at least 20,000 Hz is recommended. The recordings should ideally be made in a sound-treated room, but a quiet room, with ambient noise permanently <45 dB(A), is acceptable when a head-mounted microphone at close distance from the mouth is used (Sramkova et al. 2015). When recording voice, it is also recommended to record the background sound during the time when the examined subject is silent and determine the ambient noise level of the recording—this level should optimally be at least 10 dB lower than the sound level of the quietest voice signals to ensure quality measurements (Sramkova et al. 2015). Svec and Granqvist (2010) provide technical guidelines for selecting microphones for human voice production research (frequency response and range, dynamic range, directionality). The mouth-to-microphone distance needs to be held constant; Titze (1995) has recommended less than 10 cm (preferably 3–4 cm). A (miniature) head-mounted microphone offers a clear advantage. Off-axis positioning (45–90° from the mouth axis) reduces aerodynamic noise from the mouth in speech (Watson 1994; Sataloff 1997). Contact microphones or accelerometers, being directly in touch with the neck, work well in high-noise environments (Svec et al. 2005). Suppressing background noise and voices from other people (e.g. pupils, children) is a major issue for voice dosimetry and long-term monitoring. Sound pressure levels (SPLs) of speech can be estimated from skin vibration of the neck with acceptable accuracy when the subjects are individually calibrated. The accelerometer is totally selective and non-apparent, well suited for F0 monitoring and to some extent for SPL after adequate calibration, whereas the microphone (headset) is not completely selective, always (to some extent) visible, but it allows qualitative analysis (e.g. harmonics-to-noise ratio, singer's formant). Contactless microphones are wired or wireless. A *wireless microphone* contains a *transmitter* that sends the audio as a radio or optical signal rather than via a cable. Voice dosimeters and portable voice monitors use also accelerometers (Hunter and Titze 2010).

For routine clinical purposes, different voice/speech materials can be used.

An example of protocol for standard recording:

- /a:/ at (spontaneous) comfortable pitch/loudness, recorded 3× in order to evaluate variability of quality (Speyer et al. 2003)
- /a:/ slightly louder, in order to evaluate the possible change in quality (plasticity) and the slope of the regression line frequency/sound pressure level (Dejonckere 1998; Dejonckere and Lebacq 2001)
- A single sentence or a short standard passage

Phonetic selection can be useful, e.g. a short sentence with:

- Constant voicing (no voiceless sounds and to be spoken without interruption)
- No fricatives

Such sentences (e.g. 'We mow our lawn all year') can be analysed by the computer program for sustained vowels, and as it contains no articulation noise, there is no biasing of harmonics-to-noise computations. Computation of percentage voiceless (normal in this case is 100%) is useful for neurological voices or spasmodic dysphonia (Dejonckere 2006b; Dejonckere et al. 2012b). Further, it allows easy determination of the mean habitual fundamental speaking frequency.

Another example of a criterion for phonetic selection could be a multiplication of voice onsets, as they are critical in disturbed voices (Revis et al. 2000). Such criteria are not language-linked.

A standard reading passage should also be recorded, whenever possible. Two classic and often-used reading passages for English-speaking persons are 'the Rainbow Passage' (a phonetically selected passage including all the speech sounds of English) and 'Marvin Williams' (an all-voiced passage) (Sataloff 1997). Removal of non-voiced segments is possible a posteriori for acoustic analysis (Maryn et al. 2010a).

Long-term monitoring of voice as well as voice dosimetry has become an important issue particularly within the field of professional voice diseases. Voice dosimetry (by means of a 'voice accumulator') is a basic concept for measuring voice loading, which is the mechanical stress inflicted on the voice organ when intensively speaking or singing. It can be used, e.g. for defining 'at-risk' occupations. Long-term monitoring (by means of a 'portable voice lab') gives insight into the subject's vocal behaviour, e.g. in working environment (Manfredi and Dejonckere 2016; Cantarella et al. 2014).

6.7.3   Aerodynamics

Aerodynamic analysis of voice production includes measurement of airflow, air pressure and their relationships during phonation. By using appropriate instrumentation, a number of derived measurements can provide information of vocal efficiency.

6.7.3.1 Phonation Airflow

The simplest aerodynamic parameter of voicing is the maximum phonation time (MPT) in seconds. It consists of the prolongation of an /a:/, for as long as possible after maximal inspiration and at spontaneous, comfortable pitch and loudness. It is one of the more widely used clinical measures in voice assessment, worldwide (Hirano 1989). A prior demonstration is necessary, and three trials are required, the longest being selected for comparison to norm (Neiman and Edeson 1981). As it is an 'extreme' performance, it has been shown to be very sensitive to learning and fatigue effects. Further, in good voices, the duration of 'apnoea' (>45 s) can become the limiting factor, rather than the available air. Children show significant lower values of MPT than adults, as their lung volume is smaller (Kent et al. 1987). A reduction of possible bias—e.g. supportive respiratory capabilities compensating for poor membranous vocal fold closure—is possible by computing the ratio: averaged phonation airflow or phonation quotient (PQ) = vital capacity (ml)/MPT (s).

Vital capacity (VC) is defined as 'the volume change at the mouth between the position of full inspiration and complete expiration'. It can be measured in a reliable way by using a hand-held spirometer (Rau and Beckett 1984). VC depends, in normal subjects, on anthropometric factors and is, e.g. quite strongly correlated with height (Morris et al. 1992). It is also sensitive to lung disease. As VC is not directly related to voice quality, it is meaningful to take it in account, certainly if children are investigated.

The mean airflow rate can also be measured by using a pneumotachograph. This consists of a hand-held mouth tube (possibly connected to a mask) within which is placed a fine mesh wire screen in order to create a small resistance to airflow. This resistance results in a pressure difference across the screen that can be measured with a differential pressure transducer; the pressure difference increases with the flow. This device provides a direct measurement of the mean airflow rate (ml/s) for sustained phonation over a comfortable duration, usually 2–3 s, at the habitual pitch and intensity level, following habitual inspiration. Pathophysiological backgrounds and normative values have been reported by Hirano (1981, 1989), Verdolini (1994), Colton and Casper (1996) and Woo et al. (1987, 1994).

The averaged phonation airflow considerably varies among normal subjects, and there is a large overlapping range of values in normal and dysphonic subjects. This limits the value for diagnostic purposes (Schutte 1980). Nevertheless, when comparing glottal function before and after surgical intervention or non-surgical voice training techniques, airflow measurement may be useful in monitoring therapeutic effects (Schutte 1992), e.g. in case of paralytic dysphonia (Hirano et al. 1968; Fritzell et al. 1974; Murry and Bone 1978), or when microlaryngeal phonosurgery has been performed (Woo et al. 1994). The method is especially useful for demonstrating changes in a single test subject over time.

For comparisons (pre-/post-treatment), it is recommended to use the same kind of technique (PQ or mean airflow rate measured by a pneumotachograph).

Several dedicated devices are commercially available (e.g. the Phonatory Aerodynamic System PAS 6600 KayPENTAX, Montvale, NJ, USA) (Zraick et al. 2012). They propose various protocols, including an estimation of voicing efficiency.

6.7.3.2 Flow Glottography

Flow glottography (FLOG) consists of an inverse filtering of the oral airflow waveform. The basic tool is a high-frequency pressure transducer incorporated within an airtight Rothenberg mask (Rothenberg 1973). The inverse filtering procedure removes the resonant effects of the vocal tract and produces an estimate of the waveform produced at the vocal folds (Alku 2011) (Fig. 6.42).

The special advantage of this technique is that it differentiates and, after calibration, quantifies the leakage airflow (the continuous component of

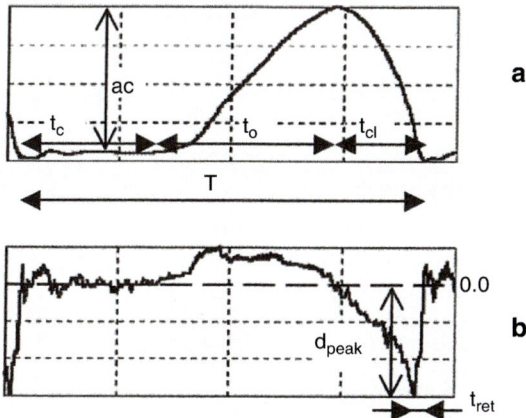

Fig. 6.42 (**a**) Flowglottogram obtained from a normal subject by inverse filtering, showing the closed time (t_c), the opening time (t_o) and the closing time (t_{cl}). In this case there is no dc flow (complete closure without leakage). (**b**) First derivative of the flowglottogram. d_{peak} is the negative peak amplitude of the derivative, at the moment of glottal closure. t_{ret} is the return phase, i.e. the time during which the derivative returns to the zero level after the instant of the negative peak. From Alku (2011) with kind permission from Springer Nature 2018

the airflow) and the pulsated airflow. Leakage airflow is an important concept: it assumes that there is an opening somewhere along the total length of the vocal folds through which air escapes. In case of leakage airflow, the plateau of the closed phase is offset from the baseline (flow = 0). Calibration is critical for reliable measurements. Flow glottography can also be used to analyse the voice onset (Dejonckere 2006a; Lebacq and Dejonckere 2019). Glottal airflow waveforms can be used for computing open, closing and speed quotients which are related to sound pressure level of the voice (Sapienza et al. 1998).

6.7.3.3 Subglottal Air Pressure

Measurements of subglottal air pressure made by using oesophageal balloons or pressure transducers and transglottal catheters, or by tracheal puncture, are semi-invasive or invasive and limited to research situations. An accurate estimation of subglottal pressure can be obtained by measuring the intra-oral air pressure produced during the repeated pronunciation of /pVp/ syllables (i.e. a vowel between two plosive consonants). A thin catheter is introduced into the mouth through the labial commissure, sealed by the lips, and not occluded by the

tongue. If there is no closure of the vocal folds, the intra-oral air pressure should be similar to the pressure elsewhere in the respiratory tract. During the production of a voiceless consonant, the vocal folds are abducted and should not impose any significant obstruction to the airflow from the lungs. Thus, the pressure behind the lips is the same everywhere and reflects the pressure available to drive the vocal folds if they were to vibrate (Rothenberg 1982; Baken and Orlikoff 2000). This technique also allows an approach to the phonation threshold pressure (PTP), the minimum pressure required to initiate phonation (Titze 1992a). Pressure is usually reported in pascal units: 1 Pa is equal to 1 Newton/m^2. 1 kPa is 10 cm of H$_2$O.

6.7.3.4 Efficiency of Phonation

Together with airflow and vocal intensity, subglottal air pressure can be used to estimate the efficiency of phonation. Obviously, reduced efficiency is expected to induce voice fatigue. Vocal efficiency is defined as the ratio of the acoustic power to the aerodynamic power and can be estimated by dividing the radiated sound pressure level of the utterance by the product of the air pressure and the airflow used to produce the utterance (Colton and Woo 1995).

6.7.4   Acoustics

Acoustic measures provide in an objective and non-invasive way a lot of information about vocal function. Increasingly, these measures have become available affordably and appear to have succeeded very well in monitoring changes in voice quality across time, e.g. before and after treatment. Acoustic measures reflect the status of vocal function but do not relate specifically to various voice disorders, because basic biomechanical changes resulting in acoustic features can be induced by various types of lesions or dysfunctions.

6.7.4.1 Visible Speech

Acoustic analysis can first be used to make the voice and speech visible, e.g. in spectrograms (Baken and Orlikoff 2000). This visual representation may be a considerable aid to the perception and description of the voice characteristics. Spectrograms are also useful for comparing normal phonation with phonation characterised by excessive noise. Commercially available software packages provide synchronised displays of the microphone signal and the spectrogram, showing the frequency distribution of acoustical energy over time. A choice can be made between narrowband filtering (frequency resolution, mainly demonstrating fundamental frequency, harmonics, interharmonic and high-frequency noise, subharmonics) and broadband filtering (temporal resolution, mainly demonstrating periodicity, but also formant location). Voice characteristics such as SPL, fundamental frequency and formant central frequency can also be displayed over time for analysis of singing voice. Visualising of fast Fourier transform (FFT) graphics (power spectrum) is usually possible, as well as long-time average spectra (LTAS). When visible speech is provided simultaneously with the voice sound, the inter-rater consistency of the perceptual quality evaluation significantly increases (Martens et al. 2007).

6.7.4.2 Acoustic Parameters

Acoustic analysis can also provide precise numerical values for many voice parameters, from averaged fundamental frequency to sophisticated calculations for noise components or tremor features. Factor analysis allows the large number of acoustic parameters to be reduced to a limited number of clusters (Dejonckere et al. 1996):

- Short-term fundamental frequency perturbation
- Short- or medium-term amplitude perturbation and voiceless segments
- Harmonics-to-noise ratio
- Long-term frequency and amplitude modulation
- Very long-term amplitude variation
- Subharmonics
- Tremor

Perturbation measures (in period and amplitude), as well as the harmonics-to-noise compu-

tations on a sustained vowel (/a:/) at comfortable frequency and intensity, appear as the most robust measures and seem to determine the basic perceptual elements of voice quality: grade, roughness and breathiness. Nevertheless, correlations with perceptual data remain usually moderate (Dejonckere et al. 1996; Wolfe et al. 1997). There are, however, arguments for combining voice samples from both continuous speech and sustained vowels in acoustic analysis of dysphonic voices (Maryn et al. 2010a). A considerable variety of mathematically based measures of perturbation has been developed. Clinically, they have led to the near universal clinical use of 'jitter' and 'shimmer' as important measurements for distinguishing normal from pathological voices (Fourcin and Abberton 2008). Jitter is computed as the mean difference between the periods of adjacent cycles divided by the mean period. It is thus an F0 (fundamental frequency)-related measurement (Fig. 6.43).

For shimmer, a similar computation is made on peak-to-peak amplitudes. Voice breaks must always be excluded. For pathological voices, the coefficients of variation of jitter and shimmer for a sustained /a/ are in the order of 20–30% for successive single trials as well as trials on different days (Speyer et al. 2004a). A general limitation is that the analysis programmes employed for acoustic analysis (and particularly for period identification) cannot (or not in a reliable way) analyse strongly aperiodic acoustic signals. Perturbation measures less than about 5% have been found to be reliable (Titze and Liang 1993), and only 'quasi-periodic' voices are suited to perturbation analysis. Therefore, visual control of the period of definition of the microphone signal is always necessary: even in regular voices, a strong harmonic or subharmonic may account for erratic values. However, recent work having recourse to realistic synthesised deviant voices with controlled jitter and noise has shown that improved acoustic programmes, using more reliable algorithms, could validly transgress the 5% limit (Manfredi et al. 2011, 2012; Dejonckere et al. 2011, 2012a). Alternatives from the field of non-linear dynamics, such as the coefficient of Lyapunov, have been proposed for analysing

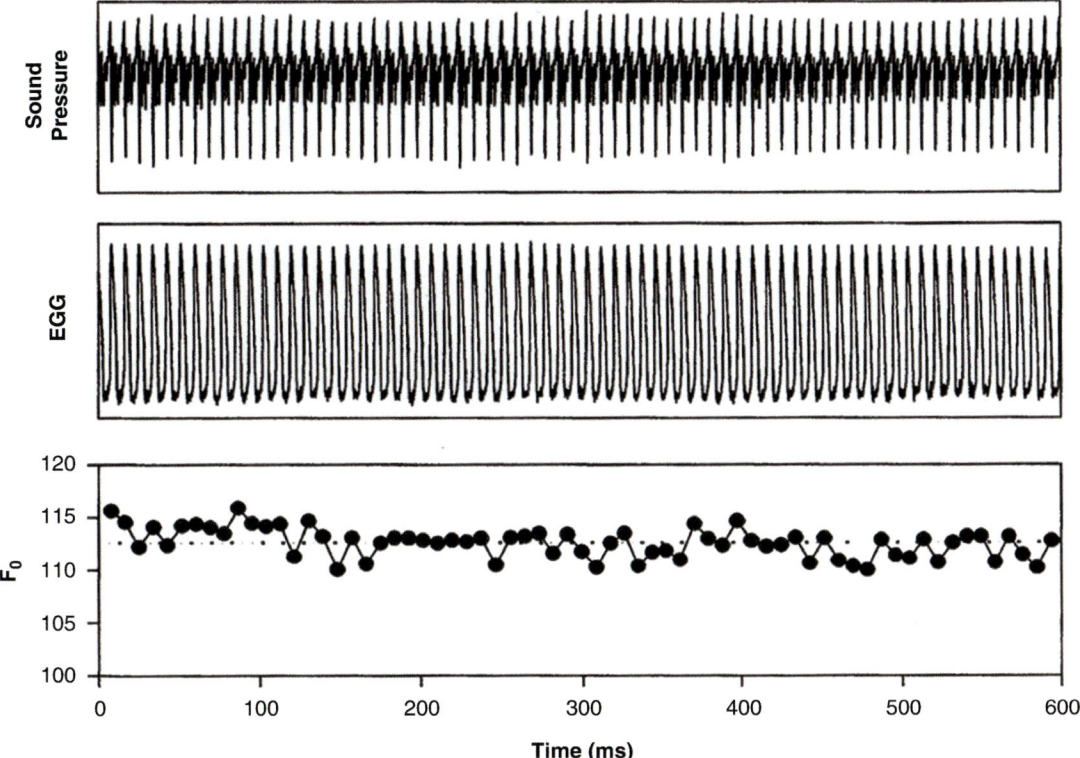

Fig. 6.43 Normal male voice, sustained /a:/: microphone signal, electroglottogram and F0 plot across time. Normal voice is characterised by slight (<1%) random variation of fundamental frequency. In most cases of pathology, this aperiodicity (jitter) increases. From Dejonckere (2010) with kind permission from Springer Nature 2018

'chaotic' or 'bifurcated' signals (Yu et al. 2000). For substitution voices, voicing quantification has also proven to be more relevant than period perturbation (Dejonckere et al. 2012c).

For signal-to-noise ratio computations (NNE (normalised noise energy), HNR (harmonics-to-noise ratio), cepstrum peak, etc.), there is currently insufficient standardisation of the optimal algorithm(s), as well as insufficient knowledge about normative values, for widely spread clinical use. The harmonics-to-noise ratio has also been found to be a parameter less suited for demonstrating the effects of therapy (Speyer et al. 2004b).

Rhinophonia is a particular resonance characteristic of the voice. It may be present without a concomitant articulation disorder. Acoustic nasometry provides objective measurements by (schematically) computing the ratio between nasal and whole voice (nasal + oral) sound pres-

sure levels (Dejonckere and van Wijngaarden 2001).

An important application of acoustic measurements is pre- and post-treatment comparisons within patients (Brockmann-Bauser and Drinnan 2011). Thus, some combined measures have been proposed, such as the 'Dysphonia Severity Index' (DSI) (Wuyts et al. 2000) and the 'Acoustic Voice Quality Index' (AVQI) (Maryn et al. 2010b). The DSI is based on the weighted combination of a selected set of voice measurements: highest frequency, lowest intensity, maximum phonation time and jitter (%). The AVQI is a multivariate acoustic measure consisting of a weighted combination of six time- and frequency-domain metrics.

6.7.4.3 Phonetography/Voice Range Profile

Basically, the phonetogram plots the dynamic range (dBA) as a function of fundamental

Fig. 6.44 Computerised phonetogram (voice range profile), with a grey scale indicating the amount of jitter (normal female voice). The more jitter, the darker the area. Horizontal axis: fundamental frequency in Hz (or musical tones on a keyboard). Vertical axis: sound pressure level, measured at 30 cm (dB A). This plot combines information about extreme possibilities of voice as well as on an aspect of voice quality. From Dejonckere (2010) with kind permission from Springer Nature 2018

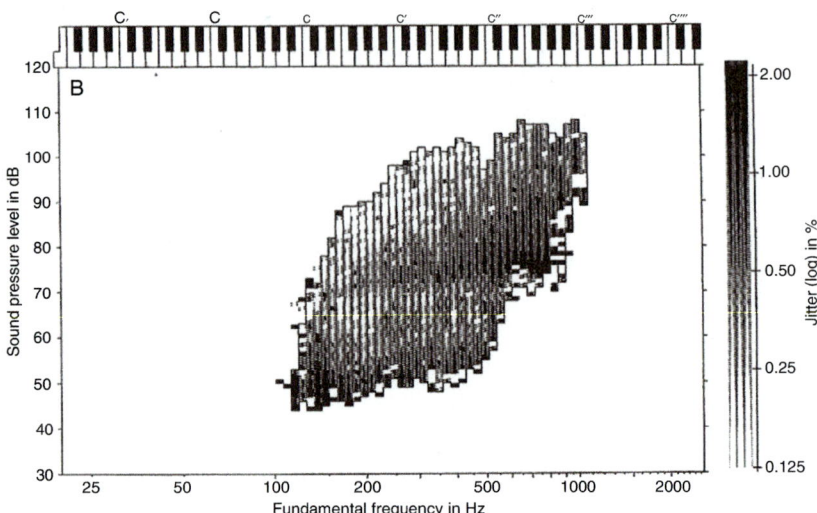

frequency range (Hz), documenting the extreme possibilities of voice. These extremes are of importance for professional voice users, especially singers (Schultz-Coulon 1990), but they must be interpreted with care (Titze 1992b) because the acoustic energy is related to spectral distribution. Normative values for children and teachers have been defined by Heylen et al. (2002).

Computerised systems make possible real-time measurement and display of fundamental frequency versus SPL and also of quality parameters such as jitter, within the whole voice area. Jitter results in various colour gradations, showing specific altered zones or register boundaries (Fig. 6.44).

Such computerised systems can also provide range profiles of current speech, possibly coupled with provocation tests, such as the task of reading at a controlled, louder intensity. These profiles are expected to be relevant for occupational voice users.

The highest and lowest frequencies and the softest intensity (dB A at 30 cm) seem most sensitive to changes in voice quality (Heylen et al. 1998; Van de Heyning et al. 1996; Wuyts et al. 2000; Speyer et al. 2003), the latter being related to phonation threshold pressure (Titze 1992a, b). The measurement of the lowest frequency allows the computation of the fundamental frequency range. Such a 'three-point range profile' can be

obtained without completing a (time consuming) whole voice range profile (Dejonckere et al. 2001). However, as these three points represent 'extreme' performances, they are, as are MPT and CV, very sensitive to learning and fatigue effects.

6.7.5 Electroglottography

Electroglottography (or electrolaryngography) (EGG) is a method for monitoring vocal fold contact, rate of vibration and perturbation of regularity during voice production (Fig. 6.45a, b).

The major advantage of electroglottography is that it does not interfere with the physiological processes of speaking or singing. The signal originates from two electrodes lightly placed on the speaker's neck at the level of the thyroid cartilage. Pitch extraction from the EGG waveform is particularly reliable—as long as there is at least partial vocal fold contact during the vibration cycle—because the waveform is unaffected by vocal tract resonances and environment noise (Fourcin et al. 1995; Dejonckere 1996). The EGG signal has been used to compute period and amplitude perturbation parameters (Fourcin and Abberton 2008; Hosokawa et al. 2014) and even as a predictor of laryngeal electromyography (Mayes et al. 2008).

Fig. 6.45 Basic principle of electroglottography (or electrolaryngography). (**a**) Top: Schematic view of current paths across the larynx, as occurring in EGG during vocal fold vibration (left, glottis closed; right, glottis open). (**b**) Bottom: Schematic electroglottographic waveform with the corresponding laryngoscopic view and a frontal section through the midportion of the glottis. Point III corresponds to minimal trans-neck impedance, which is at maximum closure of the glottis. Points I and III can always be identified with certitude on the EGG signal. From Dejonckere (2010) with kind permission from Springer Nature 2018

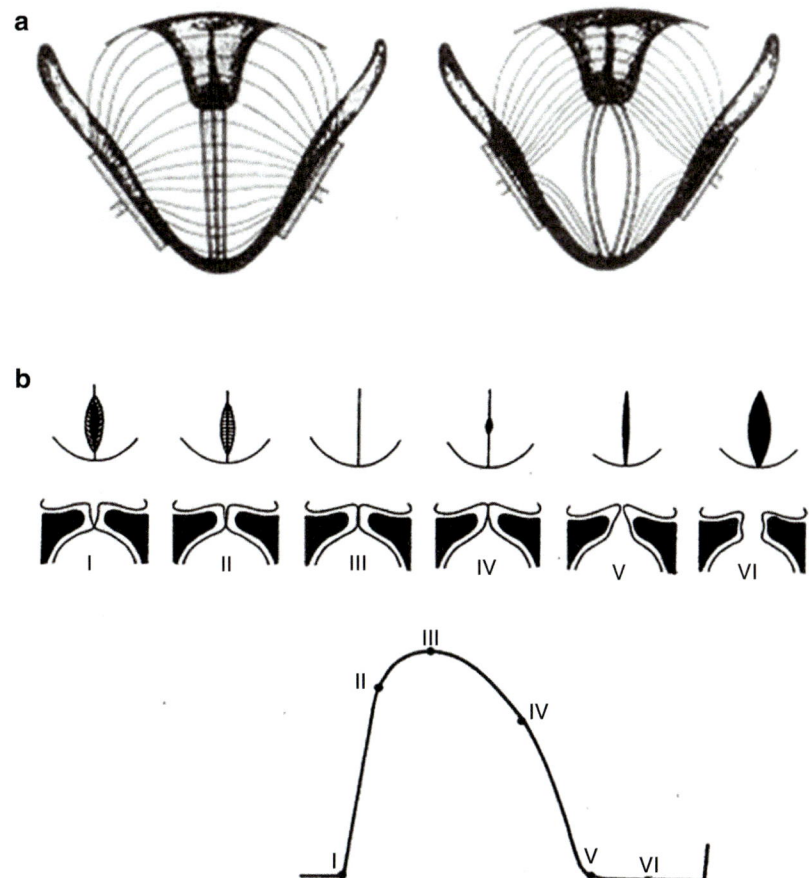

The main applications of EGG are:

- Fundamental frequency computations (range, regularity, distribution, display across time, cross plots, etc.), as long as there is a vocal fold contact
- Voice onset time
- Pre- and post-phonatory laryngeal gestures
- Closed phase information (hyper- vs. hypokinetic adduction)
- Voice range profile of spontaneous speech (falsetto excluded)
- Triggering of a stroboscopic light source

6.7.6 Electromyography

Electromyography (EMG) is an electrophysiological investigation of neuromuscular function. Main indications are mobility disorders (especially reduced mobility) (Sataloff et al. 2005). Neuromuscular pathological conditions in laryngeal muscles do not basically differ from neuromuscular pathological conditions in other muscles, so it is recommended that these investigations be performed in cooperation with a clinical neurophysiologist (Blitzer 1995; Dejonckere 1987; Dejonckere et al. 1988; Munin et al. 2000). In a supine patient with the neck extended, the cricothyroid muscle is reached by inserting the electrode off the midline close to the inferior border of the thyroid cartilage. The thyroarytenoid muscle is approached by insertion of a concentric needle electrode through the cricothyroid ligament. The needle electrode is then angled cranially 45° and laterally 20° to an approximate depth of 1.5–2 cm (Fig. 6.46).

In normal situations, the EMG signal in the vocalis muscle typically precedes (around 100–500 ms) the sound emission ('prephonatory tuning') (Fig. 6.47).

Fig. 6.46 Schematic view at the glottis level showing the needle electrode placement for laryngeal EMG. The selective approach of the posterior cricoarytenoid muscle is rarely needed

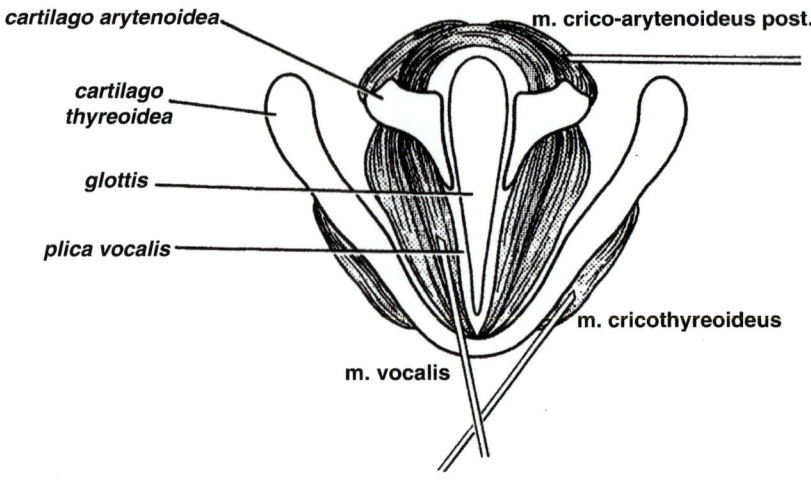

cartilago arytenoidea

m. crico-arytenoideus post.

cartilago thyreoidea

glottis

plica vocalis

m. cricothyreoideus

m. vocalis

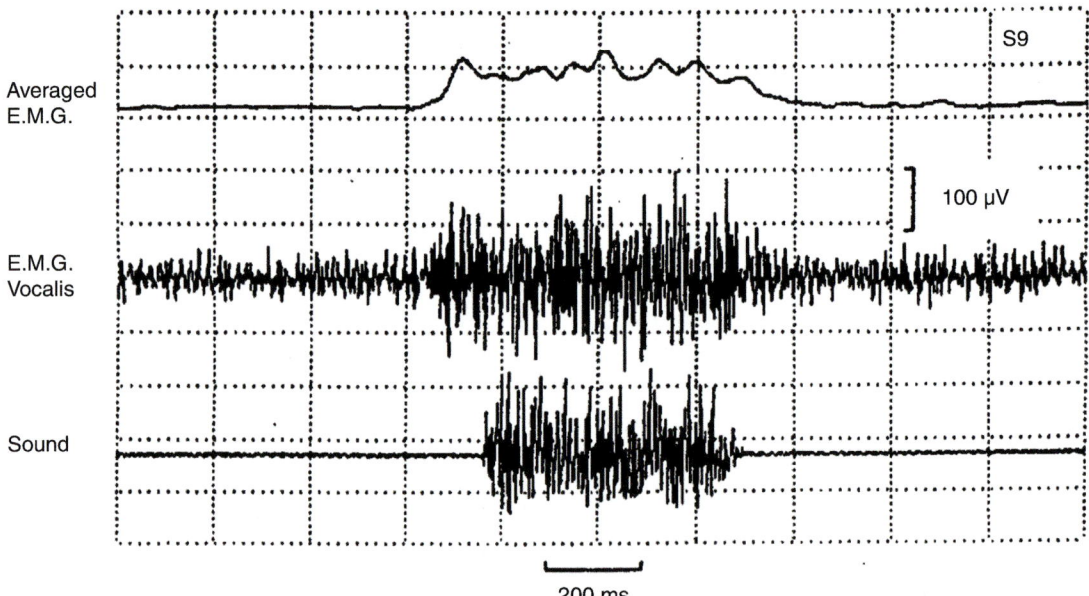

Averaged E.M.G.

S9

100 µV

E.M.G. Vocalis

Sound

200 ms

Fig. 6.47 Normal subject. The electrical activity in the vocalis muscle typically increases before the start of the vocal emission (usually 100–500 ms)

It is also possible to explore the posterior cricoarytenoid muscle (curved needle/manual rotation of the larynx or via indirect laryngoscopy with a specific needle-holder), but this is not without danger. Furthermore, this muscle is innervated by the same recurrent laryngeal nerve as the thyroarytenoid muscle but another branch of it. A classical indication for laryngeal EMG is the differential diagnosis between peripheral neurogenic and mechanical (ankylosis) reduction of vocal fold mobility. Such a question may arise, e.g. in the case of blunt and penetrating external laryngeal trauma (Schaefer 2014). The objectivity of EMG provides an additional medicolegal value. In case of unilateral vocal fold paralysis, predictors of poor prognosis for functionally meaningful recovery include fibrillation potentials (Fig. 6.48), positive sharp waves and absent or reduced voluntary motor unit potentials (Misono and Merati 2012).

Large polyphasic potentials reflect partial denervation and collateral regeneration (Fig. 6.49).

However after a few months, paradoxical reinnervation may perturb the actual functional prog-

Fig. 6.48 Pathological spontaneous activity (fibrillation potentials) in the vocalis muscle after complete denervation. Fibrillation potentials may appear as soon as 5–6 days after denervation and remain present for several years

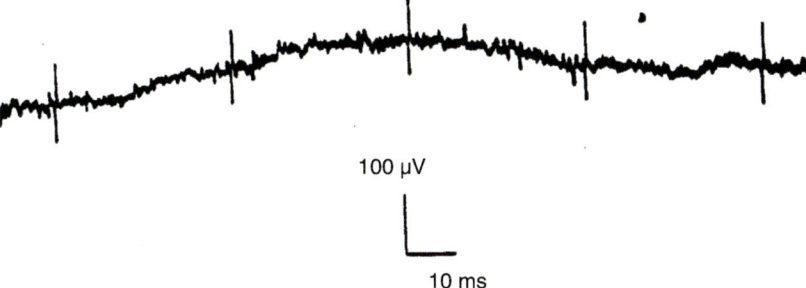

100 µV

10 ms

Fig. 6.49 Polyphasic motor unit potential in the vocalis muscle with increased duration and amplitude. Partial peripheral nerve lesion. Sprouting collaterals from intact motor units newly innervate denervated motor units but have a lower conduction velocity

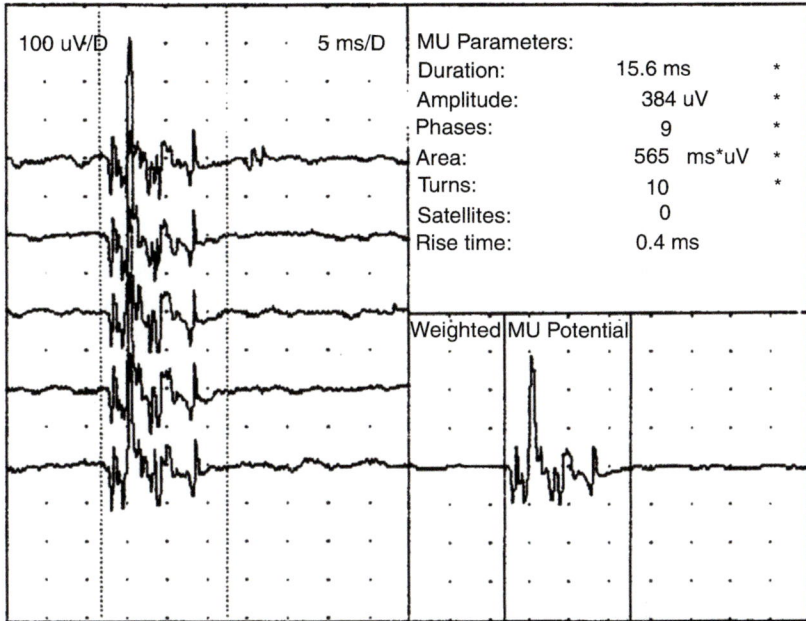

nostic value of EMG. If dedicated coated injection needles are used, EMG can be used for monitoring botulinum injections in vocal muscles. Laryngeal EMG hypercontractility during voice rest has been considered as typical in patients with Parkinson's disease and vocal complaints (Zarzur et al. 2014).

Contraindications for laryngeal EMG are the presence of dyspnoea (e.g. in a bilateral paralysis in adduction) and anticoagulant medication. Extreme care is mandatory in children. Complications are rare (vocal fold haemorrhage). An evidence-based review has been provided by Sataloff et al. (2004).

Currently the possibility of temporary injection medialisation of a paralysed vocal fold has reduced the need of a prognostic parameter. However, in future, EMG will become indispensable in context of surgical reinnervation (Dejonckere 2010).

Remark This section is based on a more detailed book chapter (Dejonckere 2010).

6.8   Voice Loading Tests

Tamás Hacki

6.8.1   Vocal Load Capacity and Vocal Loading

Vocal load capacity, which refers mainly to how long and how loud one can use the voice, is a crucial component of the phonatory ability of effective communicators. In comparison with hoarseness, which is only one of the numerous symptoms of dysphonia, restricted vocal load capacity arises as a result of several symptoms (Hacki 1996). For this reason, vocal load capacity is an important aspect of clinical assessment and voice research.

The load capacity of the phonatory system depends upon many factors, all of which are considered to be risk factors and which may be summarised as follows:

- Physiological factors
  - Constitution of the vocal organ
  - General physical condition
  - Illnesses
- Physical factors
  - Physical environment
  - Room acoustics (attenuation; resonance)
  - Speaking distance
  - Room climate, humidity
- Psychological factors
  - Personality; psychological constitution
  - Psychological condition or state
- Social factors

- Social environment
- Work-related stress
- Conversation partner (supportive; inhibiting)

In addition to general risk factors, several factors influence vocal performance immediately, for example, the current condition of the voice generators (mucosa, muscles) and respiratory structures, the respiratory and vocal technique employed at the time and the status of the patient's recovery from vocal loading. Recovery techniques include periods of rest lasting several hours as well as rapid recovery methods (such as relaxation techniques during speech).

Vocal loading is the long-term, intensive demand beyond the normal use to which the vocal organ is accustomed. The principal vocal load is the voiced aspect of spoken language. Articulation of unvoiced speech components seems to be secondary. (Complaints about vocal strain usually point towards laryngeal and respiratory fatigue.) Table 6.7

Table 6.7 Phases of vocal loading and their impact on vocal fold tissue

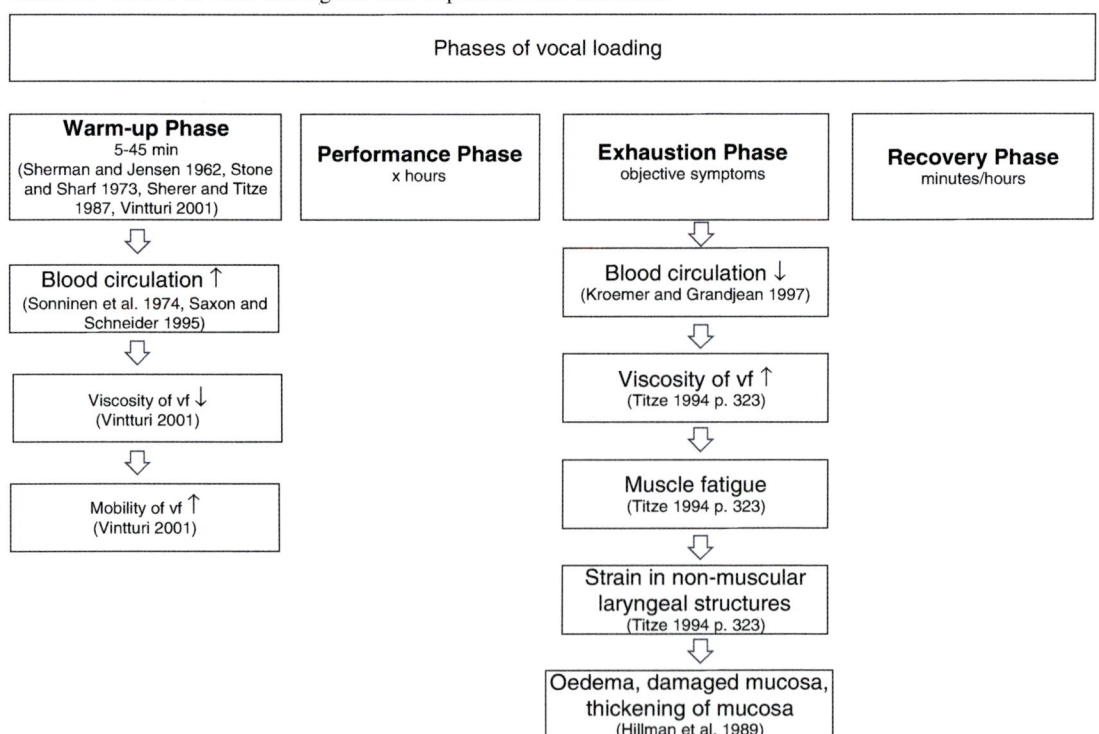

vf vocal folds (Hillman et al. 1989; Kroemer and Grandjean 1997; Saxon and Schneider 1995; Sherer and Titze 1987; Sherman and Jensen 1962; Sonninen et al. 1974; Stone and Sharf 1973; Titze 1994; Vintturi 2001) shows the physiological processes that occur during phases of vocal loading.

When one is aware of the general and immediately influential factors, the physiological processes during vocal loading (see above) as well as the many presenting symptoms, it should be clear that testing the consequences of vocal loading and ascertaining the load capacity of the voice are complicated tasks.

6.8.2 Measurement of Voice Performance or Vocal Loading 'In Vivo' and the Necessity for Vocal Load Testing

Voice performance during a working day can be recorded and analysed by using a recording device. The 'voice accumulator' of Beukers et al. (1995) measures the sound pressure level of the voice in dB(A).[1] The Ambulatory Phonation Monitor (APM) (KayPENTAX) enables the gathering and analysis of numerous vocal parameters (intensity, pitch, phonation time, etc.). Useful information about voice function and the subjective perception of the speaker can be gathered by recording (the voice) before and after a vocal load lasting several hours combined with the use of questionnaires (Laukkanen and Kankare 2006). Patients who complain about vocal fatigue generally visit their physicians hours or days after a significant vocal strain, such as teaching sessions or weekend seminars. A doctor can partially reconstruct the complaints on the basis of the history; however, key symptoms may no longer be present (e.g. acute organic alterations such as hyperaemia, surrounding oedema, damage to respiratory and laryngeal function such as glottal hypertonus, and not least, acute voice symptoms). Patients who have already had in- or outpatient treatment for vocal complaints often ask their physician if they are able to resume their vocally demanding work. This question can be best answered by conducting vocal loading tests. Such tests are also necessary when giving out medical advice on vocal abilities.

6.8.3 Vocal Loading Tests

What form can a vocal loading test take? Risk factors, such as poor room acoustics or a poor climate within a room, particular work and stress situations (see Sect. 5.1) or a vocal load of long duration, cannot be reproduced in the test situation. So how can a test be of practical value and how can the patient be supervised during the test? The creators of vocal loading tests must ensure that tests can be performed by most individuals and are comparable among individuals. Many different approaches to vocal loading tests were taken in the 1970s and early 1980s, featuring various speaking durations (20–45 min) and speech intensities (65–80 dB(A)), with and without surrounding background noise, with different mouth-microphone distances (20–50 cm) and with and without supplementary measurements (e.g. galvanic skin response, respiratory investigations, electromyography (EMG) or audio recording) (Wendler and Seidner 1996). Siegert (1987) made a recommendation for the Union of the European Phoniatricians (UEP) of a speaking duration of 20 min, target sound pressure level of 75–80 dB(A) and 30 cm distance from the microphone. The test should be conducted in the acoustic conditions of a living room. Laukkanen et al. (2004) used a text of 45 min duration, target level of 70 dB(A) and 40 cm mouth-microphone distance. In addition to these measurement parameters, the participants were asked to report their subjective symptoms before, during and after the test.

The first version of Seidner's Alternation Test ('Wechsler test') had a mouth-microphone distance of 50 cm and a 15-min duration. The second version (Seidner 2012) used a 30 cm mouth-microphone distance and 10-min duration, and this latter version proved to be more practical. In the first version, the participant reads a simple text at 70 dB(A) for 5 min and then increases to 75 dB(A) for a further 5 min, before finally returning to 70 dB(A) for 5 min. In the later version, the level varies minute by minute from 75 to 80 dB(A[1]), etc. The person being tested is notified on a monitor when his voice level is dropping below the desired value.

---

[1] A-weighting provides reduced low-frequency sensitivity compared with C-weighting.

A computer displays the following data on a graph: time course of sound level, percentage of lower deviation in sound level and time course of voice frequency. Laryngoscopy and assessment of the voice quality should take place before and immediately after vocal loading. Observation of the patient during the tests is particularly important: breathing, tension, complaints about abnormal sensations, etc. This test is recommended for the assessment of vocal capability and monitoring of therapy and as the basis for expert opinion.

Hacki (1996) developed the following test procedure: the participant phonates the vowel series u:-e:-i:-o:-a: for 20 min with a mouth-microphone distance of 30 cm. The required sound pressure level is 80 dB(C). Use of the dB(C) weighting, rather than dB(A), is to ensure that no artificial difference in output level is generated between low- and high-pitched voices. The reasons for phonating a vowel series are to test phonation more than articulation and to avoid the requirement that the person being tested concentrates on the reading of a text (they can instead monitor the sound level with an on-screen level indicator). The vowel series should be recited in a speaking voice manner, rather than in a singing voice. The output graph should display the average vocal output (expressed as energy-equivalent average level, LeqT) in real time (X-axis, time; Y-axis, sound pressure level, dB(C)) over 20 min. This value allows a comparison of the intra- and interindividual output. Laryngoscopy, stroboscopy, measurement of the average speaking frequency and an auditory assessment of voice quality (e.g. using GRBAS) (Hirano 1981) should be made before and after vocal loading. The participant should be observed during vocal loading, to ensure that he correctly follows the procedure. A questionnaire designed to measure the level of the patient's motivation and (emotional and physical) sensation during phonation should be completed after the test. Questionnaires determine the duration of any similar feelings of exertion in their daily life compared with that they felt after the test (more than 3 h would be a general indication of low-level or no pathology). Output curves from the above procedure can be classified as normal or pathological (Fig. 6.50) (Kramer et al. 1999). Normal output values (LeqT) for young participants are an average of 79 dB(C), with the lower range not below 75 dB(C) (Pabst et al. 1998). Values indicating pathology vary significantly: Kramer et al. (1998) found that voice patients who had undergone 3 weeks of voice rehabilitation had LeqT values under 70 dB(C) (averages of 67.1 dB(C) and 69.1 dB(C) for women and men, respectively). The LeqT values of 40.7% of patients had improved (in comparison with measurements taken on the initial visit to the clinic), and 15.7% had worsened.

6.8.4 Symptoms of Voice Strain

Kitzing (1981) and Seidner (2012), among others, report an elevated average speaking pitch as a typical symptom following vocal strain. Pabst et al. (1998) found an increase in the average pitch of the speaking voice of 0.7 semitones among women with normal voices (F) and 1.3 semitones in men with normal voices (M) following a 20-min vocal load at a target level of 80 dB(C). The average intensity of the speaking voices increased by 3.1 dB(A) and 3.5 dB(A) for women and men, respectively.

From our own general clinical experience after vocal loading: we take an increase in speaking pitch of more than four semitones as a sign of overly high muscle tension. Lowered speaking pitch can also be a sign of speech pathology: in such patients, we see hyperaemia or occasionally mild oedema on the edge of the vocal folds after vocal strain. A hyper- or hypotonic vibration patterns (on stroboscopy) and increase in glottal insufficiency (compared with the initial findings) are taken as a sign of intense vocal demand.

Patients claim that the effects of vocal load emerge in the resting phase. Vintturi et al. (2001) therefore investigated the effects of post-loading rest on many different parameters of phonation. Jilek et al. (2004) found that several voice parameters become worse 60 min after a vocal load of 20 min at 80 dB(C), and Echternach et al. (2013) registered deterioration in Dysphonia Severity Index (DSI) scores 60 min after vocal load. These

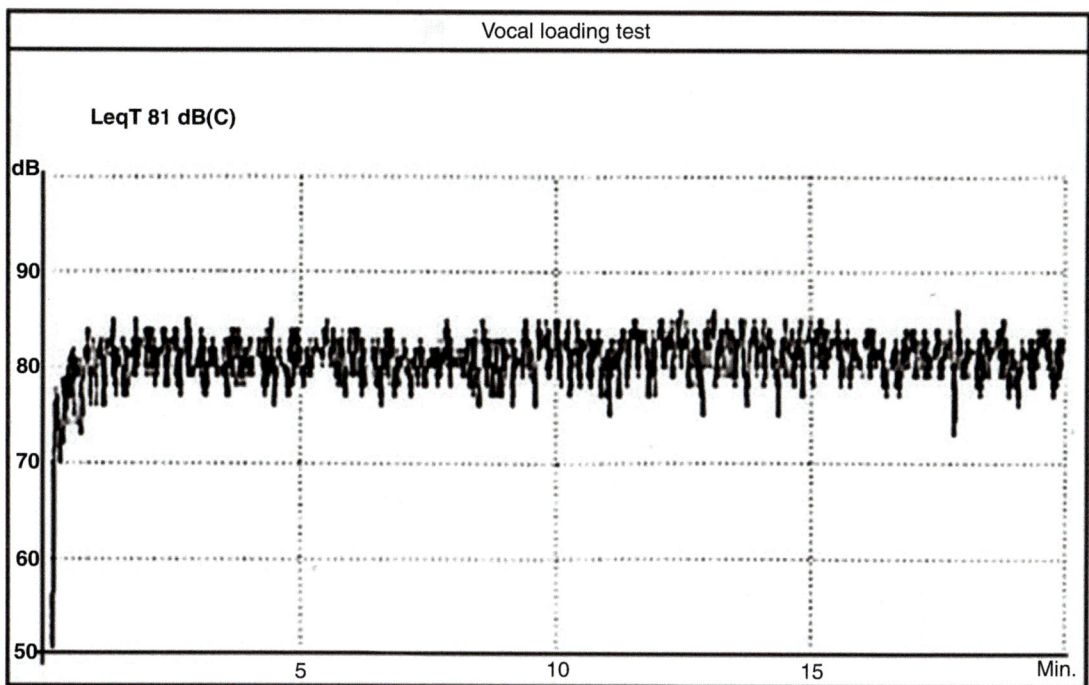

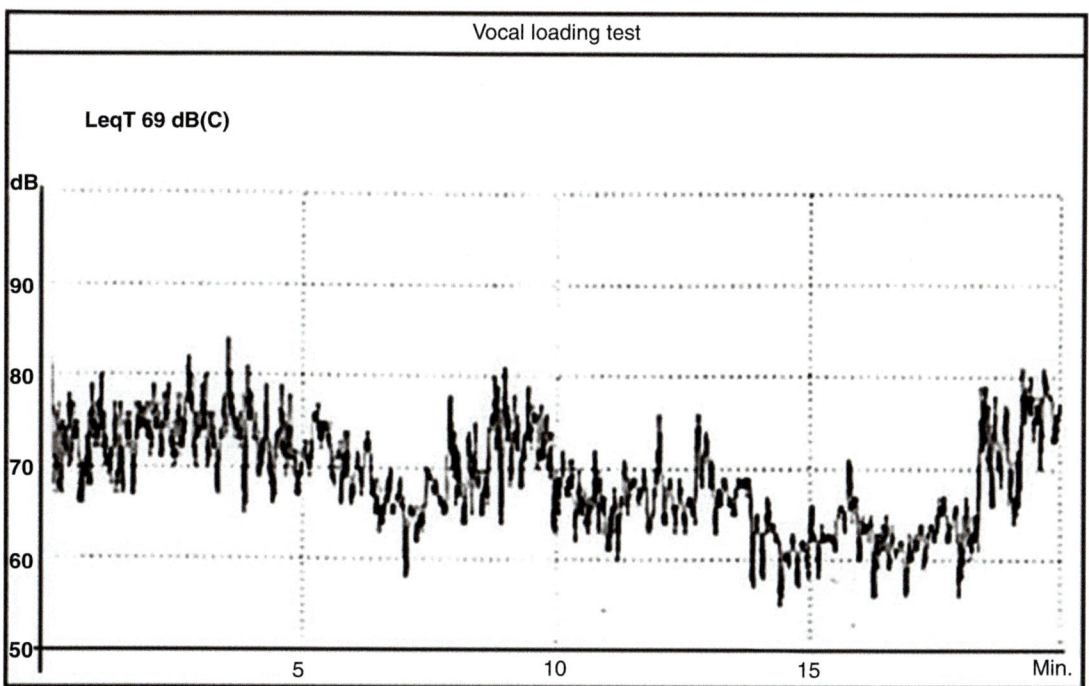

Fig. 6.50 Two types of vocal output curve (ordinate, [dB(C)]; abscissa, time [20 min]) (taken from seven presented in Kramer et al. (1999)). Above, normal homogeneous progress with warm-up phase during the first 2 min. The averaged effort (LeqT) is above average at 81 dB(C). Below, abnormal time course with total power of 69 dB(C) LeqT, indicative of pathology

results raise the question of the best time point after vocal loading for investigations to be made.

The motivation for a patient to undergo a vocal loading test is an essential and highly influential factor. Those people who themselves want to have their vocal ability tested are very differently motivated from those who are required to undergo such an examination (e.g. for questions relating to their retirement or pension). People with the latter motivation can be more easily convinced to exert vocal strain if it is made clear that only a vocal load test will provoke their reported vocal exhaustion and other symptoms.

6.8.5 Summary

Because of the complexity of the issues and the variety of symptoms of vocal strain, voice loading tests only have diagnostic value in the hands of experienced practitioners. Even here, there is a reasonable case for seeking further test improvement and appropriate standardisation.

6.9 The Usefulness of Computed Tomography and Magnetic Resonance Imaging in Investigation of the Vocal Tract

Katarzyna Karmelita-Katulska
and Matthias Echternach

6.9.1 Introduction

The mechanism of voice and speech production is a topic of interest for many disciplines such as linguistics, neurology, psychology, physiology and especially phoniatrics. Traditionally, for characterisation of voice and speech acoustics, the vocal tract shape has been studied with radiographic techniques (X-ray), but this method has certain limitations because of the ionising radiation. Radiographic studies (X-ray, computed tomography (CT)) have generally focused on bony structures (skull base, hyoid bone, etc.). MRI (magnetic resonance imaging) can clearly image the soft tissues relevant to voice and speech production (glottis, velum, lips, etc.). Nowadays, especially CT and MRI have a special role in imaging the dysfunction and certain pathologies at all stages of the voice production system, i.e. the lungs, the larynx and the vocal tract.

6.9.2 Computed Tomography

Coronal radiography and simple tomography have been used for years to observe changes in the larynx in many pathological states, but CT has become fast enough to replace these techniques. With the advent of multi-detector CT (MDCT), high-resolution reformatted coronal images are now routinely available (Baum et al. 2000; Lell et al. 2004). The advent of MDCT scanners has enabled the acquisition of images of the larynx during phonation as one volume image, and coronal reconstruction of the volume images makes it possible to observe changes in the vocal folds during phonation (Jun et al. 2005) (see Fig. 6.51a, b).

The limit of slice thickness allowing optimal imaging of the larynx is so far 1 mm. Minimal slice thickness is necessary to obtain sufficient image quality of multiplanar reformations, which require longer scan times and pose the risk of severe motion artefacts. MDCT allows an almost isotropic volume dataset to be acquired within an acceptable time interval ($\leq$10 s) (Jun et al. 2005). This is necessary for the most common scanning technique of the larynx during phonation and the Valsalva manoeuvre to show pathology of motion in the vocal folds (Fig. 6.52a, b) (Bum-Soo et al. 2008). This capability might help in identifying the correct diagnosis of vocal fold palsy (Yumoto et al. 2004). However, radiology is mostly used in order to exclude other pathologies in the recurrent nerve area.

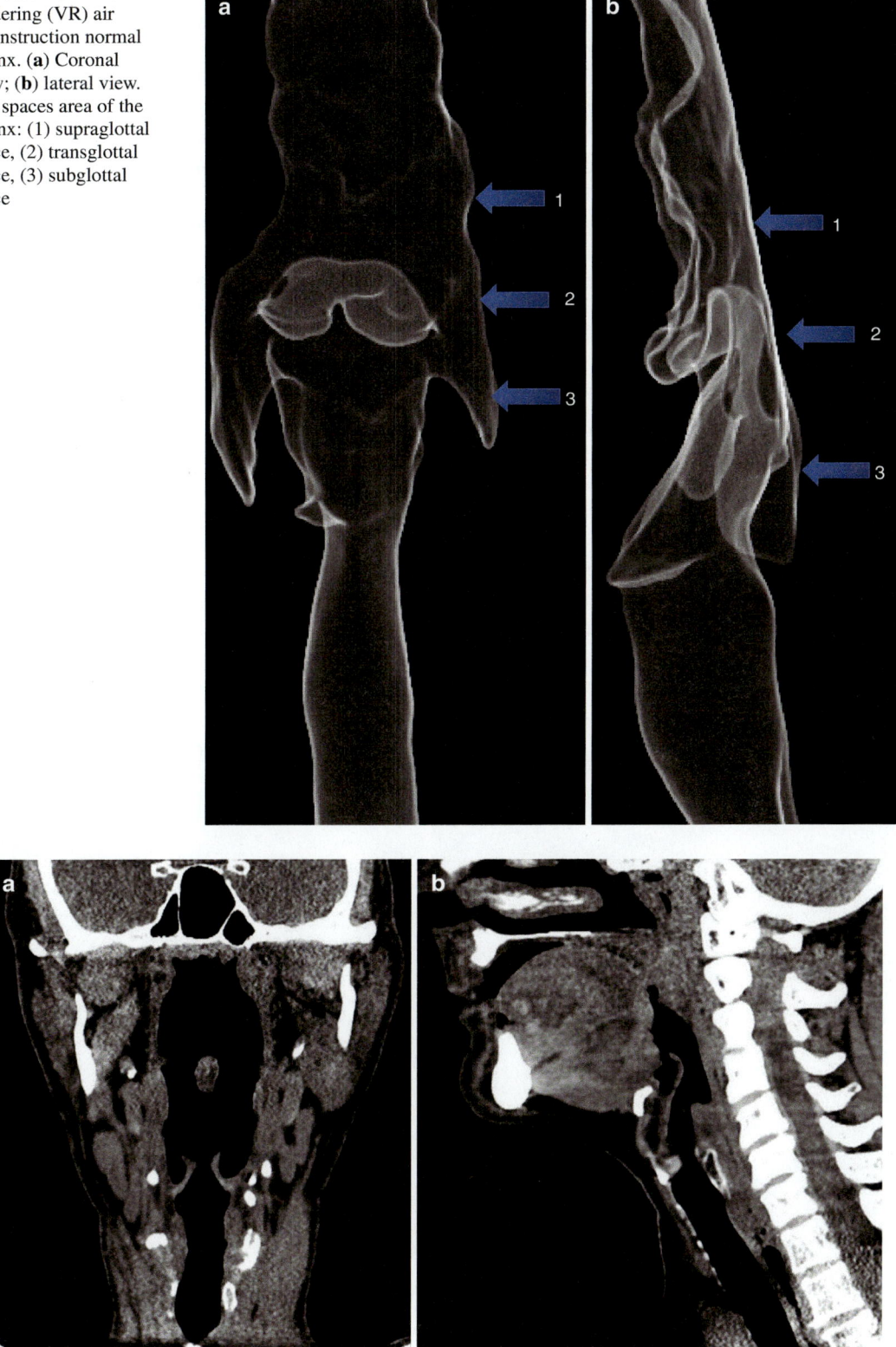

Fig. 6.51 CT volume rendering (VR) air reconstruction normal larynx. (**a**) Coronal view; (**b**) lateral view. The spaces area of the larynx: (1) supraglottal space, (2) transglottal space, (3) subglottal space

Fig. 6.52 (**a**) Coronal reconstructed CT image of the larynx during normal breathing shows the larynx at the level of the vocal cords; (**b**) sagittal reconstructed CT image of the larynx during phonation of /a/

6.9.3 Magnetic Resonance Imaging

In contrast to CT technology, magnetic resonance imaging (MRI) is a common medical imaging technique with no known health risks. A further advantage of this technology is the high quality and resolution of soft tissues (Kim et al. 2009). Since the vocal tract consists of soft tissue walls, this technology can be considered superior for imaging the vocal tract. However, a significant drawback of using MRI in voice- and speech-related studies is the long scanning time. Therefore, in recent years, great focus has been placed on the aspect of acceleration (Scott et al. 2014). Up to now, it is possible to record an entire three-dimensional dataset of the vocal tract within 11 s for analysis (Echternach et al. 2011). However, recent experiments have shown the possibility of an acceleration up to 1.3 s per vocal tract.

Nowadays, by using dynamic real-time two-dimensional MRI, the vocal tract can be analysed for functional aspects, such as voice and speech production as well as swallowing (Echternach et al. 2012). Owing to its greater representation of soft tissues, tongue, velum, lips and larynx move-ments are of crucial interest. Changes in vocal tract shape are of relevance for voice production concerning changing resonatory properties of the vocal tract and for vocal tract voice source inter-actions. Furthermore, such speech articulatory aspects as constriction and closure gestures of the tongue tip and the tongue body can also be anal-ysed. MRI movements of laryngeal inner struc-tures such as the vocal folds become a challenge, but vertical movements of the larynx can be observed during the production of some vowels and other speech sounds (Fig. 6.53a, b).

It should be mentioned, however, that all these recordings are performed from the supine position, which could have a major effect on both articulation and swallowing owing to gravitational forces. In contrast to speech, the vocal tract shape during singing is not consid-ered so much influenced by the position (Traser et al. 2013). The study of the air space of the throat and larynx during obstruction, such as in sleep apnoea, and the study of patients with a deficit of voice/speech function before and after reconstructive surgery of the larynx are impor-tant in clinical practice (Fig. 6.54a, b). There

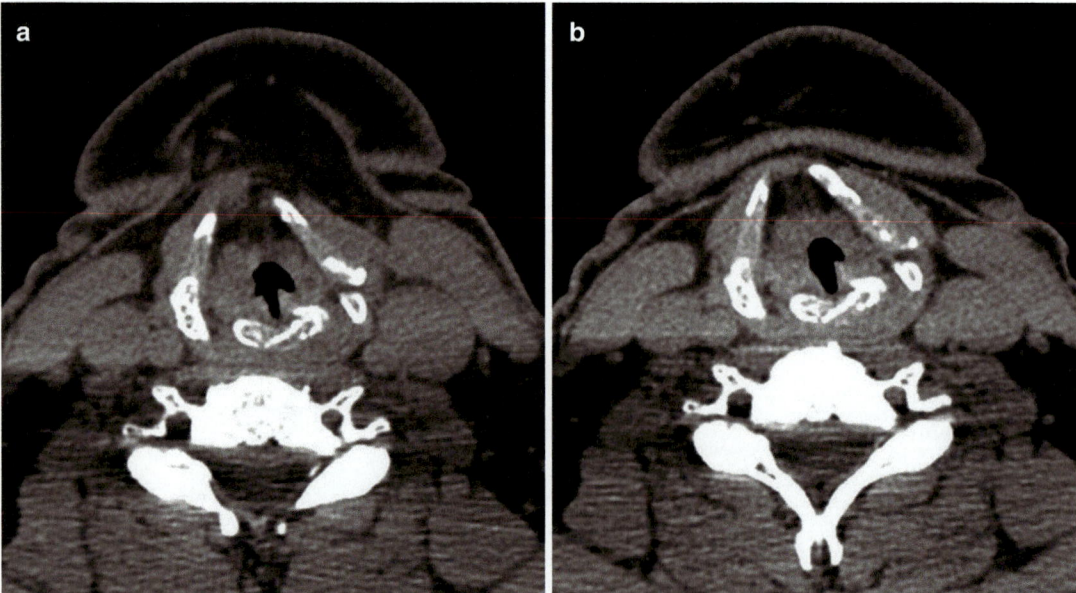

Fig. 6.53 (a) Sagittal image of a cine sequence during phonation (oe); (b) axial image

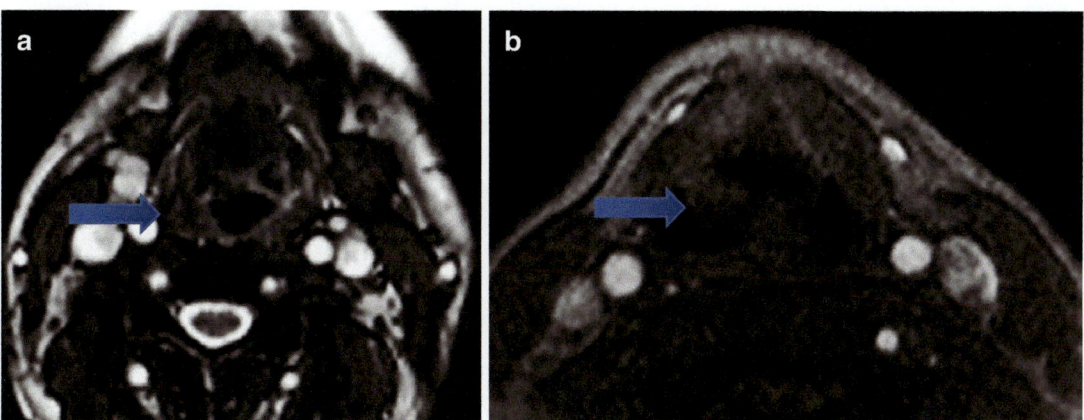

Fig. 6.54 (**a**) Axial view T2-weighted image of the larynx during normal breathing; (**b**) during phonation—on both vocal cords, small fibrotic lesions are marked by arrows

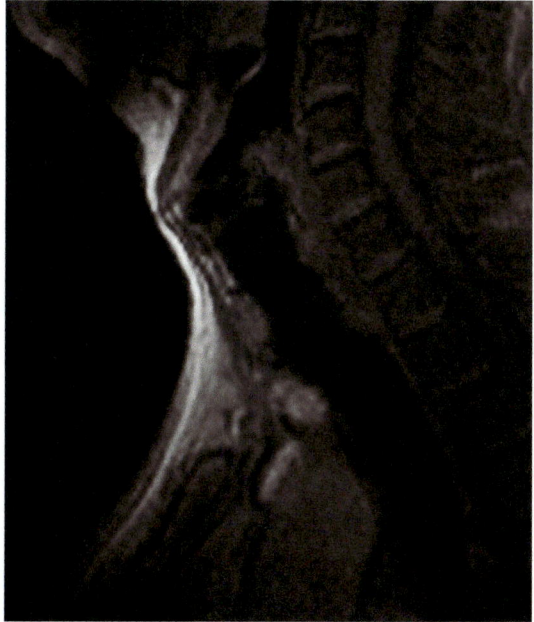

Fig. 6.55 Sagittal T1-weighted images (cine sequence) during swallowing

are many challenges for MRI of the vocal tract, such as respiration, swallowing and voice and speech movements, which require motion-insensitive imaging. All used sequences must be less sensitive to susceptibility artefacts

(Fig. 6.55). Imaging during speech processes or in non-cooperative patients demands ultrafast imaging.

6.9.4 Three-Dimensional Imaging

In recent years, three-dimensional (3D) imaging of the upper airway during sustained sound production has emerged as a promising research tool in voice production as a means to capture the full geometry of the vocal tract. As a result, these models provide improved information on the visualisation of morphological and anatomical aspects and are useful for partial measurements of the vocal tract shape in different conditions. From these 3D-MRI data, calculations of resonance can be performed on 3D printouts (Fig. 6.56) or from estimations from area functions (Echternach et al. 2015). Furthermore, this material can be used for mathematical vocal tract modelling. From MRI images, it is possible to reconstruct the vocal tract shape and volume, as well as the shape and the dimension of the nasal tract, when the velum is lowered. In addition, the shape of the oral, pharyngeal and nasal cavities can be visualised. Three-dimensional high-resolution MRI, espe-

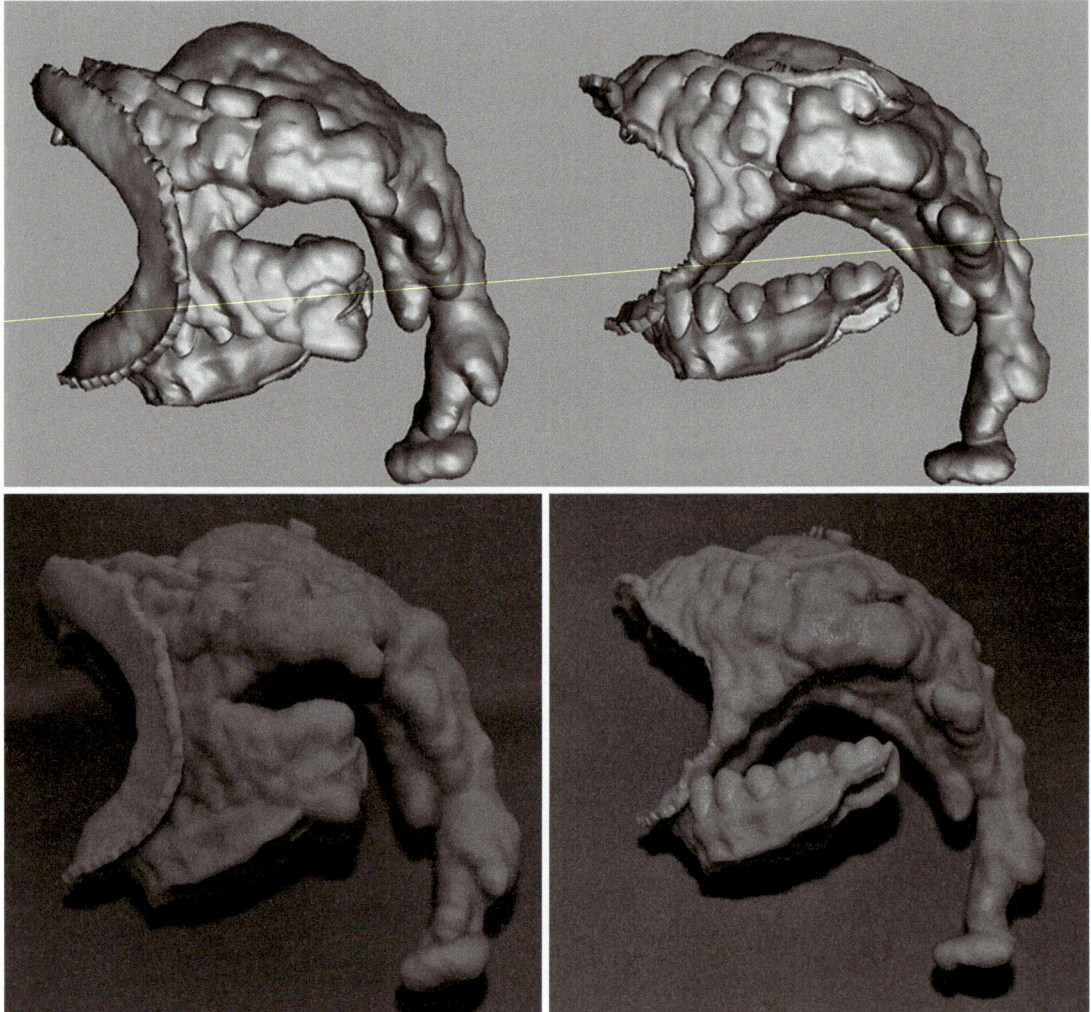

Fig. 6.56 Segmented vocal tract models from the MRI material (upper row, left, pitch C6, and right, pitch G6) and photographs of the 3D print outs (lower row, left, pitch C6, and right, pitch G6, respectively) (Reprinted with permission from Echternach M, Birkholz P, Traser L et al (2015) Articulation and vocal tract acoustics at soprano subject's high fundamental frequencies. J Acoust Soc Am 137(5):2586–2596. Copyright (2015), Acoustic Society of America). The models show the mouth on the left side. The models end at the glottal level. From these models resonatory properties of the vocal tract can be calculated

cially with parallel imaging of the upper airway, has provided valuable insights into vocal tract shaping as well as the data for the modelling of voice and speech production in different languages (Ventura et al. 2011). As a result, these computational models provide valuable information for the enhanced visualisation of morphological and anatomical aspects and are useful for partial measurements of the vocal tract shape in different conditions (Fig. 6.57). Potential use of this information can be found in medical and therapeutic applications as well as in acoustic articulatory voice and speech modelling (Baer et al. 1991).

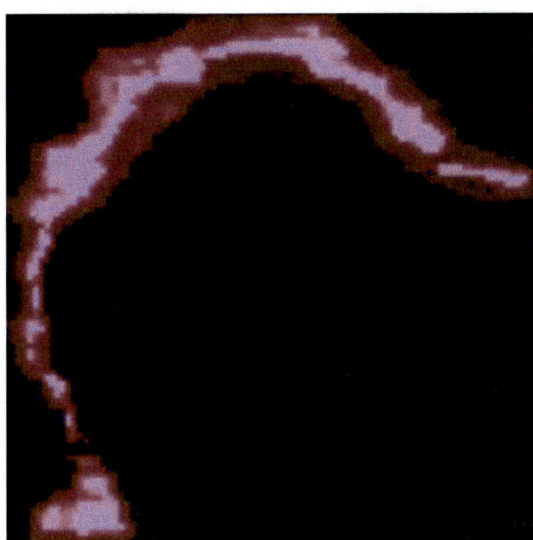

Fig. 6.57 High-resolution MRI 3D after reconstruction using parallel imaging and computer modelling of the upper airway. The shape of airspace during phonation

6.10 Ultrasound in Phoniatrics and Sonographic Examination of the Larynx

Wolfgang Angerstein

6.10.1 Ultrasound in Phoniatrics

Ultrasound application to living tissues has many advantages: it is harmless (no X-ray exposure) and non-invasive, therefore repeatable as often as necessary. Moreover, it is relatively simple and does not cause any discomfort for the patient. Therefore, it is well suited especially for children, even for small babies. And finally, it is relatively inexpensive compared with other imaging techniques such as CT or MRI.

Nowadays, mostly B-mode scans are used. In these two-dimensional images, different tissue densities are represented by different brightness grades (B = brightness) on the ultrasound screen. When a B-mode image is moved across the screen with constant velocity and the ultrasound transducer is always kept in the same place without being moved, a one-dimensional TM (time motion)-mode image results. Thus, B-mode lines in temporal order are continuously visible on the screen over the course of time.

By dividing the screen into two halves, B-mode may be combined with TM-mode. The TM-mode registers movement amplitudes of defined points at the surface of living tissues (e.g. vocal folds, epiglottis, tongue) over a period of time. The exact location of these surface points may be chosen with a cursor in the corresponding B-mode image during simultaneous recording of B- and TM-mode on the same screen.

Today, mainly high-resolution ultrasound probes with 7.5 or 19 MHz are used, either as linear array or as convex 90° resp. 100° sectorial scanners. In phoniatrics, the sonographic imaging mainly focuses on functional disturbances (dysfunctions) rather than on morphological alterations (see Table 6.8).

Table 6.8 Ultrasound in phoniatrics: spoken articulation, articulation for brass instrument playing, phonation, sucking, swallowing

Organ/region	Ultrasound technique
Lips	B-mode, colour duplex
Tongue	B-mode, TM-mode
Lateral hypopharyngeal walls, upper oesophageal sphincter	B-mode, TM-mode
Pseudoglottis (ructus)	B-mode, TM-mode
Larynx: Skeleton (ectolarynx), hyoid bone	B-mode
Vocal folds/vestibular folds (endolarynx)	Colour duplex, B-mode, TM-mode
Cervical veins (hyperfunctional dysphonia)	Colour duplex

6.10.2 Ultrasound Investigations of the Larynx

6.10.2.1 Sonographic Examination of the Larynx

The application of ultrasound to the larynx can be traced back to 1959; the first publications appeared in the 1960s (Beach and Kelsey 1969; Bordone-Sacerdote and Sacerdote 1965; Mensch 1964; Minifie et al. 1968). Sonographic examinations of the larynx are called echolaryngography, echoglottography, ultrasonoglottography, ultrasonic glottography or ultrasound glottography. The aim is an examination and documentation especially of the vocal folds but also of the ventricular folds. Their vibratory patterns during phonation can be observed and analysed. Furthermore, movements of the epiglottis, the vocal folds and the arytaenoid cartilages are visible.

Sonographic visibility of these structures is nevertheless limited by ossification of the thyroid cartilage (Bozzato et al. 2007): since the ultrasound beam is absorbed by ossified thyroid cartilage, a complete extinction of the sonographic signal or artefacts may result. Fortunately, this problem does not appear in children, because their thyroid cartilage is not yet calcified (Friedman 1997; Garel et al. 1990, 1992; Grunert et al. 1989; Raghavendra et al. 1987). Moreover,

conventional transoral or transnasal laryngoscopy is often problematic in children. Therefore, sonographic examination of the larynx (especially the vocal folds) may be a non-invasive alternative to check hoarseness and other voice abnormalities in children. In grown-ups, echolaryngography may be helpful if the larynx is hard to examine by conventional endoscopy (e.g. in patients with a strong gag reflex, with increased pharyngeal or laryngeal muscle tension or with panic attacks). Moreover, irritations of the pharynx or larynx due to endoscopy can be avoided by sonographic imaging. Although the image resolution is not as good as in MRI or CT scans, sonography of the larynx can sometimes serve as a harmless screening method even if the thyroid cartilage is already calcified.

Examples of B- and TM-mode sonography are numerous (Arruti and Poumayrac 2010; Böhme 1988a, 1989; Gomaa et al. 2013; Miles 1989; Murlewska et al. 1992; Ooi 1992; Valente et al. 1996; Zappia and Campani 2000).

The patients are usually examined when in a supine position (alternatively, they sometimes may be reclined, with their neck well extended). Since the thyroid cartilage serves both as anatomical landmark and as acoustic window (facilitating sound transmission), the ultrasound transducer is usually placed horizontally parallel to the upper margin of the thyroid cartilage (A1 in Fig. 6.58)

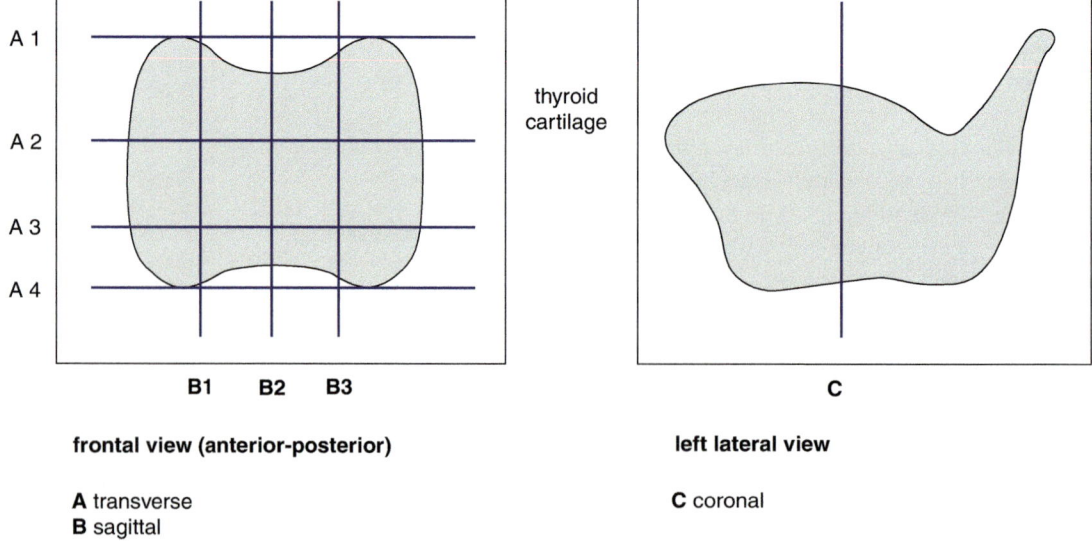

frontal view (anterior-posterior)   left lateral view

A transverse   **C** coronal
B sagittal

Fig. 6.58 Possible sectional planes for sonographic examination of the larynx

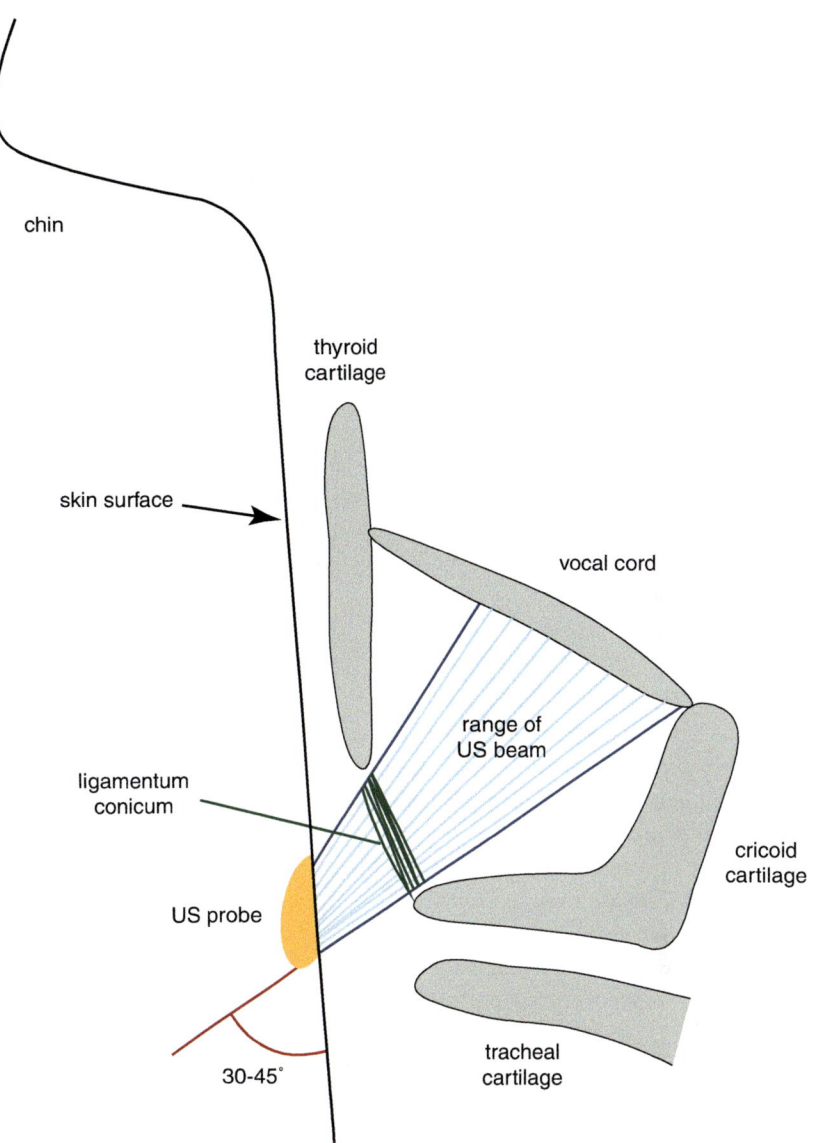

Fig. 6.59 Transverse ultrasound scanning of the glottis through the ligamentum conicum (left lateral view)

chin

thyroid cartilage

skin surface

vocal cord

range of US beam

ligamentum conicum

cricoid cartilage

US probe

30–45°

tracheal cartilage

or approximately 2 cm below the thyroid notch (A2 in Fig. 6.58) with a slight caudal inclination, thus producing transverse B-mode scans of the supraglottal and glottal regions. The scanner is then continuously moved down along the midline of the thyroid cartilage. If the scanner is placed horizontally about 1 cm below the thyroid prominence (A3 in Fig. 6.58), the ultrasound beam has an anterior-posterior direction and corresponds to the horizontal level of the vocal folds.

For transverse B-mode scans, the probe may also be positioned horizontally at the ventral side of the neck with an inclination of 30–45° against the surface of the skin. The ultrasound beam is directed upwards through the ligamentum conicum, thus hitting the caudal surface of the glottis, coming from down below in a caudo-cranial direction (A4 in Fig. 6.58, see also Fig. 6.59).

Sagittal B-mode scans of the larynx in anterior-posterior direction are possible through the midline (midsagittal planes, B2 in Fig. 6.58) or through the right and left part of the thyroid cartilage (B1 and B3 in Fig. 6.58). The ultrasound transducer is in a vertical position. In paramedian planes (B1 and B3 in Fig. 6.58), with a slight latero-medial inclination of the scanner, the recurrent laryngeal nerve may sometimes be seen as a linear structure behind or below the thyroid lobe.

For coronal B-mode scans of the glottis, the ultrasound probe is positioned vertically along the side of the neck (C in Fig. 6.58). The ultrasound beam is directed perpendicularly to the glottis, against the central parts of the thyroid cartilage and against the surface of the neck.

Movements of the vocal folds may also be observed with simultaneous B- and TM-mode registration in coronal planes. Simultaneous B- and TM-mode registration in sagittal planes shows vertical movements of the epiglottis during swallowing or phonation; simultaneous B- and TM-mode registration in transverse planes along the upper margin of the thyroid cartilage (A1 in Fig. 6.58) shows horizontal epiglottal movements.

6.10.2.2 Doppler Techniques in Larynx Investigation

By using ultrasonic Doppler techniques, voice alterations and vibratory patterns of the vocal folds during phonation can be observed. Thus, Doppler monitoring may increase the sensitivity of laryngeal B-mode examinations.

The Doppler technique rests on the principle that an echo reflected from a moving structure will be shifted in frequency in proportion to the velocity of the moving structure. At the glottal level, the Doppler frequency shift is produced by a reflection of the ultrasonic beam from the surface of the vibrating vocal folds during phonation.

The following Doppler techniques may be applied:

Pulsed Wave (PW) Method (with One Transducer) Ultrasound pulses are emitted by a transducer and reflected by the vibrating vocal folds. The reflected signal (echo) is registered by the same transducer. Thus, the time-varying displacement of the vocal folds during phonation may be calculated with the Doppler formula as Doppler frequency shift of the reflected ultrasound.

Continuous Wave (CW) Method (with Two Transducers, a Transmitter and a Receiver) Continuous ultrasound waves are transmitted laterally through the glottis with two transducers matched in frequency and located on opposite sides of the larynx. One transducer emits the ultrasound signal, which is frequency-modulated depending on vocal fold velocity and displacement during phonation. Only when the glottis is closed, the ultrasound signal is transmitted through the larynx. The ultrasonic beam passing through the vibrating vocal folds is periodically interrupted whenever the glottis is open during the vibratory cycle. This interruption depends on the fact that the acoustic impedance of air is much smaller than that of the vocal folds, and the frequency of the ultrasonic beam changes with the variations of the contact area of the vocal folds. Thus, the second transducer receives altered ultrasound waves with a frequency shift, the Doppler signal.

Duplex Sonography (Transverse B-Mode Scans Combined with PW Doppler) Duplex sonography (Böhme 1991; Schindler et al. 1990) allows an identification of the glottis even when the vocal folds are not visible in B-mode scans: during phonation, a typical Doppler frequency shift signal may be recorded that is reflected from the surface of the vibrating vocal folds. This pulsed Doppler spectrum has a positive amplitude (above the horizontal baseline), when the vibrating vocal folds are moving towards the Doppler probe. When the vibrating vocal folds are moving away from the Doppler probe, the pulsed Doppler spectrum has a negative amplitude (below the horizontal baseline). The pulsed Doppler spectrum (also called echo Doppler sonogram) shows a fundamental frequency, upper harmonics and formants in the course of time during phonation. Depending on the sample volume (which can be chosen arbitrarily), defined segments of the vocal folds may be examined. Dysphonic voices are characterised by aperiodic echo Doppler sonograms: the more dysphonic the patient, the more structures of the pulsed Doppler spectrum disappear. Also, a time difference between the onset of positive and negative pulsed Doppler spectra may occur.

Colour Duplex Sonography (Colour-Coded Transverse B-Mode Scans Combined with PW Doppler) This method detects a time difference between the onset of positive and negative pulsed Doppler spectra (Böhme 1992). When the vibrating vocal folds move towards the Doppler probe, the images are red. When they move away from the Doppler probe, the scans are dark blue. When the velocity of the vocal fold vibrations increases, the colour turns from red to orange or yellow. When the velocity decreases, the colour turns from dark blue to light blue or green. By colour Doppler imaging, vibrations of the glottal and supraglottal mucosa may be observed (Tsai et al. 2008), the effective vibration length of the vocal folds can be measured (Hsiao et al. 2002), and the vocal fold mucosal wave velocity can be calculated (Hsiao et al. 2001; Shau et al. 2001).

A thorough sonographic laryngeal examination takes between 15 min (without Doppler) and 30 min (including Doppler).

6.10.2.3 Critical Evaluation of Laryngeal Doppler Sonography

Compared with other imaging techniques for analysing vibratory patterns of the vocal folds (e.g. stroboscopy, high-speed line scanning, kymography), the spatial and temporal resolution of laryngeal Doppler sonography is not yet satisfying and needs to be improved. The same is true for voice analyses: so far the accuracy of the echo Doppler sonogram is also not satisfying (Böhme 1991; Schindler et al. 1990). Compared with conventional acoustic voice analyses (e.g. jitter, shimmer, sonography, spectrography), the pulsed Doppler spectrum is still less precise, not so reliable and therefore less meaningful in clinical routine.

At the moment, laryngeal Doppler sonography is limited to screening tests. It may also give additional, supplementary information in combination with conventional diagnostic techniques. In order to become useful for routine clinical examinations of laryngeal function and voice quality, further development and research is needed.

6.10.3 Pseudoglottis of Laryngectomised Patients

By simultaneous recording of midsagittal or transverse B-mode and corresponding TM-mode images, vibrations of the pseudoglottis during a laryngeal ructus phonation can be observed (Böckler et al. 1988; Böhme 1988b). The ultrasound probe is positioned vertically in the midline (for midsagittal scans) or horizontally (for transverse scans) at the ventral side of the neck, right below the chin and just above the tracheostoma.

During ructus phonation of different vowels, mucosal vibrations in the pharyngo-oesophageal (PE) segment are clearly visible below the root of the tongue, both in B-mode and in TM-mode scans. Each vowel has a typical, easily reproducible sonographic pattern in the TM-mode. The length of the pseudoglottis (12–18 mm) can be determined in B-mode images by distinguishing vibrating from non-vibrating mucosal tissues of the PE segment between the base of the tongue and the upper oesophagus. The mucosal vibration rates of the pseudoglottis may be determined by counting the maxima of their vibratory amplitudes in TM-mode images. Alternatively, light and dark vertical stripes caused by vibrating mucosal tissues may be counted in the TM-mode images. These sonographic vibration rates of the PE segments (42–74 Hz) are in very good accordance with the fundamental frequencies of the simultaneously recorded ructus speech sounds (44–75 Hz).

By applying special software to the B-mode scans, surface contours of the vibrating mucosal tissues can be marked interactively image by image. When these surface contours are extracted and afterwards sampled in temporal order, a pseudo-3-dimensional (pseudo-3D) reconstruction of the pseudoglottis results. The vibrating mucosal tissues can be analysed over the course of time, since the extracted B-mode contours are lined up along a temporal axis. Thus, pseudoglottal vibrations lasting for several seconds may be summarised in one illustration.

Since ultrasound beams are reflected by implanted voice prostheses, vibrations of the pseudoglottis during ructus phonation can only be observed without voice prosthesis!

6.10.4 Cervical Venous Congestion in Hyperfunctional Dysphonia

The flow of blood through the veins of the neck is dependent upon:

- Intra-pulmonary or intrathoracic changes in pressure synchronous with breathing on inspiration and expiration (pathological thoracic breathing or poorly coordinated respiration and phonation in hyperfunctional vocalisation can contribute to reduced blood flow in the jugular vein!)
- The heartbeat (physiological changes in the axis of the heart and relative position of the heart valves during systole and diastole)

Neck veins that are blocked and therefore engorged owing to strained, hyperfunctional vocalisation were described as early as 1920. This type of enlarged neck veins was not only observed in patients with hyperfunctional dysphonia but also often in woodwind and brass instrument musicians.

The cause of jugular vein distension is a distinct contraction (tension) in the sternocleidomastoid and omohyoid muscles. Figure 6.60 shows a scheme of the topographic-anatomical relationships between the jugular veins and both these muscles. The thin walls of the neck veins are easily 'squeezed' owing to these muscles' abnormal contraction, which can lead to an enormous reduction in blood circulation in the cervical veins.

The largest neck vein, the vena jugularis interna, is most easily seen on ultrasound imaging (Angerstein et al. 1993a, b). The large-calibre vena jugularis externa can also usually be displayed, especially when it is blocked and engorged through hyperfunctional vocalising.

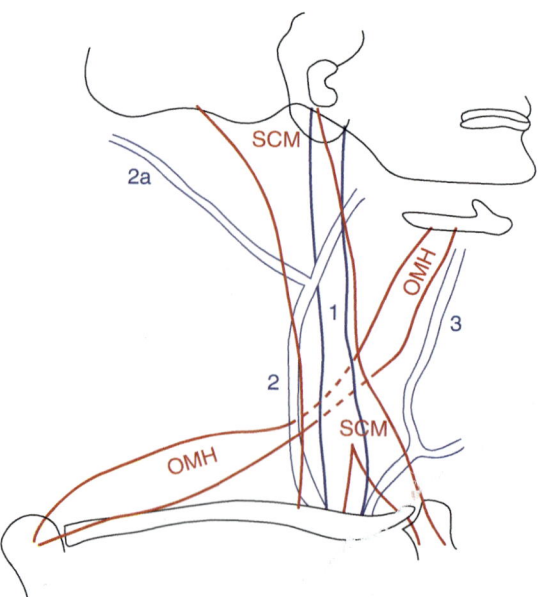

Fig. 6.60 This figure shows a schematic drawing of the topographic-anatomical relationships between the jugular veins, musculus sternocleidomastoideus and musculus omohyoideus (modified from Lanz and Wachsmuth 1955: Practical Anatomy). (1) V. jugularis interna; (2) V. jugularis externa [2a = V. jugularis externa posterior]; (3) V. jugularis anterior; *SCM* M. sternocleidomastoideus; *OMH* M. omohyoideus. Copyright with kind permission from Springer Science and Bus Media BV

A blocked vena jugularis anterior can occasionally be displayed by using sonography.

Identification of the veins in the neck is made much simpler by using the Valsalva manoeuvre (voiceless pressing) which significantly enlarges the lumen of the vein. Dilated, swollen neck veins are then significantly easier to locate. The veins on the right side of the neck are, as a rule, wider and therefore easier to recognise and investigate than those on the left. The vena jugularis interna is also positioned slightly more laterally from the arteria carotis communis on the right side than the left vein, which often overlies the artery.

The ultrasound monitor should be divided vertically in the centre line: the right side should show B-mode sectional images of the lumen of the veins; the left side should show synchronous intravenous blood flow over time (i.e. the Doppler shift frequency spectrum of the speed of the blood flow). 'Pulsed wave' (PW) Doppler signals are also used here. Depiction of the veins of the neck by using B-mode sonography with a simultaneous PW Doppler spectrum is called duplex ultrasonography. Colour-coding these signals ('colour duplex sonography') has several benefits:

- Identification of the veins is easier (especially in children).
- The direction of blood flow (away from or towards the transducer) is discernible.
- Changes in the speed of blood flow can be visualised with colour gradation.

High-resolution 7.5 MHz linear transducers are used in colour duplex sonography of the jugular vein (5 MHz is also acceptable but the resolution is better with 7.5 MHz transducers). The investigation can be performed with the patient sitting or lying supine with the head rotated 10–15° to the opposite side. One advantage of the supine position is that the jugular veins have a higher filling state and are therefore easier to locate. The seated position (with upright upper body), however, has the advantage of being the usual position in which phonation takes place (vocalisation only occasionally takes place when in a supine position!). To avoid compression of the thin-walled veins of the neck, the transducer should be pressed onto the skin of the neck as lightly as possible. A large standoff distance (approx. 5 mm) by using a sufficient amount of ultrasound gel is absolutely necessary. The Doppler probe is held over the surface of the skin at an angle of 10–45° so that the ultrasonic checking is in the antero-caudal plane. The transducer is moved from a ventral position parallel to the course of the vein being investigated (e.g. the vena jugularis interna). The arteria carotis communis and musculus sternocleidomastoideus are useful 'landmarks' to help find the vena jugularis interna. Ideally, the veins should be shown in both longitudinal and cross sections, i.e. in two planes, though it is often only possible to show them longitudinally. The head and body position should vary as little as possible during the investigation in order to minimise any position-related changes of the blood flow in the jugular veins.

The so-called Doppler gate (the locally defined area of measurement inside the lumen of the vessel) should be adjusted to the individual vessel diameter. The size of the gate and the angle between the direction of blood flow and the gate should be kept as constant as possible throughout the entire investigation. This angle varies interindividually from 30° to 45°. The best possible quality of pulsed Doppler signals can be achieved by using a low repetition frequency of the B-mode images (0–2 images per second).

Common current signals of the jugular vein can be heard during Doppler sonography, the main one of which is a low-frequency breath-like noise, synchronous with breathing, which sounds similar to a humming ('venous hum') or the howling wind. This current noise is caused by respiration-dependent pressure changes in the veins of the neck, in which fluctuations in blood flow of 10–15% occur synchronously with breathing.

An investigation of jugular vein distension by colour duplex sonography takes 10–15 min for one side of the neck, depending on how visible the veins and the quality of the Doppler blood flow signal are.

By using colour Doppler one sees a clear reduction in venous blood flow of an average 74% (up to 90% in some individual cases!) in hyperfunctional vocalisation, and the thin-walled veins of the neck can more than double in diameter in comparison with the initial values during calm breathing without phonation. Following successful logopaedic treatment of hyperfunctional dysphonia, the blood flow in the jugular veins normalises, and the diameter during phonation reduces by at least 50%! In participants with healthy voices (with no hypertonic tension of the musculus sternocleidomastoideus or omohyoideus), blood flow in the veins of the neck during physiological phonation can reduce by approximately 10% in comparison with initial values during calm breathing without phonation. Such changes of venous blood flow and diameter can be monitored during the course of therapy non-invasively and without exposure to radiation by using colour duplex sonography. Because it is non-invasive and does not require exposure to radiation, colour duplex sonography is also suitable for visualising biofeedback (hyperfunctional versus relaxed vocalisation).

References

Alku P (2011) Glottal inverse filtering analysis of human voice production—a review of estimation and parameterization methods of the glottal excitation and their applications. Sadhana 36(5):623–650. https://www.ias.ac.in/article/fulltext/sadh/036/05/0623-0650. Accessed 14 April 2019

Altenmüller E, Jabusch HC (2006a) Neurologische Erkrankungen bei Musikern. Med Welt 57:569–575

Altenmüller E, Jabusch HC (2006b) Focal dystonia in musicians: from phenomenology to therapy. Adv Cogn Psychol 2(2–3):207–220

Altenmüller E, Jabusch HC (2008) Apollos Fluch—Musikerdystonien. InFo Neurologie & Psychiatrie 5:46–53

Angerstein W, Klajman S, Neuschaefer-Rube C et al (1993a) Badanie sonograficzne szybkości przepływu krwi w zyle szyjnej wewnetrznej w hyperfunkcjonalnej dysfonii dzieciecej. (Sonographic imaging of internal jugular venous blood flow in juvenile hyperfunctional dysphonia). Otolaryngol Pol 47(3):264–269

Angerstein W, Wein B, Klajman S (1993b) Duplexsonographie der V. jugularis interna bei hyperfunktioneller Dysphonie. Sprache-Stimme-Gehör 17(1):31–34

Arcier AF, Vernay A (1994) Observation clinique: lésions musculaires labiales liées au jeu de cuivres. Médecine des Arts 8:14–19

Aronson A, Bless D (2009) Clinical voice disorders. Thieme, New York

Arruti A, Poumayrac M (2010) Ecografia laringea: una técnica alternativa en la valoración de la encrucijada aero-digestiva. Rev Imagenol 14(1):30–36

Awan SN, Roy N, Zhang D et al (2016) Validation of the Cepstral Spectral Index of Dysphonia (CSID) as a screening tool for voice disorders: development of clinical cutoff scores. J Voice 30(2):130–144

Baer T, Gore JC, Gracco LC et al (1991) Analysis of vocal tract shape and dimensions using magnetic resonance imaging: vowels. J Acoust Soc Am 90(2):799–828

Baken RJ, Orlikoff R (2000) Clinical measurement of speech and voice. Singular Thomson Learning, San Diego

Bassich C, Ludlow C (1986) The use of perceptual methods for assessing voice quality. J Speech Hear Disord 51(2):125–133

Baum U, Greess H, Lell M et al (2000) Imaging of head and neck tumors—methods-CT, spiral-CT, multislice-spiral-CT. Eur J Radiol 33(3):153–160

Beach JL, Kelsey CA (1969) Ultrasonic Doppler monitoring of vocal-fold velocity and displacement. J Acoust Soc Am 46(4b):1045–1047

Beukers R, Bierens E, Kingma H et al (1995) Voice load as measured by the voice accumulator. Folia Phoniatr Logop 47(5):252–261

Bless DM, Baken RJ (1992) Assessment of voice. J Voice 6(2):95–97

Blitzer A (1995) Laryngeal electromyography. In: Rubin JS et al (eds) Diagnosis and treatment of voice disorders. Igaku-Shoin, New York, pp 316–326

BMA (Ärztl. Sachverständigenrat beim Bundesministerium für Arbeit u. Sozialordnung) (2002) Druckschädigung der Nerven. Merkblatt zur Berufskrankheit Nr. 2106 der Anlage zur Berufskrankheitenverordnung (BKV): Bundesarbeitsblatt 11(62)

Böckelmann I, Schneyer B (2009) Arbeitsbedingte Belastungen und Erkrankungen von Musikern. Arbeitsmed Sozialmed Umweltmed 4:237–242

Böckler R, Wein B, Klajman S et al (1988) Die Ultraschalluntersuchung der Pseudoglottis bei Kehlkopflosen. HNO 36(3):115–118

Böhme G (1988a) Echolaryngographie—Ein Beitrag zur Methode der Ultraschalldiagnostik des Kehlkopfes. Laryngol Rhinol Otol 67(11):551–558

Böhme G (1988b) Ultraschalldiagnostik der phonatorischen Leistungen des Laryngektomierten. Laryngol Rhinol Otol 67(12):651–656

Böhme G (1989) Ein klinischer Beitrag zur Ultraschalldiagnostik des Kehlkopfes (Echolaryngographie). Laryngol Rhinol Otol 68(9):510–515

Böhme G (1991) Duplexsonographie des Kehlkopfes: 1. Bewegungsanalyse intralaryngealer Strukturen. Otorhinolaryngol Nova 1(6):338–342

Böhme G (1992) Duplexsonographie des Kehlkopfes: 2. Farbkodierte Bewegungsanalyse intralaryngealer Strukturen. Otorhinolaryngol Nova 2(1):43–45

Böhme G, Gross M (2001) Stroboskopie und andere Verfahren zur Analyse der Stimmlippenschwingungen. Median, Heidelberg

Boone D (1993) The Boone voice program for children, 2nd edn. Pro-Ed, Austin, TX

Boone DR, McFarlane SC, Von Berg SL (2005) The voice and voice therapy, 7th edn. Allyn & Bacon, Boston, MA

Borch DZ, Sundberg J, Lindestad PÅ et al (2004) Vocal fold vibration and voice source aperiodicity in 'dist' tones: a study of a timbral ornament in rock singing. Logoped Phoniatr Vocol 29(4):147–153

Bordone-Sacerdote C, Sacerdote G (1965) Investigations on the movement of the glottis by ultrasounds. Paper presented at the 5th International Congress on Audiology, Liège, 7–14 Sept 1965, Paper Nr. A 42, p 4

Bough D, Heuer RJ, Sataloff RT et al (1996) Intrasubject variability of objective voice measures. J Voice 10(2):166–174

Boutin H, Fletcher N, Smith J et al (2015) Relationships between pressure, flow, lip motion, and upstream and downstream impedances for the trombone. J Acoust Soc Am 137(3):1195–1209

Bozzato A, Zenk J, Gottwald F et al (2007) Der Einfluss der Schildknorpelossifikation bei der Larynxsonografie. Laryngol Rhinol Otol 86(4):276–281

Brockmann-Bauser M, Drinnan MJ (2011) Routine acoustic voice analysis: time to think again? Curr Opin Otolaryngol Head Neck Surg 19(3):165–170

Bromage S, Campbell M, Gilbert J (2005) Experimental investigation of the open area of the brass player's vibrating lips. In: Proceedings of the Forum

Acusticum, Budapest, 29 August–2 September 2005. OPAKFI, Budapest, pp 729–734

Bromage S (2007) Visualisation of the lip motion of brass instrument players, and investigations of an artificial mouth as a tool for comparative studies of instruments. PhD thesis, University of Edinburgh, Edinburgh. https://www.era.lib.ed.ac.uk/handle/1842/1966. Accessed 9 Feb 2018

Bromage S, Campbell M, Gilbert J (2010) Open areas of vibrating lips in trombone playing. Acta Acust Acust 96(4):603–613

Bumiller OE (1936) Antwort zu Frage 25 im "Fragekasten": Lippenverletzungen durch Blasinstrument. Dtsch Zahnärztl Wschr 39:295

Bum-Soo K, Kook JA, Young HP et al (2008) Usefulness of laryngeal phonation CT in the diagnosis of vocal cord paralysis. Am J Roentgenol 190(5):1376–1379

Campos FG (2005) Trumpet technique. Oxford University Press, Oxford, p 51

Cantarella G, Iofrida E, Boria P et al (2014) Ambulatory phonation monitoring in a sample of 92 call center operators. J Voice 28(3):393.e1–393.e6. https://doi.org/10.1016/j.jvoice.2013.10.002

Carding PN, Horsley IA (1992) An evaluation of voice therapy in non-organic dysphonia. Eur J Disord Commun 27(2):137–148

Chick J, Bromage S, Campbell M (2005) Transient behaviour in the motion of the brass player's lips. In: Proceedings of the Forum Acusticum, Budapest, 29 August–2 September 2005. OPAKFI, Budapest, pp 753–775

Cohen SM, Jacobson BH, Garrett CG et al (2007) Creation and validation of the Singing Voice Handicap Index. Ann Otol Rhinol Laryngol 116(6):402–406

Cohen SM, Statham M, Rosen CA et al (2009) Development and validation of the Singing Voice Handicap Index-10. Laryngoscope 119(9):1864–1869

Colton RH, Woo P (1995) Measuring vocal fold function. In: Rubin JS et al (eds) Diagnosis and treatment of voice disorders. Igaku-Shoin, New York, pp 290–315

Colton RH, Casper JK (1996) Understanding voice problems. Williams & Wilkins, Baltimore

Dacakis G, Davies S, Oates JM et al (2013) Development and preliminary evaluation of the transsexual voice questionnaire for male-to-female transsexuals. J Voice 27(3):312–320

Damsté PH (1966) Les vibrations des cordes vocales compares aux vibrations des levres d'un trombonist. J Fr Otorhinolaryngol Chir Maxillofac 4:395–396

De Bodt MS, Van de Heyning PH, Wuyts FL et al (1996) The perceptual evaluation of voice disorders. Acta Otorhinolaryngol Belg 50(4):283–291

De Bodt MS, Wuyts FL, Van de Heyning PH et al (1997) Test-retest study of the GRBAS scale: influence of experience and professional background on perceptual rating of voice quality. J Voice 11(1):74–80

Dejonckere P (2010) Assessment of voice and respiratory function. In: Remacle M, Eckel HE (eds) Surgery of larynx and trachea, vol 11. Springer-Verlag, Berlin/Heidelberg. https://doi.org/10.1007/978-3-540-79136-2_2

Dejonckere PH (1987) EMG of the larynx. Press Productions, Liège

Dejonckere PH, Knoops P, Lebacq J (1988) Evoked muscular potentials in laryngeal muscles. Acta Otolaryngol Belg 42(4):494–501

Dejonckere PH, Obbens C, de Moor GM et al (1993) Perceptual evaluation of dysphonia: reliability and relevance. Folia Phoniatr 45(2):76–83

Dejonckere PH, Remacle M, Fresnel-Elbaz E et al (1996) Differentiated perceptual evaluation of pathological voice quality: reliability and correlations with acoustic measurements. Rev Laryngol Otol Rhinol 117(3):219–224

Dejonckere PH (1996) Electroglottography: a useful method in voice investigation. In: Pais-Clemente M (ed) Voice update. Excerpta Medica, Elsevier, Amsterdam, pp 29–33

Dejonckere PH (1998) Effect of louder voicing on acoustical measurements in dysphonic patients. Logoped Phoniatr Vocol 23(2):79–84

Dejonckere PH (2000) Perceptual and laboratory assessment of dysphonia. Otolaryngol Clin N Am 33(4):731–750

Dejonckere PH, Crevier L, Elbaz E et al (2000) Clinical implementation of a multidimensional basic protocol for assessing functional results of voice therapy. In: Jahnke K, Fischer M (eds) Proceedings of the 4th EUFOS Congress, Berlin, pp 561–565

Dejonckere PH, Bradley P, Clemente P et al (2001) A basic protocol for functional assessment of voice pathology, especially for investigating the efficacy of (phonosurgical) treatments and evaluating new assessment techniques. Guideline elaborated by the Committee on Phoniatrics of the European Laryngological Society (ELS). Eur Arch Otorhinolaryngol 258(2):77–82

Dejonckere PH, Lebacq J (2001) Plasticity of voice quality: a prognostic factor for outcome of voice therapy? J Voice 15(2):251–256

Dejonckere PH, van Wijngaarden HA (2001) Retropharyngeal autologous fat transplantation for congenital short palate: a nasometric assessment of functional results. Ann Otol Rhinol Laryngol 110(2):168–172

Dejonckere PH (2006a) Aerodynamic and acoustic voice measurements. In: Benninger MS, Murry T (eds) The performer's voice. Plural Publishing, San Diego

Dejonckere PH (2006b) Critères acoustiques de fluence pour l'évaluation des dysphonies spasmodiques. Klein-Dallant C (ed) Paris, pp 157–166

Dejonckere PH, Schoentgen J, Giordano A et al (2011) Validity of jitter measures in non-quasi-periodic voices. Part I: Perceptual and computer performances in cycle pattern recognition. The effect of noise. Logoped Phoniatr Vocol 36(2):70–77

Dejonckere PH, Giordano A, Schoentgen J et al (2012a) To what degree of voice perturbation are jitter measurements valid? A novel approach with synthesized vowels and visuo-perceptual pattern recognition. Biomed Signal Process Control 7(1):37–42

Dejonckere PH, Neumann KJ, Moerman MB et al (2012b) Tridimensional assessment of adductor spasmodic dysphonia pre- and post-treatment with botulinum toxin. Eur Arch Otorhinolaryngol 269(4):1195–2003

Dejonckere PH, Moerman MB, Martens JP et al (2012c) Voicing quantification is more relevant than period perturbation in substitution voices: an advanced acoustical study. Eur Arch Otorhinolaryngol 269(4): 1205–1212

De Krom G (1995) Some spectral correlates of pathological breathy and rough voice quality for different types of vowel fragments. J Speech Hear Res 38(4):794–811

Donnet A, Dessi P, Koeppel MC (1996) Le syndrome de Satchmo. Presse Med 25(4):173

Echternach M, Sundberg J, Baumann T et al (2011) Vocal tract area functions and formant frequencies in opera tenors' modal and falsetto registers. J Acoust Soc Am 129(6):3955–3963

Echternach M, Markl M, Richter B et al (2012) Dynamic real-time magnetic resonance imaging for the analysis of voice physiology. Curr Opin Otolaryngol Head Neck Surg 20(6):450–457

Echternach M, Richter B, Traser L et al (2013) Veränderung der stimmlichen Leistungsfähigkeit durch verschiedene Stimmbelastungstests. (Change of vocal capacity due to different vocal loading tests). Laryngo-Rhino-Otol 92(1):34–40

Echternach M, Birkholz P, Traser L et al (2015) Articulation and vocal tract acoustics at soprano subject's high fundamental frequencies. J Acoust Soc Am 137(5):2586–2596

Epstein R, Hirani SP, Stygall J et al (2009) How do individuals cope with voice disorders? Introducing the Voice Disability Coping Questionnaire. J Voice 23(2):209–217

Eysholdt U, Lohscheller J (2008) Phonovibrogramm: stimmlippendynamik in einem Bild. HNO 56(12):1207–1212

Eysholdt U (2014) Heiserkeit: biomechanik und quantitative laryngoskopie. HNO 62(7):541–552

Fang-Ling L, Matteson S (2014) Speech tasks and interrater reliability in perceptual voice evaluation. J Voice 28(6):725–732

Flesch J (1925) Berufs-Krankheiten des Musikers. Ein Leitfaden der Berufsberatung für Musiker, Musikpädagogen, Ärzte und Eltern. Kampmann, Celle, pp 82–113

Fourcin A, Abberton E, Miller D et al (1995) Laryngography. Eur J Disord Commun 30:101–115

Fourcin A, Abberton E (2008) Hearing and phonetic criteria in voice measurement: clinical applications. Logoped Phoniatr Vocol 33(1):35–48

Friedman EM (1997) Role of ultrasound in the assessment of vocal cord function in infants and children. Ann Otol Rhinol Laryngol 106(3):199–209

Fritzell B, Hallen O, Sundberg J (1974) Evaluation of Teflon injection procedures for paralytic dysphonia. Folia Phoniatr 26(6):414–421

Frucht SJ, Fahn S, Greene PE et al (2001) The natural history of embouchure dystonia. Mov Disord 16(5):899–906

Frucht SJ (2009) Embouchure dystonia—portrait of a task-specific cranial dystonia. Mov Disord 24(12):1752–1762

Fussi F (2005) La voce del cantante, vol III. Omega, Torino

Gall V, Gall D, Hanson J (1971) Larynx-Fotokymografie. Arch klin exp Ohr-, Nas- u Kehlk Heilk 200(1): 34–41

Gall V, Hanson J (1973) Bestimmung physikalischer Parameter der Stimmlippenschwingungen mit Hilfe der Larynxphotokymographie. Folia Phoniatr 25:450–459

Garel C, Legrand I, Elmaleh M et al (1990) Laryngeal ultrasonography in infants and children: anatomical correlation with fetal preparations. Pediatr Radiol 20(4):241–244

Garel C, Contencin P, Polonovski JM et al (1992) Laryngeal ultrasonography in infants and children: a new way of investigating. Normal and pathological findings. Int J Pediatr Otorhinolaryngol 23(2): 107–115

Gelfer MP, Pazera JF (2006) Maximum duration of sustained /s/ and /z/ and the s/z ratio with controlled intensity. J Voice 20(3):369–379

Gerratt B, Kreiman J, Barroso NA et al (1993) Comparing internal and external standards in voice quality judgments. J Speech Hear Res 2(36):14–20

Ghirardi AC, Ferreira LP, Giannini SP et al (2013) Screening index for voice disorder (SIVD): development and validation. J Voice 27(2):195–200

Godino-Llorente JI, Osma-Ruiz V, Saenz-Lecho N et al (2010) The effectiveness of the glottal to noise excitation ratio for the screening of voice disorders. J Voice 24(1):47–56

Gomaa MA, Hammad MS, Mamdoh H et al (2013) Value of high resolution ultrasonography in assessment of laryngeal lesions. Otolaryngol Pol 67(5):252–256

Gould J, Waugh J, Carding P et al (2012) A new voice rating tool for clinical practice. J Voice 26(4):e163–e170

Gross M (1985) Larynxfotokymographie. Sprache Stimme Gehör 9:112–113

Grunert D, Stier B, Klingebiel T et al (1989) Ultraschalldiagnostik des Larynx mit Hilfe der Computersonographie. Laryngol Rhinol Otol 68(4):236–238

Hacki T (1996) Die Dysphonie und ihre Diagnostik. LOGOS 4(4):255–261

Hammarberg B (2000) Voice research and clinical needs. Folia Phoniatr Logop 52(1–3):93–102

Haynes WO, Moran MJ, Pindzola RH (2006) Communication disorders in the classroom: an introduction for Professionals in School Settings, 4th edn. Jones & Bartlett Learning, Burlington, MA, pp 267–269

Helmholtz H (1875) On the sensations of tone as a physiological basis for the theory of music. Longmans, Green and Co., London, p 146

Herbst CT, Oh J, Vydrová J et al (2015) DigitalVHI-a freeware open-source software application to capture the Voice Handicap Index and other questionnaire data in various languages. Logoped Phoniatr Vocol 40(2):72–76

Heylen L, Wuyts F, Mertens F et al (1998) Evaluation of the vocal performance of children using a voice range profile index. J Speech Lang Hear Res 41(2): 232–238

Heylen L, Wuyts FL, Mertens F et al (2002) Normative voice range profiles of male and female professional voice users. J Voice 16(1):1–7

Hillman RE, Holmberg EB, Perkell JS et al (1989) Objective assessment of vocal hyperfunction: an experimental framework and initial results. J Speech Hear Res 32:373–392

Hirano M, Koike Y, von Leden H (1968) Maximum phonation time and air usage during phonation. Folia Phoniatr 20(4):185–201

Hirano M (1974) Morphological structure of the vocal cord as a vibrator and its variations. Folia Phoniatr 26(2):89–94

Hirano M (1981) Clinical examination of voice. In: Arnold GE et al (eds) Disorders of human communication, vol 5. Springer, Wien

Hirano M (1989) Objective evaluation of the human voice: clinical aspects. Folia Phoniatr 41(2–3):89–144

Hogikyan ND, Sethuraman G (1999) Validation of an instrument to measure "voice-related quality of life" (VRQOL). J Voice 13(4):557–569

Hosokawa K, Ogawa M, Hashimoto M et al (2014) Statistical analysis of the reliability of acoustic and electroglottographic perturbation parameters for the detection of vocal roughness. J Voice 28(2):263.e9–263.e16. https://doi.org/10.1016/j.jvoice.2013.07.005

Hsiao TY, Wang CL, Chen CN et al (2001) Noninvasive assessment of laryngeal phonation function using color Doppler ultrasound imaging. Ultrasound Med Biol 27(8):1035–1040

Hsiao TY, Wang CL, Chen CN et al (2002) Elasticity of human vocal folds measured in vivo using color Doppler imaging. Ultrasound Med Biol 28(9):1145–1152

Hunter EJ, Titze IR (2010) Variations in intensity, fundamental frequency and voicing for teachers in occupational versus nonoccupational settings. J Speech Lang Hear Res 53(4):862–875

Isogai Y (1994) X-ray stroboscopy and laryngostrobography. In: Proceedings of the 3rd International Symposium on Phonosurgery, Kyoto, 26–28 June 1994. International Association of Phonosurgeons, pp 238–239

Jacobson BH, Johnson A, Grywalski C et al (1997) The Voice Handicap Index (VHI): development and validation. Am J Speech Lang Pathol 6:66–70

Jilek C, Marienhagen J, Hacki T (2004) Vocal stability in functional dysphonic versus healthy voices at different times of voice loading. J Voice 18(4):443–453

Johnson DM, Hapner ER, Klein AM et al (2014) Validation of a telephone screening tool for spasmodic dysphonia and vocal fold tremor. J Voice 28(6):711–715

Jun BC, Kim HT, Kim HS et al (2005) Clinical feasibility of the new technique of functional 3D laryngeal CT. Acta Otolaryngol 125(7):774–778

Karnell M, Melton S, Childes J et al (2007) Reliability of Clinician-Based (GRABAS and CAPE-V) and Patient-Based (V-RQOL and IPVI) documentation of voice disorders. J Voice 21(5):576–590

Kent RD, Kent JF, Rosenbek JC (1987) Maximum performance tests of speech production. J Speech Hear Disord 52(4):367–387

Kim YC, Narayanan SS, Nayak KS et al (2009) Accelerated 3D MRI of vocal tract shaping using compressed sensing and parallel imaging. Proc IEEE Int Conf Acoust Speech Signal Process 34:389–392

Kitzing P (1981) Veränderung der Sprechstimmlage bei Dysphoniepatienten in Zusammenhang mit Stimmbelastung. HNO-Praxis 6:215

Kramer H, Doleschal J, Hacki T et al (1998) Verbesserung der Stimmbelastbarkeit durch stationäre Rehabilitationsmaßnahmen. In: Gross M (ed) Aktuelle phoniatrisch-pädaudiologische Aspekte 1997/98, vol 5. Median Verlag von Killisch Horn GmbH, Heidelberg, pp 76–79

Kramer H, Pérez Álvarez JC, Hacki T (1999) Stimmleistungscharakterisierende Kurventypen im Stimmbelastungstest. In: Gross M (ed) Aktuelle phoniatrisch-pädaudiologische Aspekte 1998/99, 6th edn. Median Verlag von Killisch-Horn GmbH, Heidelberg, pp 75–79

Kreiman J, Gerratt B, Precoda K et al (1992) Individual differences in voice quality perception. J Speech Hear Res 6(35):512–520

Kreiman J, Gerratt B, Kempster G et al (1993) Perceptual evaluation of voice quality: review, tutorial, and a framework for future research. J Speech Hear Res 2(36):21–40

Kroemer KHE, Grandjean E (1997) Fitting the task to the human. 5th edn. Taylor & Francis, London

Landeck E (1974) Lippenläsionen bei Blechblasinstrumentalisten. Derm Mschr 160:762–765

Lanz T, Wachsmuth W (1955) Praktische Anatomie. Ein Lehr- und Hilfsbuch der anatomischen Grundlagen ärztlichen Handelns Vol. 1, Part 2: Hals. Springer, Berlin-Göttingen-Heidelberg, pp 28–33, 204–205, 469

Laukkanen AM, Järvinen K, Artkoski M et al (2004) Changes in voice and subjective sensations during a 45-min vocal loading test in female subjects with vocal training. Folia Phoniatr Logop 56(6): 335–346

Laukkanen AM, Kankare E (2006) Vocal loading-related changes in male teachers' voices investigated before and after a working day. Folia Phoniatr Logop 58(4):229–239

Laver J (1980) The Phonetic Description of Voice Quality. British Library Catalogue in Publication Data. Cambridge University Press, Cambridge

Laver J, Hiller S, Mackenzie Beck J (1992) Acoustic waveform perturbation and voice disorders. J Voice 6(2):115–126

Lebacq J, DeJonckere PH (2019) The dynamics of voice onset. Biomed Signal Process Control 49:528–539

Lee L, Stemple J, Glaze L et al (2004) Quick Screen for Voice and supplementary documents for pediatric voice disorders. Lang Speech Hear Serv Sch 35(4):308–319

Lell MM, Gress H, Hothorn T et al (2004) Multiplanar functional imaging of the larynx and hypopharynx with multislice spiral CT. Eur Radiol 14(12):2198–2205

Leno L (1971) Lip vibration characteristics of the trombone embouchure in performance. Instrumentalist 25:56–62

Leno L (1974) Lip vibration characteristics of the trombone embouchure in performance. Brass Bulletin 7(1):7–41

Leno L (1995) Eine Studie von (sic) Lippenvibrationen mit Highspeed-Fotographie. Schallstück 16:14–18

Leno L (2009) Lip vibration of trombone embouchures. Part1: http://www.youtube.com/watch?v=CoxnhjL MVBo&feature=channel_page. Part2: http://www. youtube.com/watch?v=UHq7vCihaXg&feature =channel_page. Part3: http://www.youtube.com/ watch?v=gmBDG_wAeS4&feature=channel_page. Accessed 6 Dec 2016

Likert R (1932) A technique for the measurement of attitudes. Arch Psychol 140:1–55

Lindestad PÅ, Södersten M, Merker B et al (2001) Voice source characteristics in Mongolian "throat singing" studied with high-speed imaging technique, acoustic spectra, and inverse filtering. J Voice 15(1):78–85

Liu S, Hayden GF (2002) Maladies in musicians. South Med J 95(7):727–734

Loock F, Lorenz M (1981) Berufskrankheiten und Berufsunfähigkeiten bei Bläsern. Arbeitshygienische Beratungsstelle der Theater und Orchester der DDR (Berlin Ost). Arbeitsmedizinische Informationen für Theater und Orchester 4:12–16

Luchsinger R (1949) Die Stroboskopie des Kehlkopfes. In: Luchsinger R, Arnold GE (eds) Lehrbuch der Stimm- und Sprachheilkunde. Springer, Wien, pp 30–36

Ma EP, Yiu EM (2001) Voice activity and participation profile: assessing the impact of voice disorders on daily activities. J Speech Lang Hear Res 44(3):511–524

Maneiro F (2014) Ruptura del músculo orbicular de los labios en un músico de viento (syndrome de Satchmo), a propósito de un caso. (Rupture of the orbicular oris muscle in a wind instrument player SATCHMO Syndrome). About a particular case. Med Segur Trab 60:779–785

Manfredi C, Giordano A, Schoentgen J et al (2011) Validity of jitter measures in non-quasi-periodic voices, Part II: The effect of noise. Logoped Phoniatr Vocol 36(2):78–89

Manfredi C, Giordano A, Schoentgen J et al (2012) Perturbation measurements in highly irregular voice signals: performances/validity of analysis software tools. Biomed Signal Process Control 7(4):37–42

Manfredi C, Dejonckere PH (2016) Voice dosimetry and monitoring, with emphasis on professional voice diseases: critical review and framework for future research. Logoped Phoniatr Vocol 41(2):49–65

Martens JW, Versnel H, Dejonckere PH (2007) The effect of visible speech in the perceptual rating of pathological voices. Arch Otolaryngol Head Neck Surg 13(2):178–185

Martin D (1942) Lip vibrations in a cornet mouthpiece. J Acoust Soc Am 13:305–308

Maryn Y, Corthals P, Van Cauwenberge P et al (2010a) Toward improved ecological validity in the acoustic measurement of overall voice quality: combining continuous speech and sustained vowels. J Voice 24(5):540–555

Maryn Y, De Bodt M, Roy N (2010b) The Acoustic Voice Quality Index: toward improved treatment outcomes assessment in voice disorders. J Commun Disord 43(3):161–174

Mauersberger R (2016) Lippenschwingungen und Stimmgebung bei Blechbläsern. Inauguraldissertation. Heinrich-Heine-Universität Düsseldorf, Düsseldorf

Mayes RW, Jackson-Menaldi C, DeJonckere PH et al (2008) Laryngeal electroglottography as a predictor of laryngeal electromyography. J Voice 22(6):756–759

Mensch B (1964) Analyse par exploration ultrasonique du mouvement des cordes vocales isolées. Comptes rendus des séances de la Société de Biologie et de ses filiales 158 = A. 116, No. 7–12. Centre National de la Recherche Scientifique/Société de Biologie. Paris, Masson 1964, pp 2295–2296 (séance du 12 décembre 1964)

Miles KA (1989) Ultrasound demonstration of vocal cord movements. Br J Radiol 62(741):871–872

Minifie FD, Kelsey CA, Hixon TJ (1968) Measurement of vocal fold motion using an ultrasonic Doppler velocity monitor. J Acoust Soc Am 43(5):1165–1169

Misono S, Merati AL (2012) Evidence-based practice: evaluation and management of unilateral vocal fold paralysis. Otolaryngol Clin N Am 45(5): 1083–1108

Moreti F, Ávila ME, Rocha C et al (2012) Influence of complaints and singing style in singers voice handicap. J Soc Bras Fonoaudiol 24(3):296–300

Morris S, Jawad MSM, Eccles R (1992) Relationships between vital capacity, height and nasal airway resistance in asymptomatic volunteers. Rhinology 30(4):259–264

Munin MC, Murry T, Rosen CA (2000) Laryngeal electromyography. Otolaryngol Clin N Am 33(4): 759–770

Murlewska A, Gryczynski M, Gadzicki M (1992) Badania ultrasonograficzne krtani. Otolaryngol Pol 46(3):238–245

Murry T, Bone RC (1978) Aerodynamic relationships associated with normal phonation and paralytic dysphonia. Laryngoscope 88(1):100–109

Nawka T, Verdonck-de Leeuw IM, De Bodt M et al (2009) Item reduction of the voice handicap index based on the original version and on European translations. Folia Phoniatr Logop 61(1):37–48

Nawka T (2012) Untersuchung des Schwingungsablaufs der Stimmlippen. In: Seidner W, Nawka T (eds)

Handreichungen zur Stimmdiagnostik. XION medical, Berlin, pp 75–98

Neiman GS, Edeson B (1981) Procedural aspects of eliciting maximum phonation time. Folia Phoniatr 33(5):285–293

Newton MJ, Campbell M, Gilbert J (2008) Mechanical response measurements of real and artificial brass player's lips. J Acoust Soc Am 123:14–20

Niimi S, Miyaji M (2000) Vocal fold vibration and voice quality. Folia Phoniatr Logop 52(1–3):32–38

Oertel M (1878) Über eine neue "laryngostroboskopische" Untersuchungsmethode des Kehlkopfes. Zbl med Wiss 16:81–82

Oertel M (1895) Das Laryngo-Stroboskop und die laryngo-stroboskopische Untersuchung. Arch Laryngol Rhinol 3:1–16

Ohlsson AC, Andersson EM, Södersten M et al (2012) Prevalence of voice symptoms and risk factors in teacher students. J Voice 26(5):629–634

Ooi LLPJ (1992) B-mode real-time ultrasound assessment of vocal cord function in recurrent laryngeal nerve palsy. Ann Acad Med Singapore 21(2):214–216

Pabst F, Seiler R, Hacki T (1998) Zur Beurteilung der Sprechstimmleistungen nach Stimmbelastungstest mittels Stimmfeldmessung. In: Gross M (ed) Aktuelle phoniatrisch-pädaudiologische Aspekte 1997/98, vol 5. Median Verlag von Killisch Horn GmbH, Heidelberg, pp 73–75

Papsin BC, Maaske LA, Mc Grail JS (1996) Orbicularis oris muscle injury in brass players. Laryngoscope 106(6):757–760

Paulsen F (2010) Mundhöhle. In: Zilles K, Tillmann B (eds) Anatomie. Springer, Berlin, pp 424–425

Pernambuco LA, Espelt A, Magalhaes HV et al (2016a) Screening for voice disorders in older adults (Rastreamento de Alteracoes Vocais em Idosos-RAVI)-Part I: Validity evidence based on test content and response processes. J Voice 30(2):246.e9–246.e16

Pernambuco LA, Espelt A, Magalhaes HV et al (2016b) Screening for voice disorders in older adults (Rastreamento de Alteracoes Vocais em Idosos-RAVI)-Part II: Validity evidence and reliability. J Voice 30(2):246.e19–246.e27

Phyland DJ, Oates J, Greenwood KM (1999) Self-reported voice problems among three groups of professional singers. J Voice 13(4):602–611

Planas J (1982) Rupture of the orbicularis oris in trumpet players (Satchmo's syndrome). Plast Reconstr Surg 69(4):690–693

Planas J (1988) Further experience with rupture of the orbicularis oris in trumpet players. Plast Reconstr Surg 81(6):975–981

Pruszewicz A (1992) Foniatria kliniczna. (Clinical phoniatrics). PZWL, Warsaw

Qiu Q, Schutte HK (2006) A new generation videokymography for routine clinical vocal-fold examination. Laryngoscope 116(10):1824–1828

Raes JP, Clement PA (1996) Aerodynamic measurements of voice production. Acta Otorhinolaryngol Belg 50(4):293–298

Raghavendra BN, Horii SC, Reede DL et al (1987) Sonographic anatomy of the larynx, with particular reference to the vocal cords. J Ultrasound Med 6(5):225–230

Rau D, Beckett RL (1984) Aerodynamic assessment of vocal function using hand-held spirometers. J Speech Hear Disord 49(2):183–188

Reinhardt DS (1973) The encyclopedia of the pivot system for all cupped mouthpiece brass instruments: a scientific text. Colin, New York

Revis J, Barberis S, Giovanni A (2000) Définition d'une mesure temporelle de l'attaque vocale. Rev Laryngol Otol Rhinol 121(5):291–296

Ricci-Maccarini A, De Maio V, Murry T et al (2013) Development and validation of the children's voice handicap index-10 (CVHI-10). J Voice 30(1):120–126

Rosen CA, Murry T (2000) Voice Handicap Index in singers. J Voice 14(3):370–377

Rosen CA, Lee AS, Osborne J et al (2004) Development and validation of the Voice Handicap Index-10. Laryngoscope 114(9):1549–1556

Rothenberg M (1973) A new inverse filtering technique for deriving the glottal airflow during voicing. J Acoust Soc Am 53(6):1632–1645

Rothenberg M (1982) Interpolating subglottal pressure from oral pressure. J Speech Hear Disord 47(2):218–224

Rozanski VE, Rehfuess E, Bötzel K et al (2015) Aufgabenspezifische Dystonie bei professionellen Musikern—Ein systematisches Review zur Bedeutung des intensiven Musizierens als Risikofaktor. Dtsch Arztebl Int 112:871–877

Sapienza CM, Stathopoulos ET, Dromey C (1998) Approximations of open quotient and speed quotient from glottal and EGG waveforms: effects of measurement criteria and sound pressure level. J Voice 12(1):31–43

Sataloff RT (1997) Professional voice. Singular Publishing Group, San Diego

Sataloff RT, Mandel S, Mann EA et al (2004) Practice parameter: laryngeal electromyography (an evidence-based review). J Voice 18(2):261274

Sataloff RT, Mandel S, Heman-Ackah YD et al (2005) Laryngeal electromyography, 2nd edn. Plural Publishing, San Diego

Sataloff RT (2005a) Clinical assessment of voice. Plural Publishing Inc, San Diego, CA

Sataloff RT (2005b) Professional voice: the science and art of clinical care. Plural Publishing Inc, San Diego, CA

Saxon KG, Schneider CM (1995) Vocal exercise physiology. Singular Publishing Group, San Diego

Schaefer SD (2014) Management of acute blunt and penetrating external laryngeal trauma. Laryngoscope 124(1):233–244

Schindler O, Gonella ML, Pisani R (1990) Doppler ultrasound examination of the vibration speed of vocal folds. Folia Phoniatr 42(5):265–272

Schneider-Stickler B, Knell C, Aichstill B et al (2012) Biofeedback on voice use in call center agents in order to prevent occupational voice disorders. J Voice 26(1):51–62

Schönhärl E (1960) Die Stroboskopie in der praktischen Laryngologie. Thieme, Stuttgart

Schultz-Coulon HJ (1990) Stimmfeldmessung. Springer, Berlin

Schuppert M, Altenmüller E (2000) Berufsspezifische Erkrankungen bei Musikern. Orchester 48:24–29

Schutte HK (1980) The efficiency of voice production. Thesis, University of Groningen, Groningen

Schutte HK (1992) Integrated aerodynamic measurements. J Voice 6(2):127–134

Schutte HK, Seidner W (2005) Physiologische Grundlagen. In: Wendler J et al (eds) Lehrbuch der Phoniatrie und Pädaudiologie, 4th edn. Thieme, Stuttgart, p 80

Scott AD, Wylezinska M, Birch MJ et al (2014) Speech MRI: morphology and function. Phys Med 30(6):604–618

Seidner W, Eysholdt U (2005) Stimme—Diagnostik. In: Wendler J et al (eds) Lehrbuch der Phoniatrie und Pädaudiologie, 4th edn. Thieme, Stuttgart, pp 115–116

Seidner W (2012) Messung der stimmlichen Belastbarkeit. In: Seidner W, Nawka T (eds) Handreichungen zur Stimmdiagnostik. XION GmbH, Berlin

Shau YW, Wang CL, Hsieh FJ et al (2001) Noninvasive assessment of vocal fold mucosal wave velocity using color Doppler imaging. Ultrasound Med Biol 27(11):1451–1460

Sherer RC, Titze IR (1987) The abduction quotient related to vocal quality. J Voice 1(3):246–251

Sherman D, Jensen R (1962) Harshness and oral reading time. J Speech Hear Res 27:172–177

Siegert C (1987) Recommendation for a standard tolerance test. Union of European Phoniatricians, Annual Bulletin, pp 46–47

Simberg S, Sala E, Laine A et al (2001) A fast and easy screening method for voice disorders among teacher students. Logoped Phoniatr Vocol 26(1):10–16

Singer K (1926) Berufskrankheiten der Musiker. Systematische Darstellung ihrer Ursachen, Symptome und Behandlungsmethoden. Hesse, Berlin, pp 130–131

Sonninen A, Damsté PH, Jol J et al (1974) Microdynamics in vocal fold vibration. Acta Otolaryngol 78:1–6

Speyer R, Wieneke GH, van Wijck-Warnaar I et al (2003) Effects of voice therapy on the voice range profiles of dysphonic patients. J Voice 17(4):544–556

Speyer R, Wieneke GH, Dejonckere PH (2004a) The use of acoustic parameters for the evaluation of voice therapy for dysphonic patients. Acta Acust united Ac 90(3):520–527

Speyer R, Wieneke GH, Dejonckere PH (2004b) Documentation of progress in voice therapy: perceptual, acoustic and laryngostroboscopic findings pretherapy and posttherapy. J Voice 18(3):325–339

Šram F, Švec J, Schutte HK (1998) Possibilities for use of videokymography in laryngologic and phoniatric practice. In: Dejonckere PH, Peters HFM (eds) Communication and its disorders: a science in progress: proceedings of the 24th congress of the International Association of Logopedics and Phoniatrics. Amsterdam, 23–27 August 1998. University press, Nijmegen, pp 256–259

Šram F, Švec J (2000) Die Tonerzeugung beim Spielen von Blasinstrumenten. In: Pahn J et al (eds) Sprache und Musik: Beiträge der 71. Jahrestagung der Deutschen Gesellschaft für Sprach- und Stimmheilkunde. Zeitschrift für Dialektologie und Linguistik: Beihefte; Heft 107. Berlin, 12–13 März 1999. Steiner, Stuttgart, pp 155–159

Sramkova H, Granqvist S, Herbst CT et al (2015) The softest sound levels of the human voice in normal subjects. J Acoust Soc Am 137(1):407–418

Stevenson S, Campbell M, Bromage S (2009) Motion of the lips of brass players during extremely loud playing. J Acoust Soc Am 125:152–157

Stone R, Scharf D (1973) Vocal change associated with the use of atypical pitch and intensity levels. Folia Phoniatr Logop 25:91–103

Story BH, Titze I (1995) Voice simulation with a body-cover model of the vocal folds. J Acoust Soc Am 97(2):1249–1260

Sullivan WG (1989) Repair of ruptured orbicularis oris in trumpet players. Plast Reconstr Surg 83:578

Sung MW, Kim KH, Koh TY et al (1999) Videostrobokymography: a new method for the quantitative analysis of vocal fold vibration. Laryngoscope 109(11):1859–1863

Švec JG, Schutte HK (1996) Videokymography: high-speed line scanning of vocal fold vibration. J Voice 10(2):201–205

Švec J, Šram F, Schutte HK (1999) Videokymografie: nová vysokofrekvenční metoda vyšetřování kmitů hlasivek. (Videokymography: a new high-speed method for the examination of vocal-fold vibrations). Otorinolaryngologie a Foniatrie (Praha) 48:155–162

Švec J, Šram F (2002) Kymographic imaging of the vocal fold oscillations. In: Hansen JHL, Pellom B (eds) Proceedings of the 7th International Conference on Spoken Language Processing. Denver, CO, 16–20 Sept 2002. Center for Spoken Language Research, Boulder, pp 957–960

Švec J, Titze IR, Popolo P (2005) Estimation of sound pressure levels of voiced speech from skin vibration of the neck. J Acoust Soc Am 117(3 Pt 1):1386–1394

Švec JG, Šram F, Schutte HK (2007) Videokymography in voice disorders: what to look for? Ann Otol Rhinol Laryngol 116(3):172–180

Švec JG, Šram F, Schutte HK (2009) Videokymography. In: Fried MP, Ferlito A (eds) The larynx, vol 1, 3rd edn. Plural Publishing, San Diego, CA, pp 253–274

Švec JG, Granqvist S (2010) Guidelines for selecting microphones for human voice production research. Am J Speech Lang Pathol 19(4):356–368

Švec JG, Šram F (2011) Videokymographic examination of voice. In: Ma EPM, Yiu EML (eds) Handbook of voice assessments. Plural Publishing, San Diego, CA, pp 129–146

Švec JG, Schutte HK (2012) Kymographic imaging of laryngeal vibrations. Curr Opin Otolaryngol Head Neck Surg 20(6):458–465

Tillmann B (1997) Farbatlas der Anatomie Zahnmedizin-Humanmedizin. Thieme, Stuttgart, p 98

Titze IR (1992a) Phonation threshold pressure—a missing link in glottal aerodynamics. J Acoust Soc Am 91(5):2926–2935

Titze IR (1992b) Acoustic interpretation of the voice profile (phonetogram). J Speech Hear Res 35(1):21–34

Titze IR, Liang H (1993) Comparison of Fo extraction models for high precision voice perturbation measurements. J Speech Hear Res 36(6):1120–1133

Titze IR (1994) Principles of voice production. Prentice Hall, Englewood Cliffs, NJ

Titze IR (1995) Workshop on acoustic voice analysis: summary statement. National Center for Voice and Speech, The University of Iowa, Denver

Titze IR, Lemke J, Montequin D (1997) Populations in the US workforce who rely on voice as a primary tool of trade: a preliminary report. J Voice 11(3):254–259

Traser L, Burdumy M, Richter B et al (2013) The effect of supine and upright position on vocal tract configurations during singing—a comparative study in professional tenors. J Voice 27(2):141–148

Tsai CG, Shau YW, Liu HM et al (2008) Laryngeal mechanisms during human 4-kHz vocalization studied with CT, videostroboscopy, and color Doppler imaging. J Voice 22(3):275–282

Unger J, Schuster M, Hecker DJ et al (2016) A generalized procedure for analyzing sustained and dynamic vocal fold vibrations from laryngeal high-speed videos using phonovibrograms. Artif Intell Med 66(C):15–28

Van de Heyning PH, Remacle M, Cauwenberge PV et al (1996) Research work of the Belgian study group on Voice disorders. Acta Otorhinolaryngol Belg 50(4):321–386

Valente T, Farina R, Minelli S et al (1996) Anatomia ecografica della laringe e delle strutture perilaringee. Radiol Med 91(3):231–237

Ventura S, Diamantino F, João M et al (2011) Imaging of the Vocal Tract Based on Magnetic Resonance Techniques. In: Ranchordas A et al (eds) Computer vision, imaging and computer graphics. Theory and applications. Springer, Heidelberg, pp 146–157

Verdolini K (1994) Voice disorders. In: Tomblin JB et al (eds) Diagnosis in speech-language pathology. Singular Publishing Group, San Diego, pp 247–306

Verduyckt I, Remacle M, Jamart J et al (2011) Voice-related complaints in the pediatric population. J Voice 25(3):373–380

Verduyckt I, Morsomme D, Remacle M (2012) Validation and standardization of the Pediatric Voice Symptom Questionnaire: a double-form questionnaire for dysphonic children and their parents. J Voice 26(4):e129–e139

Vilkman E (2004) Occupational safety and health aspects of voice and speech professions. Folia Phoniatr Logop 56(4):220–253

Vintturi J (2001) Studies on Voice Production. Academic dissertation. Medical Faculty of the University of Helsinki, Helsinki

Vintturi J, Alku P, Lauri ER et al (2001) The effects of post-loading rest on acoustic parameters with special reference to gender and ergonomic factors. Folia Phoniatr Logop 53(6):338–350

Watson C (1994) Database management of the voice clinic and laboratory. J Voice 3:99–106

Welsch U (2006) Lehrbuch histologie, 2nd edn. Urban & Fischer, München, pp 338–339

Wilken D (2009) Brass embouchures [Internet]. Chapter 1 of 6 http://www.youtube.com/user/wilktone#p/u/0/aNfZpapmLIg. Chapter 2 of 6 http://www.youtube.com/user/wilktone#p/u/1/VFi5g1tqHhE. Chapter 3 of 6 http://www.youtube.com/user/wilktone#p/u/2/AfoeACB6bA4. Chapter 4 of 6 http://www.youtube.com/user/wilktone#p/u/3/gkIi6YXy8CI. Chapter 5 of 6 http://www.youtube.com/user/wilktone#p/u/4/KVa7spYJXvY. Chapter 6 of 6 http://www.youtube.com/user/wilktone#p/u/5/ImJoiuyfJ5Y. Accessed 6 Dec 2016

Wendler J, Anders LC, Krüger H (1986) Classification of voice qualities. J Phon 14:483–488

Wendler J, Seidner W (1996) Lehrbuch der Phoniatrie und Pädaudiologie. Thieme, Stuttgart

Wilson DK (1987) Voice problems of children, 3rd edn. Williams & Wilkins, Baltimore

Wilson JA, Webb A, Carding PN et al (2004) The VoiSS and the VHI: a comparison of structure and content. Clin Otolaryngol 29(2):169–174

Wittenberg T, Tigges M, Mergell P et al (2000) Functional imaging of vocal fold vibration: digital multislice high-speed kymography. J Voice 14(3):422–442

Wolfe V, Fitch J, Martin D (1997) Acoustic measures of dysphonic severity across and within voice types. Folia Phoniatr Logop 49(6):292–299

Woo P, Colton RH, Shangold L (1987) Phonatory air flow analysis in patients with laryngeal disease. Ann Otol Rhinol Laryngol 96(5):549–555

Woo P, Casper J, Colton R et al (1994) Aerodynamic and stroboscopic findings before and after microlaryngeal phonosurgery. J Voice 8(2):186–194

World Health Organization (1971) The economics of health and disease. WHO Chron 25:20–24

Wuyts FL, De Bodt MS, Molenberghs G et al (2000) The dysphonia severity index. An objective measure of vocal quality based on a multiparameter approach. J Speech Hear Res 43(3):796–809

Yu P, Ouaknine M, Giovanni A (2000) Intérêt clinique du calcul des coefficients de Lyapunov pour l'analyse objective des dysphonies. (Clinical significance of calculating the coefficients of Lyapunov in the objective assessment of dysphonia). Rev Laryngol Otol Rhinol 121(5):301–305

Yumoto E, Oyamada Y, Nakano K et al (2004) Three-dimensional characteristics of the larynx with immobile vocal fold. Arch Otolaryngol Head Neck Surg 130(8):967–974

Zappia F, Campani R (2000) La laringe: studio ecografico anatomico e funzionale. Radiol Med 99:138–144

Zarzur AP, de Campos DA, Cataldo BO et al (2014) Laryngeal electromyography as a diagnostic tool for Parkinson's disease. Laryngoscope 124(3):725–729

Zeller HJ (1985) Therapieempfehlungen bei Beschäftigungsneuropathien und Beschäftigungsneurosen von Blechbläsern. Arbeitshygienische Beratungsstelle der Theater und Orchester der DDR (Berlin Ost). Arbeitsmedizinische Informationen für Theater und Orchester 8:1–8

Zraick RI, Smith-Olinde L, Shotts LL (2012) Adult normative data for the KAYPentax Phonatory Aerodynamic System Model 6600. J Voice 26(2):164–176

Zur KB, Cotton S, Kelchner L et al (2007) Pediatric Voice Handicap Index (pVHI): a new tool for evaluating pediatric dysphonia. Int J Pediatr Otorhinolaryngol 71(1):77–82

Prevention of Voice Disorders

7

Tadeus Nawka, Andrzej Obrębowski,
and Antoni Pruszewicz

7.1 Prevention of Voice Disorders

Antoni Pruszewicz, Andrzej Obrębowski,
and Tadeus Nawka

7.1.1 Constitutional Limits

Physiological voice production significantly depends on hygiene of the upper respiratory tract. First, an unobstructed nasal respiration should be ensured. Voice disturbances may be accompanied by deviations in the nasal cavity. Allergic reactions in the larynx resemble inflammation. Coughing attacks due to allergy put an additional burden on the voice organ.

Preliminary phoniatric vocal fitness assessment may prevent professionally induced voice disorders by assuring that a patient meets the basic requirements of fitness for a voice profession. There are contra-indications for choosing such a profession.

Absolute contra-indications include permanent paralysis of the vocal folds, laryngeal papillomas, advanced inflammatory lesions in the respiratory tract (dry and atrophic chronic inflammation of the laryngeal mucosa), severe allergic diseases, velo-palatine insufficiency and moderate or profound hearing loss.

Relative contra-indications are solid nodules and polyps of the vocal folds, relapsing inflammation in the respiratory tract and palatine tonsils, nasal obstruction, reflux disease and unilateral deafness. Obviously, the dysfunctions can be compensated for by appropriate treatment; nevertheless they can cause professional dysphonia at a high probability (Obrębowski and Pruszewicz 1996).

7.1.2 Behavioural Aspects

The use of nasal decongestants should be avoided or at least strictly limited, as it leads to paralysis of the ciliary apparatus in the mucosa. An appropriate humidification of the pharyngeal and laryngeal mucosa protects against desiccation. A dry mucosa significantly increases phonatory effort.

For prevention of voice disorders, a programme of observing vocal hygiene may be established. In

T. Nawka
Department of Audiology and Phoniatrics, Charité—
University Medicine Berlin, Berlin, Germany
e-mail: tadeus.nawka@charite.de

A. Obrębowski
Department of Phoniatrics and Audiology, Poznań
University of Medical Sciences, Poznan, Poland
e-mail: aobrebow@ump.edu.pl

A. Pruszewicz
Department of Phoniatrics and Audiology, Poznań
University of the Medical Sciences Poland,
Poznan, Poland

© Springer-Verlag GmbH Germany, part of Springer Nature 2020
A. am Zehnhoff-Dinnesen et al. (eds.), *Phoniatrics I*, European Manual of Medicine,
https://doi.org/10.1007/978-3-662-46780-0_7

this programme, voice users receive advice during consultations on how to integrate correct voice production into everyday professional life (Holmberg et al. 2001). They should experience that during phonation a decreased muscular tension within the neck is of a significant preventive importance.

In accepting principles of correct voice production, one should remember the unfavourable side-effects of certain drugs. Hormones lead to oedema and increase the muscular mass of the vocal folds. Thereby they change timbre, decrease the average frequency, and lead to loss of high notes. Anti-allergic preparations and anti-depressants induce dryness of the mucosa. In case of suspected side-effects of any medication, the physician has to look up the drug information.

The voice organ may also be negatively affected by gastro-oesophageal reflux, which irritates the posterior part of the larynx (posterior laryngitis).

In laryngitis, independent of its intensity and aetiology, the physician should not recommend whispering but to use the normal voice as far as possible. Strained whispering intensifies contraction and constriction of the supraglottal structures and activates the nonphysiological phonation mechanism (Böhme 2006), whereas a soft whisper in the form of articulation during relaxed expiration is not harmful. In many cases of vocal dysfunction evaluated by a general practitioner or laryngologist, additional phoniatric examination and diagnostics are indispensable to indicate an intervention that allows preservation or restoration of the full capacity of the organ of voice.

7.1.3 Developmental Aspects

Prevention of voice disorders in children involves multilayer procedures (see Sect. 5.16). First of all, the presence of organic lesions in the larynx should be excluded, such as papilloma, congenital webs or other anomalies. The diagnosis is far from easy, and the procedure requires several consultations to make the child acquainted with laryngological examination.

Repeated inflammation in the throat and larynx should be treated. In cases of a small but inflamed pharyngeal tonsil, adenotomy may in particular result in a radical improvement.

In children with chronic hoarseness, an audiogenic dysphonia should be excluded. Bilateral hearing loss above 40 dB HL may cause functional voice disorders.

In preventing functional voice disorders in the developmental period, the most difficult problem is to control overexcited children with the habit of using their voice above the natural intensity. As early as it is possible, the child should be taught to talk with a soft vocal attack with no hypertension of the neck muscles, with no excessive accentuation. In some cases, a conversation using voice produced without tension at a normal conversational intensity may make the child calm down. Medication to reduce psycho-motoric over-excitation, and psychological or psychiatric treatment, may also be indicated.

Teachers should set an example by using correct physiological voice production at school, since a child frequently imitates the teacher, with whom it may be emotionally linked.

Vocal training of children must be within the physiological limits of their vocal function. The musical literature as well as songs in kindergarten should be appropriate for the physiological range of the children's voices. In a choir, the possibility of individual vocal overload should be taken into account. This is particularly important during the mutation period, in which vocal training should be adjusted appropriately to its course. In principle, systematic singing lessons should start after mutation (Pruszewicz 1992).

7.1.4 Environmental Aspects: Harmful Agents

Cessation of smoking is a long-term process and not always effective. Information about the carcinogenic and circulatory risks of smoking is often more successful than explaining the unfavourable effects of smoking on the voice organ (Obrębowski 2008). Within the environment of children and youths, the habit of cigarette smoking should be combatted.

In the school environment, noise reduction supports attentiveness and concentration. A large number of pupils in the classroom, as well as poor acoustic conditions, lead the children to communicate at a high frequency and volume (Pruszewicz et al. 1974).

For teachers, an appropriate schedule of lessons with suitable distribution of teaching hours within a week should be attempted. An adequate number of pupils, air-conditioning of classrooms and application of audio-visual techniques improve teaching conditions and help to maintain vocal performance.

Mental health is assured by a conflict-free atmosphere.

7.1.5 Principal Rules

Prodromal signs of voice disturbances are transient changes in voice timbre, hoarseness in particular, vocal fatigue, the sensation of pressure or pain in the throat or in the neck following an insignificant vocal effort; they should not be ignored in general laryngological practice.

Vocal health is supported by elimination of vocal overload, such as:

- Excessively loud cries or laughs
- Prolonged screams
- Attacks of coughing
- Excessively loud singing with an infection in the respiratory tract
- Uncontrolled use of electronic voice amplifiers
- Avoidance of rooms with improper room acoustics
- Drugs affecting the vocal tract

Voice professionals should avoid burdens resulting from inappropriate use of voice such as:

- Talking for prolonged time periods with a hard voice attack
- An elevated pitch at excessive volume

- Excessively loud singing in the upper or lower range of the vocal range (Boone et al. 2005)
- Voice communication in a noisy environment (Gundermann 1970)

In the course of studies, and in particular pedagogic studies, future teachers should be made familiar with principles of correct voice production. It is worthwhile to present live examples of a proper production. Effects of the prophylactic activities markedly depend on the personality of the phoniatrician and logopedist (Gundermann 1970).

Systematic phoniatric care for voice professionals helps to identify early signs of malfunction. In such cases, voice therapy can be prescribed before the voice fails. Training of physiological principles of normal voice production with transfer into professional use may also be beneficial for those who have worked in a voice profession for some decades without supervision.

References

Böhme G (2006) Sprach-, Sprech-, Stimm- und Schluckstörungen. Urban-Fischer, Munich

Boone DR, McFarlane SC, Berg SL (2005) The voice and voice therapy. Pearson, Boston

Gundermann H (1970) Die Berufsdysphonie. Thieme, Leipzig

Holmberg EB, Hillman RE, Hammarberg B et al (2001) Efficacy of a behavioral based voice therapy protocol for vocal nodules. J Voice 15(3):395–412

Obrębowski A (ed) (2008) Narząd głosu i jego znaczenie w komunikacji spolecznej (voice organ and its importance in social communication). Wydawnictwo Naukowe Uniwersytetu Medycznego, Poznań

Obrębowski A, Pruszewicz A (1996) Zasady profilaktyki zawodowych zaburzen głosu (principles in prophylaxis of professional voice disorders). Now Lekarskie 65:1–55

Pruszewicz A (ed) (1992) Foniatria Kliniczna. PZWL, Warszawa

Pruszewicz A, Jassem W, Wacławik W (1974) Effect of noise on some acoustical parameters of speech. Folia Phoniatr 26(4):331–341

Rehabilitation and Prognosis of Voice Disorders

8

Sevtap Akbulut, Jan Betka, Viktor Chrobok,
Hanna Czerniejewska-Wolska, Felix de Jong,
Ilter Denizoglu, Ahmed Geneid, Mehmet Akif Kilic,
Nasser Kotby, Jean-Paul Marie, Sławomir Marszałek,
Andreas Müller, Tadeus Nawka, Haldun Oguz,
Arno Olthoff, Anders Overgård Jønsson,
Mette Pedersen, Antoni Pruszewicz, Barbora Řepová,
Jan Romportl, Josef Schlömicher-Thier,
Berit Schneider-Stickler, Wolfram Seidner,
Matthias Weikert, and Bożena Wiskirska-Woźnica

Electronic Supplementary Material The online version
of this chapter (https://doi.org/10.1007/978-3-662-46780-
0_8) contains supplementary material, which is available
to authorized users.

S. Akbulut
Department of Otolaryngology, Yeditepe University,
Istanbul, Turkey
e-mail: sevtap.akbulut@gmail.com

J. Betka · B. Řepová
Department of Otorhinolaryngology, Head and Neck
Surgery, Charles University in Prague and University
Hospital Motol, Prague, Czech Republic
e-mail: jan.betka@fnmotol.cz;
barbora.repova@fnmotol.cz

V. Chrobok
Department of Otorhinolaryngology and Head and
Neck Surgery, University Hospital Hradec Kralove,
Hradec Kralove, Czech Republic
e-mail: chrobok@fnhk.cz

H. Czerniejewska-Wolska
Department of Phoniatrics and Audiology,
Poznan University of the Medical Sciences Poland,
Poznan, Poland
e-mail: hannaczerniejewska@gmail.com

I. Denizoglu
Medical Park Hospital Imbatli Mahallesi,
Izmir, Turkey
e-mail: iilterdenizoglu@yahoo.com

A. Geneid
Department of Otolaryngology and Phoniatrics –
Head and Neck Surgery, Helsinki University Central
Hospital, Helsinki, Finland
e-mail: Ahmed.Geneid@hus.fi

M. A. Kilic
Department of Otolaryngology, Faculty of Medicine,
Medeniyet University, Istanbul, Turkey
e-mail: makilic@yahoo.com

N. Kotby
Otolaryngology and Phoniatrics, Ain Shams
University Cairo, Cairo, Egypt
e-mail: nkotby@cng.com.eg

J.-P. Marie
Otolaryngology, Head and Neck Surgery Department,
Centre Hospitalier Universitaire, Rouen, France
e-mail: jean-paul.marie@chu-rouen.fr

S. Marszałek
Department of Head and Neck Surgery, Poznan
University of Medical Sciences, Poznan, Poland
e-mail: marszaleksl@wp.pl

A. Müller
Department Otorhinolaryngology/Plastic Surgery,
SRH Wald-Klinikum Gera gGmbH, Teaching
Hospital of the Friedrich-Schiller-University Jena,
Gera, Germany
e-mail: andreas.mueller@wkg.srh.de

T. Nawka
Department of Audiology and Phoniatrics,
Charité—University Medicine Berlin,
Berlin, Germany
e-mail: tadeus.nawka@charite.de

H. Oguz
Fonomer, Ankara, Turkey
e-mail: drhoguz@gmail.com

A. Olthoff
Department of Otorhinolaryngology, Phoniatrics and
Pedaudiology, University Medical Center Göttingen,
Göttingen, Germany
e-mail: olthoff@med.uni-goettingen.de

A. Overgård Jønsson
University of Copenhagen, Copenhagen, Denmark
e-mail: hbk777@alumni.ku.dk

M. Pedersen
Voice Unit, The Medical Center,
Copenhagen, Denmark
e-mail: m.f.pedersen@dadlnet.dk

A. Pruszewicz
Department of Phoniatrics and Audiology,
Poznań University of the Medical Sciences Poland,
Poznan, Poland
e-mail: apruszew@wp.pl

J. Romportl
Department of Man-Machine Interaction,
New Technologies Research Centre, University
of West Bohemia, Pilsen, Czech Republic
e-mail: rompi@ntc.zcu.cz

J. Schlömicher-Thier
International Voice Center Austria (IVCA),
Neumarkt am Wallersee, Austria
e-mail: hno-schloemicher@sbg.at

B. Schneider-Stickler
Division of Phoniatrics-Logopedics, Department of
Otorhinolaryngology, Medical University Vienna,
Wien, Austria
e-mail: berit.schneider-stickler@meduniwien.ac.at

W. Seidner
Former Department for Phoniatrics and Pediatric
Audiology, University ENT Clinic Charité
(Campus Mitte), Berlin, Germany
e-mail: wolfram.seidner@charite.de

M. Weikert
Clinic St. Hedwig, Barmherzige Brüder,
Regensburg, Germany
e-mail: mweikert@bonvox.de

B. Wiskirska-Woźnica
Department of Phoniatrics and Audiology, Poznan
University of Medical Sciences, Poznan, Poland
e-mail: bozena.woznica@wp.pl

8.1 Coordination of Rehabilitative Measures

Mehmet Akif Kilic and Haldun Oguz

8.1.1 Introduction

Sometimes voice disorders may be signs of other medical problems. In such situations, voice rehabilitation may not always be managed easily by phoniatricians and logopedists. These voice disorders need to be evaluated in an interdisciplinary manner. In fact, both medical and non-medical fields of science may contribute to this process. The most important medical specialities that may contribute are phoniatrics, otorhinolaryngology—head and neck surgery in the first line—neurology, paediatrics, psychiatry, paediatric psychiatry, pulmonology, dentistry, gastroenterology, geriatrics, endocrinology, radiology, genetics and physical therapy. Among many non-medical specialities that may contribute are speech and language pathology, audiology, linguistics, developmental paediatrics, psychology, paediatric psychology, physiotherapy, acoustics, physics, biomedical sciences, pedagogy and computer information technologies.

8.1.2 Situations That May Need an Interdisciplinary Approach for Voice Rehabilitation

Total Laryngectomy and Other Major Surgery There are three approaches for voice rehabilitation following laryngectomy: oesophageal speech, tracheo-oesophageal speech and electrolaryngeal speech.

Voice quality obtained by electrolarynx is not highly satisfactory. However, it may still be preferred temporarily as a first-line rehabilitation until the use of other modalities. The patient needs to be informed about oesophageal speech and tracheo-oesophageal speech. The choice must be made together with the patient and head and neck surgeon. Primary prosthesis placement would be more convenient in case of a choice for tracheo-oesophageal speech. If oesophageal speech is tried but not found successful enough, a secondary procedure may be chosen for application of a prosthesis.

In the case of unsuccessful results, a re-consultation with the head and neck surgeon may be necessary. Hypertonicity of the pharyngo-oesophageal (PE) segment is more likely to be present. Secondary myotomy and chemo-denervation with botulinum toxin may usually serve well in patients with hypertonus.

The following list may be taken into consideration to increase the success rate in prosthetic voice rehabilitation (Hilgers and Van den Brekel 2010):

- A short myotomy of the upper oesophageal sphincter to prevent hypertonicity of the PE segment
- Suturing of the trachea in a separate fenestra in the inferior skin flap to create a stable stoma
- Sectioning of the sternal heads of the sterno-cleidomastoid muscles to prevent a 'deep' stoma
- Pharyngeal mucosa closure without tension (T-shape) to prevent pseudo-vallecula formation
- Besides total laryngectomy, all patients that would undergo a major surgery that will involve the upper respiratory or digestive system (the vocal tract) must be evaluated with a prosthodontist and the head and neck surgeon pre- and post-operatively

Neurogenic Voice Disorders If the probable diagnosis of the aetiology of unilateral vocal fold paralysis is unlikely, or if there is an involvement of other cranial nerves, it would be better to work on the case with a neurologist. If a dysphonic patient also has dysarthria, namely, dysarthro-phonia, likely diagnoses are Parkinson's disease, stroke, traumatic brain injury, amyotrophic lateral sclerosis, multiple sclerosis, myasthenia gravis or cerebral palsy. All of these entities must be considered by a neurologist.

Neurogenic spasmodic dysphonia and para-doxical vocal fold motion are two other diseases that require cooperative work with a neurologist. Details are mentioned in Sects. 5.6 and 5.8.

Psychogenic Voice Disorders Although it is not necessary for a phoniatrician to work with a psychiatrist or psychologist on all psychogenic voice disorders, in our opinion cooperation with experts in psychosomatics should always be offered to the patient. We do not treat symptoms but causes, and all phoniatricians should have basic training in psychosomatics; some psychogenic disorders such as anxiety, conversational disorder, hypochondriasis and depression may require such collaborative work.

Gastro-oesophageal Reflux Disease (GERD) and Laryngopharyngeal Reflux (LPR) GERD and LPR may cause voice disorders (Oğuz et al. 2007). However, it must also be emphasised that LPR may become an overdiagnosis for some patients. Overdiagnosis of LPR can lead to unnecessary costs and missed diagnoses. Cooperation with a gastroenterologist may be needed in cases of GERD (Thomas and Zubiaur 2013).

Consultation with a Pulmonologist Respiratory problems that are caused by bilateral vocal fold paralysis and paradoxical vocal fold motion may need differential diagnosis from lung function disturbances. Hypofunctional voice disorders may originate from a lung or chest wall pathology. Aspiration problems that are seen in vocal fold paralysis patients secondary to surgery or neurogenic dysfunction may threaten optimum lung functions. Evaluation of the patient by a pulmonologist is required in such clinical situations.

Consultation with an Endocrinologist Voice disorders especially related to vocal pitch, such as incomplete mutation or androphonia (low-pitched voice <100 Hz), are better dealt with the help of an endocrinologist. Incomplete mutation, although it is a very rare diagnosis, must be ruled out in puberphonia patients who do not benefit from voice therapy.

Voice Disorders with Motor/Posture Problems Dysarthrophonia patients who mainly present with problems of extremity mobility are usually primarily cared for by a neurologist or a specialist in physical therapy. Phoniatricians and logopedists may be involved as consultants in such disorders.

Patients with posture problems are best dealt with the help of physiotherapy, especially if their problems persist after appropriate education/counselling sessions.

Voice Disorders that Require Prosthodontic Rehabilitation Prostheses are needed to overcome resonance problems that may be caused secondarily to defects after oncological surgeries such as maxillectomy. These patients are better dealt with by consultation with a head and neck surgeon and a prosthodontist before surgery.

Prosthetic rehabilitation may become an option for cleft palate and velopharyngeal insufficiency patients for whom surgery cannot be performed.

The Role of the Phoniatrician as a Coordinator The voice patient is dealt with by a phoniatrician in the first line. The phoniatrician consults his patient with other physicians or surgeons and informs the patient in the light of these consultations and explains the needed treatment procedures. The follow-up of the phoniatrician must continue until all the treatments and procedures required by the clinical condition of the patient have ended.

Timing and Decision-Making on the Priorities, Planning the Follow-Up The timing and the order of therapy programmes, medical treatment and surgical or other invasive procedures must be dealt with primarily by the phoniatrician with collaborative interdisciplinary consensus. The order of priorities must always be decided according to the needs of the individual patient. Securing the airway and breathing first and tailoring the treatment and follow-up to increase the patient's quality of life are the main principles for a phoniatric patient.

8.2 Fundamentals, Goals and Structure of Voice Therapy

Nasser Kotby

8.2.1 Application and Administration of Voice Therapy

The main focus of this section is to highlight the mechanism of application and administration of voice therapy between the logopedist and the phoniatrician. It should be stressed that both professionals may deliver voice therapy to their patients/clients. In case there is to be a process of referral from one to the other professional, a plan of such a process is proposed and described.

8.2.1.1 Definition of Voice Therapy
Administering voice therapy requires:

- Deep understanding of vocology, including structure and function of phonation as well as the 'pathology' of phonation and the mechanism of vocal breakdown.
- Proper diagnosis of the condition! (Assessment.)
- Critical choice of the appropriate line of intervention, including not only voice therapy but also surgery and pharmacotherapy.

8.2.1.2 Categories of Voice Therapy/ Behaviour Readjustment Therapy (BRAT)

Specific Techniques in Voice
'Pushing' Exercises. These are thought to help in cases of paralytic dysphonia with a phonatory glottal gap (Froeschels et al. 1955).

The forearms are elevated and flexed in front of the chest. The patient is asked to lower (push down) the elevated forearm with considerable force while phonating a vowel. This produces a strained 'grunting sound'.

An alternative is to try, while seated on a chair, to lift oneself by pushing the arms against the seat of the chair while phonating. These 'straining' attempts are claimed to approximate the vocal folds and reduce a paralytic glottal phonatory gap. The same effect of 'straining phonation' may be achieved by pulling the interlocked fingers of both hands when held in front of the chest with flexed elbows. Attempting to pull the two hands apart strongly while producing/phonating a vowel may create that same straining phonation producing that 'grunt sound'. The pulling effort is claimed to approximate the vocal folds, not only during straining but also during phonation.

These exercises, however, are not effective in reducing a paralytic phonatory gap. Further, it is difficult to carry over this 'straining phonation' to connected speech. The pushing exercises have not stood the test of time. The management of glottal gaps follows other more effective lines of treatment, by using voice therapy and applying surgical procedures. The choice of the line of treatment depends on the course of the disease and the size of the glottal gap.

In cases of *mutational dysphonia*, one uses finger manipulation to adjust the position of the larynx in the neck, thus lowering the usually elevated larynx by external finger manipulation and pressure. This usually leads to the emergence of the deep voice. The newly produced deep voice has to be trained gradually till the patient accepts it as 'his own' voice and becomes convinced that it is the 'normal' expected voice for his growing age.

In cases of *habitual/psychogenic aphonia*, one may rely on various techniques to help the patient regain the feeling of contact of the two vocal folds in producing the 'missing' voice. The patient is instructed to feel the vibrations behind the sternum during the short attempts of induced vocalisation by using various techniques. These techniques may include:

- Coughing with hard glottal contact/attack and prolonging the phonation of a vowel after the cough.

- Humming in itself, oral or even nasalised, may help get the feeling of vibrations in the neck and upper chest, thus helping the patient experience the vocal fold contact producing these vibrations.
- Pitch gliding from lowest to the highest may guide the patient to produce a voice and help acquaint the patient with the vocal fold contact and the vibrations associated with the act of phonation.
- Inhalation phonation: this may distract the patient to produce a 'voice' in an unusual way, giving a chance for the patient to feel the contact of the vocal folds and the vibrations created by that 'phonation'.
- Auditory masking may be effective in cancelling the patient's self-monitoring and allowing the voice to emerge. Masking may be associated with 'delayed auditory feedback', which usually proves rather effective in regaining the 'missing' voice. This attempt has to be followed up by securing the continuation of that phonation and stabilising it.

The *resonance tube method* (Sovijarvi 1969; Laukkanen et al. 1995; Simberg 2000) is based on humming/phonating while having a small glass tube (5–6 mm in diameter about 27 cm long) between the closed lips. The other end of the tube is lowered in a glass of water below the water surface. The patient/subject shall hum series of vowels for a few minutes several times a day. This exercise is meant to help *vocal warming-up* in preparation for a specially demanding vocal situation, as in a classroom or giving a speech.

Diverse Non-related Methods, Mostly Focusing on Reducing Tension and Misuse of Voice

Boone (1988) lists the following:

- Reduction of voice abuse (this falls in the domain of vocal hygiene advice (Froeschels et al. 1955) rather than correcting a faulty vocal technique)
  - Relaxation, utilising various techniques
  - Head rolling

- Altering tongue position while phonating
- Laryngeal massage (Aronson 1985)
- Laryngeal stimulation
- Pitch inflexion and pitch gliding
- Inhalation phonation
- Yawn-sigh (Brodnitz 1971)
- Chant talk
- 'Burring'; phonating with the partially closed and relaxed lips

Diverse Related Methods

These are based on the particular theoretical beliefs of the author. The following techniques are mentioned for historical interest:

- Specific procedures described to correct certain vocal muscles' 'insufficiencies' (Forchhammer 1974). The exercises are claimed to strengthen the insufficient muscle or groups of muscles.
- Specific procedures to correct 'asymmetries' of laryngeal cartilage postures (Sovijarvi 1974).

Holistic Methods

These methods are devised to tackle the respiratory (pulmonary), phonatory, articulatory and gesticulatory aspects simultaneously, in a 'holistic' manner:

- The Chewing Method (Froeschels 1952). This technique is based on humming (phonating) series of vowels while chewing with a partially opened mouth with active masticatory movements. This is supposed to ease laryngeal/vocal hyperfunction. The vowel hum shall proceed gradually to articulatory movements producing connected speech.
- The Accent Method (Smith and Thyme 1978; Kotby 1995; Thyme-Frøkjaer and Frøkjær-Jensen 2001). The Smith Accent Method does not focus on giving theoretical or detailed clinical explanations of the condition of the patient. It focuses on the technical aspects of the therapy programme while continually boosting the motivation of the patient. It is a holistic approach of voice therapy both:
  - Vocally: it gives no separate attention to tension/relaxation and handles simultaneously pitch, loudness and timber.
  - Communicatively: it handles simultaneously respiratory, phonatory, articulatory and gesticulatory activities.

Despite this, minimal initial explanation to the patient is needed, to focus on few basics of vocal physiology:

- Why start with breathing exercises at the beginning of the programme? (See details below in this section.)
- Why focus on abdominal breathing? (See details below in this section.)

The technique of the Accent Method (AM) can be summarised in the following stages:

- Breathing exercises
- Phonatory exercises
- Movement exercises
  - Respiration-Adapted Phonation (Coblenzer and Muhar 1993) (please read the reference).
  - The Nasal-Reflecting Method (Pahn and Pahn 2000) (please read the reference).

It should be stressed that, despite the above-mentioned extended classification of some of the techniques and methods of voice therapy, there are many more such methods. The limitation of space in this volume does not allow referral to and describing all such methods.

8.2.1.3 Components of Voice Therapy

The voice therapy programme, whatever the technique or method, usually entails two main tasks (Kotby 1995):

- Recommendation of voice hygiene advice
- Correction of the faulty phonatory technique by the therapy technique used

Voice Hygiene Advice

This should be summarised so that the patient does not get overwhelmed. One gives only what the patient can 'digest' and apply by himself or herself without preparatory training.

It is confusing for the patients to be exposed to aspects of clinical medicine, such as the controversial role of reflux (GERD), the unconfirmed allergies and what to eat and what not to, etc. Similarly, giving advice regarding abdominal breathing, which is rather professional, is not effective. Such a physiological 'habit' can be a topic of training rather than verbal or written advice. Accordingly it is recommended that voice hygiene advice is made short, simple and easy to follow. It is summarised as follows:

- The 'Do/Do Not Do' category; avoidance of the three 'Ss':
  - *Spirits*. This usually leads to increased talkativeness. This happens in noisy surroundings. Thus the patient indulges in harmful over-talking in a noisy situation.
  - *Smoking* (active and passive). It is needless to refer to the harm it inflicts on the larynx and vocal folds.
  - *Screaming* (conscious and unconscious). The latter is defined as speaking in a noisy background and imaging that one is speaking softly while in fact the person is actually screaming to be heard against the loud background noise!
- The 'Try to' category; try to:
  - Drink more fluids/water (4–5 L per day in hot dry weather).
  - Avoid clearing the throat. This is easy to follow if fluid intake is increased and the tracheo-laryngeal secretions are becoming less sticky.
  - Avoid dry dusty places.

What about the commonly advised 'complete voice rest'? This should be seen in the frame of the following limitations:

- It has *restricted indications*.
  Complete voice rest may be applied in some selected cases:
  - During acute upper respiratory tract infections (laryngitis)
  - Following acute vocal trauma, especially in the presence of subepithelial bleeding
  - Following some types of phonosurgery

Complete voice rest including speaking is not a target in chronic voice disorders. The advice is to avoid screaming not soft talking.
- It is *difficult to follow*.
  The patient should be given advice that is possible to follow. Complete voice rest is not easy to apply in daily life, except for the restricted indications mentioned above and for limited periods of time.

Correction of Faulty Vocal Technique
This entails a dynamic integration of:

- Abdomino-diaphragmatic breathing, with active timed breath support while phonating (Kotby et al. 1993).
- Accentuated rhythmic vowel play (phonation), utilising breath control. The breathy phonation helps soften and reduce the hard glottal attack. The vowel play then proceeds to articulation (speech). The rhythms used extend from the slow largo proceeding to the relatively faster andante and allegro.
- Associated body and arm dynamic rhythmic movements. This provides a chance to apply the newly acquired vocal technique while engaged in free movements. This part of the technique suites singers and actors well.

During the therapy sessions, the *auditory feedback* of the patient is enhanced to help self-monitoring and self-correction. This feedback may be enhanced in many ways. An effective way is the frequent recording and playback of the patient's vocal performance. These recordings are to be listened to carefully with comments together with the therapist.

8.2.1.4 Indications for Voice Therapy
These include:

- Disorders of voice
  - Non-organic habitual voice disorders
  - Non-organic psychogenic voice disorders
  - Selected types of minimal associated pathological lesions (MAPLs) (Mossallam et al. 1986; Kotby et al. 1988): nodules,

contact granuloma and other early lesions, such as polyp and Reinke's oedema

- Selected types of organic voice disorders: dysplasia, small paralytic gaps (up to 2 mm) and non-organic small gaps as sometimes seen in cases of phonasthenia
- Disorders of speech
  - Dysarthria/dysarthrophonia: the therapy enhances the defective breath support and improves dysprosody and dysphonia.
  - Stuttering (fluency disorders): the therapy improves the breath control leading to better phrasing and better speech rhythms.
- Disorders of language
  - The therapy corrects the dysprosody in selected language disorders in children and adults.

8.2.1.5 Initial Protocol for Assessment of the Morphology of the Larynx/Glottis and Vocal Function

This process follows a plan of three levels of escalating objective and complex tests (Kotby 1986). The goal is to move from simple measures to more complex ones, and to move from subjective measures to objective ones, as much as possible:

- Elementary diagnostic procedures
- Clinical diagnostic aids
- Additional instrumental methods

Elementary diagnostic procedures comprise:

- Systematic and complete patient interview, suited for interpatient differentiation
- Auditory perceptual assessment (APA) by expert clinician ears, suited to interpatient differentiation
- Preliminary visual assessment of glottal pathology, mirror or scope without documentation if not available, suited to interpatient differentiation

Clinical diagnostic aids involve:

- Laryngo-videostroboscopy (Hirano and Bless 1993), suited to interpatient differentiation and intrapatient follow-up
- Laryngo-video-kymograpy (Švec et al. 2000), suited for interpatient differentiation and intrapatient follow-up
- High-speed, high-definition laryngography (Hirano and Bless 1993; Deliyski and Hillman 2010), suited to interpatient differentiation and intrapatient follow-up
- High-fidelity voice recording, suited to interpatient differentiation and intrapatient follow-up
- Radio-imaging, suited to interpatient differentiation and intrapatient follow-up

Additional instrumental measures are:

- Acoustic analysis:
  - Perturbation measures, with reservations (Kotby et al. 1998b)
  - Multi-Dimensional Voice Program (MDVP) (Deliyski and Gress 1998), suited to intrapatient follow-up
  - Voice range profile (VRP)/phonetogram (Kotby and Orabi 1995), suited to intrapatient follow-up
- Aerodynamic measures:
  - These include such simple measures as the phonatory quotient and more complex measures as the mean flow rate, subglottal pressure and sound pressure level, with extraction of the glottal indices such as efficiency and resistance (Kotby et al. 1990), suited to intrapatient follow-up
  - Flow inverse filtering (volume velocity wave/glottal area wave) (Kotby et al. 1998a), suited to intrapatient follow-up.
- Electromyography (Kotby et al. 1992), suited to interpatient differentiation and intrapatient follow-up.
- Electroglottography (Kitzing 1979), suited to intrapatient follow-up.

8.2.1.6 Voice Therapy in Association with Other Complementary Treatment Modalities for Management of Voice Disorders

This complementary line of voice therapy/treatment may be given:

- In association with pharmacotherapy
- In association with phonosurgery

The complementary voice therapy is needed to:

- Eliminate predisposing faulty vocal habits in order to avoid recurrence
- Acquaint the patient with the newly adjusted apparatus (the glottis) in order to make maximal use of the potential vocal improvement

Voice therapy in association with other intervention/treatment modalities may start:

- Actively 1 week after surgery
- Simultaneously with radiotherapy for oncological lesions of the larynx

8.2.2 Initiation and Supervision of Voice Therapy

8.2.2.1 Organisation of the Work of the Voice Therapy Team Between the Phoniatrician and the Logopedist

Voice therapy usually starts when indicated and prescribed by the phoniatrician. Phoniatricians may carry out the role of a therapist and apply the voice therapy programme. Alternatively, the patient is referred to the logopedist for voice therapy, with full case report and diagnostic categorisation, including videostroboscopy and radio imaging, when needed. The patient is referred with a proposed initial plan of intervention/therapy programme, including the duration and the frequency of sessions. The type of therapy is agreed upon in each clinic according to the prevalent and accepted method of therapy.

8.2.2.2 Agreement on the Choice of the Voice Therapy Method

The method of voice therapy is chosen according to the diagnosis and the method that is mastered and applied in any particular clinic and team (see Sect. 8.2.1.2).

8.2.2.3 Goal Setting of the Therapy Programme

Principles are:

- This should be set for each patient individually depending on the diagnosis and the patient's needs and socio-economical background.
- The goal of the therapy programme is 'normalisation' of the vocal function. This ideal goal may not always be attainable.
- The treating team should acknowledge the limiting factors and prepare the patient to accept a realistic target.

8.2.2.4 Drawing the Schedule and the Stages of the Programme and Highlighting the Task and Target of Each Stage

The schedule of the therapy programme is planned to be given:

- On an individual basis.
- Possibly to selected homogeneous groups, such as students of vocology or singing.
- In sessions of 20 minutes each.
- At a frequency of usually two sessions per week. Intensive therapy programmes of even two sessions per day may be resorted to in special situations.

The following are the stages of the voice therapy programme:

The First Stage is devoted to building rapport and heightening motivation of the patient. A simple explanation of the nature of the vocal problem, summarising the goal of the therapy programme, is needed. *Minimal initial explanation to the patient* is the goal. It is advised not to confuse the patient/client by excessive theoretical information. But the patient might need to know:

- Why breathing exercises?
  Voice is produced in the larynx by the vibrations of the vocal folds. These may be exemplified as the 'motor' of phonation. This motor needs energy, 'gasoline/petrol', which may be exemplified as the expiratory air. Thus it may

be accepted that the programme of reversing the voice problem by voice therapy should be focused in its initial phase on breathing exercises to improve breath support and expiratory control.

- Why abdominal diaphragmatic breathing? This type of breathing allows:
- Better controlled expiration
- Bigger volume of expiratory air
- Reduction of tension in the neck and shoulder muscles (where the larynx is supported by its extrinsic muscles) by bringing the 'tension' of the respiratory tract away from the clavicular/neck area to the abdominal level

The Second Stage focuses on ensuring that the patient has mastered abdomino-diaphragmatic breath support.

The Third Stage focuses on the phonatory exercises by using the accentuated vowel play in a slow rhythm, to be followed by the faster rhythms. The voice in the initial phase is produced in a breathy manner to avoid hyperfunction and hard glottal attack.

The Fourth Stage aims at 'carrying over' the healthy vocal technique that the patient has mastered to connected speech in everyday life in a stepwise manner.

The *Set-up for the Therapy Sessions* involves (Kotby 1995):

- The room, characterised by:
  - Reduction of ambient noise reaching from outside
  - Acoustic treatment of the interior of the room
  - Providing a reassuring non-distracting atmosphere
  - Air conditioning and humidity level control
- The patient's position:
  - May be recumbent at the start of the programme to master diaphragmatic breathing
  - Later: sitting, standing or even walking
- Technical aids:
  - Drum or other means to keep the tempo and rhythm. The patient should perceive and feel the tempo!

- Recording and playback of patient's voice during the therapy programme as a tool of auditory feedback with critical evaluation of the patient's recorded voice with the therapist.

8.2.2.5 Planning the Follow-Up Sessions Between the Phoniatrician and Logopedist for Assessment of Progress of the Case

The follow-up sessions are planned for each patient according to the case and depending on his or her progress in the therapy programme.

The phoniatrician and logopedist confer (through the media or even better face-to-face) to discuss the progress of the case. Issues such as lack of progress or emergence of other problems or questions regarding the time to terminate the programme are discussed.

The conference generates the decision to terminate the therapy programme or to continue or to change the treatment plan.

For the termination of the programme and the release of the patient, the assessment methodology is re-run to evaluate and document the degree of progress as well as patient satisfaction in everyday life.

8.2.2.6 Criteria for Termination of the Therapy Programme

- Patient's satisfaction in real-life situations
- Improvement of APA, as judged by the expert clinician
- Improvement of glottal picture
- Improvement of the instrumental measures

It should be noted that:

- The voice therapy programme usually takes 15–25 sessions, sometimes becoming protracted and taking up to 75 sessions.
- The aim is to 'wean' the patient as soon as possible, avoiding the patient's dependence on the therapist.

8.2.2.7 Post-therapy Guidelines for the Patient to Guarantee Continued Improvement of the Voice Condition and to Avoid Recurrence of the Vocal Problem

The guidelines for the post-therapy period should focus on, and remind the patient of, the voice hygiene advice given to the patient during the therapy programme (see Sect. 8.2.1.3).

In addition to the above-mentioned voice hygiene advice, the patient should be strongly advised to remember the following fundamentals of voice production:

- Abdomino-diaphragmatic breath support.
- No use of residual air for phonation; take a new breath. Avoid terminal fry.
- Soft glottal attack, optimal pitch.
- Rhythmic accentuated intonation of articulated speech.
- Appropriate phrasing and suitable pausing.

The patient is encouraged to contact the treating team in case of recurrence of the original symptomatology and the voice problem or the appearance of any other new related problems.

8.2.3 The Phoniatrician as a Voice Therapist

8.2.3.1 The Phoniatrician Providing and Implementing the Programme of Behaviour Readjustment Voice Therapy

See Sect. 8.2.1.2.

8.2.3.2 Patient's Homework

During the initial phase of the therapy programme, the patient is asked to apply the breathing exercises, focusing on the abdomino-diaphragmatic type of breathing. This is advised to be carried out for a period of 3–5 min to be repeated 3–5 times a day. The patient is asked to choose a calm environment at home. The patient is encouraged to avoid distraction while performing the homework. These exercises are better performed while standing (or sitting) in front of a mirror with a hand placed on the abdomen, to be able to see, hear and feel the new type of breathing thus getting a good feedback.

The homework in the more advanced phase of the therapy programme focuses on reminding the patient of the technique and encouraging following it as much as possible in everyday situations. The patient is also reminded of the voice hygiene advice.

At a later stage of the programme, and when the patients start mastering the technique, a recorded part of the therapy of about 3 min may be given to the patient to follow 2–3 times a day. The recording contains the therapist's part of the exercise followed by a silent period, of such duration that allows the patient to follow the therapist's part, just as the patient has experienced in the actual therapy session.

8.2.3.3 Carry-Over to Connected Speech in Everyday Life

The gradual stage-wise transfer from vowel play to connected speech during the therapy programme involves:

- Repeating short phrases after the therapist
- Reading aloud in front of the therapist
- Speaking with or to the therapist in a *monologue* fashion and then into the spontaneous dialogue

This stage of transfer to connected speech, which may be protracted, should continue until the new healthy vocal behaviour becomes automatic.

8.2.4 Final Assessment of the Patient Following Voice Therapy Given by the Logopedist or the Phoniatrician

8.2.4.1 Re-running the Initial Protocol of Assessment

The protocol of assessment, as mentioned in Sect. 8.2.1.5, should be comprehensive and should include some objective quantitative measures. These should allow the application of efficacy studies where rigorous control of the observations before and after intervention is mandatory (Frøkjær-Jensen and Prytz 1976; Kotby et al. 1991; Fex et al. 1994; Bassiouny 1998).

8.2.4.2 Documentation and Tabulation of the Results to Evaluate the Degree of Improvement in the Patient's Condition

The data obtained from the assessment protocol, in the initial encounter, in the follow-up session, as well as the final evaluation, are tabulated in a manner that facilitates reducing it in a manageable way in the stages of analytical and comparative statistics. Even the subjective data may be tabulated in a quasi-objective fashion. An example of this is the tabulation of the patient's self-assessment of improvement in every session. This is given in a five-step scale from very bad to very good (Kotby 1995). Several efficacy studies of the Accent Method have been published.

8.2.4.3 Assessment of the Duration and the Cost of the Therapy Programme in Comparison with the Gain of the Patient's Condition/Complaint

The effectiveness of the intervention programme refers mainly to the economical cost-effective balance of it. This has to be evaluated in a frame of reference to available coverage by existing insurance systems and the impact of the vocal disability on the patient's occupational performance. The clinical team has to develop intervention modalities that consume the least possible time span. In this respect the heightening of patient motivation to follow the programme may prove effective in reducing the duration and hence the cost of the voice therapy intervention.

8.3 Voice Therapy: A Survey of Methods and Techniques

Ilter Denizoglu

8.3.1 Introduction

Voice therapy is the treatment for a voice patient with a given voice disorder requiring behavioural methods rather than surgical methods or medication. It is the essential treatment modality of voice disorders; it may be the primary treatment modality or secondary to (during, before, after) medication or surgery. It includes techniques that directly change vocal mechanism and indirect management methods for the factors that cause vocal impairment.

Voice therapy practice mainly concerns principles of ergonomics, motor learning and behavioural treatment. Various applications in voice therapy have evolved from pedagogical approaches of arts training such as singing and theatre. These methods are then described and structured by means of physics (acoustics, aerodynamics, biomechanics, etc.) and medical principles. Any voice therapy requires an obligatory preceding physical examination by a competent physician, preferably a phoniatrician. Treatment of a patient with voice disorder is multidimensional, an haute couture team approach. The physician's responsibilities persist throughout the whole treatment process (indication, application, monitoring, termination) and the clinical survey (see Sect. 8.2).

Voice therapy cannot be defined solely as the application of a given exercise schedule; it is a tool, not the goal. Voice therapy applications can be classified into two main groups (Table 8.1) on the basis of their approaches to motor behaviour.

Indirect methods are not aimed at changing the vocal technique (i.e. the vocal motor pattern) directly; rather, they eliminate harmful habits or conditions that disturb the vocal mechanism.

Table 8.1 Classification of voice therapy applications

Voice therapy (a motor learning approach)		
8.3.2 Indirect methods	**8.3.3 Direct techniques**	
8.3.2.1 Counselling	8.3.3.1 Holistic approaches	8.3.3.2 Specific approaches

8.3.2.2 Voice rest
• Absolute voice rest
• Modified voice rest
	• Resonant therapy
	  – Resonant voice therapy (Lessac)
	  – Chant talk (Boone)
	  – Humming approach
		• Techniques used in hyperfunctional voice disorders
		  – Yawn and sigh (Boone)
		  – Laryngeal massage (Aronson)

8.3.2.3 Vocal hygiene
• Elimination of mechanical trauma
• Laryngopharyngeal reflux management
• Avoidance of irritant inhalation
• Hydration-humidification
	• Vocal function exercises (Stemple)
	• Accent Method (Smith, Kotby)
	• Source-force adjustment
	• Focusing (muscle-specific vocal exercise)
		– Confidential voice therapy (Casper)
		  – Chewing approach (Froeschels)
		  – Stretch and flow technique (Stone)
		  – Register glide
		  – Softening glottal attack

8.3.2.4 Breath support
• Abdomino-diaphragmatic breathing
• Schlaffhorst-Andersen method
• Prosody enhancement
• Breathing coordination approach
	• Vocal tract shaping
	  – Vertical laryngeal posturing
	  – Phonetic manipulations
	• Semi-obstructive vocal tract exercises
	  – Consistent backpressure
	  – Transitory backpressure
		• Techniques used in hypofunctional voice disorders
		  – Lee Silverman Voice Therapy technique
		  – Phonation by swallowing
		  – Lateral compression

8.3.2.5 Posture
8.3.2.6 Biofeedback
• Auditory biofeedback
• Visual biofeedback
• Kinaesthetic-proprioceptive biofeedback
	– Oscillatory backpressure
	  – Combined consistent and oscillatory backpressure with artificial elongation of the vocal tract (Sihvo, Denizoglu)
		– Isometric contraction (push-pull)
		• Pitch management techniques
		  – Manual manipulation
		  – Pitch gliding

8.3.2.7 Relaxation
8.3.2.8 Psychotherapy
8.3.2.9 Conscious medical hypnosis
8.3.2.10 Acupuncture-acupressure
8.3.2.11 Phytotherapy
8.3.2.12 Neuromuscular electro-phonatory stimulation
8.3.2.13 So-called alternative or complementary approaches
		– Ear training for pitch awareness
		  – Using vegetative functions
		  – Head repositioning
		• Techniques for psychogenic aphonia
		• Paradoxical vocal fold motion therapy
		• Vocal granuloma therapy
		• Ventricular dysphonia therapy
		• Transgender voice therapy

Direct methods, on the other hand, aim to change vocal mechanisms or vibration patterns directly by applying various exercises based on motor learning principles.

8.3.2 Indirect Voice Therapy Methods

Indirect voice therapy methods can also be defined as vocal ergonomics because patients are provided with different ways to use the body more efficiently through understanding the order and disorder states. Elimination of the possible external causes of voice disorder is the ultimate goal.

8.3.2.1 Counselling

The overall success rate of voice therapy depends on several factors, including the disorder being treated, the method being used and the clinician's skills. However, one of the more important factors is the patient. The patient's motivational state and coping strategies should be taken into account through the whole process. Patients need to know the nature of the problem they have. Because the vocal apparatus is *hidden inside the neck*, visual biofeedback is not possible from the vocal organ, but kinaesthetic biofeedback may help; auditory biofeedback seems to be the most reliable feedback type to monitor voice. Basic knowledge of anatomy and physiology according to the patient's personal level of awareness and data need may be provided with stroboscopic self-images of vocal folds.

Only after explaining the order can the clinician determine the disorder. The patient's side of the diagnosis depends on his knowledge and acceptance. The clinician must help the patient understand the problem and provide reasonable and realistic strategies for management. Coping strategies and readiness for behavioural change in patients determine the ultimate success of voice therapy. This depends on motivation of and adherence to strategies by the patient. Various stages can be mentioned (Prochaska and Velicer 1997) in this respect: pre-contemplation (problem not realised), contemplation (possibility of addressing the problem is considered), preparation (intending to take steps to change) and action (evident attempts to change) followed by maintenance (working to prevent relapse and consolidate gains).

Self-awareness may be awakened by simple statements. For example for a puberphonia case, after explaining the physiological events in puberty, the clinician's statement that the falsetto voice is not *the normal one* may be quite impressive. Sometimes the puberphonia patient has already developed a healthy modal voice, but the problem is about choices. The answer of the patient to the question 'Do you have another voice?' may be 'Yes but I don't like it, it is too dark'. The treatment is then only about convincing the patient to accept and use the natural sound of modal register.

Therapeutic compliance is a critical issue for the treatment outcome. To increase the patient's adherence to therapy, effective exercise instruction, choosing the proper technique (haute couture, easy-to-use and trust in the method) and feedback detection may help. Social environment counselling (family, business, school, etc.) is also important, because intensive everyday life may impair vigilance. Noisy environments may cause vocal abuse (Lombard effect) unintentionally. Treatment of childhood dysphonia should include in-house vocalisation behaviour and family training in addition.

8.3.2.2 Voice Rest

Voice rest is not used to change vocal habits. The main goal of voice rest is to give some time for recovery of traumatised tissues, especially the vocal fold mucosa (Sataloff et al. 2005a). There are two types of voice rest: absolute and modified.

Absolute Voice Rest This option is generally used post-operatively, after haemorrhage and during acute laryngitis. Any vocal act is forbidden including whisper, cough, laugh, throat clearing, etc. The duration may be between 3 and 7 days (up to 14 days), which depends on the severity of the condition.

Modified Voice Rest This variant includes different limitations and may be modified individually. There are some popular quotations for modified voice rest such as 'Arm's length rule', 'Don't say a single word for which you're not being paid' (Punt 1968) and 'Go where you want your voice to go' (Ozkan 2010).

8.3.2.3 Vocal Hygiene

Vocal hygiene is about avoiding mechanical and chemical trauma, as well as treatment by hydration and humidification.

Elimination of Mechanical Trauma Mechanical trauma is related to vocal abuse (chronic cough, fast speaker, yelling, etc.) Some methods use checklists to monitor the patient day-in and day-out such as the *Vocal Abuse Reduction Program* (Johnson 1985).

Laryngopharyngeal Reflux Management Laryngopharyngeal reflux (LPR) may alter vocal mechanism in two ways: chemical trauma-induced biomechanical change of the vocal fold mucosa and impaired sensorial biofeedback. LPR is the result of the upper oesophageal sphincter dysfunction. The upper oesophageal sphincter is composed of muscles that also affect laryngeal functions. For this reason voice therapy seems to be a therapeutic approach for the LPR treatment (Martinucci et al. 2013) in addition to medication and lifestyle-dietary alterations.

Avoidance of Irritant Inhalation Irritant inhalation is not only smoking but also may be due to volatile chemicals. This should be ascertained in advance. Smoking affects voice in several ways: impairment of kinaesthetic feedback due to a decrease in sensory input, slower mucociliary transport, thickening of mucus, Reinke's oedema and increased thickness of cover and decrease in regeneration capacity.

Exposure to Hydration and Humidification Hydration-humidification should be treated in two dimensions. Hydration may be provided by drinking 8–10 cups of water (at least 2 L) a day. The famous quotation.

Sing wet, pee pale.

Van Lawrence (1986)

helps a lot for some patients to understand and monitor water consumption. Humidification is generally harder to monitor. Use of air humidifiers in houses and work places (especially where professional voice usage exists) may help. Some strategies for speakers and singers may also work such as *tongue-tip-up breathing*. In this technique, fast inhalation is made through the mouth by elevating the tip of the tongue to the hard palate to humidify air through both sides of the moist buccal mucosa. Overuse of antihistamines and ataractics or consumption of excessive caffeine and milk may also cause dehydration and should also be taken into account.

8.3.2.4 Breath Support

Abdomino-diaphragmatic Breathing The extrinsic laryngeal muscles are mostly secondary breathing muscles, and if they work improperly for breathing, negative effects on laryngeal posture may occur, particularly in singing and professional speaking. For conversational speaking, the mode of breathing is practically irrelevant. Proper abdomino-diaphragmatic breathing prevents the secondary breathing muscles from interfering with the laryngeal posture muscles. The favourable way of managing loudness is to use subglottal pressure, not by increasing glottal resistance, trying hard and contracting the ventricular folds reflexively.

Instructions for a beginner may be as follows:

- Sit in a comfortable position.
- Put one hand on your belly and the other hand on your chest.
- Take a deep breath through your nose, and let your belly push your hand out (your upper chest and shoulders should not move upwards during inhalation).
- Breathe out through your mouth slowly at a constant rate, and do not push your shoulders downwards.

Schlaffhorst-Andersen Method Breathing is regarded in three phases: inhalation-exhalation-pause. In this sense, breathing is coordinated with body movements enhancing awareness additionally (Bessert-Nettelbeck and Saatweber 1998).

Prosody Enhancement The technique is mainly about adapting the punctuation marks into speech. Reading a text stressing the punctuation marks (comma, half breath; dot, full breath; etc.) without exceeding tidal volume limits (Rammage et al. 2001).

Breathing Coordination Approach According to Stough The exhalation process is made actively and consciously. After a forced expiration, a reflexive inspiration is triggered; then a relaxed phonation is started (Breathing Coordination Approach 2016).

8.3.2.5 Posture

Potential adverse effects of poor posture on the phonation process have been known for centuries, especially in singing pedagogy. Proper posture means a perfect balance between deep extensor muscles and flexors, which leads the body to a 'maximum muscular economy' state. The larynx is suspended from the basicranium without any direct bony attachment.

The head is the pivot point, being a powerful moment-bearing mass for the whole balance system. Forward head posture (FHP) is carrying the head forward of the centre of the shoulder, which puts increased stress on the cervico-thoracic spine and requires more work from the erector spinae muscles to maintain an erect posture. Forward head posture is one of the major posture abnormalities that effects voicing by altering the vocal tract shape, elevating vertical larynx position and disturbing the cricothyroid activity. Breathing dynamics will also change with FHP.

Various techniques such as Alexander, Feldenkrais, Yoga and Qigong exist for postural study. The basic principle is being in 'conscious awareness' of the body, which is fit, but not fixed. General rules for posture involve relaxed jaw, balanced head, ear-shoulder-hip-knee on gravity line, active spine and unlocked knees in summary.

8.3.2.6 Biofeedback

Auditory Biofeedback This option is the most powerful feedback tool for the voice system. The amplification of voice is by electronic (microphones and speakers) or analogue (HearFones®, hand around ear) methods. To decrease auditory feedback, masking can be used, especially in psychogenic aphonia. Delayed auditory feedback and looping playback may also be used as auditory feedback.

Visual Biofeedback This variant of feedback is a powerful tool for the motor learning process. Various visual feedback methods can be used in a complementary manner in voice therapy:

- Endoscopic self-images, especially laryngostroboscopic recordings (edited or real-time), make the glottal closure pattern of the patient visible. This can be used in advance to support the cognitive stage of motor learning (i.e. what the problem is, why it happened, how it is supposed to be managed, etc.).
- Acoustic analysis (user-friendly tables, streaming real-time harmonic spectrum and formants, etc.), which enables *what is heard to be seen*, may be effective, especially in professional voice users.
- Exercising in front of a mirror is a valuable feedback for posture and breathing.

Vibrotactile/Kinaesthetic-Proprioceptive Biofeedback Conscious awareness of tension in the neck can be increased. Glottal vibrations may also be used as a tool to increase awareness of the voice pattern (the spectrographic energy distribution due to the glottal closure pattern determines the resonance site). Manual palpation of suprahyoid muscle tension during phonation may also increase awareness and monitoring skills in hyperfunction.

8.3.2.7 Relaxation

Various relaxation methods (Boone 2000b) may be used for helping the voice system to turn to its *factory settings*.

Progressive Relaxation Attentional focus is first concentrated on muscle groups that can easily be controlled (tighten fist; then relax). After feeling the *weight* of tension and relaxation, the second step is to carry this feeling to the larynx to increase awareness of tightness and relaxation in the vocal organ (Jacobson 1957).

Reciprocal Inhibition Relaxation is combined with hierarchy analysis (Wolpe 1958). A preset relaxed response is carried to gradually increasing tension-producing situations. For example, the relaxed pattern used in speaking with a close friend is carried to a tenser situation (e.g. speaking to the director). The patient develops a strategy to use the relaxed voice at increasingly tense levels of hierarchy.

Stretching Exercises (Head Rotation) Sitting on a backless chair, the patient drops the head forward feeling gravity. Then rolling the head in a circular fashion very slowly; the patient feels the inactive stretch and relaxation of the neck muscles. Phonation may be added to this relaxed posture.

Open Throat Relaxation Yawning can be used to develop conscious sensations of an open throat. Negative exercise (intentionally increasing tension in the throat and then relaxing) may also help. The critical move for open throat is sustained retraction of the ventricular folds actively as in a silent laugh.

Imagination A relaxing emotional setting (imagined or experienced) may be used, such as lying on a sandy beach, floating on a lake, etc.

8.3.2.8 Psychotherapy

Various psychiatric conditions may interfere with voice problems. Psychiatric intervention or psychotherapy may be needed in specific pathologies such as psychogenic aphonia/dysphonia, performance anxiety, major depression, generalised anxiety disorder, gender identity disorder and neurotic personality.

8.3.2.9 Conscious Medical Hypnosis

Conscious medical hypnosis can be used for relaxation as well as psychogenic aphonia/dysphonia.

8.3.2.10 Acupuncture-Acupressure

Various acupuncture points are known to be related with voice production. S-10 is known as

singer's point; St9, Li18, Li15, Lu1, Lu7 and Ki6 points are also stated to affect voice in some way (Yiu and Yee-Ian Kwong 2005).

8.3.2.11 Phytotherapy

Several herbal recipes (licorice extract, slippery elm, etc.) are defined to help vocal mechanism; none of them has been proven to be effective. Nevertheless, phytotherapy may help to make the throat feel more relaxed, so that it may be easier to lower the larynx and relax the muscles. In addition, some herbs (e.g. pineapple fruit containing bromelain) may alter mucus composition and may have moisturising effect (Seidman 2006).

8.3.2.12 Neuromuscular Electro-phonatory Stimulation (See Also Sect. 8.4)

Electrotherapy by transcutaneous nerve stimulation (TENS) is defined as a therapeutic modality to change the threshold of elicitation of nerves or muscles in physical therapy. Various types of electrical current may be used for different aims (i.e. to stimulate the paralytic muscles or to relax the spasmodic muscles) (Gilman and Gilman 2008). This kind of therapy is still under controversial discussion and needs evidence-based study. Neuromuscular electro-phonatory stimulation (NMEPS) can be used in combination with direct voice therapy methods in treatment of dysphonia (Guzman et al. 2014).

8.3.2.13 So-called Alternative or Complementary Approaches

These are the approaches that may be labelled as irrational and not scientifically proven but that make the dysphonic patient feel better. Regulation, licencing and usage of alternative approaches vary from country to country. They may have placebo effect and additional sociocultural aspects especially in psychogenic aphonia. Energy therapies (bioenergy by touching the body's energy fields; magnetic field therapy), alternative medicine (traditional Chinese medicine and Ayurveda), mind-body interventions, biologically based therapies and manipulative methods may be mentioned among these approaches.

8.3.3 Direct Voice Therapy Techniques

Treatment of dysphonia by behaviour transfer through vocal exercises based on motor learning principles can be named as direct voice therapy. The cognitive phase (the patient understands what to do and why) is the first step of motor learning. Skill acquisition (the associative phase of motor learning) is the next step. Delicate motor adjustment and fine-tuning in voice production (glottal attack, glottal damping, correct registration, etc.) are important factors in this phase. Producing the most consistent and efficient voice should be monitored in various conditions (vocal pattern drift), and new strategies may be developed. The last phase of direct voice therapy is about transferring the established skill (i.e. the new phonatory pattern) into behaviour (habits in daily life), the autonomous phase.

8.3.3.1 Holistic Approaches

Holistic therapy programmes integrate all of the voice subsystems—respiration, phonation and resonance—into the rehabilitation of the voice disorder. They provide vocal hygiene counselling, attention to vocal symptoms, emotional support and direct physical exercise through manipulation of respiration, phonation and resonance. These programmes are multidimensional and may be applied to both hyperfunctional and hypofunctional voice disorders.

Resonant Therapy

The resonant voice projects well, is easy to produce and involves a sensation of vibration in the face, which refers to the so-called mask feeling. Resonant voice is characterised by ample harmonic content; the term 'resonant' does not point to resonance spaces: it is a sound that can be resonated well; it is mainly a function of the source. A high ratio of vocal output to vocal fold vibration amplitude is provided by a high maximum flow declination rate (MFDR) and lower vocal fold collision stress during vibration. Vocal folds vibrate in a slightly abducted or barely adducted position (the vocal processes stay 0.5–1 mm ahead of each other). The harmonic content

becomes richer, owing to effective closure and consequently high energy loaded in the high-frequency harmonics, and is resonated in the smaller cavities such as the nose, mouth and sinuses, which gives a feeling of a mask vibration (forward focus) on the face.

There are different approaches having similar goals.

Resonant Voice Therapy An easy and effective vibratory pattern results in increased oral vibratory sensation. Focusing on the processing of sensory information, the patient is constantly asked to monitor and concentrate on the auditory and tactile feedback. *Lessac's Y-Buzz* exercise is simply as follows: put your lips in a gentle [ʂ] position. Think of a slight yawn and hum on [y]. Keep feeling the sensation of yawn in your mouth and phonate [i]. While sustaining [i], [z] is attached to complete the Y-Buzz. Focus is carried forward, and the larynx is comfortably lowered (Lessac 1997). *Resonant voice therapy (RVT)* as presented by Verdolini-Marston et al. (1995) begins with a series of stretching and breathing manoeuvres. These may include the following: shoulders (elbows touch at the back, arms stretch in front), neck (slow rotation and side stretch), jaws (masseter massage), floor of the mouth (prevent muscle stiffness through palpation), lips (lip trills with and without voice), tongue (tongue trills and tongue manoeuvres), pharynx (yawn-sigh) and breathing (breathe out through stretching with [f] and breathe in by releasing the abdominal wall).

Following the stretching and breathing manoeuvres, a basic training gesture including a low-pitched humming (forward focus after sighing) is provided. A seven-step RVT exercise programme is applied afterwards. With sample instructions, RVT Hierarchy steps are as follows:

- RVT Hierarchy Step 1 (All Voiced): sustain a comfortable pitch with [mmamama], vary the intensity and rate, non-linguistic speech (using the same phrase), chanting and speaking specific sentences (*My mother made marmalade*).

- RVT Hierarchy Step 2 (Voiced-Voiceless Contrasts): voiceless consonant added ([mma-mapapa]) with similar exercises as the first step by using specific sentences *(My movie made Tim and Paul sad).*
- RVT Hierarchy Step 3 (Any Phrase): chant a phrase first on a predetermined note, and then over-inflect the phrase with extreme forward focus. Finally repeat the same phrase more naturally with the forward focus.
- RVT Hierarchy Step 4 (Paragraph Reading): first read a paragraph with phrase markers; then exaggerate the focus; finally repeat the same sequence without phrase markers.
- RVT Hierarchy Step 5 (Controlled Conversation): transferring the forward-focus voicing behaviour to normal conversation.
- RVT Hierarchy Step 6 (Environmental Manipulations): encouraging the patient to continue to use the new vocal pattern in various conditions (actual speaking environments, noisy café, etc.).
- RVT Hierarchy Step 7 (Emotional Manipulations): transferring the new vocal behaviour to various emotional situations (laughter, anger, etc.).

RVT hierarchy home exercises may be recommended for two 15-min periods including stretches, basic RVT gesture and a selected level of hierarchy.

Chant Talk Phonation starts with a balanced glottal attack and continues with a hymn-like monotone, high pitch. The accent is softened; vowels are sustained in a legato (connected pitch) fashion (Boone 2000a).

Humming Approach Humming is a popular method in training singing and voice therapy. Six steps are distinguished in general:

- Encourage the patient to hum in as natural a way as possible. Vegetative functions (coughing, laughing, sighing, etc.) may be used to find a way to hum freely.
- Change the loudness and pitch of the hum.

- Humming with different vowels ([hamm], [hemm], [himm], etc.).
- Hum and speak.
- Speak while imagining humming.
- Skill to behaviour transfer study.

Instant Voice Press This technique (Cooper) combines repeatedly pressing on the solar plexus (Instant Voice Jiggle Exercise 2016):

- Placing one hand on the subxiphoid region (solar plexus), with lips closed, hum while repeatedly pressing the solar plexus gently. This will cause [hmmmm] sound to break up into short bursts like 'hmm-hmm-hmm'.
- Transfer the skill to open-mouth phonation: by maintaining the same position, phonation is repeated with open mouth as [hmmaaaah].
- Transfer the skill to words: humming with counting ([hmm-hmm-one], [hmm-hmm-two], [hmm-hmm-three]).
- Open-mouth exercise without humming ([ahh-ahh-one], [ahh-ahh-two], [ahh-ahh-three]).
- Transferring that sound into normal speech without pressing.
- Skill to behaviour transfer study.

Vocal Function Exercises
These are systematic exercises (Stemple 2000) that strengthen and rebalance the subsystems involved in voice production. Exercises include maximum vowel prolongations and pitch glides using specific pitch and phonetic contexts. Four basic exercises are as follows:

- Warm-up and pose: sustain [iii] (easy, twangy, forward focus) for as long as possible on the musical note F4 for women and children and F3 for men; (this may be modified on the patient's vocal range). The goal is a clear adduction with an effective airflow rate during phonation for a stronger valve mechanism.
- Stretch: glide from the lowest pitch to the highest and sustain the high pitch. Feel the vibration on the lips or tongue (the word /knoll/ for the tongue or lip buzz using /whoop/ for the lips can be used). The goal is to improve

pitch control and flexibility by strengthening the cricoarytenoid muscle.

- Contraction: glide from a comfortable high pitch and sustain the low pitch under control. Forward focus is sustained on the low notes by twangy [iii] or using lip buzz. The goal is to strengthen the thyroarytenoid muscle by providing a clear sound at each note.
- Strong adduction: portamento (pitch sliding from one note to another) and sostenuto (sustaining a single tone) exercises with [oll] (/knoll/ without 'kn') or with [wwwuu] as long as possible on musical notes C4, D4, E4, F4 and G4. The goal is to provide a strong adduction including a balanced interarytenoid and lateral cricoarytenoid muscle contraction.

Clinicians should be aware of forward focus without tension and prevent voice breaks, improper glottal attack and breathy phonation during exercises. Patients track progress on a graph by the help of a chronometer. Once goals have been met and vocal quality has improved, a weekly programme is recommended (starting from twice the full exercises twice per day to once a week of exercise 'strong adduction' in 6–8 weeks).

Accent Method

Accentuated and rhythmic phonatory exercises are included in this technique. The accentuation can be used in both their pronunciations and related body movements (Smith and Thyme 1978; Kotby 1995):

- Abdomino-diaphragmatic respiration
- Prephonatory phase
  - First step: unvoiced unaccented consonants [ffff] and [ssss]
  - Second step: unvoiced accented consonants [ffFFF] and [ssSSS]
  - Third step: voiced accented consonants [vvVVV] and [zzZZZ]
- Phonatory phase
  - Tempo 1: vowels, largo rhythm ([yoi-yyYOOOYYY]), slow, 1 or 2 main beats in a 3-beat rhythm

- Tempo 2: vowels, andante rhythm ([yoi-yYOYYOYYOYYY]), faster, 3 main beats in a 4-beat rhythm
- Tempo 3: vowels, allegro rhythm ([yoi-yYOYYOYYOYOYYOYY]), speed increased, one unstressed vowel followed by five stressed vowels
- Articulatory phase (transfer rhythms to articulated speech)
- Rhythmic body movements

For details please see Sect. 8.2.

Source-Force Adjustment (Messa di Voce Exercise)

Messa di voce exercise is ideal and has been used effectively for a long time in singing pedagogy to establish glottal adaptation skills to subglottal pressure changes at various loudness levels. The exercise has been defined as a gradual crescendo and diminuendo while sustaining a given vowel at a comfortable pitch. In other words, phonation starts at a quiet volume, gradually and smoothly becomes louder until it reaches a high volume and then similarly becomes quiet again without changing the pitch. Normally the rules of physics will force the fundamental frequency to increase because of the higher subglottal pressure. To prevent this, the patient attempts to adjust the dynamic glottal geometry actively. This will develop the skill to balance the interactive breath force and glottal resistance.

Messa di voce is described as *the art of producing voice* by the early masters of bel canto and mostly known as the main teaching and learning principle of bel canto style. According to a statement by Reid (1965):

> The singer is able to pass freely from one register to the other, from soft to loud, from loud to soft without difficulty by the help of messa di voce.

Focusing (Muscle-Specific Vocal Exercise)

The resonance feature of a sound is defined by the type of energy transformation at the source and consequent harmonic content. Controlling the dynamic glottal geometry may be done by the kinaesthetic feedback of resonance, which is known as *placing the voice*, a well-known phenomenon in singing pedagogy (Husler and Rodd-Marling 2007). In other words, the place of the strongest vibration reflects the active muscles involved in voice production, which conversely allows the clinician to rearrange the phonation pattern.

Vocal Tract Shaping

The vocal tract (filter) and source (transglottal airflow) are continuously interacting (source frequencies depend on the filter, and the filter can both modify and resonate the source), and this phenomenon is known as the 'nonlinear source-filter theory of voice production' (Titze 2008). Vocal tract shaping, in this sense, is gaining importance as a voice therapy method.

Vertical Laryngeal Posturing In hyperfunctional voice disorders, a high vertical larynx position with tense suprahyoid-supraglottal musculature is a common finding. A comfortably low laryngeal position reduces strain in the supraglottal musculature and vocal fold tissues. There is a greater potential for creating intense sounds because the medial surfaces have a better opportunity to make contact and produce a firm glottal closure because of loosening of the vocal fold mucosa. Resonating volume is increased by a lowered larynx as a result of vocal tract elongation, hypopharyngeal enlargement (due to relaxation of pharyngeal constrictor muscles), vertically stretched and flattened ventricular folds and the pre-yawn position (anteriorly placed tongue root and palatal rise). Laryngeal lowering also reduces extrinsic laryngeal muscle overload and stress in the neck and shoulder muscles (Pehlivan and Denizoğlu 2009).

Laryngeal lowering can be achieved by a direct approach (establishing a conscious awareness of the location of the larynx at all times) or an indirect approach by various voice therapy techniques (chewing, yawn and sigh, manual manipulation, semi-obstructive vocal tract postures, etc.).

Phonetic Manipulations Vowels are acoustic results of different shapes of the vocal tract. They are said to be useful for specific goals during voice therapy, especially as supplements to a technique; for example, [u] lowers the larynx, [o] opens the throat, [i] tenses and closes the vocal folds and [a] stretches the vocal folds.

Some consonants are also helpful for therapy applications such as [l], [m], [n] and [v] for palatal lean on and positioning; [b], [d] and [g] for transitory backpressure; rolled [r] and bilabial fricative [β] for continuous oscillatory backpressure; and so on.

Semi-obstructive Vocal Tract (SOVT) Exercises

Semi-obstructive vocal tract exercises (Titze 2006; Nix and Simpson 2008) have been well-known in singing pedagogy for centuries. The main mechanism is to increase inertia of the vocal tract by applying a backpressure to the system. According to the type of the backpressure, SOVT exercises may be classified as follows:

Consistent Backpressure Consistent backpressure can be provided with or without devices:

- Artificially lengthened vocal tract assisted continuous backpressure
  - Resonance tubes of glass (Sovijarvi) (Simberg and Laine 2007) or silicone (Sihvo) (Denizoğlu 2013) provide low backpressure (wider inner diameter) and higher formant effect.
  - Drinking straws (Titze 2006) provide high backpressure and low formant effect.
- Voiced fricative consonants: [v], [z] and [j]
- Nasal consonants: [m] or humming
- Semivowels: [y] and [w]
- Hand-over-mouth exercises

Transitory Backpressure This provides high backpressure over a short duration by voiced stop consonants ([b], [g], [d]) followed by a vowel.

Oscillatory Backpressure Trills are widely used in training singing and for warming up the voice as well. Three kinds of trills are popular:

- Bilabial trill (liptrill)
- Tongue trill (rolled [r])
- Lip-tongue trill (raspberries)

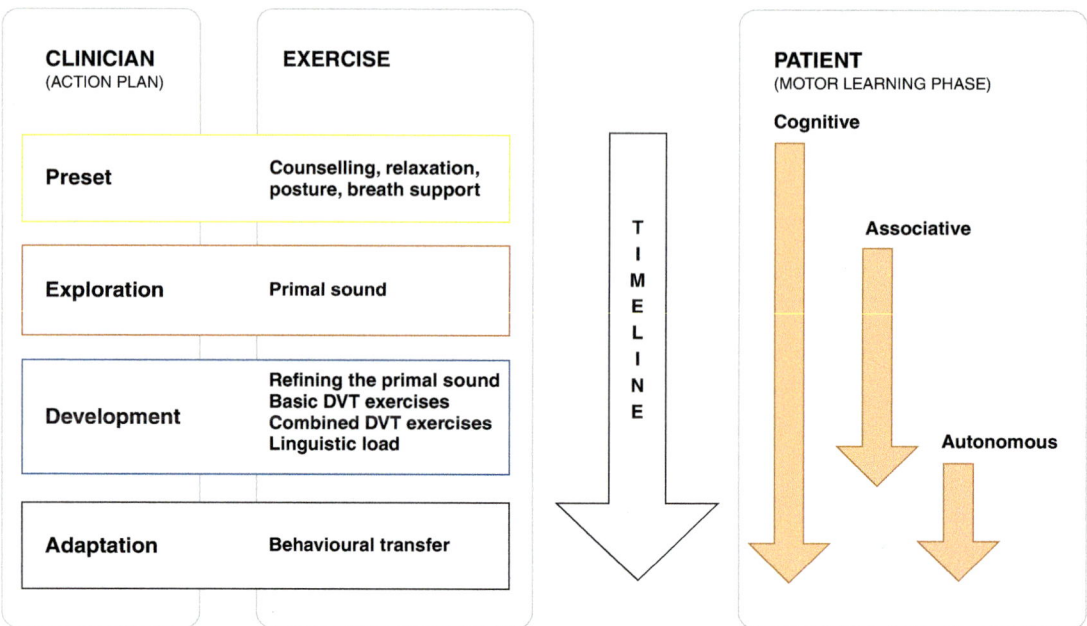

Fig. 8.1 Mind-Map of DoctorVox therapy (Denizoglu et al. 2018). Reprinted from Efficacy of Doctorvox Voice Therapy Technique for Mutational Falsetto. Denizoglu I, Sahin M, Bayrak S et al (2018) with kind permission from Elsevier

Combined Consistent and Oscillatory Backpressure with Artificial Elongation of the Vocal Tract The method of using tubes to extend and constrict the vocal tract by terminating them into a volume of water provides a combination of consistent and oscillatory backpressure to the voice system. It may be applied by different tools such as glass tubes (Simberg and Laine 2007), silicone tubes (Sihvo's LaxVox Tube) (Denizoğlu 2013) and devices (doctorVOX®, pocketVOX®, maskVOX®) (Denizoglu et al. 2018).

DoctorVox Voice Therapy (DVT) has been developed by Denizoglu but is based on Sihvo's LaxVox Method. DVT is a direct voice therapy technique that directly aims to change vocal behaviour. DVT combines phonation, resonance and breathing in a holistic approach to voice therapy. Artificially elongated vocal tract and backpressure (continuous and alternating) are the main tools. DVT provides multichannel biofeedback and enhances treatment adherence in clinical applications.

DVT is a multidimensional-multilevel treatment strategy, not an exercise of phonating into a tube submerged into a certain amount of water. It is an integrative approach for a given voice patient with three levels: the clinician's action plan, exercise patterns and the monitoring of the patient. DoctorVox Voice Therapy Technique is defined (Denizoglu et al. 2018) as a comprehensive method (Fig. 8.1). Instruction of DVT is as follows:

- **Preset**
    - Counselling: the primary concern for the patient in this phase is to understand what to do, how to do it and why. Proper and sufficient cognitive data help a lot for motor learning process.
    - Posture: take a balanced posture; *the noble posture*, which is well-known in singing pedagogy (dynamic spine, high sternum, head upright, low jaw), is ideal for both breathing and laryngeal functions. Breathing and appoggio: expiration by *lower back and lower* abdominal muscles, defocus breathing function from the upper chest and shoulders. Don't move your sternum during breathing (and phonation) as in the noble posture.
    - Relaxation: it does not define a slouched posture; it is fit-not fixed. The face, neck,

upper back and upper chest muscles are relaxed and do not interfere with laryngeal posture.

- **Bubbling without phonation**
  - Finding the primal sound is the main goal of this step.
  - Hold the device close to your rib cage.
  - Dip the tube into water (1–2 cm deep at the beginning).
  - Place the tube into the mouth between the incisor teeth and above the tongue.
  - Enclose the tube with the lips (elongate your lips as in phonating [u] to prevent air leak).
  - Inhale through the nose as in yawning or sniffing slightly.
  - Exhale into the water and try to monitor bubbling without phonation. First you can bubble in a constant rate, and then change the bubbling rate. By this way you can see, hear and monitor your breathing consciously.
- **Bubbling with phonation (finding the sound of target voice)**
  Try to hear a primal sound by various vegetative phonation manoeuvres (yawning, sighing, humming, coughing, laughing, crying, grunting, sobbing, moaning, trilling) before phonating into tube. This sound should be nonlinguistic (with no meaning).
- **Bubbling with phonation (skill acquisition)**
  Phonate into tube by this sound, add some linguistic meaning, and sustain a monotonous [huuu].
- **Skill retention**
  Various tonal exercises (sostenuto, glissando, portamento, staccato) can be used to develop the new phonatory pattern (see Sect. 1.8).
- **Behavioural transfer**
  Take the tube out, and maintain the same pattern in syllable-word-sentence-reading-conversation hierarchy.

DVT, in physical terms, adds a subsystem to the physical process of phonation (artificial elongation of vocal tract and oscillatory backpressure). The technique also provides a multichannel biofeedback, which is useful to support home exercises in a correct way by reifying the abstract concepts used in voice therapy.

8.3.3.2 Specific Approaches

Techniques that are used in specific conditions can be classified according to the pathology.

Techniques Used in Hyperfunctional Voice Disorders

Yawn and Sigh The technique (Boone and McFarlane 1993) appears to be especially effective in countering the tension symptoms of elevated larynx and constricted vocal tract that so often characterise vocal hyperfunction.

The application of the technique is as below:

- Watch the patient yawning and sighing.
- Demonstrate a yawn and explain how it feels; show figures for comparison.
- Let the patient imitate your yawn and add a sigh slightly to the end of the yawn.
- Once the yawn and sigh phonation is easily achieved, add one syllable or a word to the sigh beginning with open-mouthed vowels.
- Add a word and eventually more words on one exhalation following a yawn-sigh.
- Demonstrate the sigh phase of the exercise in detail (prolonged, easy, open-mouth exhalation with an easy phonation).
- Maintain the sigh posture with [h].
- Skip yawn-sigh and say syllables beginning with [h] ([hah], [hoh], [huh]).
- Sustain (sostenuto or glissando) vowels with the same posture ([haaaa], [hoooo], [huuuu]).
- Blend the same posture to the words beginning with open-mouth vowels.
- Maintain the relaxed phonation simply by imagining the sigh posture with conversational speech.

Laryngeal Massage The application of physical therapy (massage and osteopathy) aims to reduce tension in the upper body and to allow the larynx to relax into a more comfortable position from that which is too high because of excessive muscle contraction. In addition to muscles included in the phonation process, laryngeal joints and jaw tension are considered for manipulation. The techniques use the same mechanisms of physical therapy in general: a strained muscle is short and stiff, and when elongated by massage, it is relaxed. The procedure is applied through pressing on selected areas of the neck (especially laryngeal joints and extrinsic laryngeal muscles) with the thumb and forefinger.

The Manual Laryngeal Muscle Tension Procedure (Aronson 1990) steps are as follows:

- Focal palpation.
- Circumlaryngeal massage: moderate pressure is applied initially upon the contracted thyrohyoid space in small circles, from front to back.
- Manual repositioning of the larynx during phonation.
- This is a transient relaxation that gives auditory and kinaesthetic feedback; you must add some vocal exercises so that the patient is able to maintain easy voice production in the absence of manual manipulation.

Confidential Voice Therapy Confidential voice (Casper-Colton and Casper 1996) is a temporary breathy voice production used to help tissue recovery (especially vocal fold mucosa). It is often used in acute (short-term) voice problems and after surgery as a modified voice rest or as part of a longer-term programme that alternates periods of voice rest with more demanding voice use. Confidential voice has a light sound of voice with a soft and easy phonation. It is a breathy sound with low effort and low airflow but not a breathy whisper. Important features of the technique are:

- Pitch must not be lowered (and may be even slightly increased).
- Focus should be proper (larynx should not be pushed down).
- Mouth opening must not be reduced.
- Prosody should be preserved normal (which tends to be monotonous).

It is important to inform about the goal and rationale of the technique and warn patients that it is a transient behaviour.

Chewing Approach It is Emil Froeschels' quotation (Froeschels 1952) that:

> humans invented language by combining the various sounds they made while eating.

The main idea of the chewing approach is to make use of the more stable primary function of nutrition to stabilise the secondary function of phonation (communication). The process of chewing involves a very natural (a bit exaggerated) and free motion of the muscles of the jaw, tongue and pharynx. This method is structured on the functional relations between chewing and speaking (Froeschels 1952). The theoretical basis is considered rather speculative but in therapeutic practice has proven to be an appreciated relaxation tool for hyperfunctional phonation.

In the following the technical application is explained:

- Fulsome, appreciative chewing (with a mouth full of biscuits)
- Humming during chewing
- Closed-mouth chewing: focused voice freed from articulation
- Open-mouth chewing: phonation with slightly opened mouth
- Meaningless and meaningful syllables during chewing
- Joining [m] with [n]—[emenyem], [emenyam], [emenyim] and so on
- Adding plosives: [kyam], [pyam], [tyam] and so on
- Chewing with counting (auditory and visual feedback)
- Chewing with speaking
- Chewing with imagining speaking (skill-to-behaviour transfer)

Stretch and Flow Technique Stretch and flow phonation focuses on airflow management and aims to lower the laryngeal resistance subglottal pressure and prevent breath-holding tendencies. The model incorporates five skill levels increasing the conscious awareness about the relations between breathing and phonation. Each skill is used in a hierarchy of anxiety-producing speaking situations (from sustained sounds to repeated words up to conversational speech) (Stone and Casteel 1982).

Application of the technique includes five skill levels as below:

- Flow: control of airflow (blow without sound) encouraging patients to let unvoiced transglottal stable airflow (warm breath).
- Stretch and flow (whisper): this skill uses unimpeded voiceless transglottal airflow and slow relaxed (stretched out) articulatory movements.
- Phonate with stretch and flow: the parameter of voicing is added (gargling may be used to help) while maintaining stretched out sounds and airflow. Patients attempt not to hold their breath in conscious awareness.
- Phonate and reduce stretch: reduced stretch and increased airflow aid in regaining a more appropriate rate and preventing hyperfunctional patterns.
- Phonate and reduce airflow: fading the breathy voice quality is accomplished by asking the patient to hum or produce a louder voice without increasing extra effort.

The last step is the same as with the others, transferring the skill to behaviour.

Register Glide Hyperfunctional voice behaviour generally affects modal (chest) register (see Sect. 4.5). Fry register and falsetto register modes of phonation may stay free from the strained control patterns somehow. Fry register may be used for relaxation and maintaining a comfortably low laryngeal posture as a transient transfer phonation pattern by gliding the voice to modal register from the lowest pitches to the mid-range frequencies. Falsetto register, on the other hand, may also be used for relaxation of exaggerated downwards push of the vocal apparatus to the opposite side (Koufman and Blalock 1988).

Softening Glottal Attack Glottal attack is crucial for managing hyperfunctional vocal behaviour. It is the conjunction moment of breath force and vibration. Several techniques can be used to

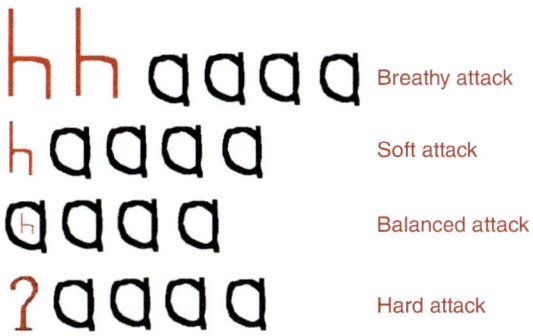

Fig. 8.2 Symbolisation of various attack types

soften, or rather balance, the glottal attack. Four types of attacks concerning breath can be distinguished (Fig. 8.2): the hard attack is a hyperfunctional uncontrolled resistive laryngeal behaviour. The breathy attack has a high prephonatory transglottal air leakage, whereas in soft attack this leakage is slightly more than effective but can be acceptable for most subjects. The most effective one is the balanced attack in which the glottal preset is similar to the one explained in resonant voice pattern (barely adducted).

Several methods may be used for balancing the glottal attack:

- Phonating vowels with [h]
    - Exaggerated [hhh] as in whisper.
    - Add vowels [hhhaaa].
    - Overdone [hhh] is faded while the patient learns to rely on kinaesthetic and auditory feedback to maintain improved voice, muscle balance and laryngeal positioning. This may be defined as the balanced attack by blending [h] with the vowel.
    - Add words to the balanced attack:
        o An easily pronounced keyword, which is a reminder of the intended vocal pattern, may be used to help skill-behaviour transfer.
        o Word pairs (hot—out) may also be used to transfer the softened attack pattern.
- Negative exercise: start with an overdone hard glottal attack, and make the patient feel the effects and kinaesthetic feedback consciously. This should be exercised for a short period,

and then gradually diminish the strain to a balanced state.

- Prephonatory pause: the patient pauses for 1 s and starts phonation afterwards. This may help to reduce prephonatory stress.
- Gliding a sustained vowel to a lower note: some patients cannot lower the pitch to a more comfortable frequency. This will make it harder to soften the glottal attack. After having a moderate pitch, the patient terminates the phonation with a soft glottal damping. The soft termination of the vowel is succeeded by another vowel at the same breath ([aaaahhhaa]).

Techniques Used in Hypofunctional Voice Disorders

Lee Silverman Voice Therapy Technique The Lee Silverman voice treatment (Ramig et al. 2001) was specifically designed for patients with Parkinson's disease. The motto is 'think louder', and the goal is to increase the effort which patients speak thereby 'pushing' the voice and making it stronger with exaggerated facial expressions. To provide enough breath support for a louder voice, patients are trained to exhale higher volumes of air out of their lungs more forcefully while simultaneously closing their vocal folds more completely. Clear articulation is also stressed during exercises.

The exercise rate is 4 days for 4 weeks. Instructions are as follows:

- 10 × [a] sustained increasingly
- 10 × glissando enlarging pitch range
- 10 × sentence with strong and loud voice
- Conversation with a decibel metre (or a software that measures loudness) for an objective feedback

Phonation by Swallowing The half-swallow—/boom/—technique (Boone) adds a phonatory task to the end of the swallowing. This may support and strengthen the glottal resistance by adding backpressure to the system. The technique has been summarised by Hedge (1996):

- Swallow, and say /boom/ as the action of swallowing is still in progress.
- Say /boom/ in a low-pitched voice.
- Say /boom/ louder and less breathy (as in telling someone off).
- Listen to recordings of two different phonations (/boom/ and habitual).
- Turn your head one side and say boom; do the same for both sides.
- Lower the chin (bending the head forwards slightly) while saying boom.
- Add sounds and words to the /boom/ (/boom-uhh, boom-one, boom-two, etc./).
- Add phrases and sentences to /boom/.
- Speak in 'boom' feeling (without saying /boom/ and swallowing) lifting the chin up and bringing the head back to the midline.

Lateral Compression In unilateral vocal fold paralysis, the thyroid cartilage may be digitally compressed from the paralytic side (or both sides) in order to help better glottal closure. The clinician may seek for the best point on the thyroid lamina to compress, for a better phonatory output.

Isometric Contraction (Push-Pull) Isometric contraction must be carefully applied in order to avoid supraglottal hyperfunction. It can be used to produce a harder glottal attack in a breathy attack. Various applications may be used to increase resistance at the glottal region (Boone 1971):

- Phonate while trying hard.
- Sit on a chair and try to lift yourself during phonation.
- Push a wall and phonate.

Pitch Management Techniques

Manual Manipulation Applying pressure externally aims to affect two pitch mechanisms: the action of the cricothyroid muscle and laryngeal elevation. Anteroposterior compression of thyroid cartilage (the Bresgen manoeuvre) reduces vocal fold tension and prevents lean-on movement (by cricothyroid action) of the thyroid cartilage. Manual laryngeal depression (pushing the thyroid notch backwards and downwards by the thumb) prevents elevation of the thyroid cartilage. Both manoeuvres prevent falsetto register and can be used to make the patient hear the chest register in puberphonia.

Pitch Gliding Finding the natural fundamental frequency may not be possible for some patients with hyperfunctional supraglottal activity and elevated larynx. Gliding from a high tone to the lowest possible frequency may lead to finding a more comfortable pitch.

Ear Training for Pitch Awareness Patients may need to be instructed about the pitch level. The results (numeric or graphical) of acoustic analysis can be shown to point out different frequencies. The clinician can imitate different pitches, defining the level of each pitch. Having the patients hear their own voices from recordings may also help. The same effect can be easily reached by having the patient cup his hands to form a channel from the mouth to one ear.

Using Vegetative Functions Reflexive phonatory behaviour is generally preserved from faulty habitual effects. Coughing, yawning, sighing, laughing, crying, grunting and sobbing are simple manoeuvres for this aim.

Head Repositioning In order to prevent falsetto register transition, the head may be repositioned (by the help of the clinician) in hyper-reflexion or hyperextension (chin-chest touch) during humming.

Techniques for Psychogenic Aphonia
Psychogenic aphonia patients generally need additional support for the treatment. It would not be proper to ignore the psychological problem or fake dysphonia. It is better to carry the voice to normal gradually, beginning with some manoeuvres with strong suggestion dominating:

- Inhalation phonation
- Masking
- Using vegetative functions (mainly coughing and laughing)
- Manual manipulation
- Conscious medical hypnosis

Paradoxical Vocal Fold Motion Therapy
After eliminating infection and reflux, a simple manoeuvre may work surprisingly well: sniff and blow. The first part of the manoeuvre is to sniff, as if slightly smelling a flower, in short breaks without purpose of inhalation. The second successive action is to blow less and less air and repeat the sniff-blow manoeuvre until the spasmodic action releases.

Vocal Granuloma Therapy
In order to prevent contact and trauma, a small gap between vocal processes may be provided by observing the larynx endoscopically while also listening to the voice of the patient. The patient is then supposed to match the endoscopic visual feedback with the auditory feedback of his own voice. This combined aural and visual approach may enable the clinician to guide the patient towards the treatment objective with precision (Leonard and Kendall 2005).

Ventricular Dysphonia Therapy
Inhalation phonation, lowered larynx techniques and SOVT exercises (see section 'Semi-obstructive Vocal Tract (SOVT) Exercises') may be used in ventricular dysphonia.

Transgender Voice Therapy
Transgender voice therapy deals with three features of voice: fundamental frequency, distribution of spectral energy and articulatory management.

Male-to-female transgender voice therapy:

- Increasing the fundamental frequency may be provided both by cricothyroid muscle action and high laryngeal position.
- Carrying the spectral energy to higher harmonics is about vocal tract shaping. Elevating vertical larynx position aids this goal.

Articulatory management is about forward action of the articulatory movements in order to create a feminine sound.

In female-to-male transgender voice therapy, the larynx is lowered, fundamental frequency is decreased by relaxing the vocal fold tension, and the articulatory movements are carried backwards to be more 'throaty' in order to create a more masculine sound.

8.3.4 Summarising Comment

Voice therapy is a multidimensional treatment approach. Clinicians need to have broad understanding, and multilayered, multidimensional and modular thinking through the whole process of treatment. This integrative model for treatment of voice disorders includes additional skills and knowledge of mechanisms of applications, stages of behavioural treatment, phases of motor learning, stages of voice therapy and steps of a given technique.

Form follows function: fundamentally, this is the central idea of voice therapy. Motion is the fourth dimension of structure; in other words, behaviour is complementarily linked to anatomy. Behaviour can be defined as the organised motion of the parts (subsystems) of the human body. Voice production is a highly complicated organised motion of subsystems, and changes in vocal behaviour can make changes in anatomy. Neural plasticity is an important part of this process: short-term changes influence the efficiency of synaptic connections and are functional. Long-term changes, on the other hand, are structural and influence the organisation and number of connections among neurons.

Therapeutic compliance is a critical issue for the treatment outcome. To increase the patient's adherence to therapy, effective exercise instruction, choosing the proper technique (haute couture, easy-to-use and trust in the method) and feedback detection may help. Exercise and feedback are the main tools in motor learning, combined with the aware intention to do better from time to time. Developing a muscle group needs muscular exercise; home exercises are part of developing a new vocal muscle pattern. This is not only for developing the strength of vocal muscles but also establishing the intended organisation among the muscles (i.e. vocal pattern) involved in voice production. The quote 'Exercise does not make perfect; it makes permanent' must be kept in mind: only correct exercise makes a perfect movement permanent.

There are numerous voice therapy methods and will be more in time. No matter how complex or simple they are, the one and the only aim of all is to reach to a target voice. Voice therapy is an agreement between the patient and the clinician to achieve and maintain the target voice. Replacement of a behaviour with a new one through motor learning happens in three phases (Fitts and Posner 1967): cognitive phase (understanding), associative phase (skill acquisition) and autonomous phase (behaviour transfer). These three phases are not separated individually; the transition between two phases may show variations among individuals.

Technique is only a tool, not the goal. Clinicians should be able to manage the action plan in this sense. During treatment, any technique can be changed; applications from various methods can be added and used together or omitted, depending on the clinician's experience and creativity concerning the patient's individual requirements. Clinical vigilance, early detection of faults and appropriate treatment are essential to improve outcomes and costs. The treatment outcome must be regarded primarily as the success of the clinician in cooperation with the patient, not the success (or failure) of the technique. Finally, the clinician should always keep in mind the Hippocratic imperative that paradigmatically reflects the spirit of the famous oath: *primum nil nocere* – first do no harm.

8.4 Neuromuscular Electrostimulation

Arno Olthoff

In the therapeutic field of phoniatricians, the application of neuromuscular electrostimulation (NMES) has to be considered for voice and swallowing disorders. Stimulation of the facial nerve follows the same principle but is not considered in this context. A German review on *Neuromuscular Electrical Stimulation Therapy in Otorhinolaryngology* has recently been published in the journal *HNO* (Miller et al. 2014).

In *dysphonia* NMES is recommended mainly for peripheral lesions of the recurrent laryngeal nerve (Garcia Perez et al. 2014; Guzman et al. 2014). Electrostimulation is applied with the intent of activating the paralysed muscle and to prevent fibrosis. In the case of vocal fold paralyses, NMES is aimed at the 'vocalis' muscle (thyroarytenoid muscle), but in functional disorders, NMES is used with the intent of increasing the muscular tone of the vocal folds. A higher tone of the 'vocalis' muscle should lead to an optimised glottal closure, less supraglottal compensation, a more efficient voice and better voice quality.

For voice therapies two commercial devices are in clinical application: Laryngoton® and Vocastim®. The first device applies electrical stimulation only after a trigger from the patient's voice. Its application reflects the voice therapy employed and is part of the therapeutic concept. The second device is used by the patient alone, who is instructed by a tape recorder. The algorithm intends to stimulate primarily paralysed and not healthy innervated muscles. In both devices surface electrodes are applied and fixed to the skin over on the vocal folds.

For *dysphagia* NMES is performed to support deglutition and its rehabilitation, e.g. in stroke patients (Lee et al. 2015; Terré and Mearin 2015; Toyama et al. 2014). The idea is to increase contractions of the pharyngeal muscles in order to support bolus transport and laryngeal elevation and to reduce penetration and aspiration. In most cases surface electrodes are used.

Reports on the benefit of NMES in voice and in swallowing rehabilitation remain contradictory. The effect of NMES on the recovery of nerves, and the possible healing with defects, also requires further knowledge. Besides the controversial peripheral neuromuscular effects of NMES, cortical modifications of the sensory-motoric representation of stimulated muscles are also discussed. Apart from an eventual peripheral or cortical impact of NMES, a therapeutic effect from a 'biofeedback' cannot be excluded.

A recommendation for or against an application of NMES cannot be given. An application 'on trial' could be an option in individual cases within a supervised therapeutic setting or within a study design.

8.5 Basic Information for the Care and Treatment of Singers

Wolfram Seidner

8.5.1 Introduction

Anyone interested in vocal health should also know something about singing and the singer's voice, which includes visits to the opera, operetta, musicals, concerts, etc., as well as practical experience of vocal study. Professional interest is good, but a positive emotional appreciation is even better, if one truly wants to understand the world of singing and song and offer successful diagnosis and treatment. It is especially recommended to make contact with an opera house (including attending rehearsals), choir, music conservatory or other such cultural institution, as one can thus better gain experience in the responsibilities of phoniatrics and voice treatment. Of course, one's clinical perspective and medical responsibility should not be neglected because of this appreciation.

It is self-evident that with singers, phoniatric responsibilities cannot be limited to exact collection of organic results. Rather, along with the indispensible voice assessment, it is necessary to take note of psychic and social circumstances, both professional and familial. There is an especially great risk to categorise singers fundamentally as emotionally unstable and not to take their complaints seriously. They are certainly accentuated in the sense of having 'interesting personality structures' and stronger emotional reactions than others; otherwise we wouldn't want to experience them as artists. But the complexity of their complaints is almost always job-specific and only infrequently expresses itself in eccentric

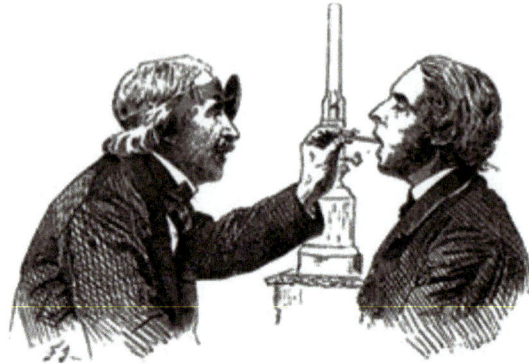

Fig. 8.3 Manuel García—laryngoscopy (Czermak 1860)

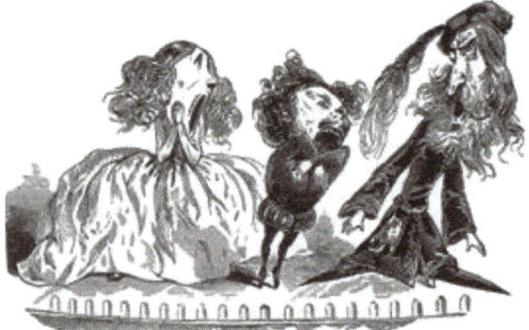

Fig. 8.4 Gustave Doré—heroic singers (Storck 1910)

behaviour. Doctors' lack of understanding of singers is often based on deficient professional competence, which is unfortunately all too often compensated for by inappropriate authoritarianism. Figures 8.3 and 8.4 mirror the arc of suspense between clinical and vocal issues.

8.5.2 Classical and Nonclassical Singing

Both categories of singing require their own understanding. Classical singing in the Western tradition (opera, oratorios, song/lied) must make do without electrical amplification, at least in opera houses and concert halls. The resonance capacity of the voice therefore plays an important role and must be rigorously built up over years of vocal technique study. This sound builds up (training of focus, placement, brilliance, 'ping', etc.) and creates the necessary resonance capacity of

the voice to fill large halls and cut through an orchestra or choir. The classical style of singing is more a physiological category than an aesthetic one, which was developed later, or possibly simultaneously. The classical singer must sing as she or he does to survive. So, it can't be discounted as 'old-fashioned' when the goal is to achieve a full, clear, resonant and flexible voice, resilient enough also to be able to sing large roles without difficulty. Moreover, certain aesthetically informed vocal techniques necessitate this production, namely, coloratura, messa di voce, trills, register, vowel blending, etc., such that vocal health is probably, but not absolutely, connected with this technique, because even the best technique cannot protect from illness, singing too often, too loud, too long or too high when the constitutional preconditions are not sufficiently observed. A full (i.e. not breathy) and clear (i.e. not rough) voice must always be the goal of all therapeutic efforts in the classical area.

In nonclassical singing, especially in pop music, these technical characteristics are not similarly required, since the voice sound is amplified by electronic equipment. Pop voice technique works to achieve a very different sound, one that is often hoarse or even pressed and screamed. From a medical perspective, it is somewhat problematical to accept hoarseness as a means of artistic expression, since it must generally always be taken seriously as a sign of illness. But questions of aesthetics are outside the realm of medical competence. The solution is to clarify a diagnosis of persistent or increasing hoarseness as soon as possible and to observe and resolve a possibly established psychological stress. When the vocal hyperfunction that often goes hand in hand with high breath pressure, marked laryngeal and vocal fold tension and forced declamation is often or exclusively used (as in pop singing), it can quickly become very dangerous for the voice. The voice is not necessarily damaged by gentle, short and controlled use of effects such as scream, rattle, growl, grunt, creak, vocal break, aspiration, etc. as long as these special vocal effects are only temporary.

'Belting', the specific means of expression used by singers, is assessed differently regarding possible vocal damage. By emphasising a calling voice function especially in the high register, the vocal strain of this sound production is less than with emphasis of declamation in the low register (chest register in women), where this sound production is only finitely possible. One must always bear in mind that constitutional predispositions are non-uniform. What one person is able to maintain effortlessly over longer periods of time in hyperfunction soon brings another singer to serious and chronic vocal damage that eventually even requires the singer to give up singing. A chronically hoarse voice that can only be produced with enhanced effort, effectively only hollering or screaming and thereby devoid of all flexibility, should better undergo intensive diagnosis and therapy than continue to be presented on stage as an artistic achievement. Gaining basic phoniatric knowledge of singing implies that every interested person should audit or even take multiple voice lessons themselves, preferably at a music school or conservatory. Only thus is it possible to understand the methods of voice teachers, who often work with strong emotions, expressive impulses and fantasy-rich metaphors and similes—unusual tools for doctors. The ends justify the means! In any case, one will realise that teaching of singing is intense work that requires much patience and that should be treated with respect. It is especially interesting to get to know the differences between classical and non-classical singing in this way. And you should definitely try singing in a choir!

8.5.3   Phoniatric Findings

In addition to detecting illness, phoniatric examinations also serve to clarify questions and problems related to singing and vocal pedagogy. Sometimes it is about judging the qualifications for voice training, or it is simply an estimation of the person's ability for specific professional jobs. Both organic and functional test results should be taken into consideration. The principal mistake lies in overvaluing the organic findings and not seeing them in relation to the functional

abnormalities, whereby functional findings do not include only the vocal fold movements but most importantly the voice sound. Balancing this relationship is especially necessary for determining the need for surgical intervention and for making far-reaching decisions in regard to actual singing engagements, as well as future professional responsibilities. The flippantly uttered observation 'Your vocal folds aren't inflamed - you can sing' should be a thing of the past.

Inherently, a carefully compiled medical history, a thorough stroboscopic examination and the perceptive auditory assessment of spoken and sung voice all take precedence over instrument-based procedures, which may be of additional importance. However, it would be a serious mistake to send singers first to a voice laboratory in order to obtain an ostensibly objective result and only later to make personal contact with them.

8.5.4   Vocal Medical History

A precise medical history is absolutely necessary for all singers. It should be an insightful consultation without any time pressure that, in addition to answering specific vocal questions, also builds trust. Of course, this goes more quickly in the case of acute complaints than it does with persistent functional disorders (e.g. dysodia) that require a very thorough examination. The vocal development must sometimes even be traced back to childhood (including the age of mutation), and the course of vocal studies must often also be scrutinised. Career-specific questions (choir? solo? career development? career setback? etc.) must include psychological and social particulars. In children with vocal damage, it is especially interesting to note if the hoarseness developed from a possible strain of the voice by excessive singing or through repeated and loud speaking or even screaming. A general medical history, together with an ENT medical history, provides a full picture of the vocal abnormalities. During the consultation, one should pay attention to voice sound, speech and manner of expression, as well as the accompanying movements (facial expressions, gestures).

8.5.5 Laryngostroboscopy

For diagnosing singers, magnifying optics and vibration analysis of the vocal folds, such as with rigid laryngostroboscopy, are indispensible. The simple laryngeal mirror is not sufficient and is only of historical interest in questions involving singers. After all, it is about obtaining a very precise assessment, especially of the moving edges of the vocal folds and of the vocal fold closure in relation to pitch and volume. Discrete changes, such as local or diffuse production of mucus ('fatigue, catarrh', noninflammatory), increased vessel visibility and functional phonation-induced vocal fold thickenings ('functional nodules', i.e. thickening of the mucous membranes just before vocal fold closure but not in respiratory position), must also be recognised, precisely diagnosed and put into relation with the voice findings. For repeated and comparative assessments, it is advantageous to use the possibilities of a digital image storage system systematically. It is obvious that a careful examination of the vocal tract must also be conducted, since pathological findings in this area could significantly impair singing.

8.5.6 Voice Assessment

The auditory assessment of the voice must take speech (unstressed in common speech or reciting numbers, stressed in a calling voice) as well as singing, both natural (song, aria) and experimental (exercises), into account. The assessment of the speaking voice can follow the RBH system, (roughness, breathiness, hoarseness) whereby additional amounts of stress, sonority and nasality are informative. Assessment of singing and singers needs special knowledge regarding specific singer-related abilities and skills, which might require a consultation with a voice teacher in certain circumstances. The documentation can take place through audio recordings (text, songs or arias) or additionally through the measurement of spoken and sung voice range profiles.

8.5.7 Dysodia

The functional disorder of the singing voice is called dysodia. It can manifest as hoarseness, but also as decreased vocal capacity (quickly fatigued, lengthy recovery), or as a reduction of certain vocal skills. What previously functioned effortlessly in terms of vocal technique now presents problems. Unfortunately, the symptoms are often falsely assessed, since important factors that could interfere with singing are either not acknowledged or taken seriously. Numerous internal and external influences that are often confluent or mutually influential can be the cause of this. Sometimes the decisive factor causing the disorder first comes to light in the course of repeated consultations or in a treatment. Among the more common causes are insufficient constitutional condition, overstress from singing or speaking, psychological factors and general inefficiency or low resistance to infection. Watch for the following: excessive demand from exhausting rehearsals, too many performances with too little rest in between or, what is also common, too short or insufficient training and wrong voice type classification. Singing too much in the upper voice range and forcing a more dramatic sound in particular lead to voice disorders. The symptoms and findings may reflect subtle singing functions. For example, the voice doesn't respond easily enough, pathological onsets occur more frequently, and piano (soft or quiet) singing is disturbed. The pitch range is reduced, and high, loud notes can only be reached with increased force. Even changes in the voice sound are possible, including a rough or breathy voice. Dullness and paraesthesia in the throat area are symptoms that must be taken seriously. In the case of specific complaints, such as difficulty in changing register, changes in vibrato or intonation problems, a voice teacher with physiological knowledge should be asked to consult. Attempts to compensate for diminished vocal ability are audible and also observable as muscular hyperfunction, especially as hypertension in the neck area, and as reflexive movements and gestures and accompanying physical movements. The treatment should be implemented causally and in certain circumstances must also intervene in the professional situation. The complaints and symptoms can often be traced to a voice technique that has been neglected for a long period of time. In this case, a systematic retraining under the direction of a competent voice teacher is strongly recommended. This also provides the opportunity to check the voice classification and possibly correct it. Speech therapy exercises only seem to make sense when there is already a certain competence in singing and the singer's voice.

8.5.8 Voices at Different Ages

Singing disorders in childhood, during puberty, in menopause and in advanced age require special diagnostic and therapeutic tools. For example, vocal rest for set periods of time is no longer recommended during voice change, since the effects of puberty can be mitigated or shortened through gentle voice use under the supervision of an experienced voice teacher. Menopause-induced voice problems often occur less frequently when vocal technique and a healthy lifestyle are maintained. Phoniatricians should also be able to help older people to sustain choir singing as an important part of their life.

8.5.9 Emergency Treatments for Singers

Phoniatric emergency treatments are almost exclusively provided to professional singers and require a basic knowledge about the upcoming artistic performance. The most common causes are head cold infections and vocal overuse (e.g. dysodia, which can lead to sudden stress-related weakness or even loss of certain vocal abilities). The earlier the treatment can begin, the less 'drastic' the measures required—in which case a close collaboration with the artistic institutions involved (e.g. theatres, arts presenters, agents, etc.) can be helpful.

Regarding the medical history, the patients themselves can be quite helpful, since they know their own abilities and available resources better than anyone and seldom exaggerate. On the other hand, they usually want to sing and rather tend to underestimate the problem and overestimate their ability. The current work situation, the difficulty of the role to be sung and the singer's current condition should all be considered in the therapeutic diagnosis.

In addition to a careful physical assessment, which is required for a complete ENT status and which cannot be limited to the larynx, it is essential to analyse briefly the sound of the speaking and singing voice. Even when a magnifying laryngostroboscopy must be performed in order to achieve an exact diagnosis of the vocal folds, the condition of the mucous membranes in the nasal and oral cavity must also be assessed, since swelling, excess mucus, paraesthesia and the after-effects thereof can also significantly restrict singing or even render it impossible. Non-inflamed vocal folds are not sufficient for professional singing! After all, distinct abnormalities in vocal fold oscillation or dry mucous membranes can cause significant discomfort. In the case of secondary organic alterations to the vocal folds ('nodules') or menstruation-related changes, larger roles should not be sung. It is especially dangerous to sing a large and heavy role when there are signs of inflammation, however insignificant.

When considering possible therapies, one must consider whether the singer will be able to sing the role in its entirety, if the performance would potentially have to be interrupted and whether or not performing is likely to cause long-term vocal damage. Ultimately, our medical responsibility is for the singer's vocal health and not for a theatre's performance schedule! An expert consultation, possibly with the participation of an experienced vocal pedagogue, together with an intense but mild anti-inflammatory treatment, vocal rest (without silent participation in rehearsals!) as well as agreements with the artistic administration are more important than the (mostly questionable) use of antibiotics or intravenous/oral corticoid applied as a 'safety chute'. These injections are certainly overrated and are usually an expression of helplessness when faced with acute singing-related problems. The exception proves the rule. The well-known laryngeal injection, by which an anti-inflammatory substance (usually an essential oil) is suddenly injected into the interior of the larynx by means of a blunt cannula, can only be valued as a kind of 'psychotherapeutic' surprise attack. The precipitously applied medicine is usually roughly coughed up, whereby no therapeutically significant dose actually reaches the vocal folds. If it is not possible to save a performance despite medical treatment, it is sometimes possible and even acceptable to use a double as an emergency solution. The role can be sung from the orchestra pit or the side stage by a vocally healthy singer, while the sick singer performs silently on the stage.

More information can be found in the books by Seidner and Wendler (2010), Dayme (2009), Nair (2007), Richter (2013), Sataloff (2005) and Sundberg and Mecke (2015).

8.6 To Sing or Not to Sing: Cancellation Policy at an International Opera Festival

Josef Schlömicher-Thier and Matthias Weikert

8.6.1 Introduction

Professional singing must be considered a high-performance sport requiring special training conditions and top physical performance (Seidner and Wendler 2004; Richter 2013; Spahn et al. 2011; Schneider-Stickler and Bigenzahn 2013). Stricken by sudden illness, the professional singer is under enormous time pressure as a premiere sets a precise deadline. There is a variety of individual factors confronting the professional singer who becomes ill while working in a theatre or festival activity, including:

- Responsibility towards members of the cast
- Anxiety of the management

- Exertion of the conductor's and director's influence
- A director who will often make the decision of recasting more difficult
- Tempting record contracts
- An audience that wishes to see a stellar performance

In such cases, the attending physician is usually and optimally a phoniatrician, as the voice specialist assumes a high degree of responsibility (Seidner 2004; Flach 1992).

It is the specialist's duty to protect the singer affected by a disorder from additional damage that could have a serious impact on the singer's further career. The specialist must also devise an effective treatment concept that will enable the patient to make full use of his voice within the shortest possible time (Seidner 2004; Schlömicher-Thier and Weikert 2003).

Unduly prolonging vocal rest as a matter of precaution risks unnecessary cancellations, involving potential sizable financial loss and even possible loss of future contracts for the singer. On the other hand, inadequate vocal rest can constitute a great danger. Finding the optimum variables in such cases requires considerable sensitivity and composure. The primary focus of this section is to report and discuss the general situation of singers and speakers in opera houses (from Regensburg and Salzburg). The data were obtained from two retrospective studies by the authors in the Austrian Voice Institute. These investigated the occupational situation of singers and actors in the theatres/festival house and music academies of Salzburg (Austria) and Regensburg (Germany). In this section we have used the masculine form of address to include both sexes but regard both female and male singers and voice users with the same degree of respect and appreciation.

8.6.2 Voice Problems

Voice problems can be divided into three groups: sudden, gradual and chronic. They can be further diversified by occupational strain and special exposure of the professional speaking and singing voice. Therefore, a vocal usage classification system was developed from numerous studies over the last 40 years (Koufman and Isaacson 1991; Schlömicher-Thier and Weikert 2003). See Sect. 5.1 for details on the vocal usage classification system by Koufman and Isaacson (1991), describing the following groups:

- Level I refers to an 'elite vocal performer' such as singers and actors.
- Level II describes a 'professional voice user' such as pedagogists, lecturers and clergy.
- Level III patients are 'nonvocal professionals' such as lawyers and doctors.
- Level IV users are 'nonvocal non-professionals' without any need for professional voice use.

Vocal problems hinder professional training or have consequences in the leisure time activity of choir singing; absence from choir rehearsals and choir performances results in personal distress. It does not, however, result in any financial loss.

This section of cancellation policy will focus on the professional voice user in Level I.

The male and female singers seen in our ENT vocal medical practice were examined in the following ways:

1. Phoniatric and performer's history in psychosocial context
2. ENT status
3. Videostroboscopy
4. Voice range profile (phonetogram)

During the examinations 1–4, a comprehensive auditory and kinaesthetic assessment of the artist's speaking and singing voice was undertaken (Richter 2013; Sataloff 2005; Wendler et al. 2005; Rubin et al. 2006; Schneider-Stickler and Bigenzahn 2013).

8.6.3   Evaluation of Professional Singers and Speakers

In an examination period extending from 1996 to 2001, we evaluated 512 singers and speakers of both genders according to the vocal usage classi-

fication system by Koufman and Isaacson (1991). Figure 8.5 represents Level I elite vocal performers, and Level II represents semi-professional voice users, i.e. singing and acting students (Level I, see yellow bar; Level II, see blue bar).

The data were split into six categories of complaints: acute, chronic, functional, psychogenic, reflux and organic. This terminology follows Sect. 4.2 by using terms which, while they may not coincide with other modern usages of the respective vocabulary, reflect the terminology used for malregulative dysphonia. It should further be noted that for reasons of data availability, in this evaluation (see Fig. 8.5), 'psychogenic dysphonia' denotes an independent entity on the same level as, and not constituting, a subgroup of regulatory dysphonia.

8.6.4   Interpretation

The diagnoses were evaluated according to the classification system by Koufman and Isaacson (1991). In these comparisons, the singers and speakers are listed without distinguishing by gender. The statistical evaluation sought to address whether there is a difference in vocal fold dysfunction complaints between the four levels of the vocal usage classification system.

The final evaluation of all the subjects can be summarised in the following manner:

- No psychogenic and functional voice disorders among the professional singers and actors of Level I.
- Prevalence of acute illnesses in professional sopranos.
- Prevalence of reflux and asthma complaints in professional singers.
- Higher occurrence of asthmatic complaints in high voices; consistent check-ups are advisable, and, when in doubt, should include the 'provocation test'.
- Prevalence of psychogenic and hyperfunctional voice disorders in the female voice.
- Clear connection between menstruation and singing strain, being the cause of the vocal fold border oedema in women (Fussi 2010; Sataloff 2005).

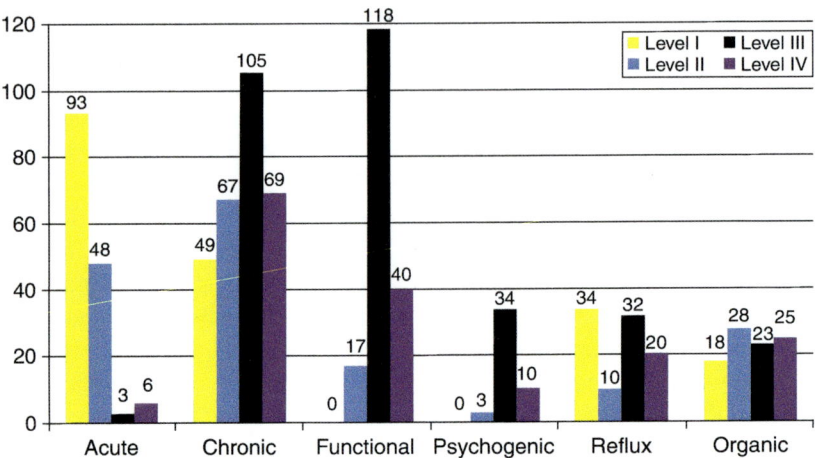

Fig. 8.5 Distribution of vocal problems among voice users without distinguishing by gender: comparison of numbers (ordinate) between L I and IV within six categories of complaint (abscissa) (*multiple and overlapping indications possible*). Voice users: professional level = L I (*yellow*) and II (*blue*), semi-professional L III (*black*) and non-professional L IV (*violet*). The numbers above the bars indicate the number of cases with the respective characteristics. Each group of bars refers to a diagnosis. Evaluation of 512 female and male singers during 1996–2001 (Schlömicher-Thier and Weikert 2003); multiple indications, number of diagnoses = 852

In conclusion, it can be stated that elite performers do not have problems in the categories 'functional' or 'psychogenic', thanks to their competence developed by consistent professional voice training. They may, however, suffer from other types of occasionally severe complaints, especially of acute problems such as laryngitis caused by the common cold, vocal fold bleeding and oedema caused by allergic rhinitis or by premenstrual voice syndrome and phonation thickenings caused by overuse of the voice. These can have serious consequences, even including the cancellation of the performance.

8.6.5 Cancellation Policy: What Should It Achieve?

Good cancellation policy should ensure that the audience, the artist/singer and the directorship enjoy a successful performance. The vocal specialist serves as a mediator between the singer and the directorship of the opera house or festival. In a circumspect approach, he needs both sides, the artist and the directorship, to trust him, in order to apply his medical exper-

tise and protect the singer's well-being. Only if the vocal specialist and the directorship collaborate with the singer's well-being in mind will it be possible to achieve an individualised, tailored solution suitable for the stage as a workplace and, finally, to satisfy the audience optimally.

Case Study 8.1

During a rehearsal, a 47-year-old mezzo-soprano suddenly lost her voice and sought consultation. She was cast in two roles during the summer festival, one in a Mozart opera and the other in a modern opera (Le Grand Macabre) by Ligeti. Rehearsals were just starting for the premieres 3 weeks later. She had been taking about 1000 mg of aspirin daily for repeated migraine attacks. A video-stroboscopic examination showed a vocal fold haematoma with a polypoid swelling on the left side (Fig. 8.6). The singer agreed that her manager should be informed. The therapy consisted of prednisolone in decreasing doses, Bromelain POS and inhalations. After a vocal rest of 10 days, the haematoma disappeared, but the polyp was still visible on the left side. The question was then whether

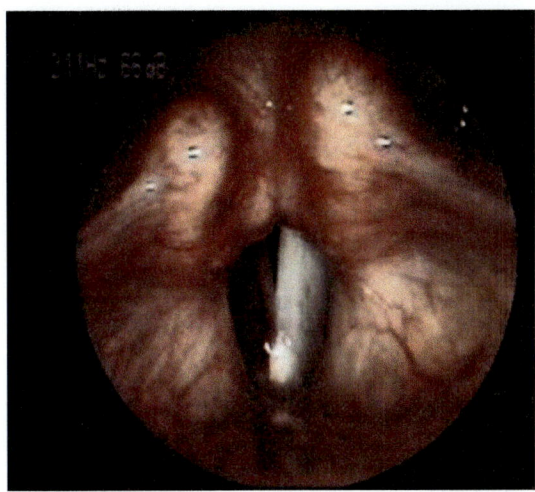

Fig. 8.6 Acute haematoma right vocal fold, accompanied by slight reflux signs of laryngeal mucosa (professional mezzo-soprano): cancellation

the singer would have to cancel her appearances in both operas or whether she could still sing the Ligeti. It was recommended that the patient should try some cautious warm-up exercises over a few hours and then an aria from the Ligeti opera. That afternoon, she sang the Ligeti aria, which required nothing above the middle register. She managed it beautifully. It was decided by the vocal specialist that she should sing the Ligeti role, but not the Mozart, which had a much higher tessitura. Thus, at least half the fee was saved.

Cancellation means that the affected artist does not perform on a particular day/evening or perhaps even on subsequent days. The artist needs an official confirmation of work disability for both the employer and the insurance company. The theatre management must prove that the financial damage was caused as a side effect by the cancellation of performances in each individual case.

Often a cancellation is the result of anxiety and uncertainty. If decisions are made in haste and without proper vocal medical assessment, considerable financial loss can result for both the opera house and the artist. This is the reality in many opera houses in the world because the staff and management do not have the courage to

explore other options of changing or maintaining a performance. Often the reason is simply that there is no vocal specialist and no phoniatrician in the opera house. The aim of this section is to show a useful arrangement for cancellation, with the goal of not burning out the artist.

A cancellation policy needs the mutual appreciation of artists and theatre management by using vocal medical procedures (Schlömicher-Thier and Weikert 2015).

8.6.6   Absolute Indications for Cancellation

These include:

- Acute infection or inflammation of the upper airways with strong harshness and the situation that no singing voice production is possible
- Infection with a high fever
- Acute vocal fold irritation with haemorrhage (Fig. 8.6)
- Acute inflammation of the larynx and the trachea that indicates acute laryngo-tracheitis with coughing
- Strong coughing due to acute bronchial asthma
- Reflux irritation of the lower hypopharynx and larynx with vomiting and accompanying gastroenteritis

Furthermore, there are indications without direct laryngeal-phoniatric causes that have a negative impact on voicing and voice control, forcing the artist/singer to cancel the performance. These include:

- Acute intravertebral disc prolapse with pain and moving problems such as knee or hip pain because of a sloping stage (Fig. 8.7).
- Acute gynaecological illness with haemorrhage, problems of pregnancy and urogenital inflammations, such as adnexitis with pain, fever and strong restriction of movement. These patients need bed rest.

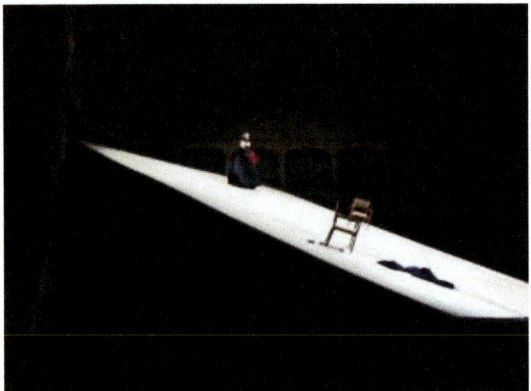

Fig. 8.7 Sloping stage in the opera

8.6.7 Relative Indications of a Possible Cancellation, Perhaps with Alteration of Performance

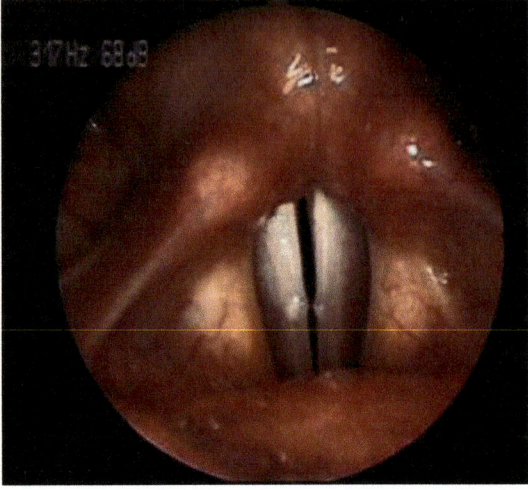

Fig. 8.8 Prenodal condition (professional soprano)

These include:

- Slight irritations after recovery time of 1 week
- Successful anti-allergic treatment, i.e. decrease of oedema of the vocal folds
- Tonsillitis and pharyngitis without irritation of the vocal folds, by successful treatment with antibiotics
- Subacute reflux laryngitis LPR: laryngopharyngeal reflux can trigger a severe laryngitis and should be treated by proton-pump inhibitors and dietary restrictions
- Prenodal condition (a tendency to thickening of the vocal folds) of female singers, e.g. at the time of premenstruation, when there is the beginning of acute vocal fold oedema, causing glissando to be restricted (Fig. 8.8)

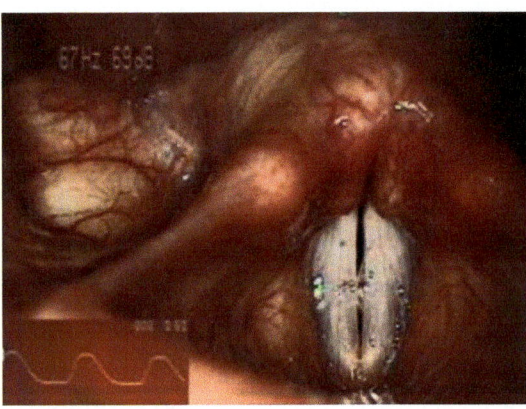

Fig. 8.9 Marginal oedema on the left side (professional soprano)

Case Study 8.2
A professional soprano, with a marginal oedema on the left vocal fold (Fig. 8.9), could get through the concert. The messa di voce (a singing technique using crescendo and decrescendo—louder and quieter—singing of a tone) was possible, but the glissando (smooth change in pitch over the individual's pitch range) was restricted. Nonetheless, her voice functioned reliably during the performance time of 4 weeks. After the production, she was treated by subsequent voice rest, medication and MLS—phonosurgery was scheduled.

What are the criteria for the final decision of relative to absolute indication of a cancellation?

Absolute indication causes the definite cancellation of performance as a rule. Relative indication means that additional time must pass before a final decision, typically 2–3 days of vocal rest. Changes to the rehearsal schedule and the modalities of the performance can and should be considered, even at an earlier stage.

8.6.8   Responsibility of Vocal and Performing Arts Medicine in the Opera and Stage

The case studies above reinforce the important function of the voice specialist. It is the specialist's primary concern to protect his patients as well as retain their trust. He must also act as a mediator between singers and management of the opera house or festival, striving to gain the confidence of both sides. Thus, he has to make as precise an estimate as possible of the patient's condition and the amount of vocal rest needed before the next performance. Overprotective 'safety advice' at every incipient infection ('Better stay at home for a week, and then we'll see how you're doing') only causes both sides to lose out: the singer loses his fee and the festival has to pay for a replacement. Only if both sides—doctor and management—collaborate in the best interests of the indisposed singer is it possible to rearrange rehearsal schedules. One possibility is for a 'standby' to sing from the orchestra pit while the indisposed singer acts out the complicated movements on stage. It is also important for the doctor to inform the artistic director as soon as possible—even if it is midnight—that a standby may be required. The burden of responsibility no longer rests with the singers, and the management gains time. In such cases, the physician in attendance assumes a high degree of responsibility: it is the specialist's duty to protect the singer affected by the disorder from additional harm, which might endanger the singer's further career (Seidner 2004; Flach 1992). He must also devise an effective concept of treatment that will enable the patient to make full use of his voice again within the shortest possible time. Any unduly prolonged precautionary vocal rest results in unnecessary cancellations, involving the risk of financial loss for the singer and endangering further contracts.

The motto here is 'Save the singer's fee, but avoid health risks'.

8.7   Initiation of Physiotherapy/ Osteopathy

Sławomir Marszałek

8.7.1   Introduction

People suffering from voice disorders are also very often affected by musculoskeletal disturbances, especially those of the muscular-fascial-ligamentous system. Therefore, to address dysphonia-related disorders and dysfunctions in the region of the musculoskeletal system effectively, a particular stress should be placed on the role of the physiotherapist and osteopath in a specialised team delivering diagnosis and therapy of vocal disorders.

When treating voice disorders, special emphasis is placed on relieving musculoskeletal tension, which particularly occurs with hyperfunctional dysphonia. Excessive extrinsic laryngeal musculature causes a pathological elevation of the larynx by shifting it upwards towards the hyoid bone. This changes phonation within the vocal tract, especially the length, tension and flexibility of the vocal folds. The tension disturbs phonatory vibration adversely, affecting the quality and capacity of voice (Marszałek et al. 2012; Van Houtte et al. 2011). For this reason a local and global pathology needs to be assessed in the cervical soft tissue, particular joints of the cervical spine and the larynx, so that a customised therapy may be applied aimed mainly to relieve musculoskeletal tension.

It needs to be underlined that a physiotherapist/osteopath should be trained in the aetiopathogenesis and management of occupational voice disorders and cooperate closely with other specialists in the voice disorder therapy team. Physiotherapeutic treatment is more general, based mainly on local and global exercises and on motor learning. Osteopathic treatment is based on precise palpatory skills and on precise manual treatment.

8.7.2 Physiotherapeutic and Osteopathic Diagnosis in Patients with Voice Disorders

8.7.2.1 Visual Examination and the Assessment of the Influence of Postural Disorders on Voice Disorders

The physiotherapist's or osteopath's competence comprises the therapy of the particular musculoskeletal system dysfunctions that have a significant impact on the occurrence and persistence of the problems with proper phonation. These patients are often observed to have postural disorders and an excessive muscle tension, which predisposes to vocal disorders, especially to hyperfunctional dysphonias. Chin protrusion increases the vocal effort and the tension of the muscles around the larynx during phonation. If this posture is not corrected, the perilaryngeal muscles become chronically overloaded during phonation and the laryngeal muscle tone elevated. An improperly positioned head, disturbed posture, body weight shifted forwards or backwards, excessive lordosis and kyphosis will all be compensated for by an excessive tension at the level of the nape and laryngeal region. The symmetry of the larynx position is similarly affected by curvature of the spine (scoliosis). Asymmetrical, rotational positioning of the cervical spine is transferred, particularly by particular layers of the cervical fascia and the upper, middle and lower pharyngeal constrictor muscles (Angsuwarangsee and Morrison 2002; Kooijman et al. 2005; Marszałek et al. 2012).

When assessing the body posture and particular asymmetries, special attention should be drawn to the ergonomics of the work of the patient with vocal disorders. Of great importance is the assessment of particular routinely made movements. This applies especially to the ways of working with a computer, playing a musical instrument, sitting at work or while driving (Marszałek et al. 2010). In conclusion, in visual assessment of a patient with voice disorders, special attention should be drawn to the position of the head and cervical spine. Particular parts of the examination are shown in Table 8.2.

Table 8.2 Visual assessment and evaluation of patients with voice disorders

View	Subject of evaluation
Front view	Symmetry of position of the head and the neck in relation to the arms and trunk
	Lifting and positioning of arms
	Possibility of asymmetry of the tonus of neck muscles and sternocleidomastoideus muscles
	Type of breathing, position of the chest
	Asymmetry of mandible position and masseter and face muscle tension
	Asymmetry in hyoid bone and larynx placing
	Range of movements in cervical spine and mandible area
Side view	Displacement gravity centre of the body forwards or backwards
	Displacement head forward in relation to the line of arms (head in protraction/retraction)
	Degree of shifting shoulder forwards in relation to the chest
	The curve of thoracic and cervical spine
	Tension of soft tissues in cervical-thoracic spine area

8.7.2.2 The Assessment of Range of Motion in the Cervical Spine and Arms Area

When assessing the muscular system of a patient suffering from voice disorders, it is important to check the scope of his or her mobility in the cervical segment of the spine. If the extent of mobility of a region being examined is below normal, the myofascial tension may be considered to be increased. The following are deemed as normal:

- In the rotation of the head, the chin should reach the line linking both shoulders (90°).
- When bent sideways, the neck should move 45° in each direction.
- When bent forwards, the chin should touch the manubrium (without opening of the mouth).
- When bent backwards, the retraction of the head should be such as to cause the forehead to form a horizontal plane (Marszałek et al. 2010).

8.7.2.3 The Assessment of Mobility in Mandible, Temporomandibular Joint and Hyoid Bone

The activity of the larynx is also adversely affected by muscular tension disorders in the temporomandibular joint region, such as malocclusion, pain in the temporomandibular joint or earlier surgery of the mandible. The above issues may induce the asymmetry of mandible position and consequent asymmetry of the muscles linking the mandible and the larynx. Asymmetrical tension and position of the hyoid bone and larynx may disturb the activity of the muscles that are directly associated with phonation. One should assess the extent of the opening of the jaw, which should be around 36–44 mm, or such as to enable three of the patient's fingers (index, middle finger, ring finger) to be placed vertically into the mouth (Marszałek et al. 2010; Lewit 2009).

8.7.2.4 Direct Manual Examination of the Larynx Area

Asymmetrical tension and position of the hyoid bone and larynx may lead to a disturbance in the activity of the muscles directly associated with phonation. The anatomical structures with a direct or indirect impact on the function and position of the larynx should be subject to palpable assessment.

When performing a direct manual examination, attention is paid to mobility disorders of particular anatomical structures, the presence of increased soft tissue tension and possible soft tissue tenderness.

Increased tension of the muscles of mastication, muscles of the mouth floor and the suprahyoid muscles contribute significantly to an excessive elevation of the larynx. In this case, the patient is examined for increased unilateral or bilateral tension and pain in the stylohyoid, mylohyoid, geniohyoid, digastric and hyoglossus muscles. It is also important to assess the position of the hyoid bone in relation to the mandible and the space between the hyoid bone and the thyroid cartilage of the larynx.

Of high significance is also the symmetry of the position of the larynx and hyoid bone in relation to each other, to the cervical spine and to the mandible. When performing a dynamic pinch grip with the thumb and index, the quality of mobility (loss or facilitation thereof) needs to be assessed for a lateral movement of the hyoid bone and the larynx in relation to the mandible and

cervical spine. A double grip—gripping the thyroid cartilage with one hand and the hyoid bone with the other—is used to assess the symmetry of lateral mobility in opposite directions. Asymmetrical mobility indicates an improper tension of the soft tissue being examined.

A further stage of the examination of anatomical structures directly associated with the larynx involves the assessment of the space between the thyroid cartilage and the cricoid cartilage. A therapist should check if the cartilages are positioned symmetrically towards each other. The space should be palpable without phonation. A dynamic, symmetrically narrowing movement should be palpable during phonation. Increased tension of the thyrocricoid muscle, as well as sternothyroid and sternohyoid muscles, makes that movement more difficult, thus affecting the quality of phonation.

When conducting a manual manipulation in the region of the larynx, particular care should be taken to avoid unintended pressure on the carotid artery and carotid bulb. It has to be remembered that this may lead to a change of blood pressure and pulse, especially with elderly patients. There is also a risk of damaging atherosclerotic plaques in the carotid artery—in this case deep manual treatment is contraindicated.

The examination and therapy related directly to the larynx and muscles in the front part of the neck should be followed by osteopathic manipulation of the cervical spine. It has to function properly to enable adequate activity and positioning of the larynx. The osteopathic examination should involve a qualitative evaluation of a global mobility of the cervical segment of the spine and the mobility of particular facet joints. If any dysfunctions are found in joints or soft tissue at a given level, the existing disorder should be normalised (Marszałek et al. 2010, 2012; Ross 1999; Rubin et al. 2000).

8.7.2.5 The Role of the Myofascial System in Voice Disorders

Interaction of cervical soft tissues is an important part of voice disorder therapy. Mobility disorders and nonphysiological increases in the tension of those structures lead to disturbances in proper functioning and positioning of the larynx. Knowledge of the functional connections and normalisation of possible mobility disorders between particular muscles, fascial layers and vertebral joints are of great significance in the therapy of patients with voice disorders.

The fascial system, understood as a weakly structured web of connective tissue, is an important part of the musculoskeletal system. It is omnipresent in the human body encompassing all systems and organs. Owing to their continuous structure, particular fascial layers allow the transfer of forces and tensions across the body.

Persistent overload, scars, tissue damage and bone fractures cause particular layers of the fascia and soft tissue to be immobilised. The resultant tissue adhesions disturb the distribution of forces and tensions in the musculofascial-ligamentous system. This, in turn, alters the range and quality of movements affected by other restrictions. They may also lead to postural changes that are relevant to dysphonia and that produce excessive muscle tension during restricted movements and phonation. To achieve a desired therapeutic outcome in dysphonia therapy, the physiotherapist or osteopath should assess the whole musculoskeletal system in the context of tissue tension transfer disorders and restrictions. The therapy of identified functional disorders of tissue mobility will enable the intensification of the treatment process. The myofascial-skeletal and visceral system should in particular be treated by a physiotherapist or osteopath as a cohesive whole that induces laryngeal functional disorders.

Owing to fascial-ligamentous interconnections within the thorax, a dynamic active contraction of the diaphragm has an impact on the cervical segment of the spine. The diaphragm is linked to the pericardium and the pleural cavity, and these are connected with, among others, the endothoracic fascia, which extends into a set of particular layers of cervical fascias that have a direct impact on the larynx. Owing to the tissue connectivity, the relaxation and activation of the respiratory diaphragm will enable the tension within the superior thoracic aperture, and consequently in the laryngeal region, to be relieved.

Interaction of cervical soft tissues is also an important part of voice disorder therapy. Mobility disorders and nonphysiological increases in the tension of those structures lead to disturbances in proper functioning and positioning of the larynx. Knowledge of the functional connections and mitigation of possible mobility disorders between particular muscles, fascial layers and vertebral joints is of great significance in the therapy of patients with voice disorders (Marszałek et al. 2010; Ross 1999; Stecco 2015).

8.7.3 Physiotherapeutic and Osteopathic Therapy of the Vocal Organ

Physical therapy involves manual therapy of the muscles and fascial structures of the neck and nape and is complementary to phoniatric treatment and voice therapy. Correct measures taken by a properly trained physiotherapist/osteopath will allow the normalisation of function of the cervical spine, muscles of the trunk, neck and larynx, thus improving the quality of voice in patients affected with vocal disorders, especially those with hyperfunctional dysphonia.

8.7.3.1 Global Myofascial Techniques in the Neck, Head and Torso Area

Before the application of manual techniques related directly to the larynx, the activities of soft tissues with indirect influence on the phonatory function need to be normalised. The improvement involves in particular the use of global manual myofascial techniques in the region of the neck and trunk:

- The application of normalisation techniques, usually those releasing the tension of the muscles responsible for mobility restriction in the above region
- The application of normalisation techniques, usually those releasing the tension of the muscles of mastication
- The application of normalisation techniques, usually those releasing the tension of the

muscles responsible for improper posture that is conducive to dysphonia (particularly hyperfunctional)

- Teaching a proper body posture in a standing and sitting position
- Education in the use of the diaphragmatic respiratory pathway and manual myofascial release of soft tissue within the abdominal fascial layers and the extrathoracic fascia (Chaitow 2010; Manheim 2009; Marszałek et al. 2010, 2012; Ross 1999)

8.7.3.2 Manual Myofascial Techniques Directly Related to the Larynx and Its Area

People with vocal disorders are often affected by tissue disorders in the region of the head, neck and shoulders. Therefore, these should be normalised by a gentle relaxation and stretching of soft tissue which is often excessively tense. The above described dysfunctions of tissues directly associated with the larynx should be normalised by using targeted techniques:

- Manual myofascial release of particular layers of the cervical fascias
- Myofascial release of the soft tissue in the region of the hyoid bone
- Normalisation of the thyrocricoid muscle and mobilisation of the space between the thyroid and cricoid cartilages
- Normalisation of the activity and mobility of cervical segment of the spine and particular facet joints (Marszałek et al. 2010, 2012; Ross 1999; Rubin et al. 2000)
- This technique decreases the tension of the internal muscles of the larynx. The therapist holds with one thumb the thyroid cartilage from below and with the other thumb the cricoid cartilage from above, and then he applies delicate pressure and stretching
- This technique stimulates the thyrohyoid muscle and because of that improves the tone. The osteopath holds with the index finger and the thumb of one hand the thyroid cartilage and with the other index finger and thumb grasps the hyoid bone. One hand stabilises the hyoid

bone, and the other moves the thyroid cartilage aside, up and down

- The therapist grasps the hyoid bone, moves it downwards and asks the patient to swallow saliva. It is a dynamic stretching of this area.

8.7.3.3 Education Regarding the Change (Normalisation) in Body Posture, Way of Breathing and Individual Coping with Stress

Patients with dysphonia should be taught to adopt models of keeping a posture with emphasis placed on the habit of maintaining a correct position of the head and ability to control a proper position of the body's centre of gravity, set up the head in the sagittal plane and control the route of deviation. The aetio-pathogenesis of these conditions often being complex and the rehabilitation of voice disorders should include elements of psychotherapy and physiotherapy, depending on the patient's individual needs. Such an interdisciplinary approach is even more important considering that the stress often causes increased tension of the nape muscle that is transferred to the extrinsic and intrinsic laryngeal and pharyngeal muscles (Kooijman et al. 2005; Marszałek et al. 2010, 2012; Ross 1999).

8.7.3.4 Self-Therapy in Patient's Active Participation in Rehabilitation

An individual assessment allows the prescription of a customised set of exercises that patients can perform on their own. This approach will permit the mitigation of the adverse impacts of the musculoskeletal overload, improper body posture and stress on voice disorders.

Patients should learn how to release and stretch their laryngeal muscles on their own. A proper education for the patient ensures that the therapy will be sustained and effective. It is important to make patients appreciate the role of the musculoskeletal system in the development of laryngeal activity disorders. Patients should be aware of the dependence of the laryngeal activity on body posture, myofascial tension and disorders of particular muscle groups. This will encourage them to develop an active and informed involvement in the therapeutic process (Marszałek et al. 2010; Ross 1999).

- The patient places the thumbs at the level of the angle of the mandible and moves them slowly to the chin
- With a flat hand, the patient presses the tender point in the trapezius muscle of the contralateral side away from the head, at the same time bending and straightening the head several times to the other side
- Active relaxation of the sternocleidomastoid muscle and cervical fascia. The patient holds the contralateral muscle between the thumb and index finger, at the same time rotating the head several times in the direction of the fixing arm
- The patient moves the head backwards and holds it for 3 s in a retraction position

8.7.4 Basic Tenets of Therapy for People with Voice Disorders Resulting from Oncological Treatment

Following cancer treatment, the musculoskeletal system is heavily affected by postsurgical or postradiation scars, tissue adhesions and radiotherapy-related tissue fibrosis. These can directly or indirectly affect the phonatory function. This usually occurs following a cancer treatment in the head and neck region involving surgery with adjuvant radiotherapy or primary radiotherapy and particularly so if the treatment is directly related to the larynx (total or partial removal of the larynx) or to the cervical lymph system, maxillary-ethmoidal massive region, mouth or salivary glands. Physiotherapy should take into account the resulting structural disorders and related dysfunctions, which tend to reduce the phonatory capabilities of the larynx and muscles responsible for phonation and articulation. Respiratory disorders, increased muscular tension and limited physical performance are often observed after a long-lasting cancer therapy associated with strong pain and restricted physical activity. These factors are significant contrib-

utors to the development of voice disorders. Physiotherapy in such cases is aimed at restoring the lost mobility and activity of particular anatomical structures directly associated with phonation and articulation. Such therapy is designed to improve the disturbed mobility and fitness of the tongue muscles, mouth floor (oral cancer), facial muscles (cancers of the parotid gland) and muscles of mastication responsible for trismus (cancers of the maxillary-ethmoidal massive). In the case of patients who have had their larynx entirely removed and who do not use any voice prosthesis, a physiotherapist should reduce the increased soft tissue tension in the region of the surgical field and the nape. This will allow the superior pharyngeal constrictor muscle and inferior constrictor muscle of pharynx to be released while facilitating the aspiration of air into the oesophagus and production of oesophageal speech.

Physiotherapy in cancer patients with voice disorders should be conducted in parallel with voice therapy.

8.8 Drug Treatment in Dysphonia: Medications and Voice

Sevtap Akbulut and Haldun Oguz

8.8.1 Drug Treatment in Dysphonia

8.8.1.1 Antihistamines

Most antihistamines, such as diphenhydramine, have anticholinergic effects that lead to dryness of the upper respiratory tract (URT) (Abaza et al. 2007; Lawrence 1987; Sataloff et al. 2005b; Thompson 1995). This results in decreased vocal fold lubrication, increased throat clearing and coughing (Alessi and Crummey 2006). Antihistamines also have a sedative effect, the severity of which varies widely with different drugs and also from person to person, which decreases the awareness of the individual about his or her own voice. Newer antihistamines such as fexofenadine, loratadine and desloratadine cause less drowsiness and often less dryness as well, but can still be bothersome (Thompson 1995; Wilken et al. 2003).

Antihistamines are found in many common and over-the-counter medications. Some sleep aids, antitussive drugs and medications recommended for dizziness and motion sickness contain antihistamines (Abaza et al. 2007; Lawrence 1987; Sataloff et al. 2005b).

8.8.1.2 Decongestants

Decongestants are effective for inhibiting nasal congestion and reducing the amount of secretions produced by shrinking mucous membranes (Thompson 1995). They are usually found in medications used for cough and for URT infections. They are often combined with antihistamines, which leads to further reduction and thickening of secretions; however, this balances the sedative effects of antihistamines. Decongestants may have mild stimulator effects on the central nervous system that may result in insomnia, tachycardia and restlessness (Abaza et al. 2007). Decongestants are not recommended for children below 2 years of age.

8.8.1.3 Mucolytic Agents

Normal mucosal secretions are extremely important for effective vocal fold vibration. Thickening of secretions may result from medications, such as antihistamines or decongestants, or by generalised dehydration. The viscosity of respiratory secretions is directly related to available body water, and there are no medications that can be a good substitute for adequate hydration. However, mucolytics may help to counteract the drying effects of antihistamines and decongestants. They can be used for treatment of thick secretions, frequent throat clearing or postnasal dripping (Abaza et al. 2007; Alessi and Crummey 2006; Sataloff et al. 2005b). Guaifenesin and acetylcysteine are the most commonly used mucolytic agents that thin mucosal secretions and act as expectorants (Oğuz and Akbulut 2013).

8.8.1.4 Antibiotics

Acute laryngitis is defined as an inflammation of the larynx lasting less than 3 weeks (Dworkin 2008; Reveiz et al. 2007). Acute URT infections, environmental factors, decreased immunological resistance and physical or psychological stress may be predisposing factors. Professional voice users tend to have laryngitis with excessive voice use (Sataloff 1981).

Acute laryngitis is generally viral in origin, most commonly with *rhinovirus, influenza virus, adenovirus* and *parainfluenza virus*. It is a self-limiting infection, symptoms of which usually resolve within 5–10 days. It has been shown that antibiotics have no effect on most cases of laryngitis (Reveiz et al. 2007; Schalen et al. 1985; Schiff 1977).

When laryngitis originates from a bacterial infection, *Streptococcus pneumoniae, Haemophilus influenzae, Moraxella catarrhalis* and *Staphylococcus aureus* are the most commonly encountered species. Amoxicillin/clavulanate, high-dose amoxicillin, cefuroxime, cefdinir, moxifloxacin, gatifloxacin, levofloxacin and telithromycin are all effective treatments (Alessi and Crummey 2006; Hol et al. 1996; Schalen et al. 1985).

8.8.1.5 Corticosteroids

Corticosteroids are potent anti-inflammatory agents that are quite helpful in acute laryngitis treatment (Sataloff 1981; Thompson 1995). There is no standard dosage and protocol of steroids for treating laryngeal oedema. Some laryngologists recommend higher doses for short periods (e.g. methylprednisolone 60 mg orally or dexamethasone 10 mg intramuscularly), while some others use it in low doses (e.g. methylprednisolone 10 mg orally) (Sataloff et al. 2005b).

Steroids must be prescribed with extreme caution. The presence of vocal fold haemorrhage and ulceration of the vocal fold mucosa should definitely be ruled out before steroid treatment (Alessi and Crummey 2006). Steroids have significant adverse effects that may occur in any patient, depending on the dosage used and the patient's metabolism and response to the medication. These include gastric irritation with a risk of ulceration and haemorrhage, insomnia, blurred vision, increased energy, increased appetite, irritability, fluid retention and mood change. They also elevate serum glucose, which requires extra caution with their use in diabetic patients (Sataloff et al. 2005b).

As corticosteroids are extremely effective in treating laryngeal inflammation, there is a tendency to abuse/overuse them, especially among singers (Sataloff et al. 2005b). *Nasal corticosteroid sprays* used for rhinitis do not seem to harm the voice, as they are not absorbed systemically and show their effect topically on the nasal mucosa. However, they may lead to mucosal drying because of their propellant ingredients (Sataloff et al. 2005b). *Inhaled corticosteroids* may cause vocal symptoms such as dysphonia, hoarseness, cough and increased throat clearing, secondary to contact irritation of the larynx (Lavy et al. 2000; Stead and Cooke 1989; Watkin and Ewanowski 1985). Prolonged use of inhaled corticosteroids can cause atrophy of the vocalis muscle and lead to Candida laryngitis (Toogood et al. 1980; Watkin and Ewanowski 1985).

8.8.1.6 Analgesics and Anti-inflammatory Agents

Acetylsalicylic acid and other nonsteroidal anti-inflammatory drugs (NSAID) may interfere with the clotting mechanism; aspirin especially leads to platelet dysfunction. The use of NSAID in professional voice users should be discouraged, as it increases the risk of vocal fold haemorrhage (Sataloff et al. 2005b; Thompson 1995). Acetaminophen may be recommended for mild to moderate pain in professional voice users.

Selective COX-2 inhibitors, a new class of NSAID, do not cause the bleeding dyscrasias seen with traditional anti-inflammatory drugs (Sataloff et al. 2005b; Verrico et al. 2003).

Narcotic analgesics and sedatives impair intellectual function and change the laryngeal sensation; they may worsen performance of singers. They may additionally cause vocal fold injury through unconscious voice abuse (Sataloff et al. 2005b).

Pain resulting from pharyngitis or laryngitis has an important protective function. Masking the pain may push the professional voice user to significant vocal damage (Lawrence 1987; Thompson 1995). Therefore, topical anaesthetics

such as benzocaine, lidocaine and analgesic throat lozenges are potentially dangerous for singers. If a singer requires analgesics taken orally or topically for relieving laryngeal discomfort, this may be a sufficient reason to postpone a performance (Sataloff et al. 2005b).

8.8.1.7 Hormones

Hormones have significant adverse effects on voice. Androgenic agents are used for treatment of endometriosis and dysmenorrhoea and for postmenopausal sexual dysfunction. They may also be included in chemotherapy regimens for breast cancer (Need et al. 1993; Pattie et al. 1998; Petit et al. 1971). The major effects of androgens on voice include lowering the fundamental frequency, vocal instability with pitch breaks and loss of high frequencies (Damste 1968; Pattie et al. 1998). These voice changes may be permanent, depending on the duration and the dosage of treatment (Boothroyd and Lepre 1990; Schlondorff 1966). Anabolic steroids that are used for treatment of osteoporosis or abused in female athletes may cause irreversible lowering of fundamental frequency (Baker 1999; Gerritsma et al. 1994; Rolf and Nieschlag 1998).

During the premenstrual period, women may exhibit vocal fatigue, decreased range and a loss of power as a result of oedema of the vocal cords (Abitbol et al. 1999). Professional voice users are particularly affected. Low-dose oral contraceptives are effective in reducing this pitch variability. Oral contraceptives with relatively high progesterone content can lead to androgen-like changes in the voice. However, voice side effects are seen in only about 5% of patients with modern low-dose oral contraceptives, and these changes are generally temporary (Amir et al. 2003; Sataloff et al. 2005b).

Oestrogen replacement therapy is effective in preventing the adverse changes in postmenopausal voice, which include lowered vocal intensity, vocal fatigue, decreased range with loss of the high tones and a loss of vocal quality (Abitbol et al. 1999). A conjugated oestrogen preparation is prescribed in combination with progesterone for hormone replacement in menopause (Sataloff et al. 2005b).

Oestrogens are sometimes used for treatment of prostatic carcinoma in men and can result in an increase of vocal pitch (Thompson 1995).

Endocrine dysfunction can lead to vocal changes, as in hypothyroidism and hypogonadism. Hypothyroidism results in a decrease in vocal efficiency because of accumulation of mucopolysaccharides in the vocal folds (Thompson 1995). Men with hypogonadism have a higher fundamental vocal frequency than normal. Hormone replacement therapy may help restore normal vocal function in all these patients (Petit et al. 1971; Sataloff et al. 2005b).

8.8.1.8 Medical Treatment in Neurological Conditions

Spasmodic Dysphonia This is an idiopathic focal dystonia of the larynx that affects the fluency of connected speech. The standard treatment of spasmodic dysphonia (SD) is intramuscular injections of botulinum toxin. The thyroarytenoid-lateral cricoarytenoid muscle complex is injected in adductor SD, while the posterior cricoarytenoid muscle is the target for abductor SD. Botulinum toxin causes a temporary paralysis of the injected muscle (Blumin and Berke 2007; Rosen and Simpson 2008a; Sulica 2004).

Parkinson's Disease This is a progressive degenerative neurological disorder in which basal ganglia are affected, creating decreased dopamine release. Breathy dysphonia, hypophonia and vocal tremor are common vocal abnormalities in Parkinson's disease with a soft, monotonic voice. For the treatment of Parkinson's disease, medications with anticholinergic properties, such as L-dopa, dopamine receptor antagonists and monoamine oxidase inhibitors, are used. The treatment of the voice component of Parkinson's disease is managed with an intensive rehabilitative voice therapy programme, Lee Silverman Voice Treatment (Blumin et al. 2004; Oğuz et al. 2006a; Ramig et al. 2001; Schulz 2002).

Essential Tremor This disease is of involuntary movement. The head, hands and vocal tract may be involved to varying degrees. Pharmacological treatment is the first-line treatment for essential tremor, but the medications used for managing it, such as primidone and propranolol, are not as effective on voice as they are on limb-based tremor. Botulinum toxin injections seem to be useful in alleviating vocal symptoms (Sullivan et al. 2003; Warrick et al. 2000).

Post-viral Vagal Neuropathy This neuropathy is noted with chronic cough with or without laryngospasm. It is thought to be related to altered laryngeal sensitivity such as in post-viral neuralgias. Gabapentin, an anticonvulsive agent, seems to be effective in treatment of this situation, as it decreases neural sensitivity (Amin and Koufman 2001; Lee and Woo 2005).

8.8.1.9 Medical Treatment in Laryngopharyngeal Reflux

Laryngopharyngeal reflux (LPR) causes objective symptoms and signs in the larynx, particularly dysphonia (Oğuz et al. 2007). Different medications are used for medical management of LPR, including antacids, histamine receptor antagonists (H2 blockers) and gastric proton-pump inhibitors (PPIs). Antacids with aluminium, magnesium or calcium preparations may be helpful for neutralisation of gastric acid. Side effects as constipation, bloating and diarrhoea, although rare, may be seen. They may also have a drying effect on the laryngeal mucosa (Abaza et al. 2007; Lawrence 1987; Sataloff et al. 2005b).

Most commonly used H2 blockers include ranitidine, famotidine, cimetidine and nizatidine. They inhibit the secretion of gastric acid from parietal cells but have limited change on the basal rate of acid production. They occasionally cause drying effect on the larynx (Abaza et al. 2007; Lawrence 1987).

PPIs suppress gastric acid production in a potent and consistent manner. All the five available compounds—omeprazole, lansoprazole, pantoprazole, rabeprazole and esomeprazole—have a similar anti-secretory potency when taken in equipotent doses. Once- or twice-daily dosing is recommended for most patients. The drugs have a low incidence of side effects, which include diarrhoea, abdominal pain, nausea, dry mouth, muscle cramps, dizziness, fatigue, headache, fungal infections and elevation of liver enzymes.

A significant improvement in reflux control is reported clinically with the addition of H2 blockers, especially given at night, to twice-daily PPI treatment (Park et al. 2005). As the positive effect of treatment on dysphonia is objectively seen at 2 months, the treatment period should be at least 3 months (Belafsky et al. 2001; Oğuz et al. 2006b).

It should be kept in mind that lifestyle modifications should be included in all therapeutic approaches for reflux. The modifications include, but are not limited to, decreased intake of fat, citrus, tomato, caffeine, chocolate, sugar and alcohol, elevation of the head of the bed, cessation of smoking and eating meals at least 2–3 h before lying down or sleeping.

8.8.1.10 Complementary and Alternative Medical Treatment Modalities

Complementary and alternative medicine covers any practice that can be used for the prevention and treatment of diseases, such as acupuncture, massage therapy, biofeedback, homoeopathy, reflexology, hypnotherapy, neuromuscular therapy, herbal supplements, naturopathy and other modalities. Conventional medicine started approximately two centuries ago, while many alternative therapies have been present for thousands of years. However there is a lack of randomised, double-blind, placebo-controlled studies evaluating their efficacy. Although healthcare professionals are hesitant to recommend complementary and alternative medical treatment modalities, there has been enormous public interest in them. Physicians should thus be aware of the strengths and limitations of complementary and alternative medical treatment modalities (Eisenberg et al. 1998; Seidman 2006).

Many *herbal products* can be used for medical purposes. Some are safe, others are potentially harmful. The quality of the product may vary from one manufacturing company to another. Whether a product contains precisely what the manufacturer claims is always a concern, as the manufacturers of herbal products are not regulated sufficiently.

People use herbal products mistakenly, confusing 'natural' with safe and effective. They may have potential side effects and may interfere with common medications. Some such common herbs are summarised in Table 8.3 (based on Sataloff et al. 2005b; Seidman 2006).

8.8.1.11 Local Medical Applications in Voice Disorders

Water, saline or other physiologically balanced solutions can be applied through a humidifier or vaporiser. Individuals living or working in a very dry environment may especially benefit from this therapy. Such treatment helps warm and humidify the vocal folds and all the tracheobronchial trees and also relaxes the larynx during the application. It should be kept in mind, though, that oral hydration is the mainstay of treatment for dehydration. Five percent propylene glycol in physiologically balanced salt solution delivered by large particle mist is helpful for lubrication in cases of laryngitis sicca after long air flights (Sataloff et al. 2005b).

Mouthwash or gargles that contain alcohol or irritating chemicals should be avoided, or they should be used only for oral rinsing. Gargling with warm saltwater solution is relaxing for the larynx.

In case of acute laryngitis, the mixture below may be used for supporting treatment:

- Rp.
- Prednisolut ex amp. 50 mg
- Bepanthene ex amp. 2500 mg
- NaCl 2500 mg
- Aqua inj. ex amp. ad 100 g
- m. f. solutio
- (for inhalation aseptic preparation)

8.8.2 Side Effects of Medications on the Voice

Most of the antihypertensive agents have various degrees of parasympathomimetic action, which result in dryness of mucous membranes (Abaza et al. 2007; Lawrence 1987; Thompson 1995). They are often combined with diuretics that cause

Table 8.3 Examples for herbal products used for medication (Based on Sataloff et al. 2005b; Seidman 2006)

Herbal product	Uses	Side effects	Interactions
Echinacea	Treatment and prevention of upper respiratory tract infections	Stimulates immune system initially, may be immunosuppressive after 8 weeks Increases urination Mild allergic reactions	Immunosuppressant drugs (corticosteroids, methotrexate, imuran)
Ginseng	Improves cognitive function Lowers blood pressure Lowers blood glucose	Bleeding Hypotension Hypoglycaemia Insomnia	Antidiabetics Coumadin and other anticoagulants Caffeine Stimulants
Ginkgo biloba	Improves cognitive function Prevents dementia Treatment of dizziness and tinnitus	Bleeding Headache Gastrointestinal irritation	Anticoagulants SSRIs MAO inhibitors Thiazide diuretics
Garlic	Lowers blood lipids Antibacterial and antimycotic effects	Bleeding Gastrointestinal upset Foetid odour	Anticoagulants Hypoglycaemics
St John's wort	Antidepressant Decreases anxiety and seasonal affective disorder	Insomnia Anxiety Photosensitivity	Antidepressants MAO inhibitors
Camomile	Decreases anxiety	Dries the mucosa of the vocal tract	
Saw palmetto	Anti-inflammatory Increases urinary flow		Diuretics
Guarana	Stimulant Increases energy	Anxiety Arrythmias Tachycardia	Stimulants Caffeine

SSRIs Selective serotonin reuptake inhibitors, *MAO* monoamine oxidase

increased viscosity of secretions secondary to dehydration. Some new antihypertensives have minimal side effects for the voice. Ganglionic blocking agents and alpha-adrenergic antagonists do not have drying effects on the vocal cords. Angiotensin-converting enzyme inhibitors also do not have drying effects, but they sometimes induce a dry cough, which can lead to vocal trauma.

8.8.2.1 Beta Blockers

Blockers such as propranolol are also used to treat hypertension. As they are sympatholytic agents, they do not result in dryness of the upper respiratory tract secretion. Small doses of beta blockers have also been used to treat performance anxiety, but they can have adverse effects on a singer's ability to sing at their best. Phoniatricians generally agree that these drugs should not be used by singers (Gates et al. 1985; Sataloff et al. 2005b).

8.8.2.2 Diuretics

Diuretics are agents that eliminate excessive fluid of the body. They are used for some diseases in which the body is unable to excrete fluids at a rate needed to maintain its fluid and electrolyte balance. They are also used in the treatment of hypertension.

They are commonly used by women for fluid retention in the premenstrual period. Decreased oestrogen and progesterone levels in the premenstrual period lead to increased circulating antidiuretic hormone. This results in fluid retention in Reinke's space and other tissues (Abitbol et al. 1999). The fluid in Reinke's space is protein bound, so diuretics cannot remobilise this fluid. Instead, diuretics cause dehydration, decreased lubrication and increased viscosity of secretions. They should not be used for vocal symptoms related to the menses (Sataloff et al. 2005b).

8.8.2.3 Sedatives

Tranquilisers are usually prescribed for pain management or for sedative purposes. Benzodiazepines, including diazepam, alprazolam, lorazepam and others, are the main ones. Other common tranquilisers are chlorpromazine, thioridazine and haloperidol. They all can cause vocal fold dryness (Abaza et al. 2007; Lawrence 1987).

Singers may use these anxiolytic drugs for trying to deal with performance anxiety. Their use should be avoided for this purpose, as they induce dryness of vocal cords. Besides this, one should be aware that mild anxiety can even enhance performance (Alessi and Crummey 2006; Sataloff et al. 2005b).

8.8.2.4 Antidepressants

Tricyclic antidepressants are strongly anticholinergic drugs causing dryness of the upper respiratory tract mucosa and resulting in hoarseness (Lawrence 1987; Lyskowski and Dunner 1980). Selective serotonin reuptake inhibitors (SSRIs), such as fluoxetine, sertraline and paroxetine, are commonly prescribed antidepressants. Even though they have weak anticholinergic effects, they cause xerostomia and can have a dehydrating effect on the larynx. Monoamine oxidase inhibitors (MAOIs) are also used in treatment of depression. They do not have a significant drying effect on the vocal folds, but they have strong adverse interactions with many medications. They should be monitored closely by a physician (Abaza et al. 2007; Lawrence 1987; Thompson 1995). Antipsychotic drugs are used for treatment of schizophrenia and other psychotic disorders. These drugs are associated with a wide range of side effects, including dry mouth and a variety of movement disorders, some of which can be distressing and irreversible.

8.8.2.5 Caffeine and Cocaine

Caffeine is a stimulant of the central nervous system carrying sympathomimetic properties. It also has a mild diuretic effect. These two properties make caffeine a dehydrating agent leading to harmful effects on a singer's voice (Akhtar et al. 1999).

Cocaine is a stimulant frequently used by singers. It causes serious damage to the nasal mucosa and results in vasoconstriction; it decreases voice control by decreasing sensorium and leads to abusive vocal habits (Fishman et al. 1971).

8.8.2.6 Vitamin C

Vitamin C (ascorbic acid) is used to prevent colds or to shorten their duration. It has been shown to be useful in limiting the duration of the common cold (Van Straten and Josling 2002), but it has a drying effect when taken in large doses, related to its diuretic effect. In addition, in large doses it may aggravate laryngo-oesophageal reflux (Sataloff et al. 2005b).

8.8.2.7 Antineoplastic Agents

Chemotherapeutic agents are usually used in combination with radiotherapy. Their typical sequelae include dry mucosa, muscle atrophy and fibrosis (van der Molen et al. 2012).

8.9 Treatment of Benign Lesions of the Larynx

Mette Pedersen, Ahmed Geneid, and Anders Overgård Jønsson

8.9.1 Introduction

The array of benign vocal fold lesions includes cysts, nodules and polyps, as well as sulci vocales and bridges of the vocal folds. The diversity of the reasons behind these lesions, being hereditary, environmental, behavioural and multifactorial, is reflected in the choice of treatment for the benign lesion encountered.

Treatment options usually include behavioural voice therapy and pharmacological treatment, as well as surgical treatment utilising cold instruments or lasers (for individual examples, see Sects. 5.4, 8.2, 8.3, 8.8 and 8.10).

With the exception of contact granulomas, the benign vocal fold lesions tend to occur in the mid-membranous vocal fold within the lamina propria (Courey et al. 1996; Gray 1989; Titze 1994).

8.9.2 Behavioural and Voice Therapy

In almost all benign lesions of vocal folds, a trial of voice therapy should be warranted (see Sects. 8.2 and 8.3). Vocal fold nodules almost always respond favourably to voice therapy, reducing in size or disappearing (Johns 2003; Holmberg et al. 2001). Voice therapy is also a valuable first-line treatment especially for those with small polyps of recent onset (Jeong et al. 2014; Klein et al. 2009; Nakagawa et al. 2012). Cysts can also respond to voice therapy (Cohen and Garrett 2007); however, there is still a need for more research on the degree of response and the kind of cyst that mostly improves with voice therapy. Contact granulomas are also known to heal with reduced hyperfunction and decreased vocal fry achieved through voice therapy. Thus, it usually results in complete disappearance of the granulomatous formation (Ylitalo and Hammarberg 2000). On the other hand, certain benign lesions such as sulcus vocalis and bridges of the vocal folds' medial edge are known to have relatively disappointing results with phonosurgery. Although voice therapy cannot be curative with these lesions, it may be useful in treating the associated phonatory dysfunction.

Lifestyle treatment should consider awareness of environmental provocations and an active response to provocations (Pedersen 2002; Pedersen 2012; Pedersen and Eeg 2012). It also includes respect for and avoiding provocation factors (dust, noise, shouting and others) (Gray and Thibeault 2002).

8.9.3 Pharmacological Treatment

Reflux medications, steroids and Botox have been used widely in the treatment of some vocal fold benign lesions (see Sect. 8.8). Interestingly, a 16-item survey mailed to all active US members of the American Academy of Otolaryngology-Head and Neck Surgery ($n = 7321$) with 16.5% response rate ($n = 1208$) showed a lack of consensus on antireflux medication and oral steroids. Patients with contact granulomas experience more pharyngeal acid reflux events than their controls (Ylitalo and Ramel 2002). Using reflux medications has been advised for patients with contact granulomas. In addition, Botox has been used successfully in treating contact granulomas (Nasri et al. 1995) and seems to be an excellent option for patients with granulomas not reacting to voice therapy.

8.9.4 Surgical Treatment

Surgery (see Sect. 8.10) is usually reserved for patients with large and old polyps and fibrotic nodules not responding to voice therapy. In addition, cysts are mostly handled surgically, with attention paid to the risk of creating atrophy if large intra-cordal cysts are removed (Johns 2003). A comparative study between the use of cold instruments and CO_2 lasers for surgical treatment of benign lesions showed no significant difference. The knowledge and experience of the phonosurgeon is the decisive factor rather than the tool used (Benninger 2000). Post-operative voice therapy has a significant role in ensuring better outcomes and less recurrence of the benign lesions. Voice rest is usually recommended after phonosurgery.

8.9.5 Future Aspects

See Sect. 4.9.

Acknowledgements Many thanks to the co-workers at The Medical Center, Copenhagen, Denmark, for helping in the completion of this section: Line Jønsson, Sanila Mahmood and Anders Jønsson.

8.10 Phonosurgery

Viktor Chrobok, Felix de Jong, and Tadeus Nawka

8.10.1 Fundamentals of Phonosurgery

8.10.1.1 Definition and Principles

Von Leden and Arnold coined the term 'phonosurgery' in 1963. In a meeting of the International Association of Phonosurgeons in Abano Terme, Italy, in 2000, phonosurgery was specified as functional surgical intervention directed exclusively or in part at improvement, restoration or preservation of the voice (and speech).

The principles of phonosurgery are based on the fundamentals of functional microanatomy and physiology of the vocal fold, specifically Hirano's body-cover theory, Gray's work on cellular space and studies on benign lesions of the lamina propria also known as Reinke's space.

The vocal folds consist of epithelium, lamina propria, skeletal muscles, nerves, vessels and cartilage. The lesions playing the most important role in the field of phonosurgery are located in the lamina propria (Zeitels and Healy 2003).

The membranous portion of the vocal folds is covered with a stratified squamous epithelium, which is the most important vibrating structure. It gives shape to the vocal folds and enables them to return to the rest position of phonatory movement.

Impaired vibratory movement of the vocal folds may be caused by the following pathological changes:

- Epithelial lesions (e.g. papillomatosis, epithelial dysplasia, chronic laryngitis, carcinoma)
- Changes of the lamina propria (e.g. Reinke's oedema, vocal nodules, polyp)
- Cysts (epidermoid cyst, retention cyst, pseudocyst)
- Sulcus, mucosal bridge
- Atrophy, scar, defect
- Vascular lesions (ectasia, varicosity, haematoma)
- Arytenoid granulations (contact granuloma, intubation granuloma)
- Anterior web (congenital, acquired, microweb)

Surgical equipment has markedly improved since the introduction of microlaryngoscopy in the 1950s: specially designed laryngoscopes, refined phonomicrosurgical instruments, powerful operating microscopes as well as the CO_2 laser coupled with advanced micromanipulators with a small spot size.

Phonosurgery encompasses a variety of elective operations; the primary goal is improving voice quality. The principles of peri-operative and post-operative care are similar for all types of phonosurgical procedures. For comprehensive descriptions, see the book on operative techniques in laryngology by Rosen and Simpson (2008b).

8.10.1.2 Peri-operative Care

Before surgery, one to two sessions of voice therapy may be useful but are not mandatory. Anticoagulation medication should be not used 7–10 days before surgery. Intravenous steroids may be used before general anaesthesia. There is usually no indication for prolonged use of steroids or antibiotics.

8.10.1.3 Post-operative Care

Conservative treatment includes hydration and continued or short-time treatment for laryngopharyngeal reflux disease, with a proton-pump inhibitor if necessary. The decision should be made on the basis of the results of the reflux symptoms index and the reflux finding score. Post-operative use of antibiotics or long-term steroids is usually not necessary.

Phonomicrosurgical procedures are followed by a period of voice rest. This period can range from as short as 2 days and extend to possibly 14 days, depending on the extent of the lesion and the degree of dissection of vocal folds, the compliance of the patient, the surgeon's philosophy and experience. Voice rest puts a heavy burden on the patient. That is why it should be prescribed prudently. There is no evidence that voice rest influences the outcome. The optimal time for initiation of voice therapy is approximately 14 days after surgery.

'Light voice use' or confidential voice therapy can be transitioned if there is adequate epithelial coverage and is usually defined as speaking with an easy, breathy, 'airy' voice (not a whisper) as if speaking 'confidentially' to someone for 5–10 min/h. This type of voice use where the vocal folds move but do not collide is often used for 7–10 days. The intention is to let the epithelium heal and cover the lamina propria without scar formation.

8.10.1.4 Management and Prevention of Complications

A variety of minor to major complications associated with phonomicrosurgery can occur in the oropharynx or larynx:

- Oropharyngeal complications are dental injuries, temporomandibular joint disorder, lingual anaesthesia, dysgeusia, paresis of the hypoglossal nerve, throat pain and rupture of the palatoglossal arch.
- Laryngeal complications include excessive oedema, vocal fold scar and granulation tissue at the operative site. Recurrence of the lesion can result in post-operative dysphonia and may require a repetition of the intervention.

The optimal management strategy for these complications includes pre- and peri-operative communication with the patient. Discussion and relationship between surgeon and patient are essential for prevention and management of complications.

8.10.2 Phonosurgical Procedures

Phonosurgery (Friedrich et al. 2007) includes phonomicrosurgery (endoscopic microsurgery of the vocal folds (Remacle et al. 2003)), laryngeal injection (synthetic and organic biological substances), laryngeal framework surgery (laryngoplasty, laryngoplastic phonosurgery, open-neck surgery that restructures cartilaginous framework of the larynx) (Nawka and Hosemann 2005) and

reinnervation of the larynx (nerve-to-nerve anastomosis, nerve-muscle pedicle reinnervation; see Sect. 8.12).

8.10.2.1 Phonomicrosurgery of the Vocal Folds

General Considerations
The patient is placed on the operating table in a supine position. The optimal head and neck position for exposure of the endolarynx with the laryngoscope is extension of the head and flexion between the neck and chest. Applying external counterpressure is useful.

Specialised laryngoscopes are required for phonomicrosurgery. New designs have improved the exposure of the anterior commissure or the larynx and its surroundings. Generally, the laryngoscope with the largest diameter should be chosen, but when the larynx is difficult to access, it is easier to expose it with a smaller laryngoscope. Laryngoscope placement is important for the success of surgery. The laryngoscope is passed through the oral cavity. The lips and tongue should be retracted. Advance the laryngoscope further under the epiglottis without folding or traumatising it, push the ventricular folds aside, and position the distal opening immediately above the vocal folds. Optimal laryngoscopic visualisation and minimal adjacent tissue injury or damage are crucial for phonomicrosurgery.

A binocular microscope with the highest magnification should be used for phonomicrosurgical procedures. The position of the microscope and laryngoscope is perfectly coaxial with the longitudinal aspect of the laryngoscope. Using a 0, 30 or 70° endoscope for visualisation in a 'three-dimensional' fashion of the endolarynx is of great value.

Instruments utilised for phonomicrosurgery include specialised blunt microelevators, cupped forceps, scissors, curved alligators, small suctions, triangular forceps or Bouchayer forceps that have been developed for retraction of the epithelium. Optimal hand control of instrumentation is achieved when the forearms of the surgeon rest on arm supports attached to the operating chair.

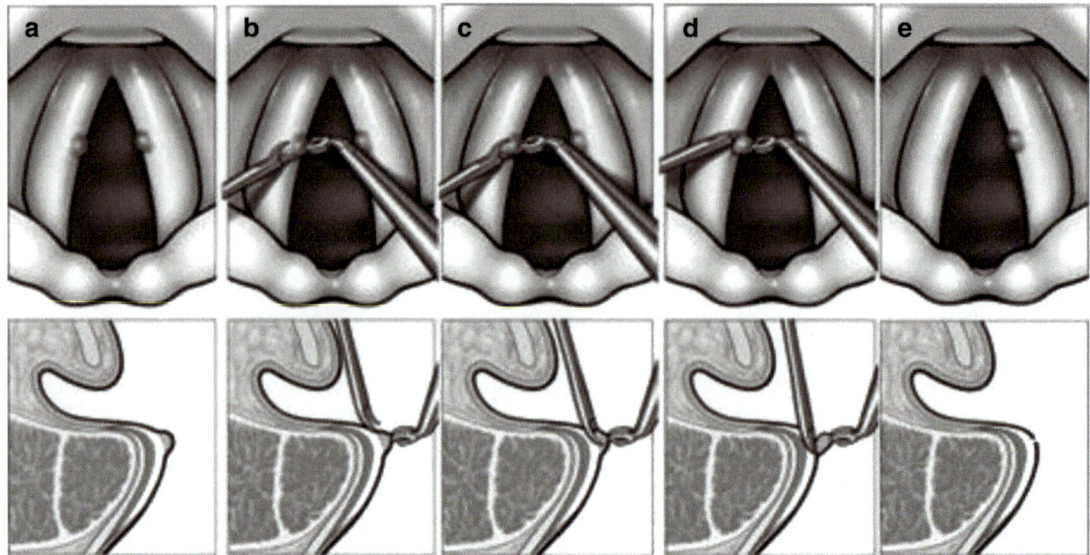

Fig. 8.10 Vocal nodule resection. The nodule (**a**) is marked by epithelial prominence. It is cut with scissors tangentially (**b–d**); the superficial lamina propria stays intact. The defect of the epithelium is minimal (**e**) (© T. Nawka, W. G. Hosemann/KARL STORZ Endoskope, Germany)

Management of Subepithelial Lesions

The main principles of precise microsurgical removal of benign vocal fold lesions are to limit dissection to the most superficial plane possible and maximise epithelial and lamina propria preservation (Zeitels and Healy 2003).

Vocal fold nodules, polyps and Reinke's oedema result from changes of the epithelium and the superficial, sometimes intermediate, lamina propria. The extensive vibration during excessive vocal load destroys the structure of the basement membrane and the superficial lamina propria. Reinke's oedema is associated with oedematous lakes in the intercellular substance, as well as fibrin and less fibronectin (Dikkers and Nikkels 1995).

Conservative removal of subepithelial pathological changes with preservation of the overlying normal epithelium and superficial lamina propria is the key aspect of most phonomicrosurgical operations. The basic principle is lifting the epithelium of the vocal folds rather than removing it. This allows healing by primary intention. The layered microstructure of the vocal folds, the pliability of the mucosa and voice quality are restored or preserved.

Nodules may be treated with voice therapy, but they will not disappear, and they will increase after high vocal load. That is why even small nodules may require phonosurgery, especially for voices that must meet high requirements. Nodules are removed completely. Their small size of 1–3 mm allows for excision without further action (Fig. 8.10).

Pedunculated polyps with a small base are excised. Large-based polyps are removed in such a way that part of the distended epithelium remains in situ and serves to cover the wound. This method is known as the microflap technique. Only redundant epithelium is removed (Fig. 8.11).

Reinke's oedema is treated on the same principle; it is removed subepithelially. The covering epithelium is incised on the superior surface of the vocal fold and dissected from the lamina propria while being largely preserved. The oedema is suctioned and kneaded. The epithelium is redraped and trimmed (Fig. 8.12).

The epithelium has to be dissected meticulously and tranquilly. An involuntary abscission of the epithelium is quite possible because it is

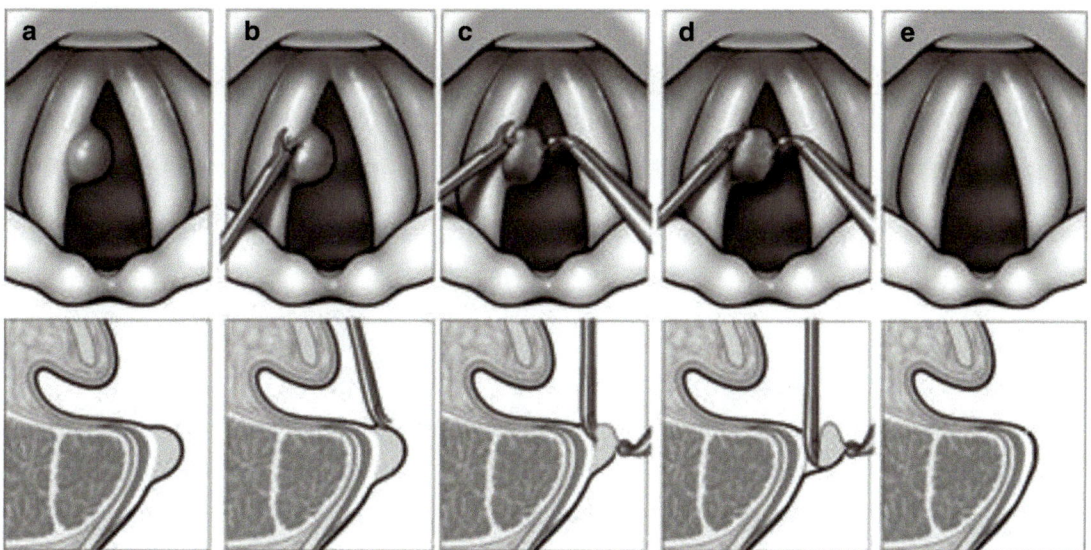

Fig. 8.11 Vocal fold polyp resection. Vocal fold polyps are epithelial swellings with a well-defined border to the surrounding sound epithelium (**a**). They are incised craniolaterally (**b**), the redundant subepithelial mass and epithelium are cut off (**c** and **d**), and the wound is covered with epithelium (**e**) (© T. Nawka, W. G. Hosemann/KARL STORZ Endoskope, Germany)

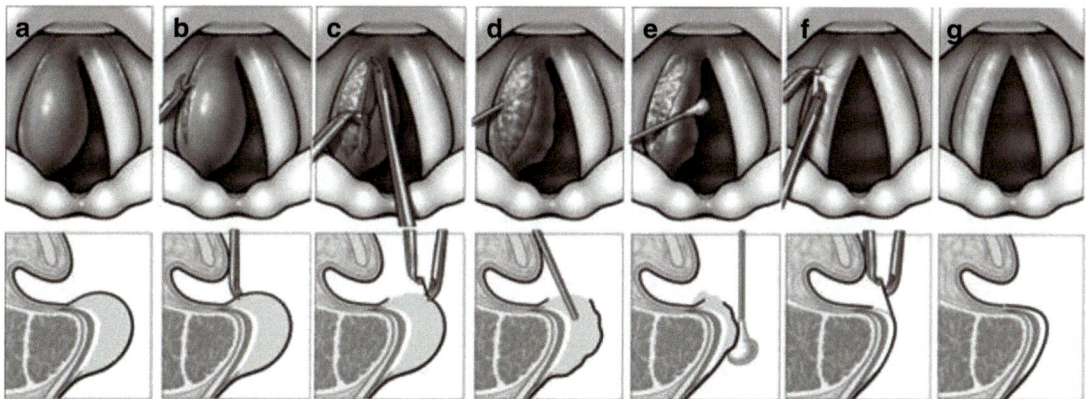

Fig. 8.12 Operation of Reinke's oedema. The epithelium covering the oedema has no definite border to the surrounding normal epithelium (**a**). On the cranial surface, the incision, or a narrow excision of epithelium, follows the arcuate line at the transition from expanded epithelium to normal-appearing mucosa (**b** and **c**). The myxoid acellular substance of the lamina propria is suctioned (**d**) or pressed out (**e**). Redundant epithelium is trimmed (**f**) and redraped so that the epithelial edges adjoin (**g**) (© T. Nawka, W. G. Hosemann/KARL STORZ Endoskope, Germany)

so thin, fragile and distended by the oedema. Wound healing leaves no scar when the lamina propria has not been damaged or removed. The epithelium closes the wound without loss of pliability, and the mucosal wave recurs during regeneration. It is better to leave some oedema covered with epithelium than to create a straight scarred vocal fold by removing too much of the epithelium.

For cysts of the vocal folds, the same principle holds true; the epithelium must be preserved (Fig. 8.13).

Retention cysts, which arise from obstructed mucous glands, have a thin epithelium that occasionally ruptures during dissection. Epidermoid cysts have a thick epithelium and are embedded in fibrous masses. They are microsurgically dissected and resected as a whole.

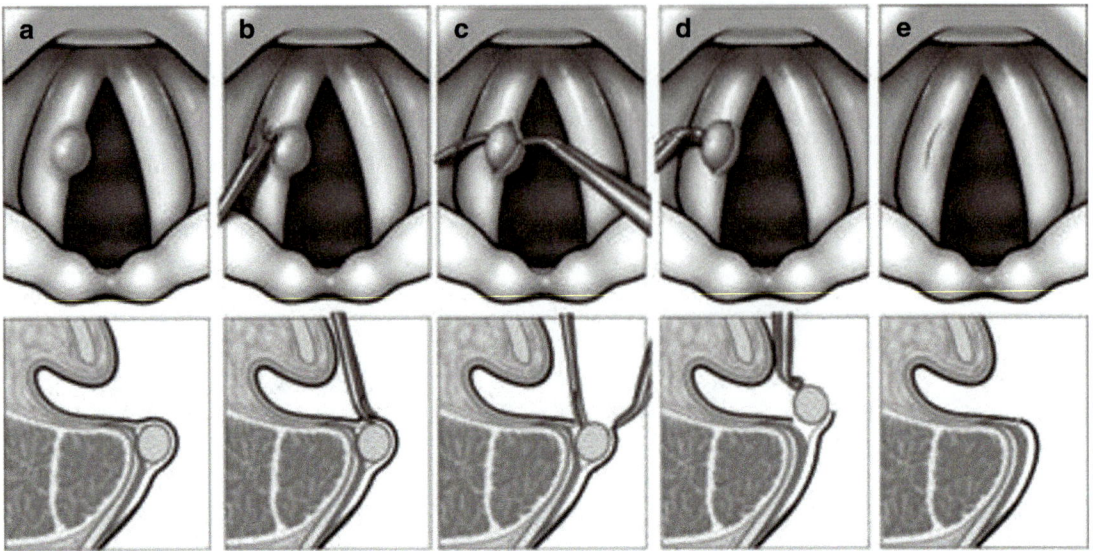

Fig. 8.13 Removing an epidermoid cyst. The epidermoid cyst has its own epithelium. It is seen through the translucent overlying normal epithelium (**a**). The incision runs laterally (**b**); the cyst is dissected (**c**) and removed with forceps (**d**). The epithelium closes at the edges of the incision (**e**) (© T. Nawka, W. G. Hosemann/KARL STORZ Endoskope, Germany)

Papillomatosis

Papilloma is a threat to the patency of the airways and can, especially in childhood, obstruct them by progressive growth in the trachea and bronchi. The usual symptom in adults is hoarseness up to aphonia. A radical resection is not possible. Papillomatosis, to date, is not curable, but it can have long periods of remission. For this reason therapy is symptomatic and should aim at maximal preservation of the superior lamina propria to maintain vocal function. Nowadays vaccination is used for prevention but also for treatment. The benefit has not been proven yet, but there is hope that recurrences of papilloma are weaker and less often.

Before ablation a subepithelial infusion with saline and adrenalin (epinephrine) distends the papillomatous epithelium and protects the deeper layers of the vocal fold, especially the lamina propria (Fig. 8.14a).

The resection is most conservative with the CO_2 laser in superpulse mode and at low power (2 W) or with a microdebrider. Bleeding and thermal damage of the lamina propria are minimised.

No matter which surgical method is used, laryngeal structures should be treated in such a way that the ablation does not go deeper than the lowest level of surrounding healthy-appearing epithelium or, in the case of papilloma spread over a plane, not below the basement membrane into the lamina propria.

Epithelial Dysplasia and Early Glottal Cancer

For resection of premalignant lesions and early cancer stages (T1), partial resection of the layered structure and the use of the CO_2 laser can lead to an optimal post-operative voice. For excision, the subepithelial infusion protects deeper layers of the lamina propria and preserves glottal voice production.

For early cancer stages, endoscopic cordectomy, performed as subepithelial cordectomy or subligamental cordectomy (Remacle et al. 2000, 2007) (Figs. 8.15 and 8.16), helps achieve a good oncological and functional outcome. By respecting oncological criteria, these tailored methods can save the phonation structures that are not infiltrated by the tumour, such as the vocal ligament, the vocalis and thyroarytenoid muscle (Fig. 8.14b).

Fig. 8.14 Subepithelial infusion to protect deeper layers of the lamina propria from thermal trauma caused by the CO_2 laser (**a**) and to help scrutinise whether or not there is an adherence of the tumour growing into deeper layers (**b**) (© T. Nawka, W. G. Hosemann/KARL STORZ Endoskope, Germany)

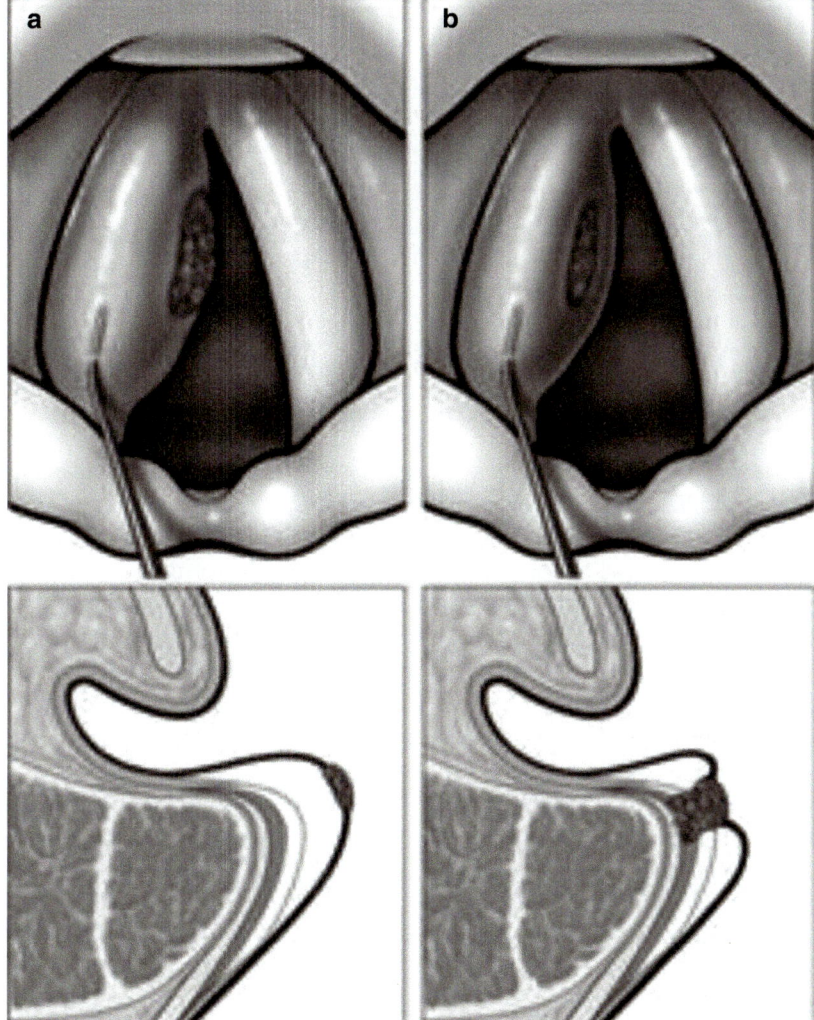

Fig. 8.15 Subepithelial cordectomy. Resection of the epithelium and the superficial lamina propria, sparing the vocal ligament and the vocalis and thyroarytenoid muscles. (**a**) Horizontal section at the glottal level, (**b**) frontal section of one vocal fold (© T. Nawka, W. G. Hosemann/KARL STORZ Endoskope, Germany)

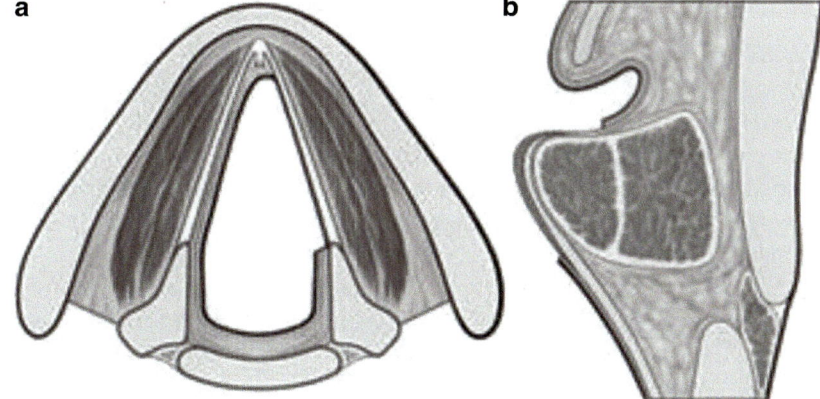

Fig. 8.16 Subligamental cordectomy. Resection of the epithelium, Reinke's space and the vocal ligament, preserving the vocalis and thyroarytenoid muscles. (**a**) Horizontal section at the glottal level, (**b**) frontal section of one vocal fold (© T. Nawka, W. G. Hosemann/KARL STORZ Endoskope, Germany)

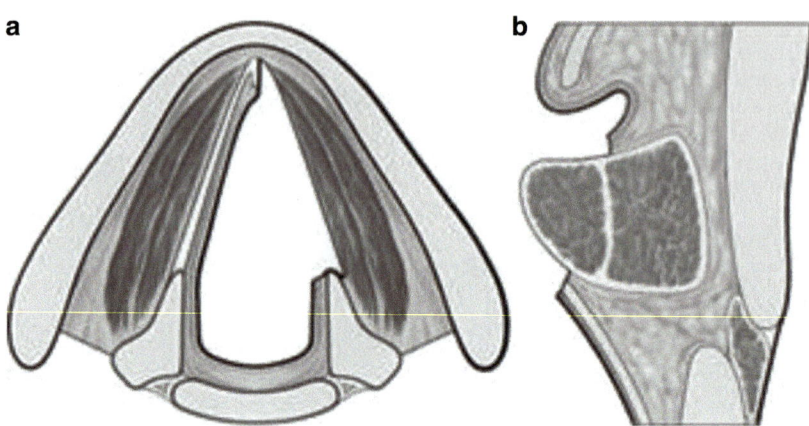

Glottoplasty

Male-to-female transsexuals require a higher speaking voice in order to be accepted. Pitch raising can be achieved by the Wendler glottoplasty technique, which is applied fairly often (Mastronikolis et al. 2013). The procedure consists of the CO_2 laser de-epithelialisation of the anterior commissure, along with the anterior third of the two vocal folds, and the suturing of the two vocal folds with one to three absorbable threads. Additionally, fibrin sealant may be applied to strengthen the stitches.

Low tones (under 132 Hz) can be eliminated by glottoplasty. However, phonosurgeons must be aware that a healthy phonatory system is disturbed. The increased pitch inevitably leads to a deterioration of vocal range and voice quality. The patients have to be informed that conservative treatment and medication with hormones may lead to a more feminine voice, too.

8.10.2.2 Phonomicrosurgery in Topical Anaesthesia

Surgery of small epithelial and subepithelial changes of the vocal folds (up to 5 mm) can be carried out on an awake patient with local anaesthesia (Nawka and Hosemann 2005). Premedication (e.g. 10 mg morphine and 0.5 mg atropine s.c. or 7.5 mg midazolam orally) is given 10 min before the intervention. The throat and the larynx are anaesthetised superficially with tetracaine, by spraying, and subsequently directly, by applying a soaked cotton swab. This procedure allows for a safe removal of nodules,

polyps, oedema, small papilloma and diagnostic biopsies with the advantage of stroboscopic and auditory voice control. These procedures are performed on an outpatient basis. The operating field is visualised via a laryngeal mirror and an operating microscope or a rigid 90° (70°) telescope. The larynx can be observed directly or on a video monitor. The correct indication and skill facilitate the precise removal of pathological changes. This technique will remain important because of the need for cost-effective outpatient procedures. It should belong to the repertoire of any phonosurgeon.

8.10.2.3 Laryngeal Injection Techniques

Laryngeal injection is one treatment modality that is used for surgery of glottal insufficiency. Vocal fold augmentation is commonly used in the following situations:

- Temporary correction of unilateral vocal fold paralysis
- Permanent correction of vocal fold atrophy (presbyphonia), vocal fold paresis (unilateral and bilateral) and unilateral vocal fold paralysis
- Trial correction of glottal insufficiency (as a diagnostic measure)
- Adjunctive vocal fold augmentation after laryngeal framework surgery
- Glottal insufficiency due to vocal fold scarring or soft tissue loss

Augmentation in direct laryngoscopy is performed in the posterior and middle part (third), laterally of the vocal fold and at 3–5 mm depth. Over-injection (15–30%) is recommended to compensate for absorption of the water-based component (fat). Injection into the superficial lamina propria (Reinke's space) should be avoided.

Augmentation substances can be divided into temporary (2–6 months) and long-lasting (permanent, 2 years or more) materials. Temporary injection materials include carboxymethylcellulose (Radiesse Voice Gel) and hyaluronic acid gel (Restylane, Hylaform). Long-lasting injection substances include autologous fat, fascia, calcium hydroxylapatite (Radiesse) and silicone (Vox Implant).

Vocal fold augmentation is preferred in cases where the overall condition of the patient raises fears of the risk of compromising the airway by oedema and haematoma. The injection can be less precise than laryngeal framework surgery, but in order to deposit the correct amount of material, it can be injected in repeated procedures. The vocal fold holds a volume of approximately 1 mL. Vocal fold augmentation is considered to have failed in achieving closure during phonation when the glottal gap is wider than 3 mm. Using autologous fat in these cases is advantageous because there is much material available and injection is continued until the vocal fold tissue does not hold any more of the injected fat and discharges the material.

8.10.2.4 Laryngeal Framework Surgery

Thyroplasty as a new phonosurgical technique was established by Isshiki, who described four types of thyroplasty: type I, lateral compression; type II, lateral expansion; type III, relaxation (shortening); and type IV, stretching (lengthening) (Isshiki et al. 1974).

At present Isshiki's techniques are generally accepted, but several new surgical modifications and different terms have been introduced. The new classification and nomenclature of laryngeal framework surgery was established by the Phonosurgery Committee of the European Laryngological Society (Friedrich et al. 2001; Isshiki 2000).

Laryngeal framework surgery (LFS) is the general term for a whole group of phonosurgical procedures; it describes surgical modification of structures of the larynx and recognises the importance of functional implications. LFS is performed in the laryngeal skeleton or inserting muscles for correction of position or tension of the vocal folds. The goal is improvement of vibratory movements of the vocal folds or reduction of unmodulated and turbulent phonatory airflow or alteration or modification of vocal pitch.

Laryngoplasty (LPL) is used for reconstruction of any part of the larynx including the vocal folds.

Thyroplasty is a subgroup of LPL, which involves only the thyroid cartilage.

The classification and indication of LFS include:

- Approximation LPL for correction of insufficient glottal closure: medialisation thyroplasty and arytenoid adduction (Figs. 8.17, 8.18 and 8.19).
- Expansion LPL for correction of vocal fold hyperadduction: lateralisation thyroplasty

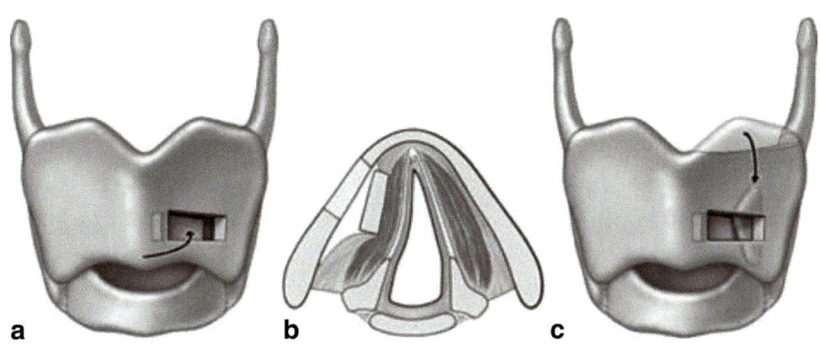

Fig. 8.17 Medialisation thyroplasty. The window is located in the lower half of the thyroid ala (**a**). The vocal fold is impressed from the side (**b**). A shim from the superior part of the thyroid cartilage secures the impressed portion (**c**) (© T. Nawka, W. G. Hosemann/ KARL STORZ Endoskope, Germany)

a   b   c

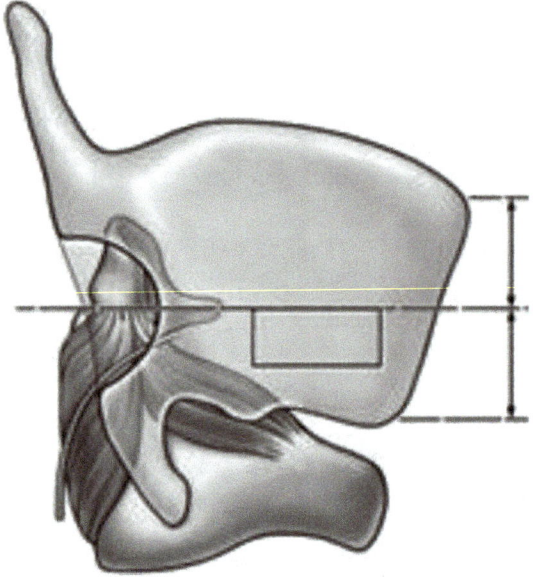

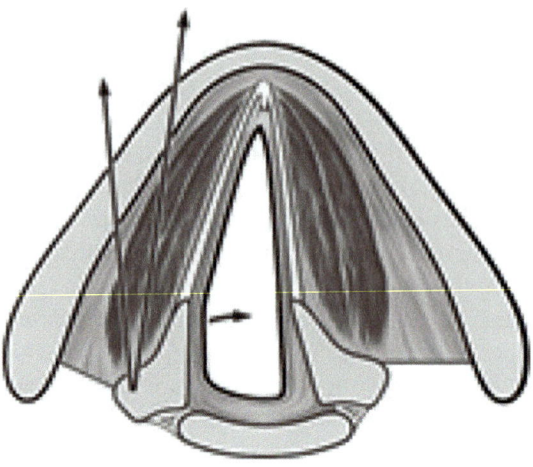

Fig. 8.18 Posterior and medialisation laryngoplasty windows (© T. Nawka, W. G. Hosemann/KARL STORZ Endoskope, Germany)

Fig. 8.19 Arytenoid adduction according to Isshiki. Luxation of the arytenoid cartilage rotates the vocal process medially, when the muscular process is pulled anteriorly. The suture is fastened at the anterior edge of the thyroplasty window. This procedure facilitates glottal closure in the membranous portion (© T. Nawka, W. G. Hosemann/KARL STORZ Endoskope, Germany)

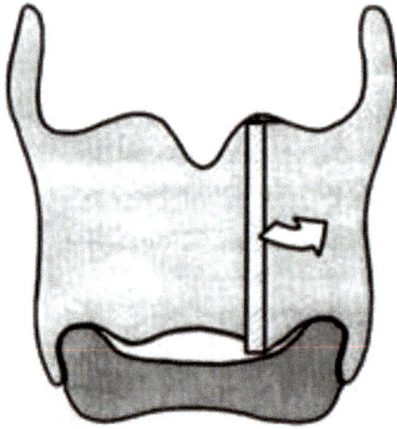

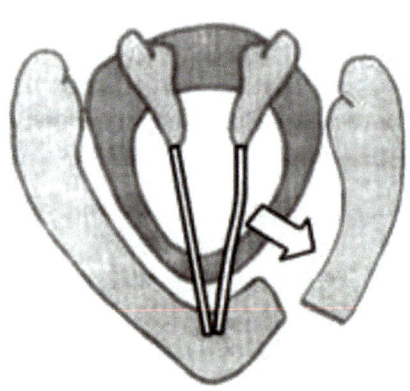

Fig. 8.20 Lateralisation thyroplasty. Lateral approach. The vocal fold is tensioned laterally (Reprinted by permission from Springer Nature: European Archives of Oto-Rhino-Laryngology. Laryngeal framework surgery: a proposal for classification and nomenclature by the Phonosurgery Committee of the European Laryngological Society. Friedrich G, de Jong FICRS, Mahieu HF et al. ©2001)

(lateral, medial approach) and vocal fold abduction (Figs. 8.20 and 8.21)

- Relaxation LPL for pathologically tightened vocal folds or too high-pitched voice: shortening thyroplasty (Fig. 8.22)
- Tensioning LPL for correcting pathologically lax vocal folds or too low-pitched voice: cricothyroid approximation (Fig. 8.23) and elongation thyroplasty (lateral, Fig. 8.24, medial approach, Fig. 8.25)

The most widely performed type of LFS is glottal narrowing procedures. There are primarily two modalities for the surgical treatment of glottal insufficiency with dysphonia or aspiration: vocal fold augmentation by injection and medialisation thyroplasty with or without arytenoid adduction. The choice of procedure often reflects the surgeon's own preference and experience. Medialisation thyroplasty and arytenoid adduction are the best procedures for

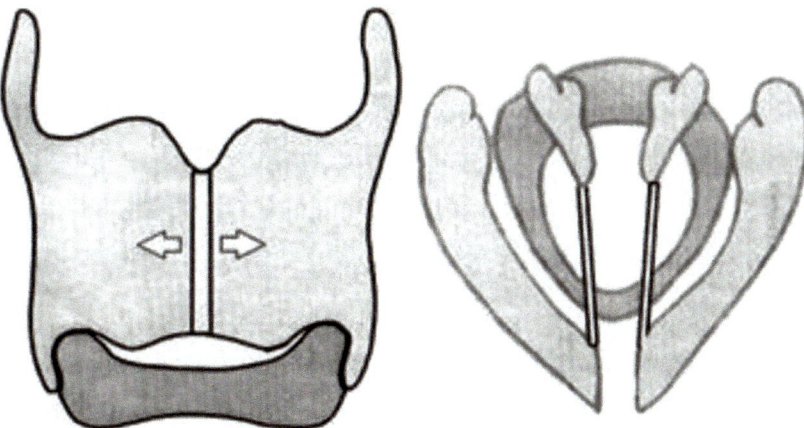

Fig. 8.21 Lateralisation thyroplasty. Medial approach. The vocal folds are separated by splitting the midline (Reprinted by permission from Springer Nature: European Archives of Oto-Rhino-Laryngology. Laryngeal framework surgery: a proposal for classification and nomenclature by the Phonosurgery Committee of the European Laryngological Society. Friedrich G, de Jong FICRS, Mahieu HF et al. ©2001)

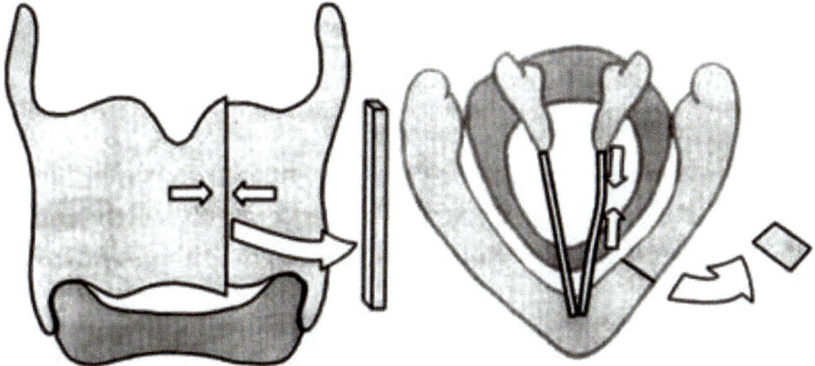

Fig. 8.22 Relaxation thyroplasty. Shortening of the framework from a lateral approach (Reprinted by permission from Springer Nature: European Archives of Oto-Rhino-Laryngology. Laryngeal framework surgery: a proposal for classification and nomenclature by the Phonosurgery Committee of the European Laryngological Society. Friedrich G, de Jong FICRS, Mahieu HF et al. ©2001)

Fig. 8.23 Cricothyroid approximation (Reprinted by permission from Springer Nature: European Archives of Oto-Rhino-Laryngology. Laryngeal framework surgery: a proposal for classification and nomenclature by the Phonosurgery Committee of the European Laryngological Society. Friedrich G, de Jong FICRS, Mahieu HF et al. ©2001)

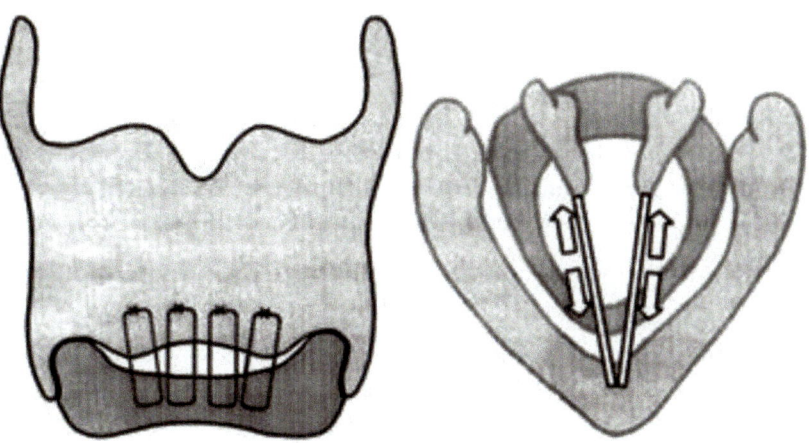

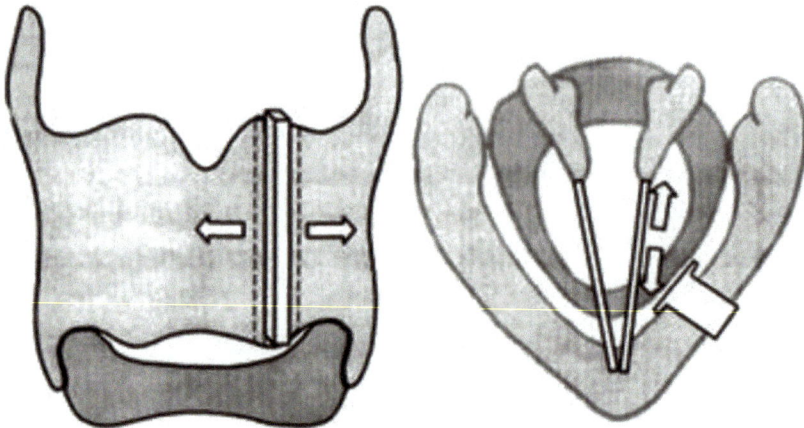

Fig. 8.24 Elongation thyroplasty, lateral approach (Reprinted by permission from Springer Nature: European Archives of Oto-Rhino-Laryngology. Laryngeal framework surgery: a proposal for classification and nomenclature by the Phonosurgery Committee of the European Laryngological Society. Friedrich G, de Jong FICRS, Mahieu HF et al. ©2001)

Fig. 8.25 Elongation thyroplasty, medial approach (Reprinted by permission from Springer Nature: European Archives of Oto-Rhino-Laryngology. Laryngeal framework surgery: a proposal for classification and nomenclature by the Phonosurgery Committee of the European Laryngological Society. Friedrich G, de Jong FICRS, Mahieu HF et al. ©2001)

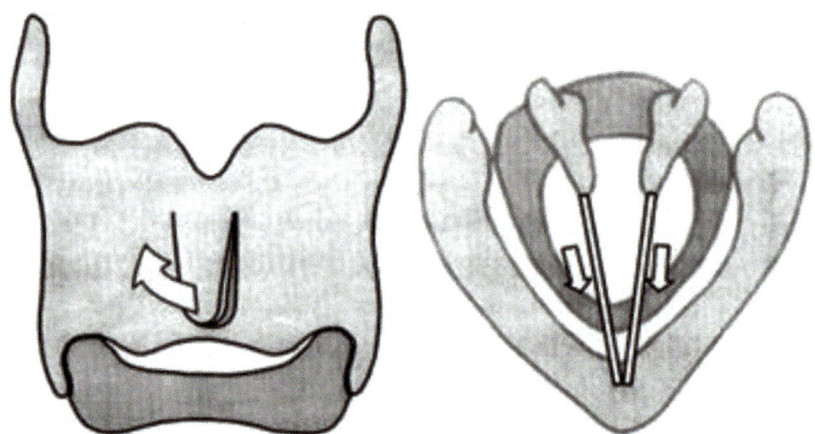

unilateral vocal fold paralysis with a large posterior glottal gap.

Different techniques and implants (silastic, Gore-Tex, hydroxylapatite, titanium) are used for achieving glottal approximation.

8.10.2.5 Prospects for the Future

Development of biomaterials is the area of research for application into superficial lamina propria in cases of scarred or non-vibrating epithelium.

Neurolaryngology deals with the electromyographic diagnostics of paralysed laryngeal muscles and justifies the selective reinnervation of the intrinsic laryngeal muscles by nerve transplants from superior parts of the phrenic nerve or from parts of the cervical ansa (see Sect. 8.12).

The selective laryngeal pacing of the posterior cricoarytenoid muscle for abduction of the vocal fold by electric stimulation is intended to reduce airway obstruction in bilateral vocal fold paralysis. It may also be indicated in cases of unilateral paralysis and spasmodic dysphonia.

8.11 Pacing in Bilateral Vocal Fold Palsies

Andreas Müller

Laryngeal Pacemaker At the end of the 1970s, when functional electrical stimulation efforts, e.g. in cardiac pacemakers, reached one of its peaks, the idea of laryngeal pacing was conceived by Zealear and Dedo (1977). Our group introduced a new concept of laryngeal neurostimulation in bilateral vocal fold palsies (bVFP) (Mueller 2011). Supported by grants and in cooperation with MED-EL Company (Innsbruck, Austria), as well as the ear, nose and throat (ENT) departments of the universities Innsbruck and Würzburg, the scientific basis for a clinical applicable laryngeal pacemaker has been established over the last 10 years. Thus minimally invasive electrodes and insertion techniques (Forster et al. 2013) as well as a stimulation device adapted to the special demands of bVFP were developed. The electrode and device stability under mechanically challenging conditions, i.e. treadmill exercise testing, among others, in race horses, has been demonstrated (Ducharme et al. 2010).

The majority of patients with bVFP after recurrent laryngeal nerve trauma suffer from some kind of pathological, mainly synkinetic reinnervation of the laryngeal muscles. This has been proven by the co-activation of abductors and adductors in laryngeal electromyography (EMG) and the lack of relevant muscle atrophy of the vocal folds in laryngoscopy. Synkinetic reinnervation preserves the contractile posterior cricoarytenoid (PCA) muscle fibres. If provisional electrical stimulation of the intramuscular recurrent laryngeal nerve branches results in selective vocal fold abduction, the patient is a candidate for laryngeal pacing even in long-lasting palsies. Besides this positive test abduction, the second important laryngeal precondition is a non-life-threatening narrowed glottal gap. General preconditions are patients free of other relevant respiratory restrictions or severe co-morbidities.

Laryngeal Pacing System In September 2012, a prospective multicentre study was started in humans for a clinical application of laryngeal pacing in bVFP, supported by the MED-EL Company. The laryngeal pacing system used (LP System, MED-EL, Austria) consisted of a 3 French LP electrode, the LP implant and the external LP processor. Implantation was carried out under general anaesthesia with larynx mask ventilation and videolaryngoscopic monitoring of the LP electrode placement. After a small horizontal skin incision over the cricoid, a disposable LP insertion tool was advanced across the upper border of the cricoid arch and drawn below the mucosa along the inner surface of the arch towards the cricoid lamina. While drilling into the lamina, the LP insertion tool delivered a continuous electrical stimulation, used to determine a 'hot spot' in the PCA (i.e. a spot that when electrically stimulated induced vocal fold abduction). Once the hot spot was found, the LP electrode was placed through the LP insertion tool, and its spiral tip was fixed into the hot spot in the PCA. The LP electrode was then tunnelled subcutaneously towards the chest wall and connected to the LP implant. After wound healing, the external processor was linked magnetically to the implant beneath the skin (Figs. 8.26 and 8.27).

Fitting Process During a fitting process, individually tailored stimulation parameters and vocal fold abducting frequencies adapted to the patient's different respiratory needs during sleep, daily routine and physical effort are found and stored in the processor. The LP processor has a single control button for switching between the stored programmes. For safety reasons implantation of the stimulation electrode was restricted to one side. After the first successful implantation in Gera (Germany), nine patients were enrolled in this study. The surgical procedure and the clinical application of the LP system were safe in all cases, and the first functional results were promising. The complete details of this study have been published in *The Laryngoscope* (Mueller et al. 2015).

In the long term, this minimally invasive approach of electrode insertion preserves the normal integrity of the larynx and is not harmful in the case of failure. In contrast to standard laser surgical glottal enlargement, laryngeal pacing is reversible and will therefore become more acceptable than any other forms of open surgery for patients suffering from iatrogenic bilateral vocal fold palsy. Laryngeal pacing seems to be inaugurating a new era of dynamic rehabilitation of the larynx in bVFP.

Fig. 8.26 Schematic drawing—woman with laryngeal pacemaker implant in situ—front view © MED-EL. Permission to use image granted by MED-EL

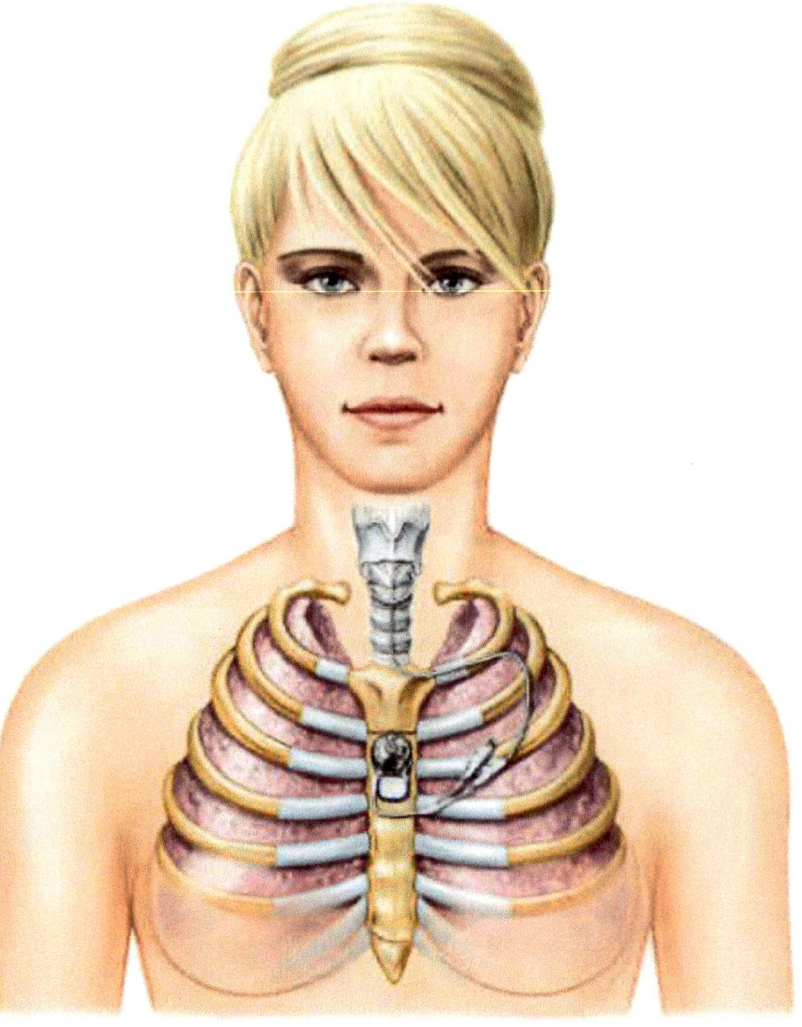

8.12 Reinnervation in Bilateral Vocal Fold Palsies

Jean-Paul Marie

In bilateral recurrent laryngeal nerve paralysis, the vocal cords are usually immobile in a paramedian position, with dyspnea but fairly good voice quality. The main problem is then to recover the abductory function to improve breathing. Classical treatments are aimed at enlargement of the larynx by endoscopic, external or mixed approaches. The consequences are usually some voice alteration and swallowing problems. The more the breathing is improved, the more the voice is altered.

To solve this problem, a number of animal experiments have been performed for decades with some success. The principle was to apply an inspiratory trigger to the abductor muscle (the posterior cricoarytenoid muscle (PCA)), often unilaterally or in some instances on both sides. The motor nerve supply was either branches from the hypoglossal nerve or roots or the main trunk of the phrenic nerve.

The reinnervation was performed by using different techniques: nerve implantation into the muscle, nerve-muscle pedicle implantation or selective nerve anastomosis.

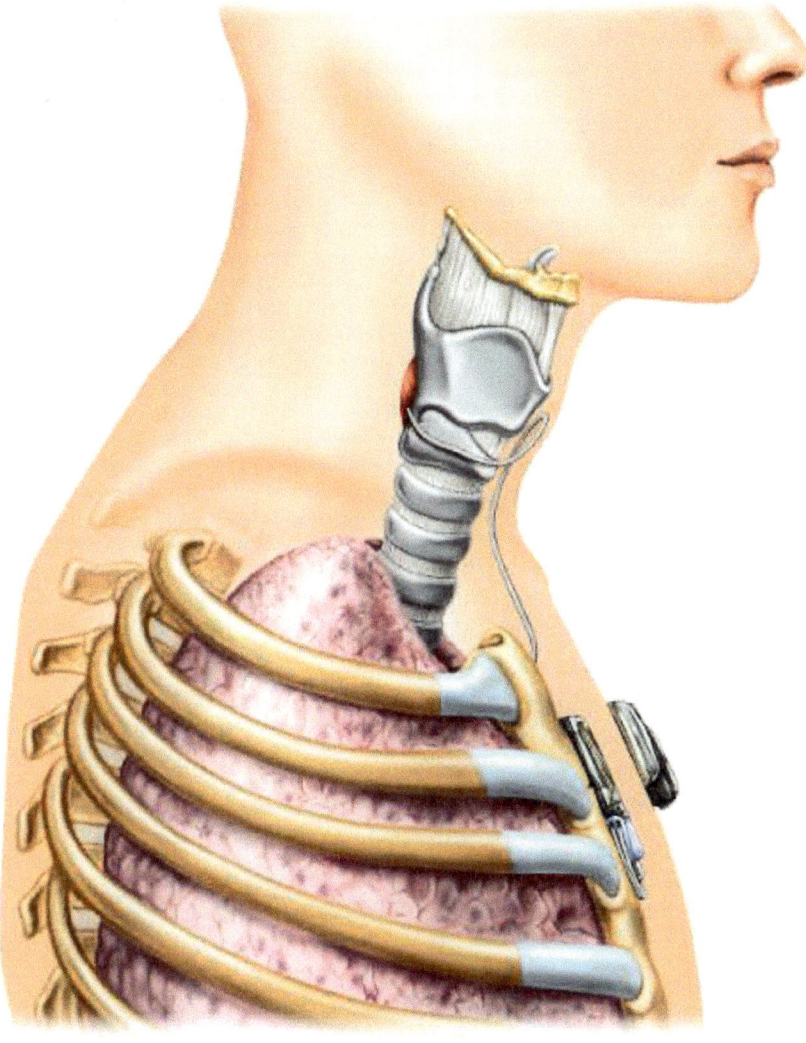

Fig. 8.27 Schematic drawing—man with laryngeal pacemaker implant in situ—lateral view © MED-EL. Permission to use image granted by MED-EL

Reinnervation by Nerve-Muscle Pedicle Technique Tucker (1978, 1982, 1989) described a nerve-muscle pedicle technique involving the ansa hypoglossi nerve supply. A piece of strap muscle was harvested with the nerve supply and implanted in the ipsilateral PCA muscle. Tucker has reported a series of 214 patients with nerve-muscle pedicle in bilateral vocal cord paralysis of which 202 had at least 2 years follow-up with 74% success. Similar success was not confirmed by other surgeons, and the technique is not currently performed today. The main criticisms were the lack of active abduction of the arytenoid and the lack of EMG inspiratory activation. The

following step was selective reinnervation by using the phrenic nerve.

Reinnervation Using the Phrenic Nerve The phrenic nerve is able to induce inspiratory activity in reinnervated muscles and has been considered an ideal nerve transfer for the PCA reinnervation. Although unilateral phrenic nerve resection is considered to be well tolerated, some effort has been made to preserve nerve supply to the diaphragm. Animal experiments and human application were performed by Crumley et al. (1980) and Crumley (1982, 1983) using the split phrenic nerve graft for PCA reinnervation. The distal part of the nerve graft was anastomosed to the abductor branch of the recurrent laryngeal nerve (RLN) inside the larynx. Although good results were obtained in animals, the first human applications did not demonstrate any active movement of the arytenoids (Crumley 1983).

Variations of Reinnervation Techniques
Variations of this technique have been described in animals by Rice (1982), Mahieu et al. (1993) and van Lith-Bijl et al. (1996, 1998). They performed an extra-laryngeal anastomosis of the phrenic nerve and sectioned the adductor branch inside the larynx to implant it inside the PCA, guiding all the axons towards that muscle. Subsequently Crumley (1984), van Lith-Bijl et al. (1997) and Marie et al. (1989) developed selective simultaneous reinnervation of adductor muscles (with the ansa) and abductor muscle (with the phrenic nerve graft) in animals, with some success.

Bilateral PCA reinnervation has been performed in humans by Zheng et al. (2002): on one side by phrenic nerve neurotisation (anastomosis of the RLN trunk and implantation of the proximal cut adductor branch of the RLN in the PCA) and on the contralateral side by the nerve-muscle pedicle technique with the ansa. Arytenoid abduction was observed in five out of six patients only on the phrenic nerve reinnervation side. More recently, Zheng has reported some success with bilateral PCA reinnervation with the left phrenic nerve (Li et al. 2013), but the lack of adductor muscle reinnervation and vocal cord atrophy may explain some partial vocal cord adduction.

New Technique We have described a new technique of bilateral selective motor reinnervation of the adductor and abductor laryngeal muscles (total motor reinnervation) (Marie 1999; Marie et al. 2000a; Marina et al. 2011) (Fig. 8.28). We have previously obtained successful results in dogs with unilateral selective reinnervation of both adductor and abductor muscles, using, respectively, the ansa hypoglossi and the phrenic nerve (Marie et al. 1989). In order to apply this technique in humans, we first studied the effects of partial phrenic nerve resection on respiration

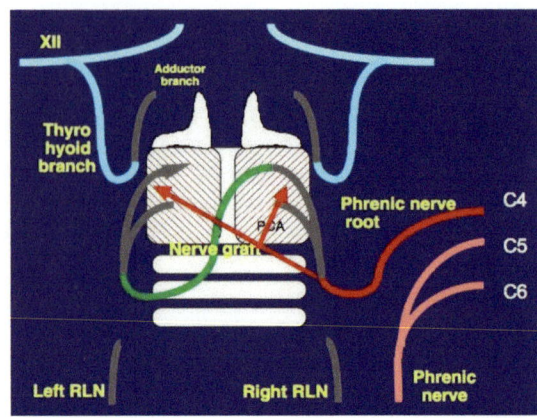

Fig. 8.28 Schematic view of total motor reinnervation of the larynx: both PCA reinnervation by the upper root of one phrenic nerve and both adductor muscle reinnervation by thyrohyoid branches of both hypoglossal nerves. The free interposition nerve graft (green), used at the beginning of our experiments, is now replaced by a Y-shaped lengthening nerve graft (red), implanted in both PCA (Marie et al. 1999, 2000a, 2001, 2007, 2006b; Marie 2009a, 2014; Marina et al. 2011). Abbreviations: *PCA* posterior cricoarytenoid muscle, *RLN* recurrent laryngeal nerve (Reprinted by permission from Springer Nature: Nerve Reconstruction. Jean-Paul Marie. In: Remacle M, Eckel HE (eds) Surgery of larynx and trachea. ©2009)

in rabbit and dog models and demonstrated that the resection of the upper phrenic nerve root had only a slight effect on respiration (Marie et al. 1997a, b, 1999, 2006a). Later, we studied the possibilities of bilateral PCA reinnervation, in order to improve the glottal opening, finally performing a total motor reinnervation of the larynx (Marie 1999). Concomitant reinnervation of adductor muscles by the thyroid branch of both hypoglossal nerves can achieve optimal supply (Marie et al. 2000b). The thyroid branch of the hypoglossal nerve is the only strap muscle supply to fire during phonation and swallowing (Marie et al. 2000c). The technique can be used in a delayed manner, even in cases of synkinesis (Marie et al. 2001).

Clinical Trial We were thus prompted to start a clinical prospective trial in humans. Below the surgical technique is summarised (Fig. 8.28).

The upper phrenic nerve root is used from one side. A free nerve-lengthening graft can be

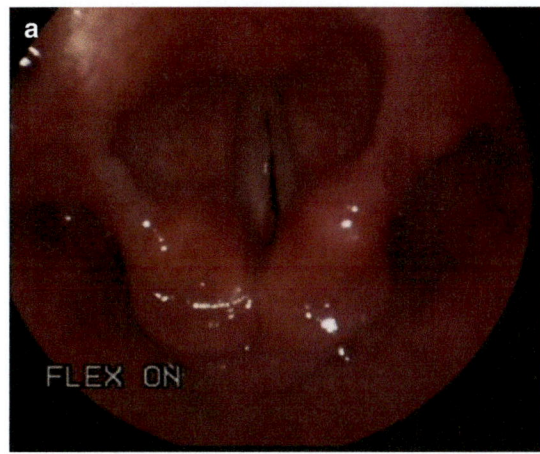

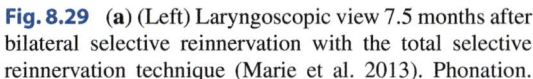

Fig. 8.29 (**a**) (Left) Laryngoscopic view 7.5 months after bilateral selective reinnervation with the total selective reinnervation technique (Marie et al. 2013). Phonation.

(**b**) (Right) Laryngoscopic view 7.5 months after bilateral selective reinnervation with the total selective reinnervation technique (Marie et al. 2013). Inspiration

provided by the superficial cervical plexus. Right- and left-sided dissection is undertaken of the thyrohyoid branch of the hypoglossal nerves (THXII) (blue). Intralaryngeal dissection of the RLN branches is performed.

The Y-shaped lengthening nerve graft is implanted inside both PCA exposed by a retrocricoid dissection. An upper transposition of the distal part of the adductor branches of the RLN is performed, and anastomosed to the THXII, on both sides. An interposition nerve graft is often necessary to avoid tension. The final step of the procedure is the anastomosis between the upper phrenic nerve root and the interposition nerve graft, in order to channel the inspiratory axonal supply to the PCA muscles. Voice recovery and improvement in ventilation should start within 6–9 months after the procedure.

To date, 49 patients have undergone this bilateral motor reinnervation with this technique, among them five children. The aetiologies were most often postsurgical injuries (after thyroidectomy) or congenital paralysis. Ten patients had previous endoscopic enlargement. Forty patients had more than 1-year follow-up.

Voice was improved or preserved in almost all cases. Thirty-five out of forty patients were decannulated, three after complementary treatment. Ventilation parameters were improved in 75% of the cases. Arytenoid abduction was observed during inspiration at least on one side in 27/40 patients, even on both sides in 16/40 patients (14/30 if there was no previous endolaryngeal scar) (Fig. 8.29a, b). In one case with previous endoscopic enlargement, breathing was improved enough to permit a secondary medialisation. Phrenic nerve function recovery was observed in most of the cases (Marie 2009a, b, 2014; Marina et al. 2011; Marie et al. 2013).

New Indications and Future Options New indications are currently in progress: rare cases of bilateral vocal fold paralysis in aperture (generally the consequence of a strongly denervated larynx) and secondary reinnervation after endoscopic procedure when the arytenoids remain passively mobile. This last indication has received ethical approval for the conducting of a new prospective trial.

In summary, the safety and reliability of this technique make it suitable as a first intention technique of treatment in cases where the voice has to be preserved and can be proposed in children.

In the future, some strategies might be used, combining reinnervation and perhaps electrical stimulation in some selective cases, in order to promote the efficiency of reinnervation (Brushart et al. 2002; Gordon et al. 2009) or to avoid atrophy of the denervated muscles before reinnervation. Moreover, some regenerative medicine techniques with stem cells might be an efficient complementary treatment.

8.13 Rehabilitation After Head and Neck Surgery

Bożena Wiskirska-Woźnica and Tadeus Nawka

8.13.1 Introduction

The treatment of malignancies is inherently complex and requires rehabilitation after the primary measures of surgical interventions, radiotherapy and chemotherapy. Early rehabilitation is particularly necessary when surgical procedures mutilate anatomical structures, as, for example, in laryngectomees, who lose their normal voice completely. Their physical and professional activity is significantly impaired and limited. Voice and speech rehabilitation improves the communication process and physical dexterity, as well as the psychic condition of patients. To restore the complex communication process is the main but not the only element of rehabilitation. Social rehabilitation at the familial, professional and environmental level is just as important.

8.13.2 Voice and Speech Rehabilitation After Total Laryngectomy

Loss of voice, speech and the defensive reflex of the larynx, as well as anosmia, rank among the most bothersome consequences of laryngectomy. After the resection, the inhaled air is no longer warmed, purified and moistened. The surgery may lead to emotional disturbances, as well as social and economic problems.

The key issue in rehabilitation of laryngectomised people is teaching them how to produce a compensatory voice and speech. There are several possible ways of communication for the laryngectomees:

- Alternative oesophageal or pharyngeal voice and speech
- Tracheo-oesophageal voice and speech by surgical creation of a tracheo-oesophageal shunt and insertion of the so-called voice prosthesis (Fig. 8.30)

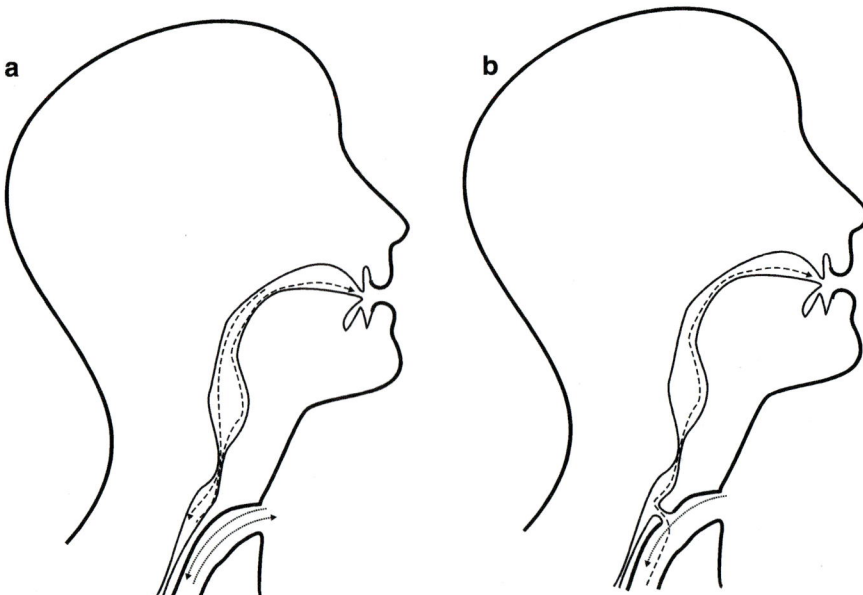

Fig. 8.30 The mechanism of voice and speech production: (**a**) oesophageal, (**b**) tracheo-oesophageal via shunt

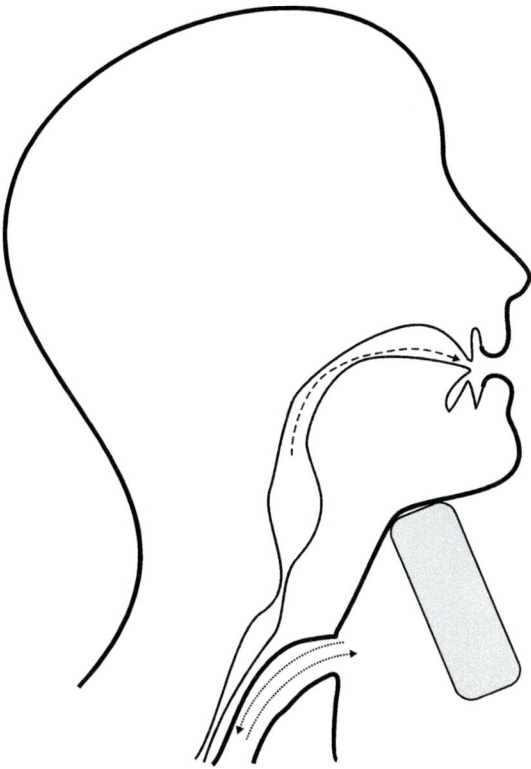

Fig. 8.31 Sound generation in the vocal tract with an electrolarynx

- Electronic speech device—the so-called artificial larynx or electrolarynx (Fig. 8.31)
- Oral-guttural pseudo-whisper, gestures, mimics or writing

The task of a phoniatrician and a speech pathologist is to help laryngectomees establish communication by means of substitute phonation. In case the laryngectomee cannot find a speech therapist or logopedist near his or her home, and does not want to go into a special rehabilitation centre, but has a computer and ability to use the Internet, telerehabilitation via the free software Skype may be a reliable tool to render continuity of the rehabilitation possible and to reduce the number of patients without rehabilitation (Galant 2017).

Transplantation of the larynx is one of the more challenging areas in modern medicine. This procedure aims to improve the quality of life rather than saving life, so the larynx transplant is considered as an elective procedure with high risks and burdens as well as benefits (Narula et al. 2011). The first successful operation was a total laryngeal transplantation performed by Marshall Strome in Ohio (USA) in 1998. The recommendation of laryngeal transplantation should only be considered for patients who have suffered irreversible injury to their larynx or patients who, because of a large benign or low-grade malignant tumour, have undergone a total laryngectomy. Because of the high risk of a second cancer in patients who have been treated for advanced laryngeal cancer, transplantation should not be considered.

8.13.2.1 Oesophageal and Pharyngeal Voice and Speech

Gutzmann was the first to describe the substitute or compensatory voice and speech in 1908, while Seeman coined the term 'oesophageal voice' in 1924. At present, patients after total laryngectomy are believed to be able to develop oesophageal or pharyngeal voice and speech, depending on the location of the pseudoglottis.

The production of the *oesophageal voice* is conditioned by the formation of the air reservoir in the upper oesophagus and the so-called pseudoglottis which produces the fundamental tone. The pseudoglottis is a sound generator in the upper oesophageal sphincter involving various anatomical structures in the area of the inferior pharyngeal constrictor muscle. The cricopharyngeal muscle plays a vital role in the formation of the pseudoglottis. Seeman recommended preservation of the area of the cricopharyngeal muscle. Radiological tests demonstrate the location of the neoglottis at the level corresponding to C5–C6 vertebrae (Fig. 8.32), with a notable bulge of the anterior and posterior wall (type I according to Pruszewicz), a bulge of only one wall (type II) or flat closure of both walls (type III) of the laryngopharynx.

The air swallowed into the oesophagus and expelled with an antiperistaltic motion causes vibration of the mucosa in the pseudoglottis with

504

Fig. 8.32 An example of location and shape of the pseudoglottis and hypopharynx after total laryngectomy (sequential pictures while swallowing contrast medium)

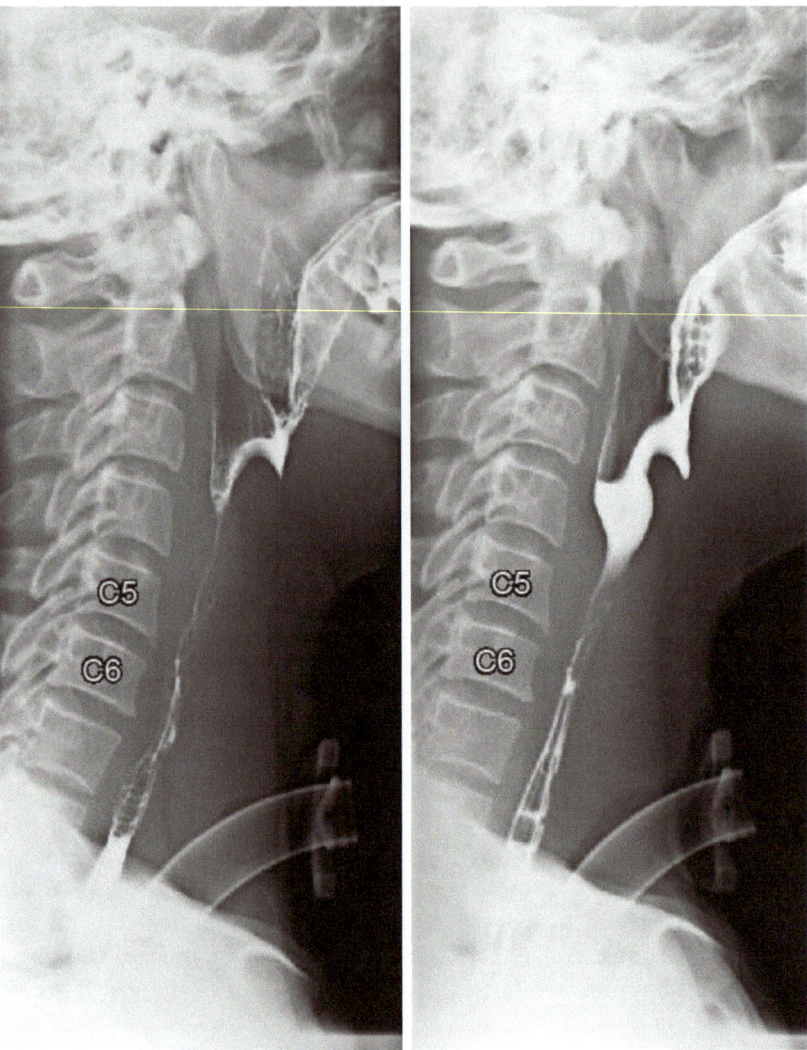

the use of the physiological reflex of burping (ructus). The ructus can be achieved in three ways:

- Inspiration into the oesophagus by drawing air through an open mouth and inclining the head backwards and sudden exhalation with accompanying loud noise during eructation of the accumulated air.
- Injection of the air by propelling it from the laryngopharynx to the oesophagus with the help of the movements of the tongue base and by provoking loud eructation.
- Swallowing air (carbonated beverages can be helpful in the beginning), thus accumulating

the air in the oesophagus, and then learning how to develop a loud ructus. The generated loud ructus as the fundamental tone is the basis for oesophageal voice and speech. After the ructus has developed in an unaltered vocal tract, the articulation of vowels and voiced stops (followed by consonant-vowel clusters and then simple words and sentences) is trained.

The next phase of rehabilitation comprises working with a speech pathologist on shaping the prosodic elements of speech, i.e. accent, rhythm, intonation and melody by reduction of primary explosive speech, attempts to connect syllables into words during one intake of air into the oesophagus, practice of speech rhythm and melody and practice of proper speech pace. Oesophageal voice is relatively low (60–80 dB), with a small range, large noise component, poor intonation and slower pace. Production is strenuous and forces laryngectomees to make frequent pauses owing to the small oesophageal volume and short phonation time.

The amount of pressure required to overcome the resistance of the pharyngo-oesophageal sphincter (Marszałek et al. 2009; Pruszewicz et al. 1992), measured with the Seeman method, is of important prognostic value (this is also true for the tracheo-oesophageal/shunt voice; see below). Pressure values between 5 and 40 mmHg are associated with good prognosis, and values 40–80 mm Hg usually signify an uncertain outcome of the rehabilitation, whereas pressure over 80 mmHg is associated with very serious difficulties in overcoming the resistance and acquiring a ructus voice. There are three invasive ways to reduce the tension of the pharyngo-oesophageal sphincter: myotomy of the inferior pharyngeal constrictor, neurectomy of the pharyngeal plexus and chemical denervation with the botulinum toxin.

The process of learning the oesophageal voice and speech ought to be initiated preoperatively. An explanatory conversation about the mechanism of substitute speech, together with a laryngectomee who can demonstrate good oesophageal speech, should take place. Respiratory and general strengthening exercises, especially for the abdominal muscles, may be recommended before surgery. The rehabilitation itself is rather long, from 6 weeks to 3–6 months, and is started usually 3 weeks after healing of the post-operative wound. The level of mastering oesophageal speech is determined with the use of the following classification: very good, good and moderate. Generally, oesophageal speech is accepted if the understandability of sentences reaches the range of 50–65%.

Pharyngeal voice (10% of substitute voice and speech) is developed when the pseudoglottis is located in the oropharynx, with the phonatory closure between the posterior wall of the phar-

ynx and the root of the tongue. The laryngopharynx becomes the substitute air reservoir, and the generated voice is croaky, strenuous, and raspy, with uneconomical use of air, but comprehensible. The ability to produce oesophageal or pharyngeal speech depends on numerous factors. The major factors impeding the development of oesophageal speech are extensive surgical resection of the laryngopharynx and the root of the tongue, hearing loss (over 50 dB), dental loss, advanced cancer, large coexisting recesses of the laryngopharynx, low intellectual level and social status, elderly age and cancer-induced coexisting depression.

As has been said, hearing loss above 50 dB significantly hinders rehabilitation of a laryngeal substitute voice. That is why an audiogram of laryngectomees and their carers should be considered before rehabilitation and a hearing aid prescribed when necessary.

8.13.2.2 Tracheo-oesophageal (Shunt) Voice and Speech

First attempts at surgical voice rehabilitation after total laryngectomy date back to the post-war period (Briani 1952) and comprise methods that aimed to develop primary and secondary voice shunts with the use of auto- and alloplastic materials. Numerous authors focused their attention on surgical methods of obtaining substitute voice (Hotz et al. 2002; Logemann 1995). The efforts of Mozolewski (1972) and Serafini and Staffieri (1976), who created cutaneous, mucosal and mucosal-muscular shunts facilitating the development of shunt speech, are particularly noteworthy. Later, shunts with the use of tracheo-oesophageal puncture and silicone prostheses were introduced (Blom and Singer 1979; Panje 1981). At present, Provox 2 is the most frequently used voice prosthesis. It is a unidirectional silicone valve, allowing the patient to direct the exhaled air from the trachea into the oesophagus and the throat, at the same time preventing foods and liquids from passing to the trachea and the lungs.

A connection between the posterior tracheal wall and the anterior wall of the oesophagus, the tracheo-oesophageal shunt, facilitates the passage of the exhaled air from the trachea into the upper oesophagus, after insertion of a so-called voice prosthesis. The air reservoir from the lungs can be used for phonation. The air passes the pharyngo-oesophageal segment (the upper oesophageal sphincter) and makes the mucosa vibrate. The resulting voice has a more distinct tone and longer phonation time than oesophageal speech. Speech has better intonation, melody and fluency. Such a voice prosthesis may be inserted during laryngectomy—primary shunt or later on secondary shunt.

There is a vast range of arguments in favour of primary surgical rehabilitation, and, indeed, such a tendency has been noted recently. The time of rehabilitation is shorter mostly because there is nearly no need of burdensome and long-lasting exercises. However, there are also drawbacks in the use of a prosthesis. The patients need a certain manual dexterity for closing the tracheostomy when speaking, they have to follow basic hygiene measures, and the replacement is necessary every 3–6 months by a physician. Otherwise fungal growth on the prosthesis develops with the consequence of valve insufficiency; the shunt may leak and lead to aspiration of saliva and food.

Factors in favour of the primary oesophageal voice include absence of an additional device and a surgical procedure, as well as additional costs. The drawbacks include a long rehabilitation process, especially the preliminary period, i.e. until ructus is mastered, a short phonation time of oesophageal voice, frequent interruptions in phonation for insufflation, less clear articulation and slightly lower voice frequency.

Thus, an individualised approach is recommended, and the following should be considered for the rehabilitation regime: whether to start with exercises aiming to develop the so-called natural voice and the oesophageal speech and proceed with the surgical creation of the secondary voice shunt only in the event of failure or to place the voice prosthesis during the laryngectomy, which is currently common practice.

8.13.2.3 Electronic Voice-Generating Devices

Attempts to use electronic prostheses should be taken only in cases where acquiring oesophageal or tracheo-oesophageal voice and speech fails, especially in the elderly, who have no chance of success in rehabilitation.

The mechanisms of action in case of electronic prosthesis, the so-called artificial larynx or electrolarynx, are based on generating vibrations of the fundamental frequency, which is modulated and transformed into articulated sounds in the vocal tract of a laryngectomee. Jaw, lip and tongue movements allow laryngectomised patients to produce audible speech sounds just as in normal speech. Electronic laryngeal prostheses may work as:

- Devices generating vibrations by using the expired air from the trachea and directing it to the oral cavity, the so-called pneumatic devices (obsolete)
- Devices generating vibrations outside the body and without the use of air, also placed in the oral cavity, e.g. the Ticchioni pipe (Pipa di Ticchioni, obsolete)
- The so-called neck vibrators, generating vibrations transferred directly to the organ of articulation by direct contact of the vibrator with the mouth floor (most common nowadays)

Recently, mini vibration generators that are placed in dental prostheses on the hard palate have been introduced in the USA.

8.13.3 Rehabilitation After Partial Laryngectomy (Larynx Preservation Surgery)

These patients present before treatment with dysphonia of varying intensity. Post-operative structural loss, depending on the extent of resection, has the greatest impact on voice quality.

In conservation laryngeal surgery with reconstruction, the most satisfactory phonatory function is obtained when the mobile parts of the larynx, the arytenoid cartilages, are preserved.

After cordectomy types according to the ELS from type I to VI and reconstructive procedures such as partial supracricoid laryngectomy with cricohyoidopexy (CHP) or cricohyoidoepiglottopexy (CHEP, method Calearo, method Sedláček),

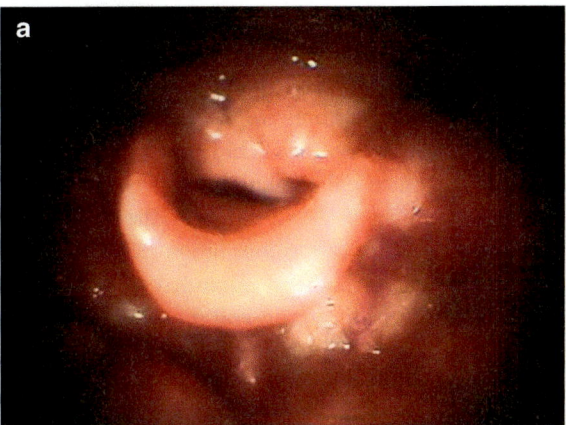 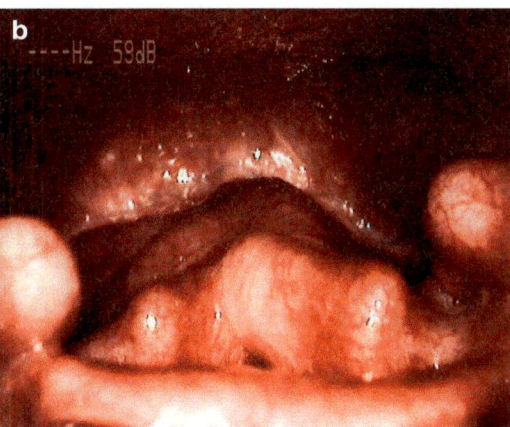

Fig. 8.33 The neoglottis (aryepiglottic phonation—contact of the aryepiglottic fold with the epiglottis) after partial supracricoid laryngectomy (**a**) and after transglottic laryngectomy according to Calearo (arytenoids conserved, contact of the arytenoid cartilages with the epiglottis) (**b**)

the voice quality depends mainly on the new level of laryngeal closure and vibrating structures which may be localised:

- At the glottal level of a structurally unaltered vocal fold and on the other side of the vestibular fold
- At the level of the laryngeal vestibule (aryepiglottic folds, arytenoid cartilages, epiglottis), resulting in the development of the aryepiglottic voice
- At the level of the vestibular folds (Fig. 8.33)

The following phonation types can result:

- Glottal phonation, with contact of the vocal folds or the neo-folds (substituted vocal fold by scar or reconstruction) at the level of the glottis
- Oblique glottoventricular phonation, with contact of an unaltered vocal fold with the opposing ventricular fold
- Ventricular phonation, with contact of both ventricular folds
- Aryepiglottic phonation, with contact of the aryepglottic fold with the laryngeal epiglottis

Supraglottal laryngectomy may not cause major disorders of the phonatory activity of the larynx; the voice can be almost normal, and complaints may be the consequence of a slight decrease in the voice range, mostly in higher

frequencies, and excessive production of thick saliva (sialorrhea). Microlaryngoscopic interventions with cold instruments (the Kleinsasser's technique) or with a laser (cordectomy or extended cordectomy, Remacle et al. 2000, 2003) lead to smaller structural changes in the larynx. Thus, good voice quality can be obtained in approximately 90% of patients with T1 and T2 carcinoma. Voice disorders and disturbances after such procedures are usually characterised by significant hyperkinesis of the external and internal laryngeal muscles. Many authors (Galetti et al. 2012; Berania et al. 2015) have reported that voice quality depends on the type of surgery performed and functional compensation, but individual compliance could mostly influence the vocal outcome.

Case Study 8.3
Vibration of a normal and a scarred vocal fold after subligamental cordectomy. The 56-year-old patient had a T1a of the right vocal fold. He underwent a laser cordectomy 5 years ago. Since then he has shown no recurrence of the tumour. The voice is moderately hoarse because of scar formation. The vocal range is severely reduced.

Case Study 8.4
Vibration of the ventricular folds alternating with the aryepiglottic folds for voice production after resection of the left vocal fold because of laryngeal cancer.

The patient had a T1a carcinoma at the age of 65. The left vocal fold had been removed completely by cordectomy type IV. One year later, he was able to produce his voice at the level of the ventricular folds alternating with the aryepiglottic folds. The voice is dominated by a rough deep sound. The vocal range is limited to soft and low notes.

Case Study 8.5

Vibration of the aryepiglottic folds for voice production after surgical treatment of a glottal carcinoma in the anterior commissure. The 49-year-old man had a carcinoma of the larynx in the anterior commissure. After five interventions, he has been tumour-free for more than 5 years. The vocal folds are shortened and completely scarred; there is an anterior synechia. Voice production is possible by vibration of the corniculate and cuneiform tubercle of the aryepiglottic folds only. Nevertheless, he is able to communicate with this voice.

The programme of phonatory rehabilitation of the voice after conservation surgeries mainly aims at reducing uneconomic hyperactivity and improving efficiency. Thus, it ought to include exercises allowing improvement of respiration, phonation, articulation and relaxation. Respiration exercises aim to increase lung capacity, teach more efficient use of air during phonation and strengthen groups of muscles that are involved in breathing. They help to achieve the proper breathing route that is most efficient during phonation. This, in turn, allows the drawing of air into the lungs and maximally lengthens the exhalation phase, resulting in breathing with the use of the intercostal muscles and the diaphragm, i.e. the diaphragmatic-costal route. Diaphragmatic-costal breathing occurs when, during inspiration, the chest cavity is evenly enlarged, with the lower part expanding during a fixed position, without the upper movement of the shoulder girdle, and with maximum flattening of the diaphragm. The inspiration should be fast and deep; the expiration ought to be long and slow. Exercises for lengthening the exhalation phase are started with phonation of the voiceless 'sss—fff—chchch and so on', with maximum relaxation of the neck muscles. Prolonged phonation is achieved by using breath support, the so-called appoggio, i.e. consciously slowing down the first third of the expiration phase, during which the lungs collapse passively after having been expanded. While exhaling the first third of lung volume, the diaphragm has to release and ascend slowly.

Basic phonation exercises include the following: conscious increase or decrease of the pharyngeal muscle tension in structurally altered conditions; production of soft phonation; establishing a voice pitch that is suitable for a given person and that allows for an easy, effortless phonation and speech; control of voice intensity; and activation of vocal resonators. The primary management includes the use of the 'm' sound with various vowels 'a-e-i-o-u' while simultaneously controlling the resonatory vibrations in the facial skeleton bones (viscerocranium) by means of touch. Another group of phonation exercises improves phonatory closure by applying the following: controlled coughing; phonation of syllables with plosives (e.g. [kik]) or vowels that are produced by involving muscle tension; exercises, based on the Froeschels's method, that cause reflexive closure of the vocal folds when uttering syllables consisting of a stop consonant and vowels, with simultaneous clapping of the hands against the chest or applying chest pressure or sudden lowering of the raised arms; and manual exercises with mechanical closure of the vocal folds by applying lateral pressure to the plate-like lamina of the thyroid cartilage or maximum rotation of the head to the side.

Articulation exercises comprise tasks that help achieve accuracy of articulating vowels and consonants, slow down the speech pace and improve phonatory-articulatory-respiratory coordination by speaking in phrases with proper breathing pauses.

Relaxation exercises are based on practising the movements of the mandible, tongue and lips, proper velopharyngeal closure and general relaxation tasks aiming to loosen the neck muscles.

8.13.4 Rehabilitative Aspects After Head and Neck Surgery

Treatment of tumours located within the oral cavity results in significant structural defects and consequent deterioration of the quality of patient life. The majority of problems is caused by the severely impaired function of chewing and swallowing. Further symptoms are limited ability to speak (articulatory disorders due to reduced movability of the peripheral organs of speech); dysgeusia; anosmia; impaired sense of touch, temperature and pain; as well as changed consistency of the saliva and significantly limited movement of the head, neck, and shoulders.

Complex rehabilitation aims to:

- Achieve optimal functional adaptation, i.e. development of proper techniques facilitating swallowing and improved mobility of a structurally changed tongue
- Improve speech comprehensibility under anatomically altered conditions, mostly by finding substitute places of articulation and exercising lip and tongue practice with the help of a speech pathologist
- Achieve emotional and social adaptation

The rehabilitation programme should encompass the mobility improvement of the mutilated tongue, tongue base and mouth floor (Matsui et al. 2007). The aims include reduction of articulatory difficulties or development of substitute articulation with the surgically altered articulation structures, slowed pace of speech, improved phonatory-articulatory-respiratory coordination, successful management of sialorrhea during articulation and exercising the chewing and the yawning (Bachher et al. 2002; Halczy-Kowalik 2006).

Early rehabilitation within the first 3 months after surgery is most effective in terms of improving the competence of articulation movements and increasing the strength and proper cooperation of muscle groups as well as of proprioceptive control.

8.13.5 Rehabilitation of Oropharyngeal Swallowing Disorders After Head and Neck Surgery

Surgical interventions for head and neck tumours may lead to difficulty in swallowing (dysphagia) due to morphological defects in the oral cavity and the pharynx and the surrounding nerves. In addition, radiotherapy, especially postsurgery, can further deteriorate swallowing by changing the biophysical properties of the affected tissues: dryness, swelling and no sensibility. Oral and pharyngeal phases of swallowing are disturbed, leading to limited food and liquid intake, poor nutrition and hydration and reduced life quality (Pruszewicz et al. 1995; Rademaker et al. 1993). Aspiration of foods and liquids, the cause of aspiration pneumonia, is the main threat of oropharyngeal dysphagia. Mechanisms to prevent aspiration are velopharyngeal closure, upward-backward tongue pushing towards the posterior wall of the pharynx and upward and forward movement of the hyoid bone with the larynx, with accompanying closing of the laryngeal inlet. Pharyngeal peristalsis, synchronised with reflexive relaxation of the superior pharyngeal constrictor muscle, enables a smooth pharyngeal phase that lasts approximately 1 s. The concept of tactile feedback assumes that the mechanism of swallowing is elicited by stimulation of afferent receptors. Proneness to aspiration is highly individual. Aspiration pneumonia is fostered by poor overall health condition, compromised immune response, lack of oral hygiene and history of pulmonary diseases. The so-called 'silent', asymptomatic aspiration is estimated to affect approximately 40% of patients (Schröter-Morasch 1996). Recurrent aspiration pneumonia is observed in 40–70% of patients after conservation laryngectomy (Miller and Eliachar 1994). Disturbances of the oropharyngeal phase of swallowing after surgical intervention for oral cavity and pharyngeal tumours are mostly connected with the prolongation of the oral phase and food accumulation (Logemann 1995).

The excision of the same structures within the oral cavity neither results in identical swallowing disorders nor guarantees the development of the same compensation mechanisms. Functional rehabilitation of swallowing in head and neck tumour cases encompasses causal, compensatory and adaptive therapy (Denk-Linnert 2006). Causal therapy exercises are designed to regulate muscle tension, to restore higher integration activities as well as to limit or eliminate pathological reflexes while simultaneously making way for physiological reflexes. Respiratory, phonatory and articulatory exercises ought to be implemented. Causal therapy consists of passive stimulation, mobilisation techniques and autonomic motor exercises (Denk-Linnert and Bigenzahn 2005). Various forms of stimulation, from stretching, rhythmic vibration, brush or thermal simulation (Logemann 1995), are applied. Mobilisation techniques, initially performed with the help of a speech pathologist, aim to elicit muscle contraction, increase muscle power and restore motor coordination. The exercises are later continued by the patient, who uses the articulation of sounds to strengthen the mechanism of closing the mouth and raising the tongue. Compensatory exercises aim to facilitate swallowing and prevent aspiration by changing the position of the body or using certain swallowing manoeuvres. Proper head position allows reducing or preventing aspiration in approximately 81% of cases (Denk-Linnert and Bigenzahn 2005).

The most common head positions include:

- Chin tuck—the airway entrance is narrowed by pushing the tongue base and the larynx backwards.
- Head back—relaxes the pharyngeal constrictor muscles and entry to the oesophagus.
- Head turn or head rotation—turning to the damaged site allows to 'switch off' the piriform sinus (Logemann 1995), which is often accompanied by the position in which the head is inclined forwards.
- Head tilt to the intact or stronger side.
- Lying down on the side or back.

Adaptive techniques include proper diet, use of special spoons and dishes for placing food in the undamaged parts of the oral cavity as well as intra-oral prostheses closing palatal defects. Swallowing rehabilitation after head and neck tumour surgery should start with a detailed conversation with the patient before the surgical procedure, explaining the extent of post-operative disturbances and ways of compensation (Pauloski et al. 2000). It requires a close cooperation of the laryngologist, phoniatrician and speech pathologist. The training ought to start after wound healing. Although proneness to aspiration varies from patient to patient, tube feeding is necessary in cases of prolonged recovery. The nasogastric feeding tube hinders the rehabilitation process and should be used no longer than 1 month. Factors that significantly influence the rehabilitation outcome include large anatomical defects, especially in the oral cavity, overall health status of patients, concomitant diseases, especially chronic pulmonary diseases, elderly age and psychological status (lack of motivation and limited cooperation with the patient). Regular rehabilitation of dysphagia after head and neck tumour surgery is an essential part of improving patients' quality of life.

8.13.6 Quality of Life in Patients After Head and Neck Surgery

The quality of life in patients treated for cancer, including oncological surgery, seems as important as the 5-year survival rate. The effects of voice rehabilitation, speech and deglutition influence their everyday life largely. The assessment of patients' life quality is also a measure of the rehabilitation outcome. Apart from biological aspects, social and emotional factors play a vital role in the process of recovery (Maune et al. 2005). Thus, scales determining the quality of life and describing individual experiences of patients connected to various diseases and conditions (*HRQOL, health-related quality of life*, Patrick and Erickson 1988; Guillemin et al. 1993; *VRQOL, voice-related quality of life*, Hogikyan and Sethuraman 1999) have found their place in the total evaluation of patient well-being and health. Psychology, oncology, phoniatrics and laryngology utilise various scales and standardised tests to measure the quality of patient life. The *University of Washington Quality of Life—head and neck cancer questionnaire (UW-QOL)* is the most tumour-specific example. This questionnaire had in version 1 9 domains (pain, activity, recreation, employment, disfigurement, speech, swallowing, chewing and shoulder function) and in version 4, 12 (pain, appearance, activity, recreation, swallowing, chewing, speech, shoulder, taste, saliva, mood, anxiety). Each of the dysfunctions may be graded from 0 (worst) to 100 (best) (Rogers et al. 2002, 2010).

The above-mentioned less detailed questionnaires on the relation between deteriorating life quality and overall health conditions include *HRQOL* and *VRQOL*. The questionnaires, comprising ten questions, measure the number of voice problems in different life situations, rated on a 5-point scale according to Likert (1, no complaints, 5, severe discomfort). Psychologists working with cancer patients use, among others, the Mental Adjustment to Cancer Scale, whereas the *Voice Handicap Index (VHI)* (see Sect. 6.2) is commonly applied in phoniatrics.

A large number of laryngectomised patients report anosmia, which is the result of absent nasal airflow, among complaints about life quality. Olfaction can be restored by performing additional muscle exercises (tongue, palate and cheeks) to produce negative intra-oral pressure that induces airflow to the nasal cavity through the nasopharynx. The 'polite yawn' technique, resembling yawning in a public situation and consisting in closed-mouth lowering and lifting of the jaw, seems to be the best method in such cases. The pressure in the oral cavity forces the air to travel through the nostrils.

A growing number of laryngectomised patients, particularly young people, have created the need to seek other forms of social rehabilitation apart from substitute voice and speech. Thus, Laryngectomee Clubs were founded in various clinical centres. Their mission is to offer access to physical, psychological, social and professional rehabilitation, as well as rehabilitation camps, social and legal service, training and workshops for rehabilitation instructors and volunteers.

8.14 Vocal Rehabilitation of Laryngectomised Patients by Personalised Computer Speech Synthesis

Jan Romportl, Barbora Řepová, and Jan Betka

8.14.1 Introduction

As voice is produced by passing air through the vocal cords, any pathology in this area might result in change of the voice quality or even in temporary or permanent voice loss. Laryngeal cancer is a generalised term that includes carcinoma of the supraglottal, glottal and subglottal structures. Squamous cell carcinoma is the most common pathology, and, despite the fact that the number of cases of laryngeal carcinoma has slightly decreased (Braakhuis et al. 2014), it is still a burning problem in cancer surgery. Although there are other perspectives in the treatment of laryngeal cancer in some of those cases, such as endoscopic laser resection or partial laryngectomies, when clinical findings are very serious, performing total laryngectomy is unavoidable to save the patient's life. Apart from many other problems related to this procedure, one of the more limiting results for the patients is that they lose their ability to produce voice. This loss significantly handicaps them and makes communication with others very problematical.

8.14.2 Text-to-Speech Synthesis

Methods and applications of computer text-to-speech (TTS) synthesis can be utilised to improve a patient's quality of life after he or she loses the ability to speak naturally using his or her own voice.

TTS system is a computer system that converts arbitrary written text into its corresponding acoustic (spoken) form in a similar (and preferably the same) way as a human would do. In other words, the input of a TTS system is text, and the output is speech. Applications of TTS systems range from email or SMS reading, telephone customer service and public announcement systems to screen readers for visually impaired and many others.

There is quite a wide range of commercial TTS systems available nowadays. Most of them generate very natural synthetic speech in a news reading style, i.e. speech that is in many cases almost indistinguishable from neutral and non-expressive speech of a real human speaker. Some of the state-of-the-art systems also offer a limited range of expressive or emotional speech features. Synthetic speech available today is thus far away from generally well known 'robotic' voices of early digital synthesisers from the 1980s. The first goal of TTS research and development—*intelligibility* of synthesised speech—was achieved almost two decades ago. The efforts in the last decade have focused mainly on the second goal—*naturalness* of synthesised speech—which is still a major open issue, especially for expressive speech. Finally, a significant part of the most recent research focuses on the third goal—*personalisation* of TTS systems, i.e. their ability to mimic voices of ordinary human speakers easily and accurately.

It is the third goal that plays a very important role for the laryngectomised patients because it enables them to keep and use their original voice, albeit in an external device.

8.14.3 Speaker Modelling

Before a TTS system can be deployed and can actually read anything, its voice or voices must be created. Like many other modern speech technologies, TTS systems utilise methods of artificial intelligence (such as machine learning, pattern recognition, automatic classification, etc.) and automatic processing of real human speech data.

A voice of a TTS system is usually based on speech recordings of a real human speaker. A collection of these speech recordings is called a *speech corpus*. In most of the standard situations (especially for commercial TTS applications), such a corpus is recorded in a sound studio by a professional voice talent who is trained to speak consistently throughout the whole recording process and who is skilled at proper pronunciation and prosody. The speaker reads aloud the sentences one by one as they are textually presented on the screen of a recording computer.

We can informally say that the more sentences the speaker is able to record, the better the resulting synthetic voice. Therefore, most of the contemporary TTS systems aiming for high synthetic voice naturalness (they utilise the so-called *unit selection* speech synthesis algorithms) usually create the voices from corpora comprising at least 10,000 recorded sentences. Even though these speech corpora are then processed by the aforementioned automatic artificial intelligence algorithms, it is still a very costly and resource-demanding process to build a new voice because it puts high demands on the speaker who often has to record the corpus full-time for several weeks. Moreover, expert manual post-processing of the speech corpus is needed as well—for example, from time to time, the speaker unconsciously reads something slightly different from what was presented to him or her in the textual form, or he or she has a specific or incorrect pronunciation in some places; so all these issues must be detected and corrected by an expert going through the corpus once it is recorded (e.g. if possible, the underlying textual form of the sentence is changed so that it conforms to what the patient actually recorded, otherwise the sentence is excluded from future processing).

A synthetic voice created this way is thus a model of the original human voice. The quality and naturalness of this model can vary significantly depending on many factors (quality of the source speaker and the corpus are among the most crucial ones), but we can say that in state-of-the-art systems nowadays, synthetic voices mimic (model) their original speakers very accurately, well capturing their characteristic speaking style and even potential pathologies in pronunciation.

For speech communication of a laryngectomised patient, it means that he or she can use (cf. Sect. 8.14.5) a device equipped with such a generic (i.e. non-personalised) TTS system, which can indeed positively influence the restoration of the patient's communication skills and social interactions. However, using the voice of some other person in everyday communication can be inconvenient for many patients as they gradually recover from their primary disease and start to resume their social and other roles interrupted by the disease; some patients even report this substitution of their own voice as embarrassing (Zahoor et al. 2011). Other studies also discuss deteriorating effects of losing personalised vocal identity, especially in cases where group membership is important (Hetzroni and Harris 1996).

Therefore, it is becoming increasingly important to endorse effective mutual interaction and cooperation between primary medical treatment processes and ongoing advances in TTS research and development, because this offers a possibility for 'digital conservation' of the patient's original voice for his or her future speech communication, a procedure called *voice banking* (or voice conservation).

8.14.4 Current Implementations of Voice Banking

The advantage of the aforementioned unit selection TTS method is its ability to generate synthetic speech almost indistinguishable from real human speech. The main drawback is—apart from its prosody and style inflexibility—the enormous demands on the quality of the speaker (cf. Sect. 8.14.3) and the size of the corpus. However, if we face the task of voice banking of a patient, we usually lack both of these. A typical interval between diagnosis of laryngeal cancer, its staging and indication for total laryngectomy

and surgery itself is approximately 2 weeks, and because the surgery is life-saving, any delay might have severe consequences. It is thus impossible to record more than several hundred sentences, and there is hardly any chance to perform the process in a professional sound studio. The patient also usually has very little or no experience with speech recording, and his or her voice in most cases is already significantly damaged at that point (strong hoarseness, improperly functioning vocal cords, etc.), which makes it quite unlikely that a standard unit selection TTS system with the patient's low-quality speech corpus could be used.

On the other hand, if the patient is fit enough to perform recording for several days with a relatively clear and healthy voice, still unaffected by the disease (a typical patient is, e.g. in an early stage of amyotrophic lateral sclerosis), at least moderate success can be achieved with the recording process. A diphone unit selection speech synthesis is offered by the project ModelTalker (Bunnell et al. 2010), which the patient can join and perform recording from his or her home (English only).

Recent progress in the field of speech synthesis research has brought the possibility of voice banking even for the patients who are about to be laryngectomised and whose disease progression does not allow for unit selection TTS. A statistical model-based speech synthesis technique called *HMM synthesis* (Hidden Markov Model synthesis, cf. (Zen et al. 2009)) offers higher synthetic voice flexibility while requiring significantly smaller speech corpora from the source speakers (patients). Moreover, HMM synthesis can be more successfully used in situations when only speech data recorded in low quality are available. This is so because the unit selection TTS synthesises speech by direct concatenation of acoustic speech units (usually phone- or syllable-sized), whereas HMM synthesis works with unit *models* statistically expressing the time sequence of acoustic data that are likely to be produced when the speech unit is uttered. We can say that HMM synthesis achieves somewhat less natural synthetic speech than unit selection for large high-quality speech corpora, but it definitely outperforms unit selection in the case of smaller medium- and low-quality speech corpora.

Initial experiments with HMM synthesis and voice banking of laryngectomised patients have been reported by Zahoor et al. (2011) for English and by Hanzlíček et al. (2012) for the Czech language. Both papers show very promising results encouraging further research and development of HMM synthesis voice banking for laryngectomised patients. The main difference between the two reports is that the former evaluates synthetic voice on the basis of a tiny set (only 7 min of speech) of very low-quality short home-made recordings of the patient (still giving relatively good results), whereas the latter aims at a long-term project of establishing standardised and professionally attended voice banking of laryngectomised patients as a part of their treatment directly at the clinic. We hold that both efforts should be combined in order to offer the best possible results to the patients. Another very important effort that must be mentioned here is the 'Edinburgh Voice Banking Project' coordinated by the Centre for Speech Technology Research at the University of Edinburgh (Yamagishi et al. 2012)—even though it aims primarily at HMM-based voice banking of motor neuron disease patients, its theoretical and practical outcomes can certainly be utilised for the laryngectomy patients as well.

The research and development effort related to the report (Hanzlíček et al. 2012) is a part of a pilot project jointly realised by the Department of Cybernetics, University of West Bohemia (CYB UWB), together with the Department of Otorhinolaryngology and Head and Neck Surgery, University Hospital Motol (ENT Motol), coordinated by the Department of Man-Machine Interaction, University of West Bohemia. The goal of this project is to build a research and development infrastructure and workflow facility for establishing a rapid voice banking and personalised TTS as a standard procedure of care and treatment of laryngectomised patients. Such a strategy can save the patients' voices in much

higher quality and improve their quality of life significantly more, than in cases of uncoordinated and hasty low-quality speech recording.

The voice banking procedure at ENT Motol is based on early identification of suitable patients when they are examined by their respective physicians. The patients are then sent to a medical doctor responsible for the project coordination at ENT Motol (this member of the clinic staff has a basic level of training in the field of speech technologies, acquired as a part of the internship at CYB UWB) who provides them with further instructions and manages the process of their recording. The recording itself takes place at an audiometric laboratory at ENT Motol, which is a sound-isolated room, and it is supervised by a trained nurse.

The recording set consists of 700 sentences selected from newspaper texts by an algorithm maximising phonetic coverage. The patients are instructed to read as many sentences as possible, by using a plain PC with a headset microphone and recording software developed at CYB UWB. The software guides the patients through the recording process and performs basic acoustic checks of the recorded sentences. The recorded corpus is then passed to CYB UWB where it is manually checked by an expert (cf. Sect. 8.14.3), and then an HMM-based synthetic voice is built by a set of semi-automatic algorithms. The whole process takes several weeks, but it can be significantly accelerated, which is mostly a matter of human resources.

So far, only informal feedback has been gathered from the involved laryngectomised patients (a formal quality-of-life study is being undertaken), but we can already say that it serves as a proof of concept because the patients and their families subjectively report a very positive attitude towards the recording process as well as towards the resulting personalised TTS system as the patients' assistive tool. Conclusions from the feedback can be summarised as follows:

- The patients complained that the sentences were too long and difficult to read without a mistake. This led to modifications of the sentence selection algorithm—the sentences will be shorter and phonetically easier to read, and the set will comprise more of them, thus making the process more convenient for the patients.

- The recording sessions were too long, and some patients experienced an enormous drop in their voice quality as they were progressing through the session, making some part of the corpus unsuitable for synthetic voice building. Therefore, the medical doctor responsible for the voice banking shall assess the patient's capability of speech recording in advance and, whenever needed, suggest more, shorter sessions separated by longer pauses.
- Some patients were interested in synthetic 'voice enhancement'. Since their voice was already so badly damaged during the process of recording, they asked if their synthetic voice model could be enhanced and restored to its healthy state. This can be partially achieved by various statistical voice modelling techniques, and further research will focus on it.
- A strategy for radically preventive voice banking should be developed. Patients whose disease has not yet developed to the stage of total laryngectomy yet but has a potential for it will be informed by their physicians of the possibility to join the voice banking programme as a pre-emptive strategy before their voice is affected by the disease. However, this issue has strong psychological and ethical implications which must be dealt with.

It is important to mention that the recovering laryngectomised patients who have not joined the programme in time (before their surgery) can still have their own personalised TTS system, as long as they are able to provide suitable speech recordings (e.g. lecture recordings, reading children's stories, etc.). However, in the case where a patient does not join the programme in time, the chances of building a satisfactory natural synthetic voice are significantly lower than in the case of the aforementioned standardised voice banking procedure, because it is quite rare for most of the patients to have really suitable speech recordings from their previous life.

8.14.5 Usage Scenarios

An important impulse for TTS systems as an assistive tool for everyday communication of laryngectomised patients has been given by the recent development and market expansion of portable computers, specifically smartphones and tablets. These devices enable the patients to have a personalised TTS system always at hand.

In addition to the overall synthetic voice quality, the most important aspect of such a TTS system application is its *user interface*, i.e. a set of features allowing the user to control textual input of the system effectively. It is quite clear that a plain text keyboard is not sufficient in many cases because it is too inconvenient and time-consuming for the patient to type in, letter by letter, all the utterances he or she wants to use in various communicative situations. Therefore, it is very useful to enhance the TTS system by a smart user interface, typically comprising adaptive and predictive keyboards (using statistical methods to offer continuation of phrases automatically while adapting to the user's typical behaviour), predefined scenarios and situations (e.g. in a shop, at the doctor's, etc.) or features of the so-called concept-to-speech synthesis (the production of synthetic speech on the basis of pragmatic, semantic and discourse knowledge, with reduced or eliminated need for textual typing, by using, e.g. graphical icons or other suitable representations, including various multimodal inputs).

The ongoing research also focuses on development of alternative TTS inputs, such as an automatic speech recognition (ASR) system modified for very silent (almost non-audible) electrolaryngeal speech produced by a specially designed electrolarynx and recorded by a non-audible murmur microphone (Hanzlíček et al. 2012). With this system, a laryngectomised patient could control the TTS system almost in the same way as those speaking normally.

However, this research is still at a very experimental level.

There is a variety of usage scenarios of personalised TTS systems for laryngectomised patients, and which is chosen depends on many factors, such as the individual attitude of the patients and their ability to learn and adapt to technologies, the success of the particular voice banking process, but also financial resources. One of the scenarios can be that a patient who joins the voice banking programme receives before the surgery a tablet with the TTS system comprising one or more generic synthetic voices. While waiting for the surgery, the patient can familiarise himself or herself with the TTS system and its user interface, and he or she can customise it to suit his or her needs. The user interface should also offer a very simplified mode of control comprising large touchscreen buttons with predefined utterances that can be used for communication with healthcare staff and family members in the first hours after surgery when the patient is still disorientated and confused and cannot type his or her own utterances.

As the patient gradually recovers, he or she can use more sophisticated features of the system and generate more complex synthesised utterances. After a period of several weeks, the patient receives the first version of his or her personal synthetic voice, which is installed on the patient's tablet. The patient can start to familiarise himself or herself with this voice and provide feedback on it while still being able to switch to the generic TTS voices if needed. The personalised synthetic voice can then be continuously improved on the basis of the patient's feedback and needs.

Acknowledgement The research leading to these results has received funding from the Norwegian Financial Mechanism 2009–2014 and the Ministry of Education, Youth and Sports of the Czech Republic under Project Contract no. MSMT-28477/2014, Project no. 7F14236, 'Naturalness in Human Cognitive Enhancement (HCENAT)'.

8.15 Indications for Tracheostomy and Tracheostoma Care

Berit Schneider-Stickler

8.15.1 Background

Tracheostomy is one of the older and more commonly performed surgical procedures. It was first documented as early as 1000 BC in Egypt. Several authors refer to the Ebers Papyrus of Egypt, dated around 1550 BC (Stock 1987). In 1620, Habicot published the first book on tracheostomy (Eavey 1998).

Tracheostoma care has traditionally been specific to specialised areas, e.g. otolaryngology and intensive care units (ICU) (Heafield et al. 1999).

The procedure has evolved from routinely being performed surgically in an operating room (surgical tracheostomy, ST) to one that has become attractive to be performed bedside in the intensive care unit (ICU) (open bedside tracheostomy, OBT) by surgeons or by anaesthesiologists/intensivists as percutaneous dilational tracheostomy (PDT).

So far it is surprising that there is so little agreement regarding such simple aspects as definition, time and type of tracheostomy, choice of tube, tracheostoma care and the removal process (decannulation).

8.15.2 Definition Tracheo(s)tomy

Tracheostomy is a surgical procedure to create an opening into the anterior wall of the trachea.

It can basically be performed in three ways:

- The opening of the trachea without any skin flap to the tracheal wall
- Surgical opening of the trachea with suturing the skin flaps onto the tracheal wall (epithelialisation)
- Permanent stoma in the neck after total laryngectomy

There is still a debate about the terminology. Both words, tracheotomy and tracheostomy, have been usually used interchangeably in the literature.

Both words have a Greek origin. Tracheotomy signifies a temporary opening of the trachea. Tracheostomy has its origin from the word *stom-* (from Greek στόμα, 'mouth'), which implies a permanent opening in the neck by suturing skin flaps onto the tracheal wall (Mitchell et al. 2013). A 'tracheostoma' is the result of both procedures: a hole in the upper anterior trachea, with trachea and larynx remaining in place, and as the result of laryngectomy.

8.15.3 Indications

The decision to perform a tracheostomy in critical patients should be adapted to each patient and pathology, balancing the situation of the patient, expected recovery process, risk of continued endotracheal intubation and surgical risk of the procedure.

Medical indications for tracheostomy include:

- Mechanical upper airway obstruction (see Table 8.4)
- Electively performed tracheostomy in major head and tumour surgeries, to avoid post-operative complications due to risk of temporary airway obstruction and swallowing problems with aspiration
- Protection of the lower airway from aspiration and access to the tracheobronchial tree for secretion removal in case of aspiration (Table 8.5)
- Respiratory failure with failure of extubation and need for prolonged ventilation (prolonged weaning) as tracheostomy reduces dead space by 50% and results in less effort in breathing and increased alveolar ventilation (Table 8.6)

Table 8.5 Protection of the lower airway from aspiration

Aetiology	Examples of pathology
Neurological	Polyneuritis, motor neuron disease, bulbar poliomyelitis, multiple sclerosis, brainstem stroke, apallic syndrome
Comatose	Head injury, brain tumour
Traumatic	Severe facial fractures

Table 8.6 Indication for tracheostomy due to respiratory failure

Aetiology	Examples of pathology
Pulmonary diseases	Acute pneumonia, exacerbation of chronic bronchitis and emphysema
Neurological diseases	Multiple sclerosis, motor neuron disease
Trauma	Severe chest injury

8.15.4 Types of Tracheostomy

Traditionally the tracheostomy has been performed in the operating room.

There are many ways to perform a tracheostomy, which can be classified into several general approaches. One common division of techniques is 'open' or surgical tracheostomy (ST), and the other is 'percutaneous' or percutaneous dilational tracheostomy (PDT). For ICU patients, the surgical tracheostomy is preferably performed under bedside conditions as open bedside tracheostomy (OBT) owing to the hazard of moving intubated critically ill patients to the operating room.

Table 8.4 Causes of mechanical upper airway obstruction as indication for tracheostomy

Aetiology	Examples of pathology
Congenital	Subglottal or upper tracheal stenosis, laryngeal synechia, laryngeal malformation, laryngeal haemangioma
Infectious	Acute epiglottitis, pseudocroup and croup coughing, Ludwig's angina
Malignant	Advanced tumour stages of larynx, pharynx, tongue and upper trachea or another oncogenesis into the upper trachea
Traumatic	Inhalation trauma of steam or smoke, blunt (stranglehold) or open (gunshot, knife) laryngeal trauma
Paralytic	Bilateral vocal fold paralysis after thyroidectomy, bulbar palsy
Obstructive	Inhaled foreign bodies in upper airway

Fig. 8.34 (**a–c**)
Common techniques of
surgical tracheostomy

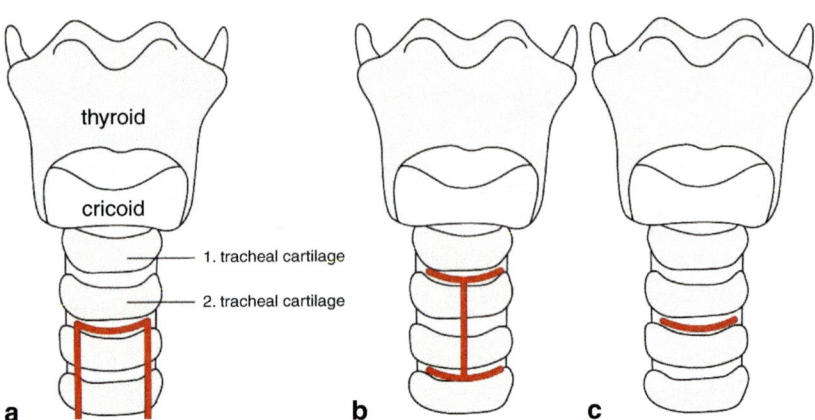

thyroid

cricoid

1. tracheal cartilage

2. tracheal cartilage

a   b   c

8.15.4.1 Surgical Tracheostomy

The surgical tracheostomy is usually performed under either general or local anaesthesia by a general surgeon/otolaryngologist/head and neck surgeon (Lindman et al. 2017).

Most common techniques of surgical tracheostomy are (Fig. 8.34):

- Surgical tracheostomy with a Björk flap (Fig. 8.34a)
- Surgical tracheostomy with an H-flap (Fig. 8.34b)
- Visor-shaped surgical tracheostomy (Fig. 8.34c)
- Tracheostomy after laryngectomy

During surgical tracheostomy, the thyroid isthmus is usually divided for better exposure of the trachea (middle tracheostomy). As an alternative, instead of transecting the isthmus, one may retract it, thus enabling better wound healing. In these cases, depending on the topographic situation, the surgeon decides upon opening the trachea above the isthmus (superior/upper tracheostomy) or below (inferior/lower tracheostomy).

The skin incision can be performed either horizontally or vertically. The horizontal incision has better cosmetic outcome after decannulation, but the vertical approach is discussed as having better functional results owing to unimpaired laryngeal elevation during swallowing and phonation.

8.15.4.2 Percutaneous Dilational Tracheostomy

The percutaneous dilational tracheostomy is by definition the placement of a tracheostomy tube with the help of commercially available sets. The technique with serial dilators was introduced by Ciaglia in 1985 (Ciaglia et al. 1985). The dilating tracheostomy forceps were developed in 1989 (Schachner et al. 1989). In 1990 Griggs introduced the use of a guidewire (Griggs et al. 1990).

The percutaneous technique of tracheostomy is meanwhile standard in many intensive care units worldwide. It completes the range of airway techniques available to anaesthesiologists and intensivists.

The most commonly used kits for percutaneous dilational tracheostomy are:

- PerkuTwist
- Blue Rhino (Ciaglia)
- Blue Dolphin (Ciaglia)

The PDT is the preferred method of anesthesiologists and performed bedside in intensive care units under general anaesthesia. Usually a bronchoscopy/endoscopy is necessary to follow the right puncture level, which should be below at least the first tracheal cartilage or even lower. The cricoid and the first or better the first two tracheal cartilages should be preserved. Fractures of a tracheal cartilage should be avoided.

8.15.4.3 Comparison of Surgical Tracheostomy and Percutaneous Dilational Tracheostomy

Both techniques, open surgical tracheostomy and percutaneous tracheostomy, have been compared intensively for the incidence of complications including bleeding, infection and tracheal stenosis. A recently published randomised clinical trial on 60 ICU patients revealed similar complications concerning copious bleeding, stomal infection, subcutaneous emphysema and airway problems (Valizade Hasanloei et al. 2014). Kettunen et al. performed a 10-year review on 616 trauma patients undergoing tracheostomy (Kettunen et al. 2014). Tracheal stenosis could be found in only four patients (1.1%) from the percutaneous group and five patients (1.9%) from the surgical group ($P = 0.509$). Thus, tracheal stenosis has not been regarded as being of high risk and should not have an impact on the decision whether to perform a surgical or percutaneous tracheostomy.

However, clinical practice shows a higher potential risk of intra- and post-operative complications (i.e. bleeding) due to the relatively blind nature of the procedure. Percutaneous tracheostomy can be performed as a bedside procedure, avoiding any risk from moving a patient to the operating theatre. Therefore, it is ideal for ICU patients. Advantages and disadvantages of percutaneous tracheostomy in comparison with surgical tracheostomy are listed in Table 8.7.

8.15.5 Early Versus Late Tracheostomy

Expected prolonged mechanical ventilation is one of the major indications for tracheostomy. Controversy regarding the optimal timing still exists. In 1989, the American College of Chest Physicians (ACCP) Consensus Conference on Artificial Airways in Patients Receiving Mechanical Ventilation argued that a tracheos-

Table 8.7 Advantages and disadvantages of percutaneous tracheostomy in comparison with surgical tracheostomy (modified after Paw and Bodenham 2004)

	Percutaneous tracheostomy in comparison with surgical tracheostomy
Advantages	• Can be performed more easily at the bedside • Avoids delays from unavailability of theatre session and surgeon • Minimal staff required • No risk from transferring patients to theatre • More cost-effective • Time effective • Better cosmetic outcome
Disadvantages	• Occasional severe major bleeding • Unproven in emergency situations • Safety in anatomical abnormalities uncertain • Safety in children unclear • Difficulties in replacing dislodged tracheal cannula early after insertion

tomy is indicated in the case of an anticipated need for mechanical ventilation longer than 21 days (Plummer and Gracey 1989). The European Consensus in 1998 followed with the recommendation to prefer a tracheostomy if the mechanical ventilation was anticipated for 10–21 days.

However, there is no common definition for what is considered early or late tracheostomy. Although inconsistent, recent studies state that early tracheostomy seems to be associated with a shorter duration of mechanical ventilation and shorter length of stay at the ICU (Griffiths et al. 2005; Higgins and Punthakee 2007; Oliver et al. 2007).

Recently, observational studies reported that tracheostomy is nowadays preferably performed on day 11 (range 5–19) after intubation (Esteban et al. 2000).

Meanwhile, early tracheostomy is defined if the procedure is performed within 4 or 5–9 days after endotracheal intubation and late tracheostomy if it is performed after 10 days (Griffiths et al. 2005; Bickenbach et al. 2011).

8.15.6 Tracheal Tube

In the literature and clinical practice, the terms tracheal tube and tracheal cannula are used interchangeably. In European countries, the term tracheal tube might be preferred.

According to indications for tracheostomy, functions of a tracheal tube include:

- Possibility of positive pressure ventilation
- Protection of aspiration
- Bypassing an upper airway obstruction
- Extraction capability in case of aspiration

The shape of a tracheostomy tube is designed to allow correct positioning into the trachea. The entry angle is of special importance, as an incorrect angle may endanger the positioning for mechanical ventilation. Further, an incorrect angle can cause irritation and trauma to the tracheal mucosa.

Tracheostomy tubes are available in a variety of lengths, diameters and materials. Special designs and a high number of additional attachments should meet individual needs of the patients.

8.15.6.1 Types and Characteristics of Tracheal Tubes

Different styles of tracheostomy cannula can be categorised as:

- Cuffed
- Uncuffed
- Fenestrated
- Variable length
- Single-lumen tubes
- Double-lumen tubes
- Subglottal suctioning

Important clinical parts of a tracheostomy cannula are demonstrated in Fig. 8.35.

It is important to know that manufacturers of tracheostomy tubes use either the outer diameter of the upper end or the inner diameter of the lower end of the outer cannula. Sizes of tubes from different manufacturs thus cannot be compared.

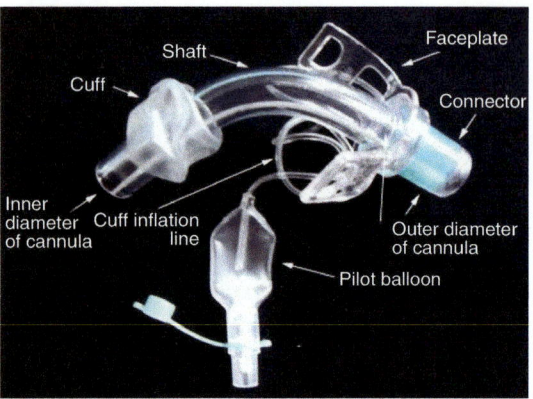

Fig. 8.35 Description of a tracheostomy cannula, in this example: Tracheotec® Vario Cuff, cuffed unfenestrated tracheostomy cannula without inner cannula. With kind permission from Company Andreas Fahl Medizintechnik-Vertrieb GmbH, Cologne, Germany

For selection of a tracheal tube size, it is important to consider whether a neonate, a paediatric or an adult patient is to be equipped. In neonates and children, several aspects have to be taken into consideration: size, weight, physical development and tracheal condition.

In women the outer diameter of the tracheal cannula should not be larger than 10 mm, in men not larger than 11 mm.

In case of a too large outer diameter of the cannula, the tracheal mucosa can be damaged; in case of a too small outer and inner diameter, higher ventilation pressure is mandatory.

According to design, material and purpose tracheostomy cannulae can be divided into:

- Metal tubes (made from silver) and medical-grade polymer tubes (made from silicone, polyvinyl chloride or other medical-grade polymer):
  - Metal tubes are made with thinner walls; thus, the inner diameter and thereby the inner volume of the tube are wider without changing the outer diameter. Disadvantages of silver tubes are stiffness and temperature sensitivity. Metal tubes are not allowed in radiotherapy.
  - Medical-grade polymer tubes are pleasantly light to wear. The material is much more elastic and adaptable with excellent

fitting, ensuring that the trachea is not placed under excessive strain. The visual advantage is transparency of the material.

- Unfenestrated and fenestrated tubes:
  The purpose of the fenestration is to allow airflow upwards for voice production. To achieve the advantage of fenestration, the patient has to use a fenestrated inner cannula; otherwise the unfenestrated inner cannula will block the fenestration. A fenestration is not mandatory to be able to phonate. Speaking is also possible with cuffed tracheal tubes if the cuff is deflated and the air can move around the tube upwards.
- Cuffed and uncuffed tracheal tubes:
  A cuffed tracheostomy tube has to be used in mechanical ventilation and in cases of the need to protect the lower airway from aspiration. The cuff pressure has to be checked thoroughly.
- Cuffed tubes with fenestrated and unfenestrated inner cannulae:
  - This type is recommended in the rehabilitation process of ICU patients if mechanical ventilation can be interrupted by spontaneous ventilation.
  - For mechanical ventilation, the fenestration of the cuffed outer cannula can be blocked by using the unfenestrated inner cannula. If the patient is able to breathe spontaneously, the fenestrated inner cannula can be used, and the cuff should be deflated.

This range of tracheostomy tubes is wide. Nevertheless, tracheostomy tubes should be ideally matched to the requirements of the individual patient.

8.15.6.2   Pressure of the Cuff

The ideal pressure of the cuff should be between 15 and 25 mm Hg in order to ensure sufficient tracheal sealing. Pressure values lower than 15 mm Hg promote the risk of aspiration, although it has been shown that a cuffed tracheal tube cannot avoid aspiration with 100% certainty.

8.15.7   Care of Tracheostomised Patients

The care of tracheostomised patients includes maximum medical care, optimum management of tracheal tube as well as the rehabilitation of voice, speaking and swallowing.

The immediate post-operative period considers standardised phase-specific effective wound treatment. The management can be simplified after epithelisation of the tracheostoma.

Although tracheostomy is one of the more commonly performed surgical procedures, standardised recommendations and guidelines for tracheostomy are quite sparse.

An interdisciplinary team collected recently published papers (Arora et al. 2008; Cetto et al. 2011; Garrubba et al. 2009; Müller and Kramer 2003; Tobin and Santamaria 2008; Kozon and Fortner 2010; Stefan et al. 2012) and developed a proposal for 'Standard Operating Procedure (SOP) of Tracheostomy Care' developed for the Vienna General Hospital and the Vienna Hospital Association. It is available on the intranet of the Vienna General Hospital (Schneider-Stickler et al. 2013). This SOP has been proven by a test phase with 60 patients, and after adaptation of the test results, the SOP has been reviewed by national and international experts. The summary of this SOP is shown in Fig. 8.36.

The SOP stresses the similarities and differences in the medical care of a freshly operated tracheostoma and a tracheostoma after epithelialisation without wound healing problems. It should simplify peristomal cleaning, antiseptic procedures, long-term skin protection, wound dressing and changing intervals of tubes. Further recommendations on suctioning and humidification are also given.

8.15.8   Complications After Tracheostomy

Complications of tracheostomy in ICU patients comprise cuff failure with insufficient tracheal sealing, subcutaneous emphysema, post-operative bleeding, accidental tube displace-

Fig. 8.36 Standard operating procedure for tracheostoma care developed by Schneider-Stickler et al. (2013). Abbreviations: *NaCl* sodium chloride, *HME* heat and moisture exchanger, *ST* surgical tracheostomy, *OBT* open bedside tracheostomy, *PDT* percutaneous dilational tracheostomy, *ICU* intensive care unit

		Freshly-operated tracheostoma	Epithelialised tracheostoma	
	Cannula	Plastic - with cuff	Plastic - without cuff (sterile) - without cuff (cleaned, disinfected)	
	Gloves	Sterile disposable gloves or unsterile disposable gloves using non-touch technique	Unused unsterile disposable gloves using non-touch technique	
	Cleaning	0.9% NaCl solution		
	Antiseptic practice	0.02% polyhexanide	Not infected: No antiseptic	Infected: Call a wound manager
	Long-term skin protection	Cavillon products		
	Wound dressing	Polyurethane foam rubber compress		
	Follow-up	- HME filter - Suture removal 10 days after tracheostomy	- HME filter	
	Change of cannula	<u>First postoperative tube change:</u> - ST/OBT: after 3 days - PDT: after 7 days		

		<u>Following tube changes:</u>
		Cuffed tube:
		  ICU: every 3 days
		  Regular ward: every 3 days in critically ill/ immunocompromised patients
		  Regular ward: every 7 days in non-ill/immunocompromised patients
		Uncuffed tube: daily		

Table 8.8 Classification of tracheal stenosis after tracheostomy and therapeutic options

Type of stenosis	Length and type		Therapy
Soft	Short segment	Apron-like	Bougienage, laser surgery
		Circular	Bougienage
	Long segment	Tracheomalacia	Tracheopexia
Rigid	<4 cm	Hour-shaped	Transverse resection (Pearson)
	>4 cm	Laryngotracheal passage	Transverse resection (Pearson) Open technique (Rethi-plasty) Closed technique

ment, self extubation and airway obstruction due to blood or encrusting of the inner tracheal cannula.

Later on, high cuff pressure and tube dislodgement can cause granuloma tissue formation and tracheal stenosis. Percutaneous dilational tracheostomy can break tracheal cartilages with following scar formation and stenosis of the trachea.

The therapeutic concept considers first of all the type and length of the tracheal stenosis (Table 8.8). The list of surgical options for reconstructive tracheal surgery is long. The table provides an overview on main therapeutic reflections.

8.15.9 Rehabilitation Process and Decannulation

One of the key components of management of tracheostomised patients is the swallowing and speech rehabilitation. The therapist has to identify and manage risk factors that put a patient at risk of aspiration, whereas the patient needs to meet sufficient nutrition and hydration.

The presence of a tracheostomy tube can have impact on laryngeal elevation and pharyngeal enlargement. Ding and Logemann (2005) performed videofluoroscopy in 623 patients after tracheostomy (cuffed/uncuffed). The authors found:

- Prolongated triggering of swallowing
- Reduced tongue functioning
- Reduced strength of tongue
- Reduced laryngeal elevation
- Reduced laryngeal protection and incomplete laryngeal closure
- Dysfunction of upper oesophageal sphincter
- Aspiration

Both authors concluded that:

- The cuff promotes laryngeal fixation and inhibits laryngeal elevation
- The cuff promotes silent aspiration
- Uncuffed tubes obstruct airway and impede reflective coughing
- After tracheostomy, more swallowing problems during oral and pharyngeal stages

Nevertheless, the equipment of a tracheostomised patient with the optimum tracheal tube shortens the rehabilitation process, enables early verbal communication, supports adequate nutrition and improves the quality of life. When the indication for the insertion of a tracheostomy tube has been resolved, the decannulation can be performed. Decannulation is by definition the permanent removal of the tracheal tube.

Criteria for decannulation can be summarised as follows:

- Successful weaning
- Patient alert, responsive and consenting
- Patient can protect airways
- No sign of pneumonia

- Normal oxygen saturation
- Patient tolerates the use of a speaking valve or digital occlusion of tracheal tube
- Reason for tracheostomy resolved

8.16   Prognosis of Voice Rehabilitation

Antoni Pruszewicz, Ilter Denizoglu, and Hanna Czerniejewska-Wolska

8.16.1 Introduction

Fundamentally, the central idea of voice rehabilitation may be defined with the words of an architect (Louis Sullivan): *form follows function.* Motion is a dimension of anatomy; moreover motion and structure are interactive complementary parts of a whole. There are two main goals in voice rehabilitation: anatomical changes (if they exist) and behavioural changes. Any attempt to compensate an anatomical defect must include a functional aspect in order to define a better prognostic outcome of voice rehabilitation. Even if phonosurgery focuses on anatomy, the main philosophy is to restore the function instead of the endoscopic appearance. So it will not be incorrect to say that the phonosurgery is a functional intervention; as the saying goes: *phonosurgery, not photosurgery.* Voice therapy is an indispensable part of the treatment process for an acceptable prognostic outcome.

Prognosis of voice rehabilitation depends on four basic elements: disorder, treatment method, clinician and the patient. Of these, the patient is likely to be the most important *prognostic factor* because the patient ought to be actively involved in (re)habilitation from the beginning to the end.

Prognostic factors that are related to voice therapy may be divided into two groups: internal (patient-related) and external (socio-environmental and clinician-related) factors.

8.16.2 Internal Factors

Internal factors are related to the patient's somatic, neuromotor and psycho-emotional conditions.

8.16.2.1 Degree (Reversibility) and Type of Anatomical or Neurological Disorder of the Primary Voice Organs

The pathology that directly effects voice production primarily determines the prognostic outcome. If the patient has irreversible anatomical or neurological lesions (major laryngeal surgeries such as type 3 cordectomy or partial laryngectomy, uni-/bilateral vocal fold paralyses, etc.), then the prognosis must be realistically assessed and the expected outcome ought to be shared with the patient.

8.16.2.2 General Health Condition and Disorders of Voice-Related Structures

The voice is a mirror that reflects the health of body and soul. Numerous pathological factors may affect phonation; some of them are listed below:

General Health Conditions Age is important from the developmental period to senescence (Kersing and Jennekens 2004); the older someone is, the greater changes in voice may be observed; regeneration capacity and tissue plasticity also decrease with age. The sex or gender of the patient may affect prognosis with their different constitution and hormonal states. Systemic neurological disorders should be well defined through diagnosis of a given voice disorder. General diseases and results of their treatment (diseases such as asthma and of the circulatory system, thyroid and renal, central and peripheral nervous system, hearing organ disturbances and the influence of drugs) also may define prognosis. The presence of absolute and relative contraindications of medications and complementary medicine for the performing voice profession should be well assessed by the clinician.

Mechanical Trauma This is the reflection of a certain amount of physical stress applied to a certain area of vocal fold tissue for a certain duration. So, not only phonating for a long time, or loud phonation for a lesser duration, but also misuse may provide a mechanical trauma to a certain area. For instance, phonation with an hourglass glottal shape creates a high mechanical trauma on the mid-membranous portion of the vocal fold mucosa. Excessive vocal load due to occupational or habitual vocal overuse is a serious deteriorating factor for the voice patient (Vilkman 2004). For call centre workers especially, teachers and some singers, sustainable professional voice depends on a logical vocal usage programme. Voice amplification, self-monitoring and brief vocal training are useful for preventing vocal overuse and misuse. Prognosis of the vocal rehabilitation also depends on daily voice use, out of work, for the occupational voice user.

Chemical Trauma Laryngopharyngeal reflux, persistent tobacco use and inhalation of various chemical vapours directly affect the biomechanical properties of the vocal folds. Reinke's oedema and changes in mucosa and mucus composition lead to changes in the biomechanical properties of vocal folds: not only the microarchitectural change of the vibrating tissue but also the behavioural shift due to altered acoustic feedback affects the phonatory pattern. A patient with Reinke's oedema should stop smoking for a better prognostic outcome.

Respiratory System Problems of the nose, sinuses, oral cavity and lungs may influence subglottal pressure (e.g. chronic obstructive pulmonary disease), alter resonance features of the vocal tract (e.g. chronic rhinosinusitis or velopharyngeal dysfunctions) or alter the biomechanical structure of the vocal folds (e.g. recurrent respiratory papillomatosis) and may each have negative effects on prognosis.

Other Factors Poor dietary habits, sleeping problems, various medications, hormonal state, excessive consumption of caffeine and alcohol and some other factors that may affect vocal use should be taken into account and be considered as prognostic factors.

8.16.2.3 Motor Learning and Neural Plasticity

Learning Styles The auditory, visual, verbal and kinaesthetics of the patients define the feedback composition that the clinician would give through the therapy process. The patient is then ready to process the familiar type of data. If the patient has an aural (auditory-musical) learning style, it helps the prognostic outcome, as it is easier to explain the target voice by auditory feedback (recorded voice, the clinician's imitation of the predicted sound of voice). In the case of a visual (spatial) learning style, it is better to choose declarative pictures or images (endoscopy, stroboscopy, anatomy charts, etc.). Verbal (linguistic) learning calls for using words, both in speech and writing. In physical (kinaesthetic) learning, the clinician may use the sense of touch or the feeling of how to phonate healthily. Patients who use a logical (mathematical reasoning and systematic remarks) type of learning may benefit from simplified explanations of physiopathological pathways including biomechanical and acoustic data.

Motor Learning Principles and Influences These constitute the main pathway for voice therapy applications (Schmidt and Lee 2014). Task orientation, motivation and focusing attention are the most important principles for motor learning that define the prognosis of the rehabilitation. The main influences on motor learning process are pre-practice, practice and feedback:

• *Pre-practice* considerations include the patients' understanding of the rationale, purpose and the technical descriptions of the vocal exercises. The clinician should model and demonstrate the expected phonatory pattern, explain the exercise by verbal instructions and stress the patient's attention to details and the outcomes.
• *Practice* contains a series of vocal exercises repeated in a predefined programme. The clinician should compose the practice programme in concordance with the motor learning process, not incidentally. Variability (blocked/random), timing and intensity of the vocal exercise should be considered in composing the action plan. Last but not least, the patient should spare time for mental practice, not only for short-term clinical outcomes but also for prevention of relapses.

• *Feedback* is another major prognostic factor in the rehabilitation process. This may be intrinsic (internal) or extrinsic (augmented). Intrinsic feedback is about the patient's self-data processing, which is formed by the auditory, visual or kinaesthetic signals that arise during or after the performance of the vocal exercise. The source of the augmented feedback may be a mechanical device (e.g. resonance tube phonation in water), a digital device (graphics of voice analysis) or another person (the clinician, family members or friends). The type of the augmented feedback may be verbal, auditory, visual or kinaesthetic. The augmented feedback supplements and guides the internal feedback (which should be monitored carefully in advance to prevent feedback dependence). The type of cognitive feedback may be partial (during exercise) or summary feedback (promotes self-monitoring and self-correction). The timing of feedback (immediate, delayed, concurrent or terminal) is another influence on motor learning.

Phase-Related Application In this integrative approach, the clinician must consider the patient's situation or motor learning phase. There are three phases (Fitts and Posner 1967) of the whole voice therapy process regarding the motor learning process for a given patient. In the cognitive phase, the clinician provides tools to make the patient understand what is wrong and what, and how and why it, is to be done for rehabilitation. The associative phase is about skill acquisition, and the last phase is transferring the new skill to a behaviour.

Neural Plasticity This is the neuro-organic reflection of the behavioural change through voice therapy. It is the ultimate outcome of vocal behaviour change, and the clinician must be aware of this steady-state phase of the rehabilitation. Acquiring a new skill and transferring it into a behaviour make functional and structural changes in the nervous system. Short-term changes are functional and can be defined as alterations in the efficiency of synaptic connections. On the other hand, long-term changes in the organisation and number of connections among neurons are structural alterations that result in remapping of the sensorymotor cortex. It has been shown by functional MRI that the acquisition of a motor skill and storage of the learning outcome make some anatomical changes to the central nervous system (Musso 1999).

8.16.2.4 Therapeutic Compliance and Adherence

It would be extremely difficult for a voice patient to acquire a new vocal skill and create a new behaviour from this phonatory pattern without receiving any prior knowledge about the skill and whether that knowledge is visual, auditory or kinaesthetic. For example, consider the primal sound which is a fairly complicated and somewhat reflexive motion of the voice system. It would be difficult indeed for a novice voice user to learn such an easy but masked skill in months, if not years. In the cognitive stage, the processing of information takes part by hearing or seeing it from a skilled person or receiving declarative knowledge about how it is performed and how it is felt or heard or even seen. The patient is actively involved in voice rehabilitation, and this reality must be shared with the patient at the beginning of the therapy.

Compliance, adherence and conformity/obedience are indispensable parts of long-term therapies, including the voice therapy process (Stephen et al. 2003), and are probably the most important patient-related factors for the prognosis. Patients ought to understand the problem, the reasons and rationale of the therapy exercises and to accept following the steps; otherwise it is too optimistic to expect a reasonable outcome. Patients who are interested in their voices, and who are motivated for vocal rehabilitation, tend to follow (focus on) treatment recommendations and voice therapy exercises to make improvements and get the best overall long-term results from treatment. Additionally, the clinician should have highly persuasive personal powers and use clinical tools in order to make the patient believe and obey the rules of the treatment for a better prognosis.

8.16.2.5 Psycho-emotional Factors (Stress, Emotion, Coping Strategies, Stages of Change)

The psycho-emotional state of the patient is critical for the prognosis of voice therapy. Psychological aspects—cooperation with the patient, his personality and susceptibility to stress conditions and voice compensation abilities in the course of rehabilitation—define the action plan of the clinician.

Coping strategies (positive/adaptive or negative/maladaptive) and psychological expressions (anxious, depressive, angry, unhappy, introvert, aggressive, theatrical, histrionic, etc.) of the patient play an important role in forming a relationship with the clinician and deciding on a specific therapy technique that will define the prognostic outcome in advance.

Changes in health behaviour have some stages according to the transtheoretical model (TTM) (Prochaska and Diclemente 1986). TTM is an integrative, biopsychosocial model to conceptualise the process of intentional behaviour change. When applying the TTM principles to voice therapy, the first stage is the pre-contemplation stage, in which the patient is not ready for (may even be defensive against) a new voice. In the contemplation stage, awareness of the bad vocal habit is increased, and the patient considers the possibility of changing. In the preparation/determination stage, a commitment is made to make a change. The action (willpower) is the next step; the patient now believes that he or she has the ability to change vocal behaviour and to become actively involved in voice therapy. The stage of maintenance involves stabilising the acquired phonatory habit (the new status quo), but relapses may occur. The last stage (transcendence) is a *new vocal personality* when the patient considers the old vocal behaviour as atypical or abnormal.

Additionally, musical abilities, articulation and expression style of speaking and education history are to be regarded as prognostic factors, especially for professional vocal performers. The action plan for the rehabilitation is structured in a multidimensional approach, including the patient's stage of change, emotional status, coping strategy for the pathology, etc. Thus, the clinician should assess and manipulate the psycho-emotional condition of the voice patient. This is also part of diagnosis and treatment process.

8.16.3 External Factors

External factors are the factors related to the social and physical environment of the voice patient.

8.16.3.1 Clinician's Skills and Capabilities

Voice therapy is not solely composed of applications of certain exercise schedules. The clinician needs to have broad understanding and multilayered/multidimensional thinking that combine mechanisms of the applications, stages of behavioural treatment, phases of motor learning, stages of voice therapy and steps of the technique through the whole process of treatment (Fig. 8.37).

Some personal features of the clinician (humanity, empathy, creativity, patience for repetitive faults and for listening, problem-solving ability, persuasive power) are critical for a successful outcome. The clinician should be open to new knowledge; he or she must continuously develop a better multidimensional approach. For singing voice therapy, additional specifications are needed for a better prognosis, which start from basic musical knowledge, including various musical styles, to a stage (solo, if possible) performance; it is a great advantage for the clinician himself to be trained for singing.

8.16.3.2 Therapy Environment

The sessions of voice therapy should be in a room that is not around noisy places; the walls should be better built from noise-proof and anechoic (hypoechoic) material. A noisy or poorly isolated room can cause distractions.

8.16.3.3 Techniques and Tools

Technique is the tool, not the goal, but the clinician should seek the best possible technique relevant to each individual. Thus, he or she should be familiar with more than one technique. In order to facilitate the rehabilitation process, various mechanical or digital tools may be used for feedback of physical support during therapy.

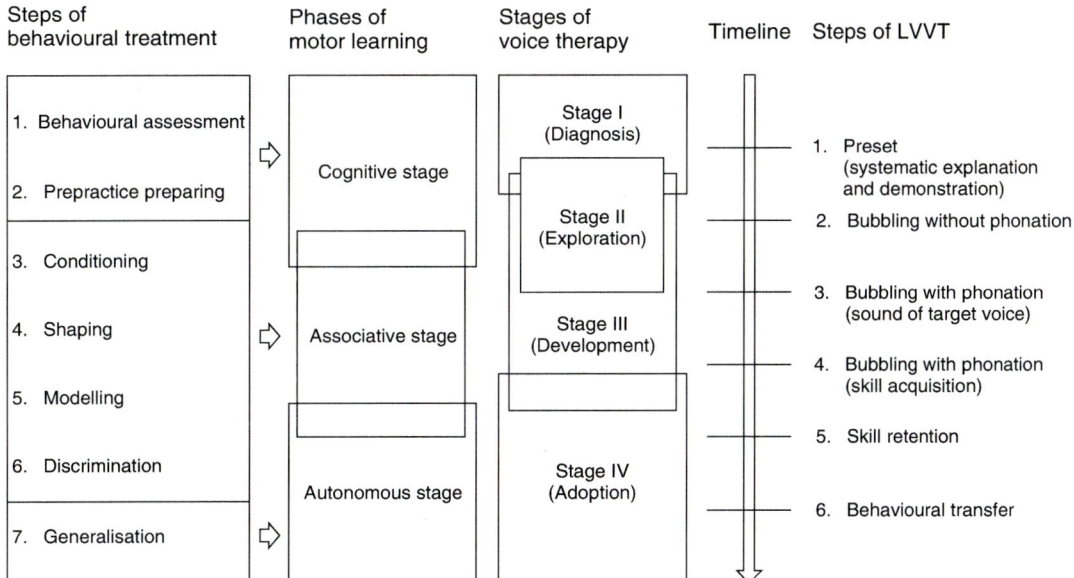

Fig. 8.37 Multidimensional understanding of voice therapy

8.16.3.4 Patient's Social Environment

The family is a dominant prognostic factor in behavioural treatment modalities. Voice has a major influence on person's image, i.e.:

> How your voice is is how the people know you.
> Boone (1994)

Clinicians should take the social environment into account. For example, a puberphonia patient will not use his new sound (generally baritone) if it is not accepted by the family and friends. Habitually, one's personal and social image is affected by voice features, and this perception (of personal image defined by voice) may be manipulated by consulting before the acoustic outcome is obtained by therapy.

8.16.3.5 Occupational Risks

These include environmental noise, poor moisture and air pollution. Excessive occupational vocal overuse must be ruled out by official authorities; otherwise it is not possible to prevent occupational injury. Termination of the rehabilitation process is also a factor that defines the prognosis. If laryngeal appearance has improved, and the patient sounds better or even feels better, rehabilitation may be terminated. One reality should be kept in mind: the prognostic outcome of voice rehabilitation is based on long-term results that are related to neural plasticity and behavioural change. Thus clinical vigilance must be continued even after the therapy applications are completed.

References

Abaza MM, Levy S, Hawkshaw MJ et al (2007) Effects of medications on the voice. Otolaryngol Clin N Am 40(5):1081–1090

Abitbol J, Abitbol P, Abitbol B (1999) Sex hormones and the female voice. J Voice 13(3):424–446

Akhtar S, Wood G, Rubin JS et al (1999) Effect of caffeine on the vocal folds: a pilot study. J Laryngol Otol 113(4):341–345

Alessi DM, Crummey A (2006) Medications: the positive and negative impact on voice. In: Benninger MS, Murry T (eds) The performer's voice. Plural Publishing, San Diego, CA, pp 153–162

Amin MR, Koufman JA (2001) Vagal neuropathy after upper respiratory infection: a viral etiology? Am J Otolaryngol 22(4):251–256

Amir O, Biron-Shental T, Muchnik C et al (2003) Do oral contraceptives improve vocal quality? Limited trail on low-dose formulations. Obstet Gynecol 101(4):773–777

Angsuwarangsee T, Morrison M (2002) Extrinsic laryngeal muscular tension in patients with voice disorders. J Voice 16(3):333–343

Aronson AF (1985) Clinical voice disorders. Georg Thieme Verlag, Stuttgart

Aronson AE (1990) Clinical voice disorders: an interdisciplinary approach, 3rd edn. Thieme-Stratton, New York

Arora A, Hettige R, Ifeacho S et al (2008) Driving standards in tracheostomy care: a preliminary communication of the St Mary's ENT-led multidisciplinary team approach. Clin Otolaryngol 33(6):596–599

Bachher GK, Dholam K, Pai PS (2002) Effective rehabilitation after partial glossectomy. Indian J Otolaryngol Head Neck Surg 54(1):39–43

Baker J (1999) A report on alterations to the speaking and singing voices of four women following hormonal therapy with virilizing agents. J Voice 13(4):496–507

Bassiouny S (1998) Efficacy of the accent method of voice therapy. Folia Phoniatr Logop 50(3):146–164

Belafsky PC, Postma GN, Koufman JA (2001) Laryngopharyngeal reflux symptoms improve before changes in physical findings. Laryngoscope 111(6):979–981

Benninger MS (2000) Microdissection or microspot CO_2 laser for limited vocal fold benign lesions: a prospective randomized trial. Laryngoscope 110(2 Pt 2 Suppl 92):1–17

Berania I, Dagenais C, Moubayed SP et al (2015) Voice and functional outcomes of transoral laser microsurgery for early glottic cancer: ventricular fold resection as a surrogate. J Clin Med Res 7(8):632–636

Bessert-Nettelbeck T, Saatweber M (1998) Therapeutical and pedagogical effects of the Schlaffhorst-Andersen Method on the singer and his voice. Logoped Phoniatr Vocol 23(Suppl 1):37–39

Bickenbach J, Fries M, Offermanns V et al (2011) Impact of early vs. late tracheostomy on weaning: a retrospective analysis. Minerva Anestesiol 77(12):1176–1181

Blom ED, Singer MI (1979) Surgical-prosthetic approaches for postlaryngectomy voice restoration. In: Keith RL, Darley FL (eds) Laryngectomee rehabilitation. College Hill Press, Houston, pp 251–276

Blumin JH, Berke GS (2007) Spasmodic dysphonia. In: Merati AL, Bielamowicz SA (eds) Textbook of laryngology. Plural Publishing, San Diego, CA

Blumin JH, Picolinsky DE, Atkins JP (2004) Laryngeal findings in advanced Parkinson's disease. Ann Otol Rhinol Laryngol 113(4):253–258

Boone DR (1971) The voice and voice therapy, 1st edn. Prentice-Hall, Englewood Cliffs, NJ

Boone DR (1988) The voice and voice therapy, 4th edn. Prentice-Hall, Englewood Cliffs, NJ

Boone DR (1994) Is your voice telling on you? How to find and use your natural voice. Singular Publishing Group Inc., San Diego, CA

Boone DR (2000a) The voice and voice therapy, 6th edn. Prentice-Hall, Englewood Cliffs, NJ, pp 175–177

Boone DR (2000b) The voice and voice therapy, 6th edn. Prentice-Hall, Englewood Cliffs, NJ, pp 210–212

Boone DR, McFarlane SC (1993) A critical view of the yawn-sigh as a voice therapy technique. J Voice 7(1):75–80

Boothroyd CV, Lepre F (1990) Permanent voice change resulting from danazol therapy. Aust N Z J Obstet Gynaecol 30(3):275–276

Braakhuis BJ, Leemans CR, Visser O (2014) Incidence and survival trends of head and neck squamous cell carcinoma in the Netherlands between 1989 and 2011. Oral Oncol 50(7):670–675

Breathing Coordination Approach (2016) Breathing coordination. Available via http://www.breathingcoordination.com/Home_Page.html. Accessed 5 Feb 2016

Briani AA (1952) Speech rehabilitation in laryngectomized by means of expired air. Arch Ital Otol Rinol Laringol 63(5):469–475

Brodnitz FS (1971) Vocal rehabilitation. A manual. American Academy of Ophthalmology and Otolaryngology, Rochester, MN

Brushart TM, Hoffman PN, Royall RM et al (2002) Electrical stimulation promotes motoneuron regeneration without increasing its speed or conditioning the neuron. J Neurosci 22(15):6631–6638

Bunnell HT, Lilley J, Pennington C et al (2010) The ModelTalker system. In: Proceedings of the 2010 Blizzard Challenge Workshop, Kansai Science City, Japan, 25 Sept 2010

Casper-Colton HC, Casper JK (1996) Understanding voice problems, 2nd edn. Williams & Wilkins, Baltimore

Cetto R, Arora A, Hettige R et al (2011) Improving tracheostomy care: a prospective study of the multidisciplinary approach. Clin Otolaryngol 36(5):482–488

Chaitow L (2010) Modern neuromuscular techniques (advanced soft tissue techniques), 3rd edn. Churchill Livingstone Elsevier, London

Ciaglia P, Firsching R, Syniec C (1985) Elective percutaneous dilatational tracheostomy. A new simple bedside procedure; preliminary report. Chest 87(6):715–719

Coblenzer H, Muhar F (1993) Atem und Stimme, 12th edn. Österreichischer Bundesverlag, Wien

Cohen SM, Garrett CG (2007) Utility of voice therapy in the management of vocal fold polyps and cysts. Otolaryngol Head Neck Surg 136(5):742–746

Courey MS, Scott MA, Shohet JA et al (1996) Immunohistochemical characterization of benign laryngeal lesions. Ann Otol Rhinol Laryngol 105(7):525–531

Crumley RL (1982) Experiments in laryngeal reinnervation. Laryngoscope 92(9 Pt 2 Suppl 30):1–27

Crumley RL (1983) Phrenic nerve graft for bilateral vocal cord paralysis. Laryngoscope 93(4):425–428

Crumley RL (1984) Selective reinnervation of vocal cord adductors in unilateral vocal cord paralysis. Ann Otol Rhinol Laryngol 93(4 Pt 1):351–356

Crumley RL, Horn K, Clendenning D (1980) Laryngeal reinnervation using the split-phrenic nerve-graft procedure. Otolaryngol Head Neck Surg 88(2):159–164

Czermak JN (1860) On the laryngoscope and the employment in physiology and medicine (Der Kehlkopfspiegel und seine Verwertung in Physiologie und Medizin). Engelmann, Leipzig

Damste PH (1968) Virilization of the voice due to anabolic steroids. Folia Phoniatr 16:10–18

Dayme M (2009) Dynamics of the singing voice, 5th edn. Springer, Berlin

Deliyski DD, Gress C (1998) Intersystem reliability of MDVP for Windows 95/98 and DOS. Paper presented at the 1998 Annual Convention of the American Speech-Language-Hearing Association, San Antonio, TX

Deliyski DD, Hillman RE (2010) State of the art laryngeal imaging: research and clinical implications. Curr Opin Otolaryngol Head Neck Surg 18(3):147–152

Denizoğlu I (2013) The Lax Vox voice therapy: method and applications. Turkiye Klinikleri J ENT Special Topics 6(2):32–40

Denizoglu I, Sahin M, Bayrak S et al (2018) Efficacy of DoctorVox voice therapy technique for mutational falsetto. J Voice. © 2018 The Voice Foundation. Published by Elsevier Inc. https://www.sciencedirect.com/science/article/pii/S0892199718300274. Accessed 14 Apr 2019

Denk-Linnert DM (2006) Funktionelle Therapie Oropharyngealer Dysphagien nach Kopf-Hals-Tumoren in Sprach-Sprech-Stimm und Schluckstörungen. In: Böhme G (ed) Sprach-, Sprech-, Stimm- und Schluckstörungen. Urban-Fisher, München-Jena, pp 402–427

Denk-Linnert DM, Bigenzahn W (2005) Oropharyngeale Dysphagien. In: Friedrich G et al (eds) Phoniatrie und Pädaudiologie. Huber, Bern, pp 169–186

Dikkers FG, Nikkels PG (1995) Benign lesions of the vocal folds: histopathology and phonotrauma. Ann Otol Rhinol Laryngol 104(9 Pt 1):698–703

Ding R, Logemann JA (2005) Swallow physiology in patients with trach cuff inflated or deflated: a retrospective study. Head Neck 27(9):809–813

Ducharme NG, Cheetham J, Sanders I et al (2010) Considerations for pacing of the cricoarytenoid dorsalis muscle by neuroprosthesis in horses. Equine Vet J 42(6):534–540

Dworkin JP (2008) Laryngitis: types, causes, and treatment. Otolaryngol Clin N Am 41(2):419–436

Eavey RD (1998) The history of tracheotomy. In: Myers EN et al (eds) Tracheotomy airway management, communication, and swallowing, vol 1. Singular Publishing Group, San Diego, pp 1–8

Eisenberg DM, Davis RB, Ettner SL et al (1998) Trends in alternative medicine use in the United States, 1990-

1997: results of a follow-up national survey. JAMA 280(18):1569–1575

Esteban A, Anzueto A, Alia I et al (2000) How is mechanical ventilation employed in the intensive care unit? An international utilization review. Am J Respir Crit Care Med 161(5):1450–1458

Fex B, Fex S, Shiromoto O et al (1994) Acoustic analysis of functional dysphonia: before and after voice therapy (accent method). J Voice 8(2):163–167

Fishman BV, McGlone RE, Shipp T (1971) The effects of certain drugs on phonation. J Speech Hear Res 14(2):301–306

Fitts PM, Posner MI (1967) Human performance. Brooks/Cole Pub. Co., Belmont, CA

Flach M (1992) Indisposition und akute Dysphonie beim Berufssänger. Laryngo-Rhino Otol 71(5):233–235

Forchhammer E (1974) Stemmens Funktioner og fejl funktioner. Munksgaard, Copenhagen

Forster G, Arnold D, Bischoff SJ et al (2013) Laryngeal pacing in minipigs: in vivo test of a new minimal invasive transcricoidal electrode insertion method for functional electrical stimulation of the PCA. Eur Arch Otorhinolaryngol 270(1):225–231

Friedrich G, de Jong FI, Mahieu HF et al (2001) Laryngeal framework surgery: a proposal for classification and nomenclature by the Phonosurgery Committee of the European Laryngological Society. Eur Arch Otorhinolaryngol 258(8):389–396

Friedrich G, Remacle M, Birchall M et al (2007) Defining phonosurgery: a proposal for classification and nomenclature by the Phonosurgery Committee of the European Laryngological Society (ELS). Eur Arch Otorhinolaryngol 264(10):1191–1200

Froeschels E (1952) Chewing method as therapy. Arch Otolaryngol 56(4):427–434

Froeschels E, Kastein S, Weiss DA (1955) A method of therapy for paralytic conditions of the mechanisms of phonation, respiration and glutination. J Speech Hear Disord 20(4):365–370

Frøkjær-Jensen B, Prytz S (1976) Registration of voice quality. Brüel Kjaer Tech Rev 3:3–17

Fussi F (2010) La Voce del Cantante. Omega Edizioni, Torino

Galant C (2017) Total laryngectomy—an experience in "telerehabilitation". Paper presented at the ENT World Congress of the International Federation of ORL Societies, Paris, 24–28 June 2017

Galetti B, Ferni F, Cammaroto G et al (2012) Vocal outcome after CO_2 laser cordectomy performed on patients affected by early glottic carcinoma. J Voice 26(6):801–805

Garcia Perez A, Hernández López X, Valadez Jiménez VM et al (2014) Synchronous electrical stimulation of laryngeal muscles: an alternative for enhancing recovery of unilateral recurrent laryngeal nerve paralysis. J Voice 28(4):524.e1–524.e7

Garrubba M, Turner T, Grieveson C (2009) Multidisciplinary care for tracheostomy patients: a systematic review. Crit Care 13(6):R177. Epub 2009 Nov 6. Review

Gates GA, Saegert J, Wilson N et al (1985) The effect of β blockade on singing performance. Ann Otol Rhinol Laryngol 94(6 Pt 1):570–574

Gerritsma EJ, Broacaar MP, Hakkesteegt MM et al (1994) Virilization of the voice in postmenopausal women due to anabolic steroid nandrolone decanoate (Decadurabolin). The effects of medication for one year. Clin Otolaryngol 19(1):79–84

Gilman M, Gilman SL (2008) Electrotherapy and the human voice: a literature review of the historical origins and contemporary applications. J Voice 22(2):219–231

Gordon T, Chan KM, Sulaiman OA et al (2009) Accelerating axon growth to overcome limitations in functional recovery after peripheral nerve injury. Neurosurgery 65(4 Suppl):A132–A144

Gray S (1989) Vocal fold physiology: acoustic, perceptual, and physiological aspects of voice mechanisms. Singular, San Diego, CA, pp 21–27

Gray S, Thibeault S (2002) Diversity in voice characteristics-interaction between genes and environment, use of microarray analysis. J Commun Disord 35(4):347–354

Griffiths J, Barber VS, Morgan L et al (2005) Systematic review and meta-analysis of studies of the timing of tracheostomy in adult patients undergoing artificial ventilation. BMJ 330(7502):1243

Griggs WM, Worthley LI, Gilligan JE et al (1990) A simple percutaneous tracheostomy technique. Surg Gynecol Obstet 170(6):543–545

Guillemin F, Bombardier C, Beaton D (1993) Cross-cultural adaptation of health-related quality of life measures: literature review and proposed guidlines. J Clin Epidemiol 46(12):1417–1432

Guzman M, Rubin A, Cox P et al (2014) Neuromuscular electrical stimulation of the cricothyroid muscle in patients with suspected superior laryngeal nerve weakness. J Voice 28(2):216–225

Halczy-Kowalik L (2006) Structural and functional conditions for creation of speech after resection of oral cancer (In Polish). In: Logopedia.T.35, Wyd. ZGPZL, Lublin, p 143

Hanzlíček Z, Romportl J, Matoušek J (2012) Voice conservation: towards creating a speech-aid system for total laryngectomees. In: Kelemen J et al (eds) Beyond artificial intelligence: contemplations, expectations, applications. Springer, Heidelberg, pp 203–212

Heafield S, Rogers M, Karnik A (1999) Tracheostomy management in ordinary wards. J Hosp Med 60(4):261–262

Hedge MN (1996) Pocket guide to treatment in speech-language pathology. Singular, San Diego, CA, p 302

Hetzroni OE, Harris OL (1996) Cultural aspects in the development of AAC users. Augment Altern Commun 12(1):52–58

Higgins KM, Punthakee X (2007) Meta-analysis comparison of open versus percutaneous tracheostomy. Laryngoscope 117(3):447–454

Hilgers FJM, Van den Brekel MWM (2010) Vocal and speech rehabilitation following laryngectomy. In: Flint

PW et al (eds) Cummings otolaryngology: head and neck surgery, 5th edn. Mosby Elsevier, Philadelphia, pp 1594–1610

Hirano M, Bless DM (1993) Videostroboscopic examination of the larynx. Singular Publishing Group Inc., San Diego, CA

Hogikyan ND, Sethuraman G (1999) Validation of an instrument to measure voice-related quality of life (V-RQOL). J Voice 13(4):557–569

Hol C, Schalen C, Verduin CM et al (1996) Moraxella catarrhalis in acute laryngitis: infection or colonization? J Infect Dis 174(3):636–638

Holmberg EB, Hillman RE, Hammarberg B et al (2001) Efficacy of a behaviorally based voice therapy protocol for vocal nodules. J Voice 15(3):395–412

Hotz MA, Baumann A, Schaller I et al (2002) Success and predictability of vox prosthesis voice rehabilitation. Arch Otolaryngol Head Neck Surg 128(6):687–691

Husler F, Rodd-Marling Y (2007) Singing. The physical nature of the vocal organ. Revised edition. Hutchinson Publishing Group, London

Instant Voice Jiggle Exercise (2016) The ISSN register. Available via http://www.voice-doctor.com/voice-disorders/instant-voice-jiggle-exercise. Accessed 28 Jan 2016

Isshiki N (2000) Progress in laryngeal framework surgery. Acta Otolaryngol 120(2):120–127

Isshiki N, Morita H, Okamura H et al (1974) Thyroplasty as a new phonosurgical technique. Acta Otolaryngol 78(5–6):451–457

Jacobson E (1957) You must relax. Mc Graw Hill Book Company, New York

Jeong W, Lee SJ, Lee WY et al (2014) Conservative management for vocal fold polyps. JAMA Otolaryngol Head Neck Surg 140(5):448–452

Johns MM (2003) Update on the etiology, diagnosis, and treatment of vocal fold nodules, polyps, and cysts. Curr Opin Otolaryngol Head Neck Surg 11(6):456–461

Johnson TS (1985) Vocal abuse reduction program. Johnson College-Hill Press, Vermont

Kersing W, Jennekens FG (2004) Age-related changes in human thyroarytenoid muscles: a histological and histochemical study. Eur Arch Otorhinolaryngol 261(7):386–392

Kettunen WW, Helmer SD, Haan JM (2014) Incidence of overall complications and symptomatic tracheal stenosis is equivalent following open and percutaneous tracheostomy in the trauma patient. Am J Surg 208(5):770–774

Kitzing P (1979) Glottografisk frekvensindikering. MAS tryckeri/Litos Reprotryck i Malmö AB, Malmö

Klein AM, Lehmann M, Hapner ER et al (2009) Spontaneous resolution of hemorrhagic polyps of the true vocal fold. J Voice 23(1):132–135

Kooijman PGC, de Jong FICRS, Oudes MJ et al (2005) Muscular tension and body posture in relation to voice handicap and voice quality in teachers with persistent voice complaints. Folia Phoniatr Logop 57(3):134–147

Kotby MN (1986) Voice disorders. Recent diagnostic advances. Egypt. J Otolaryngol 3(1):69

Kotby MN (1995) The accent method of voice therapy. Singular Publishing Group Inc., San Diego, CA

Kotby MN, Orabi AA (1995) Voice range profile as a quantitative measure of vocal function in some pathological voices. In: Kotby MN (ed) Proceedings of the XXIII World Congress of the IALP. Cairo, Aug 6–10, pp 50–53

Kotby MN, Nassar AM, Seif EI et al (1988) Ultrastructural features of vocal fold nodules and polyps. Acta Otolaryngol (Stockh) 105(5–6):477–482

Kotby MN, Barakah M, Abou El-Ella M et al (1990) Aerodynamic analysis of voice disorders. In: Sacristan T et al (eds) Proceedings of the XIV World Congress of Otorhinolaryngology, Head and Neck Surgery, Madrid, Spain, September 10–15, 1989. Kugler & Ghedini Publications, Amsterdam, pp 2041–2047

Kotby MN, El-Sady SR, Bassiouny SE et al (1991) Efficacy of the accent method of voice therapy. J Voice 5(4):316–320

Kotby MN, Fadly E, Barakah M et al (1992) Electromyography and neurography in voice neurolaryngology. J Voice 6(2):159–187

Kotby MN, Shiromoto O, Hirano M (1993) The accent method of voice therapy: effect of accentuation on F0, SPL and airflow. J Voice 7(2):319–325

Kotby MN, El Sady S, Hegazi M (1998a) Vibratory and acoustic correlates of perceived voice quality. In: Proceedings of the XXI International Annual Ain Shams Medical Congress-, March 16–19, 1998, pp 91–97

Kotby MN, Hegazi MA, El-Assal NN (1998b) Of what value are the acoustic measures of voice? In: Proceedings of the XXI International Ain Shams Medical Congress, pp 79–82

Koufman JA, Blalock PD (1988) Vocal fatigue and dysphonia in the professional voice user: Bogart-Bacall syndrome. Laryngoscope 98(5):493–498

Koufman JA, Isaacson G (1991) The spectrum of vocal dysfunction. Otolaryngol Clin N Am 24(5):985–998

Kozon V, Fortner N (2010) Wundmanagement und Pflegeentwicklungen. ÖGVP Verlag, Wien, p 49

Laukkanen AM, Lindholm P, Vilkman E (1995) Phonation into a tube as a voice training method. Folia Phoniatr Logop 47(6):331–338

Lavy JA, Wood G, Rubin JS et al (2000) Dysphonia associated with inhaled steroids. J Voice 14(4):581–588

Lawrence VL (1987) Common medications with laryngeal effects. Ear Nose Throat J 66(8):318–322

Lee B, Woo P (2005) Chronic cough as a sign of laryngeal sensory neuropathy: diagnosis and treatment. Ann Otol Rhinol Laryngol 114(4):253–257

Lee HY, Hong JS, Lee KC et al (2015) Changes in hyolaryngeal movement and swallowing function after neuromuscular electrical stimulation in patients with dysphagia. Ann Rehabil Med 39(2):199–209

Leonard R, Kendall K (2005) Effects of voice therapy on vocal process granuloma: a phonoscopic approach. Am J Otolaryngol 26(2):101–107

Lessac A (1997) The use and training of the human voice: a bio-dynamic approach to vocal life, 3rd edn. Myfield Pub, Houston, TX, p 247

Lewit K (2009) Manipulative therapy—musculoskeletal medicine. Churchill Livingstone, London

Li M, Chen S, Zheng H et al (2013) Reinnervation of bilateral posterior cricoarytenoid muscles using the left phrenic nerve in patients with bilateral vocal fold paralysis. PLoS One 8(10):e77233

Lindman JP, Morgan CE, Peralta R et al (2017) Tracheostomy technique. Drugs & diseases, clinical procedures. Available via http://emedicine.medscape.com/article/865068-technique. Accessed 28 Feb 2018

Logemann JA (1995) Dysphagia: evaluation and treatment. Folia Phoniatr Logop 47(3):140–164

Lyskowski JC, Dunner FJ (1980) Hoarseness and tricyclic antidepressants. Am J Psychiatry 137(5):636

Mahieu HF, van Lith-Bijl JT, Groenhout C et al (1993) Selective laryngeal abductor reinnervation in cats using a phrenic nerve transfer and ORG 2766. Arch Otolaryngol Head Neck Surg 119(7):772–776

Manheim CJ (2009) The myofascial release manual, 4rd edn. Slack Incorporated, Thorofare, NJ

Marie JP (1999) Contribution à l'étude de la réinnervation laryngée expérimentale; intérêt du nerf phrénique. Laryngeal reinnervation: special interest with the phrenic nerve. Dissertation, University of Rouen, France

Marie JP (2009a) Human bilateral laryngeal reinnervation: implications for transplantation. Paper presented at the American Laryngological Association (ALA) Combined Otolaryngology Spring Meetings, Scottsdale/Phoenix, Arizona, 28–29 May 2009

Marie JP (2009b) Nerve reconstruction. In: Remacle M, Eckel HE (eds) Surgery of larynx and trachea. Springer, Berlin

Marie JP (2014) Ten years' experience in selective bilateral reinnervation of the larynx in humans. Paper presented at the American Laryngological Association, Neurolaryngology Study Group, Las Vegas, 14–15 May 2014

Marie JP, Dehesdin D, Ducastelle T et al (1989) Selective reinnervation of the abductor and adductor muscles of the canine larynx after recurrent nerve paralysis. Ann Otol Rhinol Laryngol 98(7 Pt 1):530–536

Marie JP, Laquerriere A, Lerosey Y et al (1997a) Selective resection of the phrenic nerve roots in rabbits. Part I: cartography of the residual innervation. Respir Physiol 109(2):127–138

Marie JP, Tardif C, Lerosey Y et al (1997b) Selective resection of the phrenic nerve roots in rabbits. Part II: respiratory effects. Respir Physiol 109(2):139–148

Marie JP, Lerosey Y, Dehesdin D et al (1999) Experimental reinnervation of a strap muscle with a few roots of the phrenic nerve in rabbits. Ann Otol Rhinol Laryngol 108(10):1004–1011

Marie JP, Lacoume Y, Magnier P et al (2000a) Selective bilateral motor reinnervation of the canine larynx. Laryngo Rhino Otol 79:188–189

Marie JP, Laquerriere A, Choussy O et al (2000b) Thyrohyoid branch of the hypoglossal nerve in the canine; perspectives for larynx reinnervation. Paper presented at the 3rd Congress of the European Laryngological Society, Paris, 9–11 June 2000

Marie JP, Laquerriere A, Choussy O et al (2000c) Thyrohyoid branch of the hypoglossal nerve in the canine; perspectives for larynx reinnervation. Eur Arch Oto Rhin Laryngol S1, S11:257

Marie JP, Choussy O, Lacoume Y (2001) Delayed total motor reinnervation of the canine larynx. Paper presented at the "Where upper airway and digestive tract meet" Meeting, Amsterdam, 18–21 Apr 2001

Marie JP, Lacoume Y, Laquerriere A et al (2006a) Diaphragmatic effects of selective resection of the upper phrenic nerve root in dogs. Respir Physiol Neurobiol 154(3):419–430

Marie JP, Vérin E, Woisard V (2006b) Successful reinnervation of congenital bilateral vocal cord paralysis. Paper presented at the IX Congress of the European Society of Pediatric Otorhinolaryngology, Paris, 18–21 June 2006

Marie JP, Vérin E, Woisard V et al (2007) Réinnervation sélective des paralysies laryngées bilatérales en fermeture. Premiers résultats. Paper presented at the Société de Laryngologie des Hôpitaux de Paris, Paris, 24 Nov 2007

Marie JP, Bon Mardion N, Paviot A et al (2013) Bilateral functional reinnervation in bilateral vocal fold paralysis: new indications. Paper presented at the 20th IFOS Congress, Seoul, 1–5 June 2013

Marina MB, Marie JP, Birchall MA (2011) Laryngeal reinnervation for bilateral vocal fold paralysis. Curr Opin Otolaryngol Head Neck Surg 19(6):434–438

Marszałek S, Żebryk-Stopa A, Kraśny J et al (2009) Estimation of influence of myofascial release techniques on oesophageal pressure after total laryngectomy. Eur Arch Otorhinol 266(8):1305–1308

Marszałek S, Niebudek-Bogusz E, Woźnicka E et al (2010) Diagnostyka fizjoterapeutyczna i osteopatyczna w zawodowych zaburzeniach głosu. (The application of physiotherapeutic and ostheopathic diagnostics in ocuppational voice disorders). Med Pr 61(2):205–211

Marszałek S, Niebudek-Bogusz E, Woźnicka E et al (2012) Assessment of the influence of osteopathic myofascial techniques on normalization of the voice organ in patients with professional dysphonia. Int J Occup Med Environ Health 25(3):225–223

Martinucci I, de Bortoli N, Savarino E et al (2013) Optimal treatment of laryngopharyngeal reflux disease. Ther Adv Chronic Dis 4(6):287–301. https://doi.org/10.1177/2040622313503485

Mastronikolis NS, Remacle M, Biagini M et al (2013) Wendler glottoplasty: an effective pitch raising surgery in male-to-female transsexuals. J Voice 27(4):516–522

Matsui Y, Ohno K, Yamashita Y et al (2007) Factors influencing postoperative speech function of tongue cancer patients following reconstruction with fasciocutaneous/myocutaneous flaps—a multicenter study. J Oral Maxillofac Surg 36(7):601–609

Maune S, Kurz K, Meyer J et al (2005) Quality of life assessment in otorhinolaryngology. History, measures and methods. Otolaryngol Pol 59(4):489–504

Miller FR, Eliachar I (1994) Managing the aspirating patient. Am J Otolaryngol 15(1):1–17

Miller S, Kühn D, Jungheim M et al (2014) Neuromuskuläre Elektrostimulationsverfahren in der HNO-Heilkunde. (Neuromuscular electric stimulation therapy in otorhinolaryngology). HNO 62(2):131–141

Mitchell RB, Hussey HM, Setzen G et al (2013) Clinical consensus statement: tracheostomy care. Otolaryngol Head Neck Surg 148(1):6–20

Mossallam I, Kotby MN, Ghaly AF et al (1986) Histopathological aspects of benign vocal fold lesions associated with dysphonia. In: Kirchner JA (ed) Vocal fold in histopathology—a symposium. College Hill Press Inc., San Diego, CA, pp 65–80

Mozolewski E (1972) Chirurgiczna rehabilitacja g(strok)losu i mowy po laryngektomii. Otolaryngol Pol 26(6):653–661

Mueller AH (2011) Laryngeal pacing for bilateral vocal fold immobility. Curr Opin Otolaryngol Head Neck Surg 19(6):439–443

Mueller AH, Hagen R, Foerster G et al (2015) Laryngeal pacing via an implantable stimulator for the rehabilitation of subjects suffering from bilateral vocal fold paralysis: a prospective first-in-human study. Laryngoscope 126(8):1810–1816

Müller G, Kramer A (2003) In vitro action of combinations of selected antimicrobial agents and adult bovine articular cartilage (sesamoid bone). Chem Biol Interact 145(3):331–336

Musso YM (1999) Training-induced brain plasticity in aphasia. Brain 122(9):1781–1790

Nair G (2007) The craft of singing. Plural Publishing, San Diego

Nakagawa H, Miyamoto M, Kusuyama T et al (2012) Resolution of vocal fold polyps with conservative treatment. J Voice 26(3):e107–e110

Narula T, Bradley P, Carding P et al (2011) Laryngeal transplantation. Working Party Final Report. The Royal College of Surgeons of England

Nasri S, Sercarz JA, McAlpin T et al (1995) Treatment of vocal fold granuloma using botulinum toxin type A. Laryngoscope 105(6):585–588

Nawka T, Hosemann W (2005) Surgical procedures for voice restoration. GMS Curr Top Otorhinolaryngol Head Neck Surg 4:Doc14

Need AG, Durbridge TC, Nordin BE (1993) Anabolic steroids in portmenopausel osteoporosis. Wien Med Wochenschr 143(14–15):392–395

Nix J, Simpson CB (2008) Voice research and technology: semi-occluded vocal tract postures and their application in the singing voice studio. J Singing 64(3):339–342

Oğuz H, Akbulut S (2013) Ses Bozukluklarında Tedavi Seçimi. Türkiye Klinikleri J ENT Special Topics 6(2):1–9

Oğuz H, Tunç T, Şafak MA et al (2006a) Objective voice changes in non-dysphonic Parkinson's disease patients. J Otolaryngol 35(5):349–354

Oğuz H, Paksoy G, Arslan N et al (2006b) Short term effects of lansaprazol on reflux signs, symptoms and voice perturbation. Poster presented at the 3rd World Voice Congress, 19–22 June 2006, Istanbul, poster 69

Oğuz H, Tarhan E, Korkmaz M et al (2007) Acoustic analysis findings in objective laryngopharyngeal reflux patients. J Voice 21(2):203–210

Oliver ER, Gist A, Gillespie MB (2007) Percutaneous versus surgical tracheotomy: an updated meta-analysis. Laryngoscope 117(9):1570–1575

Ozkan S (2010) Personal communication. In: 5th National Audiology and Speech Disorders Congress, 23–26 September 2010, Izmir, Turkey

Pahn J, Pahn E (2000) Die Nasalierungsmethode. Matthias Oehmke, Roggentin

Panje WR (1981) Prosthetic vocal rehabilitation following total laryngectomy: the voice button. Ann Otol 90:116–120

Park W, Hicks DM, Khandwala F et al (2005) Laryngopharyngeal reflux: prospective cohort study evaluating optimal dose of proton-pump inhibitor therapy and pretherapy predictors of response. Laryngoscope 115(7):1230–1238

Patrick DL, Erickson P (1988) Assessing health-related quality of life for clinical decision making. In: Walker SR, Rosser RM (eds) Quality of life: assessment and application. MTP Press, Lancaster, UK, pp 1–22

Pattie MA, Murdoch BE, Theodoros D et al (1998) Voice changes in women treated for endometriosis and related conditions: the need for comprehensive vocal assessment. J Voice 12(3):366–371

Pauloski B, Rademaker AW, Logemann JA et al (2000) Pretreatment swallowing function in patients with head and neck cancer. Head-Neck 22(5):474–482

Paw HGW, Bodenham AR (2004) Percutaneous tracheostomy. A practical handbook, 6th edn. Greenwich Medical Media Ltd, Cambridge, p 43

Pedersen M, Beranova A, Moller S (2002) Dysphonia: medical treatment and a medical voice hygiene advice approach. Eur Arch Otorhinolaryngol 261(6):312–315

Pedersen M (2012) Laryngopharyngeal Reflux? A Randomized Clinical Controlled Trial. Otolaryngol S1:004. https://doi.org/10.4172/2161-119X.S1-004

Pedersen M, Eeg M (2012) Does treatment of the laryngeal mucosa reduce dystonic symptoms? A prospective clinical cohort study of mannose binding lectin and other immunological parameters with diagnostic use of phonatory function studies. Eur Arch Otorhinolaryngol 269(5):1477–1482

Pehlivan M, Denizoğlu I (2009) Laryngoaltimeter: a new ambulatory device for laryngeal height control, preliminary results. J Voice 23(5):529–538

Petit JC, Klein T, Rodier D (1971) Hormone therapy for advanced breast cancer with drostanolone proprionate. Bull Cancer 58(4):511–522

Plummer AL, Gracey DR (1989) Consensus conference on artificial airways in patients receiving mechanical ventilation. Chest 96(1):178–180

Prochaska JO, Diclemente CC (1986) Toward a comprehensive model of change. In: Miller WA, Heather N (eds) Treating addictive behaviors. Processes of change. Applied clinical psychology, vol 13. Springer, Boston, pp 3–27

Prochaska JO, Velicer WF (1997) The transtheoretical model of health behavior change. Am J Health Promot 12(1):38–48

Pruszewicz A, Woźnica B, Kruk-Zagajewska A et al (1992) Electromyography of cricopharyngeal muscles in patients with oesophageal speech. Acta Otolaryngol 112(2):366–369

Pruszewicz A, Obrębowski A, Woźnica B et al (1995) Ausgewählte Dysphagieprobleme in der Phoniatrie. Sprache-Stimme-Gehör 19(4):162–166

Punt NA (1968) Vocal disabilities of singers. Applied laryngology-singers and actors. Proc R Soc Med 61(11 Part 1):1152–1156

Rademaker AW, Logemann JA, Pauloski BR et al (1993) Recovery of postoperative swallowing in patients undergoing partial laryngectomy. Head Neck 15(4):325–334

Ramig LO, Sapir S, Countryman S et al (2001) Intensive voice treatment (LSVT) for patients with Parkinson's disease: a two year follow up. J Neurol Neurosurg Psychiatry 71(4):493–498

Rammage L, Morrison M, Nichol H (2001) Management of the voice and its disorders, 2nd edn. Singular Publishing Group, San Diego, CA

Reid C (1965) The free voice. Coleman-Ross Company, New York

Remacle M, Eckel HE, Antonelli A et al (2000) Endoscopic cordectomy. A proposal for a classification by the Working Committee, European Laryngological Society. Eur Arch Otorhinolaryngol 257(4): 227–231

Remacle M, Friedrich G, Dikkers FG et al (2003) Phonosurgery of the vocal folds: a classification proposal. Eur Arch Otorhinolaryngol 260(1):1–6

Remacle M, Van Haverbeke C, Eckel H et al (2007) Proposal for revision of the European Laryngological Society classification of endoscopic cordectomies. Eur Arch Otorhinolaryngol 264(5):499–504

Reveiz L, Cardona AF, Ospina EG (2007) Antibiotics for acute laryngitis in adults. Cochrane Database Syst Rev (2):CD004783. Accessed 20 Mar 2012

Rice DH (1982) Laryngeal reinnervation. Laryngoscope 92(9 Pt 1):1049–1059

Richter B (2013) Die Stimme: Grundlagen, Künstlerische Praxis, Gesunderhaltung. Henschel, Berlin

Rogers SN, Laher SH, Overend L et al (2002) Importance-rating using the University of Washington Quality of Life Questionnaire in patients treated by primary surgery for oral and oro-pharyngeal cancer. J Craniomaxillofac Surg 30(2):125–132

Rogers SN, Lowe D, Yueh B et al (2010) The physical function and social-emotional function subscales of the University of Washington Quality of Life Questionnaire. Arch Otolaryngol Head Neck Surg 136(4):352–357

Rolf C, Nieschlag E (1998) Potential adverse effects on longterm testosterone therapy. Bailliere Clin Endocrinol Metab 12(3):521–534

Rosen CA, Simpson CB (2008a) Nonsurgical treatment of voice disorders. In: Rosen CA, Simpson CB (eds) Operative techniques in laryngology. Springer, Berlin

Rosen CA, Simpson CB (2008b) Operative techniques in laryngology. Springer, Berlin

Ross S (1999) Dysphonia: osteopathic treatment. J Bodyw Mov Ther 3(3):133–142

Rubin JS, Liebermann J, Harris TM (2000) Laryngeal manipulation. Otolaryngol Chin North Am 33(5):1017–1034

Rubin JS, Sataloff RT, Korovin GS (2006) Diagnosis and treatment of voice disorders, 3rd edn. Plural Publishing, San Diego

Sataloff RT (1981) Professional singers: the science and art of clinical care. Am J Otolaryngol 2(3):262–266

Sataloff RT (2005) Professional voice. The science and art of clinical care, 3rd edn. Plural Publishing Inc, New York

Sataloff RT, Cline SE, Lyons KM et al (2005a) Voice rest. In: Sataloff RT (ed) Treatment of voice disorders, 2nd edn. Plural Publishing, San Diego CA, pp 41–45

Sataloff RT, Hawkshaw MJ, Anticaglia J (2005b) Medications and the voice. In: Sataloff RT (ed) Treatment of voice disorders. Plural Publishing, San Diego, CA

Schachner A, Ovil Y, Sidi J et al (1989) Percutaneous tracheostomy—a new method. Crit Care Med 17(10):1052–1056

Schalen L, Christensen P, Eliasson I et al (1985) Inefficacy of penicillin V in acute laryngitis in adults: evaluation from results of double-blind study. Ann Otol Rhinol Laryngol 94(1 Pt 1):14–17

Schiff M (1977) Medical management of acute laryngitis. In: Lawrence VL (ed) Transcripts of the sixth symposium: care of the professional voice. The Voice Foundation, New York

Schlömicher-Thier J, Weikert MHJ (2003) High level professional voice users vs semi-professionals and non-professionals. Poster presented at the 5th Pan European Voice Conference, Graz, Aug 2003

Schlömicher-Thier J, Weikert MHJ (2015) Acute assessment of professional singers. In: Benninger MS, Murry T (eds) The performer's voice, 2nd edn. Plural Publishing, San Diego, pp 209–222

Schlondorff G (1966) Anabolic hormones and voice disorders. Dtsch Med Wochenschr 91:555–557

Schmidt RA, Lee TD (2014) Motor learning and performance: from principles to application. Courier Companies Inc., North Chelmsford, MA

Schneider-Stickler B, Bigenzahn W (2013) Stimmdiagnostik: Ein Leitfaden für die Praxis, 2nd edn. Springer, New York

Schneider-Stickler B, Kozon V, Assadian O et al (2013) Standard operating procedure: tracheostoma care. Avaliable via http://www.meduniwien.ac.at/phon-log/sop_tracheostoma-_versorgun.pdf. Accessed 5 Feb 2017

Schröter-Morasch H (1996) Schweregradeinteilung der Aspiration bei Patienten mit Schluckstörungen. In: Gross M (ed) Aktuelle phoniatrisch-pädaudiologische Aspekte. Median Verlag, Berlin, pp 145–146

Schulz G (2002) The effects of speech therapy and pharmacological treatments on voice and speech in treatment of Parkinson's disease: a review of the literature. Curr Med Chem 9(14):1359–1366

Seidman MD (2006) Complementary and alternative medications and techniques. In: Benninger MS, Murry T (eds) The performer's voice. Plural Publishing, San Diego, CA, pp 163–176

Seidner W (2004) Phoniatrische Notbehandlung bei Sängern und Schauspielern. HNO Aktuell 12(4):143–148

Seidner W, Wendler J (2004) Die Sängerstimme. Henschel, Berlin

Seidner W, Wendler J (2010) Die Sängerstimme, 4th edn. Henschel, Leipzig

Serafini I, Staffieri M (1976) La riabilitazione chirurgica della voce e della respirazione dopo laringectomia totale. Paper presented at the 29th National Congress of the Associazione Otologi Ospedalieri Italiana, Bologna

Simberg S (2000) The resonance tube—a versatile device in voice therapy. In: Nine papers on logopedics and phoniatrics. Proceedings of the 5th Nordic Congress of Logopedics and Phoniatrics, Audiologopedisk Forening, 4–5 Feb 2000, Helsinki, Odense, pp 81–85

Simberg S, Laine A (2007) The resonance tube method in voice therapy: description and practical implementations. Logoped Phoniatr Vocol 32(4):165–170

Smith S, Thyme K (1978) Accent Metoden- en teoretiskpædagogisk fremstilling. Special-Pædagogisk Forlag, Herning

Sovijarvi A (1969) Nya metoder vid behabdlingen av röstrubbringar. Nordisk Tidskrift for Tal og Stemme 3:121–131

Sovijarvi A (1974) Therapeutic results of laryngeal asymmetric postures in dysphonic patients. World Papers in Phonetics, Tokyo

Spahn C, Richter B, Altenmüller E (2011) MusikerMedizin: Diagnostik, Therapie und Prävention von musikerspezifischen Erkrankungen. Schattauer, Stuttgart

Stead RJ, Cooke NJ (1989) Adverse effects of inhaled corticosteroids. Br Med J 298(6671):403–404

Stecco C (2015) Functional Atlas of the human fascial system, 1st edn. Churchill Livingstone Elsevier, London

Stefan H, Allmer F, Schalek K (2012) POP PraxisOrientierte Pflegediagnostik. Springer, Wien, pp 121, 186, 346, 474, 529, 536, 751

Stemple JC (2000) Voice therapy: clinical studies, 2nd edn. Singular Publishing Group, San Diego, CA

Stephen H, Kaptein AA, Pruitt S (2003) Behavioural mechanisms explaining adherence. In: Adherence to long term therapies: evidence for action. World Health Organization, Geneva, pp 125–149

Stock CR (1987) What is past is prologue: a short history of the development of tracheostomy. Ear Nose Throat J 66(4):166–169

Stone RE, Casteel RL (1982) Restoration of voice in non-organically based dysphonia. In: Filter MD (ed) Phonatory voice disorders in children. Charles C. Thomas Publisher, Springfield, pp 166–180

Storck K (1910) Musik und Musiker in Karikatur und Satire. Stalling, Oldenburg

Sulica L (2004) Contemporary management of spasmodic dysphonia. Curr Opin Otolaryngol Head Neck Surg 12(6):543–548

Sullivan KL, Hauser RA, Zesiewicz TA (2003) Essential tremor: epidemiology, diagnosis, and treatment. Neurologist 10(5):250–258

Sundberg J, Mecke AC (2015) Die Wissenschaft von der Singstimme. Wißner, Augsburg

Švec JG, Šram F, Schutte HK (2000) Videokymography in 2000: the present state and perspectives of the high-speed line-imaging technique. In: Braunschweig T et al (eds) Advances in quantitative laryngoscopy, voice and speech research. Proceedings of the 4th International Workshop. Jena, 7–8 Apr 2000. Friedrich-Schiller University, Jena, pp 57–62 (ISBN: 3-00-005636-X)

Terré R, Mearin F (2015) A randomized controlled study of neuromuscular electrical stimulation in oropharyngeal dysphagia secondary to acquired brain injury. Eur J Neurol 22(4):687–e44

Thomas JP, Zubiaur FM (2013) Over-diagnosis of laryngopharyngeal reflux as the cause of hoarseness. Eur Arch Otorhinolaryngol 270(3):995–999

Thompson AR (1995) Pharmacological agents with effects on voice. Am J Otolaryngol 16(1):12–18

Thyme-Frøkjaer K, Frøkjær-Jensen B (2001) The accent method. A rational voice therapy in theory & practice. Speechmark, Bicester

Titze IR (1994) Mechanical stress in phonation. J Voice 8(2):99–105

Titze IR (2006) Voice training and therapy with a semi-occluded vocal tract. Rationale and scientific underpinnings. J Speech Lang Hear Res 49(2):448–459

Titze IR (2008) Non-linear source-filter coupling in phonation: theory. J Acoust Soc Am 123(5):2733–2749

Tobin AE, Santamaria JD (2008) An intensivist-led tracheostomy review team is associated with shorter decannulation time and length of stay: a prospective cohort study. Crit Care 12(2):R48. Epub 2008 Apr 11

Toogood JH, Jennings B, Greenway RW et al (1980) Candidiasis and dysphonia complicating beclomethasone treatment of asthma. J Allergy Clin Immunol 65(2):145–153

Toyama K, Matsumoto S, Kurasawa M et al (2014) Novel neuromuscular electrical stimulation system for treatment of dysphagia after brain injury. Neurol Med Chir (Tokyo) 54(7):521–528

Tucker HM (1978) Human laryngeal reinnervation: long-term experience with the nerve-muscle pedicle technique. Laryngoscope 88(4):598–604

Tucker HM (1982) Nerve-muscle pedicle reinnervation of the larynx: avoiding pitfalls and complications. Ann Otol Rhinol Laryngol 91(4 Pt 1):440–444

Tucker HM (1989) Long-term results of nerve-muscle pedicle reinnervation for laryngeal paralysis. Ann Otol Rhinol Laryngol 98(9):674–676

Valizade Hasanloei MA, Mahoori A, Bazzazi AM et al (2014) Percutaneous dilatational tracheostomy and surgically created tracheostomy in ICU patients. J Cardiovasc Thorac Res 6(1):43–46

van der Molen L, van Rossum MA, Jacobi I et al (2012) Pre- and post-treatment voice and speech outcomes in patients with advanced head and neck cancer treated with chemoradiotherapy: expert listeners' and patient's perception. J Voice 26(5):664. e25–664.e33

Van Houtte E, Van Lierde K, Claeys S (2011) Pathophysiology and treatment of muscle tension dysphonia: a review of the current knowledge. J Voice 25(2):202–207

Van Lawrence L (1986) Sermon on hydration (The Evils of Dry). NATS J 42(4):22–23

van Lith-Bijl JT, Mahieu HF, Stolk RJ et al (1996) Laryngeal abductor function after recurrent laryngeal nerve injury in cats. Arch Otolaryngol Head Neck Surg 122(4):393–396

van Lith-Bijl JT, Stolk RJ, Tonnaer JA et al (1997) Selective laryngeal reinnervation with separate phrenic and ansa cervicalis nerve transfers. Arch Otolaryngol Head Neck Surg 123(4):406–411

van Lith-Bijl JT, Stolk RJ, Tonnaer JA et al (1998) Laryngeal abductor reinnervation with a phrenic nerve transfer after a 9-month delay. Arch Otolaryngol Head Neck Surg 124(4):393–398

Van Straten M, Josling P (2002) Preventing the common cold with a vitamin C supplement: a double-blind, placebo-controlled survey. Adv Ther 19(5):151–159

Verdolini-Marston K, Burke MK, Lessac A et al (1995) Preliminary study of two methods of treatment for laryngeal nodules. J Voice 9(1):74–85

Verrico MM, Weber RJ, McKaveney TP et al (2003) Adverse drug events involving COX-2 inhibitors. Ann Pharmacother 37(9):1203–1213

Vilkman E (2004) Occupational safety and health aspects of voice and speech professions. Folia Phoniatr Logop 56(4):220–253

Warrick P, Dromey C, Irish JC et al (2000) Botulinum toxin for essential tremor of the voice with multiple anatomic sites of tremor: a crossover design study of unilateral versus bilateral injection. Laryngoscope 110(8):1366–1374

Watkin KL, Ewanowski SJ (1985) Effects of aerosol corticosteroids on the voice: triamcinolone acetonide and beclomethasone dipropionate. J Speech Hear Res 28(2):301–304

Wendler J, Seidner W, Kittel G et al (2005) Lehrbuch der Phoniatrie und Pädaudiologie, 4th edn. Thieme, Stuttgart

Wilken JA, Kane RL, Ellis AK et al (2003) A comparison of the effect of diphenhydramine and desloratadine on vigilance and cognitive function during treatment of ragweed-induced allergic rhinitis. Ann Allergy Asthma Immunol 91(4):375–385

Wolpe J (1958) Psychotherapy by reciprocal inhibition. Stanford University Press, Stanford

Yamagishi J, Veaux C, King S et al (2012) Speech synthesis technologies for individuals with vocal disabilities: voice banking and reconstruction. Acoust Sci Technol 33(1):1–5

Yiu E, Yee-Ian Kwong E (2005) Acupuncture for voice disorders. In: Proceedings of 6th Pan European Voice Conference, August 31–September 3, 2005, London. British Voice Association, London, p 79

Ylitalo R, Hammarberg B (2000) Voice characteristics, effects of voice therapy, and long-term follow-up of contact granuloma patients. J Voice 14(4):557–566

Ylitalo R, Ramel S (2002) Extraesophageal reflux in patients with contact granuloma: a prospective controlled study. Ann Otol Rhinol Laryngol 111(5 Pt 1):441–446

Zahoor AK, Green P, Creer S et al (2011) Reconstructing the voice of an individual following laryngectomy. Augment Altern Commun 27(1):1–6

Zealear DL, Dedo HH (1977) Control of paralysed axial muscles by electrical stimulation. Acta Otolaryngol 83(5–6):514–527

Zeitels SM, Healy GB (2003) Laryngology and phonosurgery. N Engl J Med 349(9):882–892

Zen H, Tokuda K, Black A (2009) Statistical parametric speech synthesis. Speech Commun 51(11):1039–1064

Zheng H, Zhou S, Li Z et al (2002) Reinnervation of the posterior cricoarytenoid muscle by the phrenic nerve for bilateral vocal cord paralysis in humans. Zhonghua Er Bi Yan Hou Tou Jing Wai Ke Za Zhi (Chin J Otorhinolaryngol Head Neck Surg) 37(3):210–214

Part III

Developmental Disorders of Speech and Language

Editors: Katrin Neumann,
Antoinette am Zehnhoff-Dinnesen

Lectors: Katrin Neumann,
Jochen Rosenfeld

Basics of Developmental Disorders of Speech and Language

9

Antoinette am Zehnhoff-Dinnesen,
Doris-Maria Denk-Linnert, Mona Hegazi,
Annerose Keilmann, Christiane Kiese-Himmel,
Katrin Neumann, Sabrina Regele,
Rainer Schönweiler, and Eva Seemanova

The terminology of children's problems concerning their language development is currently being discussed internationally (Bishop et al. 2017). In particular, the abolition of the terms Specific Language Impairment or Specific Developmental Disorder of Speech and Language is proposed. The authors of this chapter are aware of the discussion, but have not yet included any changed terminology in this version of the chapter.

A. am Zehnhoff-Dinnesen · S. Regele
Clinic of Phoniatrics and Pedaudiolocis,
University Hospital Münster, Münster, Germany
e-mail: am.zehnhoff@uni-muenster.de;
sabrina.regele@ukmuenster.de

D.-M. Denk-Linnert
Division of Phoniatrics-Logopedics,
Department of Otorhinolaryngology,
Medical University of Vienna, Wien, Austria
e-mail: Doris-maria.denk-linnert@meduniwien.ac.at

M. Hegazi
ENT Department, Ain Shams University, Cairo, Egypt

A. Keilmann
Voice Care Center Bad Rappenau,
Bad Rappenau, Germany
e-mail: Keilmann@kommunikation.klinik.uni-mainz.de

C. Kiese-Himmel
Phoniatrics/Pediatric Audiological Psychology,
University Medical Center Göttingen,
Göttingen, Germany
e-mail: ckiese@med.uni-goettingen.de

K. Neumann
Department of Phoniatrics and Pediatric Audiology,
ENT Clinic, St. Elisabeth Hospital, University of
Bochum, Bochum, Germany
e-mail: Katrin.neumann@rub.de

R. Schönweiler
Department of Phoniatrics and Pediatric Audiology,
University Clinic of Schleswig-Holstein,
Campus Lübeck, Lübeck, Germany
e-mail: rainer.schoenweiler@phoniatrie.uni-luebeck.de

E. Seemanova
Department of Child Neurology, 2nd Medical
School of Charles University Prague,
Prague, Czech Republic
e-mail: Eva.seemanova@lfmotol.cuni.cz

© Springer-Verlag GmbH Germany, part of Springer Nature 2020
A. am Zehnhoff-Dinnesen et al. (eds.), *Phoniatrics I*, European Manual of Medicine,
https://doi.org/10.1007/978-3-662-46780-0_9

9.1 Definition of Developmental Disorders of Speech and Language (DDSL)

Christiane Kiese-Himmel

DDSL comprise impaired comprehension of speech and language and use of spoken or written language. Linguistic symptoms refer to phonology, lexicon, semantics, morphology and syntax; they can affect pragmatics. DDSL are one of the major reasons for referral to a paediatrician (e.g. Shevell et al. 2015), phoniatrician/pediatric audiologist, speech-language therapist or developmental psychologist; they include a wide range of atypical language development with and without an associated medical condition:

- Late talking/expressive language delay in the absence of other developmental problems
- Primary (specific) language impairments
- Secondary (non-specific) language impairments (language acquisition deficits caused by or associated with syndromes or with prematurity, maturation delay, significant organic diseases, e.g. infection diseases such as meningitis, long-lasting or permanent hearing loss, focal brain lesions during pre-, peri- and the post-natal development, mental retardation, pervasive neurodevelopmental disorders, e.g. autism spectrum disorders)
- Childhood dysphasia with Landau-Kleffner syndrome
- Mixed language disorders (e.g. a syndrome and brain injury)
- Pragmatic (communication) language disorders
- Phonological disorders before the completion of spoken language acquisition
- Developmental dyslexia (specific reading and reading comprehension impairment)
- Developmental dysgraphia (specific spelling/writing impairment)
- Language-related learning disabilities in reading and understanding written maths tasks
- Mixed disorders of verbal scholastic skills

Consequently, children with DDSL are a heterogeneous population. More boys than girls are affected. Diagnoses can overlap including cumulative effects ('comorbidity') which may be aggravated by deprivation (e.g. poverty tied to parents' low educational level), family history and growing up multilingually. In the context of DDSL, many children have difficulties in other domains such as playing, cognition and motor functions.

The objective of Sect. 9.1 is to provide an overview of the most prevalent types of childhood language disorders (including assessment and treatment) that phoniatricians are confronted with. To understand DDSL, a physician should have a broad knowledge of factors constituting age-appropriate behaviour in several domains: cognition, motor skills, auditory processing and speech and language functioning. Early identification of children with DDSL or those at risk of it and adequate early intervention can remove the symptoms and potentially avoid related problems (e.g. in communication; emotional/behavioural difficulties, disabilities in school performances) and positively influence both socialization and academic outcomes. In contrast, late-starting treatments may not improve the chances for positively modulating the trajectory of development of a DDSL.

Standardized and normed assessment instruments, especially psychometric tests with actual age- or gender-referenced norms, which evaluate the child's cognitive (and academic) abilities, are necessary for diagnosis of language delay and intellectual disability. Informal (nonstandardized) procedures and analysis of natural language samples (samples of spontaneous language through play or storytelling) are preferred diagnostic instruments for descriptive purposes. Intervention for language disorders may require the involvement of different professionals—depending on the aetiology. Speech-language pathologists are specially trained in the treatment of impaired language.

A credible prognosis for the treatment effect of an individual child can hardly be made. The outcome of language therapy will vary depending on the nature and aetiology of an individual DDSL; its medical, sometimes also psychological or occupational, therapy, as well as special education; and the time the intervention begins.

9.2 Psychomotor and Cognitive Stages of Normal Children at Different Ages

Christiane Kiese-Himmel

9.2.1 Psychomotor Developmental Stages

Psychomotor development is a very important field for the overall development of a child and academic achievement. Learning to move with adaptive control and the coordination of a sensory process with a motor activity (e.g. eye-hand coordination) guided by cognition represents psychomotor performance. Structural and functional changes in the developing brain constitute the basis for it.

The motor imitation ability for simple movements is normally present at birth, e.g. mouth opening. The oculomotor system approximates its mature state a few months after birth, and around the age of 3 months, infants are increasingly able to make accurate eye movements. When newborn reflexes disappear, psychomotor development focuses on the progressive acquisition of skills comprising both cognitive and organized patterns of motor activities. It combines thought and muscle movements and proceeds in continuing stages to achieve motor control, fine motor skills, sociability, language and self-knowledge. Physical development and growth and maturation in infancy, childhood and adolescence determine psychomotor development and constitute gross and fine motor skills from higher brain centres. Further, psychomotor development is strongly associated with environmental stimulation. Children growing up in socially disadvantaged backgrounds may be at risk of neurodevelopmental, including motor, delay, and the negative impacts of early psychosocial risks may persist into later childhood (e.g. Laucht et al. 1992, 1997; Holz et al. 2015).

The first psychomotor achievements in healthy, term-born infants involve oral contact with objects in order to determine their properties ('oral exploration') as the mouth is the first tool to experience the object world. An object is typically held in one hand and brought to the mouth, mediated by the palmar grasp reflex, in the first 3 months of age. During the third month, infants begin to develop visual control of the hand. Visually guided reaching is achieved in the course of the fourth or fifth month with subsequent activities involving the hands by grasping targets, examining, manipulating and experimenting ('manual exploration') as well as transferring objects with both hands around 6 months and exploration with index finger around 8 months. Further achievements are, among others, the following: head control about the end of the third month, rolling from the back to the front at 24 weeks; grasping thumb finger at 8 months; imitating actions on objects at 9 months; sitting without any support between 9 and 10 months (at this point, complementary bimanual activities can succeed); standing alone as well as scribbling with big arm movements at 13 months; walking without help at 14/15 months; throwing a ball or climbing on a chair at 18 months; and moving from one place to another by walking with basis control and coordination. By age 2, a child can kick a ball forwards and say his name; at 3–4 years, the child can walk backwards a few feet, stand on one leg, use child-safe scissors in one hand and draw a circle and a cross; and from 4 to 5 years, more coordinated movements help to refine psychomotor skills (e.g. walking on a balance beam, standing on one foot for 10 s, jumping backwards). Fine motor activity time involving paper and pencil activities is increasing. Between 5 and 7 years, a child can ride a two-wheel bike.

9.2.2 Cognitive Development Stages

The term 'cognition' means to understand experiences through different mental processes. They form the basis of language development. The most famous theory of cognitive development from birth to adolescence comes from the Swiss psychologist Jean Piaget (1896–1980). His theory comprises four progressive stages of learning related to chronological age and focuses on the manner in which a child engages the objects of his physical environment (constructivist perspec-

Table 9.1 Stages of cognitive development according to Piaget (1963)

Stage	Age range	Acquired competence
Sensorimotor	From birth to approximately 2 years of age	Reacting to the world by reflexes and sensorimotor activities; acquisition of 'object permanence' (objects continue to exist even when they are not to be seen)
Preoperational	Roughly 2 through 6 or 7 years of age	Developing symbol thinking, beginning of symbol employment (images, words) beyond simple motor play; language development; speech becoming more social; role-playing; egocentric thinking; incremental emergence of reasoning and logical thought
Concrete-operational	In early elementary school years through age 11 or 12	Concrete problem-solving learning to think more abstractly, e.g. understanding some reversible operations, reasoning about class inclusion and relations between classes; recognition the difference between volume and size
Formal-operational	From about ages 11 or 12 years onwards	Application of logical thought processes and abstract thinking; reasoning about hypothetical problems; deductive reasoning; systematic planning

Table 9.2 Sensorimotor stage with six substages according to Piaget (1963)

Sensorimotor stage	
Substage	Age range
1. **Neonatal reflexive behaviour**	From birth to first month
2. **First habits, primary circular reactions** (Coordinating sensation and concepts)	1–4 months
3. **Secondary circular reactions** (Intentionally coordinating sensation and concepts; repeating of an action in order to trigger a response in the environment)	4–8 months
4. **Coordination of secondary reactions**	8–12 months
5. **Tertiary circular reactions, novelty and curiosity** (Beginning trial-and-error-experimentation)	12–18 months
6. **Early representational thoughts, internalization of schemata, invention of new means** (Beginning to understand the world through mental operations instead of actions; deferred imitation)	18–24 months

tive), thereby obtaining an understanding of the world and the construction of knowledge (Table 9.1). Cognitive development derives from two processes: assimilation (new information is included into already existing cognitive structures) and accommodation (a new cognitive structure is formed). Only the first stage, the sensorimotor, comprises several substages (Table 9.2) (Kozutin 1984). The following preoperational stage (Table 9.1) is primarily characterized by the development of a symbolic mind—a fundamental milestone in cognitive functioning. By means of symbols, children are capable of gaining new types of knowledge about their world. In early elementary school years up to the age of 11 or 12, they still think in concrete terms (concrete-operational stage), and the formal-operational stage will conclude their cognitive development. Meanwhile several researchers

have hypothesized that children possess many of the aforementioned abilities at an earlier age than Piaget assumed. Moreover, Piaget did not distinguish between the constructivist framework and the stage theory, and he did not study his subjects across the whole lifespan. Thus, some alternative views of cognitive development (Neo-Piagetian theories) have emerged, in particular views relating to the educational context.

Lev S. Vygotsky (1896–1934), a Russian psychologist, defends an alternative position to Piaget while sustaining the commitment to the active learning of children (Kozutin 1984). According to Vygotsky's sociocultural developmental perspective, every developmental function evolves and emerges through social interaction with others, subsequently organized at the individual level. The psychomotor and cognitive aspects of development inherently interact throughout the lifespan.

9.3   Language Stages of Normal Children at Different Ages

Doris-Maria Denk-Linnert

9.3.1   Introduction

Typical speech and language development proceeds in stages with regularities with respect to time and content (Table 9.3). These stages in perception as well as in production always overlap and are universal among humans, but the individual developmental pace varies widely. The development takes place in five areas: prosody, phonetics/phonology, semantics/lexicon, morphology/syntax and pragmatics. The so-called milestones characterize the normal developmental course, i.e. the average age at which children should have reached specific skills (see Sect. 11.3). Knowledge of these milestones in context with linguistic, psychological, motoric and general developmental aspects is a prerequisite to recognizing developmental delays or disturbances. Normal speech and language development comprises an age-appropriate spontaneous language, normal speech activity, normal auditory speech perception and normal prosody. The available studies on the neural basis of normal language development suggest that the cerebral networks underlying language processing are already in place during early development (Friederici 2006).

In the broadest sense, speech and language development already begins in utero: at approximately 7 months of gestation, a foetus perceives, discriminates and responds to speech sounds. Early speech perception and recognition of rhythmic and prosodic characteristics of the native language appear prenatally (de Langen-Müller et al. 2011, 2012; Hennon et al. 2000; Jusczyk and Aslin 1995). Preverbal development, as noticeable to parents and others, starts at birth. Newborns already recognize and give preference to their native language (Moon et al. 2013). Prosodic characteristics are responsible for recognizing the native language (Nazzi et al. 1998).

The sensitive (critical) period for language acquisition (Ruben 1997), when the brain is best able to acquire language, lasts up to 4 (5) years of age, in parallel with brain maturation and the development of the central auditory nervous system. At the end of 13 (to 14) years, the development is completed. Preconditions for language acquisition include:

- Normal   physical-motor-mental-emotional development
- Normal intelligence
- Normal brain maturation, development of hemispheric dominance, laterality
- Normal sensory organs (especially normal hearing)
- Normal articulatory organs
- Favourable sociocultural factors

There are many theories on the mechanisms of language acquisition (evolutionary, psychological, environmental, nativistic and cognitive explanations). 'Inside-out theories' (Hockema and Smith 2009) rely on the congenital, genetically caused language ability (innate language-learning

Table 9.3 Normal speech-language development

Age (months)	Developmental stage
0–12	**Preverbal stage**
Birth–1.5	Differentiating cries
1.5–2	Cooing (first babbling phase)
4(6)–12	Babbling (second babbling phase)
9	First word understanding
10–13	First word
From month 12 onwards	**Verbal stage**
12–18	One-word utterances (one-word sentences) (holophrastic phase)
18–24	Two-word sentences (telegraphic phase)
25–36	Multiple-word sentences
37–60	More complex sentences
From month 60 onwards	Perfecting (intuitive linguistic period)

mechanism), which is the predominant cause from which language arises. 'Outside-in theories' focus on general learning mechanisms (operant conditioning with positive and negative reinforcement, imitation) and comprise cognitive and social-interactive factors. Language acquisition can be explained by a combination of behavioural (Skinner 1957) and mentalistic (Chomsky 1988) approaches of 'nurture and nature'. Under the influence of environment and experience, the innate language ability results in language acquisition. Modern explanations (e.g. emergentist coalition model) explain language as a development product that results from a combination of congenital language ability and environmental factors (Dale et al. 2015; Hollich et al. 2000).

Two phases of speech-language development can be described: preverbal and verbal phases (Table 9.3) that merge into each other. Modern theories point out that there is a continuous transition from babbling to speech production (Storkel and Morrisette 2002).

9.3.2 Preverbal Phase (First Year)

In this phase, there is no connection yet between produced speech sounds and semantic contents (Yavas 1998). Communication begins before children utter their first words. Babies react to the prosody of their parents' speech and use facial expressions, gestures, cries and other preverbal vocalizations to communicate with their parents or caregivers. Important steps of preverbal language acquisition are, among others, the sharing of a focus of attention with the parent or caregiver, the use of referential gestures and the imitation of the language babies hear in their environment. Babies recognize sounds of words before they start to understand them. Accurate perception is a necessary component of accurate production (Flege 1995). Dialogue with the parents or caregivers and the associated social interaction are essential for the acquisition of communicative skills and to drive further language development.

There are two well-known classifications of the preverbal phases that overlap (Fox-Boyer and Schäfer 2015)—that one of Stark (1980) and that

one of Oller (1980, 1999). According to Stark (1980), five stages of speech development in the first year of life can be differentiated:

- Reflexive vocalization (birth to 2 months)
- Cooing and laughter (2–4 months)
- Vocal play (4–8 months)
- Babbling with reduplicative sounds (8–10 months)
- Babbling with non-reduplicative sounds in combination with the first words (10–14 months)

Oller (1980, 1999) also describes five stages:

- Phonation (first month)
- Cooing (2–3 months)
- Expansion (4–6 months)
- Canonical babbling (6–10 months)
- Variegated babbling stage (10–12 months)

Another recent classification, the Stark Assessment of Early Vocal Development-Revised (SAEVD-R) also describes five levels of preverbal development that allow the assessment of utterances between 0 and 20 months (Nathani et al. 2006):

- Level 1: Reflexive level (first 2 months)
- Level 2: Control of phonation (1–4 months)
- Level 3: Expansion stage (3–8 months)
- Level 4: Simple canonical babbling (5–10 months)
- Level 5: Progressive forms (9–18 months)

9.3.2.1 The Crying Stage (Differentiating Cries, Reflexive Vocalization; Birth to 6 Weeks)

Cries and vegetative noises are an involuntary and biologically rooted behaviour. A newborn reflexively cries owing to hunger, pain, etc. Subsequently, crying develops to be the first form of communication (crying for attention, a need or comfort). Beginning from the fourth (fifth) week on, one can distinguish between various pleasant and unpleasant cries (indicating hunger, boredom, pain, etc.), the so-called 'modulated cry'. The sound characteristics and voice onsets differ according to the baby's intention of crying, and the caregivers can often interpret the intended message. The baby notices that a cry can bring food, comfort or companionship, i.e. the baby learns the basic rule of communication. Newborns also begin to recognize important sounds in their environment (e.g. the voice of their mother). By 6 months of age, most basic sounds of the native language can be recognized.

9.3.2.2 The Cooing Stage (Syn.: First Babbling Stage, Cooing and Laughter; 6–8 Weeks)

At the beginning of the second month, at the same time of the first smile, the baby starts to play with its articulatory organs. He or she produces cooing sounds not only reflexively. These 'first vocalizations of contentedness' are predominantly elongated vowels ('oooo', 'aaaa') and are vocal responses to the speech of others. At the end of this period, simple sequences of consonant-vowels are uttered, by producing pharyngeal, palatal or uvular sounds (Oller et al. 1999). The baby's cooing contains the basic sounds of all languages, not just those of the baby's mother language.

It has to be pointed out that even deaf babies coo. Their language development becomes deviant from normality at later ages.

9.3.2.3 The Babbling Stage (Syn.: Second Babbling Stage; 4–12 Months)

According to the milestones of normal speech development in Germany (de Langen-Müller et al. 2011, 2012, 2016), the traditional term 'second babbling stage' comprises the stages of:

- (Marginal) babbling: (4 months)
- Canonical babbling (6 months)
- Reduplicative babbling (e.g. 'baba'; 8–10 months)
- Variegated babbling (e.g. 'bada'; 8–10 months)

Like cooing, babbling provides a social reward. Babies experiment with speech sounds resulting in pitch and volume variation. Babbling infants do not articulate all the speech sounds they hear in the adult language. On the other hand, babies produce sounds that they have never heard before. Canonical babbling describes the formation of syllables consisting of consonants and vocals (e.g. 'ba'). At the age of 6 months, the baby's babbling can be attributed to the native language (Boysson-Bardies et al. 1984). A lacking verbal interaction at this age usually results in a later developmental disorder of speech, language and communication. The babbling consists of a wide variety of sounds and is defined as the combination of consonants and vowels in alternating sequences. Reduplicative babbling is characterized by the production of reduplicated syllables such as 'bababa'. Variegated babbling brings about more complex syllables or two-syllable utterances or multiple syllables with constant vocals and consonants and different intonation (Harley 2001; Nathani et al. 2006; Werker and Tees 1999). The vocalizations now take a more speech-like quality. Babbling means motor exercise and communicative function at the same time. Around 8 to 9 months, the baby starts to imitate sounds of the environment. For successful imitation, normal hearing (acoustic perception and differentiation) and normal motor skills are necessary.

9.3.2.4 First Word Understanding (9 Months)

At about 8–9 months, the baby turns and looks in the direction of sounds and listens when he or she is spoken to. The baby further pays attention to prosody and intonation or mimics the expression of parents and other persons and tries to imitate adult speech sounds. The baby understands its first words at about 9 months of age, learns about the relation between object and language, recognizes words for common items such as 'cup' or 'shoe' and begins to respond to requests (e.g. 'come here') (Grimm 2003; Bates et al. 1994). This is preparation for the production of the first word (10–12 months). An important precursor in the preverbal development of a child is the joint attention or shared attention. This happens when one individual alerts another (usually parent and child) to an object to bring it to his or her attention using eye gaze (Moore and Dunham 1995; Zollinger 2015 ('triangulation')), pointing or non-verbal or verbal indications. Both the child and the caregiver direct their attention to an object of shared interest, and both are aware of the other persons perceiving that object and showing interest in it as well.

9.3.2.5 The First Word (10–13, at the Latest 20 Months)

The preverbal phase ends with the production of the first words, starting with proto-words (word-like utterances) around the age of 10 months (see Sect. 11.3). First words are mainly nouns and refer to people of particular interest ('mama', 'dada') or objects that move ('ball', 'cat'). Verbs, adjectives, adverbs and prepositions are learned later, usually in that order. In the second year, babbled utterances and meaningful words appear side by side. Later on, linguistic expressions increase and babbling utterances decrease (Nathani et al. 2006).

Current theories and studies about phonological acquisition challenge Jakobson (1941, 1969) theory of children's speech, which states that universal contrasts are learned first in all languages ('mama', 'papa', the so-called phonological universals). Among others, Fox-Boyer and Dodd (1999), Weinrich and Zehner (2003) and Fox-Boyer (2016) have summarized modern knowledge in this field. The order of acquisition starts with vocals, followed by plosives, nasals, fricatives and affricates. Topographically front consonants precede back consonants; the /p/ and /m/ sounds appear before /k/ or /h/. Single consonants are realized before multiple consonants. A child first learns to articulate fricatives at the end of a word and plosives at the word's beginning. The production passes through a learning process and is not completely correct from the beginning.

9.3.3 Verbal Phase (from 1 Year Onwards)

A central task in the second year is the acquisition of lexicon. Word combinations bring about the beginning of productive syntactic abilities. With 2 years 90% of children can combine at least two words (Szagun 2007).

In the third year of life, basic grammatical regularities of the native language are acquired.

The emergentist coalition model is useful in explaining early speech-language acquisition and serves as a model for early intervention strategies. Speech and language are developmental products requiring these factors: sufficient language input, active engagement of the child with the input and the presence of factors that increase the odds for correctly mapping language form to meaning (Poll 2011; Hollich et al. 2000).

9.3.3.1 One-Word Sentences (Holophrastic Stage, 12–18 Months)

The stage of one-word utterances (one-word sentences) begins at about 1 year of age. One-word sentences differ from babbling vocalizations by their symbolic meaning (development of the symbol function of language). One-word utterances are also called holophrases because the toddler expresses the meaning of an entire situation by just a single word (Rupp 2013). This stage of language development interacts with cognitive development, as well as with the development of deixis and gesture. (Deixis describes the fact that words or phrases may require contextual information to convey any meaning, e.g. English pronouns, i.e. their semantic meaning is fixed, but their denotational meaning varies depending on time or place or other factors.) Eventually, one-word utterances turn into longer expressions, i.e. two-word utterances.

The toddler realizes that the acoustic string (word) and the reference (object) belong together (naming insight). Holophrases do not only name objects or persons. There is enormous ambiguity in a child's holophrases. If, for example, a toddler says 'papa', he or she may not mean 'father' exclusively but also the coat of the father or asking whether the father will come, etc. The child may declare, demand, describe or question. In conjunction with prosody, mimicry and gestures, the meaning of holophrases can be varied. Owing to the social and situational context, adults can interpret the utterances. According to the noun-bias hypothesis (Gentner 1981, 1982; Nelson et al. 1993), nouns are acquired first and make up the greatest part of the lexicon compared with other word types. In contrast, it has been observed that holophrases also comprise verbs, adjectives, relational and social-pragmatic words (Rothweiler and Kauschke 2007; Rothweiler and Meibauer 1999, Meibauer 1999). Words are frequently under-extended or overextended to inappropriate categories, e.g. all four-legged hairy creatures may be called 'dog'. At the age of 3 years, children have acquired a balanced and targeted lexicon composition (Pomnitz and Rupp 2013).

At least for English and German languages, the majority of 16- (de Langen-Müller et al. 2011, 2012, 2016) to 18- (Menyuk et al. 1995) month-old toddlers have an active lexicon of about 50 words. The receptive lexicon precedes the active one (Rothweiler and Kauschke 2007): by 13.5 months, toddlers have a receptive lexicon of about 50 words (Menyuk et al. 1995) and by 16 months already 100 words. The phase of the first 50 words starts with the first referentially used words and ends up with the beginning of the naming explosion at the age of 18 months (Kauschke 1999, Kauschke and Hofmeister 2002, Rothweiler and Kauschke 2007).

9.3.3.2 Two-Word Sentences (Telegraphic Stage, 18–24 Months)

In this period, the toddler starts to combine two words and to utter basic sentences such as 'mummy bag'; the meaning may be, e.g. 'Mummy, give me the bag', 'Mummy, where is the bag?' or 'This is Mummy's bag!' As in the previous stage, there is an enormous ambiguity in these two-word utterances. The kinds of word that are likely to be omitted are articles, prepositions, pronouns and auxiliary verbs. A toddler talking to him- or herself during this stage avoids pronouns ('baby go' instead of 'I go') and is able to understand simple instructions and questions.

At the age around 18 months, together with the combination of two words, the child's vocabulary begins to grow fast (Nelson 1973): this naming explosion or 'word spurt' represents a developmental milestone. Children usually add 10 words per day (Clark 2003). By 18 (not later than 24) months, the children utter on average at least 50 words (Menyuk et al. 1995), at the age of 24 months about 200, at the age of 30 months 500 and at

school entry 3000–5000 (Clark 2003; Rupp 2013). Interindividual differences must be considered.

Slobin (1971) found that children of approximately the same age from six different languages (English, German, Russian, Finnish, Luo and Samoan) expressed similar kinds of meanings—utterances were used to:

- Locate or name objects and people—there glass
- Request, demand or indicate a desire for people, objects or events—more milk
- Negate or indicate refusal or rejection—no wash
- Express situations or events—papa go
- Indicate possession—mama dress
- Describe—doggy big
- Question with both where questions and yes/no questions—where ball? daddy go?

In these utterances the first stages of morpheme development can be recognized:

- No morphemes are used—two woman.
- On the basis of imitation, the correct forms are sometimes used.
- Rules are being acquired and overgeneralized (overregularization)—he runned, he goed, two cats, three mans.
- The adult language is approached.

Approximately 13–20% of children (Ellis Weismer 2007) are so-called late talkers (Grimm 2003; Desmarais et al. 2008). These are defined as having an expressive vocabulary of fewer than 50 words or as lacking combinations of words at the age of 24 months. They are at risk of developing a speech-language developmental disorder. Thirty-five to fifty percent of late talkers turn out to become 'late bloomers', who catch up during the following year (until 36 months of age), whereas others end up with a specific developmental disorder of speech and language (Grimm 2003; Kauschke 2006; Schöler et al. 2007; Kühn and von Suchodoletz 2009; Sachse and von Suchodoletz 2013).

Typical deviant phonological processes (physiological speech sound deviations during speech-language development that show a specific error pattern at the age of 24–30 months) comprise, e.g. assimilations, omission of unstressed syllables, a reduction of initial consonants, backwarded articulation or deaffrication (see Sect. 11.3).

The acquisition of lexicon and grammar is mutually dependent. Many theories have been established and discarded, such as the theory of Universal Grammar by Chomsky. Nowadays a use-based approach is favoured. It is discussed whether innate (modular, nativistic) or epigenetic (recognition of regularities) factors are more important (Szagun 2013; Pinker 1991, 1994). Pinker states that a child is prepared for grammar acquisition as a spider is for web construction. The so-called semantic bootstrapping (Pinker 1984) enables children to discover syntactic rules.

A child aged 4 years can speak grammatically correct language, but grammar acquisition is not completely finished. For instance, passive sentences can only be built by 9–10 years.

9.3.3.3 Multiple-Word Sentences (25–36 Months)

With increasing age and larger vocabulary, children form longer and more complex sentences and start to use conjunctions. More complex grammar structures will be acquired: more-word sentences, negations, imperatives, questions and compound sentences. The first combinations are made with matrix sentences ('Peter falling', 'Peter cries', 'Mummy runs'). Further on, the sentences are still telegraphic although they may be quite long. Until the end of the third year, the child learns to form flexions, plurals and past forms and to use auxiliary verbs.

9.3.3.4 More Complex Sentences (37–60 Months)

From the third birthday on, development towards an adultlike grammar continues. Auxiliary verbs are being ordered correctly in questions and negatives. Grammatical markers emerge including possessive words or phrases, determiners (i.e. a word, phrase or affix that occurs together with a noun and serves to express the reference of that noun in the context) and irregular past tense verbs. A variety of early complex sentence types emerge including compound sentences, full prepositional clauses in sentences and simple infinitives. At the end of this period, later-developing morphemes are acquired.

At the age of 4, children are able to talk adequately: articulately, grammatically and semantically. They are able to use communicative language appropriately.

9.3.3.5 Perfecting ('The Intuitive Linguistic Period', 4–14 Years)

Although most of the language has been acquired in the period up to age 4–5 years, there are still many linguistic skills to be obtained. In the so-called intuitive linguistic period (Matthews 1996), larger words, a differentiated mental lexicon and longer and more complex sentences are used. There is also a further syntactic development after 4 years of age; for example, the child begins to understand passive sentences.

In this period of linguistic refinement, written language is acquired, and subsequently more sophisticated spoken and written texts are produced. Children develop further metalinguistic awareness (in the four subareas: phonological, word, syntactic and pragmatic awareness (Tunmer and Bowey 1984)) and competence. They reflect consciously upon the nature and properties of language (van Kleek 1982) and are able to talk about, analyse and think about language independent of the concrete meaning of each word. Metalingustic skills are strongly associated with reading comprehension and have also great impact on academic performance (e.g. understanding multiple meanings of words, use of irony and metaphors).

9.3.4 Normal Speech Disfluencies During Speech-Language Development

Mostly between 2.5 and 4 (5) years of age, during the intensive phases of language acquisition, a higher number of normal disfluencies (interruptions of the smooth flow of the speech) are observed in the majority (i.e. about 75%) of children (Baumgartner and Füssenich 2002). They need to be distinguished from stuttering—a term which should be strictly avoided for these normal disfluencies—and are part of normal speech-language development. They mainly consist of whole word and phrase repetitions, revisions, hesitations with interjections or incomplete sentences with change of focus (Kowal et al. 1975; Pellowski and Conture 2002). The children show neither accompanying physical behaviour as typical for stuttering (such as mimicry, limb movements or breathing irregularities) nor negative emotional reactions (such as frustration, anxiety, shame, embarrassment with talking, refusal to talk) with these disfluencies. Normal disfluencies are likely to arise from difficulties in the speech planning processes such as lexical retrieval and grammatical planning of utterances but also by interaction-relevant (pragmatic) or emotional demands (Neumann et al. 2016). Stuttering and non-stuttering children show normal disfluencies to a comparable extent, i.e. 5% (Ambrose and Yairi 1999; Pellowski and Conture 2002; Sandrieser and Schneider 2015). There is no evidence that stuttering develops from normal disfluencies (Yairi and Ambrose 2005). Girls show a tendency to suffer fewer from normal disfluencies than boys (Yairi 1981).

The following criteria characterize a normal disfluency (Schorr 1992; Guitar and Contour 2007; Bosshardt 2010; Wendlandt 2011; Neumann et al. 2016):

- Symptoms: hesitations, revisions and repetitions at the beginning of the words.
- No symptoms such as blocks, repetitions of syllables, part-word repetitions, word interruptions or sound prolongations.
- No negative reaction to dysfluencies.
- No secondary behaviour.
- Disfluent speech usually persists no longer than 6 months.
- Normal speech-language development.
- No risk factors such as a family history of stuttering.

9.4 Stages of Auditory Development in Children with Normal Hearing

Rainer Schönweiler

Speech-language development relies substantially on hearing, auditory processing and auditory perception; the stages of hearing development are outlined in Sect. 14.3.

At a gestational age of around 26 weeks, hair cells connect to the central nervous system, enabling the foetuses to hear via bone conduction (Sect. 14.3, Table 14.3) and make their first experience with 'maternal speech' and the external world (Northern and Downs 2002). Though hearing frequencies normally range between 20 Hz and 20 kHz for humans, hearing in utero is restricted to frequencies below 1 kHz, the reason behind that being the dampening effect caused by maternal tissues and the amniotic fluid. Thus, foetuses are able to perceive prosodic speech cues, while they miss acoustic information on vowel formants and consonant frequencies. This changes dramatically within 1–2 days after birth when newborns start using air conduction as the main hearing medium (Sect. 14.3, Table 14.3) and they become able to hear all speech frequencies. From this moment on, auditory feedback, and later on imitation, becomes essential for the acquisition of language and speech (Kuhl and Meltzoff 1996; Möller and Schönweiler 1999).

Throughout the post-natal stage, infants listen to their parents' speech and learn to control their own vocalizations and speech sound productions; they are able to learn any language they are presented with (Kuhl and Meltzoff 1996). A reduplicating babbling (e.g. 'bababa') which emerges at ages of 8–10 months indicates that a baby hears, because deaf babies are not able to produce it (Northern and Downs 2002).

In the infantile stage, children develop auditory processing and auditory perception abilities that permit speech understanding in a noisy environment, speech sound discrimination, dichotic listening, auditory memory and phonological awareness (Sect. 14.3, Table 14.3). Many of these abilities are required for learning at school. Children who perform poorly in tasks involving auditory discrimination of speech sounds, auditory working memory and phonological awareness are at a high risk for learning disabilities (see Sect. 15.2).

9.5 Multilingual Speech and Language Acquisition

Mona Hegazi and Katrin Neumann

9.5.1 Definition of Multilingualism

Multilingualism is a common human condition that makes it possible for an individual to function, at some level, in more than one language. The term multilingualism includes bilingualism. A child is said to be multilingual if he or she can comprehend or produce two or more languages in oral, written or sign language, with at least a basic level of functional proficiency or use. This is regardless of the age at which the languages were learned (Grech and McLeod 2012). Multilingual children are operationally defined as those children who receive regular input in two or more languages somewhere between birth and adolescence (Kohnert 2010).

Most multilinguals have a dominant language, used by the majority of people in their environment. This is usually the language of greater proficiency (Genesee et al. 2004; Paradis 2010). This language can, however, change with age, education, employment and many other factors (Baker and Prys Jones 1998; Kohnert 2004).

9.5.2 Types of Multilingualism

Multilingualism is categorized in two ways.

- According to the age of acquisition of the languages:
  - *Simultaneous acquisition* occurs when a child is raised bilingually from birth or when the second language (or third) is introduced before the age of 3 (Paradis et al. 2011).
  - *Sequential/successive acquisition* occurs when a second language (or third) is introduced after the first language is well established (although not completely acquired), generally after the age of 3 (Genesee et al. 2004).

The critical period of a transition from simultaneous to sequential language acquisition has been under debate for a long time. It has ranged from the second month of life, where a first transfer of linguistic pattern from one language to another one takes place (Genesee et al. 2004), to about 12 years (Lenneberg 1967). Nowadays, the first 3 years of life are widely accepted as the period of bilingual first language acquisition (BFLA) for the majority of children (Chilla and Haberzettl 2014).

- According to the amount of language exposure:
  - A *majority language* refers to the language spoken by the majority of people in a region.
  - A *minority language* refers to a language spoken by a minority of the population in a region.

9.5.3 Populations Exposed to Multilingualism

Conditions that foster multilingualism include (Grosjean 1996):

Migrations of Various Kinds (economic, educational, political, religious) Children may experience sequential acquisition if they immigrate to a country where a different language is spoken.

Education Sequential learning occurs if the child speaks his native language at home and, after school entry, instruction is offered in a different language.

Intermarriage Children are exposed simultaneously to two languages of the mother and father.

9.5.4   Bilingual Language Acquisition in Typically Developing Children

Simultaneous multilingual children may start talking slightly later than monolingual children. However, they still begin talking within the normal range (Meisel 2004). Those children who are exposed to two languages are able to differentiate them and have been shown to switch languages easily according to their conversation partner (Genesee 2009; Genesee and Nicoladis 2006). Young bilingual speakers may use a combination of both languages when speaking. This is considered a normal situation in bilingual language development. Children may mix grammar rules or use words from both languages in the same sentence. There is evidence that children acquiring two or more languages from birth are able to differentiate the grammatical systems of their languages without apparent effort. Moreover, the subsequent course and rate of acquisition proceed through the same developmental phases as those observed in monolingual children.

For sequential acquisition, Paradis et al. (2011) describe what a child may experience when the second language is introduced:

- The child may go through a 'silent' or 'nonverbal' period which may last up to several months. This period is necessary for the child to develop his understanding of the language (Tabors 1997). It is noted that younger children usually remain in this phase longer than older ones. Children may rely on using gestures in this period and use few words in the second language.
- A child may then begin to use short or imitative sentences and phrases. These early utterances are merely phrases he has heard and memorized. They are not constructed from the child's vocabulary set.
- Later on, the child starts to produce his own sentences incorporating his own newly learned vocabulary. With time, the child becomes more fluent but continues to make grammatical mistakes. It is noted that some of the mistakes are due to the influence of his first language.

9.5.5   Impact of Bilingualism on Language Development and Language Competence

Although it is assumed among researchers that bilingual or multilingual language acquisition occurs as frequently as monolingual language acquisition worldwide (Paradis et al. 2011), monolingualism may seem the natural or normal case of language development to parents. Hence, it is a popular assumption that exposing any child to a second (or third) language during the period of language development may hinder language growth, as well as the child's academic and intellectual development.

However, more recent research has proved that:

- Bilingual children are better able to focus their attention on relevant information, ignore distractions, stay focused, switch attention wilfully from one issue to another and hold information in mind (Poulin-Dubois et al. 2011).
- Bilingual individuals have been shown to be more creative and better at planning and solving complex problems than monolinguals (Paradis et al. 2011). Some studies have shown that bilingual speakers score higher in IQ tests than monolingual speakers (Weiten 2010).
- The effects of ageing on the brain are diminished among bilingual adults (Grosjean 1982). The higher the degree of bilingualism (measured by evaluation of the level of proficiency) in each language is, the more resistant a bilingual person is to the onset of dementia and other symptoms of Alzheimer's disease. In a study of Bialystok et al. (2007), the onset of dementia was delayed by 4 years in bilinguals compared with monolinguals with dementia.

Previous behavioural studies have supported the idea that language development is acquired in much the same way whether the child is bilingual or monolingual (Paradis 2005). However, more recent neuroimaging findings have proven that bilingual or multilingual language acquisition is associated with structural changes in the brain and with functional changes of neural activation during language processing in both hemispheres, in particular in the left inferior frontal gyrus (LIFG) and left superior temporal gyrus (LSTG). The kind and number of alterations, compared with those of monolingual individuals, depends on the age at which a second language has been acquired and differs between children with simultaneous and sequential bilingual language acquisition (e.g. Jasinska and Petitto 2013).

Among others, the following groups of children with impaired language development have been studied: children with developmental disorders of speech and language (DDSL; synonym, specific language impairment, SLI) (Paradis 2010; Gutierrez-Clellen et al. 2008), children with Down syndrome (Kay-Raining Bird et al. 2005) and children with autism spectrum disorder (ASD) (Petersen et al. 2011). The bilingual children did not demonstrate any extra delays or greater difficulties in their two languages than monolingual children in any of the studied groups. Thus, bilingualism did not have a negative effect on the children's language development, and sequential bilingual children with DDSL can also learn a second language. Although they face language-learning challenges, these are not considerably greater than those for monolingual children with the same language impairment. Multilingual children do not suffer more frequently from DDSL than monolingual ones, and multilingualism is not a cause of a DDSL (e.g. Chilla and Haberzettl 2014).

9.5.6 Issues with Assessment and Evaluation

During speech and language assessment of a multilingual child, the phoniatrician needs to determine if the child exhibits only environmentally caused language abnormalities or inconsistencies, for example, those due to an imperfectly acquired majority language, or a DDSL, i.e. a proper impairment. DDSLs always affect all languages to be acquired. Accordingly, the only reason a bilingual child would need to be provided with speech and language services is if the child has impairments in both languages.

During testing of a bilingual child, which ideally should be performed in both languages that the child has acquired, it is accepted that the child may respond in any of the languages he uses (Fierro-Cobas and Chan 2001). Testing language vocabulary and syntax should be done according to the language being tested, taking into consideration that at some stage of development, the two languages may merge with each other. The person administering the assessments must allow certain accommodations, such as additional instructions, additional trial items and training of concepts being tested (Saenz and Huer 2003; Gauthier 2012).

9.5.7 Management Issues

If bilingualism does not cause developmental disorders of speech and language, then stopping the use of one of the languages is not going to solve the problem. Instead, developmental language abnormalities need to be properly diagnosed to find their cause, and intervention needs to be started. It is important to have in mind that environmentally caused language abnormalities, for example, those due to an imperfectly acquired majority language, do not need treatment but benefit from an increase of qualitative and quantitative language input and language training programs. On the other hand, a DDSL cannot be overcome sufficiently by language training but requires language therapy (de Langen-Müller et al. 2011).

Stopping the use of the native language, in particular, causes more difficulties. Parents who stop using the native language may talk less with their child, since they may be less fluent in the other language, thus hindering natural communication. Although it is sometimes advised that each parent should constantly use one language when talking to the child (one-parent-one-language approach), provided that each language is fully mastered by this parent, it has been recognized that children will mix their languages regardless of the parents' approach

(Paradis et al. 2011). Rather, parents should speak to their child in a way that is comfortable and natural to them. Most clinical research supports the idea that intervention should be directed to one language, which is preferably the majority language (Jordaan and Yelland 2003; Zehler et al. 2003). Generalization or transfer across languages from the treated to the untreated language is expected to occur. On the other hand, there is some support for dual-language intervention plans for bilingual children (Kohnert 2008; Pena and Bedore 2009), provided there are bilingual therapists.

9.6 Epidemiology of Developmental Disorders of Speech and Language

Annerose Keilmann and Katrin Neumann

9.6.1 Objective

Epidemiological data are necessary for large-scale studies, for example, by the WHO, to provide information about the spread of a disorder and its potential causes. Moreover, they establish a basis for estimating the global and regional burden that a specific disorder brings to both the affected individuals and the society. This enables a calculation of resources that are needed to overcome the disease's negative sequelae and to plan necessary services. On a country level, epidemiological data are important for managing health services in order to prevent, identify and diagnose a disorder and to provide effective intervention and rehabilitation programs. Furthermore, they are needed for health economics and health insurance calculations on financial resources and for planning reimbursement policies.

Parents whose child is affected by a disorder often want information about its frequency of occurrence, in particular if they compare their child with other children. This also holds true for developmental language abnormalities where parents often sensitively observe siblings and other children, for example, on playgrounds

or in kindergartens. An increasing prevalence of developmental disorders of speech and language (DDSL) is a popular assumption frequently presented in the media and suspected by pedagogues and therapists. However, this assumption is not well supported. The probability that a strongly genetically caused disorder, such as a specific developmental disorder of speech and language (SDDSL), increases dramatically during a short period is rather low. Instead, a rise in public sensitivity for language abnormalities and school performance has to be taken into consideration, as well as improved options and tools for identifying and diagnosing developmental disorders of speech and language.

9.6.2 Prevalence of Late Talking and Developmental Disorders of Speech and Language

The prevalence of DDSL in general as reported for the Anglo-Saxon language area is given from 3 to 15%, mostly between 6 and 8% (Canning and Lyon 1989; Tomblin et al. 1997). Severe DDSL have to be expected in about 1% of children. The disorder affects boys more frequently than girls (Thomson and Polnay 2002). DDSL should not be confused with speech and language problems in a broader sense. For example, in an older Canadian study, *some* impairment of speech and language was observed in 16–22% of 5-year-old children (Beitchman et al. 1986).

Toddlers aged 2–3 years who demonstrate delayed onset and progression of expressive language, associated with an otherwise age-appropriate development, are denoted as 'late talkers' (Desmarais et al. 2008). Again, boys are more frequently affected than girls. In an early study (Rescorla 1989), an expressive vocabulary of fewer than 50 of the 310 target words of the Language Development Survey (LDS) and the lack of two-word combinations at 2 years of age were used as criteria for being a late talker. The prevalence reported for the Anglo-Saxon language region ranges from 2.0 to 17.5% (Horwitz et al. 2003; Reilly et al. 2007) and for Germany from 13 to 20% (Grimm 2003).

More recent research used the performance below the 10th centile on the MacArthur-Bates Communicative Development Inventory (CDI) at 24 months of age (Weismer 2007) or below the 15th centile on the LDS from 18 to 23 months of age (Rescorla and Achenbach 2002) which resulted in prevalence of late talkers of 10 or 15%.

9.6.2.1 Prevalence of Specific Developmental Disorders of Speech and Language

Specific developmental disorders of speech and language (SDDSL), also named primary developmental language disorders or specific language impairment, for which thorough diagnostics do not identify language-relevant comorbidities or conditions, represent a subset of DDSL. Their prevalence is given for the North American language area, according to the criteria of the ICD-10 or the DSM-5, to be from 5 to 8% (American Psychiatric Association 2013; Tomblin et al. 1997). For European countries, similar numbers have to be expected (Neumann et al. 2009). For SDDSL the gender distribution is reported between 1.3 and 5.9 boys to 1 girl (National Institute on Deafness and Other Communication Disorders 2008; Shriberg et al. 1999; Stromswold 1998; Tallal et al. 2001; Tomblin et al. 1997).

The most often cited study on the prevalence of specific language impairment is that of Tomblin et al. (1997), who reported a prevalence of SDDSL of 7.4% for monolingual English-speaking children of kindergarten age. For 6- and 7-year-old children, Law et al. (2000) noted median prevalence estimates of 5.5% and 3.1%, respectively. Differing from that, a higher prevalence of SDDSL has been reported for the region of Victoria in Australia with 17% (Reilly et al. 2010).

9.6.2.2 Developmental Disorders with Language-Relevant Comorbidities

In general, children with language-relevant comorbidities, such as hearing loss, genetic syndromes, intellectual disabilities, multiple handicaps, pervasive developmental disorders, autism, disorders of social functioning with onset specific to childhood and adolescence such as elective mutism or specific developmental disorders of motor functions, suffer from language disorders more frequently than typically developed children. For DDSL associated with such comorbidities, prevalence is not exactly known. According to conservative estimates, the proportion of children with diseases or conditions establishing such comorbidities in the population is given at about 3% for Germany (Kany and Schöler 2007). A considerable proportion of children have to be assumed as being threatened by a DDSL if a comorbidity—for example, a hearing loss—is not timely diagnosed and treated.

In the next subsections, exemplary studies are mentioned that deal with the coincidence of DDSL with some of the above-named comorbidities.

Language Impairment in Children with Developmental Disabilities Among disorders of children and adolescents with disabilities aged from 6 to 21 years, such as developmental delay; mental retardation; multiple disabilities; traumatic brain injury; autism; impairment of hearing, vision, speech or language; orthopaedic or other health issues; emotional disturbance; or specific learning disability in the Montana, USA, DDSL made up about 20% of those disorders in 2006/2007 according to the US Department of Education, Office of Special Education Programs (OSEP) and the State Education Agencies (SEAs). Among children aged from 3 to 5 years receiving special education, the respective value was even 60% (US Department of Education et al. 2008). Often, implications about the coincidence of DDSL and other language-relevant diseases can only be made indirectly. For example, in a study that compared communication deficits in toddlers who were diagnosed with Down syndrome and cerebral palsy, who had a history of seizures or a seizure disorder or who were born prematurely, those diagnosed with cerebral palsy evidenced significantly fewer communication impairments than children with Down syndrome and children with a history of seizures or seizure disorder (Hattier et al. 2011).

Language Impairment in Preterm Infants Language development in infants born very preterm or with very low birth weight is often compromised, even in the absence of brain damage (Charollais et al. 2010; Fernandez et al. 2010). These infants are at an increased risk of developmental language delays or language disorders that cannot be compensated for as the children age. In particular, difficulty in performing speech and language processing tasks involving complex materials indicates a problem for infants born preterm in their initial approach to language acquisition that may constrain their future language skills (Bosch 2011). For example, in a Brazilian study, 29% of very low birth weight preterm infants aged from 18 to 24 months of corrected age presented developmental language delay (Fernandez et al. 2010). Poor language skills have also been described later in life in preschoolers and teenagers who were born preterm (Charollais et al. 2010; Georgsdottir et al. 2012). Functional magnetic resonance connectivity studies in infants born preterm also suggest that the effects of preterm birth on the functional organization of language in the developing brain are both proximate (i.e. causal) and long-lasting (Kwon et al. 2016). Ethnicity and race seem to influence the cognitive and language outcome at age 18–22 months as shown in a multicentre study of Duncan et al. (2012) for extremely preterm infants.

Language Impairment in Children with Hearing Loss and Other Sensory Deficits It is well known that children with hearing impairment have a higher risk of developing speech and language disorders. For example, in a retrospective chart review of 200 children with permanent hearing loss, 61% had received speech and language evaluations, and 77% required language intervention (Wiley et al. 2011). Especially receptive language skills are impaired in case of a hearing impairment (Hansson et al. 2007; Keilmann et al. 2011). As it is obvious and reported in many studies, the probability of acquiring a language disorder depends on the severity of the hearing loss. Moeller (2000), who examined the relationship between age of enrolment for intervention of deaf and hard-of-hearing children and language outcome, reported that two

factors—age at enrolment and family involvement in the rehabilitation process—explained a significant amount of the variance in language scores obtained by the children and hence play a key role in the outcome.

Children who have visual impairment develop language normally in most cases (Keilmann 2009).

Language Impairment and Other Somatic Diseases Some other disorders not mentioned above also harbour an increased risk of a DDSL. For example, children with complex congenital heart diseases have been shown to have a significantly increased risk of difficulties in their expressive and receptive language development (Marino et al. 2012).

Ample research has been conducted to examine language development in individuals prenatally exposed to alcohol, both with and without foetal alcohol spectrum disorder (FASD). Many of these individuals tend to exhibit delays in acquisition of fundamental language skills, comprehension, language and speech development, overall language competence and knowledge of words. For example, in a study by Wyper and Rasmussen (2011), children with FASD had significantly lower scores than control children of both receptive and expressive language skills. The potential coincidence of DDSL with other FASD-related disorders such as hearing dysfunction, or craniofacial anomalies such as cleft palate or cleft lip, needs to be considered in the diagnostic process. Another environmental factor that affects language development in children with FASD is early caregiving experiences (Wyper and Rasmussen 2011).

For children with congenital cytomegalovirus infections, a high proportion of abnormalities in language development despite normal mental development is reported, for example, 32% in a Polish study (Milewska-Bobula et al. 2010).

The majority of children with autism spectrum disorders show some form of DDSL. For example, in a study of 170 diagnosed autistic children, delays in the development of speech and language skills occurred in 78% of the cases (Lian and Ho 2012). For children with both fragile X syndrome and varying degrees of autism, language measures were also correlated negatively with the severity of autism, i.e. children with more severe autism had lower language skills (McDuffie et al. 2012).

Many genetic and some non-genetic syndromes are known to be associated with a higher proportion of DDSL than typically developing children (see Sect. 9.10).

9.7 Symptomatic Profile of Specific Developmental Disorders of Speech and Language

Katrin Neumann

9.7.1 Early and Core Language Symptoms of Specific Developmental Disorders of Speech and Language

Developmental disorders of speech and language (DDSL) as defined in the current version of the International Statistical Classification of Diseases and Related Health Problems, the ICD-10 of the World Health Organization (2011), are subclassified as specific DDSL (SDDSL) and other DDSL associated with language-relevant comorbidities (DDSLC), also called non-specific DDSL. Specific DDSL, also called 'specific language impairment'

(SLI) and coded as F80 in the ICD-10, are sole developmental language disorders without any other conditions that could impair the language development of a child. DDSLC, on the other hand, are language disorders associated with other diseases or conditions that may have an impact on language development.

Only for SDDSL can specific symptoms be described precisely without any influence of confounding conditions such as a hearing loss. Therefore, this section focuses on symptoms that characterize SDDSL. For DDSLC, the symptoms are affected by the comorbidities and are not attributable to a DDSL alone. Tables 9.4 and 9.5 catalogue the expressive and receptive symptoms of an SDDSL (de Langen-Müller et al. 2012). Table 9.4 depicts early symptoms that may be observed up to the second birthday of a child; Table 9.5 demonstrates later-occurring core symptoms for the semantic-lexical, morphological-syntactic, phonetic-phonological and pragmatic levels. Symptoms described by the parents or caregivers and the symptom-related information resulting from language tests and informal examinations are both taken into consideration.

Most of the European languages are Indo-Germanic languages. Although they differ in the acquisition characteristics of the phonological systems, there are far-reaching cross-language similarities. Hence, the sequence of normal overcoming of phonological processes, i.e. physiological replacements of targeted speech sounds in childhood by simpler-to-speak ones until a sound

Table 9.4 Early language symptoms of a specific developmental disorder of speech and language (modified from de Langen-Müller et al. 2012, with kind permission from Peter Lang GmbH, Internationaler Verlag der Wissenschaften)

Expressive symptoms	Receptive symptoms
• Prelinguistic gestures are lacking	• Lacking reactions to their own names
• Late onset or lack of canonical babbling	• Social routines ('away', 'no', 'high') are not yet or poorly understood
• Only repetition of syllables (canonical babbling), no varying babbling ('lala' instead of 'lela')	• Commands are not or not appropriately followed
• Late or lacking onset of speaking	• Questions are not correctly answered despite knowledge of the correct answer
• No or only single, idiosyncratic words	• Initially often autistic or compulsive seeming behaviour as expression of an impaired speech perception
• First words much later than 15 months	• Sometimes echolalia
• At 24 months production of fewer than about 50 words (late talker), no making up for a delay until 36 months	*Note: Because of the redundancy of communicative situations, receptive deficits are only unreliably recognizable for caregivers and always need a specific examination at single linguistic levels*
• Slowed course or stagnation of language development	
• Concern of caregivers because of language development of the child	

Table 9.5 Core language symptoms of SDDSL at distinct linguistic levels after 24 months of age as identified by the patient's history, informal examinations and language tests (modified from de Langen-Müller et al. 2012, with kind permission from Peter Lang GmbH, Internationaler Verlag der Wissenschaften)

Linguistic level	Symptoms
Vocabulary (lexicon) Semantics	Poor receptive (passive) or expressive (active) vocabulary or age-inappropriate vocabulary The child • Speaks only a few words (poor vocabulary) • Learns new words only slowly (slowed increase of vocabulary) • Has difficulties in word retrieval • Makes naming errors or averts naming • Uses passe-partout words (make, do) • Often replies with commonplace phrases (Oh really? O.K.) • Replies in an unspecific way (yes/no/don't know) *More detailed symptoms and test results* • Poor vocabulary (lexemes) or meaning (semantic) concepts • Unsecure interconnections and structuring (semantic fields and relations) • Impaired storage or access to word forms • No age-appropriate performance in word production or perception • Low lexical variety • Only restricted fast mapping possible (quick adjustment of an unknown word form to an unknown referent, e.g. quick learning of the new word 'dog' and finding its correct meaning out of a large number of possible meanings when meeting a dog which nibbles on a bone and understanding implicitly that 'dog' is neither the bone nor the nibbling nor the colour, the tail or the snout of the dog (Grimm and Weinert 2002)) • Unstructured vocabulary • Abnormal composition of the vocabulary, deficits may be specific for a word class (e.g. verbs)

Morphology syntax	Impaired ability to understand and apply the morpho-syntactic rules of the native language; stagnation of the grammatical development
	• Expressive level
	  – Problems in using the morphological (i.e. case, tense, number and genus markings, subject-verb congruency, verb flexion) and syntactic (i.e. word position, in particular of verbs, subordinate clauses) rules of the native language
	  – Later restrictions of the narrative and text-grammatical abilities
	• Receptive level
	  – Problems in the perception of complex sentence structures and W-questions (Who? Where? Why?) or of the function of morphological markings
	More detailed symptoms
	• Length of utterance too short for the age
	• Lacking or wrong word markings
	• Rare structures which are untypical of normal language acquisition, i.e. phenomena that occur during normal language acquisition but are no longer age-appropriate
	• Children between 2 and 3 years of age:
	  – No word combinations at 24 months
	  – Only one-word or two-word utterances at 28–36 months
	  – Wrong word position and word sequence (e.g. verb in second position in Germanic languages at 36 months)
	• Children between 3 and 4 years of age:
	  – Degraded sentence structures, grammatical markings and omitted function words
	• Children between 4 and 5 years of age:
	  – Only simple main clauses, lacking of subordinate clauses and obligatory constituents
	• Children older than 5 years:
	  – Superficially correct syntactic structures but only few complex sentence structures
	  – Rigid, inflexible sentence structures
	  – Difficulties in making an experience or a process understandable

(continued)

Table 9.5 (continued)

Linguistic level	Symptoms
Phonology	Impaired ability to receive and organize phonemes in a target language and to retrieve and use them adequately (phonological disorder)[a] • E.g. elision, substitution, permutation of sounds • Poor phoneme inventory • Non-overcome/age-inadequate phonological processes (use of wrong phonological rules or of rules that belong to earlier developmental stages) • Problems in the retrieval and combination of phonemes to sound sequences and words • Abnormal word accentuation
Pragmatics	Lacking competence to understand and use language appropriately in a communicative situation[b] • Qualitative and situation-related restriction of communicative and dialogue competencies • Striking echolalia • Difficulties in understanding of speech acts • Problems in the use of non-verbal communicative means, e.g. non-modulated or suspect eye contact • Problems in the organization of narratives • Difficulties with turn-taking • Difficulties of older children in making an experience or a process understandable

[a]The term 'specific speech articulation disorder' as used in the ICD-10 (F80.0) is an umbrella term for any disturbance of the speech sound production that lies below the normative range, considering the intelligence and developmental age of a child. It covers both phonetic and phonological disorders, isolated or in combination. But only phonological impairments belong to SDDSL and are addressed here, because a phonetic disorder is the lack of ability to produce a sound (mechanically/articulatory) and does not belong to SDDSL. Moreover, for specific speech articulation disorders the term 'dyslalia' has been used formerly. This term, however, stems from a period where no distinction between phonetic and phonological deficiencies had been made. Because it is unclear which of either difficulty is meant with dyslalia, the term has been omitted. Hence, only the terms 'phonological' and 'phonetic' disorder are used here. Phonological impairments may profoundly affect the language development of a child and therefore always belong to SDDSL (Chiat and Roy 2008)

[b]A diagnostic distinction of a pragmatic deficiency as a symptom of an SDDSL from other primary disorders is necessary

and its application in a language has been acquired properly, is similar in different languages. Therefore, the following list demonstrates the sequence of overcoming of phonological processes in German exemplarily (Fox-Boyer 2016:

• Up to 2.5 years:
  – Elision of final consonants (table → *tabe*)
  – Forward displacement of the velar nasal sound (anger → *anner*)
  – Plosivation (sun → *dun*)
  – Glottal replacement /r/ (robber → *hobber*)
• Up to 3.0 years:
  – Deletion of nonstressed syllables (banana → *nana*)
  – Deaffrication of /pf/ and /ts/ (Mitsubishi → *Misubishi*)
• Up to 3.5 years:
  – Forward displacement of /g/ and /k/ (garden → darden; cup → *tup*)

  – Backward displacement of /sch/ (sheep → *çeep*)
• Up to 4.0 years:
  – Reduction of consonant clusters (snow → *now*)
  – Assimilations (Maria → *Mamia*)
• Up to 4.5 years:
  – Voicing (tone → *done*)
  – Devoicing (vase → *fase*)
• Up to 5 years:
  – Forward displacement of /ʃ/ and /ç/ to /z/ (school → *sool*)

9.7.2 Differential Diagnoses and Associated Disorders

From a superficial evaluation of symptoms, often SDDSL cannot be distinguished from other language abnormalities or conditions or diseases affecting language development. These factors may hamper a diagnostic classification. In particular non-pathological language abnormalities that do not require a treatment may occur additionally to an SDDSL. Therefore, in order to formulate a correct diagnosis (caution, an SDDSL is an exclusion diagnosis), the following differentiations have to be made on the basis of the symptoms [see Tables 9.6 and 9.7 and the subsequent passage on environmental (sociogenic) language abnormalities]:

Table 9.6 Differential diagnoses and potential SDDSL-associated findings that have to be taken into consideration when diagnosing an SDDSL (modified from de Langen-Müller et al. 2012, with kind permission from Peter Lang GmbH, Internationaler Verlag der Wissenschaften)

Differential diagnoses	Potential SDDSL-associated findings
SDDSL is not caused by the following disorders:	But SDDSL may be associated with organic and developmental psychopathological findings

Sensory disorders
• Hearing disorders (H90.–)/deafness (H 91.9):
  – Recurrent otitis media with effusion and conductive hearing loss
  – Other acquired hearing loss
  – Congenital/neonatal sensorineural or conductive unilateral or bilateral hearing loss (H90.0–H90.4), ear malformations
  – Combined hearing loss (H90.5)
• Other sensory disorders, e.g. vision disorders/blindness (H53–H54)
	• Occasionally occurring otitis media: may indicate a comorbidity; therefore in case of an SDDSL a repeated assessment of hearing is necessary
	• Limitations of the verbal short-term memory and of central auditory processing

Pervasive developmental disorders (F84) • Childhood autism (F84.0) • Atypical autism (F84.1) • Rett syndrome (F84.2) • Other childhood disintegrative disorders (F84.3) • Asperger syndrome (F84.5)	• Combination with mild, non-predominant other developmental abnormalities such as mild specific developmental disorders of scholastic skills (F81) or of motor function (F82)
Mental retardation (F70–F79) *Multi-handicaps* *Genetic syndromes* (see Sect. 9.10)	• Mild non-verbal abnormalities with normal IQ
Neurological disorders such as • Developmental neurological disorders, e.g. mild forms of cerebral palsy • Acquired aphasia (R47.0), childhood aphasia • Landau-Kleffner syndrome (F80.3; acquired childhood aphasia with epilepsy; onset of the disorders accompanied by EEG abnormalities in the temporal lobe)	• Subtle structural/functional abnormalities of the brain • Lacking asymmetry and lateralization/hemispheric dominance • (Focal) neurological deficit

Conduct and emotional disorders (F90–F98)
• Hyperkinetic disorders
• Anxiety disorders
• Attachment disorders
• Elective mutism (F94.0)
	• Problems of social interaction
	  – Negative experience of communication
	  – Low self-esteem
	• Conduct abnormalities/disorders with low social contact, drawback, depression, school refusal or aggressiveness as possible social consequences or accompanying symptoms

Environmental language abnormalities • Neglect: frequently language abnormalities of socially deprived children, twins who are often on their own, children from lower, less-educated social classes	• Psychosocial factors that influence treatment effects and course of an SDDSL negatively • SDDSL of multilingual children affects all languages

Table 9.7 Further differential diagnostic needs (modified from de Langen-Müller et al. 2012, with kind permission from Peter Lang GmbH, Internationaler Verlag der Wissenschaften)

SDDSL also have to be differentiated from:
• Disturbed motor functions
– Malformation or impairment of the articulation organs
– Disturbed oral speech motor functions by cleft palate
– Other organic diseases of the articulators
• Specific developmental disorders of motor function (F82)
– Clumsy child syndrome
– Developmental coordination disorder
– Developmental dyspraxia, childhood apraxia of speech
– Specific developmental disorder of oral motor function (synonym, orofacial disorder, myofunctional disorder, F82.2)
– Phonetic disorder (synonym, speech disorder, speech sound disorder, articulation disorder)
– An interdental or addental sigmatism, as it occurs frequently in preschoolers, is in most cases not caused by a phonological disturbance but by a phonetic abnormality
• Speech fluency disorders
– Stuttering (F98.5)
– Cluttering (F98.6)
• Voice disturbances (R49)
• Central auditory processing disorders (CAPD) (F80.20)
• Specific developmental disorders of scholastic skills (F81)
– Specific reading disorder (F81.0)
– Specific spelling disorder (F81.1)
– Specific disorder of arithmetical skills (F81.2)
– Mixed disorder of scholastic skills (F81.3)

- Differential diagnoses (other diseases, comorbidities)
- Potentially SDDSL-associated findings that may also be of importance for other language abnormalities
- Solely or additionally occurring environmentally related language abnormalities that do not need language therapy such as:
  - Sociogenically caused deviations from the normal language development due to lacking input
  - Language abnormalities during bi- or multilingual language acquisition

9.7.3 Environmental (Sociogenic) Language Abnormalities

Oral language acquisition requires in addition to congenital species-specific abilities the presence of a sufficient and informative offer of verbal communication in a target language. Children use the verbal input of their environment to approach the target language. Environmental conditions may thus influence language develop-ment positively or negatively. A negative influence may lead to similar language-associated abnormalities such as an SDDSL on the symptoms' surface or, for example, in the case of social deprivation, to language and communication abnormalities related to attachment disorders (F94.1, F94.2). The following environmental (socially related) language abnormalities have to be distinguished from an SDDSL:

Sociogenically Caused Deviations from the Normal Language Development Owing to Lacking Input Language abnormalities due to lack of input, neglect or wrong language role models do not require a language therapy but language-stimulating training (Neumann and Euler 2013). They may aggravate a present DDSL.

Language Abnormalities During Bi- or Multilingual Language Acquisition Bi-/multilingual children (see Sect. 9.5) sometimes show peculiarities during language acquisition that result from an interference between the languages on the phonetic-phonological, semantic-lexical and morphological-syntactical levels. They do not represent a DDSL. Children who grow up in a positive multilingual environment do not have more frequent DDSL than monolingual children. SDDSL of bi-/multilingual children always affect all languages (Håkansson et al. 2003; Paradis et al. 2003). The acquisition of more than one language does not additionally complicate the language acquisition of children with DDSL who grow up with a simultaneous bilingualism.

DDSL are to some extent language-specific, i.e. depending on the complexity and the age at which certain structures have to be acquired; for example, different grammatical abilities may be affected across languages (Leonard 2000; Paradis et al. 2003).

9.7.4 Developmental Language Delay/Late Talkers

Developmental language retardations have to be classified, dependent on the age of the child, as developmental language delay - late talkers up to the third birthday - or as DDSL, from the third birthday on (Kiese-Himmel 2008). According to the UEP (1987), a developmental language delay is a delay of at least 6 months from the age norm of the normal language development. The term can be misunderstood, because it suggests that the language abnormality is only a transient developmental retardation. This occurs however only during early language acquisition, whereas later on a substantial delay is in most cases paralleled by a contentual deviation from the normal language development and hence is a DDSL. Therefore, the term is used in Germany, for example, only for children between their second and third birthdays (de Langen-Müller et al. 2012).

The definition of the term late talker differs somewhat in the literature. According to most authors, it depicts children without any primary abnormality, who produce up to their second birthday fewer than 50 words and no word combinations (Desmarais et al. 2008). For other authors late talkers are children who have not produced their first words by 18 months (Bishop et al. 2012). The prevalence of late talkers has been reported as 2.0–17.5% for Anglo-Saxon countries (see Sect. 9.6).

Some late talkers make up for the delay between their second and third birthdays—late bloomers. In a literature review, 75% of children diagnosed as late talkers at 18 months of age were reported to move into the normal range on standardized language measures by 3 years of age (Paul and Roth 2011). But an illusionary recovery is also possible with recurrent problems, frequently in phonological awareness but also in morphosyntax, a short time before school entry. Other authors have reported that about half to two thirds of late talkers fail to make up for the delay completely until the 36th month of life or end up with a DDSL (Kauschke 2003; Sachse and von Suchodoletz 2009). In particular, a child with a language delay at an age of 2 years has a very low probability of making up for it if he or she has a deficient language perception and if the educational status of her parents is low. Compared with normally developed children, late talkers have a 20-fold increased probability for language abnormalities at kindergarten age. At school entry age, 16% of the former late talkers suffered from an SDDSL, and an additional 18% showed mild language deficits in a study of Kühn and von Suchodoletz (2009). About 20% of late talkers examined by Rice et al. (2008) were diagnosed with a DDSL at 7 years of age (Rice et al. 2008). Buschmann et al. (2008) observed cognitive developmental delays and autistic symptoms of late talkers at the age of 24 months. All these findings point to the necessity of a thorough diagnostics and follow-up of late talkers.

9.8 Aetiology and Pathogenesis of Developmental Disorders of Speech and Language

Katrin Neumann

9.8.1 Introduction

The aetiology of developmental disorders of speech and language (DDSL) differs between specific developmental disorders of speech and language (SDDSL), where other language-relevant disorders or disturbances are excluded and other DDSL associated with language-relevant comorbidities (DDSLC), where the comorbidity is the reason for the language disorder, either alone or with additional factors that also underlie SDDSL, i.e. predominantly language-specific genetic influences (Neumann et al. 2009). Therefore, in the following subsections, aetiology and pathogenesis are separately described for SDDSL and the most important comorbidities of DDSLC.

9.8.2 Aetiology of Specific Developmental Disorders of Speech and Language (SDDSL)

SDDSL, in the ICD-10, the International Statistical Classification of Diseases and Related Health Problems (World Health Organization 2016), coded as F80, may not be referred causally to neurological or sensory disorders, genetic syndromes, malformations such as cleft palate, mental retardation, pervasive developmental disorders, multiple disabilities, conduct and emotional disorders or socioculturally caused environmental language abnormalities. In other words, SDDSL are diagnosed by exclusion ('assumption of normality') (de Langen-Müller et al. 2012).

9.8.2.1 Genetic Factors

Genetic factors are recognized as being the main cause of SDDSL (SLI Consortium 2002). The hypothesis of a polygenic-multifactorial inheritance with involvement of a 'major' gene and a gender-dependent threshold is favoured (Lewis et al. 1993; Monaco 2007; Newbury et al. 2002). In family aggregation studies (Lahey and Edwards 1995; Tallal et al. 2001; Tomblin 1989) and in twin studies (Bishop et al. 1995; Lewis and Thompson 1992; Tomblin and Buckwalter 1998), a familial clustering of SDDSL has been shown. Several gene loci have been identified by linkage analyses and are applicable to large groups of children with SDDSL. In a study of the SLI consortium (SLI Consortium 2002), linkages between SDDSL and gene loci at 16q and 19q

have been found. Bartlett et al. (2002) reported linkages with chromosomal regions 13q and 2p. Neither study showed coherence with the chromosomal region 7q, which has been described for the *KE family*.

9.8.2.2 Behavioural-Genetic Studies

Behavioural-genetic studies, in particular twin and adoption studies, may quantify how much variance (diversity) in a population related to language competence may be referred to genetic variability and how much to environmental influences. A thorough review and meta-analysis of behavioural-genetic studies including linkage studies (Stromswold 2001) and further studies (Bishop et al. 2006; Hayiou-Thomas 2008) have shown that genetic factors are responsible for a considerable part of the variance in developmental language disabilities but only for a small part of the variance of language competence of subjects with normal language development. Hence, genetic factors are the main reason of the language competence of children with DDSL.

9.8.2.3 Environmental Factors

Environmental factors, in particular social determinants of the language environment, have much less influence on the occurrence of SDDSL, and the influence of the family-specific environment is—except for the extent of the vocabulary—obviously negligible. With caution it may be stated that poor language stimulation by the family, in particular by the mother, is not a primary cause of an SDDSL (Leonard 1987). Sachse and von Suchodoletz (2009) observed in late talkers that, in addition to deficits in speech perception, poor school education of the parents in particular reduced the probability of their children's catching up the delay by the age of 3 years and predicted an SDDSL. It is unequivocal that institutionalized children, with whom only poor social interaction takes place; twins, who are often on their own; and children from families with many children, in particular those from socially disadvantaged groups, all exhibit developmental language deviations more often than others (Grimm 2003). The parental socio-economic status (income-to-needs ratio, family income) was not an influential factor for the appearance of an SDDSL in several large studies (among others National Institutes of Health). However, maternal sensitivity and depression, and whether the mother was married, have been shown as possibly influential, whereas maternal education has been evaluated controversially (Botting et al. 2001; La Paro et al. 2004; Stanton-Chapman et al. 2002).

9.8.2.4 Neurolinguistic Perspective

From a neurolinguistic perspective, deficient cerebral processing and representation of language may be causal for SDDSL. If mechanisms of language processing do not function effectively, the input cannot be used effectively. Hence, language acquisition runs slower and is more troublesome. Abnormalities causal for an SDDSL may also occur at the cognitive level (weakness of domain-non-specific information processing), the perceptual level (disturbed basal and higher functions of sensory processing, in particular of auditory processing) and the biological level (abnormal development and lateralization of cerebral structures and genetic factors). None of these hypotheses is sufficiently proven empirically so far or fit all children with SDDSL (de Langen-Müller et al. 2012).

Currently, predominantly genetically determined developmental factors are assumed to be causal for SDDSL, possibly with some psychosocial and environmental factors working epigenetically. Therefore, and because the aetiology of SDDSL is only identified for subgroups of children, a causal therapy of SDDSL is not available so far. Hence, the intervention focuses on specific language symptoms, independent of the assumed causality.

9.8.3 Aetiology of Other Developmental Disorders of Speech and Language Associated with Language-Relevant Comorbidities (DDSLC or Non-specific DDSL)

For DDSL associated with comorbidities, the proportion of the language impairment that is caused by the additional underlying disease or disturbance is not easy to separate from a possible SDDSL component. It has to be assumed that the same hereditary factors, which are mainly causal for SDDSL, may also contribute to complex language impairment in some children with language-relevant comorbidities, but the extent and nature of this proportion is hard to assess because it interferes with the components of the underlying condition.

9.8.3.1 Developmental Disorders of Speech and Language Associated with Mental Retardation (ICD-10: F70–F79)

The prevalence of intellectual disabilities for European countries ranges from 3 to 7% of the population (for Germany 0.4% with IQ values up to ≤50 and 2.5–2.9% with IQ values >50–70) (Langen 2006; Maulik and Harbour 2010). Causes are genetic factors resulting in brain diseases and—to a lesser degree—acquired cerebral injuries such as alcohol embryopathy. In most cases (up to 75%), the causes for intellectual disabilities remain unidentified. The largest cause of mental retardation (about 15%) is Down syndrome (Bower and Petterson 2001). For most subjects with an intellectual disability, oral communication is disturbed or—less often—impossible.

9.8.3.2 Developmental Disorders of Speech and Language Associated with Hearing Loss or Central Auditory Processing Disorders (ICD-10: H90–H91; F80.20)

Hearing disorders are the most prominent comorbidities of DDSLC. In case of mild hearing loss, language deficits are often counterbalanced by compensatory strategies and speaking does not appear abnormal to other people. For children with severe hearing loss, DDSLCs are common. Their extent and pattern depend on the time of diagnosis and treatment of the hearing loss, the language talent of a child and the familial background (Moeller 2000). With timely and modern hearing intervention and rehabilitation, many children develop normal language abilities (Kiese-Himmel 2003).

Disturbed middle ear ventilation because of age-related anatomical characteristics of the Eustachian tube, a smaller tympanum and frequent infections of the upper airways, otitis media, and blocking of the pharyngeal ostium of the Eustachian tube by secretion or enlarged adenoids are typical conditions at toddler and preschool ages. From the first to the third year of life, about 10–30% of children have been reported to suffer from middle ear effusion with resulting conductive hearing loss; at preschool ages the value is still 10–20% and at school age 5–10% (Fiellau-Nikolajsen 1983; Northern and Downs 2002). A reduced Eustachian tube pressure may also cause a mild conductive hearing loss ranging from 10 to 30 dB; in case of a middle ear effusion, the hearing loss mostly ranges from 20 to 50 dB (Schönweiler 1992).

Specific diseases such as Kartagener syndrome, an autosomal recessive genetic ciliary disorder comprising the triad of sinusitis, situs inversus and bronchiectasis or a primary ciliary dyskinesia (PCD; same symptoms as Kartagener syndrome but without situs inversus) also lead to chronic middle ear effusion. The genetic defect causes, among other conditions, a disturbed action of cilia lining the lower and upper respiratory tract, sinuses, Eustachian tube and middle ear. Congenital or, in the neonatal period, acquired permanent hearing disorders are predominantly associated with sensorineural hearing loss. Their prevalence in Europe ranges from 1 to 3 per 1000 newborns. About 10–30% of permanent hearing loss in children has a late onset or runs progressively. Causes for permanent infant hearing loss are genetic factors, pre-, peri- or postnatal infections such as congenital CMV infection, syndromes, craniofacial malformations and ototoxic impairments, e.g. caused by aminoglycosides.

Because of both the typical recurrent or fluctuating middle ear-caused hearing loss and the occurrence of fluctuating and progressive sensorineural or mixed hearing loss, singular audiograms often do not reflect the conditions for language development well, and repeated measurements may be useful for estimating the hearing profile over a longer period and for the reduction of obtainable audio-verbal learning

pattern for a child. Hence, for a middle ear effusion persisting longer than 3 months, draining ear tubes and eventually an adenectomy are recommended (Deutsche Gesellschaft für Phoniatrie und Pädaudiologie 2005).

In a study of 1300 German-speaking preschoolers with DDSL, hearing loss was diagnosed in 48% (Schönweiler 1992). In the age group up to 4 years—the most important period of language development—more than half of the children were hard of hearing. In 95% hearing loss was a mild conductive hearing loss fluctuating about 20 dB. Results of meta-analyses examining the relationship between otitis media with effusion and language development found either low effects (Casby 2001) or no to very small negative associations (Roberts et al. 2004). However, these reviews have been criticized because of systematic errors and do not seem to be generalizable for children with increased risk for a DDSL or language-relevant comorbidities.

According to Schönweiler (1992), a mild hearing loss may also:

- Cause phonological misperceptions
- Reduce the comprehension of new words
- Affect the perception of unstressed syllables, particularly at word-end positions
- Lead to morphological errors and contextual misinterpretations together with pragmatic disturbances

Unilateral hearing loss as caused by hereditary factors, malformations, trauma, otosclerosis, disturbed tympanic ventilation, cholesteatoma or infections may also be associated with distorted language development and may affect scholastic skills later on (Lieu 2013).

Central auditory processing difficulties are frequently associated with DDSL (Tallal 1980). An interface between the auditory and language systems is the phonological storage component of the auditory working memory, the phonological loop (Baddeley 1992). It stores and rehearses speech-based information and is necessary for the acquisition of both native and second-language vocabulary. This loop enables a child to keep longer, not yet analyzed language portions in the phonological working memory and is an important predisposition for the production and retrieval of phonemes and the development of vocabulary, syntax, morphology as well as reading and spelling skills. Hence, the acquisition of a lexicon and grammar is closely related to this memory system. Children with DDSL perform significantly worse in the phonological working memory than peers with normal language development (Grimm 2003; Hasselhorn and Werner 2000).

9.8.3.3 Developmental Disorders of Speech and Language Associated with Other Sensory Disorders and Multiple Disabilities

Blindness with or without residual vision (visus ≤2%), with a prevalence of 4–5 per 1000 newborns, is a frequent sensory disorder and may influence language development at the beginning. Its causes are hereditary malformations of the eye and the optic nerve, inflammation and impairment of the immature retina (retinopathia praematorum) or of the visual cortex in preterm babies. Most of the affected children have normal language development. Sometimes, however, the disturbed acquisition of the precursor abilities, such as the absence of referential eye contact, hinders early language development. Nevertheless, the subsequent language acquisition of blind children of normal intelligence resembles that of typically developed children with some minor qualitative deviations. This is interpreted as a result of adaptive compensatory strategies of children and parents (Perez-Pereira and Conti-Ramsden 1999).

For children with multiple disabilities, whether they are of genetic or non-genetic in origin, such as Down or Landau-Kleffner syndromes, the severity of the language impairment depends on the specific combination of physical and intellectual disabilities. The specific aetiology of some exemplary language-relevant syndromes is described in Sect. 9.8.3.6. A large synopsis of language-related syndromes is given in Sect. 9.10.

9.8.3.4 Developmental Disorders of Speech and Language Associated with Pervasive Developmental Disorders (ICD-10: F84)

Pervasive developmental disorders comprise, among others, childhood autism; atypical autism; Rett syndrome; other childhood disintegrative disorders such as dementia infantilis, disintegrative and symbiotic psychoses and Heller syndrome; overactivity disorders associated with mental retardation and stereotyped movements; and Asperger syndrome. They are characterized by qualitative deviations in social interactions and communication patterns and by a restricted, stereotypical, repetitive repertoire of interests and activities. In a study of Schönweiler (1994), 20% of children with language impairment had global developmental retardation.

Rett syndrome (see also Sect. 9.8.3.6) is a seizure syndrome that nearly exclusively affects girls but in combination with the Klinefelter syndrome can affect boys. After the first to second year of life, both cognitive and language abilities are lost (e.g. object permanence) leading to a severe impairment of language and communication.

The causes of autism are not clear up to now. The most probable cause is a pre-, peri- or postnatal brain injury. Anomalies of chromosomes 3, 7 and 15 and the X chromosome are discussed. Five per 10,000 children are affected. The gender proportion is about 4:1 boys/girls (Grimm 2003). About half of the autistic children do not acquire oral language; language development of the other half is strongly delayed and qualitatively aberrant. This does not hold true for children with Asperger syndrome, a mild form of autism that affects ~3.6 per 1000 children aged from 7 to 16 years. Here, language development is nearly undisturbed, although speech may appear formal and pedantic with a peculiar prosody (Ehlers and Gillberg 1993).

For hyperactive disturbances with reduced intelligence and movement stereotypies (ICD-10: F84.4), an ill-defined disorder of uncertain nosological validity, a severe mental retardation (IQ <35) is combined with problems of hyperactivity, attention deficits and stereotypical behaviour. Language impairment is obligatory and contributes to a specific or global developmental retardation.

9.8.3.5 Speech and Language Abnormalities Associated with Disorders of Social Functioning with Onset Specific to Childhood and Adolescence Such as Selective Mutism (ICD-10: F94.0)

Selective mutism is not a speech or language disorder but a communication disorder due to a psychically caused speech arrest. Speech and language abilities are normal in most cases. The communication may run normally or almost normally under specific circumstances (i.e. in a certain group of subjects or with a specific individual). A prevalence of selective mutism from 0.5 to 0.7 per 1000 children at early school age is reported (Schwartz and Shipon-Blum 2005).

9.8.3.6 Developmental Disorders of Speech and Language Associated with Syndromes

Many syndromes (clusters of symptoms, genetically caused in most cases) are associated with DDSLC. Subsequently, some language-relevant syndromes are listed exemplarily with a focus on their aetiology and pathogenesis. For a comprehensive systematic list of language-affecting syndromes with focus on their symptoms, see Sect. 9.10.

Landau-Kleffner Syndrome Also called *infantile acquired aphasia*, *acquired epileptic aphasia* or *aphasia with convulsive disorder*, the Landau-Kleffner syndrome (LKS) is a rare childhood neurological syndrome characterized by acute or progressive loss of the receptive and expressive language abilities of a child and development of an aphasia paralleled by the appearance of paroxysmal electroencephalographic (EEG) activity, in particular sleep-activated EEG paroxysms predominating over the temporal or parieto-occipital regions (Pearl et al. 2001). It affects both Broca's area and Wernicke's area, i.e. cerebral regions that control speech motor planning and comprehension of speech. Usually it emerges from the ages of 3 to 7 years with a sex ratio of 1.7–2:1 males to females. In most cases, the reasons for LKS are unknown. It may appear secondary to other diseases such as low-grade brain tumours, closed-head injury, neurocysticercosis, demyelinating diseases or a vasculitis of the central nervous system (Neiman and Seyffert 2016). Also genetic causes are assumed (Myers and Scheffer 1993).

Angelman Syndrome (AS) This neurodevelopmental disorder is caused by genomic imprinting, i.e. by a deletion or inactivation of genes on the maternally inherited chromosome 15, while the paternal chromosome, which may be of normal sequence, is imprinted and therefore silenced. The usual maternal contribution to a region of chromosome 15 is lost mostly by a deletion of a segment of the chromosome and less often by a uniparental disomy, translocation or single gene mutation in that region. Its sister syndrome, the Prader-Willi syndrome, is caused by a similar loss of paternally inherited genes and maternal imprinting. AS is characterized by severe intellectual and developmental disability, sleep disturbance, seizures, jerky movements such as hand flapping, frequent laughter or smiling, a happy demeanour and DDSLC.

Cri du Chat Syndrome This syndrome, also named *chromosome 5p deletion syndrome*, *5p-* (5p minus) or *Lejeune's syndrome*, is characterized by a partial deletion, a missing part of the short arm of chromosome 5 (also called 5p monosomy or partial monosomy). About 90% of cases are caused by a sporadic deletion; the remaining 10–15% are due to unequal segregation of a parental balanced translocation. The 5p monosomy, which usually has the more severe symptoms, is often accompanied by a trisomic portion of the genome. The disorder is characterized by a high-pitched cry similar to that of a cat; severe cognitive, speech and motor delays; microcephaly; low birth weight; muscular hypotonia; swallowing and sucking problems; drooling; behavioural problems such as hyperactivity;

aggression; tantrums; repetitive movements; specific facial features (widely set eyes, low-set ears, small jaw, rounded face); and sometimes heart defects.

22q11.2 Deletion Syndrome This syndrome is also known as *DiGeorge syndrome or anomaly, velocardiofacial syndrome (VCFS), Shprintzen syndrome, conotruncal anomaly face syndrome (CTAF)* or *Takao syndrome, Sedlackova syndrome, Cayler cardiofacial syndrome, strong syndrome, congenital thymic aplasia or thymic hypoplasia*. These syndromes have in common a high frequency of hemizygous deletions of chromosome 22q11.2 (Kobrynski and Sullivan 2007). 22q11.2 deletion is the most common microdeletion syndrome. The majority of patients share a large (>3 Mb [Mb: megabase pairs, a length of DNA/RNA comprising 1,000,000 base pairs]) hemizygous deletion of 22q11.2. The remaining patients either have smaller deletions that are nested within the 3 Mb typically deleted region or have rare deletions other than in the typical regions (Shaikh et al. 2000). The majority of deletions occur sporadically as de novo lesions, which indicates a high mutation rate within this genomic region. The prevalence of this autosomal dominant inherited syndrome is about 1:4000 (Shaikh et al. 2000). A 22q11 deletion may be associated with high level of functioning, but in most cases it is characterized by a malfunction of many organ systems such as cognitive impairment, brain morphological changes, DDSLC, cleft palate, facial abnormalities, hypoparathyroidism and hypocalcaemia, thymic aplasia and cardiac abnormalities such as truncus arteriosus and tetralogy of Fallot (Kobrynski and Sullivan 2007).

Fragile X Syndrome This syndrome, also named *Martin-Bell syndrome* or *Escalante's syndrome*, is a common form of inherited intellectual disability and belongs to the leading causes of autism. It results from a mutation of the *fragile X mental retardation 1 (FMR1) gene* on the X chromosome, which is most commonly an increase in the number of CGG trinucleotide repeats in the 5′ untranslated region of *FMR1* (Santoro et al.

2012). It is inherited in an X-linked dominant pattern with possibly reduced penetrance but not following the traditional attribution to dominant or recessive. Its prevalence ranges from 1/2400 to 1/27,000 depending on the population (Peprah 2012). It occurs in about 1 of 3600 males and 1 of 4000–6000 females, the latter mostly less affected than males. The syndrome is associated with mental retardation ranging from mild to severe; autism in 50% of the cases; variable DDSLC symptoms; physical characteristics such as an elongated face, large or protruding ears or large testicles (macro-orchidism); and behavioural characteristics such as stereotypic movements (e.g. hand flapping), hyperactivity or attention deficits and social anxiety (Garber et al. 2008; McLennan et al. 2011).

Prader-Willi Syndrome (PWS) This syndrome is caused by a functional loss of genes deleted or not expressed from a specific region of the paternal chromosome 15 (q 11–13). Parent-specific gene activation (when some genes are active only on the paternal copy of the chromosome) plays the major role in the occurrence of PWS. In about 70% of patients, critical genes in chromosome 15 are lacking because the genes on the paternal copy have been deleted and the genes on the maternal copy are inactive. In 25% of cases, two copies of chromosome 15 are inherited from the mother (maternal copies) instead of one copy from each parent (maternal uniparental disomy). In rare cases of PWS, a translocation or a mutation or another defect may inactivate genes on the paternal chromosome 15 (Genetics Home Reference 2014). Some genes with functional loss in PWS encode small nucleolar RNAs (snoRNAs). The loss of a particular group of *snoRNA genes*, known as the *SNORD116 cluster*, seems to account for the PWS symptoms.

In most cases PWS is not inherited, in particular if caused by a deletion in the paternal chromosome 15 or by maternal uniparental disomy. The underlying genetic changes occur at random during the formation of eggs and spermatozoa or in early embryonic development. Patients typically have no history of PWS in their family. PWS prevalence estimates range from 1 in 8000 to 1 in

25,000, with the most frequently reported figure being 1 in 10,000 live births (Genetics Home Reference 2014).

The multiphasic syndrome is characterized by low muscle tone and poor feeding in infancy and in the second stage by hyperphagia (an uncontrollable drive to eat), combined with weight gain on fewer calories, short stature, incomplete sexual development, cognitive disability, behavioral problems and a chronic feeling of hunger that can lead to excessive eating and life-threatening obesity (Prader-Willi Syndrome Association, 2016) but also by DDSLC symptoms.

Opitz G/BBB Syndrome (G/BBB: Initials of the Families First Diagnosed with the Syndrome) This syndrome, also called *hypertelorism-hypospadias syndrome, hypertelorism with oesophageal abnormalities and hypospadias, hypospadias-dysphagia syndrome, Opitz BBB syndrome, Opitz-Frias syndrome, Opitz G syndrome* or *Opitz syndrome*, causes several abnormalities along the midline of the body and occurs either as X-linked or as a less frequent autosomal dominant form. The X-linked syndrome is caused by mutations in the *MID1 gene*, which encodes midline-1 protein production. Its lack causes a disturbed cell division and migration (Lu et al. 2013). This form of the syndrome with its X-linked pattern of inheritance affects males more than females (it is unlikely that both X chromosomes carry the mutation), who mostly show only a hypertelorism or no symptoms at all. The rare autosomal dominant Opitz/GBBB syndrome is caused by a mutation of the *SPECC1L gene*, which is close to the 22q11.2 region. This mutation leads to a disorganization of microtubules and a disturbed migration of cells to their proper location, in particular during facial development. Some patients do not have any of the described genetic changes (Genetics Home Reference 2015).

The incidence of X-linked Opitz G/BBB syndrome is reported as 1 in 10,000 to 50,000 males (probably under-diagnosed); that of the autosomal dominant form is unknown. It is part of a larger condition—the 22q11 syndrome—the incidence of which is about 1 in 4000 (see above). Characteristics of the Opitz G/BBB syndrome are hypertelorism and laryngeal, tracheal or oesophageal abnormalities, such as laryngeal cleft with resulting dysphonia, dysphagia or dyspnoea, occasionally leading to recurrent pneumonia or life-threatening breathing problems. Furthermore, genital abnormalities in males may occur that also cause problems in the urinary tract, such as hypospadias, cryptorchidism or an underdeveloped or bifid scrotum. Mild intellectual disability and developmental delay has been reported in about 50% of cases together with delayed motor skills, e.g. walking, DDSLC and learning difficulties. Autistic spectrum disorders with impaired communication and socialization skills may also occur. Cleft lip or cleft palate affects about half of the patients. Cardiac defects, imperforate anus and cerebral malformations such as hypo- or agenesis of corpus callosum are less common. Specific facial features such as a prominent forehead, widow's peak hairline, flat nasal bridge, thin upper lip and low-set ears may be present (Genetics Home Reference 2015; Lu et al. 2013).

Smith-Lemli-Opitz Syndrome (SLO Syndrome) This syndrome, also named *7-dehydrocholesterol reductase deficiency* or *RSH syndrome*, is caused by mutations in the *DHCR7 gene*, which encodes the enzyme 7-dehydrocholesterol reductase. The enzyme mediates the production of cholesterol. Cholesterol is necessary for embryonic development and for the production of several hormones and digestive acids. Furthermore it is a structural component of cell membranes and myelin. In the Smith-Lemli-Opitz syndrome, a low cholesterol level caused by lack of 7-dehydrocholesterol reductase together with an accumulation of potentially toxic byproducts of cholesterol in the blood, nervous system and other tissues is assumed to disrupt the growth and development of several body systems (Genetics Home Reference 2007).

The syndrome is inherited in an autosomal recessive manner. Its prevalence is given with 1 in 20,000 to 1 in 60,000 newborns. It is most frequent in whites of European ancestry, particularly people from Central European countries such as Slovakia and the Czech Republic (Genetics Home Reference 2007). For symptoms see Sect. 9.10.

Rett Syndrome This syndrome is an X-chromosomal dominant inherited, post-natal occurring encephalopathy of the grey matter of the brain (see also Sect. 9.8.3.4). It almost exclusively affects females. It is caused in most cases by mutations of the *MECP2 gene* on the long arm of the X chromosome. Its course and severity is determined by the location, type and severity of the *MECP2* mutation and the process of random X-inactivation. The syndrome is regarded as part of a spectrum of *MECP2*-related disorders that include classical Rett syndrome, variant Rett syndrome, *MECP2*-related severe neonatal encephalopathy, PPM-X syndrome and *MECP2* duplication syndrome. For the Rett syndrome, more than 200 mutations have been identified. In 99% of cases, these mutations occur sporadically as de novo mutations. Hence, in most cases Rett syndrome is not an inherited disorder (National Organization for Rare Disorders (NORD) 2015). The syndrome affects about 1 in 10,000 live female births (Neul et al. 2010).

First symptoms occur typically after a 6- to 18-month period of regular appearing development. However, in this period mild symptoms might also occur such as muscular hypotonia and slow head growth.

Core symptoms of the typical Rett syndrome are:

- A partial or complete loss of acquired purposeful hand skills
- A partial or complete loss of acquired spoken language
- Gait abnormalities with either dyspraxia or absence of the ability to walk
- Stereotypic hand movements such as hand wringing/squeezing, clapping/tapping, mouthing and washing/rubbing automatisms

Atypical forms of the syndrome need to show only two of the core symptoms but have to include at least five of the following symptoms, which may be also observed in the classical form (Neul et al. 2010):

- Breathing disturbances when awake
- Bruxism when awake
- Impaired sleep pattern
- Abnormal muscle tone
- Peripheral vasomotor disturbances
- Scoliosis/kyphosis
- Growth retardation
- Small cold hands and feet
- Inappropriate laughing/screaming spells
- Diminished response to pain
- Intense eye communication ('eye pointing')

Both the classical and the atypical form of the syndrome are characterized by a period of regression followed by recovery or stabilization. Some of the symptoms resemble autism. Seizures may occur.

Regarding language development, the areas of productive and partially receptive language competence and cognitive abilities become increasingly lost from the seventh month to the second year of life, and autistic traits may occur. Children with Rett syndrome either may produce only a few words or completely lose their ability to communicate verbally. They tend to non-verbally communicate by gestures, touching items and voluntary eye movements. Other possible language-relevant symptoms are mental retardation, brain malformations, ataxia, hand stereotypies and apraxia.

Williams-Beuren Syndrome This multisystem neurodevelopmental disorder, also named *Williams' syndrome*, usually occurs sporadically owing to its location within a highly repetitive, unstable genomic region that is prone to unequal crossover during meiosis. Cases of dominant inheritance have been described. It is most often caused by a hemizygous deletion of the chromosomal region q11.23 on the long arm of chromosome 7, with a consequential loss of chromosomal material spanning 1.5–1.8 megabases and containing 26–28 genes, among them the *LIMkinse-1 gene* (*LIMK1*) and the *elastin gene* (*ELN*) (Nikitina et al. 2014).

It is a microdeletion disorder or contiguous gene deletion disorder leading most probably to hypo-expression of gene products (Pober 2010). The syndrome affects approximately 1 in 7500 to 1 in 20,000 persons (Martens et al. 2008). Overall, the Williams-Beuren syndrome is associated with a distinctive, 'elfin' facial appearance and a flat nasal bridge, an unusually cheerful demeanour and ease with strangers, a developmental delay combined with initial language abnormalities and later strong language skills related to the cognitive status, severe visuospatial impairment, cardiovascular problems and transient high blood calcium. For more symptoms see Sect. 9.10.

9.8.3.7 Developmental Disorders of Speech and Language Associated with Specific Developmental Disorders of Motor Function (F82)

The motor development of a child is closely related to its development of cognitive functions. Gross motor skills (general strength of body and limbs, coordination of movements) have to be distinguished from static and fine motor skills (mimics, manual dexterity). For language development the orofacial fine motor skills are important. Motor clumsiness and disturbed fine, static and gross motor skills are often observed in DDSL (Powell and Bishop 1992). It is unclear so far whether there is any causal relation between the two. Below-average motor skills have been reported to occur more frequently in children with DDSL than in healthy children (overall, 40%; fine motor skills, 10–17%; gross motor skills, 13%; gross and fine motor skills together, 32–37%; orofacial myofunctional developmental abnormalities, 42% (Keilmann et al. 2005; Nickisch 1988; Schönweiler 1992, 1994)). Frequent neuromotor abnormalities and a higher proportion of lefthanders have been reported for children with DDSL (Noterdaeme et al. 1999).

In a study of Schönweiler (1994), hearing loss was the most frequent comorbidity of DDSL (50%), followed by orofacial myofunctional abnormalities (42%), gross and fine motor skills (33%) and global developmental disorders including intellectual disabilities (i.e. IQ <85 in each of two non-verbal intelligence tests: 19%). In about half of the cases, there were two comorbidities present and in a separate quarter three of them. This indicates the multifaceted nature of a DDSL and the necessity to search for comorbidities before diagnosing an SDDSL.

9.9 Genetics of Developmental Disorders of Speech and Language

Sabrina Regele, Antoinette am Zehnhoff-Dinnesen, Katrin Neumann and Eva Seemanova

The development of speech and language of children may be hampered significantly by hearing impairment; intellectual disability; pervasive, neurological or motor disorders; language-relevant syndromes; or adverse environmental factors. If normal patterns of language acquisition are disturbed from the early stages of development on, without the presence of one of the named organic or psychic factors, a specific developmental disorder of speech and language (SDDSL), according to the definition of the World Health Organization in the International Statistical Classification of Diseases and Related Health Problems ICD-10 (2016), has to be assumed (Bishop 2006; Tager-Flusberg and Cooper 1999). SDDSL have predominantly genetic causes. An SDDSL or specific language impairment (SLI) is coded in the ICD-10 as F80. Its prevalence in preschool children is reported at 5–7% (Law et al. 2000; Tomblin et al. 1997).

With the help of twin studies and adoption studies, a statement can be made about the extent to which language skills are based on genetic or environmental factors. Genetic factors are responsible for a considerable part of the variance in disorders of speech and language and for a smaller part of the variance in the language skills of speech- and language-unimpaired persons. Apart from vocabulary, the influence of the environment appears to be low in SSDSL. The parental socio-economic status is not an influencing factor, whereas maternal sensitivity, family status and depression in mothers are such factors (Neumann et al. 2009).

Four methodological approaches have been used to investigate genetic factors: family aggregation studies, twin studies, pedigree analysis and molecular genetic studies. Stromswold (1998) performed a family aggregation study and found a positive family history in 46% of SSDSL group members compared with 18% in the control group. In twin studies conducted by Bishop et al. (1995), Lewis and Thompson (1992) and Tomblin and Buckwalter (1998), a significantly higher pairwise match for identical twins than dizygotic twins was identified. Possible inheritance pattern of SDDSL were investigated in several pedigree analyses. Such analyses, however, are not easy to conduct, because SSDSL symptoms may change with patients' ages, and symptoms can vary among individuals (Neumann et al. 2009).

In several molecular genetic studies, candidate genes have been described. The most well-known gene that contributes to the manifestation of speech and language disorders is the *FOXP2 gene* (chromosome 7q31). A British research group (Lai et al. 2000, 2001) has analysed a unique three-generation pedigree, the KE family. This British family of Pakistani origin showed severe speech and language impairments. The disorders were characterized by severe orofacial dyspraxia and impairment of spoken and written language. An unrelated individual, patient CS, who exhibited the same phenotype, showed a chromosomal translocation on chromosome 7. The affected gene on chromosome 7q31 was called *FOXP2*. *FOXP2* is a transcription factor of the forkhead box (FOX) family that regulates the expression of almost 1000 other genes. *FOXP2* not only has

an influence on the development of the central nervous system but also on the development of other organs, such as the lungs, heart and oesophageal muscles (Haesler et al. 2004; Shu et al. 2007). *FOXP2* regulates the gene *CNTNAP2* (contactin-associated protein-like 2) on chromosome 7q35 (Vernes et al. 2008), among other functions. *CNTNAP2* plays a role in the development of the central nervous system. There is a significant association between single nucleotide polymorphisms of *CNTNAP2* and the ability to repeat non-words in children with SLI (Vernes et al. 2008). Moreover, there is an association with autistic disorders, schizophrenia, epilepsy and attention deficit hyperactivity disorder (ADHD) (Alarcon et al. 2008; Elia et al. 2010; Friedman et al. 2008).

The SLI Consortium 2002 examined 98 British families with specific language impairment and identified mutations on 16q23-24(SLI1) and on 19q13(SLI2) associated with it. *ATP2C2* and *CMIP* on chromosome 16q were identified as the causal genes. An association between the gene *DAKP3* on chromosome 19p13.3 and early expressive vocabulary has been suggested (St. Pourcain et al. 2014). Different phenotypes for SLI1 and SLI2 were described by the SLI Consortium (2002, 2004) and in a multivariate genome scan (2007), showing linkage to SLI1 and SLI2 and non-word repetition (SLI Consortium 2002, 2004; Monaco 2007). In another genome-wide association meta-analysis of two large cohorts, a significant association was found between the *ABCC13* gene on chromosome 21q11.2 and non-word repetition (Luciano et al. 2013).

In the genome-wide linkage study from Bartlett et al. (2002), 13q21 was identified as a reading-based phenotype of SDDSL. However, evidence for linkage on 16q and 19q was not replicated in that study. Reading disabilities and SDDSL share candidate genes and risk factors. *KIAA0319*, *CNTNAP2* and *CMIP* are examples of these common risk genes for dyslexia and SDDSL (Newbury et al. 2011). There is coincidence in the clinical manifestations of autism spectrum disorders and DSSL. Common gene loci for both diseases have been identified on chromosome 7 q31 and chromosome 13 q21 (Bradford et al. 2001; Li et al. 2005).

A high incidence of SDDSL is described in a Chilean population from Robinson Crusoe Island, probably due to consanguineous marriage and ancestry from colonizing families. Mutation in the *NFXL1 gene* was found to be causal for SDDSL cases in this population. Mutations in this gene have also been detected in four SDDSL cases in the United Kingdom (Villanueva et al. 2015). *ATP13A4* on chromosome 3q25.29 is another candidate gene (Kwasnicka-Crawford et al. 2005). It is assumed

to be involved in calcium regulation. A single gene located on 12p13.31–q14.3 was suggested as being causal for auditory processing difficulties associated with a language impairment in a three-generation German family (Addis et al. 2010). The gene *ROBO2* modulates the proliferation of central nervous system progenitors (Borrell et al. 2012). Mutations in *ROBO2* have been linked to deficits in expressive vocabulary in infancy.

In summary, many different candidate genes have been described as being involved in aetiology of heterogeneous developmental language disorders (see Table 9.8). An interaction of certain genes with environmental factors may also

Table 9.8 Candidate genes for specific developmental disorders of speech and language

Gene	Chromosome	Phenotype	Reference
FOXP2	7q31	Developmental verbal dyspraxia Impairment in expressive and receptive language	Lai et al. (2000) Lai et al. (2001) Li et al. (2005)
ATP2C2	16q24.1 (SLI1)	Non-word repetition deficit (deficits in phonological short-term memory)	SLI Consortium (2004) Newbury et al. (2009)
CMIP	16q23.2 (SLI1)	Non-word repetition deficit (deficits in phonological short-term memory) Deficits in reading	SLI Consortium (2004) Newbury et al. (2009) Newbury et al. (2011)
	19q13 (SLI2)	Deficit in non-word repetition Impairment of expressive and receptive language	Monaco (2007)
	13q21 (SLI3)	Deficits in reading	Bartlett et al. (2002) Bartlett et al. (2004) Bradford et al. (2001)
CNTNAP2	7q35 (SLI4)	Non-word repetition deficit (deficits in phonological short-term memory) Impairment of expressive and receptive language Deficits in reading	Vernes et al. (2008) Newbury et al. (2011)
ATP13A4	3q25-29	Impairment of expressive and receptive language	Kwasnicka-Crawford et al. (2005)
ABCC13	21q11.2	Non-word repetition deficit	Luciano et al. (2013)
	12p13.31-q14.3	Auditory processing deficit Speech delay	Addis et al. (2010)
ZNF385D	3p24.3	Impairment of receptive und expressive language Deficits in reading	Eicher et al. (2013)
COL4A2	13q34	Impairment in receptive and expressive language Deficits in reading	Eicher et al. (2013)
NDST4	4q26	Oral language deficits	Eicher et al. (2013)
NFXL1	4p12	Grammatical (morpho-syntactical) deficits Impairment of receptive language	Villanueva et al. (2015)
ROBO2	3p12.3	Deficits in expressive vocabulary in infancy	St. Pourcain et al. (2014)
KIAA0319	6p22	Impairment of expressive and receptive language Deficits in reading	Newbury et al. (2011) Rice et al. (2009)

contribute to the occurrence of DDSL. To find language-related genes, it is also important to consider language difficulties present in cognitive and syndromic disorders and to investigate above-average language abilities (Graham and Fisher 2015).

In cases of DDSL associated with other diseases that establish language-relevant comorbidities (DDSLC), genetic causes may also be at work. Because they are predominantly related to the comorbidity, they depend on the kind and expression of the disease, for example, in the case of Down syndrome of genetically caused hearing loss. Because of the diversity of comorbidities, their genetic underpinnings are not mentioned here in detail but in Sect. 9.10. Notably, in some DDSLC cases, the genetic conditions of SDDSL may additionally be present. Clinically, the part of the DDSL that is caused by the comorbidity cannot readily be discerned from the component that is caused by the SDDSL condition in such children (Neumann et al. 2009), but genetically this might be the case in the near future, at least for some cases.

9.10 Syndromes Associated with Developmental Disorders of Speech and Language

Sabrina Regele, Eva Seemanova, Katrin Neumann, and Antoinette am Zehnhoff-Dinnesen

A syndrome is a non-random characteristic association of anomalies and features due to the same aetiology. Usually, neither all symptoms described for a syndrome are present at once in one individual, nor is one symptom alone pathognomonic for a syndrome. The name of the syndrome is frequently either ascribed to the scientist or physician who identified and described the condition in an initial publication or it is an acronym for the leading features of the syndrome.

The aetiology of the syndromes is one of the following:

- Teratogenic embryopathies—non-genetic phenocopies
- Monogenic disorders due to mutation of one gene
- Chromosomal aberrations due to numerical or structural disturbances of one or more chromosomes
- Polygenic disorders due to a combination of factors that are responsible for a genetic predisposition, making the individual sensitive to deleterious environmental agents. Only a combination of predisposition and environmental influence results in manifestation of multifactorial-determined disorders.

All these syndromes can affect the cognitive development, the development of the auditory system, the morphogenesis of orofacial structures or the neurological and muscular development relevant for the perception or production of language. It is important to be aware of the genetic and molecular heterogeneity of most syndromes (autosomal dominant or recessive forms, gonosomal forms, point mutations, microdeletions, microduplications, imprinting centre disturbances, uniparental hetero-/iso-disomy, paternal or maternal) and to differentiate between the mutations occurring de novo and those inherited from a healthy parent carrier of the mutation (autosomal recessive, gonosomal recessive or chromosomal balanced translocation, incomplete expression and penetrance). Most cases of numerical chromosomal aberrations are due to new mutations with no risk to relatives and unrelated to structural chromosomal aberrations that with high probability are inherited from one carrier parent or both parents.

The following Tables 9.9, 9.10, 9.11, 9.12, 9.13, and 9.14 include the incidence, prevalence, language deficits, usual cognitive status and clinical manifestations of common genetic syndromes associated with language impairment. Figures 9.1, 9.2, 9.3, 9.4, and 9.5 show the visual diagnosis of the most common syndromes.

574

Table 9.9 Numerical chromosomal aberrations

	Karyotype	Incidence prevalence	Language deficits	Intelligence mean IQ	Clinical manifestations
Klinefelter	47,XXY 48,XXXY 49,XXXXY (20% of cases)	1:660 males (prevalence) **Most common numerical chromosomal aberration**	– Delayed language development – Impairment of receptive and expressive language – Deficits in auditory processing and processing of speech tempo	Normal	**Physical appearance** Tall stature, eunuchoidism **Organ-related manifestation** – Primary testicular failure, hypergonadotropic hypogonadism, infertility – Increased risk of developing breast cancer (Aksglaede et al. 2013; Bojesen et al. 2003; Girardin et al. 2009; Hong and Reiss 2014; Van Assche et al. 1996)
Down	46,XX,t(21;14) 46,XY,t(21;14) (translocation) 46,XX/47,XX,+21 46,XY/47,XY,+21 (mosaic)	1:1000 (prevalence) **Most common aneuploidy of autosomal chromosomes**	– Late and slow development of both vocabulary and grammar – Impairment of receptive and expressive language (receptive language is better than expressive language) – Anomalies in articulatory organs and motor control – Utterances are often short but mostly informative and pragmatically functional	50	**Physical appearance** Short stature, brachycephaly, wide hands, single transverse palmar crease, increased space between large and second toes, downward slant of the eyelids medially, epicanthal folds, flat face, hypertelorism, flat nasal bridge, ear dysplasia, fissured tongue, macroglossia, high-arched palate, micrognathia **Organ-related manifestation** – Cardiac anomalies (atrioventricular defects, ventricular septal defects) – Duodenal/anal/oesophageal stenosis or atresia, Hirschsprung disease – Vestibular malformations, conductive, mixed or sensorineural hearing loss – Increased incidences of leukaemia, hypothyroidism, celiac disease, diabetes mellitus, Alzheimer's disease – Severe refractive errors, cataracts, strabismus – Obstructive sleep apnoea, constricted nasopharynx, congenital subglottic stenosis – Renal and urinary tract malformations, cystic dysplastic kidney (Arumugam et al. 2015; Kajimoto et al. 2007; Megarbane et al. 2013)
Superfemale (Trisomy X)	47,XXX	1:1000 female newborns (incidence) **Most common female chromosomal abnormality**	– Impairment of receptive and expressive language	85–90	**Physical appearance** Tall stature, epicanthal folds, hypotonia and clinodactyly **Organ-related manifestation** – Seizures – Renal and genitourinary abnormalities – Premature ovarian failure (Nielsen and Wohlert 1991; Otter et al. 2012; Tartaglia et al. 2010b)

				IQ	
Supermale	47, XYY	1:1000 male newborns (incidence)	– Delayed language development – Impairment of receptive and expressive language	Normal to slightly low normal	**Physical appearance** Tall stature, hypertelorism, macrocephaly **Organ-related manifestation** – Seizures, tremor, hypotonia – Asthma – Increased testicular volume (Hong and Reiss 2014; Nielsen and Wohlert 1991)
Tetrasomy of the X chromosome	48,XXXX	About 40 cases known so far	– Delayed language development – Impairment of receptive and expressive language	60	**Physical appearance** Short stature, epicanthic folds, hypertelorism, clinodactyly, radioulnar synostosis (Linden et al. 1995; Schoubben et al. 2011)
Pentasomy of the X chromosome	49,XXXXX	About 25 cases known so far	– Delayed language development – Impairment of receptive and expressive language	50	**Physical appearance** Short stature, hypertelorism, epicanthic folds, microcephaly, upward-slanting palpebral fissures, depressed/broad nasal bridge, short neck **Organ-related manifestation** – Congenital heart defects (persistent ductus arteriosus/ventricular septum defect) – Skeletal anomalies (hip dysplasia, subluxation of several joints) (Linden et al. 1995; Schoubben et al. 2011)
Turner	45,X Different types of mosaics exist	1:2500 (prevalence) live-born females **Most common chromosomal aberration in spontaneously aborted foetuses**	– Deficits in speech fluency	95–102	**Physical appearance** Short stature, nail hypoplasia, multiple pigmented nevi, oedema of the hands or feet, lymphedema, nuchal folds, low hairline, low-set ears, small mandible, high-arched palate **Organ-related manifestation** – Ovarian dysgenesis – Left-sided cardiac anomalies – Progressive sensorineural hearing loss – Thyroid and gastrointestinal involvement – Renal anomalies (Barrenas et al. 2000; Bondy and Turner Syndrome Study Group 2007; Hong and Reiss 2014; Jacobs et al. 1990; Mazzocco 2006; Temple and Shephard 2012)

(continued)

Table 9.9 (continued)

	Karyotype	Incidence prevalence	Language deficits	Intelligence mean IQ	Clinical manifestations
Edwards	47,XX, +18 47,XY, +18	0.8:10,000 (prevalence) **Median survival from 2.5 to 14.5 days**	Impairment of receptive and expressive language for survivors Verbal communication is very limited to a few single words – Speech perception is better than expressive language	Mental retardation	**Physical appearance** Microretrognathia, blepharophimosis, orofacial clefts, low-set ears, absence of external auditory canal, preauricular appendages **Organ-related manifestation** – Kidney disorders – Cardiac defects – Encephalocele (Braddock et al. 2012; Hsu et al. 2016)
Patau	47, XX,+13 47, XY,+13	1:5000 to 1:20,000 (incidence) **Only 5% survive 6 months**	Verbal communication is very limited to a few single words – Speech perception is better than expressive language	Mental retardation	**Physical appearance** Microcephaly, flat faces, short nose and lips, increased distance between upper lips and nose, bushy eyebrows, micrognathia, retrognathia, cleft palate, cleft lips **Organ-related manifestation** – Holoprosencephaly, myelomeningocele – Respiratory and heart defects – Incomplete development of the optic and olfactory nerves – Hearing loss – Genital malformations, scoliosis (Braddock et al. 2016; Spagnoli et al. 2015)
Trisomy 8 (Warkany)	Most cases are mosaic forms: 46,XX/47,XX,+8 46,XY/47,XY,+8	1:25,000 to 1:50,000 (incidence)	– Delayed language development – Impairment of expressive language	Mild mental retardation	**Physical appearance** Deformed skull, prominent forehead, high-arched palate, low-set, dysplastic ears, long and slender trunk, plantar/palmar furrows, distinctively abnormal toe posture **Organ-related manifestation** – Ureteral-renal anomalies – Vertebral anomalies, narrow pelvis – Absent or dysplastic patellas, joint contractures (Agrawal and Agrawal 2011; Ptok and Morlot 2009; Riccardi 1977)

| Trisomy 9 | 46,XX/47,XX+9 46,XY/47,XY+9 Survivors present normally as mosaic forms or partial trisomy 9p | Around 125 cases known so far | – Delayed language development
 – Impairment of receptive and expressive language
 – Rarely achieving the ability to speak single words | Mild to serve mental retardation | **Physical appearance**
 Dysplasia of terminal phalange, cyanosed hands and feet, clawlike nails, high and broad forehead, small eyes, horizontal or downslanted palpebral fissures, large nose, large mouth with downturned angle, lower lip, micrognathia, narrow and high-arched palate, mandibular retrognathism, microdontia
 Organ-related manifestation
 Heart defects (ventricular/atrial septal defect, persistent ductus arteriosus, right-sided placement of the heart, hypoplastic left heart syndrome)
 – Undescended testes, hypospadias
 Dandy-Walker syndrome (DWS, a rare group of congenital human brain malformations), enlargement of the ventricles, holoprosencephaly
 – Loose joints, scoliosis
 – Kidney and urinary tract anomalies
 (Arnold et al. 1995; Bruns and Campbell 2015; Patil et al. 2014) |

Table 9.10 Structural chromosomal aberrations

	Deletion	Duplication	Incidence prevalence	Language deficits	Intelligence mean IQ	Clinical manifestations
Monosomy 1p36	1p36		1:5000 to 1:10,000 (prevalence)	– Impairment of expressive language (few isolated words or first word combinations)	Severe to profound retardation	**Physical appearance** Straight eyebrows, deep-set eyes, epicanthal folds, midface retrusion, wide nasal bridge, long philtrum, pointed chin, late-closing anterior fontanel, microbrachycephaly, posteriorly rotated and low-set ears, brachy-/camptodactyly **Organ-related manifestation** – Seizures, structural brain abnormalities – Congenital heart defects – Eye/vision problems – Hearing loss – Skeletal anomalies, hypotonia – Abnormalities of the external genitalia – Renal and gastrointestinal anomalies – Hypothyroidism (Battaglia 1993)
Wolf-Hirschhorn	4 p		1:50,000 (incidence)	– Speech is mostly limited to guttural or disyllabic sounds	44	**Physical appearance** Greek warrior helmet appearance, prominent glabella, widely spaced and protruded eyes, short philtrum and downturned corners of the mouth, micrognathia, clefts of lip and palate, dysplastic ears, periauricular tags, microcephaly **Organ-related manifestation** – Seizures – Congenital heart diseases – Sensorineural hearing loss, ophthalmic defects – Skeletal anomalies – Renal defects (Antonius et al. 2008; Fisch et al. 2008; Paradowska-Stolarz 2014)
Cat cry/cri du chat	5p		1:37,000 (incidence)	– Cat-like cry as an infant – Delayed language development – Better receptive than expressive language – Lacking of word production to short sentences at the age of 4.5–5.5 years	Moderate to severe retardation	**Physical appearance** Microcephaly, round faces, hypertelorism, epicanthal folds, downslanting palpebral fissures, broad nasal bridge, low-set ears, preauricular tags, downturned corners of the mouth, short neck, micrognathia, dental malocclusion, growth deficiency **Organ-related manifestation** – Hyperacusis, sensorineural hearing loss – Myopia, strabismus, cataracts, optic nerve abnormalities – Hypoplasia or agenesis of the corpus callosum, periventricular leukomalacia, abnormalities of white matter, myelination, cerebral or cerebellar atrophy or both, hydrocephalus – Cardiovascular, gastrointestinal, renal and genitourinary anomalies (Cornish and Bramble 2002; Jose-Ramon et al. 2015; Nguyen et al. 2015)

| Williams-Beuren | 7q11.23 | 1:7500 to 1:20,000 (incidence) | About 55 | – Conspicuous, abnormal speech pragmatics
– Delayed language development (first words at age of 2–3 years)
– Articulation problems
– Low lexical development (deficits in long-term memory)
– *Early language acquisition:* echolalia, difficulties in word retrieval
– *Preschool ages:* omission of function words (telegram style), confusion of the grammatical gender
– *Older children:* Speak fluently, enjoy speaking eloquent, extroverted bright and well-languaged creating new words (sometimes leading to overestimation of their cognitive abilities)
– *Adulthood:* regular spontaneous speech | **Physical appearance**
Cocktail party personality without social anxiety *young children:* pixie-like, with a flat nasal bridge, short upturned nose, periorbital puffiness, long philtrum and delicate chin older children and *adults:* coarse features, with full lips, a wide smile and a full nasal tip
Organ-related manifestation
– Hyperacusis, sensorineural hearing loss
– Vascular stenosis, hypertension, valve abnormality
– Intracardiac lesion, stroke, type I Chiari malformation
– Unusually shaped primary teeth, malocclusions
– Hypercalcemia, hypothyroidism
– Osteopenia or osteoporosis, glucose intolerance or diabetes mellitus
– Early onset of puberty
– Gastroesophageal reflux, diverticular disease, rectal prolapse
– Celiac disease, structural renal anomalies, bladder diverticula, recurrent urinary tract infections, nephrocalcinosis
(Lumaka et al. 2016; Mohan and Mittal 2011; Pober 2010) |

(continued)

Table 9.10 (continued)

	Deletion	Duplication	Incidence prevalence	Language deficits	Intelligence mean IQ	Clinical manifestations
WAGR W: Wilms' tumour A: Aniridia G: Genitourinary abnormalities R: Mental retardation	11p13		1: 500,000 to 1: 1,000,000 (prevalence)	– Delayed language development	35–70	**Organ-related manifestation** – Sporadic aniridia (absence of iris) – Genitourinary abnormalities – Wilms' tumour nephropathies (cancer of the kidneys typically occurring in children, rarely in adults) – Brain abnormalities – Pancreatitis (Diacono et al. 2012; Fischbach et al. 2005; Shetti et al. 2015; Tezcan et al. 2015)
Prader-Willi	15q 11–13 Paternal deletion		1:10,000 to 1:30,000 (prevalence)	– Delayed language development – Abnormal or impaired articulation, rhinophonia – Deficit in oral fluency Restricted vocabulary, predominant use of content words, lacking function words, morphological markings, erroneous syntax	70	**Physical appearance** Obesity, small hands and feet, scoliosis, growth retardation, hypotrophy in infancy **Organ-related manifestation** – Diabetes mellitus – Muscle hypotonia – Cryptorchidism (Griggs et al. 2015)

| Angelman | 15q 11–13 (maternal deletion) | 1:15,000 (prevalence) | – Delayed language development
– Lacking babbling during baby and toddler period
– Striking mouth/chewing movements, insufficient control of the oral muscles (tongue protrusion), hyper-salivation
– Severely restricted speech production but preserved ability to learn alternative communication strategies
– Vocabulary on average one to six words up to complete speech arrest
– Phonologically incorrect, semantically unprecise used words
– Good speech perception competence | Severe mental retardation | **Physical appearance**
Brachycephaly, mandibular prognathism, wide mouth, widely spaced teeth, frequent bouts of laughter and joyous facial expressions, an easily excitable personality
Organ-related manifestation
– Seizures, abnormal EEG patterns
– Hypermotoric, frequent hand flapping and mouthing actions (e.g. chewing)
– Overall impaired balance
(Peters et al. 2011; Sachdeva et al. 2015; Wilson et al. 2011) |
| Smith-Magenis | 17p11.2 | 1:15,000 to 1:25,000 (prevalence) | – Delayed language development
Impairment of receptive and expressive language (receptive language skills better than expressive language) | Mild-to-moderate mental retardation | **Physical appearance**
Short stature, brachydactyly, cleft lip/palate
Organ-related manifestation
– Congenital heart disease
– Renal defects
– Hearing loss
– Eye abnormalities
(Elsea and Girirajan 2008) |

(continued)

Table 9.10 (continued)

	Deletion	Duplication	Incidence prevalence	Language deficits	Intelligence mean IQ	Clinical manifestations
Deletion 18 p	18p		1:50,000 (incidence)	– Delayed language development – Impairment of receptive and expressive language	Borderline to severe mental retardation	**Physical appearance** Short stature, ptosis, strabismus, hypertelorism, protruding ears, broad and flat nose, high-arched palate, micrognathia, abnormal central incisors **Organ-related manifestation** – Muscular hypotonia – Panhypopituitarism, growth hormone deficiency (Wester et al. 2006)
Deletion 18q	18q		1:40,000 (incidence)	– Delayed language development – Impairment of receptive and expressive language (expressive language development is more affected than perceptive)	Moderate to severe mental retardation	**Physical appearance** Brachycephaly, frontal bossing, deep-set eyes, midface hypoplasia **Organ-related manifestation** – Seizures, hypotonia – Genitourinary abnormalities (hypospadia, cryptorchidism, genital hypoplasia, shawl scrotum) (Cody et al. 2007)
Alagille syndrome	JAG1 (20p12.2) NOTCH2 (1p12)		1:70,000 (prevalence)	– Delayed language development	Normal to mild retardation	**Physical appearance** Broad forehead, pointed chin, triangular face, deep-set eyes, posterior embryotoxon, anterior segment abnormalities of the eyes, upslanting palpebral fissures, prominent ears, straight nose **Organ-related manifestation** – Biliary atresia – Dysplastic kidneys – Congenital heart disease (peripheral pulmonary stenosis, tetralogy of Fallot) – Vertebral malformations (butterfly vertebrae, fusion of adjacent vertebrae, spina bifida occulta) (Ahn et al. 2015; Spinner et al. 1993; Tanteles et al. 2015)

Syndrome	Gene/location	Incidence	Speech and language	IQ	
DiGeorge syndrome	Tbx1 (22q11.21)	1:2000 to 1:4000 (incidence) **Most common microdeletion syndrome**	– Impairment of receptive and expressive language – Rhinophonia aperta due to velopharyngeal insufficiency	70–84	**Physical appearance** Long face, malar flatness, craniosynostosis, nasal malformations, hypertelorism, ptosis, epicanthal folds, posterior, embryotoxon, loose or sagging skin of the upper or lower lids, cleft lip and palate, protuberant ears; preauricular tags, narrow external auditory meati **Organ-related manifestation** – Congenital heart disease (tetralogy of Fallot) – Immunological defects – Neonatal hypocalcaemia – Seizures (Digilio et al. 2013; Jerome and Papaioannou 2001; McDonald-McGinn et al. 1993; Mlynarski et al. 2016)
Goldenhar (Oculo-auriculo-vertebral)	1p22.2–p31.1 5q13.2 5p15 12p13.33 14q31.1–q31.3 15q24.1 22qter 22q11.2 10p14–p15 14q23.1 22q11.1–q11.21	1:5600 (incidence)	– Impairment of receptive and expressive language – Impaired articulation – Hypernasality	Normal	**Physical appearance** Ear anomalies (preauricular tags, dysplasia, anotia, microtia), hemifacial microsomia, facial asymmetry (right side appears more frequently involved than the left side), orofacial clefts, ocular defects **Organ-related manifestation** – Conductive or sensorineural hearing loss or both – Congenital heart defects (ventricular septal defect, tetralogy of Fallot, dextrocardia, transposition of great arteries, double-outlet right ventricle) – Genitourinary and cerebral malformation (Bartlett et al. 2002; Beleza-Meireles et al. 2014; Girardin et al. 2009; Van Lierde et al. 2004)

Table 9.11 Autosomal dominant disorders

	Gene/chromosome regions	Incidence prevalence	Language deficits	Intelligence mean IQ	Clinical manifestations
Noonan	PTPN11(12q24) SOS1 (2p22.1) CBL (11q23.3) BRAF (7q34) RAF1 (3p25) SHOC2 (10q25) MAP2K1 (15q22.31) RIT1 (1q22) NRAS (1p13.2) KRAS (12p12.1) RRAS (19q13.33)	1:1000 to 1:2500 (incidence)	– Delayed language development – Impairment of receptive and expressive language	85	**Physical appearance** Short stature; hypertelorism; ptosis; downslanting palpebral fissures; low-set, posteriorly rotated ears **Organ-related manifestation** – Heart defect – Recurrent otitis media, sensorineural hearing loss – Multiple skeletal anomalies – Various skin manifestations (Ekvall et al. 2015; Sharland et al. 1992; Tartaglia et al. 2010a' van der Burgt 2007)
Neurofibromatosis type 1 Von Recklinghausen disease	NF1(17q11.2)	1:3000 (prevalence)	– Impairment of receptive and expressive language – Motor dyspraxia, speech disfluency (neurogenic stuttering) – Hypernasality – Reading and writing problems	Normal (but 30–60% have learning problems)	**Physical appearance** Cutaneous neurofibromas, Café-au-lait pigment spots, intertriginous freckling, Lisch nodules **Organ-related manifestation** – Optic pathway glioma, congenital glaucoma (Cosyns et al. 2010; Klein-Tasman et al. 2014; Li et al. 2015)
ECC (Ectrodactyly, Ectodermal Dysplasia, Clefting)	EEC1 (7q11.2-21.3) EEC3 (3q27-29) (EEC2 no longer exists)	More than 300 cases known so far	– Impaired language acquisition due to hearing loss and cleft lip/palate	Normal	**Physical appearance** Ectrodactyly (split hand/foot malformation), ectodermal dysplasia (dry skin, sparse hair, dystrophic nails, hypoplastic teeth, lacrimal duct obstruction), facial clefts (clefting may affect the lip or palate) **Organ-related manifestation** – Hearing loss – Anomalies of the kidney (recurrent urinary tract infections, vesicoureteral reflux) – Decreased/absence of sweat glands (overheating, hyperthermia) (Barrow et al. 2002; Koul et al. 2014)

Syndrome	Gene (locus)	Prevalence/incidence	Speech/language	Cognition	Physical appearance
Waardenburg type 1	PAX3 (2q36.1)	1:20,000 to 1:40,000 (prevalence)	– Delayed language development	Normal	**Physical appearance** White forelock/early greying of the scalp hair, pigmentary disturbances of the iris, medial eyebrow, flare, heterochromia, iridium, brilliant blue irises, dystopia canthorum, broad nasal root, prominent columella, leukoderma (localized loss of skin pigmentation) **Organ-related manifestation** – Sensorineural hearing loss (Milunsky 1993)
Beckwith-Wiedemann	11p15.5	0.07:1000 (prevalence)	– Impaired articulation	Normal	**Physical appearance** Cleft palate, maxillary hypoplasia, microcephaly, prominent occiput, flattened nasal dorsum, downward slanted palpebral fissures, anterior linear earlobe creases, posterior helical ear pits, facial flame nevus (forehead), macroglossia, gigantism (Heggie et al. 2013)
Treacher Collins/ Franceschetti-Zwahlen-Klein	TCOF1 (5q32) 60% of cases being spontaneous, 40% familial POLR1C (6p21.1) POLR1D (13q12.2)	1:50,000 (incidence)	– Delayed language development – Hypernasality or hyponasality	Normal	**Physical appearance** Microcephaly, dental malocclusion, anterior open bite, widely spaced teeth, high palate, hypoplasia of the zygomatic complex, cleft palate, inferolateral orbital cleft, absence of lid lashes medial to the defect, colobomas of the lower eyelids, atresia of the external auditory canal(s) **Organ-related manifestation** – Bilateral conductive hearing loss – Narrow upper airways (Dauwerse et al. 2011; Plomp et al. 2016; Trainor et al. 2009)
Apert syndrome	FGFR2 (10q26)	1:65,000 (prevalence)	– Impairment of receptive and expressive language – Hypernasality	Low to normal	**Physical appearance** Syndactyly of the hands and feet, acrobrachycephaly, intrauterine fusion of the coronal suture, high broad forehead, flat face, low-set ears, ear abnormalities, hypertelorism, downslanting palpebral fissures, cleft palate, bifid uvula **Organ-related manifestation** – Conductive and sensorineural hearing loss – Abnormalities of the central nervous system (ventriculomegaly, hydrocephalus, deficient or absent septum pellucidum, agenesis of the corpus callosum, limbic malformations) – Cardiovascular, respiratory, gastrointestinal, genitourinary anomalies – Skeletal malformations (Breik et al. 2016; Huang et al. 2004; Shipster et al. 2002)

(continued)

Table 9.11 (continued)

	Gene/chromosome regions	Incidence prevalence	Language deficits	Intelligence mean IQ	Clinical manifestations
Charge C: Coloboma H: Heart defects A: Atresia (choanal atresia) R: Retarded growth and development G: Genital abnormalities E: Ear anomalies	CHD7 (8q12.2)	1:15,000 to 1:17,000 prevalence	– Delayed language development	Normal to serve mental retardation	**Physical appearance** Short stature; square face; broad, prominent forehead prominent nasal bridge and columella; flat midface; short webbed neck; sloping shoulders; hypoplastic nails; clinodactyly; polydactyly; brachydactyly; joint hyperflexibility; contractures; protruding jaw; overbite; wide ears with little or no lobe; prominent antihelix; unilateral or bilateral facial palsy **Organ-related manifestation** – Heart defects (tetralogy of Fallot, perimembranous ventricular septal defect, double-outlet right ventricle, AV canal defects) – Unilateral or bilateral coloboma of the iris, retina-choroid – Genitourinary abnormalities (micropenis and cryptorchidism) – Sensorineural/conductive hearing loss unilateral or bilateral choanal atresia/stenosis – Cleft lip or palate – Oesophageal atresia/tracheoesophageal fistula – Renal anomalies (solitary kidney, hydronephrosis, renal hypoplasia) – Mild to severe T-cell deficiency – Cerebral anomalies (corpus callosum agenesis) – Anomalies of the olfactory tracts and bulbs (Lalani et al. 1993; Martire et al. 2016)
Sotos	NSD1 (5q35)	100 cases known so far	– Delayed language development – Impairment of receptive and expressive language	78	**Physical appearance** Overgrowth in childhood; large occipitofrontal circumference; long, narrow face; prominent forehead and chin; downslanting palpebral fissures; arched eyebrows **Organ-related manifestation** – Cardiac (dilatation of the ascending aorta) – Genitourinary anomalies – Seizures – Connective tissue laxity (joint hyperextensibility) – Scoliosis (Hood et al. 2016; Sheth et al. 2015)

| Cornelia de Lange | NIPBL (5p13.2) 60% RAD21 (8q24.11) SMC3 (10q25.2) (HDAC8 (Xq13.1) SMC1A (Xp11.22) X-linked dominant pattern) | 1:20,000 to 1:40,000 (incidence) | – Delayed language development
– Impairment of expressive language (substitution or elision of consonants)
– Dyspractic speech
– Lexical abilities better than syntactical ones
– Less intentional communicative behaviour | 53 | **Physical appearance**
Microcephaly, confluent eyebrows, long curly eyelashes, short neck with low anterior and posterior hairlines, long philtrum, thin lips, micrognatia, small nose with low bridge, low-set ears, crescent-shaped mouth, hirsutism
Organ-related manifestation
– Skeletal anomalies
– Congenital diaphragmatic hernia
– Cardiac, respiratory, genitourinary abnormalities
– Gastro-oesophageal dysfunction
– Ophthalmologic anomalies
(Deardorff et al. 1993; Liu and Krantz 2009; Parisi et al. 2015; Uzun et al. 2008) |

Table 9.12 Autosomal recessive disorders

	Gene chromosome regions	Incidence prevalence	Language deficits	Intelligence mean IQ	Clinical manifestations
Smith-Lemli-Opitz	DHCR7 (11q13.4)	1:950,000 (prevalence Canada)	– Language is rarely developed – Severe intellectual disability associated with absent speech – Speech production at the level of two-word utterances, not able to accomplish complex verbal tasks	From borderline to severe intellectual disability	**Physical appearance** Microcephaly; narrow forehead; short nose; capillary haemangiomas over the nasal root; low-set, posteriorly rotated ears; ptosis; epicanthal folds; micrognathia; high and narrow hard palate; cleft palate; polydactyly; 2–3 toe syndactyly **Organ-related manifestation** – Congenital heart defects – Gastrointestinal malformations (Hirschsprung, pyloric stenosis) – Renal anomalies – Cerebellar hypoplasia, hypoplasia of corpus callosum – *Males*: hypospadia, bilateral cryptorchidism, undervirilization of the genitalia, blind vaginal pouch and rudimentary uterus in 46 XY individuals – *Females*: hypoplasia of the labia minora and majora, bicornuate uterus, septate vagina (Nowaczyk 1993; Nowaczyk and Irons 2012)
Nijmegen breakage	NBN (8q21–24)	Around several hundred cases known so far	– Delayed language development – Impairment of receptive and expressive language	Borderline mental retardation in 45% Moderate mental retardation in 20%	**Physical appearance** Short stature, microcephaly, sloping forehead, receding mandible, prominent nasal root and nose, large ears, upward slant of the palpebral fissures, irregular skin pigmentation (hyper- or hypo-pigmented) **Organ-related manifestation** – Ovarian failure – Increased risk of lymphoma (Chrzanowska et al. 2012; Gupta and Nagarkar 2009)
Sjögren-Larsson	ALDH3A2 (17p11.2)	<0.4:100000 (prevalence)	– Delayed language development – Impairment of receptive and expressive language – Dysarthria	Moderate mental retardation	**Physical appearance** Microcephaly, short stature, hypertelorism, dental enamel hypoplasia, widely spaced teeth **Organ-related manifestation** – Congenital ichthyosis – Spasticity in the extremities – Crystalline retinopathy – Leukoencephalopathy – Epileptic seizures – Peripheral neuropathy (Fuijkschot et al. 2009, 2012; Tanteles et al. 2015)

Table 9.13 Gonosomal dominant disorders

	Gene chromosome regions	Incidence prevalence	Language deficits	Intelligence mean IQ	Clinical manifestations
Charcot-Marie-Tooth Type CMTX1	GJB1 (Xq13.1)	1:2500 (incidence) **One of the more common genetic neurological disorders** Males are usually more affected than females	– Dysarthria	Normal	**Physical appearance** Muscular atrophy, foot drop and deformity **Organ-related manifestation** – Motor and sensory neuropathy, ataxia – Visual impairment Symptoms develop in late childhood, adolescence and early adulthood (Barisic et al. 2008; Ionasescu et al. 1992; Siskind et al. 2009)

Table 9.14 Gonosomal recessive disorders

	Gene chromosome regions	Incidence	Language deficits	Intelligence mean IQ	Clinical manifestations
Fragile X (Martin-Bell syndrome)	FMR1 (Xq27.3)	1:4000 to 1:5000 (incidence)	– Delayed language development – Ranging from subtle communication deficits up to complete lacking of language structures – Difficulties in word retrieval – Echolalia, perseverations and self-talk – Heavily impaired grammar and articulation	30–50 **Most frequent form of inherited intellectual disability**	**Physical appearance** Elongated face, large head, prominent forehead and chin, protruding ears, soft and smooth cutis, pubertal macro-orchidism, obesity **Organ-related manifestation** – Mitral valve prolapse – Strabismus – Gastroesophageal reflux, recurrent otitis media – Joint laxity, hypotonia – Periventricular heterotopia, epilepsy **Most common known genetic cause of autism spectrum disorder** (Arvio 2016; Crawford et al. 2001; Fernandez et al. 2015; Lee et al. 2015; McLennan et al. 2011; Saul and Tarleton 1993)

(continued)

Table 9.14 (continued)

	Gene chromosome regions	Incidence	Language deficits	Intelligence mean IQ	Clinical manifestations
Coffin-Lowry	RPS6KA3 (Xp22.12)	1:50,000 to 1:100,000 (incidence)	– Delayed language development – Males: limited vocabulary to lacking language development	Males: severe to profound retardation Heterozygous females: normal to profound retardation	Physical appearance Microcephaly, short stature, coarse face, prominent forehead, short hands, hyper-extensible fingers, thick eyebrows, widely spaced eyes, depressed nasal bridge, wide mouth, thick vermilion of the lips, prominent ears **Organ-related manifestation** – Epileptic seizures – Cardiac abnormalities (mitral, tricuspid and aortic valves), cardiomyopathy – Progressive kyphoscoliosis – Dental anomalies with delayed eruption and premature loss – Sensorineural hearing loss – Increased intraventricular, subarachnoid spaces, abnormalities of the corpus callosum (Hanauer and Young 2002; Pereira et al. 2010; Rogers and Abidi 1993)
FG Syndrome (Opitz-Kaveggia)	MED12 (Xq13) Most common cause	Around one hundred cases known so far	– Delayed language development – Impairment of receptive and expressive language – Deficits in communication skills	Moderate to severe retardation	**Physical Appearance** Craniosynostosis, macrocephaly, long face, tall forehead, prominent ears, downslanting palpebral fissures, hypertelorism, full upper eyelids broad, flat thumbs and halluces, partial syndactyly **Organ-related manifestation** – Agenesis or hypoplasia of the corpus callosum – Hypotonia – Anal fistula, stenosis and atresia, pyloric stenosis – Congenital cardiac anomalies, renal cysts and urolithiasis – Skeletal anomalies (joint contractures) (Graham Jr. et al. 2010; Graham and Schwartz 2013; Schwartz et al. 2007)

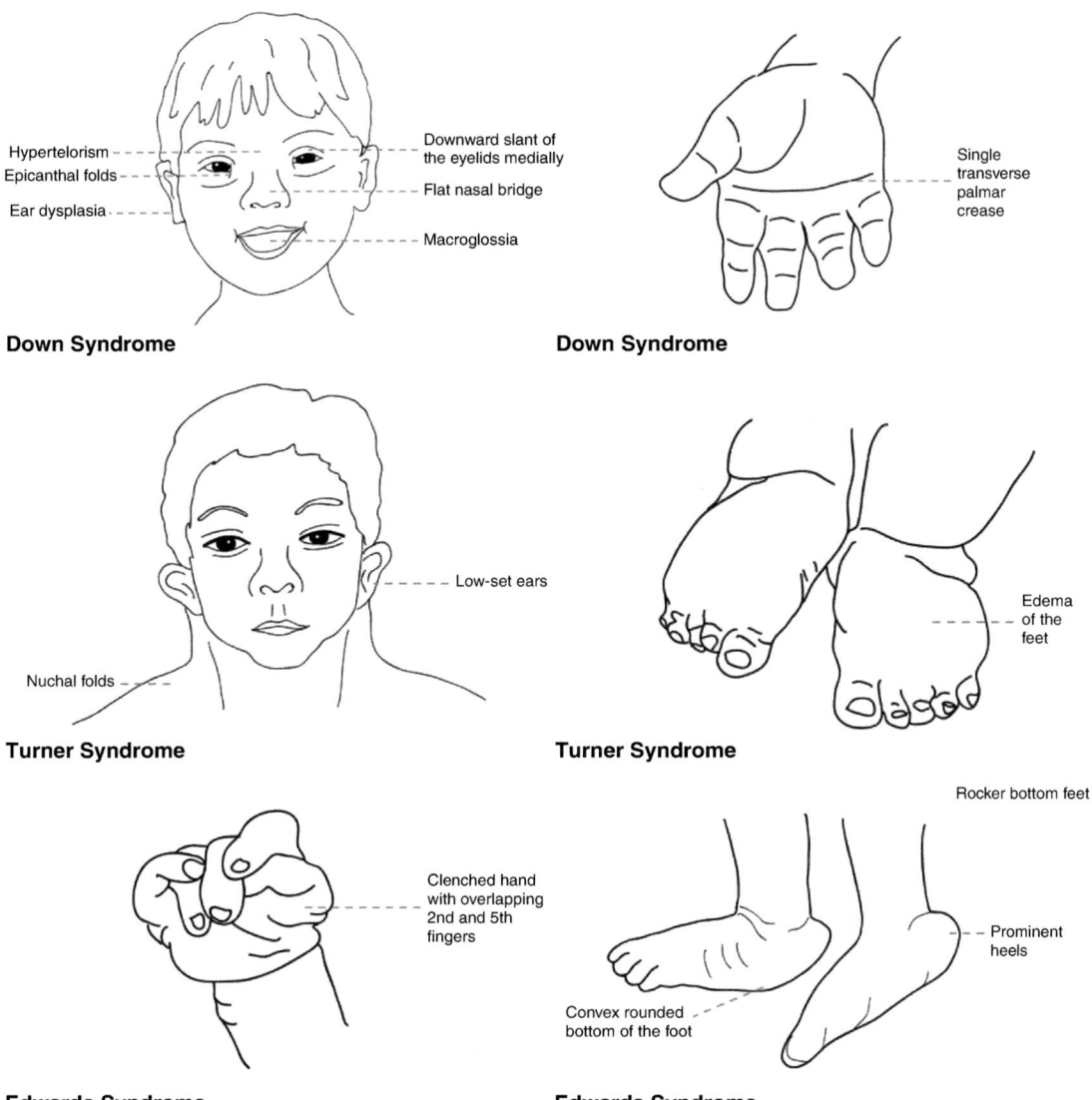

Fig. 9.1 Visual diagnosis of the most common syndromes with numerical chromosomal aberrations

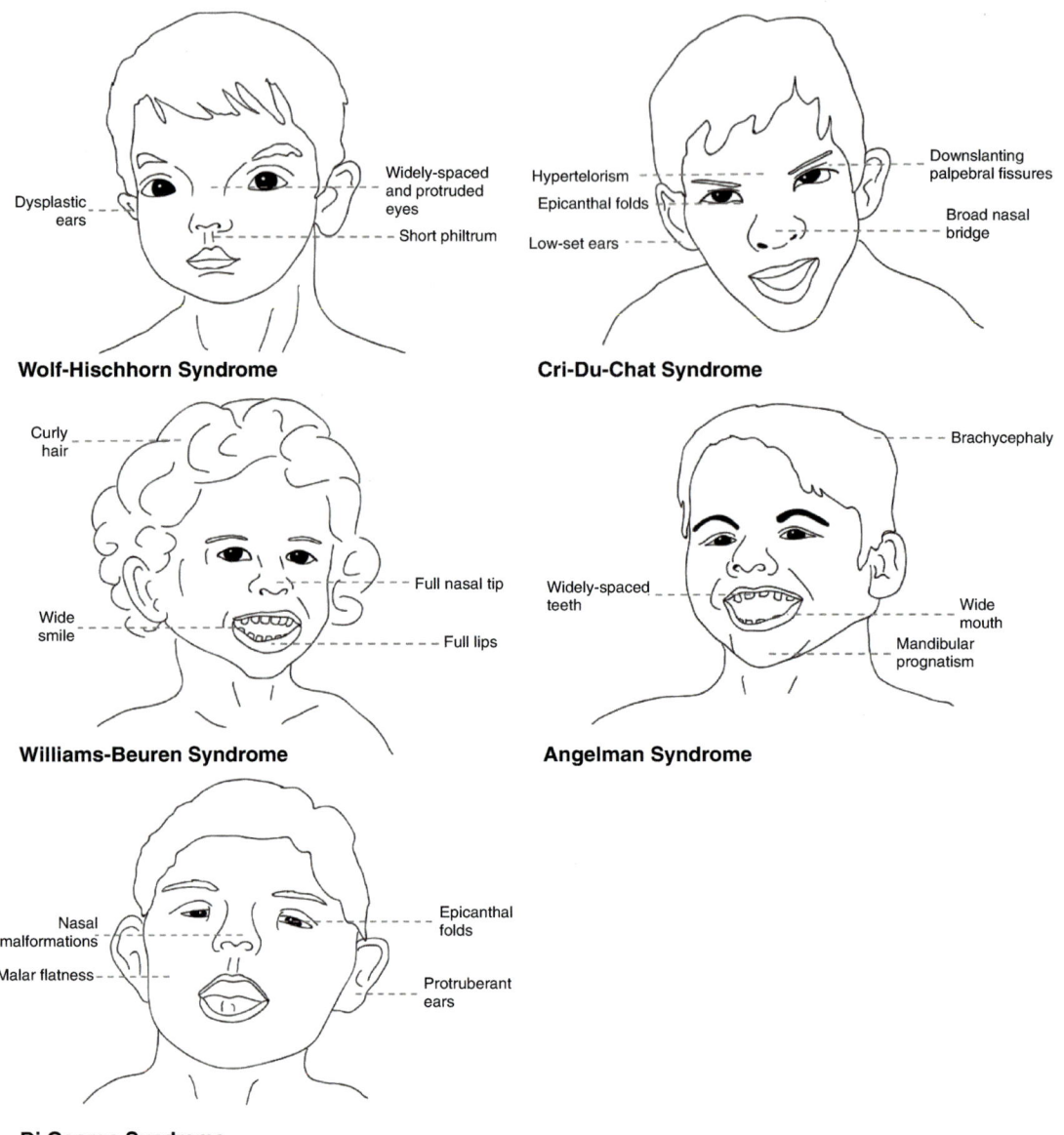

Wolf-Hischhorn Syndrome

Dysplastic ears

Widely-spaced and protruded eyes

Short philtrum

Cri-Du-Chat Syndrome

Hypertelorism

Epicanthal folds

Low-set ears

Downslanting palpebral fissures

Broad nasal bridge

Williams-Beuren Syndrome

Curly hair

Wide smile

Full nasal tip

Full lips

Angelman Syndrome

Brachycephaly

Widely-spaced teeth

Wide mouth

Mandibular prognatism

Di George Syndrome

Nasal malformations

Malar flatness

Epicanthal folds

Protruberant ears

Fig. 9.2 Visual diagnosis of the most common syndromes with structural chromosomal aberrations

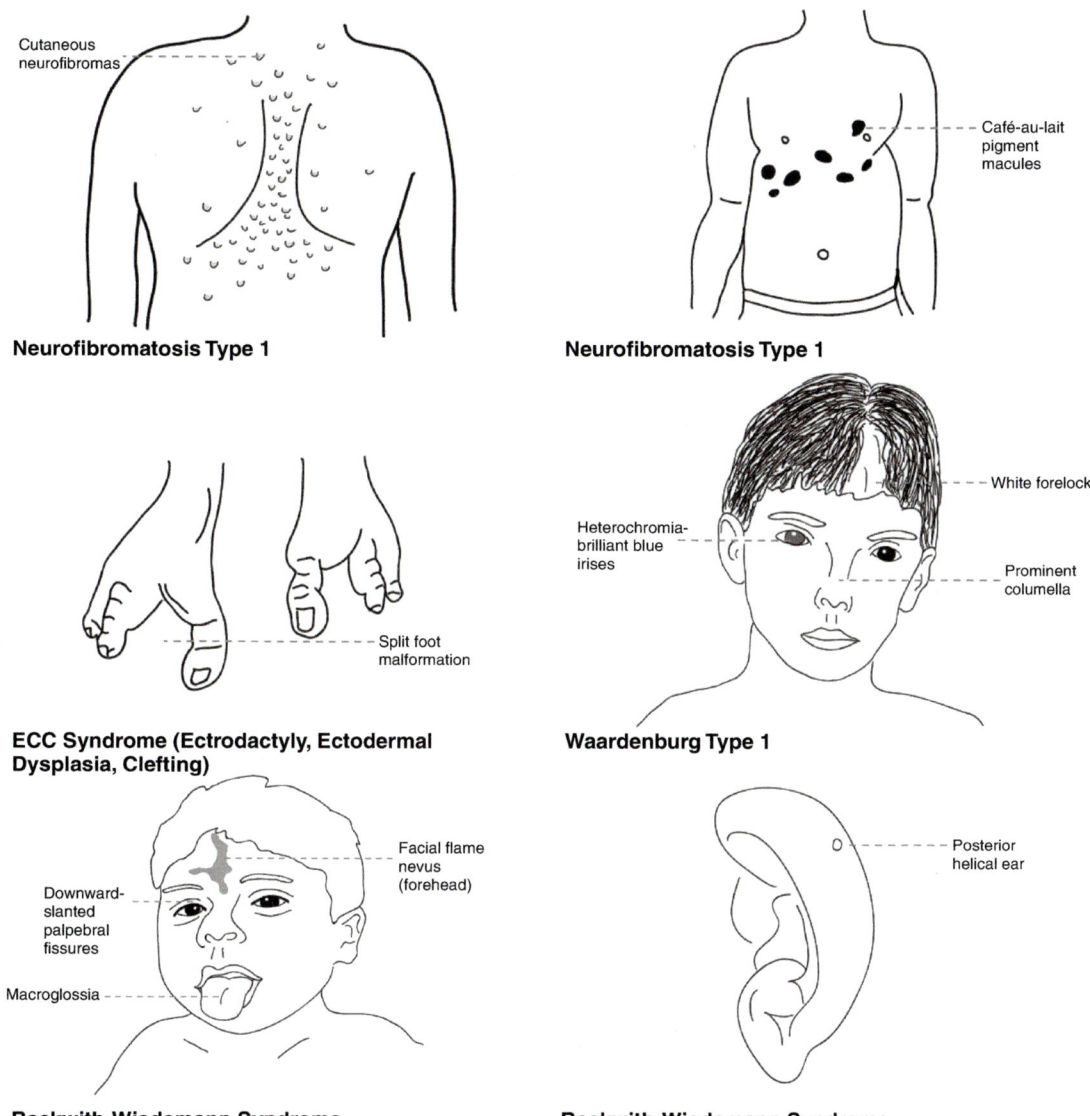

Fig. 9.3 Visual diagnosis of the most common syndromes with autosomal dominant inheritance

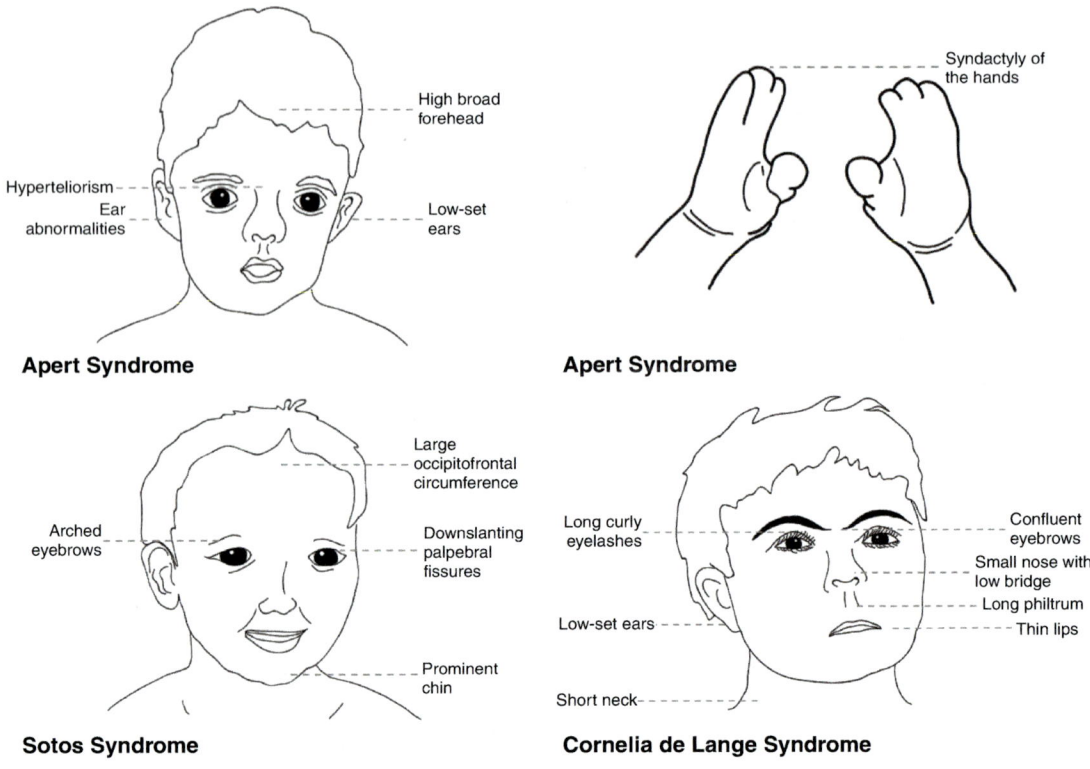

Apert Syndrome

Apert Syndrome

High broad forehead

Hyperteliorism

Ear abnormalities

Low-set ears

Syndactyly of the hands

Sotos Syndrome

Large occipitofrontal circumference

Arched eyebrows

Downslanting palpebral fissures

Prominent chin

Cornelia de Lange Syndrome

Long curly eyelashes

Confluent eyebrows

Small nose with low bridge

Long philtrum

Low-set ears

Thin lips

Short neck

Fig. 9.3 (continued)

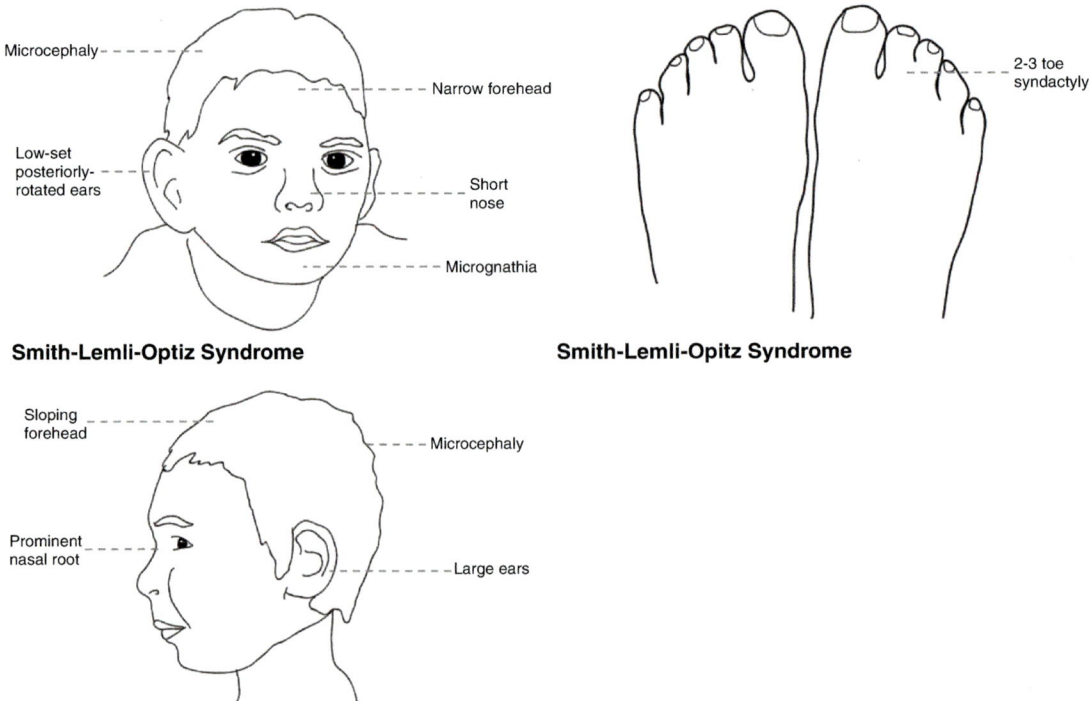

Smith-Lemli-Optiz Syndrome

Microcephaly

Narrow forehead

Low-set posteriorly-rotated ears

Short nose

Micrognathia

Smith-Lemli-Opitz Syndrome

2-3 toe syndactyly

Nijmegen Breakage Syndrome

Sloping forehead

Microcephaly

Prominent nasal root

Large ears

Fig. 9.4 Visual diagnosis of the most common syndromes with autosomal recessive inheritance

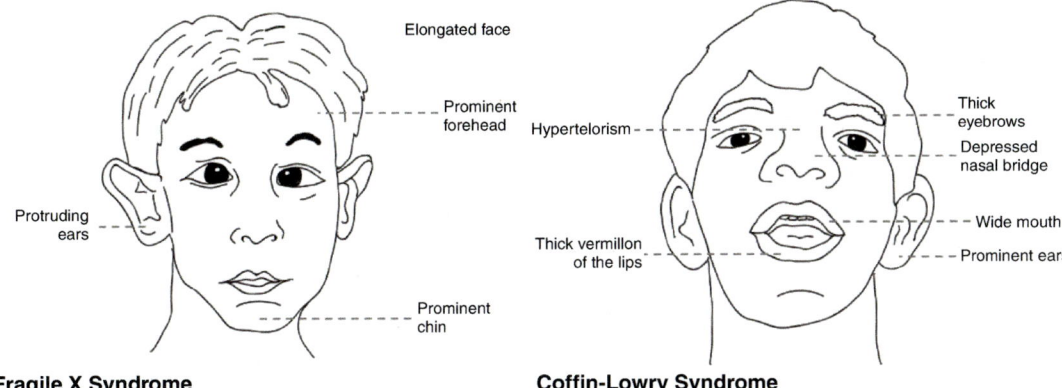

Fig. 9.5 Visual diagnosis of the most common syndromes with gonosomal recessive inheritance

References

Addis L, Friederici AD, Kotz SA et al (2010) A locus for an auditory processing deficit and language impairment in an extended pedigree maps to 12p13.31-q14.3. Genes Brain Behav 9(6):545–561

Agrawal A, Agrawal R (2011) Warkany syndrome: a rare case report. Case Rep Pediatr 2011:437101. https://doi.org/10.1155/2011/437101

Ahn KJ, Yoon JK, Kim GB et al (2015) Alagille syndrome and a JAG1 mutation: 41 cases of experience at a single center. Korean J Pediatr 58(10):392–397

Aksglaede L, Link K, Giwercman A et al (2013) 47,XXY Klinefelter syndrome: clinical characteristics and age-specific recommendations for medical management. Am J Med Genet C Semin Med Genet 163C(1):55–63

Alarcon M, Abrahams BS, Stone JL et al (2008) Linkage, association, and gene-expression analyses identify CNTNAP2 as an autism-susceptibility gene. Am J Hum Genet 82(1):150–159

Ambrose NG, Yairi E (1999) Normative disfluency data for early childhood stuttering. J Speech Lang Hear Res 42(4):895–909

American Psychiatric Association (2013) Diagnostic and statistical manual of mental disorders DSM-5 (R), 5th edn. American Psychiatric Association, Arlington

Antonius T, Draaisma J, Levtchenko E et al (2008) Growth charts for Wolf-Hirschhorn syndrome (0-4 years of age). Eur J Pediatr 167(7):807–810

Arnold GL, Kirby RS, Stern TP et al (1995) Trisomy 9: review and report of two new cases. Am J Med Genet 56(3):252–257

Arumugam A, Raja K, Venugopalan M et al (2015) Down syndrome—a narrative review. Clin Anat 29(5):568–577

Arvio M (2016) Fragile-X syndrome—a 20-year follow-up study of male patients. Clin Genet 89(1):55–59

Baddeley A (1992) Working memory. Science 255(5044):556–559

Baker C, Prys Jones S (1998) The encyclopedia of bilingualism and bilingual education. Multilingual Matters Inc., Toronto

Barisic N, Claeys KG, Sirotkovic-Skerlev M et al (2008) Charcot-Marie-Tooth disease: a clinico-genetic confrontation. Ann Hum Genet 72(Pt 3):416–441

Barrenas M, Landin-Wilhelmsen K, Hanson C (2000) Ear and hearing in relation to genotype and growth in Turner syndrome. Hear Res 144(1–2):21–28

Barrow LL, van Bokhoven H, Daack-Hirsch S et al (2002) Analysis of the p63 gene in classical EEC syndrome, related syndromes, and non-syndromic orofacial clefts. J Med Genet 39(8):559–566

Bartlett CW, Flax JF, Logue MW et al (2002) A major susceptibility locus for specific language impairment is located on 13q21. Am J Hum Genet 71(1):45–55

Bartlett CW, Flax JF, Logue MW et al (2004) Examination of potential overlap in autism and language loci on chromosomes 2, 7, and 13 in two independent samples ascertained for specific language impairment. Hum Hered 57(1):10–20

Bates E, Marchman V, Thal D et al (1994) Developmental and stylistic variation in the composition of early vocabulary. J Child Lang 21(1):85–121

Battaglia A (1993) 1p36 deletion syndrome. In: Pagon RA et al (eds) GeneReviews(R). University of Washington, Seattle

Baumgartner S, Füssenich I (eds) (2002) Sprachtherapie mit Kindern, vol 3, pp 204–289

Beitchman JH, Nair R, Clegg M et al (1986) Prevalence of speech and language disorders in 5-year-old kindergarten children in the Ottawa-Carleton region. J Speech Hear Disord 51(2):98–110

Beleza-Meireles A, Clayton-Smith J, Saraiva JM et al (2014) Oculo-auriculo-vertebral spectrum: a review of the literature and genetic update. J Med Genet 51(10):635–645

Bialystok E, Craik F, Freedman M (2007) Bilingualism as a protection against the onset of symptoms of dementia. Neuropsychologia 45(2):459–464

Bishop DVM (2006) What causes specific language impairment in children? Curr Dir Psychol Sci 15(5):217–221

Bishop DVM, North T, Donlan C (1995) Genetic basis of specific language impairment: evidence from a twin study. Dev Med Child Neurol 37(1):56–71

Bishop DVM, Laws G, Adams C et al (2006) High heritability of speech and language impairments in 6-year-old twins demonstrated using parent and teacher report. Behav Genet 36(2):173–184

Bishop DV, Holt G, Line E et al (2012) Parental phonological memory contributes to prediction of outcome of late talkers from 20 months to 4 years: a longitudinal study of precursors of specific language impairment. J Neurodev Disord 4(1):3

Bishop DVM, Snowling MJ, Thompson PA at al (2017) Phase 2 of CATALISE: a multinational and multidisciplinary Delphi consensus study of problems with language development: Terminology. J Child Psychol Psychiatry 58(10):1068–1080

Bojesen A, Juul S, Gravholt CH (2003) Prenatal and postnatal prevalence of Klinefelter syndrome: a national registry study. J Clin Endocrinol Metab 88(2):622–626

Bondy CA, Turner Syndrome Study Group (2007) Care of girls and women with Turner syndrome: a guideline of the Turner Syndrome Study Group. J Clin Endocrinol Metab 92(1):10–25

Borrell V, Cardenas A, Ciceri G et al (2012) Slit/Robo signaling modulates the proliferation of central nervous system progenitors. Neuron 76(2):338–352

Bosch L (2011) Precursors to language in preterm infants: speech perception abilities in the first year of life. Prog Brain Res 189:239–257

Bosshardt HG (2010) Frühintervention bei Stottern: Behandlungsansätze für Kinder im Vorschulalter. Hogrefe, Göttingen

Botting N, Faragher B, Simkin Z et al (2001) Predicting pathways of specific language impairment: what differentiates good and poor outcome? J Child Psychol Psychiatry 42(8):1013–1020

Bower CL, Petterson B (2001) Intellectual disability in Western Australia. J Paediatr Child Health 36(3):213–215

Boysson-Bardies B, Sagart L, Durand C (1984) Discernible differences in the babbling of infants according to target language. J Child Lang 11(1):1–15

Braddock B, McDaniel J, Spragge S et al (2012) Communication ability in persons with trisomy 18 and trisomy 13. Augment Altern Commun 28(4):266–277

Braddock SR, South ST, Schiffman JD, Longhurst M, Rowe LR, Carey JC (2016) Braddock-Carey syndrome: a 21q22 contiguous gene syndrome encompassing RUNX1. Am J Med Genet A 170(10):2580–2586. https://doi.org/10.1002/ajmg.a.37870. Epub 2016 Aug 23.

Bradford Y, Haines J, Hutcheson H et al (2001) Incorporating language phenotypes strengthens evidence of linkage to autism. Am J Med Genet 105(6):539–547

Breik O, Mahindu A, Moore MH et al (2016) Central nervous system and cervical spine abnormalities in Apert syndrome. Childs Nerv Syst 32(5):833–838

Bruns DA, Campbell E (2015) Twenty-five additional cases of trisomy 9 mosaic: birth information, medical conditions, and developmental status. Am J Med Genet A 167A(5):997–1007

Buschmann A, Jooss B, Rupp A et al (2008) Children with developmental language delay at 24 months of age: results of a diagnostic work-up. Dev Med Child Neurol 50(3):223–229

Canning PM, Lyon ME (1989) Young children with special needs: prevalence and implications in Nova Scotia. Can J Educ 14(3):368–380

Casby MW (2001) Otitis media and language development: a meta-analysis. Am J Speech Lang Pathol 10(3 Pt 1):65–80

Charollais A, Stumpf MH, Beaugrand D et al (2010) Évaluation à 6 ans du langage de l'enfant né grand prématuré sans paralysie cérébrale: étude prospective de 55 enfants [Evaluation of language at 6 years in children born prematurely without cerebral palsy: prospective study of 55 children Article in French]. Arch Pediatr 17(10):1433–1439

Chiat S, Roy P (2008) Early phonological and sociocognitive skills as predictors of later language and social communication outcomes. J Child Psychol Psychiatry 49(6):635–645

Chilla S, Haberzettl S (2014) Handbuch Mehrsprachigkeit. Reihe Sprachentwicklung und Sprachentwicklungsstörungen. (Handbook multilingualism. Series language development and developmental language disorder). Elsevier, München

Chomsky N (1988) Language and problems of knowledge. MIT Press, Cambridge

Chrzanowska KH, Gregorek H, Dembowska-Baginska B et al (2012) Nijmegen breakage syndrome (NBS). Orphanet J Rare Dis 7:13

Clark EV (2003) First language acquisition. Cambridge University Press, Cambridge

Cody JD, Sebold C, Malik A et al (2007) Recurrent interstitial deletions of proximal 18q: a new syndrome involving expressive speech delay. Am J Med Genet A 143A(11):1181–1190

Cornish K, Bramble D (2002) Cri du chat syndrome: genotype-phenotype correlations and recommendations for clinical management. Dev Med Child Neurol 44(7):494–497

Cosyns M, Vandeweghe L et al (2010) Speech disorders in neurofibromatosis type 1: a sample survey. Int J Lang Commun Disord 45(5):600–607

Crawford DC, Acuna JM, Sherman SL (2001) FMR1 and the fragile X syndrome: human genome epidemiology review. Genet Med 3(5):359–371

Dale PS, Tosto MG, Hayiou-Thomas ME et al (2015) Why does parental language input style predict child language development? A twin study of gene–environment correlation. J Commun Disord 57:106–117

Dauwerse JG, Dixon J, Seland S et al (2011) Mutations in genes encoding subunits of RNA polymerases I and III cause Treacher Collins syndrome. Nat Genet 43(1):20–22

de Langen-Müller U, Kauschke C, Kiese-Himmel C et al (eds. in equal authorship) (2011) Diagnostik von Sprachentwicklungsstörungen (SES), unter Berücksichtigung umschriebener

Sprachentwicklungsstörungen (USES) (Synonym: Spezifische Sprachentwicklungsstörungen (SSES)) Interdisziplinäre S2k-Leitlinie. Register-Nr: 049/006. Available via: http://www.awmf. org/uploads/tx_szleitlinien/049-0061_S2k_ Sprachentwicklungsstoerungen_Diagnostik_2013-06-abgelaufen_01.pdf. Accessed 11 April 2018

de Langen-Müller U, Kiese-Himmel C, Neumann K et al (equal authorship) (2012) Diagnostik von (umschriebenen) Sprachentwicklungsstörungen. [Diagnostics of (specific) developmental disorders of speech and language.] [German]. Peter Lang, Frankfurt am Main

de Langen-Müller U, Kiese-Himmel C, Neumann K et al (equal authorship) (2016) Diagnostik von Sprachentwicklungsstörungen (SES), unter Berücksichtigung umschriebener Sprachentwicklungsstörungen (USES). Interdisziplinäre S2k-Leitlinie, 2011/ in Revision 2016, AWMF-Registernummer 049-006

Deardorff MA, Noon SE, Krantz ID (1993) Cornelia de Lange syndrome. In: Pagon RA et al (eds) GeneReviews(R). University of Washington, Seattle

Desmarais C, Sylvestre A, Meyer F et al (2008) Systematic review of the literature on characteristics of late-talking toddlers. Int J Lang Commun Disord 43(4):361–389

Deutsche Gesellschaft für Phoniatrie und Pädaudiologie (2005) S2-Leitlinie: Periphere Hörstörungen im Kindesalter, AWMF-Registernummer 049/010[S2-guideline: peripheral hearing disorders in infancy and childhood, AWMF registry number 049/010.] [German]. Available via http://www.awmf.org/leitlinien/detail/ll/049-010.html. Accessed 4 May 2014

Diacono D, Fagbemi A, Puleston J et al (2012) Bezafibrate to prevent relapsing pancreatitis in WAGR syndrome. BMJ Case Rep 2012. https://doi.org/10.1136/bcr-2012-006413

Digilio MC, Luca AD, Lepri F et al (2013) JAG1 mutation in a patient with deletion 22q11.2 syndrome and tetralogy of Fallot. Am J Med Genet A 161A(12): 3133–3136

Duncan AF, Watterberg KL, Nolen TL et al (2012) Effect of ethnicity and race on cognitive and language testing at age 18-22 months in extremely preterm infants. J Pediatr 160(6):966–971

Ehlers S, Gillberg C (1993) The epidemiology of Asperger syndrome. A total population study. J Child Psychol Psychiatry 34(8):1327–1350

Eicher JD, Powers NR, Miller LL et al (2013) Genome-wide association study of shared components of reading disability and language impairment. Genes Brain Behav 12(8):792–801

Ekvall S, Wilbe M, Dahlgren J et al (2015) Mutation in NRAS in familial Noonan syndrome—case report and review of the literature. BMC Med Genet 16:95

Elia J, Gai X, Xie HM et al (2010) Rare structural variants found in attention-deficit hyperactivity disorder are preferentially associated with neurodevelopmental genes. Mol Psychiatry 15(6):637–646

Ellis Weismer S (2007) Typical talkers, late talkers, and children with specific language impairment: a language endowment spectrum? In: Paul R (ed) Language disorders from a developmental perspective: essays in honor of Robin S. Chapman. Erlbaum, Mahwah, pp 83–101

Elsea SH, Girirajan S (2008) Smith-Magenis syndrome. Eur J Hum Genet 16(4):412–421

Fernandez LV, Goulart AL, Santos AM et al (2010) Neurodevelopmental assessment of very low birth weight preterm infants at corrected age of 18-24 months by Bayley III scales. J Pediatr (Rio J) 88(6):471–478

Fernandez RM, Pecina A, Lozano-Arana MD et al (2015) Clinical and technical overview of preimplantation genetic diagnosis for fragile X syndrome: experience at the University Hospital Virgen del Rocio in Spain. Biomed Res Int 2015:965839. https://doi.org/10.1155/2015/965839

Fiellau-Nikolajsen M (1983) Epidemiology of secretory otitis media. A descriptive cohort study. Ann Otol Rhinol Laryngol 92(2 Pt 1):172–177

Fierro-Cobas V, Chan E (2001) Language development in bilingual children: a primer for pediatricians. Contemp Pediatr 18(7):79–98

Fisch GS, Battaglia A, Parrini B et al (2008) Cognitive-behavioral features of children with Wolf-Hirschhorn syndrome: preliminary report of 12 cases. Am J Med Genet C Semin Med Genet 148C(4):252–256

Fischbach BV, Trout KL, Lewis J et al (2005) WAGR syndrome: a clinical review of 54 cases. Pediatrics 116(4):984–988

Flege JE (1995) Second language speech learning: theory, findings, and problems. In: Strange W (ed) Speech perception and linguistic experience: issues in cross-language research. York Press, Baltimore, pp 233–277

Fox-Boyer A, Dodd B (1999) Der Erwerb des phonologischen Systems in der deutschen Sprache. Sprache-Stimme-Gehör 23:183–191

Fox-Boyer A (2016) Kindliche Aussprachestörungen, 7th edn. Schulz-Kirchner Verlag, Idstein

Fox-Boyer A, Schäfer B (2015) Die phonetisch-phonologische Entwicklung von Kleinkindern. In: Sachse S (ed) Ringmann S, Siegmüller G (series eds) Handbuch Spracherwerb und Sprachentwicklungsstörungen. Bd. I Kleinkindphase. Urban & Fischer, München, Jena, pp 39–62

Friederici AD (2006) The neural basis of language. Development and its impairment. Neuron 52(6):941–952

Friedman JI, Vrijenhoek T, Markx S et al (2008) CNTNAP2 gene dosage variation is associated with schizophrenia and epilepsy. Mol Psychiatry 13(3):261–266

Fuijkschot J, Maassen B, Gorter JW et al (2009) Speech-language performance in Sjogren-Larsson syndrome. Dev Neurorehabil 12(2):106–112

Fuijkschot J, Theelen T, Seyger MM et al (2012) Sjogren-Larsson syndrome in clinical practice. J Inherit Metab Dis 35(6):955–962

Garber KB, Visootsak J, Warren ST (2008) Fragile X syndrome. Eur J Hum Genet 16(6):666–672

Gauthier C (2012) Language development in bilingual children. A research paper submitted in partial fulfillment of the requirements for the Master's Degree, Southern Illinois University, Carbondale

Genesee F (2009) Early childhood bilingualism: perils and possibilities. J Appl Res Learn 2(Special Issue):1–21

Genesee F, Nicoladis E (2006) Bilingual acquisition. In: Hoff E, Shatz M (eds) Handbook of language development. Blackwell, Oxford, pp 324–342

Genesee F, Paradis J, Crago M (2004) Dual language development and disorders: a handbook on bilingualism and second language learning. Brookes, Baltimore

Genetics Home Reference (2007) Smith-Lemli-Opitz syndrome. Available via https://ghr.nlm.nih.gov/condition/smith-lemli-opitz-syndrome. Accessed 10 Sept 2016

Genetics Home Reference (2014) Prader-Willi-syndrome. Available via https://ghr.nlm.nih.gov/condition/prader-willi-syndrome#genes. Accessed 10 Sept 2016

Genetics Home Reference (2015) Opitz G/BBB syndrome. Available via https://ghr.nlm.nih.gov/condition/opitz-g-bbb-syndrome. Accessed 10 Sept 2016

Gentner D (1981) Some interesting differences between nouns and verbs. Cogn Brain Theory 4:161–178

Gentner D (1982) Why nouns are learned before verbs: linguistic relativity versus natural positioning. In: Kuczai SA (ed) Language development, vol 2: language, thought and culture. Lawrence Erlbaum, Hillsdale, pp 301–334

Georgsdottir I, Erlingsdottir G, Hrafnkelsson B et al (2012) Disabilities and health of extremely low-birthweight teenagers: a population-based study. Acta Paediatr 101(5):518–523

Girardin CM, Lemyre E, Alos N et al (2009) Comparison of adolescents with Klinefelter syndrome according to the circumstances of diagnosis: amniocentesis versus clinical signs. Horm Res 72(2):98–105

Graham SA, Fisher SE (2015) Understanding language from a genomic perspective. Annu Rev Genet 49(1):131–160

Graham JM Jr, Schwartz CE (2013) MED12 related disorders. Am J Med Genet A 161A(11):2734–2740

Graham JM Jr, Clark RD, Moeschler JB et al (2010) Behavioral features in young adults with FG syndrome (Opitz-Kaveggia syndrome). Am J Med Genet C Semin Med Genet 154C(4):477–485

Grech H, McLeod S (2012) Multilingual speech and language development and disorders. In: Battle D (ed) Communication disorders in multicultural and international populations, 4th edn. Elsevier, St. Louis, pp 120–147

Griggs JL, Sinnayah P, Mathai ML (2015) Prader-Willi syndrome: from genetics to behaviour, with special focus on appetite treatments. Neurosci Biobehav Rev 59:155–172

Grimm H (2003) Störungen der Sprachentwicklung. Grundlagen—Ursachen—Diagnosen—Intervention—Prävention [Disorders of language development. Objectives—Causes—Diagnoses—Intervention—Prevention]. Hogrefe, Göttingen

Grimm H, Weinert S (2002) Sprachentwicklung. In: Oerter R, Montada L (eds) Entwicklungspsychologie, 5th completely revised edn. Beltz, Weinheim, p 528

Grosjean F (1982) Life with two languages. Harvard University Press, Cambridge

Grosjean F (1996) Living with two languages and two cultures. In: Parasnis I (ed) Cultural and language diversity and the deaf experience. Cambridge University Press, Cambridge

Guitar B, Conture EG (2007) The child who stutters: to the pediatrician, revised 4th edn. (Publication No. 23). Stuttering Foundation of America, Memphis

Gupta D, Nagarkar A (2009) Speech impairment in Nijmegen breakage syndrome: a rare anomaly. Int J Pediatr Otorhinolaryngol 73(6):873–875

Gutierrez-Clellen V, Simon-Cereijido G, Wagner C (2008) Bilingual children with language impairment: a comparison with monolinguals and second language learners. Appl Psycholinguist 29(1):3–20

Haesler S, Wada K, Nshdejan A et al (2004) FoxP2 expression in avian vocal learners and non-learners. J Neurosci 24(13):3164–3175

Håkansson G, Salameh EK, Nettelbladt U (2003) Measuring language development in bilingual children: Swedish-Arabic children with and without language impairment. Linguistics 41(2):255–288

Hanauer A, Young ID (2002) Coffin-Lowry syndrome: clinical and molecular features. J Med Genet 39(10):705–713

Hansson K, Sahlén B, Mäkki-Torkko E (2007) Can a 'single hit' cause limitations in language development? A comparative study of Swedish children with hearing impairment and children with specific language impairment. Int J Lang Commun Disord 42(3):307–323

Harley TA (2001) The psychology of language, 2nd edn. Psychology Press, New York

Hasselhorn M, Werner I (2000) Zur Bedeutung des phonologischen Arbeitsgedächtnisses für die Sprachentwicklung. [The meaning of the phonological working memory for the language development] [German]. In: Grimm H (ed) Enzyklopädie der Psychologie, Serie Sprache, Band 3: Sprachentwicklung. [Encyclopedia of psychologie, series language, vol 3: language development]. Hogrefe, Göttingen, pp 363–378

Hattier MA, Matson JL, Sipes M et al (2011) Communication deficits in infants and toddlers with developmental disabilities. Res Dev Disabil 32(6):2108–2113

Hayiou-Thomas ME (2008) Genetic and environmental influences on early speech, language and literacy development. J Commun Disord 41(5):397–408

Heggie AA, Vujcich NJ, Portnof JE et al (2013) Tongue reduction for macroglossia in Beckwith Wiedemann syndrome: review and application of new technique. Int J Oral Maxillofac Surg 42(2):185–191

Hennon E, Hirsh-Pasek K, Michnick Golinkoff R (2000) Die besondere Reise vom Fötus zum spracherwerbenden Kind. In: Grimm H (ed) Sprachentwicklung.

Enzyklopädie der Psychologie. Themenbereich C, Serie III, 3rd edn. Hogrefe, Göttingen, pp 41–103

Hockema SA, Smith LB (2009) Learning your language, outside-in and inside-out. Linguistics 47(2):453–479

Hollich GJ, Hirsh-Pasek K, Golinkoff RM et al (2000) Breaking the language barrier: an emergentist coalition model for the origins of word learning. Monogr Soc Res Child Dev 262:1–138

Holz NE, Boecker R, Hohm E et al (2015) The long-term impact of early life poverty on orbitofrontal cortex volume in adulthood: results from a prospective study over 25 years. Neuropsychopharmacology 40(4):996–1004. https://doi.org/10.1038/npp.2014.277. Epub 2014 Oct 15

Hong DS, Reiss AL (2014) Cognitive and neurological aspects of sex chromosome aneuploidies. Lancet Neurol 13(3):306–318

Hood RL, McGillivray G, Hunter MF et al (2016) Severe connective tissue laxity including aortic dilatation in Sotos syndrome. Am J Med Genet A 170A(2):531–535

Horwitz SM, Irwin JR, Briggs-Gowan MJ et al (2003) Language delay in a community cohort of young children. J Am Acad Child Adolesc Psychiatry 42(8):932–940

Hsu TY, Lin H, Hung HN et al (2016) Two-dimensional differential gel electrophoresis to identify protein biomarkers in amniotic fluid of Edwards Syndrome (Trisomy 18) pregnancies. PLoS One 11(1):e0145908

Huang F, Sweet R, Tewfik TL (2004) Apert syndrome and hearing loss with ear anomalies: a case report and literature review. Int J Pediatr Otorhinolaryngol 68(4):495–501

Ionasescu VV, Trofatter J, Haines JL et al (1992) X-linked recessive Charcot-Marie-Tooth neuropathy: clinical and genetic study. Muscle Nerve 15(3):368–373

Jacobs PA, Betts PR, Cockwell AE et al (1990) A cytogenetic and molecular reappraisal of a series of patients with Turner's syndrome. Ann Hum Genet 54(Pt 3):209–223

Jakobson R (1941) Kindersprache, Aphasie und allgemeine Lautgesetze. Uppsala, Almqvist & Wiksell

Jakobson R (1969) Kindersprache, Aphasie und allgemeine Lautgesetze. Suhrkamp, Frankfurt

Jasinska KK, Petitto LA (2013) How age of bilingual exposure can change the neural systems for language in the developing brain: a functional near infrared spectroscopy investigation of syntactic processing in monolingual and bilingual children. Dev Cogn Neurosci 6:87–101

Jerome LA, Papaioannou VE (2001) DiGeorge syndrome phenotype in mice mutant for the T-box gene, Tbx1. Nat Genet 27(3):286–291

Jordaan H, Yelland A (2003) Intervention with multilingual language impaired children by South African speech-language therapists. J Multiling Commun Disord 1(1):13–33

Jose-Ramon CF, Lizett CC, Daniel TL et al (2015) A systematic review of the oral and craniofacial manifestations of cri du chat syndrome. Clin Anat 9(5):555–560

Jusczyk PW, Aslin RN (1995) Infants' detection of the sound patterns of words in fluent speech. Cogn Psychol 29(1):1–23

Kajimoto M, Ichiyama T, Akashi A et al (2007) West syndrome associated with mosaic Down syndrome. Brain Dev 29(7):447–449

Kany W, Schöler H (2007) Fokus: Sprachdiagnostik. Leitfaden zur Sprachstandsbestimmung im Kindergarten. [Focus: language diagnostics. Guidelines for language assessment in kindergarten]. Cornelsen Scriptor, Mannheim

Kauschke C (1999) Der Erwerb des frühkindlichen Lexikons—eine empirische Studie zur Entwicklung des Wortschatzes im Deutschen. Narr, Tübingen

Kauschke C (2003) Sprachtherapie bei Kindern zwischen 2 und 4 Jahren—ein Überblick über Ansätze und Methoden. [Language therapy of children between 2 and 4 years of age—an overview about approaches and methods] In: de Langen-Müller U, et al (eds) Früh genug, zu früh, zu spät? Modelle und Methoden zur Diagnostik und Therapie sprachlicher Entwicklungsstörungen von 0 bis 4 Jahren [Early enough, too early, too late? Models and methods for diagnostics and therapy of developmental language disorders between 0 and 4 years of age]. Prolog, Cologne, pp 152–183

Kauschke C (2006) Late talker. In: Siegmüller J, Bartels H (eds) Leitfaden. Sprache—Sprechen—Stimme—Schlucken. Urban & Fischer, Munich, pp 65–68

Kauschke C, Hofmeister C (2002) Early lexical development in German: a study on vocabulary growth and vocabulary composition during the second and third year of life. J Child Lang 29(4):735–757

Kay-Raining Bird E, Cleave P, Trudeau N et al (2005) The language abilities of bilingual children with Down Syndrome. Am J Speech Lang Pathol 14(3):187–199

Keilmann A (2009) Sehstörungen und visuelle Wahrnehmungsstörungen. In: Keilmann A et al (eds) Sprachentwicklungsstörungen. Huber, Bern, pp 127–129

Keilmann A, Braun L, Schöler H (2005) Welche Rolle spielt das Merkmal Intelligenz bei der Diagnostik und Differenzierung sprachentwicklungsgestörter Kinder? [Diagnosis and differentiation of children with language development disorders. What role can be attributed to intelligence?] [German]. HNO 53(3):268–284

Keilmann A, Kluesener P, Freude C et al (2011) Manifestation of speech and language disorders in children with hearing impairment compared with children with specific language disorders. Logoped Phoniatr Vocol 36(1):12–20

Kiese-Himmel C (2003) Characteristics of children with permanent mild hearing impairment. Folia Phoniatr Logop 55(2):70–79

Kiese-Himmel C (2008) Entwicklung sprach- und kommunikationsgestörter Kinder, am Beispiel von "Late Talkers" und Kindern mit spezifischen Sprachentwicklungsstörungen. [Development of children with language and communication disorders as shown for late talkers and children with specific developmental disorders of speech and language] In: Hasselhorn M, Silbereisen RK (eds) Entwicklungspsychologie des Säuglings- und Kindesalters. 4. Ausgabe. Enzyklopädie der Psychologie. Themenbereich C: Theorie und Forschung. Serie V: Entwicklungspsychologie. [Developmental psychology of infancy and childhood, 4th edn. Encyclopedia of psychology. Subject area C: theory and research. Series V: developmental psychology]. Hogrefe, Göttingen, pp 693–730

Klein-Tasman BP, Janke KM, Luo W et al (2014) Cognitive and psychosocial phenotype of young children with neurofibromatosis-1. J Int Neuropsychol Soc 20(1):88–98

Kobrynski LJ, Sullivan KE (2007) Velocardiofacial syndrome, DiGeorge syndrome: the chromosome 22q11.2 deletion syndromes. Lancet 370(9596):1443–1452

Kohnert K (2004) Processing skills in early sequential bilinguals. In: Goldstein B (ed) Bilingual language development and disorders in Spanish-English speakers. Brookes, Baltimore, pp 53–76

Kohnert K (2008) Language disorders in bilingual children and adults. Plural, San Diego

Kohnert K (2010) Bilingual children with primary language impairment: issues, evidence and implications for clinical actions. J Commun Disord 43(6):456–473

Koul M, Dwivedi R, Upadhyay V (2014) Ectrodactyly-ectodermal dysplasia clefting syndrome (EEC syndrome). J Oral Biol Craniofac Res 4(2):135–139

Kowal S, O'Connell DC, Sabin EJ (1975) Development of temporal patterning and vocal hesitations in spontaneous narratives. J Psycholinguist Res 4(3):195–207

Kozutin A (1984) Thought and language, revised edition. The MIT, Cambridge

Kuhl PK, Meltzoff AN (1996) Infant vocalizations in response to speech: vocal imitation and developmental change. J Acoust Soc Am 100(4 Pt 1):2425–2438

Kühn P, von Suchodoletz W (2009) Ist ein verzögerter Sprechbeginn ein Risiko für Sprachstörungen im Einschulungsalter? [Is a delayed speech onset a risk for a language disorder at school entry age?]. Kinderarztl Prax 80(5):343–348

Kwasnicka-Crawford DA, Carson AR, Roberts W et al (2005) Characterization of a novel cation transporter ATPase gene (ATP13A4) interrupted by 3q25-q29 inversion in an individual with language delay. Genomics 86(2):182–194

Kwon SH, Scheinost D, Vohr B et al (2016) Functional magnetic resonance connectivity studies in infants born preterm: suggestions of proximate and long-lasting changes in language organization. Dev Med Child Neurol 58(4):28–34

La Paro KM, Justice L, Skibbe LE et al (2004) Relations among maternal, child, and demographic factors and the persistence of preschool language impairment. Am J Speech Lang Pathol 13(4):291–303

Lahey M, Edwards J (1995) Specific language impairment: preliminary investigation of factors associated with family history and with pattern of language performance. J Speech Lang Hear Res 38(3):643–657

Lai CS, Fisher SE, Hurst JA et al (2000) The SPCH1 region on human 7q31: genomic characterization of the critical interval and localization of translocations associated with speech and language disorder. Am J Hum Genet 67(2):357–368

Lai CS, Fisher SE, Hurst JA et al (2001) A forkhead-domain gene is mutated in a severe speech and language disorder. Nature 413(6855):519–523

Lalani SR, Hefner MA, Belmont JW et al (1993) CHARGE syndrome. In: Pagon RA et al (eds) GeneReviews(R). University of Washington, Seattle

Langen EG (2006) Geistige Behinderung. In: Siegmüller J, Bartels H (eds) Sprache—Sprechen—Stimme—Schlucken. Urban & Fischer, München, Jena, pp 170–214

Laucht M, Esser G, Schmidt MH et al (1992) "Risikokinder": Zur Bedeutung biologischer und psychosozialer Risiken für die kindliche Entwicklung in den beiden ersten Lebensjahren "Risk children": the importance of biological and psychosocial risks for child development in the first two years of life. Prax Kinderpsychol Kinderpsychiatr 41(8):274–285

Laucht M, Esser G, Schmidt MH (1997) Developmental outcome of infants with biological and psychosocial risks. J Child Psychol Psychiatry 38(7):843–853

Law J, Boyle J, Harris F et al (2000) Prevalence and natural history of primary speech and language delay: findings from a systematic review of the literature. Int J Lang Commun Disord 35(2):165–188

Lee M, Won J, Lee S et al (2015) Benefits of physical exercise for individuals with Fragile X Syndrome in humans. J Lifestyle Med 5(2):35–38

Lenneberg EH (1967) Biological foundations of language. Wiley, New York

Leonard LB (1987) Is specific language impairment a useful construct? In: Rosenberg S (ed) Advances in applied psycholinguistics (1): disorders of first-language development. Cambridge University Press, Cambridge, pp 1–39

Leonard LB (2000) Specific language impairment across languages. In: Bishop DVM, Leonard LB (eds) Speech and language impairments in children: causes, characteristics, intervention, and outcome. Taylor & Francis, Philadelphia, pp 115–129

Lewis BA, Thompson LA (1992) A study of developmental speech and language disorders in twins. J Speech Hear Res 35(5):1086–1094

Lewis BA, Cox NJ, Byard PJ (1993) Segregation analysis of speech and language disorders. Behav Genet 23(3):291–297

Li H, Yamagata T, Mori M et al (2005) Absence of causative mutations and presence of autism-related allele in FOXP2 in Japanese autistic patients. Brain Dev 27(3):207–210

Li H, Liu T, Chen X et al (2015) A rare case of primary congenital glaucoma in combination with neurofibromatosis 1: a case report. BMC Ophthalmol 15:149

Lian WB, Ho SK (2012) Profile of children diagnosed with autistic spectrum disorder managed at a tertiary child development unit. Singap Med J 53(12):794–800

Lieu JE (2013) Unilateral hearing loss in children: speech-language and school performance. B-ENT (Suppl 21):107–115

Linden MG, Bender BG, Robinson A (1995) Sex chromosome tetrasomy and pentasomy. Pediatrics 96(4 Pt 1):672–682

Liu J, Krantz ID (2009) Cornelia de Lange syndrome, cohesin, and beyond. Clin Genet 76(4):303–314

Lu T, Chen R, Cox TC et al (2013) X-linked microtubule-associated protein, Mid1, regulates axon development. Proc Natl Acad Sci U S A 110(47):19131–19136

Luciano M, Evans DM, Hansell NK et al (2013) A genome-wide association study for reading and language abilities in two population cohorts. Genes Brain Behav 12(6):645–652

Lumaka A, Lukoo R, Mubungu G et al (2016) Williams-Beuren syndrome: pitfalls for diagnosis in limited resources setting. Clin Case Rep 4(3):294–297

Marino BS, Lipkin PH, Newburger JW et al (2012) Neurodevelopmental outcomes in children with congenital heart disease: evaluation and management: a scientific statement from the American Heart Association. Circulation 126(9):1143–1172

Martens MA, Wilson SJ, Reutens DC (2008) Research Review: Williams syndrome: a critical review of the cognitive, behavioral, and neuroanatomical phenotype. J Child Psychol Psychiatry 49(6):576–608

Martire B, Panza R, Pillon M et al (2016) CHARGE Syndrome and Common Variable Immunodeficiency: a case report and review of literature. Pediatr Allergy Immunol 27(5):546–550

Matthews A (1996) Linguistic development. Avaliable via https://aabs.files.wordpress.com/2007/03/childlinguisticdevelopment.pdf. Accessed 20 Oct 2017

Maulik PK, Harbour CK (2010) Epidemiology of intellectual disability. In: Stone JH, Blouin M (eds) International encyclopedia of rehabilitation. Available via http://cirrie.buffalo.edu/encyclopedia/en/article/144/. Accessed 4 May 2014

Mazzocco MM (2006) The cognitive phenotype of Turner syndrome: specific learning disabilities. Int Congr Ser 1298:83–92

McDonald-McGinn DM, Emanuel BS, Zackai EH et al (1993) 22q11.2 deletion syndrome. In: Pagon RA, Adam MP, Ardinger HH (eds) GeneReviews(R). University of Washington, Seattle

McDuffie A, Kover ST, Abbeduto L et al (2012) Profiles of Receptive and expressive language abilities in males with comorbid fragile X syndrome and autism. Am J Intellect Dev Disabil 117(1):18–32

McLennan Y, Polussa J, Tassone F et al (2011) Fragile X syndrome. Curr Genomics 12(3):216–224

Megarbane A, Noguier F, Stora S et al (2013) The intellectual disability of trisomy 21: differences in gene expression in a case series of patients with lower and higher IQ. Eur J Hum Genet 21(11):1253–1259

Meibauer J (1999) Über Nomen-Verb-Beziehungen im frühen Wortbildungserwerb. In: Meibauer J, Rothweiler M (eds) Das Lexikon im Spracherwerb. Francke, Tübingen, pp 184–207

Meisel J (2004) The bilingual child. In: Bhatia T, Ritchie W (eds) The handbook of bilingualism. Blackwell Publishing Ltd, Oxford, pp 91–113

Menyuk P, Liebergott JW, Schultz MC (1995) Early language development in fullterm and premature infants. Lawrence Erlbaum, Hillsdale

Milewska-Bobula B, Zebrowska J, Olszaniecka M et al (2010) Evaluation of intellectual development of children following congenital, mildly symptomatic cytomegalovirus (CMV) infection. A prospective study. Med Wieku Rozwoj 14(4):370–373

Milunsky JM (1993) Waardenburg syndrome type I. In: Pagon RA et al (eds) GeneReviews(R). University of Washington, Seattle

Mlynarski EE, Xie M, Taylor D et al (2016) Rare copy number variants and congenital heart defects in the 22q11.2 deletion syndrome. Hum Genet 135(3):273–285

Moeller MP (2000) Early intervention and language development in children who are deaf and hard of hearing. Pediatrics 106(3):E43

Mohan B, Mittal CM (2011) Supravalvular aortic stenosis in William's syndrome. Ann Pediatr Cardiol 4(2):213–214

Möller S, Schönweiler R (1999) Analysis of infant cries for the early detection of hearing impairment. Speech Comm 28(3):175–193

Monaco AP (2007) Multivariate linkage analysis of specific language impairment (SLI). Ann Hum Genet 71(Pt 5):660–673

Moon C, Lagercrantz H, Kuhl PK (2013) Language experienced in utero affects vowel perception after birth: a two-country study. Acta Paediatr 102(2):156–160

Moore C, Dunham P (1995) Joint attention: its origins and role in development. Lawrence Erlbaum Associates, Mahwah

Myers KA, Scheffer IE (1993) GRIN2A-related speech disorders and epilepsy. In: Pagon RA et al (eds) GeneReviews(R). University of Washington, Seattle. NBK385627

Nathani E, Ertmer DJ, Stark RE (2006) Assessing vocal development in infants and toddlers. Clin Linguist Phon 20(5):351–369

National Institute on Deafness and Other Communication Disorders (2008) Statistics on voice, speech, and language. Available via http://www.nidcd.nih.gov/health/statistics/vsl.asp#2. Accessed 17 July 2016

National Organization for Rare Disorders (NORD) (2015) Rett syndrome. Available via http://rarediseases.org/rare-diseases/rett-syndrome/. Accessed 10 Sept 2016

Nazzi T, Bertoncini J, Mehler J (1998) Language discrimination by newborns: toward an understanding of the role of rhythm. J Exp Psychol Hum Percept Perform 24(3):756–766

Neiman ES, Seyffert M (2016) Acquired epileptic aphasia. Available via http://emedicine.medscape.com/article/1176568-overview. Accessed 7 Aug 2016

602

Nelson K (1973) Structure and strategy in learning to talk. Monogr Soc Res Child Dev 149(38):1–2

Nelson K, Hampson J, Shaw LK (1993) Nouns in early lexicons: evidence, explanations and implications. J Child Lang 20(1):61–84

Neul JL, Kaufmann WE, Glaze DG et al (2010) Rett syndrome: revised diagnostic criteria and nomenclature. Ann Neurol 68(6):944–950

Neumann K, Euler HA (2013) Kann ein Sprachstandsscreening zwischen Sprachförder- und Sprachtherapiebedarf trennen? [Is a language screening for children suited to distinguish between the necessity for treatment or education?]. In: Redder A, Weinert S (eds) Sprachförderung und Sprachdiagnostik—interdisziplinäre Perspektiven [Language training and language diagnostics—interdisciplinary perspective]. Waxmann, Münster

Neumann K, Keilmann A, Rosenfeld J et al (2009) Leitlinien der Deutschen Gesellschaft für Phoniatrie und Pädaudiologie zu Sprachentwicklungsstörungen bei Kindern (gekürzte Fassung). [Guidelines of the German Society of Phoniatrics and Pediatric Audiology on developmental speech and language disorders of children] [German]. Kindh Entwickl 18(4):222–231

Neumann K, Euler HA, Bosshardt HG et al (2016) (Hrsg.: Deutsche Gesellschaft für Phoniatrie und Pädaudiologie). Pathogenese, Diagnostik und Behandlung von Redeflussstörungen. Evidenz- und konsensbasierte S3-Leitlinie, AWMF-Registernummer 049-013, Version 1. Available via http://www.awmf.org/leitlinien/detail/ll/049-013.html. Accessed 1 Sept 2016

Newbury DF, Bonora E, Lamb JA et al (2002) FOXP2 is not a major susceptibility gene for autism or specific language impairment. Am J Hum Genet 70(5):60–71

Newbury DF, Winchester L, Addis L et al (2009) CMIP and ATP2C2 modulate phonological short-term memory in language impairment. Am J Hum Genet 85(2):264–272

Newbury DF, Paracchini S, Scerri TS et al (2011) Investigation of dyslexia and SLI risk variants in reading- and language-impaired subjects. Behav Genet 41(1):90–104

Nguyen JM, Qualmann KJ, Okashah R et al (2015) 5p deletions: current knowledge and future directions. Am J Med Genet C Semin Med Genet 169(3):224–238

Nickisch A (1988) Motorische Leistungen bei Kindern mit verzögerter Sprachentwicklung. Folia Phoniatr (Basel) 40:147–152

Nielsen J, Wohlert M (1991) Chromosome abnormalities found among 34,910 newborn children: results from a 13-year incidence study in Arhus, Denmark. Hum Genet 87(1):81–83

Nikitina EA, Medvedeva AV, Zakharov GA et al (2014) Williams syndrome as a model for elucidation of the pathway genes—the brain—cognitive functions: genetics and epigenetics. Acta Nat 6(1):9–22

Northern JL, Downs MP (2002) Hearing in children, 5th edn. Lippincott Williams & Wilkins, Baltimore, Philadelphia, pp 127–206

Noterdaeme M, Schnöbel E, Amorosa H (1999) Neuromotorische Auffälligkeiten bei sprachentwicklungsgestörten Kindern. [Neuromotor abnormalities in children with developmental language disorder] [German]. Sprache-Stimme-Gehör 23: 155–158

Nowaczyk MJM (1993) Smith-Lemli-Opitz syndrome. In: Pagon RA et al (eds) GeneReviews(R). University of Washington, Seattle

Nowaczyk MJ, Irons MB (2012) Smith-Lemli-Opitz syndrome: phenotype, natural history, and epidemiology. Am J Med Genet C Semin Med Genet 160C(4):250–262

Oller DK (1980) The emergence of sound of speech in infancy. In: Yeni-Komshian GH, Kavanagh JK et al (eds) Phonology, vol 1: production. Lawrence Erlbaum, New York, pp 93–112

Oller DK, Eilers RE, Neal AR et al (1999) Precursors to speech in infancy: the prediction of speech and language disorders. J Commun Disord 32(4):223–247

Otter M, Schrander-Stumpel CT, Didden R et al (2012) The psychiatric phenotype in triple X syndrome: new hypotheses illustrated in two cases. Dev Neurorehabil 15(3):233–238

Paradis J (2005) Grammatical morphology in children learning English as a second language: implications of similarities with specific language impairment. Lang Speech Hear Serv Sch 36(3):172–187

Paradis J (2010) The interface between bilingual development and specific language impairment. Appl Psycholinguist 31(2):227–252

Paradis J, Crago M, Genesee F et al (2003) French-English bilingual children with SLI: how do they compare with their monolingual peers? J Speech Lang Hear Res 46(1):113–127

Paradis J, Genesee F, Crago M (2011) Dual language development and disorders: a handbook on bilingualism & second language learning. Paul H. Brookes Publishing, Baltimore

Paradowska-Stolarz AM (2014) Wolf-Hirschhorn syndrome (WHS)—literature review on the features of the syndrome. Adv Clin Exp Med 23(3):485–489

Parisi L, Di Filippo T, Roccella M (2015) Behavioral phenotype and autism spectrum disorders in Cornelia de Lange Syndrome. Ment Illn 7(2):5988. https://doi.org/10.4081/mi.2015.5988

Patil S, Rao RS, Majumdar B (2014) Chromosomal and multifactorial genetic disorders with oral manifestations. J Int Oral Health 6(5):118–125

Paul R, Roth FP (2011) Characterizing and predicting outcomes of communication delays in infants and toddlers: implications for clinical practice. Lang Speech Hear Serv Sch 42(3):331–340

Pearl PL, Carrazana EJ, Holmes GL (2001) The Landau-Kleffner syndrome. Epilepsy Curr 1(2):39–45

Pellowski MW, Conture EG (2002) Characteristics of speech disfluency and stuttering behaviors in 3- and 4-year-old children. J Speech Lang Hear Res 45(1):20–34

Pena E, Bedore L (2009) Bilingualism in child language disorders. In: Schwartz RG (ed) Handbook of child language disorders. Psychology Press, New York, pp 281–307

Peprah E (2012) Fragile X syndrome: the FMR1 CGG repeat distribution among world populations. Ann Hum Genet 76(2):178–191

Pereira PM, Schneider A, Pannetier S et al (2010) Coffin-Lowry syndrome. Eur J Hum Genet 18(6):627–633

Perez-Pereira M, Conti-Ramsden G (1999) Language development and social interaction in blind children. Psychology Press, East Sussex

Peters SU, Kaufmann WE, Bacino CA et al (2011) Alterations in white matter pathways in Angelman syndrome. Dev Med Child Neurol 53(4):361–367

Petersen J, Marinova-Todd SH, Mirenda P (2011) An exploratory study of lexical skills in bilingual children with Autism Spectrum Disorder. J Autism Dev Disord 42(7):1499–1503. https://doi.org/10.1007/s10803-011-1366-y

Piaget J (1963) The origin of intelligence in the child. Norton, New York

Pinker S (1984) Language learnability and language development. Harvard University Press, Cambridge

Pinker S (1991) The rules of language. Science 253(5019):530–535

Pinker S (1994) The language instinct: the new science of language and mind. Penguin Books, London

Plomp RG, van Lieshout MJ, Joosten KF et al (2016) Treacher Collins Syndrome: a systematic review of evidence-based treatment and recommendations. Plast Reconstr Surg 137(1):191–204

Pober BR (2010) Williams-Beuren syndrome. N Engl J Med 362(3):239–252

Poll GH (2011) Increasing the odds: applying emergentist theory in language intervention. Lang Speech Hear Serv Sch 42(4):580–591

Pomnitz P, Rupp S (2013) Lexikonentwicklung. In: Ringmann S, Siegmüller J (eds) Handbuch Spracherwerb und Sprachentwicklungsstörungen. Schuleingangsphase. Elsevier, Munich, p 25

Poulin-Dubois D, Blaye A, Coutya J et al (2011) The effects of bilingualism on toddlers' executive functioning. J Exp Child Psychol 108(3):567–579

Powell RP, Bishop DVM (1992) Clumsiness and perceptual problems in children with specific language impairment. Dev Med Child Neurol 34(9):755–765

Prader-Willi Syndrome Association (2016) About Prader-Willi syndrome. Available via http://www.pwsausa.org/about-pws/. Accessed 7 Aug 2016

Ptok M, Morlot S (2009) Sprachentwicklungsstörung bei Mosaik-Trisomie 8. Language development impairment and trisomy 8 mosaicism. HNO 57(7):685–689

Reilly S, Wake M, Bavin EL et al (2007) Predicting language at 2 years of age. A prospective community study. Pediatrics 120(6):1441–1449

Reilly S, Wake M, Ukoumunne OC et al (2010) Predicting language outcomes at 4 years of age: findings from Early Language in Victoria Study. Pediatrics 126(6):e1530–e1537

Rescorla L (1989) The language development survey: a screening tool for delayed language in toddlers. J Speech Hear Disord 54(4):587–599

Rescorla L, Achenbach TM (2002) Use of the language development survey (LDS) in a national probability sample of children 18 to 35 months old. J Speech Lang Hear Res 45(4):733–743

Riccardi VM (1977) Trisomy 8: an international study of 70 patients. Birth Defects Orig Artic Ser 13(3C):171–184

Rice ML, Taylor CL, Zubrick SR (2008) Language outcomes of 7-year-old children with or without a history of late language emergence at 24 months. J Speech Lang Hear Res 51(2):394–407

Rice ML, Smith SD, Gayan J (2009) Convergent genetic linkage and associations to language, speech and reading measures in families of probands with Specific Language Impairment. J Neurodev Disord 1(4):264–282

Roberts JE, Rosenfeld RM, Zeisel SA (2004) Otitis media and speech and language: a meta-analysis of prospective studies. Pediatrics 113(3 Pt 1):238–248

Rogers RC, Abidi FE (1993) Coffin-Lowry syndrome. In: Pagon RA et al (eds) GeneReviews(R). University of Washington, Seattle

Rothweiler M, Kauschke C (2007) Lexikalischer Erwerb. In: Schöler H, Welling A (eds) Sonderpädagogik der Sprache. Handbuch Sonderpädagogik. Hogrefe Verlag, Göttingen, pp 42–57

Rothweiler M, Meibauer J (1999) Das Lexikon im Spracherwerb: ein Überblick. In: Meibauer J, Rothweiler M (eds) Das Lexikon im Spracherwerb. UTB Francke, Tübingen, pp 9–31

Ruben RJ (1997) A time frame of critical/sensitive periods of language development. Acta Otolaryngol (Stockh) 117(2):202–205

Rupp S (2013) Semantisch-lexikalische Störungen bei Kindern, Praxiswissen Logopädie. Springer, Berlin, Heidelberg. https://doi.org/10.1007/978-3-642-38019-8_2

Sachdeva R, Donkers SJ, Kim SY (2015) Angelman Syndrome: a review highlighting musculoskeletal and anatomical aberrations. Clin Anat 29(5):561–567

Sachse S, von Suchodoletz W (2009) Prognose und Möglichkeiten der Vorhersage der Sprachentwicklung bei Late Talkers [Prognosis and options for the language development of late talkers]. Kinderarztl Prax 80(5):318–328

Sachse S, von Suchodoletz W (2013) Sprachverständnis bei Late Talkers. HNO 61(11):937–943

Saenz T, Huer M (2003) Testing strategies involving least biased language assessment of bilingual children. Commun Disord Q 24(4):184–193

Sandrieser P, Schneider P (2015) Stottern im Kindesalter, 4th edn. Thieme, Stuttgart

Santoro MR, Bray SM, Warren ST (2012) Molecular mechanisms of fragile X syndrome: a twenty-year perspective. Annu Rev Pathol 7:219–245

Saul RA, Tarleton JC (1993) FMR1-related disorders. In: Pagon RA et al (eds) GeneReviews(R). University of Washington, Seattle

Schöler H, Welling A, Borchert J et al (2007) Sonderpädagogik der Sprache. Hogrefe Verlag, Göttingen

Schönweiler R (1992) Eine Untersuchung an 1300 Kindern zur Inzidenz und Therapie von Hörstörungen bei kindlichen Sprachstörungen [Examination of 1,300 children for incidence and therapy of hearing disorders in pediatric speech disorders] [German]. Laryngorhinootologie 71(12):637–643

Schönweiler R (1994) Synoptische Betrachtung der Ergebnisse an 1300 sprachentwicklungsverzögerten Kindern aus ätiopathogenetischer, audiologischer und sprachpathologischer Sicht [Synopsis of results with 1,300 children with language developmental delay from the etiopathogenetic, audiologic and speech pathology viewpoint] [German]. Folia Phoniatr Logop 46(1):18–26

Schorr U (1992) Störungen der Redefähigkeit. In: Grohnfeldt M (ed) Handbuch der Sprachtherapie, vol 5. Marhold, Berlin

Schoubben E, Decaestecker K, Quaegebeur K et al (2011) Tetrasomy and pentasomy of the X chromosome. Eur J Pediatr 170(10):1325–1327

Schwartz RH, Shipon-Blum EDO (2005) "Shy" child? Don't overlook selective mutism. Contemp Pediatr 22(7):30–39

Schwartz CE, Tarpey PS, Lubs HA et al (2007) The original Lujan syndrome family has a novel missense mutation (p.N1007S) in the MED12 gene. J Med Genet 44(7):472–477

Shaikh TH, Kurahashi H, Saitta SC et al (2000) Chromosome 22-specific low copy repeats and the 22q11.2 deletion syndrome: genomic organization and deletion endpoint analysis. Hum Mol Genet 9(4):489–501

Sharland M, Burch M, McKenna WM et al (1992) A clinical study of Noonan syndrome. Arch Dis Child 67(2):178–183

Sheth K, Moss J, Hyland S et al (2015) The behavioral characteristics of Sotos syndrome. Am J Med Genet A 167A(12):2945–2956

Shetti AN, Dhulkhed VK, Gujrathi AD et al (2015) Anesthetic management of a patient with Wilms tumor, aniridia, genital anomalies and mental retardation syndrome undergoing right nephrectomy. J Anaesthesiol Clin Pharmacol 31(2):280–281

Shevell MI, Majnemer A, Rosenbaum P et al (2015) Profile of referrals for early childhood developmental delay to ambulatory subspecialty clinics. J Child Neurol 16(9):645–650

Shipster C, Hearst D, Dockrell JE et al (2002) Speech and language skills and cognitive functioning in children with Apert syndrome: a pilot study. Int J Lang Commun Disord 37(3):325–343

Shriberg LD, Tomblin JB, McSweeny JL (1999) Prevalence of speech delay in 6-year-old children and comorbidity with language impairment. J Speech Lang Hear Res 42(6):1461–1481

Shu W, Lu MM, Zhang Y et al (2007) Foxp2 and Foxp1 cooperatively regulate lung and esophagus development. Development 134(10):1991–2000

Siskind C, Feely SM, Bernes S et al (2009) Persistent CNS dysfunction in a boy with CMT1X. J Neurol Sci 279(1–2):109–113

Skinner BF (1957) Verbal behavior. Appleton-Century-Crofts, New York

SLI Consortium (2002) A genomewide scan identifies two novel loci involved in specific language impairment. Am J Hum Genet 70(2):384–398

SLI Consortium (2004) Highly significant linkage to the SLI1 locus in an expanded sample of individuals affected by specific language impairment. Am J Hum Genet 74(6):1225–1238

Slobin DI (1971) Psycholinguistics. Scott Foresman, Glenview

Spagnoli C, Kugathasan U, Brittain H et al (2015) Epileptic spasms and early-onset photosensitive epilepsy in Patau syndrome: an EEG study. Brain Dev 37(7):704–713

Spinner NB, Leonard LD, Krantz ID (1993) Alagille syndrome. In: Pagon RA et al (eds) GeneReviews(R). University of Washington, Seattle

St. Pourcain B, Cents RA, Whitehouse AJ et al (2014) Common variation near ROBO2 is associated with expressive vocabulary in infancy. Nat Commun 5:4831

Stanton-Chapman TL, Chapman DA, Bainbridge NL et al (2002) Identification of early risk factors for language impairment. Res Dev Disabil 23(6):390–405

Stark RE (ed) (1980) Stages of speech development in the first year of life, vol 1: production. Academic, New York

Storkel HL, Morrisette ML (2002) The lexicon and phonology: interactions in language acquisition. Lang Speech Hear Serv Sch 33(1):24–37

Stromswold K (1998) Genetics of spoken language disorders. Hum Biol 70(2):297–324

Stromswold K (2001) The heritability of language: a review and metaanalysis of twin, adoption, and linkage studies. Language 77(4):647–722

Szagun G (2007) Das Wunder des Spracherwerbs. So lernt ihr Kind sprechen. Beltz Verlag, Weinheim, Basel

Szagun G (2013) Sprachentwicklung beim Kind, 5th edn. Beltz Verlag, Weinheim, Basel

Tabors P (1997) One child, two languages. Paul H Brookes Publishing, Baltimore

Tager-Flusberg H, Cooper J (1999) Present and future possibilities for defining a phenotype for specific language impairment. J Speech Lang Hear Res 42(5):1275–1278

Tallal P (1980) Auditory processing disorders in children. In: Levinson P, Sloan C (eds) Auditory processing and language. Clinical and research perspectives. Grune & Stratton, New York, pp 81–100

Tallal P, Hirsch LS, Realpe-Bonilla T et al (2001) Familial aggregation in specific language impairment. J Speech Lang Hear Res 44(5):1172–1182

Tanteles GA, Nicolaou M, Patsia N et al (2015) A rare cause of pruritic ichthyosis: Sjogren-Larsson syndrome in the first reported patients of Cypriot descent. Eur J Dermatol 25(5):495–496

Tartaglia M, Zampino G, Gelb BD (2010a) Noonan syndrome: clinical aspects and molecular pathogenesis. Mol Syndromol 1(1):2–26

Tartaglia NR, Howell S, Sutherland A et al (2010b) A review of trisomy X (47,XXX). Orphanet J Rare Dis 5:8

Temple CM, Shephard EE (2012) Exceptional lexical skills but executive language deficits in school starters and young adults with Turners syndrome: implications for X chromosome effects on brain function. Brain Lang 120(3):345–359

Tezcan B, Rich P, Bhide A (2015) Prenatal diagnosis of WAGR syndrome. Case Rep Obstet Gynecol 2015:928585. https://doi.org/10.1155/2015/928585

Thomson C, Polnay L (2002) Community paediatrics, 3rd edn. Elsevier, Edinburgh

Tomblin JB (1989) Familial concentration of developmental language impairment. J Speech Hear Disord 54(2):287–295

Tomblin JB, Buckwalter PR (1998) Heritability of poor language achievement among twins. J Speech Lang Hear Res 41(1):188–199

Tomblin JB, Records NL, Buckwalter P et al (1997) Prevalence of specific language impairment in kindergarten children. J Speech Lang Hear Res 40(6):1245–1260

Trainor PA, Dixon J, Dixon MJ (2009) Treacher Collins syndrome: etiology, pathogenesis and prevention. Eur J Hum Genet 17(3):275–283

Tunmer WE, Bowey J (1984) Metalinguistic awareness and reading acquisition. In: Tunmer WE et al (eds) Metalinguistic awareness in children: theory, research and implications. Springer, Berlin, pp 144–168

UEP Commission Speech and Language (1987) UEP-report. Annu Bull UEP 5:37–44

US Department of Education, Office of Special Education Programs (OSEP), State Education Agencies (SEAs) (2008) Report of children with disabilities for ages 6 through 21 EDFacts reporting system by age and disability for SY 2006-2007 (OSEP006C). Available via http://s3.amazonaws.com/zanran_storage/www.opi.mt.gov/ContentPages/50933027.pdf. Accessed 17 July 2016

Uzun H, Senses DA, Uluba M et al (2008) A newborn with Cornelia de Lange syndrome: a case report. Cases J 1(1):329

Van Assche E, Bonduelle M, Tournaye H et al (1996) Cytogenetics of infertile men. Hum Reprod 11(Suppl 4):1–24; discussion 25–26

Van der Burgt I (2007) Noonan syndrome. Orphanet J Rare Dis 2:4

Van Kleek A (1982) The emergence of linguistic awareness: a cognitive framework. Merrill-Palmer Q 28(2):237–266

Van Lierde KM, Van Cauwenberge P, Stevens I et al (2004) Language, articulation, voice and resonance characteristics in 4 children with Goldenhar syndrome: a pilot study. Folia Phoniatr Logop 56(3):131–143

Vernes SC, Newbury DF, Abrahams BS et al (2008) A functional genetic link between distinct developmental language disorders. N Engl J Med 359(22):2337–2345

Villanueva P, Nudel R, Hoischen A et al (2015) Correction: exome sequencing in an admixed isolated population indicates NFXL1 variants confer a risk for specific language impairment. PLoS Genet 11(6): e1005336

Weinrich M, Zehner H (2003) Phonetische und phonologische Störungen bei Kindern. Springer, Berlin, Heidelberg

Weismer ES (2007) Typical talkers, late talkers, and children with specific language impairment: a language endowment spectrum? In: Paul R (ed) The influence of developmental perspectives on research and practice in communication disorders: a Festschrift for Robin S. Chapman. Erlbaum, Mahwah, pp 83–102

Weiten W (2010) Psychology: themes and variations. Wadsworth Cengage, Learning

Wendlandt W (2011) Sprachstörungen im Kindesalter, 6th edn. G. Thieme, Stuttgart

Werker JF, Tees RC (1999) Influences on infant speech processing: toward a new synthesis. Annu Rev Psychol 50:509–535

Wester U, Bondeson ML, Edeby C et al (2006) Clinical and molecular characterization of individuals with 18p deletion: a genotype-phenotype correlation. Am J Med Genet A 140A(11):1164–1171

Wiley S, Arjmand E, Meinzen-Derr JK et al (2011) Findings from multidisciplinary evaluation of children with permanent hearing loss. Int J Pediatr Otorhinolaryngol 75(8):1040–1044

Wilson BJ, Sundaram SK, Huq AH et al (2011) Abnormal language pathway in children with Angelman syndrome. Pediatr Neurol 44(5):350–356

World Health Organization (2010/2011) International statistical classification of diseases and related health problems, 10th Revision. Available via http://www.who.int/classifications/icd/en/. Accessed 26 Apr 2014

World Health Organization (2016) International statistical classification of diseases and related health problems, 10th Revision (ICD-10)-WHO, Version for 2016. Available via http://apps.who.int/classifications/icd10/browse/2016/en. Accessed 10 Sept 2016

Wyper KR, Rasmussen CR (2011) Language impairments in children with fetal alcohol spectrum disorders. J Popul Ther Clin Pharmacol 18(2):e364–e376

Yairi E (1981) Disfluencies of normally speaking two-year-old children. J Speech Lang Hear Res 24(4):490–495

Yairi E, Ambrose NG (2005) Early childhood stuttering for clinicians by clinicians. Pro-Ed, Austin

Yavas M (1998) Phonology: development and disorders. Singular, San Diego

Zehler A, Fleischman H, Hopstock P et al (2003) Policy report: summary of findings related to LEP and SPED-LEP students (Report submitted to USDE, OELA). Development Associates, Arlington

Zollinger B (2015) Die Entdeckung der Sprache, 9th edn. Haupt Verlag, Bern

Special Kinds of Developmental Disorders of Speech and Language

10

Ulrike Becker-Redding, Katrin Neumann, and Rainer Schönweiler

10.1 Subtypes of Developmental Disorders of Speech and Language

Rainer Schönweiler and Katrin Neumann

10.1.1 Terminology of Subtypes of Developmental Disorders of Speech and Language

A variety of terms are used to refer to children who do not speak adequately for their age, including such speech vs. language disorder, delay vs. impairment, primary or specific as opposed to non-specific or secondary language disorders. As a result, permutations of these terms are often not used consistently, although a clear physiological and aetiological classification is highly desirable.

U. Becker-Redding
Praxis für Logopädie, Bochum, Germany
e-mail: logopaedie-becker-redding@gmx.de

K. Neumann
Department of Phoniatrics and Pediatric Audiology,
ENT Clinic, St. Elisabeth Hospital, University of
Bochum, Bochum, Germany
e-mail: Katrin.neumann@rub.de

R. Schönweiler
Department of Phoniatrics and Pediatric Audiology,
University Clinic of Schleswig-Holstein,
Campus Lübeck, Lübeck, Germany
e-mail: rainer.schoenweiler@phoniatrie.uni-luebeck.de

Usually, the term 'speech disorder' is used for articulatory problems, while 'language disorder' or 'language impairment' (LI) includes structural or systemic problems of language acquisition (de Langen-Müller et al. 2013). The terms 'disorder' and 'impairment' mean deviations in the quality, quantity and time course of language acquisition regardless of age, while 'delay' implicates a pure harmonic delay of more than 6 months, i.e. that both language quantity and quality closely match that of a healthy child at least 6 months younger (UEP 1987). The term 'delay' is commonly used until the age of 3 years, when a comprehensive language test could be performed to unravel the patterns of errors that justify the term 'disorder' and when the typical period, during which late talkers usually may make up for their delay, has passed (Kiese-Himmel 2008; Schöler and Scheib 2004). The terms 'specific language disorder' (SLD) and 'specific language impairment' (SLI) are the most often used terms, at least in association with a 'primary' aetiology without comorbid conditions.

Developmental speech-language disorders are categorised in the International Statistical Classification of Diseases and Related Health Problems, the ICD-10 of the World Health Organization (2011). In its current version, they are called 'developmental disorders of speech and language' (DDSL) and are subclassified as specific DDSL (SDDSL; synonymous with 'specific language disorder' (SLD) and 'specific language

© Springer-Verlag GmbH Germany, part of Springer Nature 2020
A. am Zehnhoff-Dinnesen et al. (eds.), *Phoniatrics I*, European Manual of Medicine,
https://doi.org/10.1007/978-3-662-46780-0_10

impairment' (SLI)) and other DDSL. Because the latter are associated with language-relevant comorbid diseases, they may be called 'DDSL associated with language-relevant comorbidities' (DDSLC; synonymous with 'secondary' or 'non-specific DDSL'). For specific (or primary) developmental disorders of speech and language (SDDSL), codes according to the ICD-10 taxonomy are subsumed under categories F80.1 to F80.9, more precisely under F80.0–F80.2 (de Langen-Müller et al. 2013) (there are some weaknesses in the ICD-10 classifications). DDSL as associated with comorbidities (DDSLC; secondary DDSL) may be classified as F80.9, F83 or F89. Additionally, the comorbid diseases receive their own ICD-10 codes, e.g. H90.3 for bilateral sensorineural hearing loss. Because adverse social conditions are not a disease and do not require medical intervention, they are not listed in the ICD-10 code. Genetic factors are the main reasons for SDDSL. At the present state of research, however, it is difficult or impossible to make a causal attribution of a specific gene pattern to an individual SDDSL.

10.1.2 Changes in Prevalence Reports

Recently, in a couple of countries, for example, in Germany, the period prevalence of developmental speech-language disorders in infants and preschool children per year has been reported to approach 20% or even more. Respective data are, for example, collected and periodically published by governmental working groups in North Germany (e.g. Thyen et al. 2015). They contradict former well-based reports of 6–8% DDSL prevalence from Anglo-Saxon countries (Canning and Lyon 1989; Thomson and Polnay 2002). This current reporting trend of prevalence might be biased because it is not very probable that a highly genetically caused disorder such as a DDSL increases dramatically in prevalence within years. Often, in these reports, 'speech-language disorders' are assumed by evaluating 'surface' symptoms rather than by a valid test-based diagnosis of a DDSL. Subsequently, the reported prevalence increase might be due to vague diagnostic criteria

resulting in 'overdiagnosis' and 'overtreatment'; in fact up to 25% of preschool children in Germany— or even more—receive speech-language therapy. These counts exceed the data from other countries two- to threefold.

Another potential bias causing high prevalence is that frequently the test outcomes for single linguistic subdomains are simply added or seen as single results instead of being weighted according to their prognosis. As to 'overtreatment', a high proportion of children may receive treatment owing to the lack of interventional alternatives or to parental and social desires, such as for migrant children who have not acquired the common language sufficiently. Moreover, numbers of children diagnosed with DDSL could have risen over the years from increased awareness, emphasis and need for language proficiency in schools and for vocational training, study and jobs. The assumption that the increasing prevalence is biased has support from the fact that most children treated for speech and language disorders approach normal language levels at school ages (see Fig. 10.1), whereas high-quality long-term studies show that a 'true' DDSL population scores significantly lower than a control population in articulation and expressive and receptive language tests and has lower educational and occupational outcomes, whether they are treated or not for their DDSL, even 28 years after the first diagnosis (Felsenfeld et al. 1992, 1994). The high prevalence may, however, also be caused by transiently occurring comorbidities, such as fluctuating hearing loss due to recurrent otitis media, which require the attention of phoniatricians and other medical professionals. Finally, it cannot be excluded that genome-environment interplay changes the prevalence of developmental speech-language disorders over time.

10.1.3 Types of Comorbid Conditions

'Comorbid conditions' refer to diseases that with a high probability occur along with DDSL as reported by high-standard studies. Profound hearing loss is a typical example of such a 'comorbid condition', often being even the main reason for a speech-language delay or disorder, if unaided.

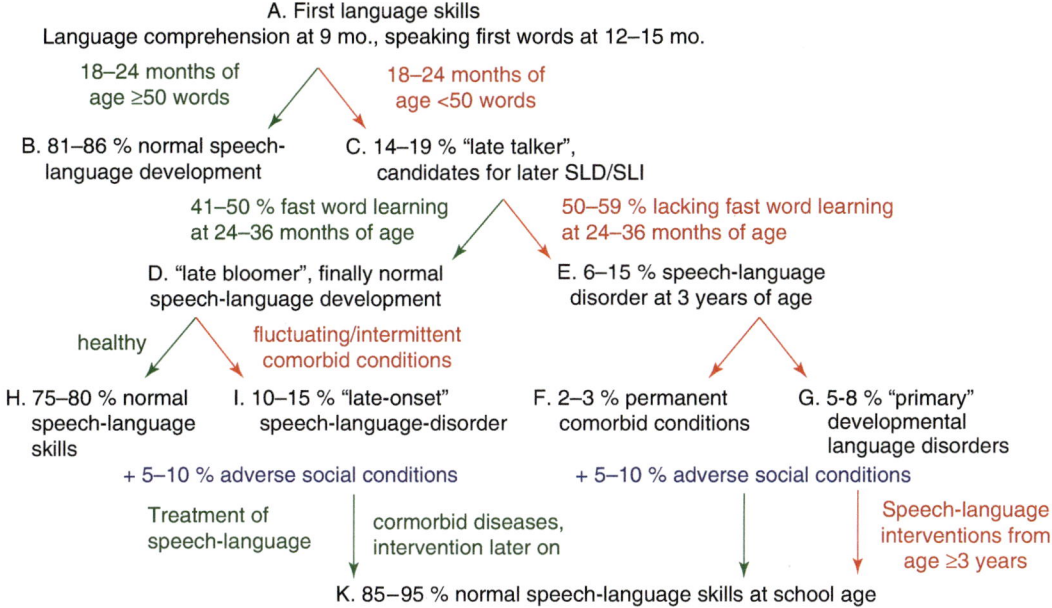

A. First language skills
Language comprehension at 9 mo., speaking first words at 12–15 mo.

18–24 months of age ≥50 words

18–24 months of age <50 words

B. 81–86 % normal speech-language development

C. 14–19 % "late talker", candidates for later SLD/SLI

41–50 % fast word learning at 24–36 months of age

50–59 % lacking fast word learning at 24–36 months of age

D. "late bloomer", finally normal speech-language development

E. 6–15 % speech-language disorder at 3 years of age

healthy

fluctuating/intermittent comorbid conditions

H. 75–80 % normal speech-language skills

I. 10–15 % "late-onset" speech-language-disorder

F. 2–3 % permanent comorbid conditions

G. 5-8 % "primary" developmental language disorders

+ 5–10 % adverse social conditions

+ 5–10 % adverse social conditions

Treatment of speech-language

cormorbid diseases, intervention later on

Speech-language interventions from age ≥3 years

K. 85–95 % normal speech-language skills at school age

Fig. 10.1 Subtypes of primary and secondary speech-language disorders at different developmental ages

The impact of a comorbid condition on speech and language development depends much on its severity and disease progression over time and on the individuals' idiosyncratic (mental) capacity to compensate for such a condition. For instance, many children with a mild conductive hearing loss may not experience a speech-language delay, whereas children with a developmental delay or other risk factors may do.

The impact of mild conductive hearing loss—often fluctuating in presence and severity—and developmental speech-language delay or disorder has been a matter of debate for three decades. Several meta-analyses of studies aiming at quantifying such an impact have demonstrated effect sizes below significance (e.g. Paradise et al. 2005; Rosenfeld et al. 2011), but the underlying studies contained substantial flaws in methodology (Schönweiler 2006), indicating that no robust conclusion pro or contra ventilation tubes (grommets) or pro and contra early versus late insertion could be drawn. Therefore, guidelines on the treatment of otitis media with effusion by insertion of grommets do not follow these meta-analyses (Rosenfeld et al. 2013a). Rather, they recommend that clinicians determine if a child with recurrent acute otitis media, or with

otitis media with effusion of any duration, is at increased risk for speech, language or learning problems from the otitis. Such risks could stem from baseline sensory, physical, cognitive or behavioural factors—e.g. permanent hearing loss independent of otitis media with effusion, suspected or confirmed speech and language delay or disorder, autism-spectrum disorder or other pervasive developmental disorders, syndromes or craniofacial disorders (including cognitive, speech or language delays, cleft palate or developmental disorders). For children classified 'at risk', earlier examination of hearing and speech-language development and earlier insertion of grommets have been recommended (Rosenfeld et al. 2004, 2013b), with the expectation of improved speech-language outcome, even if no scientific proof for this exists at present. This recommendation is underscored by reports that children with such a risk benefit more from ventilation tubes in their speech, language, learning and school performance outcome than children without risk factors (Rosenfeld et al. 2011).

The negative impact of comorbid diseases, e.g. of hearing disorders, developmental delay, oral motor disorders and others, is outlined by various guidelines and also in this book. In terms of duration and potential for improvement, comorbid conditions can be classified as fluctuating/intermittent and permanent types. Examples of fluctuating/intermittent comorbid conditions are periods of otitis media with effusion and cases of hospitalisation due to severe illness or family crises. Examples of permanent comorbid conditions are sensorineural hearing loss, seizure disorders with developmental delay and genetic disorders.

A third category, 'sociogenic' or 'environmental' language *abnormalities* that are caused by adverse social conditions such as poor language stimulation or language abnormalities during multilingual language acquisition with low input in the common language, does not count as a 'medical' comorbid condition. Consequently, they do not require medical treatment but a language-stimulating input of sufficient quality and quantity (e.g. early literacy, language-stimulating conversation, narratives; see Sect. 12.2). It has to be taken into consideration, however, that DDSL may coincide with such adverse conditions, and it is challenging but necessary for a phoniatrician to discern a DDSL from the sociogenically caused language abnormalities in order to make an appropriate recommendation for intervention.

10.1.4 Subtypes of Developmental Disorders of Speech and Language at Different Ages

Which type of primary or secondary speech-language disorder is found in a differential diagnostic procedure depends, in part, on the individual developmental age (Fig. 10.1). First verbal skills usually appear around the age of 10 months when infants begin to understand first words (Fig. 10.1A) (de Langen-Müller et al. 2013). Between 18 and 24 months of age, they typically acquire up to 50 words, provided that speech is developing within the realm of what is considered normal language development (Fig. 10.1B). Those struggling with language development at the age of 2 are called 'late talkers'. These children carry an increased risk for the later diagnosis of a DDSL (developmental

language disorder, Fig. 10.1C) (de Langen-Müller et al. 2013; Desmarais et al. 2008). About 41–50% of 'late talkers' finally catch up to peers at the age of 3 years ('late bloomers', Fig. 10.1D). If they still fall behind their peers in speech and language skills at the age of 3 years, they could be classified as having a DDSL (Fig. 10.1E) (de Langen-Müller et al. 2013). About one third of these children may have a 'secondary' disorder due to permanent comorbid conditions, suggesting the need for a causal therapy (Fig. 10.1F). The remaining two thirds may be classified as having a SDDSL and need a speech-language intervention (Fig. 10.1G).

Children showing normal speech and language development (Fig. 10.1B, D) may either continue in this development (Fig. 10.1H) or may be affected by later illness. If such a late-onset illness, e.g. fluctuating hearing loss, late-onset hearing loss or diseases of the central nervous system, hinders speech-language development, the affected children may develop a DDSLC (secondary speech-language disorder) despite having had a good start (Fig. 10.1I). Because both DDSL and sociogenic language abnormalities are more prevalent in socially weak regions, the occurrence of both disturbances may underlie regional differences. Finally, the majority of children treated for speech and language disorders develop 'normal' speech and language skills by the time they start school (Fig. 10.1K).

10.1.5 Comorbid Conditions, Differential Diagnoses and Adverse Social Conditions

In the following, comorbid conditions, differential diagnoses and adverse social conditions are explained.

10.1.5.1 Hearing Disorders
Permanent sensorineural or conductive types of hearing loss, whether aided or not, are certainly well-known comorbid conditions and may be seen as the main reason for DDSLC (secondary speech-language disorders). This is because hearing loss reduces the quantity and quality of linguistic information necessary for language

acquisition. As a general rule, the higher the degree of hearing loss, the higher the risk of a speech-language disorder (Northern and Downs 2002). Therefore, children with a bilateral moderate or profound hearing loss often show significantly reduced language abilities compared with children with a bilateral mild hearing loss. However, one should keep in mind that even mild hearing loss may establish a huge barrier to the child's ability to acquire language (Paradis et al. 2003), so that it makes sense that children with mild and minimal hearing loss (bilateral or even unilateral pure tone thresholds between 16 and 25 dB) are fitted with hearing aids. Whether fluctuating/intermittent (not permanent) hearing loss due to otitis media with effusion (OME) has a negative impact on speech-language development has been subject of controversial debate. Many of the North American paediatric cohort studies failed to confirm such an impact; however, as the critics rightly pointed out, all these studies were plagued by serious methodological flaws (Schönweiler 2004). Certainly, hearing loss significantly increases the risk for a speech-language disorder if there are additional comorbid medical conditions, developmental disorders or deprivation (de Langen-Müller et al. 2013; Northern and Downs 2002; Rosenfeld et al. 2013a; Schönweiler 1994, 2004).

10.1.5.2   Other Sensory Deficits

Loss of vision has been shown to cause at maximum some delay in the early phase of language acquisition; however, it is not a true comorbidity of a DDSL (de Langen-Müller et al. 2013; Neumann et al. 2008).

10.1.5.3   Developmental Disorders and Mental Retardation

Speech-language disorders and delay can be observed as part of many developmental disorders (e.g. autism-spectrum disorders), mental retardation and syndromes (specifically genetic syndromes) (de Langen-Müller et al. 2013). Typically, speech and language skills, judged from observed test results, match the individual developmental scores. Such a developmental profile is consistent with the observed speech-language delay being secondary in nature (de

Langen-Müller et al. 2013; Schönweiler 2004). In many syndromes, a developmental delay is often combined with a hearing disorder or another sensory deficit. If untreated, speech and language screening results can be much worse than expected from non-verbal developmental test results.

10.1.5.4   Disorders and Diseases of the Central Nervous System

Comorbid neurological diseases may increase the risk for a secondary speech-language disorder. Examples of such diseases are cerebral palsy, structural malformation of the brain (e.g. agenesis of the corpus callosum) and abnormal functional findings (e.g. lacking development of hemispheric dominance) (de Langen-Müller et al. 2013).

10.1.5.5   Risk Factors at Birth and Preterm Birth

In general, risk factors at birth and premature birth per se are not causes for developmental speech and language disorders. However, they establish a risk factor, and their impact depends on the severity of the adverse perinatal conditions and the presence of comorbidities. In particular, children with gestational age under 28 weeks at birth and those with birth weight below 1100 g have been shown to be at an increased risk for hearing disorders (Jimenéz et al. 2008; Rieger-Fackeldey et al. 2010; Robertson et al. 2009), other sensory deficits (Marston et al. 2007), developmental delay, developmental language delays or language disorders (see Sect. 9.6). In clinical practice protocols, most infants at risk are monitored for many diseases and developmental delay, including congenital and late-onset hearing loss as well as speech-language delay or disorder, regardless of the individual risk.

10.1.5.6   Differential Diagnoses

Landau-Kleffner syndrome is an acquired childhood *aphasia*, but not a typical developmental language disorder, although it is classified as ICD 10 F80.3. It is accompanied by paroxysmal abnormalities on the EEG, and in the majority of cases also by epileptic seizures, which symptoms, if anticonvulsive treatment is successful, could to an extent be similar to those of a secondary speech-language disorder.

Elective mutism can sometimes be observed as a result but not a cause of a primary or secondary speech-language disorder. Speech-language disorders may lead to social interaction disorders, low self-esteem, social withdrawal, depressive mood and aggressiveness.

10.1.5.7 Adverse Social Conditions

Adverse social conditions are considered to be a frequent environmental non-medical cause of speech-language abnormalities. They do not establish a disease but nonetheless need to be addressed by medical professionals, predominantly by counselling and training parents to promote speech and language development of their child. Twins sometimes talk to each other in a 'secret language', but this is not a medical problem and can be solved by educational modifications in the family. Multilingual education (see Sect. 9.5) is another non-medical condition that may be associated with speech-language *abnormalities* but does not cause speech-language *disorders*. It is important to note that symptoms of a DDSL are typically observed in all languages spoken by the child (Håkansson et al. 2003; Paradis et al. 2003).

10.2 Developmental Verbal Dyspraxia

Ulrike Becker-Redding

10.2.1 Definition

According to the American Speech-Language-Hearing Association (2007)

> Childhood Apraxia of Speech (CAS) is a neurological childhood … speech sound disorder in which the precision and consistency of movements underlying speech are impaired in the absence of neuromuscular deficits (e.g., abnormal reflexes, abnormal tone). CAS may occur as a result of known neurological impairment, in association with complex neurobehavioral disorders of known or unknown origin, or as an idiopathic neurogenic speech sound disorder. The core impairment in

planning or programming spatiotemporal parameters of movement sequences results in errors in speech sound productions and prosody.

The voluntary movement of the musculature involved in speech production seems to be impaired or even impossible, while movement of the same muscles appears normal, apart from articulation (Morley et al. 1954). CAS has to be differentiated from oral apraxia, the former referring to a verbal behaviour, the latter to oral movements apart from speech.

10.2.2 Terminology

Various terms are in use for CAS throughout the Anglo-Saxon literature, such as 'developmental verbal dyspraxia of speech' (DVD), 'verbal dyspraxia', 'speech dyspraxia', 'developmental articulatory dyspraxia' (DAD) or 'developmental apraxia of speech' (DAS). More recently, the term 'childhood apraxia of speech' (CAS) has been preferred with the argument that the term 'developmental' may suggest that this disorder is part of an overall developmental delay that the children will outgrow, but this is not the case. On the contrary, the disorder exists from early childhood on, and there is only little progress in speech motor skills development without a specific therapy approach (American Speech-Language-Hearing Association 2007).

10.2.3 Prevalence

As with other complex neurobehavioural disorders, the prevalence of CAS is reported as having increased during the past decade (American Speech-Language-Hearing Association 2007). This, however, is probably not a true increase but caused by factors such as a growing sensibility of the problem, better assessment procedures and raised attention to the language proficiency of children. As sources and types of studies vary, so do the figures currently available in the research literature. One preliminary population estimate, based solely on clinical referral data, is that CAS occurs in 0.1–0.2% of children (Shriberg et al. 1997). For specific genetically at-risk groups, higher prevalence figures have been reported, e.g. for children with galactosaemia, a 180-fold risk corresponding to a prevalence of 1.8% has been reported (Shriberg et al. 2011).

10.2.4 Symptoms of Childhood Apraxia of Speech

Recent research indicates that no validated list of diagnostic features of CAS is available that differentiates this symptom complex from other types of childhood speech sound disorders. Nevertheless, there are three segmental and suprasegmental features (core markers) that have gained consensus among researchers (American Speech-Language-Hearing Association 2007). These are:

- Inconsistent errors in consonants and vowels in repeated productions of syllables and words
- Lengthened and disrupted coarticulatory transitions between sounds and syllables (the movement of articulators between phoneme targets, whereby the transition shares the articulatory and acoustic characteristic of both phonemes; gradual changes from the first phoneme target to the second one)
- Inappropriate prosody, especially in the realisation of lexical or phrasal stress

At least one of these features has to be present to justify the diagnosis of CAS. In addition to the three core features, characteristic anomalies frequently noted are:

- Unintelligible speech.
- Lack of sufficient consonant repertoire; mostly vowels are uttered.
- Single phonemes can be produced but not combined into syllables or words.
- Increased error frequency with increased length or complexity of utterances.
- No or limited ability of verbal imitation.
- Oral groping when attempting sound production.
- Struggle behaviour when attempting to imitate speech or speak.
- Vowel distortions that are not caused by oral motor weakness.

- Receptive language (comprehension) significantly better than expressive language (verbal output).
- Abnormal intra-oral sensory perception (hyper- or hyposensitivity) including oral stereognosis.

The case history frequently indicates:

- Late onset of speech/language, first words frequently after 18 months, no typical developmental increase by age 36 months or later.
- 'Quiet' babies, limited or no canonical babbling.
- Clear words might be blurted out but cannot be produced upon imitation.
- General awkwardness or clumsiness.

The communication behaviour may show the following characteristics:

- Non-verbal compensatory strategies such as gesturing, facial movements or descriptive sounds might be used for communication.
- Awareness of the disorder, frustration with its own speaking, refusal to repeat or to speak.

Additional problems occurring with CAS can be oral (non-speech) dyspraxia, fine or gross motor dyspraxia and difficulties in sensory, in particular tactile, perception. The model depicted in Fig. 10.2 describes the various functions that occur when processing and producing a verbal message during speech-language development. Children with CAS have deficits in three of the speech motor production areas, i.e. programming, storing and planning (American Speech-Language-Hearing Association 2007). Hence a CAS is a primarily expressive speech-language disorder.

Reading the diagram of Fig. 10.2 clockwise from the acoustic input (bottom left), the following general processing stages are encountered as (explanations of Stackhouse and Wells slightly modified by the author):

- *Peripheral Auditory Processing*: The input sound is analysed for its component physical attributes of frequency and intensity and rates of change thereof.

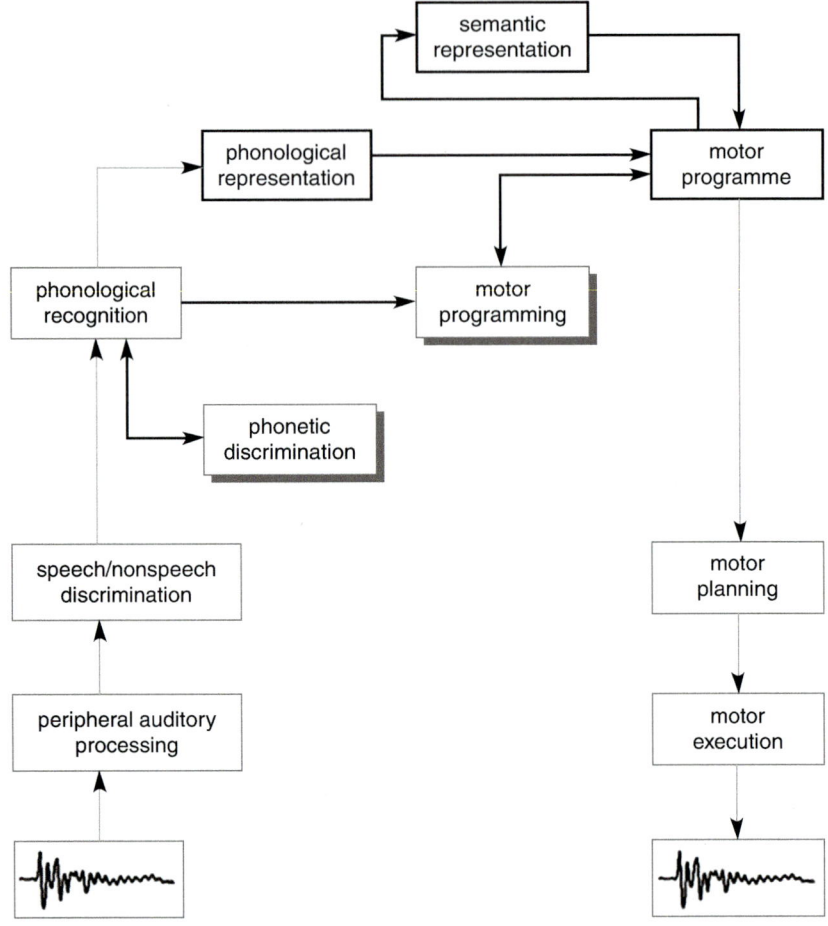

Fig. 10.2 Speech processing model according to Stackhouse and Wells (1997). Copyright with kind permission by John Wiley and Sons

- *Speech/Non-speech Discrimination*: The input sound is classified as speech or non-speech before any attempt is made at word recognition.
- *Phonological Recognition*: Speech sounds are classified as belonging to a language which is either familiar or not. The phonological features of the familiar language are identified according to their phonological features (phonemes, phoneme clusters, syllabic structures).
- *Phonetic Discrimination*: Process of denoting any perceptible distinction between one speech sound and another, irrespective of whether the sounds are phonemes or allophones (variants of a phoneme). Phonetic features that do not belong to familiar language patterns are not processed further.
- *Phonological Representation*: The equivalent of the phonological input lexicon, where

whole words have a previously stored entry according to their sound and syllable features.
- *Semantic Representation*: Cerebral storage of word meaning.
- *Motor Programme*: It is the equivalent of the phonological output lexicon, where the motor commands required for the production of the targeted speech sounds, syllables and words are stored, also defined as articulatory targets or gestures. Children with CAS have significant problems with storing the correct motor programme, especially its sequence (American Speech-Language-Hearing Association 2007).
- *Motor Programming*: Here internal sound representations can be deliberately manipulated to produce words not previously known. This is relevant for the imitation of new or unknown words and also requires functions to process

the length and sequence of the verbal material. Children with CAS have difficulties with imitation; problems increase especially with length of the speech material (American Speech-Language-Hearing Association 2007).

- *Motor Planning*: Motor programmes from either the lexical or nonlexical routes prepare a specific sequence of speech sounds as well as intonation, speed and rhythm. The final result is a 'single utterance plan', which is then turned into muscular activation patterns at the motor execution. This area is particularly difficult for children with CAS (American Speech-Language-Hearing Association 2007).
- *Motor Execution*: Articulatory (phonatory) gestures required for the accurate pronunciation of the word are produced as muscle action. Although children with CAS seem to have problems in executing speech motor commands, most theoretical concepts regard the problems of the speech production difficulties in CAS further 'upstream' than the actual execution of the motor plan (American Speech-Language-Hearing Association 2007). By contrast, children with dysarthria show difficulties in motor execution. In children with CAS, however, typically the quality of speech production seems rather to be influenced by the problems in the three areas described above (motor programme, motor programming, motor planning).

10.2.5 Assessment

There is no generally accepted diagnostic procedure for CAS (American Speech-Language-Hearing Association 2007). A few tests, usually available in North America, are predominantly based on the clinical symptomatology. The most promising domains for a sensitive and specific identification of CAS are maximal performance in multisyllabic productions and prosody. There is a wide agreement that children with CAS are best identified and assessed by medical professionals (phoniatricians, logopedists, speech-language pathologists) trained for or experienced with the disorder. Potentially co-occurring disorders, especially oral dyspraxia, need to be identified or excluded.

The following diagnostic tests or tasks are recommended by the author:

- Speech-language assessment with standardised and normed tests: CAS children display a significant (at least 6 month) discrepancy between receptive and expressive language skills, with the receptive skills being appropriate for the age or cognitive level of the child.
- Verbal imitation tasks with phonemes, syllables and words of increasing length or phonological complexity: children with CAS show a significant increased error rate.
- Determination of consistency through repeated imitation of words: inconsistency in children with CAS.
- Determination of the diadochokinetic rate by using syllable sequences of one (puh-puh-puh), two (puh-tuh-puh-tuh-puh-tuh) and three syllables (puh-tuh-kuh- puh-tuh-kuh-puh-tuh-kuh): children with CAS are unable to perform this test properly.
- Automatised speech, e.g. counting: speech sound production is more consistent than for spontaneous speech or picture-naming tasks in children with CAS.

From the described assessment tools, together with the information gained from the developmental case history and the behavioural aspects described earlier, the diagnosis of CAS can be made, rejected or may be suspected.

10.2.6 Treatment

Neither the lack of a definite diagnosis of CAS nor the young age of a child should restrain therapists from starting a CAS-tailored intervention. At times the final diagnosis is only confirmed through successful therapy. Parent counselling is an important constituent of the treatment. Although robust evidence is lacking, the earlier the onset of treatment, i.e. under 3 years of age, the more favourable the prognosis seems to be. Therapeutic approaches standard for phonetic or phonological speech sound disorders have been shown to be of little effectiveness (Maas et al. 2014). Instead, treatment should be performed by therapists trained for or specialised in the therapy of CAS.

Three kinds of treatment approaches that focus directly on improving speech production can be recommended to date:

- *Motor programming approaches* utilise motor-learning principles, including the need for many repetitions of speech movements in order to support the child in acquiring and automatising skills of an accurate and consistent production of sounds and sound sequences (Maas et al. 2014).
- *Sensory cueing approaches* involve the use of the child's senses (e.g. vision, touch), as well as gestures to cue (or self-cue) some aspects of the targeted speech sounds. Cueing is often used in conjunction with another approach such as motor programming (Hall 2000).
- *Rhythmic (prosodic) approaches*, such as melodic intonation therapy (Helfrich-Miller 1994), use prosodic patterns (melody, intonation, rhythm and stress) to improve functional speech production.

Crucial for all treatment approaches is a sufficient dosage, i.e. an adequate frequency, intensity and duration of therapy and practising. An appropriate treatment dosage for CAS is reasoned from the principles of motor learning (McNeil et al. 1997). Facing the need for repetitive production practice in speech motor disorders such as CAS, intensive and individualised treatment appears to be required. Several research studies have supported the need for three to five individual sessions per week as opposed to the traditional and less intensive one to two sessions per week (American Speech-Language-Hearing Association 2007). For younger children, the frequency and length of sessions need to be adjusted to their age; shorter and more frequent sessions are recommended. Caretakers should be instructed to work as co-therapists in order to ensure regular and intensive training. The overall duration of intervention is expected to be at least 2–3 years, depending on the severity of the disorder, the treatment continuity and the child's age at therapy start.

References

American Speech-Language-Hearing Association (2007) Childhood apraxia of speech. Technical Report. Available via http://www.asha.org/policy/TR2007-00278/. Accessed 19 July 2017

Canning PM, Lyon ME (1989) Young children with special needs: prevalence and implications in Nova Scotia. Can J Educ 14(3):368–380

de Langen-Müller U, Kauschke C, Kiesel-Himmel C et al (eds in equal authorship) (2013) Diagnostik von Sprachentwicklungsstörungen (SES), unter Berücksichtigung umschriebener Sprachentwicklungsstörungen (USES). Available via http://www.awmf.org/uploads/tx_szleitlinien/049-0061_S2k_Sprachentwicklungsstoerungen_Diagnostik_2013-06_01.pdf. Accessed 27 Jan 2014

Desmarais C, Sylvestre A, Meyer F et al (2008) Systematic review of the literature on characteristics of late-talking toddlers. Int J Lang Commun Disord 43(4):361–389

Felsenfeld S, Broen PA, McGue M (1992) A 28-year follow-up of adults with a history of moderate phonological disorder: linguistic and personality results. J Speech Hear Res 35(5):1114–1125

Felsenfeld S, Broen PA, McGue M (1994) A 28-year follow-up of adults with a history of moderate phonological disorder: educational and occupational results. J Speech Hear Res 37(6):1341–1353

Håkansson G, Salameh EK, Nettelbladt U (2003) Measuring language development in bilingual children: Swedish-Arabic children with and without language impairment. Linguistics 41(2):255–288

Hall PK (2000) A letter to the parent(s) of a child with developmental apraxia of speech. Part IV: treatment of DAS. Lang Speech Hear Serv Sch 31(2):179–181

Helfrich-Miller KR (1994) A clinical perspective: melodic intonation therapy for developmental apraxia. Clin Commun Disord 4(3):175–182

Jimenéz MAM, Servera GC, Roca JA et al (2008) Seguimiento de recién nacidos de peso menor o igual a 1.000g durante los tres primeros años de vida. An Pediatr (Barc) 68(4):320–328

Kiese-Himmel C (2008) Entwicklung sprach- und kommunikationsgestörter Kinder, am Beispiel von "Late Talkers" und Kindern mit spezifischen Sprachentwicklungsstörungen. In: Hasselhorn M, Silbereisen RK (eds) Enzyklopädie der Psychologie. Themenbereich C: Theorie und Forschung. Serie V: Entwicklungspsychologie des Säuglings- und Kindesalters, 4th edn. Hogrefe, Göttingen, Bern, Toronto, Seattle, pp 693–730

Maas E, Gildersleeve-Neumann C, Jakielski KJ et al (2014) Motor-based intervention protocols in treatment of childhood apraxia of speech (CAS). Curr Dev Disord Rep 1(3):197–206

Marston L, Peacock JL, Calvert SA et al (2007) Factors affecting vocabulary acquisition at age 2 in children born between 23 and 28 weeks' gestation. Dev Med Child Neurol 49(8):591–596

McNeil MR, Robin DA, Schmidt RA (1997) Apraxia of speech: definition, differentiation, and treatment. In: McNeil MR (ed) Clinical management of sensorimotor speech disorders. Thieme, New York, pp 311–344

Morley ME, Court D, Miller H (1954) Developmental dysarthria. Br Med J 1(4852):8–10

Neumann K, Keilmann A, Kiese-Himmel C et al (2008) Leitlinien der Deutschen Gesellschaft für Phoniatrie und Pädaudiologie zu Sprachentwicklungsstörungen bei Kindern. Available via http://www.dgpp.de/cms/media/download_gallery/SES%20lang.pdf. Accessed 16 May 2017

Northern JL, Downs MP (2002) Hearing in children, 5th edn. Lippincott Williams & Wilkins, Baltimore, Philadelphia, pp 1–31, 65–89

Paradis J, Crago M, Genesee F et al (2003) French-English bilingual children with SLI: how do they compare with their monolingual peers? J Speech Lang Hear Res 46(1):113–127

Paradise JL, Campbell TF, Dollaghan CA et al (2005) Developmental outcomes after early or delayed insertion of tympanostomy tubes. N Engl J Med 353(6):576–586

Rieger-Fackeldey E, Blank C, Dinger J et al (2010) Growth, neurological and cognitive development in infants with a birth weight < 501 g at age 5 years. Acta Paediatr 99(9):1350–1355

Robertson CM, Watt MJ, Dinu IA (2009) Outcomes for the extremely premature infant: what is new? And where are we going? Pediatr Neurol 40(3):189–196

Rosenfeld RM, Culpepper L, Doyle KJ et al (2004) Clinical practice guideline: otitis media with effusion. Otolaryngol Head Neck Surg 130(5 Suppl):S95–S118

Rosenfeld RM, Jang DW, Tarashansky K (2011) Tympanostomy tube outcomes in children at-risk and not at-risk for developmental delays. Int J Pediatr Otorhinolaryngol 75(2):190–195

Rosenfeld RM, Schwartz SR, Pynnonen MA et al (2013a) Clinical practice guideline: tympanostomy tubes in children. Otolaryngol Head Neck Surg 149(1 Suppl):S1–S35

Rosenfeld RM, Schwartz SR, Pynnonen MA et al (2013b) Clinical practice guideline: tympanostomy tubes in children—executive summary. Otolaryngol Head Neck Surg 149(1):8–16

Schöler H, Scheib K (2004) Desiderate und Thesen zur Diagnostik bei Sprachentwicklungsstörungen. Sprache Stimme Gehör 28(1):37–41

Schönweiler R (1994) Synoptische Betrachtung der Ergebnisse an 1300 sprachentwicklungsverzögerten Kindern aus ätiopathogenetischer, audiologischer und sprachpathologischer Sicht. Folia Phoniatr Logop 46(1):18–26

Schönweiler R (2004) Mittelohrschwerhörigkeit und Sprachentwicklung: Korrelation, Kausalität und Konsequenzen (conductive hearing loss: correlation, causality, and consequences). Laryngorhinootologie 83(11):757–758

Schönweiler R (2006) Zeitige Einlage von Paukenröhrchen sinnlos? Sprache Stimme Gehör 30(2):85–86

Shriberg LD, Aram DM, Kwiatkowski J (1997) Developmental apraxia of speech: I. Descriptive perspectives. J Speech Lang Hear Res 40(2):273–285

Shriberg LD, Potter NL, Strand EA (2011) Prevalence and phenotype of childhood apraxia of speech in youth with galactosemia. J Speech Lang Hear Res 54(2):487–519

Stackhouse J, Wells B (1997) Children's speech and literacy difficulties 1: a psycholinguistic framework. Whurr Publishers Ltd, London

Thomson C, Polnay L (eds) (2002) Community paediatrics, 3rd edn. Elsevier, Edinburgh

Thyen U, Brehm S, Bethge S et al (2015) Untersuchungen der Kinder- und Jugendärztlichen Dienste und der Zahnärztlichen Dienste in Schleswig-Holstein Schuljahr 2014/2015. Publication of the "Ministerium für Soziales, Gesundheit, Wissenschaft und Gleichstellung des Landes Schleswig-Holstein". Available via https://www.schleswig-holstein.de/DE/Landesregierung/VIII/Service/Broschueren/Broschueren_VIII/Gesundheit/schuleinguntber2015.pdf?__blob=publicationFile&v=2. Accessed 16 May 2017

UEP (1987) Commission speech and language. UEP-Report. Annu Bull UEP 5:37–44

World Health Organization (2010/2011) International statistical classification of diseases and related health problems, 10th Revision. Available via http://www.who.int/classifications/icd/en/. Accessed 22 Jan 2017

Diagnosis and Differential Diagnosis of Developmental Disorders of Speech and Language

11

Tahany AbdelKarim Elsayed, Wolfgang Angerstein,
María Bielsa Corrochano, Dirk Deuster,
Andrea Joe Embacher, Uta Hanning, Mona Hegazi,
Christiane Kiese-Himmel, Ben A. M. Maassen,
Barbara Maciejewska, Ana Martínez Arellano,
Peter Matulat, Katrin Neumann,
Thomas Niederstadt, Karen Reichmuth,
Jochen Rosenfeld, Rainer Schönweiler,
Melanie Vauth, Adam P. Vogel, and Dagmar Weise

The authors Mona Hegazi and Barbara Maciejewska have
contributed equally to Sect. 11.9.

T. AbdelKarim Elsayed
Speech-Language Pathology and Psychology,
Salmiya, Kuwait

W. Angerstein
Phoniatrie und Pädaudiologie, Univ.-Klinikum
Düsseldorf, Düsseldorf, Germany
e-mail: angerstein@med.uni-duesseldorf.de

M. Bielsa Corrochano
Clinica Foniatria Y Logopedia Bielsa,
Talavera de la Reina, Spain
e-mail: info@foniatriabielsa.com

D. Deuster · A. J. Embacher · P. Matulat
K. Reichmuth · M. Vauth
Clinic of Phoniatrics and Pedaudiology, University
Hospital Münster, Münster, Germany
e-mail: deusted@ukmuenster.de; andrea.
embacher@ukmuenster.de; matulat@uni-muenster.
de; karen.reichmuth@ukmuenster.de;
melanie-jasmin.vauth@ukmuenster.de

U. Hanning
Department of Neuroradiological Diagnostics and
Intervention, University Hospital Hamburg,
Hamburg, Germany
e-mail: uhanning@uni-muenster.de

M. Hegazi
ENT Department, Ain Shams University, Cairo, Egypt

C. Kiese-Himmel
Phoniatrics/Pediatric Audiological Psychology,
University Medical Center Göttingen,
Göttingen, Germany
e-mail: ckiese@med.uni-goettingen.de

B. A. M. Maassen
Center for Language and Cognition Groningen
and Department of Neurosciences/BCN,
University Medical Center Groningen, University
of Groningen, Groningen, The Netherlands

Department of Neurosciences/BCN, University
Medical Center Groningen (UMCG), Groningen, The
Netherlands
e-mail: b.a.m.maassen@rug.nl

B. Maciejewska
Department of Phoniatrics and Audiology,
Poznan University of Medical Sciences,
Poznan, Poland
e-mail: barbaramaciejewska@ump.edu.pl

A. Martínez Arellano
Clinica Foniatria Y Logopedia, Pamplona, Spain
e-mail: anamarellano@medena.es

K. Neumann
Department of Phoniatrics and Pediatric Audiology,
ENT Clinic, St. Elisabeth Hospital, University of
Bochum, Bochum, Germany
e-mail: Katrin.neumann@rub.de

T. Niederstadt
Department of Clinical Radiology, University
Hospital Münster, Münster, Germany
e-mail: tnieders@uni-muenster.de

J. Rosenfeld
Abteilung Gehör-, Sprach- u. Stimmheilkunde,
Kantonsspital St.Gallen, St. Gallen,
Switzerland
e-mail: jochen.rosenfeld@kssg.ch

© Springer-Verlag GmbH Germany, part of Springer Nature 2020
A. am Zehnhoff-Dinnesen et al. (eds.), *Phoniatrics I*, European Manual of Medicine,
https://doi.org/10.1007/978-3-662-46780-0_11

R. Schönweiler
Department of Phoniatrics and Pediatric Audiology,
University Clinic of Schleswig-Holstein, Campus
Lübeck, Lübeck, Germany
e-mail: rainer.schoenweiler@phoniatrie.uni-luebeck.de

A. P. Vogel
Centre for Neuroscience of Speech, The University
of Melbourne, Parkville, VIC, Australia
e-mail: vogela@unimelb.edu.au

D. Weise
Abteilung Neuropädiatrie, Universitätsmedizin
Göttingen, Göttingen, Germany
e-mail: dweise@med.uni-goettingen.de

11.1 Diagnostic Interview with Parents

Rainer Schönweiler

If a child is referred to a speech-language specialist for a suspected speech-language disorder or delay, a comprehensive diagnostic interview is the most important step to elucidate the nature of the problem and to select appropriate tests from the many existing (de Langen-Müller et al. 2011; Schönweiler 1993; Tomasello 2000). During the oral part of the interview, the chronological and developmental age of the child should be taken into account (de Langen-Müller et al. 2011; Schönweiler 1993). A standard test battery may not cover individual symptoms of a child such as a specific reduction of consonant clusters or a morphological grammar error. In this case, a diagnostic interview provides valuable hints on the selection of an appropriate, individually tailored test procedure to confirm or exclude the error.

An accurate record of the complaints and symptoms uttered during the first visit that had initiated the consultation of the speech-language specialist is important and serves as base for comparison during follow-up visits. The oral part of the interview assesses information on current complaints and medical history. In addition, questionnaires or forms may be used and filled in by parents or other caregivers either before the first visit or in the waiting area. A physician should not expect the parents to understand all the questions right; it is better to take time to discuss the answers point by point and add the missing information.

Other valuable sources of information are prior medical records, letters and other documents related to previous treatments and examinations. Parents should be asked to bring along all available relevant documents and materials, such as CT images or X-rays, to their first and, may be, also later appointments either as copies for the medical documents or in order to copy them if needed.

If a developmental disorder or delay of speech and language is the main reason for the visit, the interview should start with questions addressing the time of the first appearance of characteristic speech-language skills as remembered by the parents as well as examples of the child's present communicative abilities. If other caregivers are involved in parenting, their impressions should be added to the protocol of this interview. For future counselling of such cases, it is important to enquire about which person—caregiver or professional helper—has initiated the visit and which symptom or combination of symptoms has been the main reason for the visit. In other words, one should start with questions characterizing communication and symptoms of a suspected speech-language disorder (de Langen-Müller et al. 2011; Tomasello 2000). Questions should address either the developmental speech-language level a child has reached for his or her chronological age related to the expected stages of typical language development or acquired skills related to the actual developmental age if an intellectual or general developmental delay is present or suspected (Table 11.1), especially for premature children.

Exemplary questions are: At what age did the child utter words such as 'Mom', 'Pa', names of siblings or 'No'? At what age did the first two-word sentence come? How many words does the child speak at present? Did the parents count the number of words, or—much better—did they make a list of

Table 11.1 Questions characterizing speech-language abilities arranged by developmental stage and age

Level of language development	Ability	Percentile 50 (milestones) (references)	Percentile 90 (cornerstones) (references)	Suggested question for parents and caregivers
Vocalization	Reduplicating babbling	6 months (Gerken 1994; Largo et al. 1986; Oller et al. 1999; Papoušek and Papoušek 1989; Penner 2000)	8–10 months (Largo et al. 1986; Oller et al. 1999)	At what age did your child use doubled syllables such as 'baba'?
Phonetic and phonological level	Correct articulation of all speech sounds except sibilants	4 years and 6 months (Fox 2006; Fox and Dodd 1999; Schäfer and Fox 2006)		At what age did your child speak vowels and consonants correctly (except sibilants)?
Semantic and receptive lexical level	First language comprehension	9 months (Bates et al. 1994)		At what age did your child first understand words such as 'no' or names?
Expressive lexical level	Speaking first words	13 months (Bates et al. 1994, 1995; Kauschke 1999; Menyuk et al. 1995)	18–20 months (Largo et al. 1986)	At what age did your child speak its first word(s)?
	Speaks 'mama' ('mom', 'mum', 'mummy') or 'papa' ('pop', 'dad', 'daddy')	10–15 months (Zollinger 2004)	18–20 months (Largo et al. 1986)	At what age did your child first call you 'mama' ('mom', 'mum', 'mummy') or 'papa' ('pop', 'dad', 'daddy')?
	Speaks roughly 50 words	18 months (Kauschke 1999; Menyuk et al. 1995)	24 months (Szagun and Steinbrink 2004)	At what age did your child speak 50 words? Did you make a list of the words?
	Hierarchical organizing of words	3 years (McGregor et al. 2002; McGregor and Waxman 1998)		At what age did your child know 'apple' as a fruit or 'carrot' as a vegetable?
Morphological and syntactic level (grammar)	Uses two-word sentences	18–24 months (Clahsen 1986; Tomasello 2000; Weissenborn 2000)	25–26 months (Kauschke 1999; Menyuk et al. 1995)	At what age did your child first combine two words?
	Uses three-word sentences	24–30 months (Clahsen 1986; Kauschke 1999; Szagun and Steinbrink 2004)	No data	At what age did your child first combine up to three words to a sentence?
	Uses questions	30–36 months (Clahsen 1986; Penner and Kölliker-Funk 1998; Rothweiler 2002; Weissenborn 2000)	No data	At what age did your child first use a sentence as a question?
	Uses subordinate clauses	36 months (Rothweiler 1999, 2002)	No data	At what age did your child first use a subordinate clause?
Pragmatic level	Respects turn-taking in conversations	2 years (Karmiloff and Karmiloff-Smith 2001)		At what age did your child respect turn-taking in a conversation?
	Organizes themes in conversations	3 years (Karmiloff and Karmiloff-Smith 2001)		At what age was your child able to tell you something that happened?
Fluency	Speaks without word repetitions, prolongations, blocks and remarkable coping strategies			Does your child speak fluently most of the time? (Note that word repetitions at age around 3 are 'normal')

words their child uses or has used at certain developmental milestones such as the second birthday?

It is also important to know whether parents apply any strategies to improve the communicative abilities of the child. It might be helpful to demonstrate a typical example of corrective feedback (improved repetition of an utterance) or parallel talk (parent parallels the child's actions verbally and repeats utterances of the child correctly and unobtrusively without requiring answers to questions): Is one of these methods known by the parents?

A developmental speech-language disorder can be suspected if answers at one or more subscales of the developmental language scale have been found to be below the normative developmental age of the child. The respective answers in a diagnostic interview also help to choose appropriate tests to confirm the diagnosis of a speech-language disorder.

The next step of the interview is to take an accurate record on the medical history (Table 11.2). Typically, the clinician starts to ask for birth-related information including gestational age at birth, premature conditions, risk indicators and neonatal screening results, specifically neonatal hearing screening (Schönweiler 1993; Tomasello 2000). In many countries, such information is kept in previous medical records. The next questions address the presence of ear and hearing problems, such as episodes of acute otitis media or periods of otitis media with effusion and other typical causes of late-onset hearing loss (Schönweiler 1993; de Langen-Müller et al. 2011) that may affect the development of speech and language (de Langen-Müller et al. 2011; Schönweiler 2004). The clinician needs to ask for syndromes, malformations such as cleft palate and other chronic diseases. Some of these conditions require physical examination following the interview. Further questions should address the motor skills including feeding history and oral-motor functioning, furthermore the nutrition status, the cognitive, memory play and visual skills as well as the child's daily activities (Tomasello 2000).

The interview continues with questions on recent treatments and otherwise interventions (Schönweiler 1993; Tomasello 2000). For instance, a child may have undergone surgery for otitis media with effusion, cleft lip or palate and cardiac defects. In cases of severe illness or complications, a child may have been hospitalized for a long time. In particular, a phoniatrician should ask whether ear surgery has been performed and whether the adenoid glands or the tonsils have been removed or if such a surgery is planned.

Questions should also focus on recent diagnostic examinations, counselling, trainings and other remediation services including their quality and quantity. Have the parents already been counselled on linguistic enrichment principles such as narrative reading and corrective feedback? If a training or therapy is ongoing, it should be asked for the kind of professionals involved, the methods used and the total amount and frequency of sessions administered so far. If no treatment is running, the physician should ask whether the child is in a 'wait-and-see' phase at current. Parents should be also asked whether a child is under medication and if so to provide details such as generic names and dosages. Furthermore, information is needed about diagnostic and therapeutic steps that have already been planned by other professionals.

In order to assess the familial risk of speech, language and hearing disorders, it is important to document the health history of family members (Table 11.3). A useful starting point may be to ask if members of the family suffer from speech-language disorders, dyslexia, fluency disorders or hearing loss. If affirmed more information should be gathered, for example, on receipt of speech-language services, participation in special educational programmes because of a disability or the use of hearing aids.

Questions should also address the child's emotional and social development and environmental situation (Schönweiler 1993; Tomasello 2000). It should be asked whether a child lives at home, together with the family, or if she or he grows up with a single parent or in a home where one parent is often absent or where grandparents or other caregivers overtake the care. Information should be gained also on the presence and number of siblings, their age and the position of the child in the

Table 11.2 Medical history in children with a suspected speech-language disorder

Topic	Diagnoses	Related question	Treatments and therapeutic interventions	Related questions
Birth	Preterm birth, low birth weight, hypoxia, hyperbilirubinemia, risk factors for DDLS	At what gestational age was the child born? Was the birth 'normal' or 'complicated'? What exactly happened? What was the result of the neonatal hearing screening test?	Stay at neonatal intensive care unit (NICU), blood transfusion, oxygen, extracorporeal membrane oxygenation (ECMO), aminoglycosides	After birth, was your child in hospital for a long period? What kind of treatment did your child receive?
Hearing	Congenital hearing loss, periods of serous or mucous otitis media with effusion, acute otitis media, mastoiditis, auditory deprivation, meningitis, encephalitis, cerebral insult, head trauma	Does your child suffer from a permanent hearing loss or ear infection? When was it diagnosed?	Ear surgery, hearing aids, cochlear implants, bone conduction implants, middle ear implants, educational programme for hard-of-hearing children	Does your child wear hearing aids or an implant? Did your child undergo ear surgery?
Malformations	Craniofacial abnormalities such as cleft lip, cleft palate, preauricular or neck fistulas, malformations of the auricula, preauricular lobes, stenosis or atresia of the outer ear canal, facial dysmorphia such as hypertelorism or epicantus; other malformations concerning, for example, the brain, heart, kidneys, liver or limbs	Does your child suffer from a malformation?	Surgical treatment	Has your child received a surgical treatment? How long did he or she stay in hospital?
Speech-language development	Developmental language delay (late talker); developmental disorder of speech and language (DDSL), subclassified in specific (or primary) DDSL and DDSL with language-relevant comorbidities (DDSLC or unspecific or secondary DDSL); speech fluency disorder	See Table 11.1, column 'Suggested questions for parents and caregivers'	Counselling on linguistic enrichment and corrective feedback, training interventions, educational programmes	Have you already been counselled on how to facilitate the speech-language abilities of your child? Has your child already received a speech-language therapy? Does your child attend an educational programme? Or is your attitude 'wait and see'?
Psychomotor, oromotor and cognitive development	Developmental disorder or delay, cerebral palsy (CP), seizure disorders, dyspraxia, ataxia	Does your child suffer from any developmental delay or disorder?	Training, educational programmes	What kind of training therapies or services does your child receive, e.g. physiotherapy? Does your child attend an educational programme? Or is your attitude 'wait and see'?
Other diseases	For example, hypothyreosis	Did neonatal screening or follow-up examinations reveal any other diseases?	Medical treatment	Does your child need medication? Which ones and what dosages?

Table 11.3 Interview on family history of speech, language and hearing disorders, developmental delay and intellectual retardation

Topic	Relevant diagnoses	Related questions
Speech and language	Developmental language delay (late talker); developmental disorder of speech and language (DDSL), either specific (or primary) DDSL or DDSL with language-relevant comorbidities (DDSLC or unspecific or secondary DDSL); speech fluency disorder	Do members of the family suffer from a speech-language disorder, dyslexia or fluency disorder?
Hearing	Congenital hearing loss (conductive or sensorineural), ear malformation (e.g. preauricular fistulas or lobes, ear canal atresia)	Do members of the family suffer from hearing loss? Did or do members of the family wear hearing aids or a hearing implant? Did members of the family receive a surgical correction of an inborn ear abnormality?
Psychomotor, oromotor and cognitive skills	Developmental disorder or delay, cerebral palsy (CP), seizure disorders, dyspraxia, ataxia	Did or do members of the family suffer from neurological or psychiatric diseases? Did or do family members receive a special education because of a disability?

sequence of siblings. Furthermore, it should be asked about the daily care for the child, for example, whether she or he attends a kindergarten.

Questions of the diagnostic interview should be carefully formulated in order to avoid embarrassing the parents. For example, medically important questions on consanguinity, professional qualifications and educational background of the parents might sometimes be perceived to be personal or intrusive and might cause discomfort. Sometimes parents are not prepared to answer certain questions immediately. It might be appropriate then to return to relevant questions later after the clinician had gained more trust from the parents.

11.2 Questionnaires on Child Development

Jochen Rosenfeld

11.2.1 Definition

Questionnaires are instruments for targeted assessment of one or more developmental domains of a child. In the context of early childhood development, they are often used for the detection of developmental risks in terms of secondary prevention. They are considered an effective and reasonable method for the screening for developmental peculiarities.

11.2.2 Construction Principles

For parent questionnaires, which assess the developmental status of children, various question-answer formats are used: in partially standardized questionnaires, the questions usually are uniform, and the answers of the interviewees are open (open-ended questions). This format is used in questions on a child's history such as pregnancy, delivery or medication.

In standardized questionnaires, the questions are expressed uniformly too, but the answers are predetermined (closed-ended questions). Possible predetermined types of answer for closed-ended questions are dichotomous (two possible answers, e.g. for yes/no questions) or polytomous answers (more than two predetermined answers). The scaling (measure) of answers to questions, based on the level of measurement (Trochim 2006), can be nominal (e.g. gender), ordinal (e.g. highest educational level) or by interval (e.g. age).

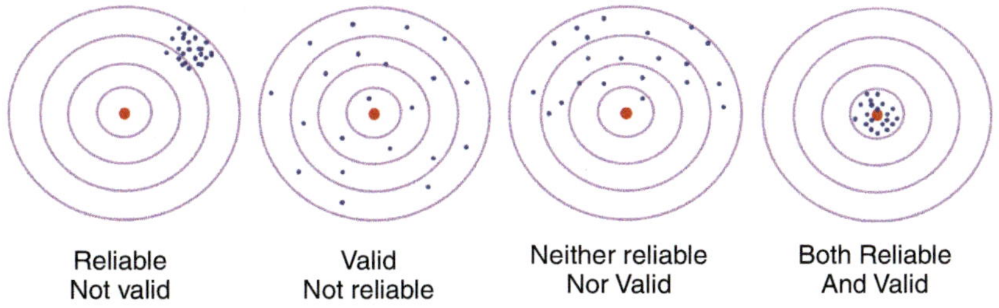

Reliable
Not valid

Valid
Not reliable

Neither reliable
Nor Valid

Both Reliable
And Valid

Fig. 11.1 Relationship between validity and reliability of psychometric tests (From Trochim and Donnelly (2007). The Research Methods Knowledge Base, 3E. © 2007 Custom Solutions, a part of Cengage, Inc. Reproduced by permission. www.cengage.com/permissions)

11.2.3 Quality Criteria

Standardized questionnaires have to fulfil the primary quality criteria of well-designed tests and assessments:

- Validity for psychometric tests according to the American Educational Research Association, American Psychological Association and National Council on Measurement in Education (2014)

  …the degree to which evidence and theory support the interpretations of test scores.

- Reliability according to Trochim (2006) the consistency and repeatability of measures, which are interdependent (Fig. 11.1)
- Objectivity, the independence of a test result from general conditions and confounding factors such as environmental conditions or examiners

If they rely on normative data, the representativeness of the validation sample (e.g. examined population) is fundamental. Relevant secondary quality criteria are the acceptance by respondents (e.g. comprehensibility, reasonability), economics (e.g. costs, investigation time, analysis time) and usefulness (e.g. consequences such as early intervention for a child who has been classified as being impaired).

11.2.4 Limitations

Partially standardized questionnaires with open-ended questions offer the respondent more freedom to answer questions according to the individual situation and therefore to describe the reality as closely as possible. They have the downside, however, that a standardized evaluation is not possible unless a post hoc assignment of answers to standard formats is done, in order to enable generalization. On the contrary, standardized questionnaires are sometimes criticized because their predetermined answers may appear schematic and misleading or miss the individually appropriate answer, so that the specific situation of the respondent cannot be fully described. Nevertheless, on the whole they reveal the more reliable and trustworthy results and are the main tools of psychometric tests, for example, in psychology. Sources of potential error can hamper data evaluation, such as skipping questions because they are not clear, doubtful answers due to unclear questions or unintended response bias (e.g. extreme responding, social desirability bias, acquiescence bias).

11.2.5 Implications

Questionnaires on child development either refer to various developmental domains such as motor, cognitive, socio-emotional and language (e.g. Ages and Stages Questionnaires (ASQ-3), Squires et al. 2009; Parents' Evaluation of Developmental Status (PEDS), Glascoe 1999; Parents' Evaluation of Developmental Status—Developmental Milestones, Brothers et al. 2008) or to one domain (e.g. MacArthur-Bates communicative development inventories, Fenson et al. 2007; Language Development Survey, Rescorla 1989; Parent

Language Checklist, Burden et al. 1996; Structured Screening Test, Laing et al. 2002). They are often used as screening instruments for assessment of developmental risks. For-parent questionnaires especially have proven of value, as these can be filled in at home or in the waiting room of a doctor's office. Mostly, only little time is required from the medical staff to analyse the results. If they are atypical, elaborate diagnostics should follow.

11.3 Assessment of the Developmental Speech and Language Status of Children

Katrin Neumann

11.3.1 Normal Language Development: The Concept of Milestones and Border Stones

For the proper evaluation of the language status of a child, knowledge of the distinct age-appropriate developmental targets of the acquisition of a specific language is necessary. As for other domains of infant and child development, the concept of milestones and borderline stones is useful for characterizing important steps in the acquisition of the native language for each linguistic domain (Kliegman et al. 2011). As demonstrated in Table 11.4 for the example of German language acquisition, milestones indicate at which average age a child has reached domain-specific levels of competence. Border stones are distinct developmental targets that are reached by 90% of all normally developed children by a certain age (Michaelis 2004).

11.3.2 Diagnostics of Developmental Disorders of Speech and Language

For the diagnosis of developmental disorders of speech and language (DDSL), the separation of specific developmental disorders of speech and language (SDDSL) and DDSL with comorbidities has to be taken into consideration. Hence the first step of the diagnostic process is to seek comorbidities, because SDDSL is an exclusion diagnosis. Furthermore, DDSL have to be distinguished from socioculturally caused environmental language abnormalities, which do not need treatment but language input and training (see Sect. 9.8).

11.3.2.1 Analysis of Spontaneous Speech

The analysis of spontaneous speech is an important tool in the diagnostics of developmental language deficits, and it complements language tests. It is based on the observation of the child during a guided game or a dialogue, mostly with adults (parents or examiner). It is important to create situations that stimulate the child to communicate. Speech and language-related behaviour and utterances of the child have to be documented. Video recordings may be helpful for language and interaction analyses and may also provide information on the parental communicative behaviour and style. From such informal observations, important information about phonetic-phonological, semantic-lexical, morphologic-syntactical and pragmatic-communicative abilities of a child can be gained. Furthermore, prosody, speech fluency and motivation to speak and to communicate as well as joyfulness of speaking may be analysed. For the evaluation of the spoken utterances, speech competence (the mastery of the speech-language systems) has to be distinguished from performance (the demonstration of the competence while communicating). Speech-language diagnostics aims to elicit as much as possible competence via performance within a short time (Neumann et al. 2009).

For a more thorough analysis of spontaneous speech, a detailed transcription, coding and analysis of language samples can be gained from audio or video recordings. Computer programs may be useful here, such as the Systematic Analysis of Language Transcripts (SALT) (Miller et al. 2011; SALT Software 2014) and the Computerized Language Analysis (CLAN)

Table 11.4 Time course of the normal German language acquisition (modified according to de Langen-Müller et al. 2012, with kind permission from Peter Lang GmbH, Internationaler Verlag der Wissenschaften)

Domain	Stage of development	Milestone (average age)	Borderline stone (age at 90th percentile)
Early language perception	Interest in human language ('eavesdropping')	Prenatally, first weeks of life	
	Perception of rhythmic and prosodic features of mother tongue	Prenatally, first weeks of life	
Development of vocalization	Crying	Birth	
	Cooing	Sixth to eighth week	
	Marginal babbling (testing of sound production)	Fourth month	
	Canonic babbling (syllables of consonants and vowels, e.g. *ba*)	Sixth month	Eighth to tenth month
	Reduplicated babbling (doubling of syllables, e.g. *baba*)	Eighth to tenth month	11th to 15th month
	Varying babbling (e.g. *bada*)	Eighth to tenth month	
Acquisition of the phonological system	Elementary sound inventory	12th month	
	Simple syllable structures (mostly open syllables)		
	Starting organization of the phonological system (use of sounds of the target language)	18th month	
	Starting to overcome phonological processes (systematic developmental changes of pronunciation of the target language)	2.5–4.5 year of life	
	Development of phonological awareness: detect syllables; 'clap' syllables; detect rhymes; detect initial sounds	About third year of life	
	Development of phonological awareness: detect and localize phonemes (smallest contrasting unit regarding meaning in the sound system), segmentation, analysis and synthesis of sounds into words	About fifth year of life	
Acquisition of vocabulary	Starting to understand words	Ninth month	
	Understanding approximately 50 words	16th month	
	Pre-forms of naming (situation-dependent proto-words)	Tenth month	
	Purposeful usage of *mama* and *papa*	Tenth to 15th month	18th to 20th month
	Production of the first words (one-word utterances)	13th to 20th month at latest	18th to 20th month
	Production of at least 50 words	18th to 24th month at latest	24th month
	Vocabulary spurt	18th to 21th month	
	Stage 1: personal/social words (*yes*, *hello*), relational words (*there*, *on*), onomatopoeia, proper names, some nouns	12th to 18th month	
	Stage 2: noun growth, start of verb acquisition	19th to 30th month	
	Stage 3: verb growth, function words (*because*), pronouns	30th to 36th month	
	Overextensions and underextensions (e.g. *dog/bow-wow* for naming all animals)	Second year of life	
	Acquisition of the hierarchical organization of the mental lexicon; understanding semantic relations	Third year of life till school age	
	Acquisition of word formation: compounding (composition, e.g. *front door*) + derivation (e.g. *heat → heater*; *sun → sunny*)	Second to fifth year of life	

(continued)

Table 11.4 (continued)

Domain	Stage of development	Milestone (average age)	Borderline stone (age at 90th percentile)
Acquisition of grammar	Production of word combinations (two- or more-word utterances)	18th to 24th month at latest	25th to 26th month
	Increase of utterance length: at the age of 3 years, approximately 3 words per utterance on average	Third year of life	
	Production of simple syntactic structures	Third year of life	
	Decrease of omissions of obligatory constituents (e.g. subject)	Third year of life	
	Decrease of omissions of function words	Third to fourth year of life	
	Verbs in second position (*Lisa cake eat → Lisa eats cake* or *What eats Lisa?*)	30th to 36th month	
	Use of variable sentence types: declarative sentence, interrogative sentence, exclamatory sentence	30th to 36th month	
	Occurrence of subordinate clauses	36th month	
	Use of the definite article (*the*)	30th to 36th month	
	Correct subject-verb congruency (*I eat—she eats*)	Second to third year of life	
	Acquisition of the German case system, accusative at first, dative later	36th month to school entry age	
	Acquisition of the plural system	Second to sixth year of life	
	Acquisition of tempus markers	Third year of life	
	Temporary grammatical overextensions (*I runned away.*)	Third to fourth year of life	
Development of conversational and narrative abilities	Eye contact with primary attachment figure	Third month	
	Early expression of communicative intentions via looking, gestures and vocalizations	First year of life	
	Triangular eye contact	Ninth month	
	Establishing shared focus of attention		
	Adherence to turn-taking rules	Second year of life	
	Child relates to conversation partner in dialogue	18th month	
	Organization of topics in dialogue	Third year of life	
	Development of narrative competence; increasing coherence (content-related) and cohesion (formal connection of text elements) in narration	36th month to early school age	
	Understanding irony and metaphors	Sixth year of life	
Literary language acquisition	Logographic stage (recognition of frequent words)	Preschool age, early elementary school age	
	Alphabetic stage (linkage between sounds and letters)	Early elementary school age	
	Orthographic stage (learning of orthographic rules)	Elementary school age	

Program (MacWhinney 1995), which is a part of the Child Language Data Exchange System (CHILDES 2014), a database of speech audio files and text transcriptions in more than 20 languages serving as a central repository for first-language acquisition data (CHILDES 2014). Transcripts are necessary to calculate, for example, the mean length of utterances (MLU). This is a measure of linguistic productivity and language proficiency in children. It is the average number of morphemes per utterance contained in a sample of 100 utterances. The MLU is a benchmark of language acquisition, a good marker of DDSL, and may predict the further reading abilities of children (Bishop and Adams 1990; Rice et al. 2010). However, because the usefulness of MLU is questioned, it should not be used as the only diagnostic measure of language proficiency in children.

11.3.2.2 Examination of the Developmental Speech and Language Status with Informal and Nonstandardized Procedures

For a rough, informal evaluation of the phonetic-phonological, semantic-lexical and pragmatic competence of a child, simple test tools such as picture cards are suitable. Grammatical abilities might also be judged by using pictures that stimulate the production of specific grammatical structures, such as 'Brush your teeth!' to elicit the imperative or 'This is one apple, and these are two…?' for eliciting information on plural production (Neumann et al. 2011). The informal judgement of the types of language-related competence of a child requires the knowledge from professionals on the age-appropriate developmental targets (milestones) for each tested linguistic level (see Table 11.4).

11.3.2.3 Language Tests

The assessment of language skills should be performed with valid and normed tests, in order to get, as far as possible, examiner-independent, reproducible and reliable results. The use of only such tests enables the comparison of an individual test result with normal values, its interpretation and a differentiated evaluation of a child's language developmental status compared with the age norm. Comprehensive language tests that examine all or at least some linguistic levels have to be distinguished from tests that analyse only one type of competence, for example, vocabulary. The scores of single subtests of comprehensive tests ought not to be interpreted separately for different linguistic domains (grammar, vocabulary, etc.); otherwise such tests would reveal more children suspected of a DDSL than its prevalence (Neumann et al. 2011). In other words, if many subtests are performed, the probability is high by chance alone that at least one of them would indi-

cate a deficit, which may lead to overdiagnosis. Therefore, a weighting system is required that evaluates test results according to the severity and prognosis of the specific deficiency.

Principles of the Interpretation of Test Values
Test results may be available as raw values or standardized values. Raw values are related to scores that result from an assignment prescription of a test. This could be, for example, the number of correct results in a language test or a sum score in a questionnaire test based on Likert scales ranging from 0 (does not fit at all) to 5 (fits perfectly). Raw values are useful (a) when related to reaching a cutoff value and as a base for (b) different categories (e.g. below average, average, above average) and (c) further transformations, e.g. in standardized values. Standardized values, on the other hand, are easier to interpret than raw values.

> *Example*: A child has performed a speech perception test and has solved 6 of 10 items correctly. At first glance this suggests a quite good test result, which, however, may be oversimplified and wrong, because from the reference values it is clear that in the normative sample all children are able to solve five items correctly, and the majority of subjects even at least six items. A transformation of the raw value '6' into a standardized value, for example into the 10th percentile (to be interpreted roughly as: 90% of the subjects of the normative sample have solved more items) or a value that is even more related to the distribution of the normative values, such as the intelligence quotient, indicate a rather 'below average' result in this example (Petermann and Macha 2005).

A classical test construction is based on standard scales. For the tests applied during the assessment of DDSL/SDDSL, percentile scales, z scales, T scales, C scales and intelligence scales are used most frequently (Fig. 11.2). Standard scales enable the identification of the position of an examined child relative to a control sample. This requires an empirically gained reference frame from a sufficiently large, representative control sample. The named scales relate a test value to the average of the standard distribution and to the variance of the latter in order to answer the question: Is, or by how much is, the test score above or below the average?

The standardized values shown in Fig. 11.2 follow this sequence: (a) The average value of a

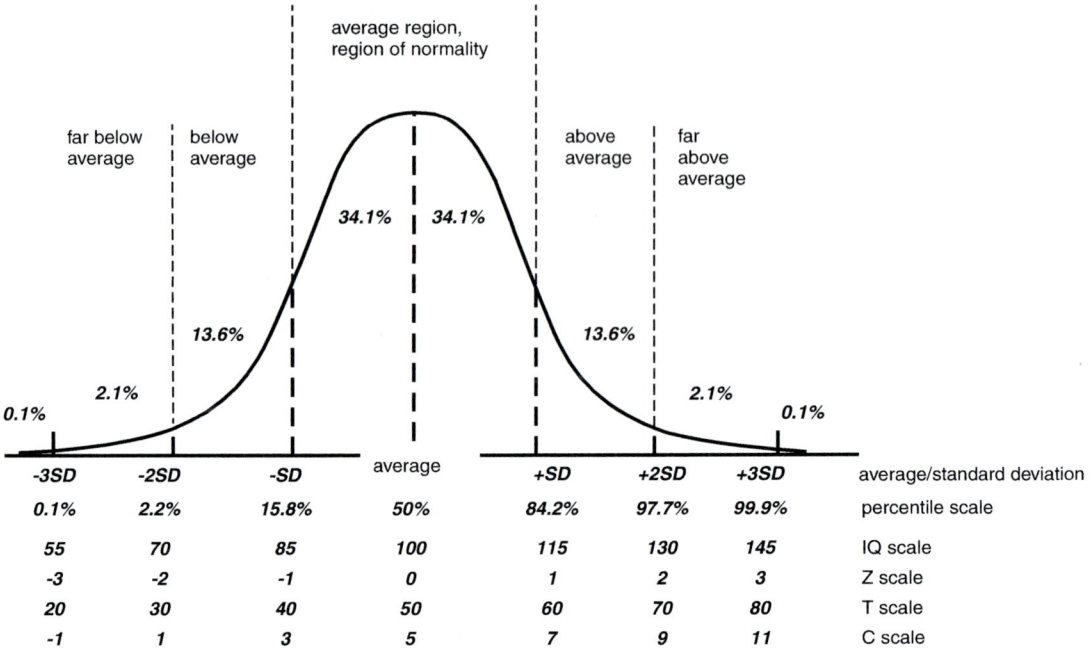

Fig. 11.2 Principles of generation of standard values and frequently used standard scales for the assessment of DDSL/SDDSL. Percentile, *z*-, *T*-, *C*- and intelligence (IQ) scales: selected standard values in a normal distribution (Gaussian curve) and convention of their interpretation (modified according to Petermann and Macha (2005) with kind permission from the authors)

distribution is identified. (b) A numerical value according to the chosen scale is attributed to the average. The percentile scale attributes the percentage of 50 to the average of the scale; the IQ scale, the IQ value 100; the *z* scale, the *z* value 0; the *T* scale, the *T* value 50; and the *C* scale, the value 5. (c) In order to interpret a test score, the spread of the distribution is of interest, in particular the distance between the average and the standard deviation (SD), because the test values on a specific scale are related to the SD. For example, the IQ scale subdivides the distance between the average and one standard deviation into 15 scale units (an IQ value of 85 represents an intelligence that deviates 1 SD from the average downwards; an IQ of 70 indicates a deviation of 2 SD from the average downwards). The *T* scale attributes 10 points to the distance of the SD from the average. In this way each of the scales enables the quantification of direction and extent of a deviation from the average by a scale value.

The percentages given on the Gaussian bell curve of a normal distribution are useful for ori-entation. They indicate the proportion of subjects of a sample (e.g. the norming sample) which is in the respective performance range. Between −1 and +1 SD lie about 68.2% of all subjects, i.e. more than two thirds. Below −1 SD are located the worst 15.8% of the subjects of the normative sample related to the values of a specific test; below −2 SD, the worst 2.2%; and below −3 SD, the worst 0.1%.

Related to those reference values, the performance in a certain test can be interpreted. The region between −1 and +1 SD from the average is regarded as the average or normal region (~68.2% of all subjects), i.e. a *T* value of 43 or an IQ of 91 is 'average'. The deviation of a test value of more than one but not more than two SD from the average may be interpreted as 'below average' or 'above average' (13.6% of subjects are located on each side of the average distribution). The 'below average' region is often considered as a region of risk. Thus, a *T* value of 35 or the 12th percentile is 'below average' and an IQ value of 125 'above average'. Deviations of more than ±2 SD from the average may be named 'far below/above average' (2.2% on each side). A *T* value of 26 or the second percentile is thus 'far below average' and an IQ < 70 as well (regarded an intellectual disability), and an IQ > 130 is 'far above average' (intellectual giftedness) (Petermann and Macha 2005).

Diagnostic Criteria for Specific Developmental Disorders of Speech and Language Four diagnostic criteria are defined for the diagnosis of an SDDSL (F80.1 and F80.2) according to the International Statistical Classification of Diseases and Related Health Problems, the ICD-10 of the World Health Organization (2011), slightly modified by Dilling et al. (2008) and de Langen-Müller et al. (2012). They are based on the discrepancy between the language skills of a child and the age-related normative values and on the assumption of normality. According to this assumption, neurological, sensory, emotional, social or physical disorders, which could explain the language problems, are lacking. There is no reduced intelligence (IQ < 85, as measured with a nonverbal intelligence test).

- Perceptive and expressive language skills, as assessed from standardized and normed tests, are 1.5–2 SD below the age-dependent normative values at one or more than one language/communicative level.
- The expressive and receptive language skills, as assessed by structured behavioural and linguistic analyses, are considerably below the average abilities of the age norm.
- The use and understanding of nonverbal communication are within the age norm.
- The assumption of normality is justified.

Additionally, the ICD-10 defines a double discrepancy criterion between cognitive and language competence: for an SDDSL diagnosis, language perception or language production of a child is below the level appropriate for his or her age. Additionally, the receptive/expressive language competence is 1–1.5 SD below the nonverbal IQ that is at least average (IQ ≥ 85) (see criteria 1 and 4). This criterion is, however, under debate.

A diagnostic algorithm as shown in Fig. 11.3 demonstrates the steps of an interdisciplinary

diagnostics of a (S)DDSL and the subsequent interventions. If there is suspicion of an age-inappropriate language development, audiological assessment of the hearing of a child is inevitable. Thereafter, the language competence is assessed. A subsequent differential diagnostics does not follow a fixed scheme but depends on the specific symptoms (de Langen-Müller et al. 2012). If there is suspicion of an SDDSL, possible comorbidities have to be excluded.

11.3.2.4 Screening Tests for the Developmental Speech and Language Status

Parent questionnaires have been shown to be a useful screening for the language development status of young children (Dale 1991). Universal or regional screening tests at kindergarten or pre-school ages, i.e. short and easy to perform and to analyze language tests, have been implemented in some European regions. They aim at the detection and support of children with language abnormalities by either language therapy or training, in order to ensure sufficient language competence at school entry. In most cases such screening can distinguish between children who have language abnormalities and those who do not. Only a few screening tests, such as the German Kindersprachscreening (KiSS.2), trichotomize between (a) normally developed children, (b) children who have sociogenically caused language abnormalities and who require language training and (c) those who are suspect for having a DDSL and need therapy (Neumann and Euler 2013).

In order to evaluate the validity of a screening, the proportion of children who fail it (REFER, screening-positive) and of those who pass it (PASS, screening-negative) have to be evaluated by comparing the results of the screening and those of reference language tests (gold standard) in a sufficient large, unselected sample of screened children. Furthermore, the proportion of false and correct positives (REFER rate) and false and correct negatives (PASS rate) have to be calculated (Table 11.5). From these values, sensitivity and specificity of the screening may be calculated, the most important validity criteria. Specificity measures the ability of language screening to detect children with normal

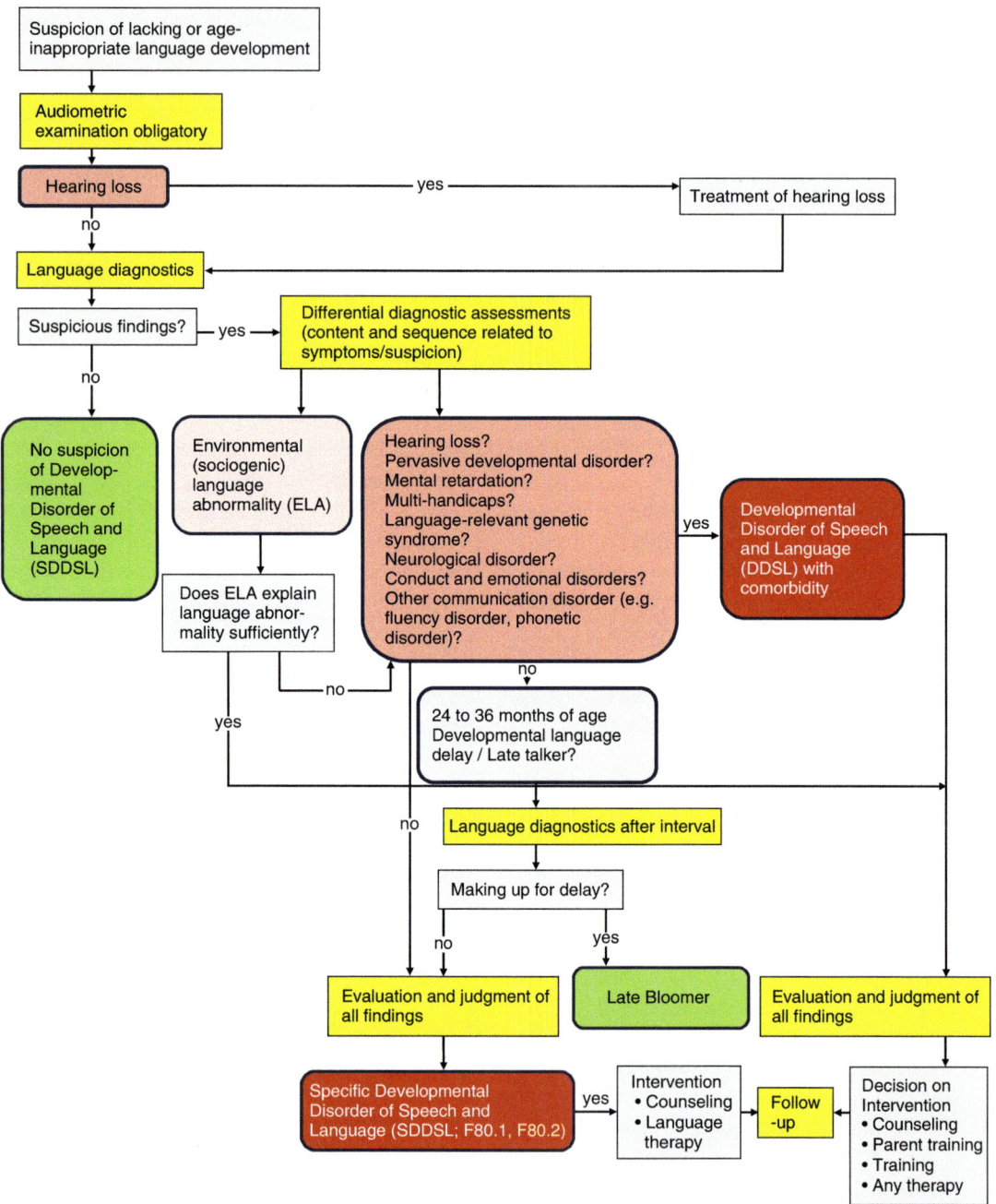

Fig. 11.3 Diagnostic algorithm for developmental disorders of speech and language (modified according to de Langen-Müller et al. 2012, with kind permission from Peter Lang GmbH, Internationaler Verlag der Wissenschaften)

language development correctly, and the sensitivity indicates the ability to identify children with language abnormalities correctly.

Sensitivity and specificity of screening are related to each other. This can be demonstrated by a receiver operating characteristic (ROC)

curve, which shows the ability of screening to distinguish between two conditions such as PASS and REFER (Fig. 11.4).

For a PASS/REFER decision, a cut-off criterion has to be defined. Cut-off values may be derived from the prevalence of a disease. If the

Table 11.5 Agreement between the results of language screening and diagnostic language assessment with language tests

		Diagnostic tests		
		DDSL (D+)	No DDSL (D−)	Total
Screening	REFER (S+)	**cp**	fp	cp+fp
	PASS (S−)	**fn**	rn	fn+cn
	Total	cp+fn	fp+rn	cp+fp+cn+fn

S+ screening-positive, *S−* screening-negative, *D+* diagnostics-positive, *D−* diagnostics-negative, *cp* correct positive, *cn* correct negative, *fp* false positive, *fn* false negative

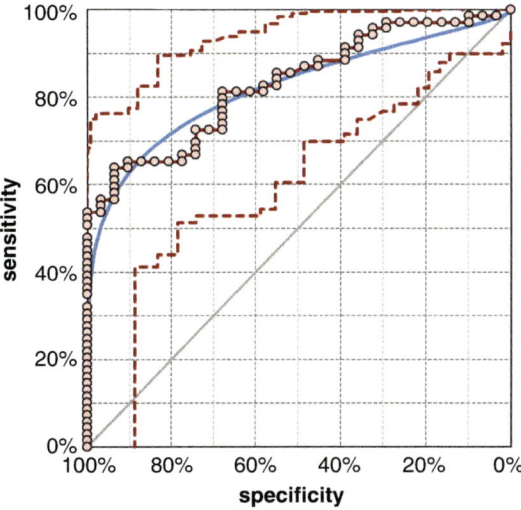

Fig. 11.4 Hypothetical ROC curve of a screening procedure. Because for ROC analyses the original proportions of false positives have been used, which are 1-specificity, the *x*-axis values descend from 100. The figure demonstrates an ROC curve (circles), a trend curve assuming a normal distribution of the data (blue curve), the upper and lower 95% confidence limits (dashed red lines) and the diagonal (grey line). The predictive power of a screening starts above the diagonal. The larger the AUC, the higher the validity of the screening. An increase in specificity in the decision algorithm of the screening results in a decrease of the sensitivity. An ideal curve would run rectangularly along the *y*-axis and the upper borderline of the diagram. Image adapted from Keller (2014) with kind permission of Dr. Thomas Keller

prevalence of SDDSL is given as 4–7% and that of DDSL with comorbidity estimates at least 3%, then diagnostic testing for DDSL should not reveal much more than 10% of children in a normal population who fail it, which is between −1 and −2 SD (see 'Diagnostic Criteria' in Sect. 11.3.2.3). For screening the borderlines have to be extended, because a certain number of false positives (children who do not pass the test but have no DDSL) have to be accepted in order to minimize the number of false negatives (children who pass the test despite a DDSL). The cut-off value of a screening depends on a trade-off between the proportion of false negatives that is acceptable and that of false positives, which would increase the number of children who have to undergo follow-up diagnostics. It seems reasonable that screening should reveal about 15% of children who do not pass it in order to get the (at maximum) 10% of children who really have a DDSL from subsequent diagnostics.

The real language status of a child and the screening result for a given cut-off point can be compared in a contingency table (Table 11.5). In ROC curves the value pairs of specificity and sensitivity of a screening are drawn for all possible cut-off values. The area under the curve (AUC) indicates the validity of a screening. The more it approaches 1, the higher the validity.

Language screening programs are crucial because (a) children without language abnormalities are easier to detect than those with abnormalities (Law et al. 2000), (b) the language development for each specific linguistic competence has large variance and (c) there is often only poor evidence for a sufficient validity of a reference tests. Therefore, sensitivities and specificities of language screening that do not lie below 80% are assumed by convention to be acceptable (Petermann and Macha 2005; Plante and Vance 1994).

11.3.2.5 Examples of Language Screening, General and Specific Speech-Language Tests and Developmental Tests that Include Language Subtests

Tables 11.6, 11.7 and 11.8 show examples of valid and standardized language screening and general speech, language and developmental tests, which also include language subtests, for German- and English-speaking Europe.

Table 11.6 Screenings, general developmental language tests and (The spelling x;y years in the table means x years and y months of age.) language-covering general developmental tests for German- and English-speaking Europe for the evaluation of a risk for a DDSL and other developmental disorders or delays

Method	Aim	Age-related test (year;month)					
		≤12 months	12–24 months	25–36 months	3–5 years	6–10 years	≥11 years
Screenings Parent questionnaires	Evaluation of a risk	ELFRA 1 (1;0) PLS-5 ST (0–7;11) MBCDI (0;8–3;1)	ELFRA 2 (2;0) ELAN (1; 4–2;2) FRAKIS (1;6–2;5) SBE-2-KT (1;9–2;0)[a,b] CDI (1;3–5;11) PLS-5 ST (0–7;11) LDS (1;6–2;11) MBCDI (0;8–3;1)	ELAN (1;4–2;2) SBE-3-KT (2;8–3;4) CDI (1;3–5;11) PLS-5 ST (0–7;11) LDS (1;6–2;11) MBCDI (0;8–3;1)	KiSS.2 (4;0–4;5)[b] SSV (3;0–5;0) LSV (4;0–6;5) BISC (preschool age) HASE (4;0–6;11) ETS 4-8 (4;0–8;11) CDI (1;3–5;11) PLS-5 ST (0;0–7;11) NSST S (3;0–7;11) LiSe-DaZ (3;0–6;11)[b]	ETS 4-8 (4;0–8;11) NSST S (3;0–7;11) LiSe-DaZ (3;0–6;11)[b]	
General developmental language tests and language-covering general developmental tests	Evaluation of a deviation from the age norm	PLS-5 (0;0–7;11) BISD III (0;1–3;6)	BISD III (0;1–3;6)	SETK-2 (2;0–2;11) PDSS (2;0–6;11) TELD, −2, −3 (2;0–7;11) NRDLS (2;0–7;5) WJ-III (2;0–90;0) BISD III (0;1–3;6) Vineland-II (0;0–90;0)	SETK 3-5 (3;0–5;11) PDSS (2;0–6;11) P-ITPA (4;0–11;0) BUEVA (4;0–5;11) HSET (3;0–9;0) TELD, −2, −3 (2;0–7;11) TOLD (4;0–17;11) NRDLS (2;0–7;5) CELF (5;0–21;0) CELF-P (3;0–6;11) WJ-III (2;0–90;0) BISD III (0;1–3;6) ITPA-3 (5;0–12;11) LiSe-DaZ (3;0–6;11)[b] TOLD-P:4 (4;0–8;11) Vineland-II (0;0–90;0) WRAT-4 (5;0–94;0)	PDSS (2;0–6;11) P-ITPA (4;0–11;0) BUEVA (4;0–5;11) SET 5-10 (5;0–10;11) HSET (3;0–9;0) TELD, −2, −3 (2;0–7;11) TOLD (4;0–17;11) NRDLS (2;0–7;5) CELF (5;0–21;0) CELF-P (3;0–6;11) WJ-III (2;0–90;0) ITPA-3 (5;0–12;11) LiSe-DaZ (3;0–6;11)[b] TOLD-P:4 (4;0–8;11) TOLD-I:4 (8;0–17;11) Vineland-II (0;0–90;0) WRAT-4 (5;0–94;0)	LTB-J (grade 9–10) TOLD (4;0–17;11) CELF (5;0–21;0) WJ-III (2;0–90;0) ITPA-3 (5;0–12;11) TOLD-I:4 (8;0–17;11) Vineland-II (0;0–90;0) WRAT-4 (5;0–94;0)

[a]Available in 34 languages

[b]Also suited for bi- and multilingual children

Table 11.7 Examples of specific language tests examining distinct linguistic skills for German- and English-speaking Europe

Diagnostic fields	Competence	Age-related test (year;month)					
		≤12 months	12–24 months	25–36 months	3–5 years	6–10 years	≥11 years
Basal or precursor functions							
	Verbal/phonological working memory				HASE (4;0–6;11) BISC (preschool age) Mottier (4;0–16;0) KiSS.2 (4;0–4;5) ETS 4–8 (4;0–8;11) AWMA (4;0–22;0) SSV (3;0–5;11)	HASE (4;0–6;11) BISC (preschool age) Mottier (4;0–16;0) AWMA (4;0–22;0) ETS 4–8 (4;0–8;11) MÜSC (first 5 school weeks)	AWMA (4;0–22;0) Mottier (4;0–16;0)
	Oral-motor skills			Check lists (e.g. Garliner; Giel & Tillmanns-Karus; Kittel)	Check lists (e.g. Garliner; Giel & Tillmanns-Karus; Kittel)	Check lists (e.g. Garliner; Giel & Tillmanns-Karus; Kittel)	
	Phonological awareness				TPB (4 to about 7 years) BISC (preschool age) ETS 4–8 (4;0–8;11	TPB (4 to about 7 years) MÜSC (first 5 school weeks) ETS 4–8 (4;0–8;11)	
Language competence							
Phonetics/ phonology	Articulation		PLAKKS-II (1;6–5;11)	PLAKKS-II (1;6–5;11) PDSS (2;0–6;11) GFTA-2 (2;0–21;11)	AVAK (children) PLAKKS-II (1;6–5;11) PDSS (2;0–6;11) KiSS.2 (4;0–4;5) TDA (3;0–8;0) GFTA-2 (2;0–21;11) PAT (3;0–8;11)	PDSS (2;0–6;11) TDA (3;0–8;0) GFTA-2 (2;0–21;11) PAT (3;0–8;11)	GFTA-2 (2;0–21;11)
	Phoneme discrimination			PDSS (2;0–6;11)	PDSS (2;0–6;11) KiSS.2 (4;0–4;5) Mottier (4;0–16;0)	PDSS (2;0–6;11) Mottier (4;0–16;0) BLDT (end of second grade)	

(continued)

Table 11.7 (continued)

Diagnostic fields	Competence	Age-related test (year;month)					
		≤12 months	12–24 months	25–36 months	3–5 years	6–10 years	≥11 years
Grammar	Morphology Perception			PDSS (2;0–6;11)	SETK 3–5 (3;0–5;11) PDSS (2;0–6;11) TROG-D (3;0–10;11) KiSS.2 (4;0–4;5) NSST (3; 0–7; 11 years) NRDLS (2; 0–7; 5) TTFC-2 (3;0–12;11) TOLD-P:4 (4;0–8;11)	PDSS (2;0–6;11) NSST (3;0–7;11) TROG-D (3;0–10;11) TTFC-2 (3;0–12;11) TOLD-I:4 (8;0–17;11) TOLD-P:4 (4;0–8;11)	TTFC-2 (3;0–12;11) TOLD-I:4 (8;0–17;11)
	Production		FRAKIS (1;6–2;5)	PDSS (2;0–6;11)	SETK 3–5 (3;0–5;11) ESGRAF-R (4–16 years) PDSS (2;0–6;11) KiSS.2 (4;0–4;5) NSST (3;0–7;11) TOLD-P:4 (4;0–8;11)	ESGRAF-R (4–16 years) PDSS (2;0–6;11) NSST (3;0–7;11) TOLD-I:4 (8;0–17;11) TOLD-P:4 (4;0–8;11)	ESGRAF-R (4;0–16;0) TOLD-I:4 (8;0–17;11)
	Syntax Perception			TSVK (2–8 years) PDSS (2;0–6;11) NRDLS (2;0–7;5)	TSVK (2;0–8;0) TROG-D (3;0–10;11) MSVK (5 year-end of first grade) SETK 3–5 (3;0–5;11) PDSS (2;0–6;11) KiSS.2 (4;0–4;5) NSST (3;0–7;11) NRDLS (2;0–7;5) TTFC-2 (3;0–12;11) TOLD-P:4 (4;0–8;11)	TSVK (2;0–8;0) TROG-D (3;0–10;11) MSVK (5 year-end of first grade) PDSS (2;0–6;11) NSST (3;0–7;11) NRDLS (2;0–7;5) TTFC-2 (3;0–12;11) TOLD-I:4 (8;0–17;11) TOLD-P:4 (4;0–8;11)	TTFC-2 (3;0–12;11) TOLD-I:4 (8;0–17;11)
	Production		ELFRA 2 (2;0) FRAKIS (1;6–2;5)	PDSS (2;0–6;11) NRDLS (2;0–7;5)	SETK 3–5 (3;0–5;11) PDSS (2;0–6;11) KiSS.2 (4;0–4;5) NSST (3;0–7;11) NRDLS (2;0–7;5) TOLD-P:4 (4;0–8;11)	PDSS (2;0–6;11) NSST (3;0–7;11) NRDLS (2;0–7;5) TOLD-I:4 (8;0–17;11) TOLD-P:4 (4;0–8;11)	TOLD-I:4 (8;0–17;11)

Semantics and vocabulary	Semantics	ELFRA 1 (1;0)		PDSS (2;0–6;11) NRDLS (2;0–7;5) PPVT III (2;6–90;0)	Teddy-Test (3;0–8;6) MSVK (5 year-end of first grade) PDSS (2;0–6;11) KiSS.2 (4;0–4;5) NRDLS (2;0–7;5) PPVT III (2;6–90;0)	Teddy-Test (3;0–8;6) MSVK (5 year-end of first grade) NRDLS (2;0–7;5) PPVT III (2;6–90;0) TOLD-I:4 (8;0–17;11)	PPVT III (2;6–90;0) TOLD-I:4 (8;0–17;11)
Vocabulary	Perception (passive)	ELFRA 1 (1;0)		PDSS (2;0–6;11) PPVT III (2;6–90 years) NRDLS (2;0–7;5)	PDSS (2;0–6;11) KiSS.2 (4;0–4;5) TTFC-2 (3;0–12;11) CREFT-3 (5;0–89;11) PPVT III (2;6–90;0) NRDLS (2;0–7;5)	PDSS (2;0–6;11) CREFT-3 (5;0–89;11) TTFC-2 (3;0–12;11) TOLD-I:4 (8;0–17;11) NRDLS (2;0–7;5)	PPVT (14;0–60;0) CREFT-3 (5;0–89;11) TOLD-I:4 (8;0–17;11) TTFC-2 (3;0–12;11) PPVT III (2;6–90;0) PPVT German version (13;0–90;0)
	Production (active)	ELFRA 1 (1;0)	ELFRA 2 (2;0) ELAN (1;4–2;2) FRAKIS (1;6–2;5)	PDSS (2;0–6;11) NRDLS (2;0–7;5)	AWST-R (3;0–5;6) PDSS (2;0–6;11) KiSS.2 (4;0–4;5) CREFT-3 (5;0–89;11) NRDLS (2;0–7;5)	WWT 6–10 (6;0–10;0) PDSS (2;0–6;11) CREFT-3 (5;0–89;11) NRDLS (2;0–7;5) TOLD-I:4 (8;0–17;11)	CREFT-3 (5;0–89;11) TOLD-I:4 (8;0–17;11)
Pragmatics/communication			Vineland-II (0;0–90;0) Das pragmatische Profil (0;0–10;0)	Vineland-II (0;0–90;0) Das pragmatische Profil (0;0–10;0)	MSVK (5 year-end of first grade) KiSS.2 (4;0–4;5) Vineland-II (0;0–90;0) Das pragmatische Profil (0;0–10;0)	MSVK (5 year-end of first grade) Vineland-II (0;0–90;0) Das pragmatische Profil (0;0–10;0)	Vineland-II (0;0–90;0)

Table 11.8 Register of examples of language screening tests, general and specific language tests and language-covering developmental tests for German- and English-speaking Europe

Test	Language	References
AVAK	German	Hacker D, Wilgermein H (2001) AVAK-Test mit CD-ROM Analyseverfahren zu Aussprachestörungen bei Kindern, 2nd. edn CD-ROM 2006) Reinhardt, München
AWMA	English	Alloway TP (2007) Automated working memory assessment (AWMA). Pearson, Oxford. Available via www.psychcorp.co.uk/product.aspx?n=1343&s=1492&cat=1356&skey=3909. Accessed 7 June 2014
AWST-R	German	Kiese-Himmel C (2005) Aktiver Wortschatztest für 3-bis 5-jährige Kinder – Revision. Beltz, Göttingen
BISC	German	Jansen H, Mannhaupt G, Marx H et al (2002) Bielefelder Screening zur Früherkennung von Lese-Rechtschreibschwierigkeiten. 2nd revised edn. Hogrefe, Göttingen
BISD III	English	Bayley N (2006) Bayley scales of infant and toddler development, 3rd edn. Harcourt Assessment Inc., San Antonio
BLDT	German	Niemeyer W (1976) Bremer Lautdiskriminationstest 2. Klasse BLDT, Herbig, Bremen
BUEVA	German	Esser G, Wyschkon A (2002) BUEVA – Basisdiagnostik umschriebener Entwicklungsstörungen im Vorschulalter. Hogrefe, Göttingen
CDI	English	Ireton H (1992) Child Development Inventory. Behavior Science Systems, Inc., Minneapolis Ireton H, Glascoe FP (1995) Assessing children's development using parents' reports: the Child Development Inventory. Clin Pediatr (Phila) 34(5):248–255
CELF	English	Semel E, Wiig E, Secord W (1995) Clinical evaluation of language fundamentals, 3rd edn. The psychological corporation, Harcourt Brace & Company, San Antonio
CELF-P	English	Wiig EH, Secord W, Semel E (1998) Clinical evaluation of language fundamentals – preschool (CELF-preschool). The psychological corporation, Harcourt Brace Jovanovich, San Antonio
CREFT-3	English	Wallace G, Hammill DD (1994) Comprehensive receptive and expressive vocabulary test, 3rd edn (CREFT-3). Pro-Ed, Austin
Das Pragmatische Profil	German	Dohmen A, Dewart H, Summers S (2009) Das Pragmatische Profil – Analyse kommunikativer Fähigkeiten von Kindern. Elsevier, München
ELAN	German	Bockmann AK, Kiese-Himmel C (2006) ELAN—Eltern Antworten. Beltz, Göttingen
ELFRA	German	Grimm H, Doil H (2006) ELFRA – Elternfragebögen für die Früherkennung von Risikokindern, 2nd revised edn. Hogrefe, Göttingen
EOWPVT-R	English	Gardner MF (2000) Expressive one-word picture vocabulary test – revised (EOWPVT). Academic Therapy, Novato
ESGRAF-R	German	Motsch HJ (2018) ESGRAF-R Testmanual: Evozierte Sprachdiagnose grammatischer Fähigkeiten, 2nd revised edn. Reinhardt, München
ETS 4-8	German	Angermaier M (2007) Entwicklungstest Sprache 4 bis 8 Jahre (ETS 4-8). Pearson Assessment, Frankfurt
FRAKIS	German	Szagun G, Stumper B, Schramm SA (2007) Fragebogen zur frühkindlichen Sprachentwicklung und FRAKIS-K (Kurzform). Pearson, Frankfurt
GFTA-2	English	Goldman R, Fristoe M (2000) Goldman-Fristoe Test of Articulation-2 (GFTA-2). American Guidance Service, Circle Pines
HASE	German	Schöler H, Brunner M (2008) HASE – Heidelberger Auditives Screening in der Einschulungsdiagnostik, 2nd revised edn. Westra, Wertingen
HSET	German	Grimm H, Schöler H (1991) Heidelberger Sprachentwicklungstest (HSET), 2nd revised edn. Hogrefe, Göttingen
ITPA-3	English	Hammill DD, Mather N, Roberts R (2001) Illinois test of psycholinguistic abilities, 3rd edn (ITPA-3). Pro-Ed, Austin
KISS.2	German	Euler HA, Holler-Zittlau I, van Minnen S et al (2010) Psychometrische Gütekriterien eines Kurztests zur Erfassung des Sprachstandes vierjähriger Kinder. HNO 58(11):1116–1123 Neumann K, Holler-Zittlau I, Euler HA (2011) Kinder-Sprach-Screening "KiSS". Available via https://soziales.hessen.de/gesundheit/kinder-sprachscreening-kiss. Accessed 7 June 2014

Table 11.8 (continued)

Test	Language	References
LDS	English	Rescorla L (1989) The language development survey: a screening tool for delayed language in toddlers. J Speech Hear Disord 54:(4)587–599
LiSe-DaZ	German	Schulz P, Tracy R (2012) LiSe-DaZ. Linguistische Sprachstandserhebung – Deutsch als Zweitsprache. Hogrefe, Göttingen
LSV	German	Götte R (1976) Landauer Sprachentwicklungstest für Vorschulkinder LSV. Beltz, Weinheim
LTB-J	German	Barwitzki K, Hofbauer C, Huber M et al (2008) LTB-J - Leipziger Testbatterie zur Messung des formal-sprachlichen Entwicklungsstandes bei Jugendlichen. BBW, Leipzig
MBCDI	English	Fenson L, Marchman VA, Thal DJ et al (2007) MacArthur-Bates communicative development inventories: user's guide and technical manual, 2nd edn. Paul H. Brookes Publishing, Baltimore
Mottier	German	Kiese-Himmel C, Risse T (2009) Normen für den Mottier-Test bei 4- bis 6-jährigen Kindern. HNO 57(9):943–948 Risse T, Kiese-Himmel C (2009) Der Mottier-Test. Teststatistische Überprüfung an 4- bis 6-jährigen Kindern. HNO 57(5):523–528
MSVK	German	Elben CE, Lohaus A (2000) Marburger Sprachverständnistest für Kinder MSVK. Hogrefe, Göttingen
MÜSC	German	Mannhaupt G (2006) Das Münsteraner Screening zur Früherkennung von Lese- und Rechtschreibschwierigkeiten (MÜSC). Cornelsen, Berlin
NRDLS	English	Edwards S, Letts C, Sinka I (2011) The New Reynell Developmental Language Scales (NRDLS). GL Assessment, London
NSST	English	Lee, Lee LL (1969) Northwestern syntax screening test. Northwestern University Press, Evanston
NSST S	English	Ratusnik DL, Klee TM, Ratusnik CM (1980) Northwestern syntax screening test: a short form. J Speech Hear Disord 45(2):200–208
PDSS	German	Kauschke C, Siegmüller J (2009) Patholinguistische Diagnostik bei Sprachentwicklungsstörungen, 2nd edn. Elsevier, Heidelberg
PAT	English	Pendergast K, Dickey SE, Selmar JW et al (1984) Photo articulation test. Stoelting, Chicago
PPVT III	English	Dunn LM, Dunn LM (1997) Examiner's manual for the Peabody Picture Vocabulary Test-third edition (PPVT-III). American Guidance Service, Circle Pines
	German	Bulheller S, Dunn LM, Dunn LM et al (German edition) (2003) Peabody Picture Vocabulary Test: (PPVT); Manual. Swets Test Services, Frankfurt
P-ITPA	German	Ballaschk K, Hänsch S, Esser G (2010) P-ITPA. Potsdam-Illinois Test für Psycholinguistische Fähigkeiten. Hogrefe, Göttingen
PLAKSS-II	German	Fox A (2014) PLAKSS-II Psycholinguistische Analyse kindlicher Sprechstörungen-II, 1st edn. Pearson, Frankfurt
PLS-5	English	Zimmerman IL, Steiner VG, Pond RE (2011) PLS-5 Preschool Language Scales, 5th edn. Pearson, San Antonio
PLS-5 ST	English	Zimmerman, IL, Steiner VG, Pond RE (2011) Preschool Language Scale-5 Screening Test, 5th edn. (PLS-5 Screening Test). Pearson, San Antonio
Prüfbögen zur Mundmotorik	German	Garliner D (1989) Myofunktionelle Therapie in der Praxis - Gestörtes Schluckverhalten, gestörte Gesichtsmuskulatur und die Folgen - Diagnose, Planung und Durchführung der Behandlung. Hütig, Heidelberg Giel B, Tillmanns-Karus M (2004) Kölner Diagnostikbogen für Myofunktionelle Störungen. modernes lernen, Dortmund Kittel AM (2009) Myofunktionelle Therapie, 9th revised edn. Schulz-Kirchner, Idstein
SBE-2-KT	German	Suchodoletz Wv, Sachse S (2009) Sprachbeurteilung durch Eltern, Kurztest für die U7 (SBE-2-KT). Available via http://www.kjp.med.uni-muenchen.de/download/SBE-2-KT.pdf. Accessed 7 June 2014 Suchodoletz Wv, Sachse S (2009) Sprachbeurteilung durch Eltern, Kurztest für die U7 (SBE-2-KT), non-normalized translation in 33 languages. Available via https://www.kjp.med.uni-muenchen.de/download/SBE-2-KT.pdf. Accessed 13 April 2018

(continued)

Table 11.8 (continued)

Test	Language	References
SBE-3-KT	German	Suchodoletz Wv, Kademann S, Tippelt S (2009) Sprachbeurteilung durch Eltern, Kurztest für die U7a (SBE-3-KT). Available via http://www.kjp.med.uni-muenchen.de/download/SBE-3-KT.pdf. Accessed 7 June 2014
SET 5-10	German	Petermann F, Metz D, Fröhlich LP (2010) SES 5-10. Sprachstandserhebungstest für Kinder im Alter zwischen 5 und 10 Jahren. Hogrefe, Göttingen
SETK-2	German	Grimm H, Aktas M, Frevert S (2000) Sprachentwicklungstest für zweijährige Kinder SETK-2. Hogrefe, Göttingen
	German	Grimm H, Aktas M, Frevert S (2010) Sprachentwicklungstest für drei- bis fünfjährige Kinder SETK 3-5, 2nd revised edn. Hogrefe, Göttingen
SSV	German	Grimm H, Aktas M, Kießig U (2003) Sprachscreening für das Vorschulalter SSV. Kurzform des SETK 3-5. Hogrefe, Göttingen
Teddy-Test	German	Friedrich G (1998) Teddy-Test. Hogrefe, Göttingen
TDA	English	Templin MC, Darley FL (1969) The Templin-Darley tests of articulation; a manual and discussion of articulation testing, 2nd edn. Bureau of Educational Research and Service, Division of Extension and University Services, University of Iowa, Iowa City
TELD, TELD-2, TELD-3	English	Hresko WP, Reid DK, Hammill DD (1981) Test of early language development. Pro-Ed, Austin, TX
TTFC-2	English	McGhee RL, Ehrler DJ, DiSimoni F (2007) Token test for children-second edition (TTFC-2). Pro-Ed, Austin, TX
TOLD-P:4	English	Newcomer PL, Hammill DD (2008) Test of Language Development-Primary, 4th edn (TOLD-P:4). Pro-Ed, Austin
TOLD-I:4	English	Hammill DD, Newcomer PL (2008) Test of Language Development-Intermediate, 4th edn (TOLD-I:4). Pro-Ed, Austin
TPB	German	Fricke S, Schäfer B (2011) Test phonologischer Bewusstheitsfähigkeiten, 2nd edn. Schulz-Kirchner, Idstein
TROG-D	German	Fox AV (2008) TROG-D - Test zur Überprüfung des Grammatik-Verständnisses, 3rd edn. Schulz-Kirchner, Idstein
TSVK	German	Siegmüller J, Kauschke C, van Minnen S et al (2010) Test des Satzverständnisses bei Kindern. Eine profilorientierte Diagnostik der Syntax. Elsevier, Heidelberg
Vineland-II	English	Sparrow SS, Balla DA Cicchetti DV (2005) Vineland Adaptive Behaviors Scales, 2nd edn (Vineland-II). American Guidance Service, Circle Pines
WJ-III	English	Woodcock RW, McGrew KS, Mather N (2001) Woodcock-Johnson-III Tests of achievement. Riverside Publishing, Itasca
WRAT-4	English	Wilkinson GS, Robertson GJ (2006) Wide Range Achievement Test - fourth edition (WRAT-4) professional manual. Psychological Assessment Resources, Lutz
WWT 6-10	German	Glück CW (2007) WWT 6-10. Wortschatz- und Wortfindungstest für 6- bis 10-Jährige. Urban & Schwarzenberg, München

11.4 Oral-Motor Examination Protocol

Ana Martínez Arellano and
María Bielsa Corrochano

11.4.1 Introduction

The orofacial system consists of bony, nervous and muscular components. As in all mammals, the primary functions of this orofacial system are food intake (sucking, eating, drinking, biting, swallowing) and breathing. Furthermore, its potential for mimicry is an important communication means. In humans it additionally serves a secondary function: speech sound production. For children, the structural and functional adequacy of the oral-motor system provides the basis for the development of all the named functions.

An oral-motor examination, as part of the phoniatric assessment in cases of developmental speech, language and swallowing abnormalities, helps to verify normal patterns as well as organic or functional deficits underlying *phonetic* (mechanical and acoustical forming of speech sounds) speech sound disorders and swallowing problems in childhood. This examination together with an assessment of the status of speech sound development as described in Sect. 11.5 should be used systematically in order to enable a distinction between *phonetic* and *phonological* (linguistic) components of speech sound abnormality or disorder.

After a parental interview on the clinical history of their child, focusing on the development of the primary functions and oral perception, oral-motor examination includes the exploration of the following orofacial components and their interplay, in order to

> determine their structural and functional adequacy for speech
>
> Nicolosi et al. (2003)

and swallowing: lips, jaws, teeth, tongue, hard palate, soft palate and pharynx. It should comprise the following aspects:

- Inspection of the structure and muscle tone at rest, assessing size, symmetry, shape and possible presence of scars, clefts or other anomalies of the specific orofacial components
- Examination of oral functions during the performance of specific oral movements, observing muscle tone, coordination and extent of mobility

The results of the above-named examinations provide relevant information about the possible causes of speech sound disorders and swallowing problems of the children examined. With respect to differential diagnoses, this examination also serves as a decision-making ('pass/fail') procedure (American Speech-Language-Hearing Association (ASHA) 2004) to initiate further comprehensive assessments if cardinal symptoms of specific disorders are found, such as dysglossia, central speech motor processing disorders (dyspraxia, dysarthria) or peripheral or central swallowing disorders (ASHA 2004). In the following key aspects of an oral-motor examination, potential methods and possible observations are listed.

Constituents of an oral-motor examination protocol:

- Clinical history
- Test instruments and materials
- Inspection of the orofacial structures and evaluation of muscle tone at rest
- Examination of oral function in motion
- Interpretation

11.4.2   Clinical History

Clinical history should include questions regarding:

- Pregnancy and birth: foetal distress, natural or assisted childbirth, prematurity, damaging or deleterious factors.
- Age of acquisition of developmental skills (walking, early speech, micturition/faecal control). If these functions are delayed, a potential developmental retardation has to be taken into consideration.
- Feeding, diet and food intake: natural, artificial (e.g. tube feeding), type of bottle nipple, difficulties in sucking, mastication, age of weaning, coughing or choking while or after eating/drinking, aspiration of food or liquid into the lungs (chronic respiratory failure, pneumonia).
- Development of oral perception: intensity of oral exploration in the first year of life; tolerance/acceptance of varying food consistencies and food tastes/flavours.
- Diseases of ear, nose and throat.
- Parafunctions: dummy/pacifier (type, frequency, age of weaning), digit or object sucking, labial or lingual sucking, nail biting, bruxism, snoring, dribbling.

11.4.3   Test Instruments and Materials

In order to carry out the examination, a source of frontal light and basic examination materials are needed: gloves, tongue depressors, small mirror for mirror-fogging test and nasal speculum or nasal fibrescope. For the evaluation of swallowing and chewing, solid, semisolid and liquid aliments are used.

11.4.4 Inspection of the Orofacial Structure and Muscle Tone at Rest

Assess the size, symmetry, shape and possible presence of scars, clefts or other anomalies of each orofacial structure as below.

11.4.4.1 External Orofacial Examination

Facies:
- Facial malformations or other anomalies, e.g. hypo-/hypertelorism, epicanthus

Lips:
- Structure: size, symmetry, lingual frenulum, scars, clefts
- Function:
  - Resting position: lips open or closed, hypo- or hypertonus
  - Closure: complete, incomplete

Nose/Nostrils:
- Examination using the nasal speculum or nasal fibrescope and a small mirror for:
  - Structure: size, form variants, malformations, deviation of nose or nose septum, hyper- or hypoplasia of nasal conchae, width of nostrils, nasal entrance and ducts
  - Function: nasal airway obstruction, mucus, mucosal swallowing

Temporomandibular Joint:
- Structure: symmetry of the mandibular branches, protrusion or retraction/hypoplasia of mandibula
- Function: degrees of freedom and extent of movement

11.4.4.2 Intraoral Examination

Tongue:
- Structure: form and size such as macroglossia, microglossia, scars, symmetry

- Function: muscular tone, position at rest (protrusion, support on the palate, support on incisors interdental), motility, fasciculation, deviation

Cavum Oris and Pharynx:
- Structure: dental status, status of palate and pharyngeal tonsils (hypertrophy, status after adeno-/tonsillectomy or tonsillotomy, scars), status of mucosa (mucus, swelling, infections), salivary cysts
- Function: closure of mouth, muscular tone, hypersalivation, velopharyngeal insufficiency

Hard Palate:
- Structure: malformations or abnormalities such as clefts or fissures, scars, fistulae, form deviations (flat or 'Gothic')
- Function: closure between the mouth and nose, mouth closure

Soft Palate:
- Structure: malformations or abnormalities such as clefts, bifid uvula, short, long or deviating uvula
- Function: velopharyngeal insufficiency, hypernasal speech, nasal regurgitation during swallowing

Teeth and Occlusion:
- Structure: dental status (decayed, missing or filled teeth, dental diastema, malposition) for the primary dentition (deciduous teeth) and for the permanent dentition.
- Function: occlusion. The child is requested to bite and to show her or his teeth.
  - Anteroposterior match: Class I (normocclusion), Class II (distocclusion), Class III (mesiocclusion)
  - Vertical match: normal bite, open bite (anterior, lateral), overbite
  - Transversal match: crossbite (uni- or bilateral), lateral deviation

11.4.5 Examination of Functionality

Lips:
- In order to examine mobility, the child is requested to make the following movements:

lifting, stretching, lateralization, vibration (lip flapping) and kissing. The child's ability to perform these movements and the muscular tone and strength with which they are performed are assessed for:

- Tone and strength: hypotonus, hypertonus
- Mobility: normal, difficult/restricted in a certain direction, very limited, impossible
- Closing: complete, incomplete, impossible

Tongue:
- For examining mobility the child is requested to stretch his or her tongue out; to raise, lower and lateralize it; and to press it against the cheeks from inside the mouth. The tone is examined by using a tongue depressor, asking the child to press against it. In babies and young children, the examination is completed by tactile stimulation of the mouth mucosa and the tongue:
  - Mobility: stretching out, upwards (touching nose), downwards, right, left, rotation
  - Tone and strength: hypotonus, hypertonus
  - Lingual frenulum: normal, shortened (ankyloglossia)

Temporomandibular Joint:
- For examining mobility the child is requested to open and close his or her mouth and to complete lateral motions. Muscle tone is evaluated by palpating the joints bimanually:
  - Mobility: opening (normal, difficult/restricted in certain directions, very limited, impossible), symmetry of closure
  - Dysfunctions: cracking, bruxism, clicks, blockage

Soft Palate:
- In order to evaluate sufficient velopharyngeal closure of the soft palate, the child is requested to vocalize a word with the plosive /c/ (e.g. cuckoo, Coca-Cola). Breath noise (rhinophonia aperta) indicates lacking or incomplete velopharyngeal closure. Furthermore, vowel sounds are examined, for example, of /u:/ or /a:/. A nasal component (airy noise) indicates a functional rhinophonia aperta.

Chewing and Swallowing:
- The child's myofunctional maturity is evaluated according to her or his age. Food intake (chewing and drinking), oral preparation and swallowing should be observed. Possible findings are:
  - Chewing with open mouth
  - Gathering of saliva at the corners of the mouth or on the lips
  - Food remaining in the mouth after swallowing
  - Drooling, dribbling of saliva or food
  - Movement forward of the tongue while speaking, chewing and swallowing (tongue thrust), tongue pressure on teeth, lateral tongue pressure, lingual interposition between teeth
  - Head movements, effort in perioral muscles
  - For babies: adaptation to the bottle nipple
  - For infants and young children: licking a spoon

11.4.6 Interpretation

By interpreting the results of the examination for an individual child, the causes for developmental speech sound and swallowing disorder as named in the following can be differentiated. Other disorders, which should either be excluded or considered as potential diagnoses that need further assessment, are listed below:

11.4.6.1 Phonological Speech Sound Disorder

In the case of a speech sound disorder or abnormality, a phonological cause or at least a component has to be assumed, if the organic and myofunctional adequacy of the orofacial system is given and other potential comorbidities (including hearing loss) are excluded. In this case, the phonological developmental status must be examined closely as described in Sect. 11.5.

11.4.6.2 Phonetic Speech Sound Disorder

Orofunctional causes: immaturity or imbalance of orofacial functions and oral senses without organic abnormalities (including normal hearing); functional inadequacy such as hypotonus of orofacial muscles, poor coordination of oral-motor sequences, often associated with abnormal development of food intake or oral perception (e.g. limited acceptance of a sufficient variety of food flavours or consistencies)

Mechanical causes: for example, a missing tooth, diastema, velopharyngeal insufficiency

In cases of insufficient velopharyngeal closure and excessive nasal component of speech sounds (rhinophonia aperta), careful differential diagnosis is essential because several underlying causes are possible (e.g. neurological; organic; functional) (Grunwell 1993); see also Part I, Speech Disorders (Dysglossia/Nasality/Velopharyngeal Insufficiency), Volume 2.

In the following, differential diagnoses of speech sound and swallowing disorders that may involve orofacial muscle dysfunctions are listed with respect to organic and functional as well as peripheral and central causes:

- *Speech sound disorders* due to hearing impairment (see Part IV, Disorders of Hearing Development).
- *Dysglossia*: a speech sound disorder due to an organic affection of articulation organs (lips, tongue, palate, teeth, jaw, vocal folds) caused by oro- or craniofacial malformations, paralyses, injuries, tumours, muscle disorders or surgery (e.g. cleft lip or palate, macroglossia, scars); see Part I, Speech Disorders (Dysglossia/Nasality/Velopharyngeal Insufficiency), Volume 2.
- There is evidence that a shortened lingual frenulum (ankylogossia) may affect breastfeeding and can be treated by surgical procedures. However, there is insufficient evidence that it affects speech sound development or that surgery improves articulatory development of a child. Therefore, frenulotomy or frenuloplasty is not recommended for improvement of speech sound disorders in cases of ankyloglossia (Francis et al. 2015).
- *Speech-language-relevant syndromes*: oro- or craniofacial malformations or abnormalities are often symptoms of a syndrome and should be diagnosed comprehensively (see Sect. 9.10).
- *Functional (peripheral) swallowing disorders*: orofacial dysfunctions/myofunctional disorders with orofacial muscle imbalance and difficulties in motor coordination and sequencing lead to insufficient oral preparation of swallowing, tongue thrust, malocclusion, mouth breathing, retardation in the development of oral perception and oral hyper-/hypo-sensibility; see Part I, Speech Disorders (Dysglossia/Nasality/Velopharyngeal Insufficiency), Volume 2.
- *Central swallowing disorders*: coughing or choking during or after eating/drinking; penetration or aspiration of food or liquid into the lungs; recurrent episodes of pneumonia; raised temperature (as early sign of subclinical pneumonia); substantial/rapid weight loss with no clear cause (Nicolosi et al. 2003); see Part VI, Swallowing Disorders including Rehabilitation of Tumour Patients, Volume 2.*Oral dyspraxia*: inability to plan and perform an oral-motor task on purpose; symptoms:

  groping, trial-and-error behaviour; purposeful programming of muscular movement while involuntary movements remain intact.

  Nicolosi et al. (2003)

- *Childhood apraxia of speech* (CAS), also termed developmental verbal dyspraxia, is regarded as a special form of oral dyspraxia and needs diligent assessment (see Sect. 10.2).
- *Dysarthria*: a

  motor speech disorder due to impairment originating in the central or peripheral nervous system…
  Usually part of a more generalised neurological impairment…

- (e.g. cerebral palsy)

  Respiration, articulation, phonation, resonation and/or prosody may be affected; volitional and automatic actions, such as chewing and swallowing and movements of the jaw and tongue may also be deviant.

  Nicolosi et al. (2003)

See Part IV, Acquired Motor Speech Disorders (Dysarthria, Dyspraxia), Volume 2.

11.5 Assessment of Speech Sound Development

Karen Reichmuth and Melanie Vauth

11.5.1 Speech Sound Disorders (SSDs) in Children

The assessment of speech sound development is obligatory for comprehensive speech and language evaluation of a child with communication concerns or whenever an SSD is suspected (ASHA 2016).

> Speech sound disorders (SSD) is an umbrella term…
> (introduced by the ASHA in 2004)…referring to any combination of difficulties with perception, motor production and/or the phonological representation of speech sounds and speech segments… that impact speech intelligibility.
>
> ASHA (2016)

SSDs constitute the largest group of communication difficulties amongst young children. In English-speaking countries, the prevalence of SSDs in childhood (3–11 years) varies from 3 to 15% (for an overview see McLeod et al. 2013). SSDs in children can be of known (e.g. organic) or unknown aetiology (McLeod et al. 2013); those of unclear origin represent the largest portion (Fox-Boyer et al. 2016). Organic causes of an SSD are hearing impairment, orofacial dysfunction (myofunctional disorder), craniofacial anomalies such as cleft palate or other dysglossia, genetic or non-genetic syndromes and neurological impairment or diseases (e.g. cerebral palsy leading to dysarthria or apraxia) (ASHA 2016). Genetically based SSDs identified by familial clustering of SSDs are also included. For SSDs with unknown causes, several risk factors are discussed (e.g. repeated otitis media, deficits in phonological working memory, delayed phonological development) (Fox-Boyer et al. 2016). Childhood apraxia of speech (CAS) depicts an outlier in the field of

SSD (for details see Sect. 10.2). Neurological causes are hypothesized without the evidence of neurological findings associated with the disorder (Fox-Boyer et al. 2016).

Following aetiology and psycholinguistics, the classification of SSDs in children with developmental speech and language disorders should broadly distinguish three subgroups: phonetic disorders, phonological disorders and neurological motor-speech disorders (see Fig. 11.5 for overview and Table 11.9 for closer definitions). Speech sound abnormalities due to dysphonia, psychogenic speech disorders that mimic other speech disorders (Duffy 2016), speech fluency disorders such as stuttering and cluttering and prosodic abnormalities are excluded from the classification outlined here. For a critical review on various classification and more details of SDDs, see Dodd (2014).

> Children with speech sound disorders can have difficulties with perception, articulation/motor production, phonological representation of speech segments (consonants and vowels), phonotactics (syllable and word shapes) and prosody (lexical and grammatical tones, rhythm, stress, and intonation) that may affect speech intelligibility and acceptability.
>
> International Expert Panel on Multilingual Children's Speech (2012)

Differential diagnosis is needed but often difficult to provide, owing to the large heterogeneity of speech sound disorders. Mixed profiles (phonetic and phonological abnormalities) are also common (Strand and McCauley 2008; Navasivayam et al. 2013). Mandatorily, organic causes should initially be detected or excluded (including hearing tests and oral-motor examination). Especially in cases of excessive nasal components of speech (hypernasality), differential diagnosis is essential because several underlying serious causes are possible for insufficient velopharyngeal closure (e.g. neurological, organic, functional, sensory). In case of uncertainty, a referral to a neuro-pediatrician for excluding a neurological cause is obligatory.

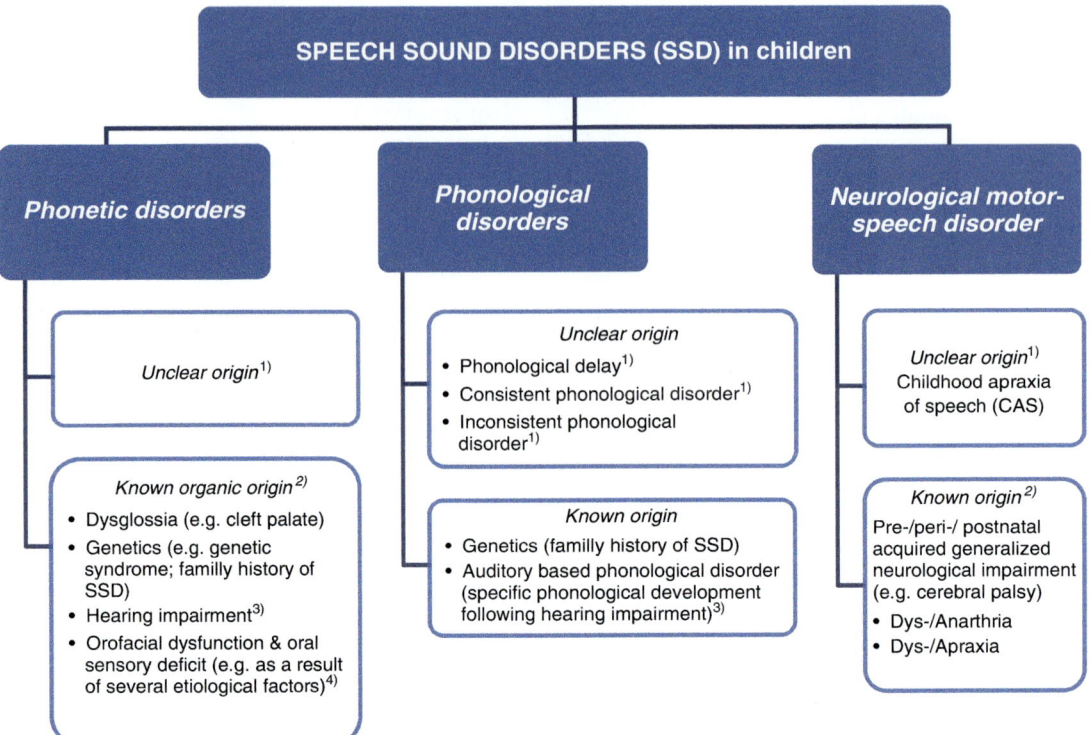

Fig. 11.5 Classification of speech sound disorders (SSD) in children based on etiology and psycholinguistics developed by Reichmuth and Vauth. (1) The five subgroups from the classification of speech sound disorders of unclear origins are from Dodd (2005), Fox-Boyer et al. (2016). (2) Excluding functional dysphonia and speech fluency disorders. (3) For diagnostic and treatment reasons, Reichmuth (2018) underlines the necessity to classify speech sound disorders in hearing-impaired children as a both phonetic and phonologi- cal disorder. (4) Several aetiological factors are known to foster the emergence of orofacial dysfunction and sensory deficits: e.g. preterm birth, organic reasons for persisting mouth breathing, oral habits and tongue thrust (Bigenzahn 2003); see also Part I, Speech Disorders (Dysglossia/ Nasality/Velopharyngeal Insufficiency), Volume 2. The organic origin does not always become obvious. So orofacial dysfunction and sensory deficits can be subsequent or co-occurring symptom as long as the origin is not known

Table 11.9 Characteristics of SSD subtypes (Overview developed by Reichmuth and Vauth)

Subgroup	Definition
Phonetic disorder	General inability to perform correctly the articulatory movements required to produce a certain phone (isolated or in word); maintained ability to realize phonological information correctly if a hearing impairment is excluded
Of unknown origin	
– (without evident organic reason)	• Substitutions or distortions of the same sounds in isolation and in all phonetic contexts during imitation, elicitation and spontaneous speech tasks (e.g. lateral lisp) (Dodd 2014); affects around 12% of all children with SSDs of unknown origin (Dodd 2014)
Of known origin	
– Orofacial dysfunction	• Oral sensory deficits; orofacial dysbalance; orofacial hypotonus: for example, tongue thrust, an oral myofunctional phenomenon that can affect production of some sounds, e.g. /s/, /z/, /sh/, /ch/ and /j/ (ASHA 2016), and may cause multiple interdentality of other alveolar sounds (e.g. t, l, n) (see Part I, Speech Disorders (Dysglossia/Nasality/ Velopharyngeal Insufficiency), Volume 2)
– Dysglossia	• Structural causes: e.g. craniofacial malformations such as cleft palate or macroglossia influence the ability to perform correct articulatory movements; both articulation and resonance (e.g. nasal component, hypernasality) may be affected; maintained ability to realize phonological information correctly if a hearing impairment is excluded (see Part I, Speech Disorders (Dysglossia/Nasality/Velopharyngeal Insufficiency), Volume 2)
– Hearing impairment	• Peripheral hearing loss; sensory-input-caused limitations in speech sound development, which can be reduced by early identification (e.g. by newborn hearing screening) and treatment (hearing devices) of the hearing loss (see also 'phonetic-phonological disorder in hearing-impaired children' in this table)

Table 11.9 (continued)

Subgroup	Definition
– Genetic (e.g. syndromes)	• Genetic causes lead to diverse aspects of organic origins of SSDs (e.g. dysglossia, hearing loss, orofunctional deficits); syndrome-specific SSD expression, e.g. in Down syndrome, Pierre Robin syndrome, Franceschetti syndrome
Phonological disorder	Defined as failure of the correct use of the linguistic component of a speech sound (phoneme); inability to process or deficiency in processing phonological information correctly and to use a phoneme linguistically correctly in words, even though the isolated performance of the phone is possible
Of unknown origin	
– Phonological delay	• Prolonged use (at least 6 months) of at least one (formerly) physiological phonological process of normal speech sound development (see Table 11.10) (Fox-Boyer et al. 2016; Dodd 2014); isolated performance of the phone is (often) possible
– Consistent phonological disorder	• Consequent use of at least one pathological phonological process (Fox-Boyer et al. 2016; see also Dodd 2014); isolated performance of the phone is (often) possible
– Inconsistent phonological disorder	• Inability to pronounce repeatedly a specific word identically; a high rate of inconsistency >40% (in a given wordlist of 25–30 words) (see also Dodd 2005, 2014; Fox-Boyer 2014); isolated performance of the phone is (often) possible
Of known origin	
– Genetic	Family history of SSD
– Phonetic-phonological disorder in hearing-impaired children	• Overall influence of the hearing loss on the phonological acquisition often leads to specific, mostly consistent, phonological processes (even when hearing devices are fitted): structural simplification such as deletion of (weak) syllables and final consonants, nasalization of vowels and vowel shift; structural simplification such as deletion of speech sounds or weak syllables and assimilation as well as systemic simplifications such as stopping of fricatives (see Table 11.10)
Neurological motor-speech disorders	
Of unknown origin	
– Childhood apraxia of speech (CAS; synonym: verbal developmental dyspraxia)	• Failure of central oral or verbal motor planning functions are assumed (see Sect. 10.2 for details) without obvious neurological impairment; inadequate intonation (e.g. word stress and prosody); speech characterized by inconsistency, oromotor symptoms (e.g. difficulty in sequencing of articulatory movements), slow speech rate, disturbed prosody, short length of utterance, poorer performance in imitation than in spontaneous speech production (Dodd 2014); predominant use of vowels; reduced use of consonants; adiadochokinesis (inability to execute repetitions of rapidly changing articulatory movements)
Of known origin	
– Dysarthria	• Motor-speech disorder due to impairment of the central or peripheral nervous system; respiration, articulation, phonation, resonation or prosody may be affected; volitional and automatized motor actions such as jaw and tongue movements in chewing and swallowing may also be deviant; usually part of a neurological impairment, e.g. cerebral palsy (Nicolosi et al. 2003); see Part IV Acquired Motor Speech Disorders (Dysarthria, Dyspraxia), Volume 2
– Dyspraxia	• Impaired capacity to programme the position of speech musculature and the sequencing of muscle movements (respiratory, laryngeal and oral) for the volitional production of phones as part of a neurological impairment, e.g. cerebral palsy; involuntary production of the same phone or movement is possible, e.g. cerebral palsy (Nicolosi et al. 2003; see Part II)

11.5.2 About Speech Sounds: Linguistic Fundamentals for Assessment

Every language has its specific inventory of speech sounds (for details on 57 languages, see Speech Accent Archive, Weinberger 2015). The way children develop the proper articulation of speech sounds (phonetics) and their correct linguistic use in language (phonology) follows physiological processes.Accordingly, speech sounds in a certain language are determined by these two components:

- The *phonetic component* emphasizes the specific physical and articulatory characteristics of each speech sound.
- In this sense speech sounds are called *phones*. The regular development of a child's phonetic inventory depends on normally developed speech organs, as well as normal hearing and oral-motor control. In this context the acquisition of the correct use of phones is an *aspect of speech development*. Speech sounds are usually subclassified into two broad groups: consonants and vowels. See Fig. 11.6 for an example of the phonetic inventory of consonants in English from the Speech Accent Archive (Weinberger 2015). See Fig. 11.7a, b for vowel charts of Jones (1972, adapted) and the International Phonetic Association (IPA 1999).The *phonological component* emphasizes the linguistic aspect speech sounds have in language as *phonemes*. A phoneme is the

shortest arbitrary unit of sound in a given language.

Nicolosi et al. (2003)

- It distinguishes the meaning of one word from another in the particular language: e.g. the use of the phonemes /t/ or /p/ distinguishes

between the word *cut* and *cup*. So the acquisition of the correct linguistic use of phonemes is an *aspect of language development*.

11.5.3 Considering the Framework for Assessing Speech Sound Development

Traditionally, immature speech motor skills were considered to cause SSD. As a consequence, investigating oral and speech motor movements with informal protocols is still one of the standard methods in assessing speech sound disorders. This traditional reduction of phonetic analysis only provides a gross quantitative measure of speech sound development (Dodd 2014; Fox-Boyer et al. 2016). For treatment recommendations this procedure does not provide a sufficient classification. It is, for example, well documented that phonological SSD nonverbal oral-motor training does not lead to an improved competence in speech sound use or to better sound intelligibility (e.g. Dodd 2014; Powell 2008). Specific phonological treatment is necessary. By contrast, traditional articulation therapy is most successful in phonetic disorders, but only

Consonants (Pulmonic)

	Bilabial	Labiodental	Dental	Alveolar	Postalveolar	Retroflex	Palatal	Velar	Uvular	Pharyngeal	Glottal
Plosive	p b			t d				k g			
Nasal	m			n				ŋ			
Trill											
Tap or Flap											
Fricative		f v	θ ð	s z	ʃ ʒ						h
Affricate					tʃ dʒ						
Lateral fricative											
Approximant				ɹ			j				
Lateral approximant				l							

Where symbols appear in pairs, the one to the right represents a voiced consonant. Shaded areas denote articulations judged impossible.

Fig. 11.6 Native phonetic inventory—English: the consonants found in most native English dialects are demonstrated. Source: Speech Accent Archive, Weinberger (2015) Speech Accent Archive, for English, adapted from Ladefoged (2006). Matrix of consonants: consonants are determined by three parameters according to the manner of formation—(a) place of articulation (*x*-axis), (b) mode of articulation (*y*-axis) and (c) use of voice (voiced/voiceless), e.g. [t] vs. [d] (definition adapted from Nicolosi et al. 2003). The worldwide convention is to transcribe phones according to the International Phonetic Alphabet (IPA). Republished with permission of South-Western College Publishing, a division of Cengage Learning, from A Course in Phonetics. Ladefoged P. 5th edition. Thomson Wadsworth, Boston © 2006

a

VOWELS

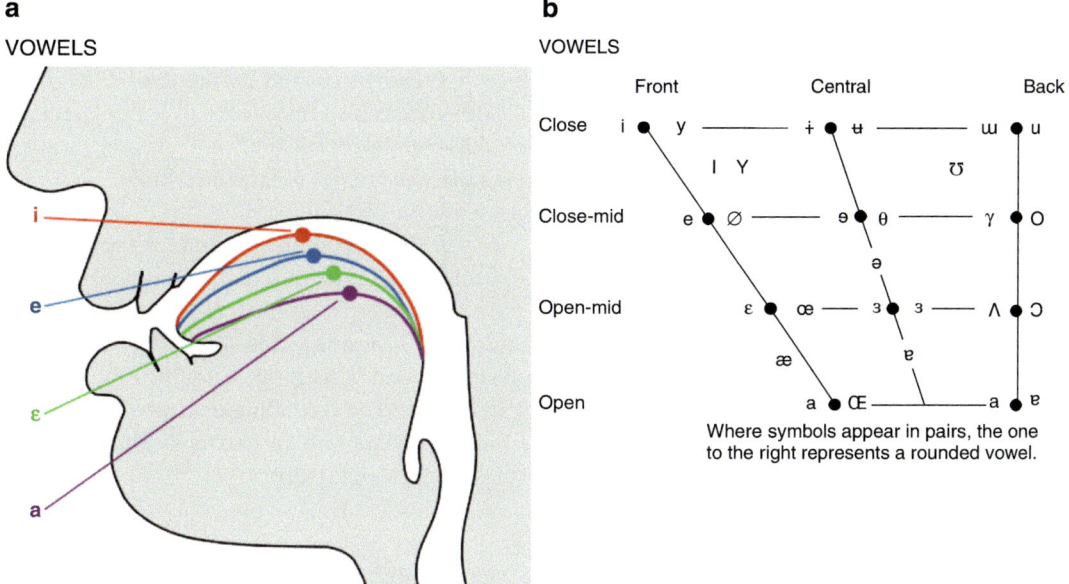

b

VOWELS

Where symbols appear in pairs, the one to the right represents a rounded vowel.

Fig. 11.7 (**a**) Cardinal tongue position regarding tongue height (vertical dimension) and tongue backness (horizontal dimension) for different vowels (i, e, ɛ, a; see Fig. 11.7b). Adapted by Ishwar and LadyofHats, based on Jones (1972). Image URL: https://de.wikipedia.org/wiki/Datei:Cardinal_vowel_tongue_position-back(png).svg. Covered by Creative Commons Attribution-ShareAlike 3.0 licence. (**b**) Schematic vowel diagram from the International Phonetic Alphabet representing the three main features to describe vowels: (1) In the vertical dimension vowels are arranged according to the degree of aperture of the mouth and jaw (from open to closed vowels) and the tongue *height* relative to the roof of the mouth. (2) In the horizontal dimension, vowels are arranged according to the position of the tongue in the mouth during the articulation (tongue *backness*: front, central, back). (3) The rounding of the lips during articulation determinates rounded from unrounded vowels (*roundedness*). The worldwide convention is to transcribe vowels according to the International Phonetic Alphabet (IPA) (definition adapted from IPA 1999; 2015; Nicolosi et al. 2003; Ladefoged 2006)

12% of SSDs of unknown origin in children are classified as purely phonetic disorders (Dodd 2014). Another example is the treatment of SSD in hearing-impaired children, which traditionally focuses on auditory training. From a psycholinguistic perspective, these children also need phonological treatment targets to establish their phonological system, despite the influence of their sensory-based limitations (Reichmuth 2018). So, differential diagnostics are needed to identify the nature of a child's speech sound disorder in order to select an appropriate treatment approach (Strand and McCauley 2008; Namasivayam et al. 2013; Dodd 2014). The structure of the diagnostic process for identifying SSDs should provide a well-based diagnosis enabling recommendations for efficient and evidence-based treatment. It has to be based on the best available evidence of therapy efficiency and effectiveness.

The contemporary theoretical framework coming from psycholinguistic research on SSD permits a broader look at children's developing speech sound processing with regard to phonological aspects of speech sounds, input and output difficulties or deficits in memory functioning. The two most noted psycholinguistic models are those of Stackhouse and Wells (1997) and Dodd (2005, 2014). Following Dodd (2005, 2014) and others (Fox-Boyer et al. 2016), cross-linguistic research on SSDs of unclear origin (i.e. excluding hearing impairment, dysglossia, dysarthria) are classified into five subgroups (marked in Fig. 11.5). Reasons for phonological disorders are delayed phonological development, e.g. due to repeated otitis media, and deficits in perceiving phonological information correctly, leading to consequent phonological disorders or severe deficits in phonological working memory, causing inconsequent phonological disorders (Dodd 2014; Fox-Boyer et al. 2016).

11.5.4 Cross-Linguistic Features in Normal Speech Sound Acquisition

Summarizing cross-linguistic studies on normal speech sound acquisition in 24 languages, McLeod (2012b) described the following cross-linguistic features in normal speech sound acquisition:

- Vowels, nasals, and plosives appear to be the *earliest sounds* to be produced by children. Children produce more sounds and greater articulatory variation as they grow older. McLeod (2012b)
- *Intelligibility* of speech rises continuously during the first 5 years of age. A guideline of Coplan and Gleason (1988) for expected conversational intelligibility levels of typically developing children is recommended by the ASHA (2016): 1 year, 25% intelligible; 2 years, 50% intelligible; 3 years, 75% intelligible; and 4 years, 100% intelligible.
- The *age of acquisition of consonants*, defined by the age when most children (90% or 75% by convention) are able to pronounce a consonant as does an adult and shows a wide diversity across languages. Nevertheless the 90% criterion of correct consonant production is reached in 5-year-olds cross-linguistically, whereas 2-year-olds produce consonants correctly at least 70% of the time (McLeod 2012b).
- *Common mismatches* are

  sounds children typically produce before they achieve the adult target.
  McLeod (2012b)

Some similarities are found across such sounds, but generally they differ between languages. For example, common mismatches for /s/ are (examples from McLeod 2012b):

- /s/—plosive consonant, e.g. [t] in many languages such as in English, Dutch, Finnish, Hungarian and Portuguese
- /s/—lateralized fricative, e.g. [ɬ] in Greek
- /s/—palatal consonant, e.g. palatalization in Japanese and [ʃ] in Israeli Hebrew

Typically, children's sound changes during speech development follow certain phonological error patterns, defined as *physiological phonological processes*. See Table 11.10 for these systemic and structural simplifications, which can be observed cross-linguistically in preschool children attempting to produce adultlike utterances (McLeod 2012b).

- In cases of *systematic simplifications*, the error pattern is conditioned by one phonological feature of the speech sound itself or its phoneme category, regardless of its position in the word. So fricatives are systematically replaced by a stop consonant, for example, and therefore the phonological error pattern is called *stopping* (see Table 11.10).
- In cases of *structural simplifications*, the error pattern is conditioned by word structure, phoneme surrounding and intonation. With the tendency to delete final consonants, even though they can be correctly pronounced in another position of the word, for example, the phonological error pattern is called 'final consonant deletion' (see Table 11.10).

11.5.5 Assessment Procedure of Speech Sound Disorders

A screening procedure of the developmental speech sound status for detecting an SSD has to fulfil the usual validity criteria for a screening, such as appropriate sensitivity and specificity. If a screening has failed or in cases of suspicion of an SSD, a comprehensive assessment should follow, examining the speech sound disorder in depth in order to classify the SSD subgroup (ASHA 2016).

Following international guidelines (ASHA 2004, 2016), the diagnostic procedure of a

Table 11.10 Physiological phonological processes in speech development (cross-linguistic)

Physiological phonological processes in speech development (cross-linguistic)[a]	Description of the phonological processes[b]	Example[b]
Systemic simplifications		
– Backing	Substitution of any nonvelar consonant by a velar	For example, tub= tʌg
– Fronting	Tendency to replace velar or palatal consonants by alveolar, bilabial or labiodental consonants	For example, velar fronting: cot = tot For example, palatal fronting: mash= mæs
– Stopping	Replacement of fricatives […] with a stop consonant	For example, soup= dup
– Devoicing	Substitution of a voiced consonant by a voiceless consonant	For example, big= bɪk
– Voicing	Voicing of voiceless consonants	For example, pen= bɛn
Structural simplifications		
– Assimilation/consonant harmony	Tendency to create internal symmetry within words; a process whereby a child changes one or more phonemes to match production features of other sounds or characteristics of an utterance	For example, velar assimilation: duck= gək For example, labial assimilation: top= bop
– Cluster reduction	Reduction of a consonant cluster to a single consonant	For example, spoon = pun
– Initial consonant deletion	Deletion of the initial consonant of a syllable or word	For example, house= aʊs
– Final consonant deletion	Reduction of consonant-vowel-consonant (CVC) words or syllables to a consonant-vowel (CV) form	For example, pig= pɪ
– Reduplication	Syllable duplication, doubling	For example, kitty= tɪ tɪ
– (Weak) syllable deletion	Dropping of unstressed syllables	For example, telephon= təfon

[a]McLeod (2012b)
[b]Description and examples from Nicolosi et al. (2003)

child with SSD should include the following assessments:

- History
- Oral-motor examination (see Sect. 11.4)
- Observation and documentation of spontaneous speech
- Judgement of intelligibility
- Examination with a naming test
- Stimulability of isolated phones
- Examination of speech perception
- Proving of phonological consequence in words
- Conclusion of assessment

11.5.5.1 History
Following the ASHA (2016), the case history typically includes gathering information about the:

- Family's concerns about the child's speech
- History of middle ear infections
- History of speech, language or literacy difficulties in the family
- Languages used in the home
- Primary language spoken by the child

Further information such as on oral sensory and functional development is gathered by the clinical history, e.g. on the birth, feeding, etc., which is part of the oral-motor examination (see Sect. 11.4).

11.5.5.2 Oral-Motor Examination

The oral-motor examination assesses the structural and functional adequacy of the speech movements (Nicolosi et al. 2003). The recommended procedure is outlined in Sect. 11.4. It should be applied regularly in order to supplement the assessment of the speech sound developmental status, to detect organic causes of an SSD and to enable distinctions between *phonetic* (articulatory movements) and *phonological* (linguistic) components of a speech sound disorder.

11.5.5.3 Observation and Documentation of Spontaneous Speech

The observation of spontaneous speech constitutes a relevant part of speech sound assessment. Spontaneous speech samples of the child during a dialogue or play activity provide an impression of the error patterns and the intelligibility of the child's speech. Moreover, the severity of the SSD and its influence on communicational behaviour and success can be observed. Severe to profound SSDs may lead to frequent conversational breakdown. Following the framework of the International Classification of Disability and Functioning in its children and youth version (ICF-CY; WHO 2007), the ASHA (2004) recommends appreciating the limitations of a child's activity and participation in social life caused by the SSD. Regarding this, parental concerns and burdens have also to be considered in the assessment.

11.5.5.4 Intelligibility

A judgement of a child's intelligibility is a useful indicator of the severity of its speech problem. It should be done by the examiner and may be supported by the impression of family members or other related persons. It is a subjective, perceptual judgement, based on how much of the child's spontaneous speech is understood by the listener. In order to guarantee comparability, it should

be assessed from a Likert scale. Intelligibility is often used to determine the need for intervention and to evaluate the progress of a therapy (ASHA 2016).

> A child of three years of age or older who is unintelligible is generally recognized as a candidate for treatment.
>
> Bernthal et al. (2013)

The *Intelligibility in Context Scale (ICS)* (McLeod 2012a, b) is recommended as a seven-item screening measure of children's speech intelligibility. It is designed for parents who rate the child's speech intelligibility for a range of communicative partners on a Likert scale (0–5). It is available free online in 60 languages, thus also enabling an assessment of speech intelligibility in multilingual children. In preschool children aged 4–5 years and 5 months, for example, the application of the ICS revealed significant differences between children whose parents had concerns about their child's speech and those who did not (McLeod et al. 2015). First data on bilingual children show that the ICS scores are robust across languages (McLeod et al. 2015).

11.5.5.5 Examination with a Naming Test

Single-word picture elicitation by the use of naming tests is standard for speech assessments in many languages. However, the use of well-validated, reliable and normed naming tests is still not established (McLeod and Verdon 2014). Besides single-word testing, the ASHA (2016) recommends the analysis of an additional speech sample of connected speech (e.g. story telling). The error analysis is aimed at determining whether the individual displays primarily phonetic speech production deficits or deficits associated with phonological constraints (ASHA 2004; Dodd 2005).

The construction of naming tests follows segment-orientated or process-orientated criteria (Fox-Boyer et al. 2016):

- *Segment-orientated assessment.* This focuses exclusively on the phonetic aspects of speech sound development by testing the correct articulation of every phone in single words. The result reveals a child's phonetic inventory and an independent analysis of speech sound error types (e.g. deletions, omissions, substitutions, distortions, additions or a description of atypical articulation). For assessing the *phonetic inventory* of children, the language-specific construction of the inventory (see Speech Accent Archive (online) for 57 languages, Weinberger 2015) and the language-specific course of phone development (normative data) should build the diagnostic basis for distinguishing age-adequate errors in the test performance from age-inadequate errors.

For a more comprehensive assessment, a relational analysis process-orientated testing is needed.

- *Process-orientated assessment.* This enables the analysis of the underlying phonological system of the child's speech sound development to explain the observed error pattern from a phonological perspective. Phonological error patterns are systemic or structural simplifications (see Table 11.9 for an overview) (McLeod 2012b; ASHA 2004). For assessing the correct or incorrect linguistic use of phonemes in children, the language-specific course of phoneme development (normative data) should establish the basis for distinguishing age-adequate errors and phonological processes (see Table 11.9) from the prolonged use of age-inadequate phonological processes and problems to overcome them.

Relying only on segment-orientated testing does not fulfil contemporary requirements for classifying SSDs, especially for the deduction of specific treatment recommendations (Fox-Boyer et al. 2016; Dodd 2014).

As to quality assurance of tests, McLeod and Verdon (2014) included 98 instruments designed to assess children's speech sound production in languages other than English in a review (62 had

been commercially published, 17 had been published in journal articles and 19 were informal assessments). Thirty of the commercially published assessment tests were available for in-depth analysis. These tests encompass the assessment of speech sounds for 17 languages other than English (Cantonese, Danish, Finnish, German, Greek, Japanese, Korean, Maltese-English, Norwegian, Pakistani-heritage languages, Portuguese, Putonghua (Mandarin), Romanian, Slovenian, Spanish, Swedish, Turkish). According to the review, about half (53%) of these assessment tests are norm-referenced with large variability in the size of the normative sample. These norm-referenced tests are listed in Table 11.11. The other assessments are criterion-referenced.

McLeod (2012c) further offers an unevaluated online collection of speech sound assessment instruments, templates and tests for 36 languages. It includes

> published tests and word lists that can be used to assess children's articulation and phonology in languages other than English.
>
> McLeod (2012c)

But a critical evaluation of test quality should be done by the professionals before they are used. As for all psychometric tests, adequate psychometric properties (e.g. validity, objectivity, reliability, norming) of tests to assess articulation (speech motor performance) and phonology (phonological error patterns) need to be fulfilled and documented. However, test construction and quality often do not fulfil these requirements (e.g. McCauley and Strand 2008; Kirk and Vigeland 2014; McLeod and Verdon 2014).

For high standards of assessment, normative data for each language regarding phonetic and phonological speech sound development are indispensable. Aiming at this target, test developers and researchers in the field need to improve the quality of available tests in order to increase the reliability and validity of speech sound assessment, because many tests do not fulfil classical criteria of test construction (see review of Flipsen and Ogiela 2015 for psychometric criteria for good test construction).

Table 11.11 Norm-referenced assessment tools of the speech sound developmental status of children for different languages

Assessed language	Name of assessment	Age range (years; months)	Phones *(segmental-oriented)*	Phonological processes *(process-orientated)*	Other areas relevant for SSD
Cantonese[a]	*Hong Kong Cantonese Articulation Test* (Cheung et al. 2006)	2;6–5;6	+	–	–
English[a,b]	*Diagnostic Evaluation of Articulation & Phonology (DEAP)* (Dodd et al., UK-edition, 2016 & US-edition, 2006)	3;0–6;11/8;11	+	+	Inconsistency of phonological processes; oromotor assessment
English[a,b]	*Toddler Phonology Tests (TPT)* (McIntosh and Dodd 2011)	2;0–2;11	+	+	–
Finnish	*Fonologiatesti* (Kunnari et al. 2012)	2;0–6;11	+	–	–
German	*Patholinguistische Diagnostik von Sprachentwicklungsstörungen* (Kauschke and Siegmüller 2009, 2nd ed.)	2;0–6;11	+	+	Perception; prosody; oromotor assessment
German[b] (incl. Austrian & Swiss-German)	*Psycholinguistische Analyse kindlicher Aussprachestörungen-II PLAKKS-II* (Fox-Boyer 2014)	2;6–8;0	+	+	Inconsistency of phonological processes
Greek	*Assessment of Phonetic & Phonological development* (Panhellenic Association of Logopedists 1995)	2;6–6;0	+	–	–
Korean	*Assessment of Phonology & Articulation for children* (Kim et al. 2007)	2;6–6;5	+	+	–
Korean	*Urimal Test of Articulation & Phonology* (Kim and Shin 2004)	2;0–6;11	+	+	–
Maltese-English[a]	*Maltese-English Speech Assessment* (Grech et al. 2011)	2;0–6;0	+	+	Stimulability, inconsistency of phonological processes; oromotor assessment
Pakistani[a] heritage languages: Mirpuri, Punjabi, Urdu	*Bilingual Speech Sound Screen: Pakistan heritage Languages* (Stow and Pert 2006)	1;4–7;11	+	+	
Putonghua	*Putonghua Segmental Phonology Test* (So and Jing 2000)	2;0–6;11	+	–	–
Spanish[a]	*Bilingual English-Spanish Assessment* (Peña et al. 2014)	4;0–6;11	+	–	–
Spanish[a]	*Contextual Probes of Articulation Competence: Spanish* (Goldstein and Iglesias 2006)	3;0–8;11	+	+	–
Spanish[a]	*Spanish Preschool Articulation Test* (Tsugawa 2002)	Not specified	+	–	–

Table 11.11 (continued)

Assessed language	Name of assessment	Age range (years; months)	Areas assessed		
			Phones *(segmental-oriented)*	Phonological processes *(process-orientated)*	Other areas relevant for SSD
Swedish	*Svenskt Artikulations-och Nasalittets Test* (Lohmander et al. 2005)	2;8–10;2	+	+	Oromotor assessment
Turkish	*Ankara Artikülasyon Testi* (Ege et al. 2004)	2;6–12;11	+	–	–
Turkish	*Türkçe* Sesletim-Sesbilgisi Testi (Topbaş 2004/2005)	1;3–14;3	+	+	Perception; oromotor assessment

Modified according to McLeod and Verdon (2014)
[a]Manual in English included
[b]Two English and one German assessment tools added by the section authors

11.5.5.6 Stimulability of Isolated Phones

Eliciting isolated phones enables the examiner to evaluate the degree of a child's ability to produce or imitate a previously misarticulated phone correctly. This procedure provides information about the speech motor skills of the child and the level of cueing that seems to be necessary to achieve the best speech sound production (e.g. auditory model; auditory and visual model; tactile cues) (ASHA 2016). Standards for the testing procedures are given by Glaspey and Stoel-Gammon (2007). Some test batteries include stimulability subtests (see Table 11.11) (ASHA 2016).

It is assumed that a good ability of sound imitation predicts the acquisition of a sound with or without intervention; this may help the selection of appropriate cues and therapy targets and may predict the improvement by an SSD therapy (ASHA 2016). This holds true at least for phonetic disorders and childhood apraxia of speech (CAS), but for phonological disorders, testing the speech sound stimulability is of questionable predictive value with respect to treatment necessity and success.

11.5.5.7 Speech Perception Testing

A child's fundamental linguistic and auditory perceptual abilities or limitations for acquiring correct phoneme use is examined by testing its speech sound discrimination (another part of auditory speech perception is tested by speech audiometry).

The following test constituents are recommended (ASHA 2016; Nicolosi et al. 2003):

- Auditory speech sound discrimination: the basic auditory ability to differentiate paired speech sounds with minimal contrasts in syllables or words without lip reading; assessment requires a same-different response (e.g. /jam/ vs. /jam/; /cam/ vs. /jam/).
- Phoneme discrimination by picture identification: the auditory and linguistic ability to discriminate slight phonemic contrast of phonemes in minimal word pairs without lip reading; assessment requires the identification of one picture out of two to four by pointing (e.g. house/mouse/louse).

Children with phonetic SSD and normal hearing should perform properly in these tasks, whereas children with phonological SSD and healthy hearing often show difficulties. In cases of abnormal test results, further examinations are used to determine if errors are related to a generalized perceptual problem (Bernthal et al. 2013).

Children with hearing impairment often have limitations in speech sound perception. Diagnostic procedures of these children should allow the examiner to determine which speech sounds are properly understood and whether hearing devices are well-fitted and functioning. Auditory discrimination tasks may help to evaluate which phonemic contrasts are audible for the child and which speech sounds must be cued visually throughout therapy.

11.5.5.8 Proving of Phonological Consistency in Words

This examination is needed in cases of a phonological disorder. To identify whether a phonological error occurs consistently (in all naming trials of a word the same phonological process is used) or inconsistently (the use of phonological processes in a word differs in the repeated naming procedure), certain criteria for test material are needed. Fox-Boyer et al. (2016) summarize the following international criteria for designing a speech test that focuses on phonological process analysis including the assessment of consistency:

- The test includes about 100 items.
- All phonemes are tested in different positions in the word up to four times.
- Items vary in number of syllables, structure of syllables and word stress.
- Normative data allow the differentiation of a developmental delay of speech sound acquisition and a speech sound disorder.

11.5.5.9 Conclusion of Assessment

The assessment of the speech sound developmental status of a child should result in:

- Diagnosis and subclassification (see Fig. 11.5 and Table 11.9) of a speech sound disorder
- Description of the characteristics and severity of the disorder (mild-severe-profound)
- Identification of factors that might contribute to the speech sound disorder
- Referral to other professionals or further comprehensive assessment as needed
- Parental guidance by giving information and advice about the SSD of their child
- Recommendations for specific intervention targets based on the classified SSD
- Planning follow-up assessments in order to control the outcome of an SSD intervention

(see Dodd 2005 for treatment targets of phonological disorders)

11.6 Objective Speech Motor Analysis in Children

Ben A. M. Maassen and Adam P. Vogel

11.6.1 Introduction

Speaking is the most complex motor performance humans can conduct. Approximately 100 muscles are involved, which together have to control intricately time-aligned movements. Complex series of such movements result in an utterance, that is, an acoustic speech signal with specific qualities that can be understood by the listener. Because of the intricate complexity of our speech production system, the quality of single speech movements cannot be evaluated in isolation, but need the background of the neurological and motor processes involved in speech production.

11.6.2 Process-Orientated Approach

The production of speech is controlled by systems and strategies that include the planning and preparation (or *programming*) of movements and the execution of these programs to result in muscle contractions and structural displacements (Kent 2000). It is well known that—for a native speaker of English—pronouncing a word in a foreign language (such as the French 'cathédrale') is more difficult than pronouncing an equally complex word in one's native language (the English 'cathedral'). Repetitions of such a word would be less consistent in the foreign than in the native language. It can be concluded that the quality of speech movements depends not only on the auditory and neurophysiological motor control functions but to a large extent also on the higher-level control strategies. For the motor control of speech, these higher levels are the language functions: vocabulary, sentence pro-

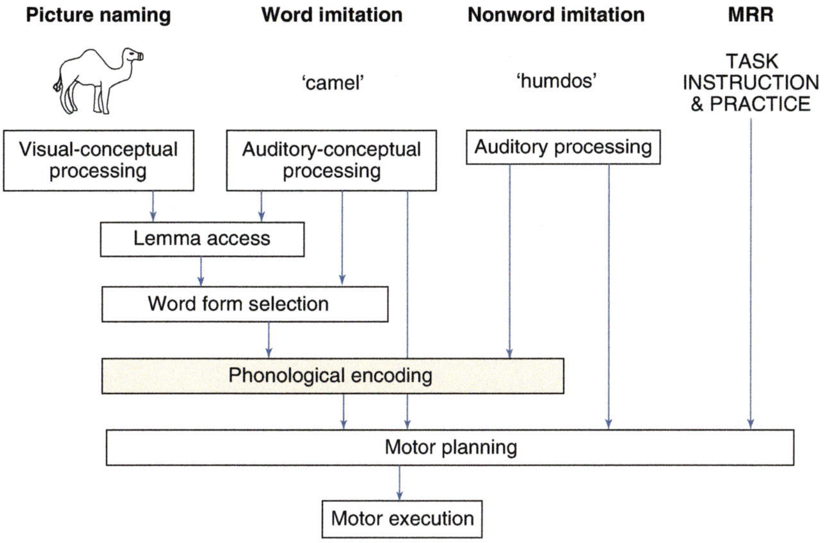

Fig. 11.8 Elicitation tasks for a process-orientated speech production analysis (source: Maassen and Terband 2015, with kind permission from Wiley and Sons)

duction processes and phonological skills. There is abundant evidence that persons with apraxia of speech, for example, produce better speech quality when producing familiar and overlearned utterances (like spontaneous, emotional phrases) than linguistically more complex and completely new utterances. Therefore, in clinical practice, speech assessment in children is based on different tasks of varying complexity and analyses of performance contrasts between tasks (Fig. 11.8).

Manipulation of speech conditions, followed by comparison of speech performance under different conditions, allows for a *process-orientated diagnosis*. For example, non-word imitation tasks assess the quality of the auditory-motor stream of speech production: how well can the child programme and execute speech movements that result in the same auditory template as the presented model. The motor strategies involved are based on auditory targets. In contrast, picture naming requires retrieval of the auditory-articulatory word form stored in long-term memory, followed by planning and programming the speech movements according to an internal model.

In clinical motor-speech evaluations, it is not uncommon to elicit non-speech movements for the assessment of neuromuscular functions. Examples are the maximum repetition-rate (MRR), a.k.a. diadochokinetic (DDK) task, such as /pʌpʌpʌ.../, /tʌtʌʌtʌ.../ and /pʌtʌkʌ.../, or maximum sound prolongation, such as /aaaa..../ or /sssss.../, to assess coordination of respiratory, vocal and articulatory functions. The role and benefit of the assessment of non-speech oral movements are controversially discussed with respect to many oral-motor disorders, and thus determining the clinical value of these movements requires careful definitions and task descriptions (Kent 2015).

Therefore, a process-orientated model is required for the clinical interpretation of speech performance. Below, the available methods are described for assessing speech performances objectively: perceptual judgement, acoustic analysis, physiological measurements and kinematic measurements.

11.6.2.1 Perceptual Analysis

Listener-based evaluation of speech production remains the standard process for describing output in clinical practice. This also is largely true for experimental descriptive work to evaluate how speakers sound at a single time point. The attraction of perceptual judgement is clear. It is relatively straightforward for clinicians to apply in clinical settings. A widely accepted terminology allows clinicians and researchers to describe a patient across broad speech subsystems of articulation, prosody, voice quality and respiration. For cases with concomitant speech and language deficits, transcription is essential for accurate differential diagnosis of phonological (language) versus articulation (speech) disorders in children and phonemic versus phonetic contrasts in adults (e.g. frontotemporal dementia (Poole et al. 2017)).

A specific method based on perceptual judgement is a phonetic transcription, in which speech is transcribed with help of the International Phonetic Alphabet (IPA 2015), followed by analyses that consist of counting occurrences of particular sound productions. Several studies have shown that broad phonetic transcription that uses the basic symbols without diacritics[1] can reliably be made by trained speech-language pathologists, but the percentage correspondence between two transcribers drops to 25% when diacritics are also included (Vieregge and Maassen 1999).

Thus, most phonetic transcriptions in fact are phonemic transcriptions (transcriptions of the phonemes contained in an utterance), which implies that they are applied for research and diagnosis of phonological (Hodson and Paden 1991) or higher language disorders rather than of motor-speech disorders. However, several studies have demonstrated the use of transcriptions for studying childhood apraxia of speech (CAS). Such comprehensive studies analysing segmental error patterns have been conducted by Maassen et al. (1997), Thoonen (1998) and Thoonen et al. (1994). Phonetic transcriptions of consonants produced in word and pseudo-word imitation tasks revealed overall increased substitution and omission rates for the children with CAS in comparison with children with normal speech. Because errors in these studies were quantified, it was possible to make a *speech profile* by correcting for overall error rate. It was found that, while children with CAS produce a higher rate of phoneme anticipations, perseverations and metatheses (i.e. syntagmatic errors[2]) than control subjects, after correction for the overall higher error rate, the *relative* number of syntagmatic and paradigmatic errors appears identical for both groups. In general, the error profiles showed very few differences between groups, suggesting that the speech of children with CAS can be characterized by a high rate of 'normal' slips of the tongue. However, the children with CAS showed specifically a low percentage of retention of place of articulation in words and inconsistency with respect to feature realization and feature preference. These two characteristics, high rate of place-of-articulation errors and inconsistency, stood out as possibly diagnostic for CAS.

11.6.2.2 Hardware Options for Speech and Voice Assessment

Speech samples can be recorded by using a variety of hardware options (see Vogel and Morgan (2009) for hardware/software and Svec and Granqvist (2010) for microphones), with the quality of those recordings in part determined by the acoustic measurements of interest. A push to use ubiquitous devices such as smartphones in clinical and experimental settings has led to validation studies comparing low-quality (but easy to use) hardware and high-quality (but potentially cumbersome, expensive or difficult to use) configurations (Lin et al. 2012; Manfredi et al. 2016; Vogel and Maruff 2008; Vogel et al. 2014). Current evidence highlights the limitations of smartphones for measures of perturbation (i.e. voice quality) but confirms their utility in other contexts (i.e. listener-based ratings, less fine-grained acoustic analysis such as frequency, intensity or timing). Briefly, when considering whether recording hardware is suitable for the purpose, an examiner should consider why they are using the equipment, how portable it needs to be, costs and whether the equipment should

---

[1]Diacritics are symbols to indicate slight deviance of sound articulation; examples are aspiration of a plosive [e.g. /tʰ/] or more centralized articulation of a vowel [e.g. /ë/].

[2]As defined by Thoonen et al. (1994), syntagmatic errors are related to the context, such as anticipations, perseverations and transpositions; paradigmatic errors are speech sound errors of place, manner or voice, not induced by the context.

be calibrated and those undertaking subsequent analysis of recordings require further training (Vogel and Morgan 2009).

11.6.2.3 Acoustic Analysis of Speech and Voice

Acoustic analysis of speech is an objective method for describing speech output. The nature of motor-speech production dictates a multi-parameter approach to analysis. As for listener-based ratings, analysis can focus on measures of *timing*, *intensity*, *quality* and *frequency*. Examples of acoustic measures of timing include inter-word intervals, percentage of silence within a sample or speech rate (see Vogel et al. (2012) for their application). Intensity can be explored through measurements of spectral tilt (differences in power across the spectrum, e.g. the alpha ratio (Vogel et al. 2010)) or measurements of sound pressure (e.g. decibels). There is a variety of voice quality measurements including cepstral analysis (see Vogel et al. (2017) for its application), measures of perturbation such as jitter and shimmer, as well as summative parameters such as the harmonics-to-noise ratio. Frequency can be described in the context of its fundamental (acoustic equivalent of pitch) and formants (resonant frequencies of the vocal tract). There are many software options available to examiners. They differ in accuracy and algorithms deployed to describe the signal (Burris et al. 2014; Tsanas et al. 2014), usability and cost (Vogel and Morgan 2009), with some high-quality free options (e.g. *Praat*, http://www.fon.hum.uva.nl/praat/, Boersma and Weenink 2014).

11.6.2.4 Stimuli and Elicitation of Speech Samples

Assessments for identifying strengths and weaknesses (characterization) of a speaker's speech profile require a different methodological approach to assessments designed to measure changes in speech over time, resulting from treatment or disease progression (see Vogel and Maruff (2014) for review of consideration of these issues). Characterization of speech is needed for recognizing targets for therapy and for providing differential diagnosis. It can be adequately

achieved in one session by examiners eliciting a variety of speech tasks designed to provide a diagnosis. Assessment protocols for characterization can include a combination of connected speech tasks (e.g. monologue or conversation, picture description, reading or automated tasks such as counting), sustained vowels (e.g. prolonged /a:/), alternating motion rate tasks (e.g. diadochokinesis), non-word tasks or repetition of words increasing in length and complexity.

To determine whether speech has changed from a baseline assessment, we need to know what it sounds like when it is stable. Assessments detecting change should be sensitive to impairment and be stable in the absence of any modifications in performance. To avoid changes in function resulting from repeated assessment (i.e. practice, motivation, physiological voice fluctuations (Vogel and Maruff 2014)), protocols should be concise, easy to complete and sensitive to impairment, have alternative forms for mitigating the impact of familiarity/practice and incorporate factors such as time of day, mental health and motivation of the speaker (Vogel et al. 2011).

11.6.2.5 Physiological and Kinematic Assessment of Motor Speech

The value of instrumental assessments of speech is questionable in clinical assessments. The time demand, cost and expertise required to administer tests can be prohibitive, and interpretation does not typically suit clinical assessment time frames. In a research context, however, physiological or kinematic tools can provide information on the underlying mechanisms influencing output.

The muscular control of speech can be investigated by physiological protocols including electromyography (EMG) of the tongue (e.g. genioglossus) or larynx (e.g. cricothyroid) (Hardcastle 2006). EMG records the electrical activity of muscles either via surface electrodes or intramuscular sensors. Data can provide understanding of muscle activation (e.g. duration and site of activation) during speech tasks. The utility of EMG as a diagnostic or therapeutic tool is challenged by our relatively limited knowledge of the subtle and complex nature of speech musculature. The value of surface

EMG in particular is further limited by varying degrees of sensitivity in relation to relevant muscle activation (Stepp 2012). With increased knowledge on suitable innervation locations, EMG may in the future provide a viable treatment modality for treatment in some motor-speech disorders.

Electropalatography (EPG) measures tongue-to-palate contact from sensors embedded within a palatal plate worn by the speaker. EPG data include both temporal and spatial information on tongue placement and are represented visually (Gibbon and Lee 2016). The visual image can be used by assessors to describe aspects of articulation, differentiating domains of impairment (Folker et al. 2010), or by patients as a feedback tool to adjust their own speech (Morgan et al. 2007). Similar to EPG, electromagnetic articulography (EMA) provides information on the consistency and stability of movement patterns relating to speech by measuring the action of articulators within a 3D space. Speakers wear a helmet with transmitter coils attached to anatomical sites relevant for the investigation, commonly the upper and lower lip, jaw, tongue tip and body (Fig. 11.9). The generated data can provide an understanding of the underlying

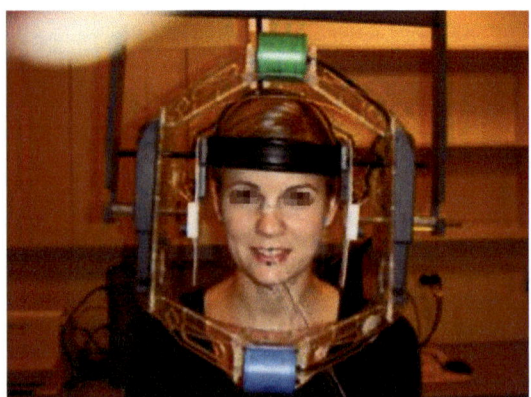

Fig. 11.9 Electromagnetic articulography (EMA; Courtesy of Dr. Joanne Folker; Carstens Medizinelektronik GmbH, Germany). Note: The sensor coils attached to the lips, nose and tongue generate a current that is inversely proportional to the cube of the distance to each of three induction coils (behind the subject, not shown here), from which their position in the midsagittal plane can be calculated. More recent versions of this equipment allow for 3D localization

movements associated with different speech disorders (Folker et al. 2011; Shellikeri et al. 2016; Terband et al. 2011) by providing data on deviations from the midline and the velocity of tongue movements in connected speech.

11.6.2.6 Neuroimaging Studies

Imaging modalities such as magnetic resonance imaging (MRI) can provide information on the underlying neurological control of motor-speech production. Recent reviews point to a relative absence of experimental work describing the structural and functional outcomes of motor-speech disorder in children (Liégeois et al. 2014; Morgan et al. 2016). In the pediatric context, there is currently no evidence to suggest that right-sided lesions are more likely to result in dysarthria or left-hemisphere lesions in apraxia of speech (Liégeois and Morgan 2012). Importantly, persistent dysarthria, rather than an impairment that resolves spontaneously, is thought to be the result of bilateral lesions (Morgan et al. 2013). In adult populations, our understanding of the neural correlates of motor-speech production is largely drawn from the stroke literature. Recent evidence in apraxia highlights the importance of the left precentral gyrus (Itabashi et al. 2016) and reduced bilateral premotor connectivity relative to severity in apraxia (New et al. 2015). Corollary evidence from studies of patients with neurodegenerative diseases such as dementia points to a breakdown within the speech networks connecting premotor planning areas to temporal language regions (Ballard et al. 2014; Mandelli et al. 2014). Evidence from dysarthria studies also highlights the role of subcortical and cerebellar regions in precise speech motor control and modification (Morgan et al. 2016; Urban 2013).

11.6.3 Concluding Remarks

We have described objective methods for the assessment of speech motor symptoms in children at different levels of the communication chain from the brain of the speaker to the ears of the listener and beyond. Speech disorders can be described in neurological, structural, physiological, acoustic and auditory terms. As argued in the introduction, proper interpretation of measurement data requires a speech production model and comparison of speech performances under different conditions, so-called *process-orientated* diagnostics.

11.7   Assessment of the Cognitive and General Developmental Status of Children

Christiane Kiese-Himmel

11.7.1   Introduction

Linguistic as well as cognitive abilities develop in mutual interdependence. Consequently, infants with delayed or disordered language development will achieve age-appropriate verbal intellectual functioning later than normal, and infants with delayed cognitive development, more specifically with cognitive deficits (e.g. limited capacity in phonological working memory, perceptual weaknesses), will learn language later.

There are also many genetic syndromes with behavioural phenotypes that affect language acquisition, given their association with learning disabilities or mental disability (significantly subaverage in intellectual functioning from IQ < 85), or a general developmental delay. Moreover, infants with foetal alcohol exposure often have impaired mental functioning and language learning problems. Children with other developmental disorders of speech and language associated with language-relevant comorbidities (synonym: nonspecific language impairment) often do not perform age-appropriately on measures of nonverbal intelligence. By definition, children with specific developmental disorders of speech and language (synonym: specific language impairment) display a significant discrepancy (two standard deviations or more below the average for their age) between receptive (or expressive) language abilities and age-level nonverbal intelligence and an average or higher psychometric intelligence. A valid and reliable assessment of a child's cog-

nitive abilities and aptitude is the base for future clinical examinations and provides baseline data to monitor the effects of intervention.

11.7.2   Types of Diagnostic Assessment Approach

The *examiner* (usually a *qualified developmental* or *clinical psychologist*) has to be aware of the specific clinical question of the phoniatrician/pedaudiologist. This question determines the selection of the approach:

- Screening for developmental delay (before further assessment)
- Broad and in-depth assessment

as well as the assessment tools such as:

- Clinical interview
- Parental report
- Behavioural checklist/questionnaire
- Observational assessment
- Normed and standardized test
- Test battery.

Normally, an intelligence test has to be administered to obtain an idea of a child's cognitive development status, which means his or her ability to solve problems by perception, verbal and nonverbal reasoning. There are many different types of test for measuring intelligence.

11.7.3   Pre-assessment Information

A pre-, peri- or postnatal risk factor may limit (early) cognitive achievement of a child, and multiple risk factors may have cumulative effects on his or her development. Therefore, before testing a child, the examiner should obtain information on the history of the child (mainly history of maternal, pregnancy and perinatal conditions; (extremely) low birth weight; postnatal pathological conditions; physical developmental milestones; family history concerning hearing, language, academic difficulties; socio-economic status of the family) and results of physical examinations, additional existing diagnoses and medications, treatment histories or information from other professionals. Non-medical professionals (e.g. teachers) should only be contacted for information if parents/caregivers have given written permission.

11.7.4 General Principles for Psychometric Procedures in the Clinical Setting

An infant (till 1 year), a toddler (ages 1–3 years) or a preschooler (ages 3–5 years) has limited concentration, a short attention span, short interest levels and insufficient abilities to regulate its own behaviour compared with older children.

- The individual assessment should consequently take place in a neutral assessment context, be interesting for the child and be of a rather brief duration. It is recommended to take breaks or to perform several diagnostic sessions, if necessary.

Furthermore, the child's ability to interact and react adequately with an unknown person in an unfamiliar environment without the presence of a parent or another family member is relevant to the assessment situation.

- Since many children perform better in the presence of individuals to whom they have close relations, the examiner should provide or permit their presence (except in certain child-protection assessment situations in which a parent tends to interfere or to offer solutions to the child).
- The examiner should introduce himself or herself in the entry phase and describe the purpose of the meeting ('pre-diagnostic interaction').

The examiner has to bear in mind that tests have to be administered carefully in order to avoid diagnostic errors and to produce a reliable result that reflects the true level of cognitive functioning.

- The examiner must be informed about the methods of intellectual assessment and the theoretical underpinnings of the assessment tools, their characteristics, psychometric properties and limitations (e.g. handicaps accommodating assessment), be familiar with these and experienced with the tools. In general, the examiner should be experienced in working with children.
- Most importantly, aspects addressing the sensory integrity status and special needs such as motor disabilities of the child have to be taken into account. The latter are presumptions for a proper interpretation of the results in the context of all available information.
- Estimation of the general cognitive developmental stage should begin with demands or items that are within the child's capability. The examiner has to follow the instructions, examination and analysis procedures carefully, particularly the order in which the subtests have to be administered; to conduct the assessment tools accurately, in a fair and ethical manner; and to assure confidentiality. It is a breach of ethics for a psychologist to administer an intelligence test without the child's full understanding.
- Finally, the examiner should have the clinical skills required to interpret the assessment data appropriately, to synthesize them with all other available information into an overall picture and to communicate their relevance to other professionals (e.g. therapists) as well as family members in a sensitive way.

11.7.5 Aim of Psychometric Procedures

The main objective of psychometric procedures is the assessment of the general developmental status, more specifically the cognitive status (including the general intelligence level), in making classification and placement according to test scores, differential diagnosis or educational decisions and support needs. This is necessary to ascertain whether the child is at risk of cognitive developmental delay or exhibits:

- A major isolated development problem
- A broad developmental delay up to a global retardation
- Some cognitive weaknesses
- A reduced verbal intelligence quotient (IQ)
- A learning disorder (IQ 70–84 according to ICD-10)
- A mental retardation (mild, IQ 50–69; moderate, IQ 35–49; severe, IQ 20–34; profound, IQ < 20)
- An intelligence score average or above normal ('high-ability' children).

The diagnosis involves testing and evaluation. Individual testing is much more reliable than testing in a group, but no single test can identify who is mentally handicapped. Multiple scores and several criteria must be combined in order to make this judgement—as for judging 'high-ability' children—given that genetic and contextual factors interact. In the light of brain plasticity during early childhood, cognitive disabilities may be modulated by environmental factors, such as the social or educational context, with consequences for the cortical development.

Amongst children with impaired cognitive functioning, other psychological problems often emerge. Subsequently, the child's pattern of strengths and weaknesses of cognitive competence has to be identified as a marker for his or her:

- Further developmental course
- Therapy, training or another intervention success
- Special education needs
- Academic achievements and school performance.

11.7.6 Selected Examples of Assessment Tools

Infancy and childhood diagnostic assessments focus on special domains or on a broad range of development. The supposed cognitive developmental level at which the child functions and his or her history both influence his or her understanding of the tasks. Therefore, diagnostic instruments should be selected on the basis of the child's chronological age, medical and developmental history and their validity, reliability and user-friendliness (quick and easy to administer). Furthermore, the presence or absence of up-to-date standards or norms should be considered for the selection. Intelligence tests are the best available tools for revealing a child's cognitive functioning. The most popular assessment tools have been adopted from US, British or Dutch instruments.

11.7.6.1 Age Ranges
Infancy and Toddler Age An infant or toddler with suspected language disability has to be assessed via a well-standardized, norm-referenced, valid and reliable *developmental scale*. It should be complemented by a description of the individual's functional difficulties and a *caregiver's evaluation of development and behaviour*, which has been shown to be as accurate as those administered by professionals in identifying children with developmental problems (Glascoe and Dworkin 1995).

Childhood A child should first be assessed with a *nonverbal intelligence test* offering optimal psychometric properties in order to avoid problems in understanding and following instructions ('culture-fair assessment'). Most behavioural tests require a spoken response. Therefore, a verbal assessment may not be appropriate for children whose reduced speech intelligibility will invalidate the interpretation of responses. A language-free measure is also suitable for children with hearing loss, developmental disorder of speech and language, autism or test anxiety; for children from linguistically and culturally diverse backgrounds (e.g. migrant children); and for children who are difficult to test. Testing should be complemented by measures completed by parents (e.g. questionnaires).

11.7.6.2 Early Childhood Assessment Tools
Early childhood assessment tools are, for example, the single administered, norm-referenced *Bayley Scales of Infant and Toddler Development* (current version: *Bayley III*) from 1 to 42 months (Bayley 2006, 2014) or the *Griffiths Mental*

Development Scales Revised from 2 to 8 years (Luiz et al. 2006). They measure, amongst other abilities, sensorimotor intelligence, receptive and expressive language and social-emotional behaviour, whereas intelligence tests focus more on cognitive abilities. That is, the skills evaluated by infant scales are not the same as those measured by psychometric intelligence tests. A useful adjunct to intelligence tests is measurement of cognitive processes underlying performance in intelligence tests, such as working memory capacity which is the base, amongst others, for an increase of other cerebral capacities, for example, the mental lexicon.

11.7.6.3 Example of Measures of Intelligence

Intelligence tests evaluate different components of mental functioning and assess cognitive development. A good example of *measures of intelligence* is the standardized and norm-referenced *Kaufman-Assessment Battery for Children (K-ABC*; Kaufman and Kaufman 1983) for children aged 2.5 through 12.5 years, which permits testing of hearing- or speech-language-impaired individuals or those with limited English proficiency. It comprises a multidimensional cognitive processing approach with items of little cultural content. A composite mental score results from the areas of 'sequential' versus 'simultaneous' information processing, investigated by several subtests. Furthermore, an achievement score and a nonverbal intelligence score can be calculated. In the meantime, a revision was published (*K-ABC-II*; Kaufman and Kaufman 2004) to make the test appropriate for a wider age (from 3 to 18 years) and for a wider range of abilities. The subtests are organized in three levels (ages 3; 4–6; 7–18 years). The *K-ABC-II* is—like the *K-ABC*—founded on Luria's neuropsychological model corresponding to learning abilities, sequential vs. simultaneous processing and planning ability and on the psychometric Cattell-Horn-Carroll approach of long-term and of short-term memory, visual processing, fluid reasoning and crystallized abilities (McGrew 2005). It yields a nonverbal composite and a mental processing fluid-crystallized index plus individual scale scores. Melchers and Melchers published the German version *K-ABC-II* (2015).

11.7.6.4 Latest Revisions of the Snijders-Oomen Nonverbal Intelligence Tests

Another example concerns the latest revisions (Tellegen and Laros 1993) of the popular *Snijders-Oomen Nonverbal Intelligence Tests: SON-R 2.5-7* comprising six subtests with separate total scores for the spatial performance and for the reasoning scale (Tellegen et al. 1998, 2009) and *SON-Revised 5.5-17* with seven subtests without a memory test, but with abstract reasoning and concrete reasoning tests, spatial tests and perceptual tests (Snijders et al. 1989). Both tests also provide a total intelligence score that indicates how an infant or a child performs in comparison with other children of the same age; and both tests are well suited for use with children of ethnic minorities (Tellegen and Laros 2005) as well as for mentally retarded, hearing- or speech-language-impaired and autistic children, because they do not need spoken language in administration. The *SON* tests are used in several countries, and test manuals are published in several languages. For example, a standardization of the SON-R 2.5-7 has been conducted in the Netherlands, Germany, the United Kingdom, Denmark, France, the Czech Republic, Portugal, Slovakia and Romania.

11.7.6.5 General Intelligence Functioning

The approach used in the family of the popular *Wechsler Intelligence Scale for Children* is based on the general intelligence functioning (highest 'g' loading), e.g. the *Wechsler Intelligence Scale for Children-IV* with an age range of 6 years to 16 years and 11 months (*WISC-IV*; Wechsler 2003), adapted for some European countries, e.g. Spain and the UK in 2004 and Germany in 2011. It comprises ten core subtests and five additional subtests that can be summed to provide four indices and one full scale IQ. Thus, it is a multi-trait/multi-method test. In the meantime, the fifth edition with 14 subtests has been published (*WISC-V*

Integrated; Wechsler 2014); it is considered as a powerful upgrade for better understanding of a child's cognitive processes and for choosing of appropriate interventions.

The *Wechsler Preschool and Primary Scale of Intelligence* was originally developed by Wechsler in 1967 for preschoolers and young children (2 years 6 months to 7 years 7 months old). The test, now replaced by the *WPPSI-IV* (Wechsler 2012) with new processing speed subtests and reduced expressive language requirements, is available in many other European languages, e.g. Danish, Dutch, English (UK), Finnish, French, German, Icelandic, Italian, Lithuanian, Norwegian, Portuguese, Slovenian, Spanish and Swedish. Subtests exist for two age bands: 2 years 6 months to 3 years 11 months and 4 years 0 month to 7 years 7 months. For both, three levels of results are offered: full scale, primary index scale (verbal comprehension index; visual-spatial index; working memory index; fluid reasoning index; processing speed index) and ancillary index scale levels (vocabulary acquisition index; nonverbal index; general ability index; cognitive proficiency index).

11.7.6.6 Nonverbal Matrices

The nonverbal *Raven's Progressive Matrices* (measuring general intelligence) require the ability to recognize shapes/figures and their relationships, e.g. in childhood and for persons of limited intellectual ability. The brief intelligence measure *Coloured Progressive Matrices* (*CPM*), a 36-item test, has an age range from 5 to 11 years and the *Standard Progressive Matrices* (*SPM*) from 6 years to 16 years 0 month and from 17 years 0 month years of age upwards, a 60-item test used in measuring abstract reasoning and fluid intelligence. They are all unidimensional tests, but a useful nonverbal measure of overall cognitive functioning, and provide an overall intelligence score (Raven et al. 2004).

11.7.6.7 Alternative Testing Approaches

In addition, there are a number of alternative testing approaches and methods for estimating general cognitive developmental stage (e.g.

neuropsychological-based assessment; learning tasks; informal play-based assessment) and more individually administered tests of intelligence that could not all be named and described in this brief overview.

11.7.7 Assessment Results

The assessment of both the child's cognitive processing abilities and of intelligence in an individually administered test indicates the intellectual level and profile as well as any delay or risk. This assessment information must be evaluated by the examiner in order to ensure that the results are valid and reliable and to determine a diagnosis (in combination with all clinical data) including both management and conclusions such as prognostic implications.

11.7.8 Forward Look

Frequently, re-evaluation ('follow-up') and consideration of environmental and biomedical variables are necessary:

- To identify whether a child has caught up his or her delay(s)
- To locate patterns of development (e.g. continuity; discontinuity; spurts; atypical)
- To monitor the further development processes in children at (high) risk (e.g. in case of preterm birth; very low-birth weight; persistent hearing impairment).

Nevertheless, high correlations between developmental infant assessment and the measurement of intelligence at later ages should not be expected, because intelligence is not a unitary construct. Comorbidity may be relevant for outcomes of cognitive development even when the nonverbal IQ is normal. Intelligence is also correlated with functional literacy and socioeconomic status, and children who underachieve in educational systems may suffer a decline in their intelligence.

11.8 Assessment of Emotion, Behaviour and Attention in Language Disorders

Peter Matulat and
Tahany AbdelKarim Elsayed

11.8.1 Introduction

Children with developmental disorders of speech and language (DDSL) often show co-existing behavioural and attentional abnormalities. A proper diagnosing of DDSL therefore has to take into consideration whether such abnormalities are present and to what extent they influence the communicative, social and academic performance of a child.

A proper diagnosis includes the decision on which of the individual components of this complex disorder needs intervention (medical, psychological treatment or educational support) and which component has priority in treatment. This section describes the association between DDSL and behavioural and attentional abnormalities and proposes exemplary assessment tools for making a safe diagnosis of behavioural and attention disorders associated with DDSL.

11.8.2 Attention Disorders and Disorders of Speech and Language

Attention deficit/hyperactivity disorders (ADHD) and specific developmental disorders of speech and language (DDSL) are both common neurodevelopmental disorders that have a negative impact on children across social and educational domains and that create family and social burdens extending beyond the affected individual (Barkley 2006; Biederman et al. 2004). The onset of such disorders normally takes place at an early age, and they often persist throughout the person's life (Ebejer et al. 2012). Before the age of 5, it is difficult to diagnose, because most young infants are easily deflectable and impulsive. The worldwide-pooled prevalence of ADHD in children is estimated to be 5.3% with no significant difference between Europe and North America (Polanczyk et al. 2007; Willcutt 2012). The disorder affects approximately five times as many boys as girls (Novik et al. 2006).

DDSL is one of the disorders that frequently co-occur with ADHD (Sciberras et al. 2014). It even has been reported as the most frequent comorbidity for ADHD, occurring in 6.7–11.5% of cases (Rosenbaum and Simon 2016). In a literature review, co-occurrence rates of ADHD and DDSL ranging from 5% to almost 95% have been reported (Redmond 2016). Children with ADHD have more deficits in receptive and expressive language and memory than typically developed children (DaParma et al. 2011).

The high co-occurrence of ADHD and DDSL raises the question of a common neuropsychological cause (Mueller and Tomblin 2012). In fact, neuropsychological and genetic studies have found similarities between both nosological entities beyond entity-specific findings (Boada et al. 2012). These similarities mainly relate to working memory and the ability to inhibit prepotent responses as part of the 'executive functions', which mediate problem-solving actions (for more information see paragraph 'Theory-Driven Diagnosis of Attention Disorders' below).

One must be careful not to interpret high comorbidity numbers as implying a common cause. For example, a high comorbidity rate could result from different operational definitions of speech and language disorders used in studies by various professional groups (psychiatrists, speech and language pathologists, psychologists) (McGrath et al. 2008). In addition, Willcutt et al. (1999) emphasize that comorbidity seems to be the rule rather than the exception in developmental disorders in childhood. Seventy to 90% of children diagnosed with ADHD meet the criteria for at least one additional diagnosis.

Differential-diagnostic considerations are important for diagnosing DDSL, because several similar neuropsychological deficits may overlap with those of the disease or interfere with it.

11.8.3 Behaviour-Driven Diagnosis of Attention Disorders

According to the current versions of the *Diagnostic and Statistical Manual of Mental Disorders* (DSM-5) (American Psychiatric Association 2013) and the International Classification of Diseases (ICD-10) (World Health Organization 1993), which has a slightly narrower definition, attention deficit/hyperactivity disorders (ADHD) are chronic neurodevelopmental disorders characterized by inattention, impulsivity and hyperactivity in at least two settings and lasting more than 6 months. Some symptoms must be present before the age of 12. There are three subtypes of ADHD: the combined type, the predominantly inattentive type and the predominantly hyperactive/impulsive type.

In both classifications (DSM-5 and ICD-10), the formal clinical diagnosis of attention disorders is primarily based on the symptomatology, i.e. predominantly based on the behaviour of a child. Attention impairment is thought to be the central deficit, and subtypes are assumed to represent each of the specific characteristics.

For diagnosis of an ADHD, a child must show at least six symptoms of inattention or six symptoms of impulsive or hyperactive behaviour having a direct negative impact upon social and academic/occupational activities or both (DSM-5 2013). For adults and adolescents aged 17 years or older, only five symptoms are required.

The symptoms of inattention are (American Psychiatric Association 2013) when a child:

- Fails to give close attention to details or makes careless mistakes in schoolwork
- Has difficulty sustaining attention in tasks or play activities
- Does not seem to listen when spoken to directly
- Does not follow through on instructions and fails to finish school work
- Has difficulty organizing tasks and activities
- Avoids or is reluctant to engage in tasks that require sustained mental effort
- Often loses things
- Is easily distracted by extraneous stimuli
- Is forgetful in daily activities

The hyperactive-impulsive symptoms are (American Psychiatric Association 2013) when a child:

- Fidgets with or taps its hands or squirms in its seat
- Leaves its seat in situations when remaining seated is expected
- Runs about or climbs in situations where it is inappropriate
- Is often unable to play or engage in leisure activities quietly
- Is often 'on the go' acting as if 'driven by a motor'
- Talks excessively
- Blurts out answers before questions have been completed
- Has difficulty awaiting turn
- Interrupts or intrudes on others

The DSM-5 introduced a new requirement for the diagnosis of ADHD in children. From behavioural observations the severity of the disease is assessed as mild, moderate or severe, depending on the number of symptoms and the impairment of functioning. The clinical assessment involves the evaluation of information gathered from the child, the parents, other family members and educators/teachers. It should only be made by appropriately qualified professionals (NICE 2008).

The following examinations are included in various national guidelines (Kavanagh et al. 2014):

- A clinical and psychosocial assessment of the person with the focus on behaviour and symptoms in the different domains and settings
- A developmental and psychiatric history
- The assessment of the person's mental state

Clinical assessment should include clinical examinations, (semi-)structured clinical interviews and behavioural observations. A diagnosis based on rating scales, inventories and checklists or observations alone is considered insufficient. Rating scales and checklists are useful diagnostic instruments

(Alloway et al. 2009) but on their own are not sufficient for the diagnosis of an attention disorder (Bezdjian et al. 2009). A list of clinical practice tools for children is available on the website of the National Resource Center on ADHD of the organization Children and Adults with Attention-Deficit/Hyperactivity Disorder (CHADD 2017).

The examination of the patient should include the assessment of vision, hearing and motor function, as well as the exclusion of neurodevelopmental disorders or cognitive impairment. Information on frequently co-existing psychiatric disorders (oppositional defiant and conduct disorders, anxiety, coordination problems, depression) (Steinhausen et al. 2006; Taylor et al. 2004) should also be assessed. There are currently no standardized psychometric tests that can diagnose ADHD (Taylor et al. 2004).

11.8.4 Theory-Driven Diagnosis of Attention Disorders

The theory-driven definition focuses on cognitive or neuropsychological factors of disturbed attention (Barkley 1997). It claims that attention is not a uniform entity but has to be viewed as a multicomponent construct (Posner and Peterson 1990). Barkley's theory of ADHD is the most supported one (Willcutt et al. 2005). Barkley suggested that children with ADHD have a core impairment in their response inhibition. This has a secondary effect on the four intermediate executive functions named below and leads to poor control and difficulties with timing, flexibility and persistence, as well as to problems with goal-orientated behaviour. Behavioural inhibition is the ability to stop an initial or ongoing response and to redirect oneself to goal-orientated behaviour. In order to inhibit a response to an event, it is necessary to interrupt an ongoing action, to win time and to protect this period of time from disturbances (interference control).

The executive functions involved in this process are:

- Working memory
- Self-regulation of affect/motivation/arousal
- Internalization of speech
- Reconstitution

Working memory is important for monitoring behaviour. It refers to the ability to retain and manipulate information in the short term and to be able to generate and evaluate mental representations of the past (retrospection) and future (prospection). Self-regulation of affect, motivation and arousal points to the importance of these factors for emotional self-control and social perspective taking (i.e. understanding the feelings of others) in goal-directed behaviour. Internalization of speech refers to the ability to use internally generated speech to guide one's behaviour and actions (Alderson-Day and Fernyhough 2015). Reconstitution refers to the ability to analyse behaviour, achieve verbal and behavioural fluency, to have goal-directed behavioural creativity and to perform mental simulations of behavioural possibilities. Psychometric examination concepts have been developed for individual subfunctions of the above concept, on the basis of these theoretical considerations.

There is some empirical evidence that children with ADHD perform worse than control groups in tests of response inhibition, such as go/no-go paradigm tests and the stop-signal paradigm test (both of which test impulse control) as well as in continuous performance tests (testing sustained and selective attention). The stop-signal task (SST) (Logan 1994) and the continuous performance test (CPT) (Conners 2004; Soreni et al. 2009) are commonly used in practice. Working memory is often tested by using memory span tests (Engle et al. 1999), for example, the backwards digit-span or letter-span task.

A lack of endurance and poor or few interactions with peers may be indicative of self-regulation problems of affect, motivation and arousal. The absence of responses to verbal instructions and delay in the development of self-directed speech relate to problems with the internalization of speech. A verbal fluency test (e.g. COWAT, Benton and Hamsher 1976; Loonstra et al. 2001) can be used to test difficulties in reconstitution. Henry and Beatty (2006) showed that these kinds of tests are sensitive to cognitive dysfunction in executive functions. The ability to tell stories (Tannock et al. 1993) and act creatively (Healey and Rucklidge 2008) may be impaired in children with ADHD. According to measures of ideational fluency are very important because they test fluency at a higher conceptual level than word fluency tests. Ideational fluency is seen as a distinct cognitive ability (Vannorsdall et al. 2012) and seems to be independent of IQ (Brown 2006). In ideational fluency tests, the child has to recite words as quickly as possible, following specified rules.

11.8.5 Emotional and Behavioural Problems and Disorders of Speech and Language

More than half of children with diagnosed speech and language problems also have an emotional or behavioural disorder (EBD) (Benner et al. 2002). Stevenson et al. (2011) found that children with language disorders were four times more likely to manifest a problematic behaviour than typically developed children, according to parental reports. The researchers re-examined children they had initially studied at 3 years of age and found that behavioural problems such as social withdrawal, inattention or negativity and psychiatric disorders persisted in 8-year-olds (Carson et al. 1998; Stevenson et al. 2011). According to Hollo et al. (2014), many children with EBD also have an undiagnosed speech and language disorders that strongly impinge upon their long-term psychosocial and academic development (Cohen et al. 2013; Conti-Ramsden and Botting 2008; Yew and O'Kearney 2013).

As children reach adolescence, demands on language competence increase, and language skills become even more crucial for establishing and maintaining social relationships. Inadequate communication may cause misunderstandings, increase conflicts and lead to deterioration in the quality of friendships, leaving children and adolescents at risk of stress, loneliness and mental health problems (Durkin and Conti-Ramsden 2010; Leonard et al. 2011). Adolescents with language impairments may see themselves as less socially accepted than their typically developing peers and may also be perceived as withdrawn and unsociable by their peers and teachers (Im-Bolter et al. 2013).

The assessment of emotional and behavioural problems usually follows the diagnostic criteria defined in the DSM-5 (American Psychiatric Association 2013) or ICD-10 (World Health Organization 1993). Questionnaires and (semi-) structured interviews are often used. Give an overview of the commonly used parent- and caregiver-report tests for the assessment of younger children.

The Child Behavioural Checklist (CBCL/6-18) is a commonly used instrument to assess the behavioural profile of children aged 6–18 years. It has been translated into many languages and has scored well for reliability in the following empirical syndrome scale scores (Achenbach and Rescorla 2001):

- Aggressive behaviour
- Rule-breaking behaviour
- Social problems
- Attention problems
- Anxious/depressed
- Withdrawn/depressed
- Thought problems
- Somatic complaints

In addition, six DSM-orientated scales are also available, which are very consistent with DSM-5 (Achenbach and Rescorla 2001) categories:

- Depressive problems
- Anxiety problems
- Somatic problems
- Attention deficit/hyperactivity problems
- Oppositional defiant problems
- Conduct problems

A preschool version of the CBCL (CBCL/1½–5) is available (The ASEBA Approach 2017).

11.9 Neurological Examination of Children: Basics

Mona Hegazi, Barbara Maciejewska, Katrin Neumann and Dagmar Weise

11.9.1 Introduction

Neurological evaluation is an integral part of the assessment protocol of an abnormal language development of children in cases of suspected neurological disorders or general developmental abnormalities. It includes a parental interview, a general physical examination and a detailed neurological examination. The latter involves an examination of the cranial nerves, the motor and sensory systems and additional neurological tests when necessary. A detailed neurological evaluation reflects the developmental status of the central nervous system and may identify indicators for brain lesions or abnormal cerebral functions. Phoniatricians should know and recognize common neurological symptoms of children and consult neuro-pediatricians when needed.

11.9.2 Clinical History with Respect to Neurodevelopmental Disorders

A detailed child's history should include the following information:

- Pregnancy, perinatal and neonatal history: Apgar score, birth weight, prematurity, infections
- Developmental history: child's age at acquisition of developmental milestones such as social smiling; head control; rolling over; maintaining a sitting position; walking independently; babbling; vocal play and use of first words; phrases and sentences; toilet training; self-feeding and dressing
- Presence of neurological symptoms or complaints in general: nature, duration, permanent or episodic (e.g. seizure) occurrence; maintained, progressive or resolving course; localization to a specific anatomical region
- Symptoms related to specific neurological disorders such as cerebral palsy: impaired coordination; muscle tone; spasticity; weakness; tremor; developmental disorders of speech and language; loss of vision or hearing; diffi-

culties in sensation; motor developmental delay, e.g. inability to roll over, sit, crawl or walk; disturbed cognitive functions; seizure; and dysphagia
- Impact of the diagnosed or suspected neurological disorder on cognition, behaviour and language, the degree to which activities of daily life are compromised and if any medication, treatment or rehabilitation is applied or has been given in the past
- Family history: parental consanguinity; number and gender of siblings; position in the sequence of children; maternal age at delivery and family history of neurological; systemic and other disorders including hearing loss, developmental language disorders, intellectual disability and dyslexia

11.9.3 General Physical Examination

This should include:

- Height, weight, head circumference and blood pressure
- General appearance, dysmorphia and skin examination for neurocutaneous lesions
- Examination of the midline of the back and neck for sacral dimples, tufts of hair or other signs of spinal dysraphism
- General abdominal and chest examination

11.9.4 Detailed Neurological Examination

11.9.4.1 General Appearance
- Dysmorphia
- Body position: supine, symmetrical and with flexion of all limbs
- Skin exam: neurocutaneous lesions such as cafè-au-lait macules, which may indicate a neurofibromatosis; angiofibrosis or shagreen patches in case of tuberous sclerosis and other mucocutaneous lesions

- Location of the hair whorl: may signify presence of cerebral malformations
- Palmar creases: typical for several genetic syndromes such as Down syndrome
- Midline of the back and neck: exam for sacral dimples, tufts of hair or other signs of spinal dysraphism
- Unusual body odour: may be present in several neurometabolic disorders (Swaiman 2012; Michelson and Shu 2012; Fenichel 2009)

11.9.4.2 Spontaneous Position

- A healthy infant lies supine, with flexion of the limbs.
- Muscle tone assessment of limbs and in the head-neck-trunk axis: movements need to be symmetrical (Swaiman 2012; Michelson and Shu 2012; Fenichel 2009).

11.9.4.3 Skull and Cranial Nerve Examination

- The shape of the skull and the head circumference (microcephaly, macrocephaly, craniosynostosis) and the bulging and tension of the anterior and posterior fontanelle should be assessed at first.
- In infants and young children, squint and nystagmus, pupillary size and reaction to light, extra-ocular movements as well as facial asymmetries and facial mimic should be noted. Temporalis and masseter muscles can be tested during sucking.
- The jaw reflex, glabellar reflex, gag reflex and palmomental reflex need to be evaluated.
- The child's response to a bell or by recalling a whispered word can be observed, and the auropalpebral reflex should be checked (closure of the eye in response to loud noises).
- In older children detailed cranial nerve examination is performed assessing the function of all cranial nerves (I–XII) (Swaiman 2012; Michelson and Shu 2012; Fenichel 2009).

11.9.4.4 Motor System

- Posture and abnormal movements: opisthotonus, abducted hips or 'frog-sign', myoclonus, cerebellar tremor and choreo-athetotic movements.

- Muscle state: muscle atrophy, pseudohypertrophy (bulky appearance but with weakness) and fasciculations.
- Muscle tone: passive muscle tone is assessed by testing the resistance of passive movements in the joints while the infant is awake and not crying.
- Muscle power: this is tested by observing the response to simple manoeuvres such as retrieving a toy. The following grading system is used for assessing muscle strength according to the Lovett scale:
  - 0 No muscle contraction, no movement
  - 1 Flicker or trace of contraction visible or palpable
  - 2 Active movement without gravity
  - 3 Active movement against gravity
  - 4 Active movement against gravity with some resistance
  - 5 Active muscle contraction against full resistance, normal, full strength (for age)

11.9.4.5 Reflexes (Movement Automatisms)

Examples are shown in Table 11.12.

Newborn and Infant Reflexes (Primitive Reflexes) The primitive reflexes (also called infantile, infant or newborn reflexes) are a group of motor reflexes found in newborns. These automated movements are mediated at the spinal cord or brainstem levels. They do not require cortical involvement and disappear over time. They develop in utero and are usually present at birth. These reflexes are patterned, consistent and involuntary movements that help to make the baby aware of his or her body and surroundings (Zafeiriou 2004; Berger 2007). They build the fundament for conscious movements.

The roles of primitive reflexes are:

- To assist the birthing process
- To help the newborn to adjust to a life outside the womb when his or her nervous system is not fully developed
- To assist the baby to move and build up motor and cognitive skills

Table 11.12 Developmental reflexes and reactions, procedure of elicitation and response onset, integration and significance (based on Fenichel 2009; Zafeiriou 2004; Berger 2007; Blomberg and Dempsey 2011; Goddard 2005)

Reflex	Method of eliciting stimulus	Expected response	Duration	Significance—abnormal indication
Sucking	Touching the baby's mouth or upper lip	Sucking rhythmical movements of the lips	Birth to 1 year	Weak or immature sucking ability or lacking reflex in immature/premature babies; reflex reappears in advanced and diffuse cerebral atrophy
Moro (startle)	With the child in the supine position, apply a loud noise or an unpredictable sudden movement of the baby's body	Symmetrical rapid abduction and then extension of the arms with the opening of hands (similar to hugging), legs and head extend; subsequently the shoulders adduct, the elbows and fingers flex	Birth to 4–6 months	Asymmetry may indicate a brain lesion or peripheral nerve injury, e.g. paresis, paralysis

Blinking	Shine bright light in eyes	Eyelids close	From birth on throughout life	Absence indicates pure light sensation
Acoustic blink	Create loud noise around child	Both eyes blink	From birth on throughout life	Absence indicates hearing loss
Flexor withdrawal	With the child supine, and the lower extremities in an extended position, press a stimulus to the sole of the foot	Stimulated limb is withdrawn (hip and knee flexion)	Birth to 2 months	Persistence denotes brain damage such as cerebral palsy
Extensor thrust	With the child supine and the lower extremities in flexed position, apply pressure against the sole of the foot	Reflex extension of the leg muscles	Birth to 2 months	Persistence denotes brain damage such as cerebral palsy
Galant	While the child lies in prone position, stroke along one side of the spine—the dorsal paravertebral skin especially lumbar region	Lateral flexion or outward rotation of the hip towards the irritated side	Birth to 4–6 months	Lack of the reflex—damage of the spinal cord in thoracic segments Asymmetrical reaction—pyramid paresis/paralysis

(continued)

Table 11.12 (continued)

Reflex	Method of eliciting stimulus	Expected response	Duration	Significance—abnormal indication
Palmar grasp	Stimulate the skin of the palmar surface of the infant, for example, by placing a finger in the infant's hand	Infants fingers flex around the finger or an object in a grasp	Birth to 5–6 months	Persistence indicates cerebral dysfunction
Plantar grasp	Stroking the sole of the foot	Flexion of the toes and the foot	Birth to 5–6 months	Absence indicates spastic cerebral palsy
Rooting	Touch or stroke the cheek or lips (corner of the mouth) laterally	Head and mouth are turned towards the same side touched and a sucking motion is done	Birth to 2 months	Persistence indicates cerebral dysfunction

Placing

Support the child upright, the dorsum of the foot is placed against the edge of the table

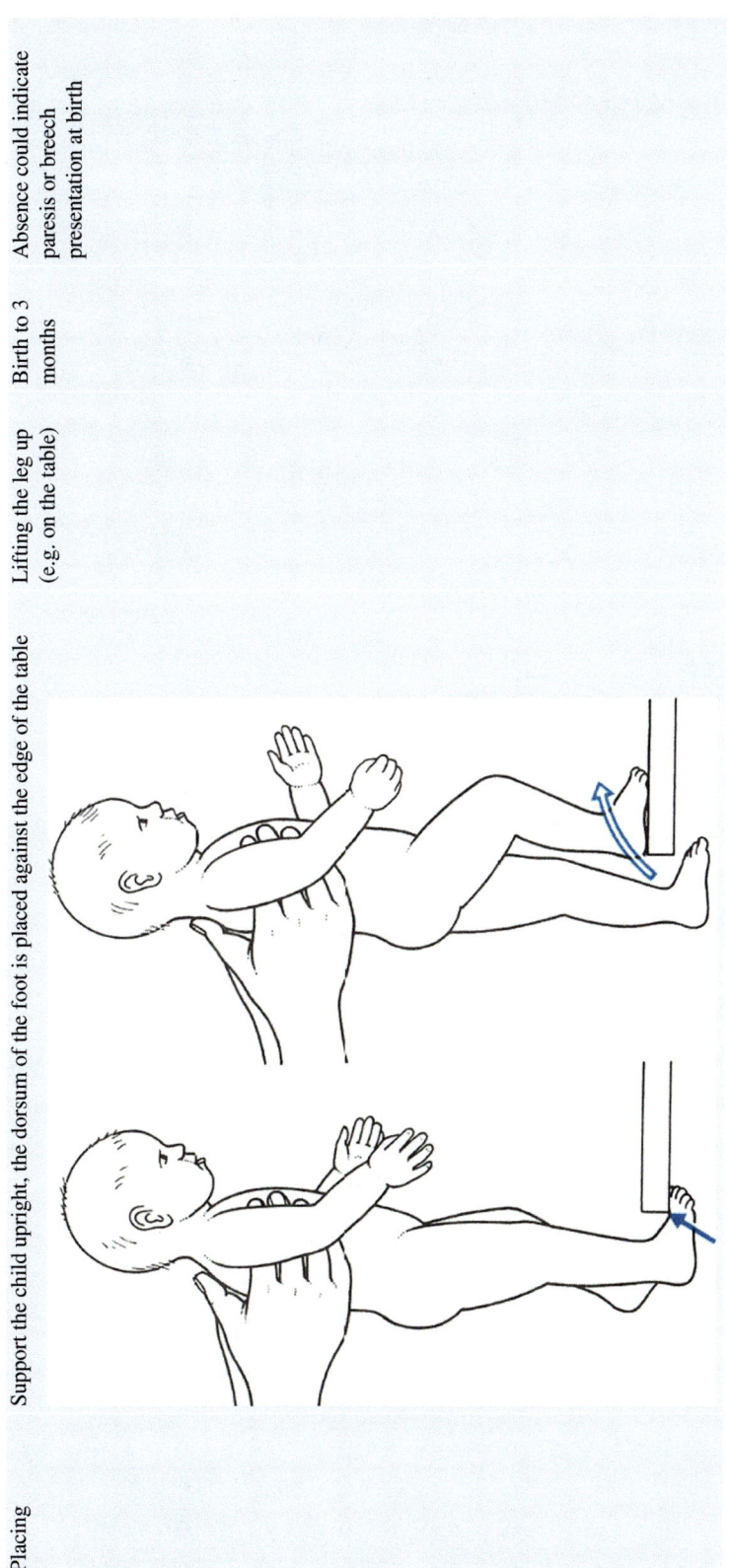

Lifting the leg up (e.g. on the table)

Birth to 3 months

Absence could indicate paresis or breech presentation at birth

(continued)

Table 11.12 (continued)

Reflex	Method of eliciting stimulus	Expected response	Duration	Significance—abnormal indication
Primitive walking/ stepping	The child is held under the arms in vertical position with feet touching a solid surface and then leaned forward and the feet are pressed on the surface	Alternate flexion and extension of the legs (as if walking)— rhythmical alternating steps	Birth to 3–4 months	Absence could indicate paresis or cerebral palsy
Palmomental reflex	Stroke the thenar eminence in a proximal to distal direction using a sharp object (causing discomfort not pain)	Ipsilateral or bilateral contraction of the mentalis muscle	Birth to 3 months	Reappearance indicates processes that disrupt normal cortical inhibitory pathways and thus affection of frontal lobes (frontal release sign)
Rotation test/ dolls's eye/ vestibulo-ocular reflex	Rotate child from one side to another	Eyes turn in direction of rotation	Birth to 11–14 days	Vestibular problem or eye muscle paresis

Labyrinthine head righting	While the child is in the vertical position and blindfolded, tilt the child anteriorly, posteriorly or vertically	The head is orientated vertically and is maintained steadily	From birth to 2 months on throughout life	Allows controlling the head position irrespective of gravity
Asymmetrical tonic neck/fencer	With body supine, gently turn the head to one side	Extension of the limbs on the side of the face and flexing of the arm and leg of the other side (fencing position)	Birth to 6 months	Persistence impedes active rolling and the development of hand-eye coordination; can indicate major cerebral palsy

(continued)

Table 11.12 (continued)

Reflex	Method of eliciting stimulus	Expected response	Duration	Significance—abnormal indication
Symmetrical tonic neck	With a child prone over the examiner's knee or placed in quadruped position on the floor, flex the child's head forwards (tonic neck I)	Flexion of the infant's head forwards causes flexion of the arms and extension of the legs (tonic neck I) Extension of the head backwards leads to extension of the arms and flexion of the legs (tonic neck II)	From 2/3 months to 6/9 months	Persistence impedes vertical positioning such as crawling on hands and knees, sitting without support
	and then extend the head backwards (tonic neck II) (not shown)			
Babinski/plantar reflex	Firmly stroke along the lateral surface of the plantar foot surface from the heel to the fifth toe	Upward extension (dorsiflexion) of the big toe towards the top of the foot and fanning of the other toes	Up to about 2 years of age	Persistence beyond 2 years indicates upper motor neuron lesion, unilateral persistence—possible cerebral palsy

| Landau reflex | Hold the child horizontally in a prone position in the air | Infant maintains a convex arc position with the head raised and arms extended and spine and hips extended in sequence | From 6 months to 2.5 years | The appearance of this reflex breaks up the total flexion pattern seen at birth |
| | | When the infant's head is flexed by the examiner, the extension of the hips disappears | | Failure to integrate means over-reactiveness to stimulation or vestibular problems |

(continued)

Table 11.12 (continued)

Reflex	Method of eliciting stimulus	Expected response	Duration	Significance—abnormal indication
Parachute reflex (protective extension reaction forward)	Suspend the baby in the horizontal prone position and then drop him or her a short distance onto a soft surface—head first; suddenly lower the infant as in falling	Arms extend and hands open in a defensive mechanism to protect the head	From 8 months on throughout life	Upper extremity pyramidal tract dysfunction, asymmetrical response—sign of hemiparesis

Neonatal neck righting	With child supine, flex his head and rotate it slowly to one side	The whole body (shoulders, trunk and pelvis) move towards the side to which the head is turned	Birth to 6 months	Early in development the infant uses the reflex for transition between supine, lying on the side and eventually prone positions
Neonatal body righting	With body supine, flex one leg up towards the chest and rotate (adduct) the leg across the body	Infant's body follows the direction of pelvic, move towards the side to which the leg is turned	From 6 to 12 months	Assists the child in rolling between supine and prone It allows rotation of one part of the body before the other, helping sitting and standing from supine position without rolling over to prone
Positive supporting reaction (magnetic reaction)	Place a finger on the sole of the foot	Limb extension that follows the finger as it is withdrawn	Birth to 4–5 months	Consists of those reflex muscular contractions whereby the body is supported against gravity
Negative supporting reactions	Standing Stretch of extensor muscle	Consists of inhibition of the extensor muscles and unfixing of the joints that thus enable the limb to be flexed and moved into a new position (disappearance of positive supporting reaction)	Birth to 4 months	Presence of positive supporting (+) after 8 months is abnormal. Also excessive flexion (−) is abnormal after 4 months
Tonic labyrinthine prone reflex	While child is prone, lift him up to evaluate the presence of flexor tone	Tonic flexion of the body	Birth to 6 months	Persistence impedes normal rolling patterns, balance and gross motor skills

(continued)

Table 11.12 (continued)

Reflex	Method of eliciting stimulus	Expected response	Duration	Significance—abnormal indication
Tonic labyrinthine supine reflex	While child is supine, lift the child to sitting to observe for extensor tone	Tonic retraction of the shoulders and extension of the body	Birth to 6 months	Persistence impedes normal rolling patterns, balance and gross motor skills
Supine or prone lying	While the child lies supine or prone on a tilt board, with arms and legs extended, tilt the board to one side	Righting of head and thorax, abduction and extension of arm and leg on the raised side (equilibrium reaction), protective reaction on the lowered side of board	From 6 months on throughout life	Cerebral cortex dysfunction
Four-foot kneeling	While child is in quadruped position, tilt him to one side	Righting of head and thorax (body flexes on the side of the tilt), abduction and extension of the arm and the legs on the raised side (equilibrium reaction), protective reaction on the lowered side	From 8 months on throughout life	Lacking indicates cerebral cortex dysfunction
Sitting	While child is seated, pull or tilt him to one side		From 10 months on throughout life	Lacking indicates cerebral cortex dysfunction
Kneel standing	While child is in kneel-standing position, pull or tilt him to one side		From 18 months on throughout life	Lacking indicates cerebral cortex dysfunction
Hopping reactions	With child in standing position and held by the arms, move the child backwards, forwards or to one side	Righting of head and thorax, hopping steps in the opposite direction of the tilt to maintain equilibrium	From 18 months on throughout life	Lacking indicates cerebral cortex dysfunction
Optical righting reflex	Hold child with armpit in a suspended position and then change position of the head from side to side	Eyes will move to the same side as head	From 1 to 2 years on throughout life	Lacking indicates cerebral cortex dysfunction

Figures with kind permission from Prof. Rainer Lietz (1996)

The primitive reflexes can be divided into three groups:

- The multisensory reflex—the Moro reflex (0–4 months).
- Primitive reflexes of position that affect all four limbs include the:
  - Tonic labyrinthine reflex (TLR) (0–6 months)
  - Asymmetrical tonic neck reflex (ATNR) (2–6 months)
  - Symmetrical tonic neck reflex (STNR) (3–6 months)
- Primitive tactile reflexes, triggered by touch and include:
  - The suck-swallow reflex (0–12 months)
  - Stepping/primitive walking (0–2 months)
  - The placing reflex (0–3 months)
  - The palmomental reflex (0–3 months)
  - The palmar reflex (0–4 months)
  - The plantar reflex (0–8 months)
  - The rooting reflex (0–3 months)
  - The Galant reflex (0–6 months)
  - The Babinski reflex (0–18 months)

The primitive reflexes are observed in normal infants in response to particular stimuli, but it is impossible to evoke them in neurologically intact adults. These reflexes disappear owing to the maturation-associated development of the frontal lobes (Mazurkiewicz-Beldzińska 2017). Gradually, as the primitive reflexes retreat or are integrated, conscious voluntary movements are established. In a typically developing child, paralleled by cortical maturation and myelinisation, most of these reflexes are integrated, i.e. they are replaced by voluntary motor skills, controlled by upper levels of the brain motor processing. They disappear within or after the first year of life and transit to mature responses. If a baby is unable to inhibit the primitive reflexes within the appropriate time window, his or her motor development is delayed, making it more difficult to follow the inborn program. Such a delay is a stumbling block of the brain maturation (Blomberg and Dempsey 2011), causing problems with gross and fine motor coordination and sensory perception (Mazurkiewicz-Beldzińska 2017; Goddard 2005).

A child may retain the primitive reflexes for some of the following reasons: low birth weight, premature birth, severe illness, trauma or injury in infancy, decreased ability to explore environment in early months.

Postural Reflexes When the primitive reflexes are integrated, postural reflexes develop. These reflexes ensure the unconscious control of posture, balance and coordination in the active and static individual (Zafeiriou 2004; Berger 2007; Goddard 2005). They are mainly responsible for the reflective maintenance of the body's posture when its position is altered by movement and ensure that the body remains upright and aligned. Because gravity effects on the body trigger these responses, these reflexes usually start to develop after birth. They help in carrying the maturing child through the developmental milestones of head control, rolling, sitting, crawling and standing.

Most of the postural reflexes arise in the midbrain, i.e. they are mediated from a higher cerebral level than the primitive reflexes, and thus their appearance signifies a maturation of the nervous system. The shift from primitive to postural reflexes is a gradual process with some overlap. Usually the postural reflexes are established by the age of 3.5 years. Typically, they are maintained throughout life but may decay with age, allowing the primitive reflexes to reappear (Swaiman 2012; Berger 2007; Blomberg and Dempsey 2011; Goddard 2005).

Postural reflexes are divided into two groups:

- Righting reflexes: for example, neck righting reflex, labyrinthine head righting reflex (LHRR), body righting reflex, Landau reflex (6 months to 2.5 years)
- Equilibrium reactions: parachute reflex (from 8 months on throughout life)

The movement automatisms mentioned above can be checked in three basic positions in infants:

- The supine position (rooting reflex, Moro reflex, ATNR)
- The prone position (Galant reflex, STNR)
- The holding position (Landau reflex, parachute reflex)

Classification of Reflexes According to Integration Centres in the Central Nervous System These are:

- Infant reflexes: e.g. suck-swallowing, defaecation and urinating reflexes are essential for a newborn's survival immediately after birth;

their centres are located in the brainstem and the spinal cord. The reflexes are automatic till the cortex centres take control of these processes.

- Spinal reflexes: they include flexor withdrawal, extensor thrust, crossed extension and the Galant reflex, deep tendon reflexes (the biceps (C5-6), triceps (C6-8), brachioradialis (C5-6), patellar (L2-4) and ankle (L1-2) reflexes) and superficial reflexes (such as the plantar reflex (S1), the superficial abdominal reflex (T7-T12), comprising reflexes of the upper abdominal (T8, 9) and lower abdominal quadrants (T11, 12) and the cremasteric reflex (L1-2)).
- Brainstem reflexes: these reflexes are static-postural reflexes; their persistence denotes delayed CNS maturation. They include the asymmetrical tonic neck reflex (0–6 months), symmetrical tonic neck reflex (0–6 months) and tonic labyrinthine reflex (prone and supine) (0–4 months) (Mazurkiewicz-Beldzińska 2017).
- Midbrain reflexes: these reflexes, combined with the equilibrium reflexes, enable the child to roll over, to sit up and to get on her or his hands and knees. They include the neck righting reflex (0–6 months), the body righting reflex (6–18 months) and the labyrinthine righting reflex (from 2 months on throughout life).
- Cortical equilibrium reactions: these are movement responses to maintain equilibrium or balance. They include supine and prone lying (from 6 months on throughout life), four-foot kneeling (from 8 months on throughout life), sitting (from 10 months on throughout life), kneel standing (from 15 months on throughout life) and the hopping reflex (from 18 months on throughout life). Maturation of equilibrium reactions brings the individual to the human bipedal stage of motor development. The next higher level of motor activity can be reached only when a proper reaction at the lower level has been created. Therefore, the reflexes are needed to achieve the next higher level of motor activity. Their occurrence indicates normal muscle tone and the body's adaptation in response to changes of the centre of gravity. They emerge together with the postural reaction of righting from 6 months on.

11.9.4.6 Cerebellar System

The examination of the cerebellar system includes the testing of rapid alternating movements (diadochokinesis), finger-to-nose and heel-to-shin tests as well as the Romberg sign.

11.9.4.7 Locomotion

Crawling and gait in older children: gait is best assessed by observing the patient walking barefooted with the legs and feet exposed. Pathological examples are circumduction gait (hemiparesis), broad-based ataxic gait (cerebellar disorder), steppage gait (high stepping) (peripheral neuropathy) and waddling gait (myopathy).

11.9.4.8 Sensory System

- Light touch: tested by pinprick
- Joint position sense (proprioception): measures the child's ability to perceive the position of a joint with his or her vision occluded and minimal external cues, tested by asking the child to replicate a joint position accurately with the opposite extremity or describing the position verbally
- Vibration sense: tested by tuning fork
- Higher cortical functions: examined by two-point discrimination, stereognosis and graphesthesia (see Sect. 11.10)

11.9.4.9 Additional Diagnostic Tests

See Sects. 9.9, 9.10, 3.1 and 16.22 for genetic examination; Sects. 11.16, 16.21 and 1.15 for neuroimaging such as magnetic resonance imaging (MRI) and computed tomography (CT); and Sects. 11.12–11.14 for metabolic tests and electroencephalography.

11.10 Developmental Milestones and Assessment of Tactile and Kinaesthetic Perception

Christiane Kiese-Himmel and
Andrea Joe Embacher

11.10.1 Introduction

The body senses are crucial for the development of the body's various communication systems. Usually, the senses work together and form the basis for learning and memory. The brain receives signals from the senses controlling the body, its position and its movement. The body also serves as a channel for expression ('body language'). Tactile information is, for example, vital for blind people (e.g. Braille symbols) and for deaf-blind people using tactile signing. All this implies a normal hand function. Kinaesthesis is necessary for motor planning, i.e. organizing and synthesizing of movements such as those for speaking and articulation (Debuschewitz et al. 2004). For example, a refined proprioception (experience of movement and muscle tension) is necessary for controlling the position and movements of the tongue, an important sensorimotor organ, in order to produce speech sounds. In turn, problems with language and visual-spatial skills are often associated with poor somatic sensory processing. Language-impaired children as well as those with resolved developmental language deficits (with normal nonverbal intelligence and without gross neurological findings) demonstrate tactile-kinaesthetic deficits (Kiese-Himmel and Kruse 1998; Kiese-Himmel and Schiebusch-Reiter 1999). Substantial correlations have been found between tactile-kinaesthetic perception and selected language facets (Götze et al. 2001; Kiese-Himmel et al. 2015). Thus, it seems that haptic perception involving the integration of cutaneous and proprioceptive information may be a link between symbolic representations (e.g. object words) and nonlinguistic representations (Kiese-Himmel 2008). Müürsepp et al. (2011) showed that deviations in haptic perception are very common in boys with minor to moderate expressive-specific language impairments. These are only some reasons why tactile and kinaesthetic perception is of great importance for phoniatrics and pedaudiology.

11.10.2 Fundamentals of Somatosensory Sensation

Tactile-kinaesthetic perception is part of the somatosensory system including tactile perception (cutaneous sensibility), kinaesthesis (pro-

prioception) and haptic perception (active touch). The skin, as the largest and most complex sensory organ of the human body, constitutes the tactile modality of the somatosensory system (e.g. Purves et al. 2004). The skin integument consists of two dependent layers, the epidermis and dermis (corium), containing four types of cutaneous mechanoreceptors and specialized nerve endings in the glabrous (hairless) skin (Fig. 11.10):

- The slowly adapting Ruffini corpuscles (for moderate static touch, stretching of the skin)
- The slowly adapting Merkel's disks (for light static touch)
- The quickly adapting Pacinian corpuscles (for pressure and vibration)
- The quickly adapting Meissner corpuscles (sensitive to light dynamic touch, gentle fluttering).

Rapidly adapting receptors responding briefly to stimuli allow the adjustment of grip and force, especially fingertip force. For example, a smooth object requires a greater grip force than a rough one, and dynamic control of fingertip force is essential for small and fragile objects. The mechanoreceptors that respond to a stimulus do not only differ in their rate of adaptation but also in their morphology and in the size of the skin area they are dispersed over (small or large receptive field size over which the application of a stimulus excites a primary afferent fibre). Additionally, there are subcutaneous tissues and numerous free endings (unencapsulated dendrites of a sensory neuron) throughout the skin operating as receptors reacting to thermal or painful stimuli, as well as thermoreceptors that allow the sensation of 'cold' or 'warm'. Nociceptors provide the sensation of pain caused by harsh physical, chemical or thermal stimuli. The hairy skin contains hair follicle sensors responding to hair displacement and free endings for receiving sensations.

The neural processing of somatosensory stimulation—starting after the activation of peripheral receptors in the skin—is highly complex. A rough sketch: the stimuli will be transduced into electrical signals and transmitted via the centrally projecting axons of the dorsal root gan-

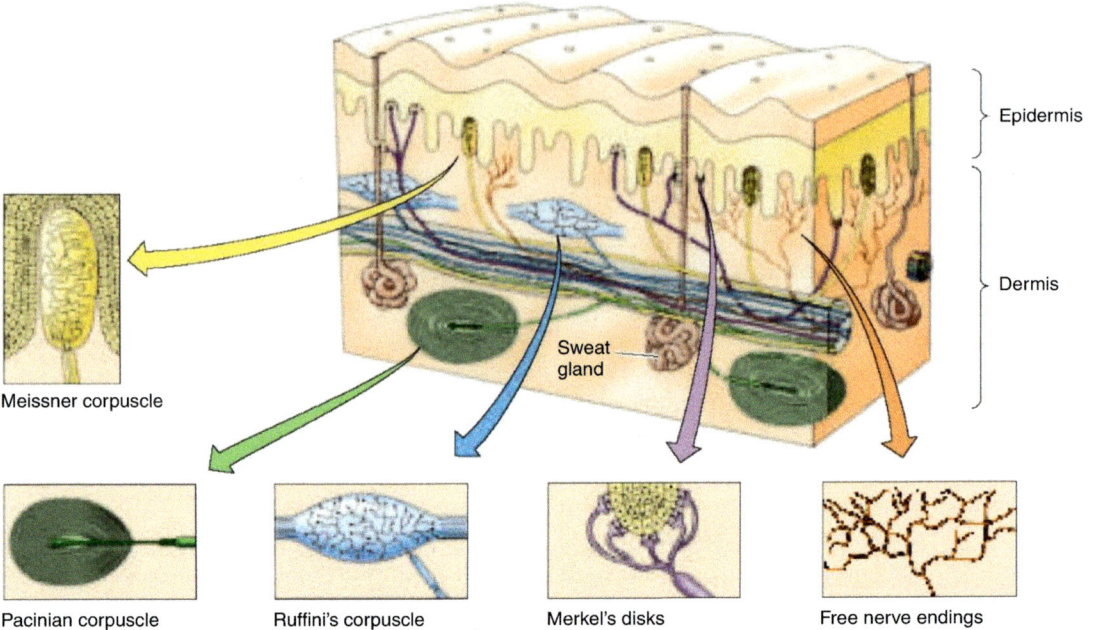

Fig. 11.10 The skin harbours a variety of morphologically distinct mechanoreceptors. This diagram represents the smooth, hairless (also called glabrous) skin of the fingertip (Purves et al. 2004). With kind permission from Sinauer Associates, Inc.

glion cells to convey sensory impulses to the spinal cord, from here to neurons in the brainstem nuclei (second-order cells) to specific nuclei in the thalamus (third-order neurons), and finally to the parietal lobe of the cerebral cortex. Within the spinal cord, the smaller nerve fibres (responsible for pain and temperature) form the lateral spinothalamic pathway, and the large myelinated nerve fibres carrying mechanosensory information from the body constitute the lemniscal tract (information of the face is carried by the trigeminal somatic sensory pathway to the central nervous system). The signals in the peripheral afferents ascend the medial-lemniscal pathway, processing information in parallel and serially, until they reach the somatosensory cortices where they are transformed into perception (Fig. 11.11). In addition, top-down processes such as attention, motivation and expectation may modify perception.

The somatosensory system comprises a widespread cortical network; streams of information from different nerves are processed and integrated. The dorsal stream (dorsal column-medial lemniscus pathway) projects to the primary somatosensory cortex (SI) in the posterior parietal cortex (Brodmann areas 3a, 3b, 1, 2) showing complex responses that are important in motor planning or motor performance as in grasping an object. The SI has direct access to the primary motor cortex, aids in guiding movements and gives sensory feedback for motor control. Because of a crossing-over of the ascending somatosensory fibre tracts, the SI receives the whole somatosensory input of the contralateral side of the body. Somatic receptors on left side of body go to the right cerebral hemisphere and vice versa, both for the anterolateral and the dorsal pathways.

The somatic representations of different body regions are cortically mapped. It is important to have in mind that the somatotopic maps do not reflect the correct proportions of the skin areas. The 'sensory homunculus' of each brain hemisphere shows a distorted representation of the (contralateral) body side because the amount of the cortical area is a function of the density of

Fig. 11.11 General organization of the somatic sensory system (Purves et al. 2004). With kind permission from Sinauer Associates, Inc.

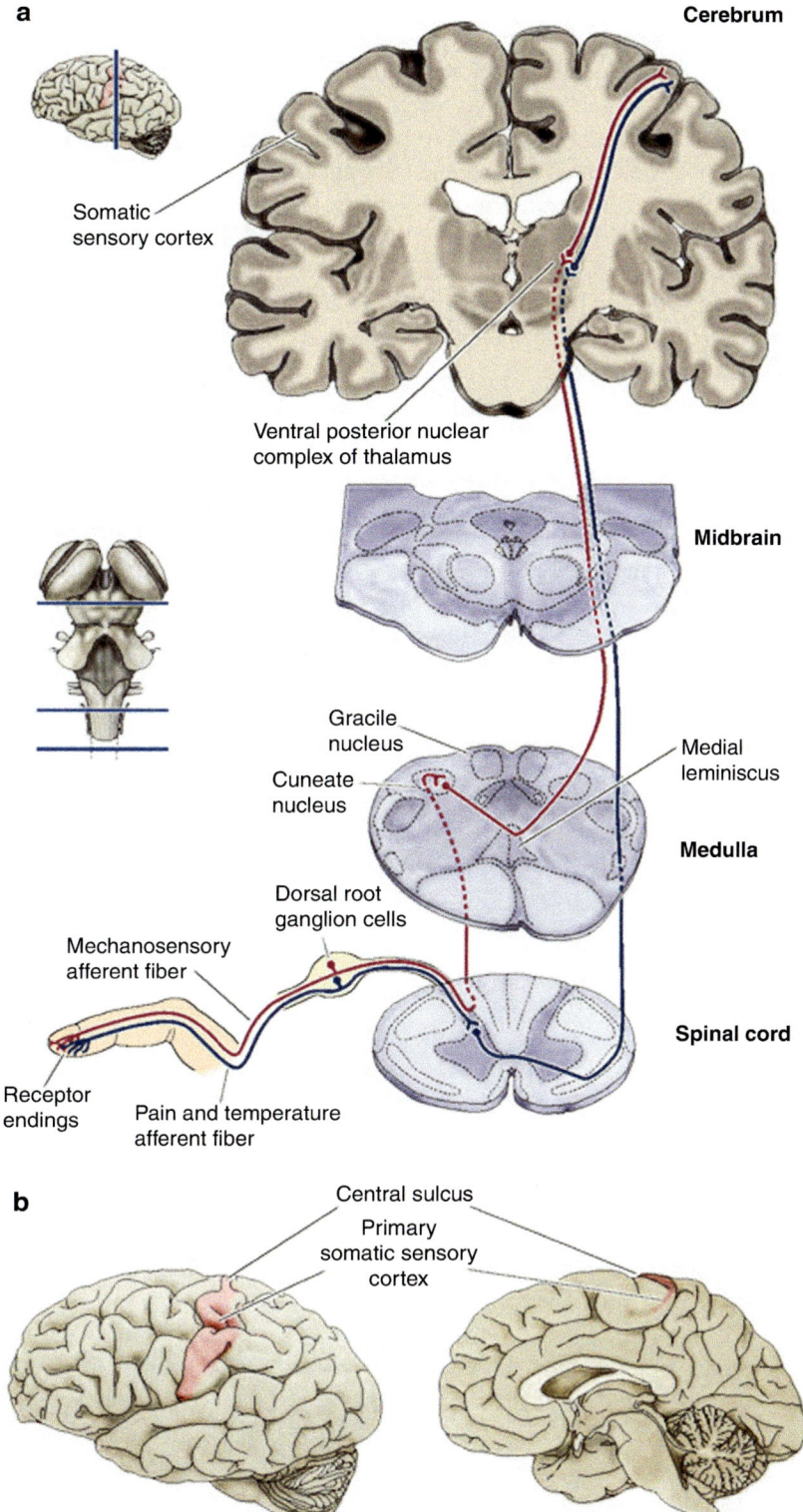

innervation. Thus, sensorial areas of the genitals, tongue, lips and fingertips of the thumb and index finger are extensively represented and greater than other sensorial body parts. Somatic sensory information is distributed from the SI to other cortical fields, e.g. the secondary somatosensory cortex (SII) located in the Sylvian fissure, serving more general aspects of sensation. Representations of tactile information can interact with information from the visual and/or auditory system (bimodal perception respectively intermodal relations).

11.10.3 Tactile and Haptic Perception

Sensibility Sometimes (rather rarely), two types of cutaneous sensibility ('epicritic'; 'protopathic')—first studied by Head (1905)—are distinguished in the scientific literature instead of the physiological approach of linking cutaneous receptors with specific sensory qualities.

Protopathic sensibility, which is responsible for the perception of extremes of temperature and pain, triggers a protective reaction such as avoidance, escape, defense or attack. This response must be extremely rapid in order to protect the perceiver from injury in an emergency situation ('protective sensibility'). Humans use the somatosensory system not only passively for detecting touch (mechanoreception) but also actively in exploring object properties (i.e. size, shape, geometry, hardness, texture, slipperiness, weight, temperature) and in manipulating an object (e.g. Kiese-Himmel 2006). Thus, *epicritic sensibility* ('functional sensibility'), which is responsible for the perception of light touch, fine tactile stimuli and fine temperature, needs more time in detecting such stimuli. For this, proprioceptors support a dynamic representation of stimuli in contact with the skin without vision, called *haptics* (e.g. Grunwald and Beyer 2001; Grunwald 2008).

Haptics This ability involves the integration of spatial-temporal patterns. Haptics or active touch—in contrast to passive touch (also known as superficial sensation)—is mostly performed by the hands moving over an object ('the sensorimotor hand'). Active touch is used in object recognition or identification of object properties. Several 'haptic exploratory procedures' performed by special hand movements and grasping strategies (Lederman and Klatzky 1987) are distinguished (e.g. pressure, rubbing the fingers, enclosure with the hands, lateral motion, static contact, unsupported holding, contour following, bimanual coordination). Exploratory procedures and object properties are related, and the type of hand movement is influenced by an object dimension required to obtain. 'Pressure' will be selected to obtain information about the hardness of an object. The hand and mouth are used as sensory organs specifically for stereognostic tasks, extracting spatial information by active exploration. Thus, a distinction is made between manual and oral stereognosis. Oral stereognosis is the ability to perceive and recognize the form of a solid object in the oral cavity by using touch to provide cues about its texture, size and spatial properties. Manual stereognosis is defined as the investigation of common objects and their properties by palpation.

Tactile Spatial Resolution (Tactile Acuity) Touch provides precise spatial information to the brain. The spatial resolution of this information is correlated with the size of the corresponding representation in the SI. *Two-point discrimination*—a measure of spatial resolution—is the local ability to differentiate between two tactile stimuli applied at the same time at two points of the body of a blindfolded subject ('minimal interstimulus distance'). It refers to the activation of two separate populations of neurons and is said to be an index of sensory ageing (Shimokata and Kuzuya 1995) because it declines with increasing age (for both sighted and blind objects).

The number of touch corpuscles in the skin of an adult human varies from 7 to 135 per square centimetre (Zimmer 2012). As a result, there are differences in mechanosensory discrimination across the body surface. The receptive fields are smaller in body regions with high perceptual spatial resolution. Mechanoreceptors are very densely packed in the tip of the tongue, the lips and the fingertips, especially in the thumb and

Fig. 11.12 Two-point discrimination thresholds (mm) (Purves et al. 2004). With kind permission from Sinauer Associates, Inc. Variation in the sensitivity of tactile discrimination as a function of location on the body surface, measured here by two-point discrimination. (After Weinstein 1968)

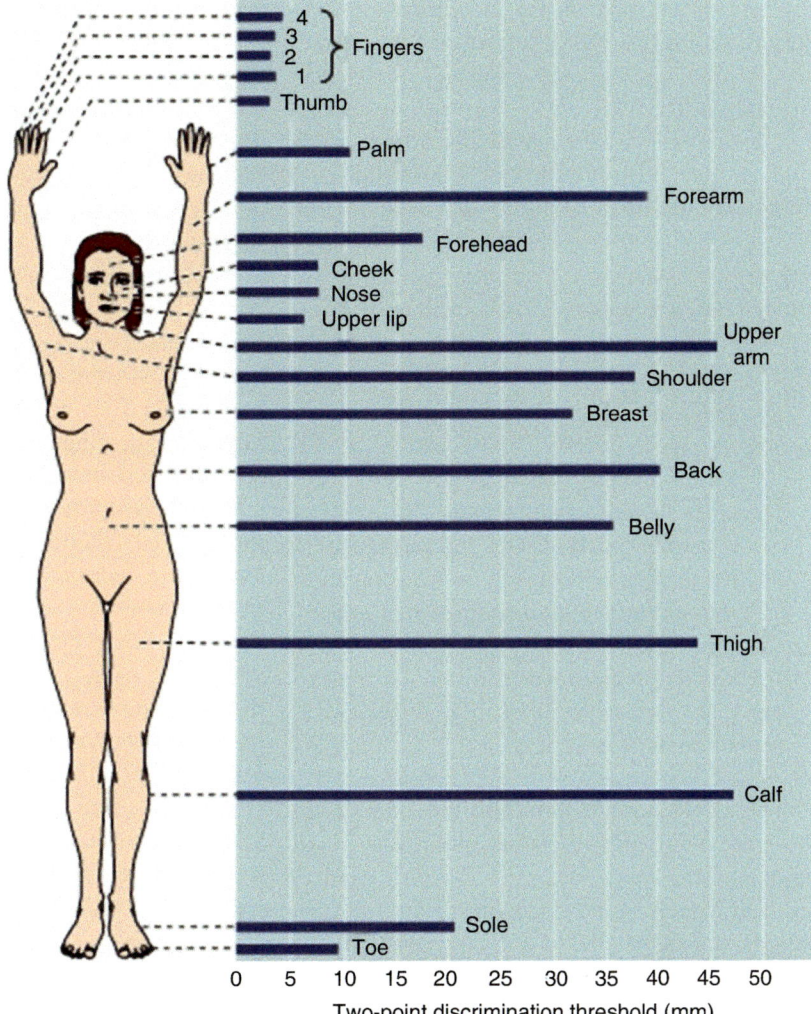

index finger, the regions with the highest spatial resolution of the human body. Perceptual spatial resolution is low in the thigh and calf region as well as in the skin of the back. The tactile discrimination threshold in the fingertips is 1–2.5 mm, in the palm 5–10 mm and in the forearm about 40 mm (Fig. 11.12).

11.10.4 The Kinaesthetic (Proprioceptive) Modality

The continuous combination of tactile and moving stimuli, which is fundamental for the development of various brain functions, is managed by the kinaesthetic (proprioceptive) modality.

Proprioception describes the perception of non-visually experienced movements, i.e. the unconscious ability to move and control parts of the body. Proprioceptors (kinaesthetic sensors) do not respond to external stimuli as do the cutaneous receptors, located on the body surface. This contrast describes the difference between 'interoception and exteroception'.

The proprioceptors of the musculoskeletal and locomotor systems lying in deeper somatic structures located in muscles, joints and joint capsules are distributed all over the body. Sensation comes from deeper tissues, muscle spindles, Golgi receptors, Pacinian and Ruffini corpuscles, as well as from free nerve endings. Ruffini corpuscles are located in ligaments, tendons and articular capsules and provide information for the central nervous system allowing conscious perception ('sensation') of joint position, movement velocity or articular movements. There also exists unconscious sensory information, such as that one arising from muscles (tone, posture, coordination) and ligaments.

Several sub-modalities are included in proprioception that enable control over movements and their coordination. The integrated processing of all those sensory signals enable the body representation:

- The *sense of position*, focusing on the awareness of body position, the location of the extremities and position of the joints in space
- The *sense of movement*, focusing on an aspect of a movement such as direction and speed
- The *sense of force*, focusing on the perception of the amount of muscular force that is used for a movement
- The *sense of tension*, focusing on the level of muscular tension required to generate a particular movement.

The *vestibular system* (with a receptor site in the inner ear) has widespread interactions with other sensory modalities contributing to body- and self-awareness and expanding to emotion processing, mental health and social recognition (see Lopez 2016). Both proprioceptive and vestibular inputs are integrated in head and body movements through space and in balance control. Moreover, the vestibular system provides a stable frame of reference for sensory comparison in the case of divergent responses of other sensory modalities such as the visual modality. Apart from the topic of this section, it should be noted that hair cells in the cochlea are the most sensitive mechanoreceptors, transducing air pressure waves into nerve signals and sending them to the brain.

11.10.5 Development of Somatosensory Modalities

Touch is the first sense functioning in utero. As early as the eighth week of pregnancy, typical developing human embryos are able to react to a gentle touch of their upper lip by responding with bodily movements. The palms of the hands are sensitive to touch in the tenth or 11th week of post-conceptual age. At 12th weeks, the foetus can close her or his fingers and thumb. By 15th–17th weeks, sensibility of the abdomen and buttocks is present. The movement sense is prenatally functional in humans from the 28th week of gestation on.

Early tactile stimulation of a newborn is vital for his or her calming and wellbeing ('social touch') because it gives him or her a feeling of security (Montague 1995). Newborns begin to explore their environment actively immediately after birth by using their hands and mouth to touch surfaces and objects (Bushnell and Boudreau 1991). Developmental trajectories of sensory and motor hand function are well documented (e.g. Jones and Lederman 2006). Perception of temperature and size solely with the hands is present very early, perception of texture and hardness at about 6 months, perception of weight at about 9 months and perception of shape after 10 months of age, linked to the dexterity of the fingers. Precision gripping between thumb and index finger starts around 10 months; improvement of grasping proceeds in parallel with the maturation of the neural pathways. Preterm infants may have mild problems in sensory responsiveness (Case-Smith et al. 1998). In preterm infants—independent of postnatal age—manual tactile discrimination of shape information has been reported as being present at a postconceptional age of 34 weeks (Lejeune et al. 2014).

Hatch and Maietta (1991) claim that the quality of touching and physical activities within the first year of life forms the basis of communicative development. Encouraging physical activity may thus support the development of language. Hendrickson et al. (2015) assessed the temporal dynamics of vision and action that infants are using to evaluate the underlying word representations that guide his or her responses. They showed that children who were faster at processing words were also those who exhibited better haptic performance. Kiese-Himmel (2005, 2007, 2008) considered haptic discrimination experiences as a precursor for higher cognitive processes such as conceptual categorization underlying symbolic development in infants, e.g. in the natural acquisition of open-class content words.

Hirschfeld et al. (2012) found a decrease in pain sensitivity with increasing age over a period of a year in children between 6 and 16 years of age. Pain perception seems to be influenced by developmental changes during puberty (Blankenburg et al. 2011).

Taylor et al. (2016) described in a systematic review how different somatosensory modalities develop in typically developing individuals between birth and 18 years, and they concluded that the pattern of somatosensory development varies depending on the evaluation tool used as well as the somatosensory function being measured. Haptic recognition, touch detection (discrimination) and proprioception improve from young children at the age of 3 years to young adults (Dunn et al. 2015). The somatosensory system matures till adolescence, together with the finger dexterity. Nevertheless, the sense of touch is a function of life span development and changes. Haptic recognition of unfamiliar objects is a demanding task in old age, because the covariation between individual sensory performance and general cognitive functioning in old age increases (Kalisch et al. 2012).

11.10.6 Assessment and Evaluation Tools of Tactile-Kinaesthetic Perception in Children

There are different procedures to assess tactile-kinaesthetic perception, comprising qualitative and quantitative methods in addition to a parent-reported interview ('developmental sensory history'):

- Standardized questionnaires; sensory rating scales
- Developmental psychological motor scales, profiles and tests
- Observation including observational protocols of tactual playing activities (e.g. finger painting; drawing with shaving cream; blowing bubbles), sensorized toys for measuring

manipulation capabilities, grasping actions and forces
- Videotaping and analysis of hand movements in haptic exploration tasks
- Tactile-kinaesthetic psychometric tests
- Hand function evaluation (e.g. Jebsen-Taylor Test)
- Neurological, electrophysiological/(neuro-)physiological (e.g. stimulation of the median nerve; somatosensory evoked event-related potentials; functional magnetic resonance mapping), psychophysical and (neuro-)psychological examinations

Open clinical judgement is required as supplementary overall assessment, although it is based on a subjective (not evidence-based) evaluation.

Limb position sense and kinaesthesis can be checked individually at clinical examination.

For assessing responsiveness in exploring individual sensory development related to tactile-kinaesthetic stimuli, the structured parent's rating scale (*Diagnostischer Elternfragebogen zur taktil-kinästhetischen Responsivität im frühen Kindesalter, DEF-TK*; Kiese-Himmel 2000) comprising 32 items is a useful German language tool. It provides normative data for two age groups (for children aged 1 year, 3 months to 3 years, 11 months and aged 4 years, 0 months to 7 years, 11 months).

Furthermore, sensibility assessments may be performed by using threshold or functional tests. For example, the spatial resolution can be evaluated by measuring *two-point discrimination thresholds* simultaneously touching the skin with the two spikes of an aesthesiometer ('simultaneous two-point discrimination') or of a sliding aesthesiometer (time-varying stimuli: 'dynamic two-point discrimination'). If the points are perceived as separated, the distance between them is reduced in small steps until the smallest distance that is recognized as separate is reached. Assessment of sensibility by functional tests is influenced by age, practice, fatigue and stress (Purves et al. 2004).

The standardized German *Entwicklungstest 6-6-Revision* (Petermann and Macha 2013) from 6 months to 6 years (75 months of age) contains a subtest named 'Handmotorik' in the scale 'Fine Motor Skills'. This subtest determines whether targeted grasping and releasing, manipulation and use of objects are age-typical. The US-American *Peabody Developmental Motor Scales* (*PDMS-2*; Folio and Fewell 2000) covering an age span from birth through age 5 contains a subtest 'Object Manipulation' (24 items, given to children ages 12 months and older) measuring a child's movements needed to catch, throw and kick a ball. In addition, there is a subtest 'Grasping' (26 items) starting with the ability to hold an object with one hand and progressing up to actions involving the controlled use of the fingers of both hands to button and unbutton garments. Normative data for subtest raw scores (standard scores, percentile ranks, age equivalents) are provided.

A *haptic exploration task* (manual stereognosis) provides information about tactile discrimination and exploration procedures in the absence of vision. Everyday objects or natural ones such as chestnuts, dried beans, walnuts or stones can be used for exploration. An assessment can also be performed by observing the child's spontaneous handling of toys, monitoring the exploratory procedures and comparing those with sensorimotor trajectories. Larger objects or sheets are used for an exploration by using the feet. Oral stereognosis is measured by using test pieces of defined geometrical forms (e.g. circular, oval, rectangular, star or rhomboid forms) that are placed on the tongue. The person being examined has to discriminate between them or identify their shapes by drawing or writing a description of them. With such tests, for example, an orofacial myofunctional therapy may be evaluated by detecting residual perceptive deficits (comparison of pre- and post-treatment measurements).

The standardized German *Göttingen Developmental Test of Tactile-Kinaesthetic Perception* is available for children aged 3 years, 6 months to 6 years (*TAKIWA*; Kiese-Himmel 2003) including seven subtests: two-point discrimination; pressure sensitivity; touch localization in hands and forearm, uni- and di-haptic finger identification, stereognosis of object properties, object stereognosis and graphesthesia. Norms are provided for each subtest and for the

sum score. The evaluation can be supplemented by test scores of the US-American *Sensory Integration and Praxis Tests* (*SIPT*; Ayres 1996) comprising 17 brief subtests requiring children to perform different sensory tasks (amongst others tactile and kinaesthetic tests) as well as motor tasks. Any of the individual tests can be administered separately. Norms are provided for each test for children from the ages of 4 to 8 years, 11 months.

In the clinical literature, there are many evaluation tools for hand function. Thus, *hand function* can be measured by the widely used *Jebsen-Taylor Hand Function Test* (Jebsen et al. 1969) or by hand grip dynamometry in adults (e.g. *Hand Grip Strength Test*, Roberts et al. 2011). The Jebsen-Taylor Test consists of seven subtests: writing; simulating page turning; picking up small common objects; simulated feeding; stacking draughts/checkers; picking up large, light objects; and picking up large, heavy objects. The non-dominant hand is tested before the dominant hand. On the basis of the Jebsen-Taylor Test, Beagley et al. (2016) have offered preliminary norms in evaluating hand dexterity of typically developing Australian children aged 5–10 years. Culicchia et al. (2016) provide an adaption and validation of the Jebsen-Taylor Test in a healthy Italian population of six small age groups (6–19; 20–29; 30–39; 40–49; 50–59; 60–87 years of age). Normative data for hand grip strength in a representative longitudinal cohort study of people originally aged 18 years and more were collected in Australia by Massy-Westropp et al. (2011). Roughly, a low gripping force contributes to a reduced functional capability, but it should be noted that the dynamometer or the measurement protocol used may differ.

In the USA, Royeen and Fortune (1990) presented a 26-item self-reporting screening scale: *The Touch Inventory for Elementary-School-Aged Children* (*TIE*) with normative data (percentiles) to detect tactile defensiveness—a somatosensory impairment. Additionally, Bennett and Peterson (1995) reported that using information both from mothers (completing a modified version of the TIE) and children might provide a more complete picture of tactile defensiveness of a child. Because diagnostic instruments to identify somatosensory impairments are beyond the scope of this article, neurological, electrophysiological/(neuro-)physiological, psychophysical and (neuro-)psychological examinations are not described in this section.

Overall, for a comprehensive assessment, a combination of different tools is needed.

11.10.7 At a Glance

The functioning and different modalities of the somatosensory system are necessary for someone to interact with the outside world as well as with his own body. They play a unique role in the interaction of the senses, sensory experiences and sensorimotor integration. The somatic sensory modalities have a sustainable effect on the development of a human. The resulting perceptions are largely dependent on spinal and cerebral processing that relies on specialized neural systems of afferent impulses and efferent feedback control. Unfortunately, there are only a few reliable actual standardized psychometric tests in the field of child development for measuring somatosensory performance including passive touch, proprioception and haptic abilities. On the other hand, there are more evaluation tools available for use in clinical practice.

11.11 Interpretation of the Results of Logopedic/Speech-Language Pathologist Examinations

Dirk Deuster

11.11.1 Using Standardized Test Procedures in the Examination of Linguistic Levels

To evaluate the language development of a child, knowledge of the normal language development (see Sect. 9.3) and its standard values (see Sect. 11.3) are required and essential. Therefore, standardized examination procedures are useful for evaluation because they provide information on the individual test result in comparison with that of the normal group. Depending on the developmental age of the child, various standardized test procedures in different languages for each linguistic level are available (see Sect. 11.3).

Usually, besides the analysis of spontaneous speech, a logopedic/speech-language pathologist (SLP) examination includes these standardized test procedures for language evaluation and presents the results in T values or percentile ranks when applicable. However, in some children it will not be possible to use such test procedures, for example, in children with severe emotional or cognitive deficits or when a symptomatic profile does not fit an existing test procedure. In these cases, an exclusive subjective estimation of the language status or use of informal and non-standardized procedures, with or without additional subtests of standardized test procedures, is often carried out. Although this is possible, in principle it should be justified in each individual case, and the results need a particular interpretation by the phoniatrician.

11.11.2 Interpretation and Prerequisites for the Interpretation of the Results of Logopedic/SLP Examinations

As a prerequisite for interpretation of the results of logopedic/SLP examinations, the phoniatrician has to know the:

- Clinical findings including audiometric tests
- Common standardized test procedures for language testing (scope of application, construction, standard values) and the manuals of the applied tests

It is highly desirable for the SLP to know a child personally from a consultation, in order to gain an overall impression of his or her general and developmental status or to perform informal tests and evaluate the level of communicative behaviour including spontaneous speech. However, this is sometimes not possible, e.g. if a medical opinion has to be rendered only from the medical documentation.

When interpreting the findings, the phoniatrician has to:

- Judge the appropriateness of the test procedures.
- Consider the results of each linguistic level separately, as well as in general, by weighting the tests results of the single linguistic levels, e.g. phonological disorders have a relative good spontaneous prognosis compared with that of an impairment of speech perception or of (passive) vocabulary (von Suchodoletz 2009).
- Determine the severity of the language impairment (concerning several or single linguistic levels).
- Match the results of logopedic/SLP examinations with her or his own estimation of language development of the child.
- Interpret the results in context with the general, psycho-motoric and emotional development of the child.

Only when taking account of these points is the phoniatrician able to decide which support measure is necessary for the child (e.g. speech and language therapy, remedial or special needs education) (de Langen-Müller et al. 2013; Schöler and Scheib 2004).

11.12 Laboratory Examinations of Developmentally Delayed Children

See Part I, Chap. 3, Sect. 3.3

11.13 Objective Analysis by Cortical Potentials, Basics on Electroencephalography (EEG)

See Part I, Chap. 3, Sect. 3.3.

11.14 Clinical Neurophysiology

See Part I, Chap. 3, Sect. 3.3.

11.15 Sonography of the Tongue During Articulation

Wolfgang Angerstein

11.15.1 Introduction

The human tongue has two main functions:

- Primary functions (life essential, evolutionarily older):
- Chewing, swallowing (bolus forming, control and transport), other sensory perception including temperature (thermoception), kinaesthetic sense (proprioception), pain (nociception), vibration (mechanoreception), tasting (gustatoception, chemoception), touching (tacitoception, syn. epicritic sensibility)
- Secondary function (not life essential, evolutionarily younger):
- Articulation, both during running speech (i.e. spoken articulation) and during brass instrument playing (i.e. brass articulation)

These tongue functions can be investigated thoroughly by sonography, as reported in a vast number of publications since Kelsey et al. (1969) and Minifie et al. (1971).

11.15.2 Examination Methods

Nowadays, tongue movements are mostly investigated by using B-mode scans (Stone 2005). In these two-dimensional sectional images, individual tissue densities are represented on the monitor as different levels of brightness (B). If a B-mode sectional image of a constant velocity moves over the monitor but the transducer remains in the same position, a one-dimensional time motion

(TM) image results (Stone 2005). Thus, movements of random points of the B-mode sectional image become visible on the monitor. If the monitor is split into two halves, B-mode scans and TM-mode images can be displayed simultaneously. In TM-mode, the amplitudes of movement at defined points of the tongue surface are continuously displayed over a given period of time. The exact location of the surface points can be determined in the corresponding B-mode image by using a cursor: when the cursor intercepts the tongue surface in a B-mode scan, the amplitude of movement of this particular point of intersection is recorded in a time-dependent manner in TM-mode. The two-dimensional B-mode image is typically displayed on the left side of a split monitor and the one-dimensional TM-mode on the right side.

The most common transducers used at current are 5 or 7.5 MHz transducers with a 90° or 100° sector. The transducer (which is usually convex for adults and linear for children) is placed submentally lengthwise underneath the floor of the mouth, after generous application of ultrasound gel to improve the coupling and increase the standoff distance. Usually, the transducer is held by the examiner, bearing in mind that it may slip during articulation and swallowing movements. The alternative—fixation of the head by using a specially constructed, complicated apparatus—might be too demanding for the patient. Moreover, if the head is fixed, natural, comfortable speech and swallowing are not possible. It is also worth considering that a child whose head is fixed will usually not comply with testing, so tongue sonography in children should preferably be performed with the patient's head free to move.

Tongue sonography is performed while the patient is sitting. Tongue movements are monitored at a frequency of 25 images per second by real-time video recording. Ultrasound investigations allow the assessment of tongue movements which are not visible from the outside when the mouth is closed. Because the mesopharynx usually contains a layer of air between the tongue and the hard palate that completely reflects ultrasound at the tissue-air border, depiction of the

tongue surface and its movements is possible by using B-mode sectional images.

If the transducer is positioned lengthwise submentally in the midline, midsagittal B-mode scans of the tongue surface are recorded (Stone 2005). The tip of the tongue is always displayed on the left side of the screen, the root of the tongue on the right side and the surface or dorsum of the tongue in the upper section of the screen (see Fig. 11.13). When the transducer is turned submentally by 45° (so that it is crosswise to the lengthwise position), coronary sectional images of the tongue surface are obtained (see Fig. 11.14). Thus, two planes of the tongue can be examined sonographically.

Various software programmes have been developed since the late 1980s by which the contours of the tongue dorsum can be digitally captured with interactive image processing systems in order to extract them from the B-mode ultrasound images ('automatic contour tracking') (Wein et al. 1988; Watkin and Rubin 1989; Wein 1990; Unser and Stone 1992; Akgul et al. 1999; Li et al. 2005; Stone 2005; Lindner et al.

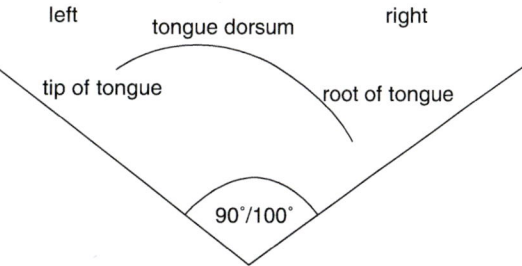

Fig. 11.13 Mediosagittal ultrasound B-mode scan of the tongue surface (scheme)

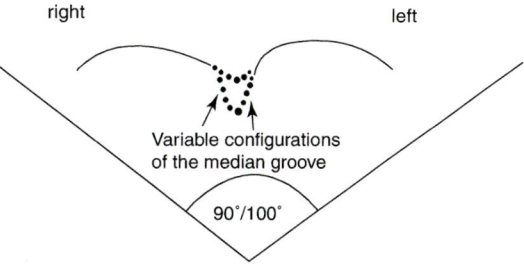

Fig. 11.14 Coronal ultrasound B-mode scan of the tongue surface (scheme)

2007). Amongst other techniques, these programmes use greyscale-value difference analyses (Parthasarathy et al. 2005; Lindner et al. 2007). If the contours of the tongue dorsum are automatically extracted from B-mode ultrasound images in regular time intervals (e.g. every 30 or 40 ms) and plotted along the Z axis of an X-Y-Z coordination system, a pseudo-three-dimensional reconstruction of the tongue surface in the course of time is obtained (Wein et al. 1988; Watkin and Rubin 1989; Wein 1990; Lindner et al. 2007). Numerous reports on temporal (time-dependent) pseudo-three-dimensional reconstructions of tongue dorsum movements for spoken (Wein et al. 1988; Watkin and Rubin 1989; Wein 1990) and brass (Lindner et al. 2007) articulation have been published.

Several computer-assisted software algorithms are available for 'real' three-dimensional reconstructions of the tongue surface in all three spatial planes during the articulation of vowels and consonants (Stone and Lundberg 1996; Stone 2005; Bressmann et al. 2005a, b, c).

11.15.3 Possible Diagnostic Applications

For scanning the tongue in routine phoniatric consultations, two-dimensional B-mode sonography is used almost exclusively. Here, functional disturbances of tongue movements (such as myofunctional disorders) and neurogenic disorders of tongue movements (such as systemic neurological diseases or hypoglossus nerve paralysis) are of phoniatric relevance. Visualization of morphological tongue alterations (such as carcinoma or scarring following partial tongue resection with or without reconstructive plastic surgery) is more often applied in adults by otorhinolaryngologists.

During vowel and consonant articulation, the contours of the tongue surface can be easily displayed in real time by using midsagittal B-mode ultrasound sectional imaging (Shawker and Sonies 1984; Stone et al. 1987; Bigenzahn et al. 1988; Wein et al. 1990a, b, 1991). A characteristic configuration of the tongue dorsum is shown for each vowel. In coronary B-mode ultrasound

sectional imaging, a median V-shaped groove is shown on the tongue surface when /s/ is correctly articulated (Wein et al. 1991; Angerstein 1994). This median groove allows air flow from the hypopharynx to the teeth and lips. In cases of lateral sigmatism, the groove is localized on the right (dextral lateral sigmatism) or left (sinistral lateral sigmatism) lingual border instead of in the middle of the tongue surface (Wein et al. 1991). Correct or inaccurate /s/-articulation can be sonographically documented in this manner.

By appropriate positioning of the cursor in midsagittal B-mode scans, movements of the tongue surface can be precisely measured and documented at any user-defined point with regard to frequencies and amplitudes (Böckler et al. 1989; Angerstein 1994). During articulation of /r/, the frequency and amplitude of the tip of the tongue can be clearly displayed (Böckler et al. 1989). The use of TM-mode to measure and document the frequency of vibration and the amplitude of movement of the frontal section of the tongue during the production of Spanish /r/ phonemes (monovibrant, multivibrant) is phonetically interesting (Neuschaefer-Rube et al. 1999). Frequencies and amplitudes of the tip of the tongue during coarticulation of a consonant and the vowel /a/ can be best investigated in TM-mode by articulating the syllable chain /la-la-la/ and of the tongue root by articulating /ka-ka-ka/ or /ga-ga-ga/ (Angerstein 1994). It is important to watch out for signs of fatigue, such as uncoordinated or dysrhythmic frequency or amplitude changes. The syllable chains /pa-ta-ka/ (in which the middle vowel /a/ is combined with the anterior consonant /p/, the middle consonant /t/ and the posterior consonant /k/), /mi-ma-mu/ or /miau/ (in which the soft consonant /m/ is combined with the anterior vowel /i/, the middle vowel /a/ and the posterior vowel /u/) can be used to investigate co-articulatory movements of the tongue surface in TM-mode. By using these techniques, frequencies and amplitudes of surface movements at the tip, in the middle and at the root of the tongue can be measured and documented (Böckler et al. 1989; Angerstein 1994).

Symptoms of fatigue (irregularities in frequency or amplitude of tongue dorsum movements) in dysarthric patients with systemic neurological disease (Shawker and Sonies 1984; Svensson 1990; Angerstein 1994) or in patients with hypoglossus nerve paralysis (Böhme 1990) are of particular interest to phoniatricians when using B-mode and TM-mode imaging.

Lingual searching movements related to speech apraxia can also be documented with midsagittal B-mode scans, especially through pseudo-three-dimensional reconstructions of tongue surface contours over time (Wein et al. 1993). In laryngectomized patients with ructus speech (oesophagus voice), typical tongue movements related to inhalation or injection of air into the oesophagus can be observed by midsagittal B-mode sectional imaging (Svensson 1991).

Not only spoken articulation but also brass articulation (movements of the tongue surface related to playing a brass instrument) can be analysed and video documented by using midsagittal B-mode scans with simultaneous TM-mode recording (Angerstein 2003; Angerstein et al. 2009; Zielke et al. 2010, 2012; Zolotas and Bird 2010). Pseudo-three-dimensional reconstructions of tongue surface contours in the course of time are also possible during brass articulation (Lindner et al. 2007). Tongue sonography may be important for brass instrument players in order to assess various playing techniques (such as the tremolo-like movement of the tip of the tongue similar to the articulation of a rolling /r/, known as flutter-tonguing, or the double strike of the tongue, as in /te-te/, /ta-ta/ or /ti-ti/, known as double-tonguing), myofunctional disorders and embouchure dystonia (dystonia of the perioral and labial musculature which have been recognized as occupational diseases affecting brass instrument players). The relationship between spoken articulation (e.g. American or Japanese vowels) and brass articulation (e.g. clarinet or trumpet playing) is striking when the tongue surface contours are compared in midsagittal B-mode sectional images (Gardner 2010; Gardner and Stone 2010; Suzuki 2011): the contours of the tongue surface when playing clarinet or trumpet have great similarities with the contours when articulating particular vowels (/a/, /o/, /e/).

Interrelations between tongue positions used by brass instrument players and their native lan-guage are also apparent: most probably, brass musicians use different tongue dorsum contours depending on their first (mother) language while playing identical series of notes! By using video recordings of midsagittal B-mode scans, Heyne and Derrick (2014, 2015) were able to demonstrate that different configurations of the tongue surface are used even when identical series of notes are played and that this is apparently dependent on the native language of the musician.

11.15.4 Visual Biofeedback for Speech Rehabilitation and Brass Instrument Training

Midsagittal B-mode ultrasound sectional imaging can be used not only for diagnostic purposes but also therapeutically in order to provide visual biofeedback, both for speech rehabilitation (Bigenzahn et al. 1988) and for the training of brass articulation. This technique is particularly suitable for children because it is non-invasive and does not require radiation.

Patients must adapt their tongue shapes as closely as possible to contour patterns which are shown to them (either marked with a cursor on the monitor or displayed on a second control monitor) (Shawker and Sonies 1985; Böckler 1990). Thus, patients learn the correct articulation of vowels and consonants under visual control. This ultrasonographic support has been reported to be especially beneficial—even long term— for patients with bilateral profound hearing loss when auditory feedback was lacking despite the use of hearing aids (Shawker and Sonies 1985; Klajman et al. 1988; Böckler et al. 1988; Böckler 1990; Böhme 1990; Bernhardt et al. 2005; Bacsfalvi and Bernhardt 2011), possibly useful in case of contraindication of cochlea implantation. Therapy-resistant phonetic or phonological disorders affecting single phonemes (e.g. the substitution of /r/ by /w/) can also be successfully treated using midsagittal B-mode scans (Shawker and Sonies 1985). Several authors reported that lateral sigmatism was corrected by coronary B-mode ultrasound sectional imaging, where patients were able to match their own tongue contours to the models provided by their therapists (Böckler et al. 1990; Böhme 1990).

Moreover, lingual B-mode scans are particularly useful in developing the correct tongue positions for brass articulation (Gardner 2010). Therefore, this visual biofeedback technique is also recommended for brass instrument teachers.

11.16 Magnetic Resonance Imaging of the Brain

Uta Hanning and Thomas Niederstadt

11.16.1 Introduction

The last decade has seen explosive growth in the use of magnetic resonance imaging (MRI) to explore structural and functional brain development in children. In particular, with the inven-

tion of new technologies, including voxel-based morphometry and functional MRI, a precise investigation of brain regions classically associated with language function is feasible. Broca's area in the posterior frontal lobe and Wernicke's area in the temporal lobe are the most relevant regions centrally involved in language functions (Fig. 11.15).

Beyond these classical language regions, advances in cognitive neuroscience have led to the formulation of an interactive dual-stream model of auditory language processing. It assumes two interacting streams or pathways of the cerebral architecture, a dorsal and a ventral pathway, in long association fibre tracts, to which the fasciculus arcuatus/fasciculus longitudinalis superior belongs (*dual-stream model* (Hickock and Poeppel 2015)). There is neuroradiological evidence for the existence of those pathways and the abnormalities they show in cases of lesions associated with language impairment (Almairac

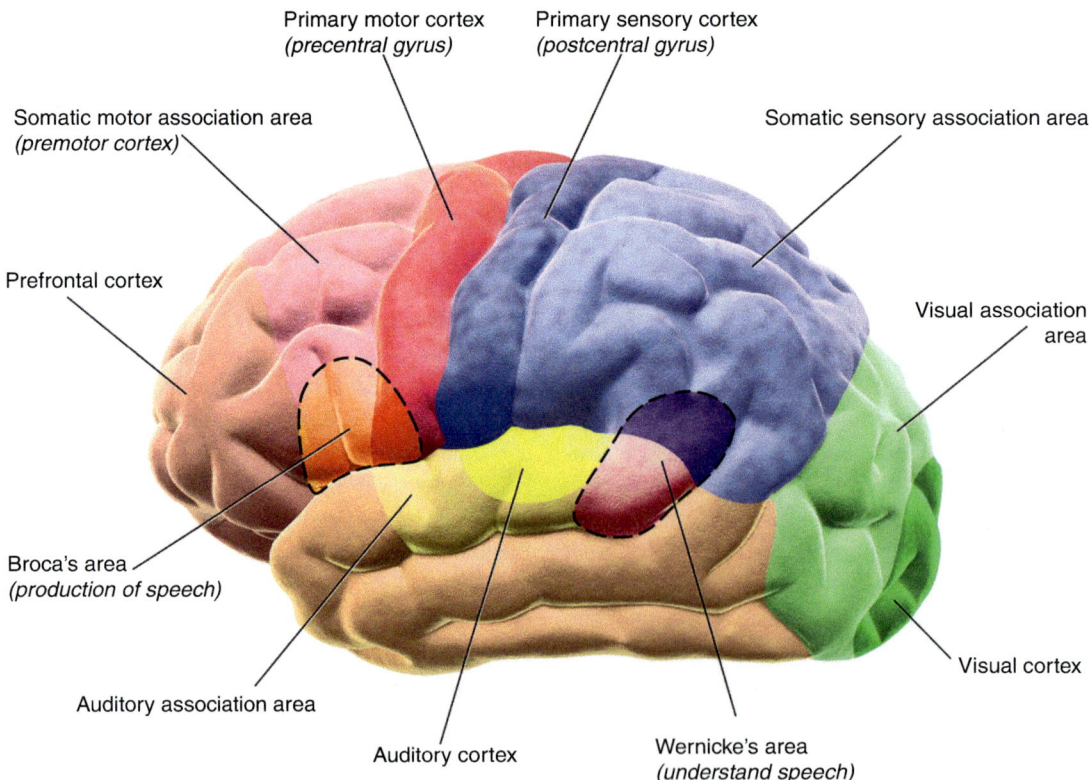

Fig. 11.15 Motor and sensory regions of the cerebral cortex (Blausen.com staff 2014)

et al. 2015) and other speech-language abnormalities such as stuttering (Kell et al. 2009).

Phoniatricians ordering MRI should be aware of the following basic principles, advantages and challenges of pediatric MRI.

11.16.2 Basic Principles of MRI

MR applies strong magnetic fields and nonionizing radio-frequency (RF) energy to generate a signal from the body. The technique is based on the magnetic characteristics of protons in anatomical nuclei. Because two thirds of the atoms in the human body consist of hydrogen, most medical applications use the hydrogen nucleus for imaging.

When a patient is positioned within a MRI scanner, a strong magnetic field is generated around the area to be imaged. As the hydrogen nuclei act as small magnets, they align themselves parallel or antiparallel to the direction of the field. The field strength of the external magnetic field is measured in units of Tesla. A radio-frequency pulse (RF pulse) that has the same frequency as the involved protons is then applied, which transfers energy to the protons. This results in the disturbance of the alignment of these hydrogen nuclei. If the RF pulse is switched off, the nuclei are reorientated to equilibrium and a lower energy state. In this process of nuclear relaxation, the excited hydrogen atoms release a radio-frequency signal, which can be recorded and displayed.

The contrast between different tissues is determined by the rate at which excited atoms return to the equilibrium state; for instance, an object emitting a strong signal appears bright, while objects giving a weak signal or none appear dark.

11.16.3 Advantages and Challenges of MRI

Advantages and challenges of MRI comprise:

- No involvement of ionizing radiation.
- Flexible and fast imaging method.

- Compatibility with certain implanted medical devices; titanium implants and modern stapes are compatible and pacemakers are contraindications.

Under controlled conditions, 1.5-T MRI can be performed in patients with cochlear implants. Modern CIs have a rotating magnet that aligns along the magnetic field lines. If the large CI-related artefacts are to be prevented, which may disturb the interpretation of the image, the magnet may be removed under local anaesthesia for the imaging procedure and reinserted later on. Patients should be counselled regarding the risk of internal magnet movement that may occur in up to 15% of cases (Carlson et al. 2015).

11.16.4 Varieties of Magnetic Resonance Images

There are three general MR imaging techniques, *structural imaging*, *functional imaging (fMRT)* and *diffusion tensor imaging (DTI)*, for exploring language disorders.

11.16.4.1 Structural Imaging/Voxel-Based Morphometry

Structural images are like a 'snapshot' of the brain at a certain time. Generally these scans are of quite high resolution (1 mm^3 of tissue) and, for instance, can be applied to reconstruct the cortex in order to measure its thickness in different locations. Voxel-based morphometry is a new imaging approach that affords exploration of local differences in brain anatomy (volume, shape and position), on the basis of a procedure of statistical parametric mapping.

Findings Structural MRI imaging of children with developmental disorders of language usually appear normal upon visual inspection. One of the exceptions are developmental malformations, e.g. polymicrogyria, characterized by an excessive number of small gyri on the surface of the brain. It is more a descriptive diagnosis than a disease itself and may be a part of a developmental disorder. The extremely rare occurring bilateral peri-

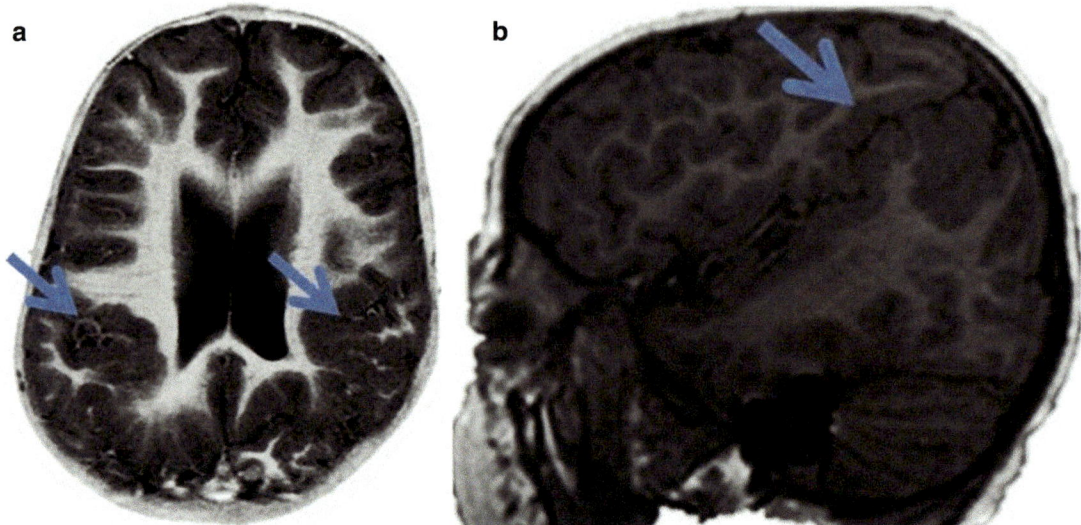

Fig. 11.16 Bilateral perisylvian syndrome with bilateral perisylvian polymicrogyria (**a**) axial T1-weighted IR-sequence (**b**) 3D-T1-weighted image

sylvian syndrome (BPS) is associated with polymicrogyria located in the perisylvian region (Fig. 11.16). Patients usually suffer from delayed language and motor development and oropharyngeal dysfunction (Guerreiro et al. 2002).

Nevertheless, subtle structural abnormalities, such as degree of myelinisation and neuronal size, are only detectable with more sophisticated techniques, such as voxel-based morphometry. In developmental disorders of speech and language, cortical and subcortical anomalies have been reported with a notable degree of anatomical heterogeneity except in the superior temporal gyri (Liegeois et al. 2014).

One of the studies reported reduced grey matter in the right temporal gyri and left posterior superior temporal region (Badcock et al. 2012). Contrariwise, another study described an increased regional volume within a right perisylvian area (Soriano-Mas et al. 2009) (Fig. 11.17). Interestingly, these regions correspond to the classical language areas such as Broca's and Wernicke's region.

11.16.4.2 Functional MRI (fMRI)

Functional MRI (fMRI) is a functional imaging technique based on a MRI technology that calculates neuronal activity by identifying associated changes in cerebral blood flow. This technique works because neuronal activation and cerebral blood flow are coupled. When an area of the brain is activated, for example, during language perception, planning and execution processes, blood flow to that region also increases.

The most commonly used fMRI method is the blood-oxygen-level-dependent (BOLD) contrast. This technique is based on the phenomenon that the ratio of oxygenated to deoxygenated haemoglobin in the blood is related to energy use by brain cells. For this reason fMRI can be used to assess and compare the pattern of functional activation of brain regions during different cognitive and motor tasks. Functional MRI in children requires special precautions owing to the risk of movement, preparation of the child and task design (de Guibert et al. 2011).

Findings Only a few fMRI studies have investigated the activation patterns of children with developmental disorders of speech and language while performing different task panels for language mapping (de Guibert et al. 2011). Hypoactivation of the posterior superior temporal gyri is the main consistent finding (Liegeois et al. 2014). Furthermore, a recently published study

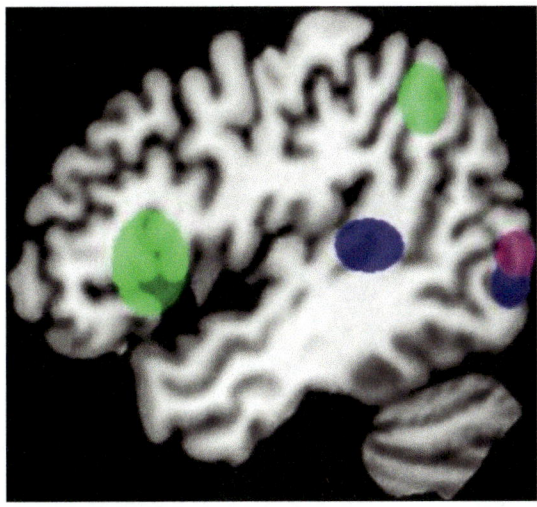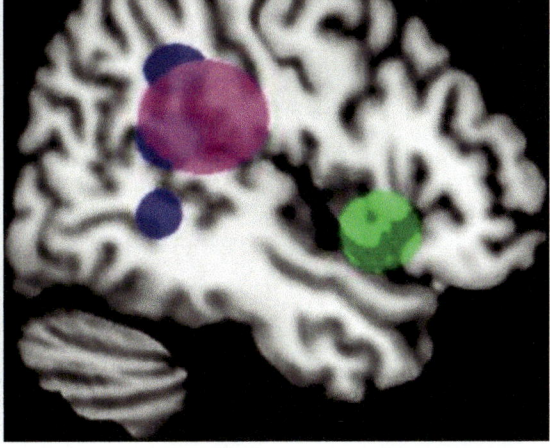

Fig. 11.17 Morphological grey matter (GM) in individuals with developmental disorders of speech and language (Liegeois et al. 2014)/specific language impairment (Badcock et al. 2012; Soriano-Mas et al. 2009). Modified according to Liegeois et al. (2014), Open access by Creative Commons Attribution License. *Colour code*: GM volume decreases, Badcock et al. (2012) blue; GM increases, Badcock et al. (2012) green; Soriano-Mas et al. (2009) purple

reported a lack of functional lateralization in major language regions and consequently an atypical lateralization of language function in core language areas (de Guibert et al. 2011). The results from fMRI studies of developmental disorders of speech and language remain inconsistent, which may be caused by the heterogeneity of developmental language impairment.

11.16.4.3 Diffusion Tensor Imaging (DTI)

Diffusion tensor imaging (DTI) is based on the facts that water molecules move randomly (Brownian motion) and show a different diffusion around white and grey matter, so that water moves quickly along white matter pathways and slowly through grey matter. DTI allows the measurement of constricted movement of water molecules and in the end enables the virtual reconstruction of the orientation and location of white matter tracts. The hypothesis behind DTI is that findings may indicate an early pathological change in the cerebral fibre microstructure.

Findings Children with developmental language disorders showed a reduced fractional

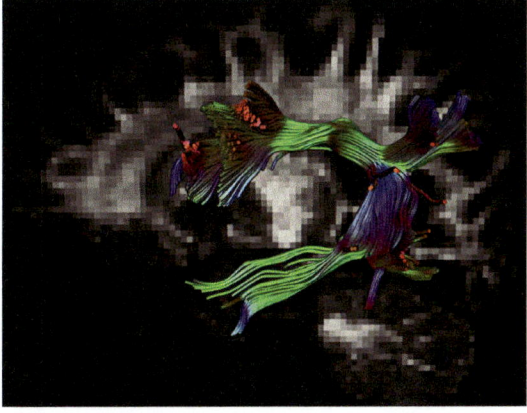

Fig. 11.18 DTI of the superior longitudinal fascicle (Verhoeven et al. 2012). Copyright with kind permission from Oxford University Press

anisotropy (a measure of white matter microstructure) in the superior longitudinal fascicle (Verhoeven et al. 2012). It is one of the major language white matter tracts and can be regarded as the key language tract connecting the caudal temporal cortex and inferior parietal cortex to locations in the frontal lobe, mainly the classical Broca's and Wernicke's area (Fig. 11.18).

References

Achenbach TM, Rescorla LA (2001) Manual for the ASEBA school-age forms & profiles. University of Vermont, Research Center for Children, Youth, & Families, Burlington

Akgul YS, Kambhamettu C, Stone M (1999) Automatic extraction and tracking of the tongue contours. IEEE Trans Med Imaging 18(10):1035–1045

Alderson-Day B, Fernyhough C (2015) Inner speech: development, cognitive functions, phenomenology, and neurobiology. Psychol Bull 141(5):931–965

Alloway TP, Gathercole SE, Holmes J et al (2009) The diagnostic utility of behavioral checklists in identifying children with AD(H)D and children with working memory deficits. Child Psychiatry Hum Dev 40(3):353–366

Almairac F, Herbet G, Moritz-Gasser S et al (2015) The left inferior fronto-occipital fasciculus subserves language semantics: a multilevel lesion study. Brain Struct Funct 220(4):1983–1995. https://doi.org/10.1007/s00429-014-0773-1

American Educational Research Association, American Psychological Association, National Council on Measurement in Education (2014) Standards for educational and psychological testing. American Educational Research Association, Washington, DC

American Psychiatric Association (2013) Diagnostic and statistical manual of mental disorders, 5th edn. American Psychiatric Association Publishing, Arlington

American Speech-Language-Hearing Association (ASHA) (2004) Preferred practice patterns for the profession of speech-language pathology [preferred practice patterns]. Available via https://www.asha.org/policy/PP2004-00191/. Accessed 5 Dec, 12 Dec 2015/28 May 2016

American Speech-Language-Hearing Association (ASHA) (2016) Practice portal for clinical topics: speech sound disorders: articulation and phonology. Available via www.asha.org/Practice-Portal/Clinical-Topics/Articulation-and-Phonology. Accessed 3 Sept 2016

Angerstein W (1994) Ultraschallgestützter Untersuchungsgang zur Beurteilung der Zungenbeweglichkeit. Sprache-Stimme-Gehör 18:80–84

Angerstein W (2003) Sonography of the tongue while playing the didgeridoo. Musikphysiol Musikermed 10(1):14–15

Angerstein W, Isselstein A, Lindner C et al (2009) Ultrasound examinations of the tongue while playing wind instruments. Musikphysiol Musikermed 16(1):7–8

Ayres AJ (1996) Sensory integration and praxis tests, 3rd edn. Western Psychological Services, Los Angeles

Bacsfalvi P, Bernhardt BM (2011) Long-term outcomes of speech therapy for seven adolescents with visual feedback technologies: ultrasound and electropalatography. Clin Linguist Phon. 25(11–12):1034–1043. https://doi.org/10.3109/02699206.2011.618236

Badcock NA, Bishop DV, Hardiman MJ et al (2012) Co-localisation of abnormal brain structure and function in specific language impairment. Brain Lang 120(3):310–320. https://doi.org/10.1016/j.bandl.2011.10.006

Ballard KJ, Savage S, Leyton CE et al (2014) Logopenic and nonfluent variants of primary progressive aphasia are differentiated by acoustic measures of speech production. PLoS One 9(2):e89864. https://doi.org/10.1371/journal.pone.0089864

Barkley RA (1997) Behavioral inhibition, sustained attention, and executive functions: constructing a unifying theory of AD(H)D. Psychol Bull 121(1):64–94

Barkley RA (2006) Attention-deficit hyperactivity disorder: a handbook for diagnosis and treatment, 3rd edn. Guilford Press, New York

Barkley RA, Edwards G, Laneri M et al (2001) Executive functioning, temporal discounting, and sense of time in adolescents with attention deficit hyperactivity disorder (ADHD) and oppositional defiant disorder (ODD). J Abnorm Child Psychol 29(6D):541–556

Bates E, Marchman V, Thal D et al (1994) Developmental and stylistic variation in the composition of early vocabulary. J Child Lang 21(1):85–121

Bates E, Dale P, Thal D (1995) Individual differences and their implications for theories of language development. In: Fletcher P, MacWhinney B (eds) The handbook of child language. Basil Blackwell, Oxford, pp 96–152

Bayley N (2006) Bayley scales of infant and toddler development, 3rd edn (Bayley-III). Administration manual, Harcourt, San Antonio

Bayley N (2014) Bayley scales of infant and toddler development, 3rd edn (Bayley-III). Pearson Assessment, Frankfurt/Main (German version: Reuner G, Rosenkranz J (eds))

Beagley SB, Reedman SE, Sakzewski L et al (2016) Establishing Australian norms for the Jebsen Taylor Test of Hand Function in typically developing children aged five to 10 years: a pilot study. Phys Occup Ther Pediatr 36(1):88–109

Benner GJ, Nelson JR, Epstein MH (2002) Language skills of children with EBD: a literature review. J Emot Behav Disord 10(1):43–59

Bennett JW, Peterson CQ (1995) The touch inventory for elementary-school-aged children: test-retest reliability and mother-child correlations. Am J Occup Ther 49(8):795–801

Benton AL, Hamsher K (1976) Multilingual aphasia examination. AJA Associates, Iowa City

Berger D (2007) Primitive reflexes and righting reactions. A look through the lens of survival, emotions and memory. Available via https://daveberger.net/daves-articles/primitive-reflexes-and-rightingreactions-a-look-through-the-lense-of-survival-emotions-and-memory/. Accessed 5 May 2018

Bernhardt B, Bacsfalvi P, Gick B et al (2005) Exploring the use of electropalatography and ultrasound in speech habilitation. J Speech Lang Pathol Audiol 29(4):169–182

Bernthal J, Bankson NW, Flipsen P (2013) Articulation and phonological disorders. Pearson Higher Education, New York

Bezdjian S, Baker LA, Lozano DI et al (2009) Assessing inattention and impulsivity in children during the Go/NoGo task. Br J Dev Psychol 27(2):365–383

Biederman J, Monuteaux MC, Doyle AE et al (2004) Impact of executive function deficits and attention-deficit/hyperactivity disorder (AD(H)D) on academic outcomes in children. J Consult Clin Psychol 72(5):757–766

Bigenzahn W (2003) Orofaziale Dysfunktionen im Kindesalter, 2nd revised edn. Thieme, Stuttgart

Bigenzahn W, Gritzmann N, Höfler H (1988) Artikulations- und Schluckbewegungen der Zunge in der Real-time-Sonographie. Zentralbl HNO 135:137

Bishop DV, Adams C (1990) A prospective study of the relationship between specific language impairment, phonological disorders and reading retardation. J Child Psychol Psychiatry 31(7):1027–1050

Blankenburg M, Meyer D, Hirschfeld G et al (2011) Developmental and sex differences in somatosensory perception - a systematic comparison of 7- versus 14-year-olds using quantitative sensory testing. Pain 152(11):2625–2631

Blausen.com staff (2014) Medical gallery of Blausen Medical 2014. Wikiversity J Med 1(2). https://doi.org/10.15347/wjm/2014.010. ISSN 2002-4436

Blomberg H, Dempsey M (2011) Movements that heal: rhythmic movement training and primitive reflex integration. BookPal, Coopers Plains

Boada R, Willcutt EG, Pennington BF (2012) Understanding the comorbidity between dyslexia and attention-deficit/hyperactivity disorder. Top Lang Disord 32(3):264–284

Böckler R (1990) Medizinische Grundlagen des Ultraschallverfahrens bei der Anwendung zur Artikulationsanbahnung. HÖRPÄD 44:15–17

Böckler R, Wein B, Neumann H et al (1988) Zungensonographische Unterstützung der Anbahnung des /k/-Lautes bei einem gehörlosen Kind. HÖRPÄD 42:337–343

Böckler R, Wein B, Klajman S (1989) Ultraschalluntersuchung der aktiven und passiven Beweglichkeit der Zunge. Folia Phoniatr 41(6):277–282

Böckler R, Wein B, Wild A et al (1990) Sonographische Unterstützung der logopädischen Behandlung des Sigmatismus lateralis. Sprache-Stimme-Gehör 14:117–119

Boersma P, Weenink D (2014) Praat: doing phonetics by computer. Available via http://www.fon.hum.uva.nl/praat/. Accessed March 2017

Böhme G (1990) Ultraschalldiagnostik der Zunge. Laryngol Rhinol Otol 69(7):381–388

Bressmann T, Heng CL, Irish JC (2005a) Applikations of 2D and 3D ultrasound imaging in speech-language pathology. J Speech Lang Pathol Audiol 29(4):158–168

Bressmann T, Thind P, Uy C et al (2005b) Quantitative three-dimensional ultrasound analysis of tongue protrusion, grooving and symmetry: data from 12 normal speakers and a partial glossectomee. Clin Linguist Phon 19(6–7):573–588

Bressmann T, Uy C, Irish JC (2005c) Analysing normal and partial glossectomee tongues using ultrasound. Clin Linguist Phon 19(1):35–52

Brothers KB, Glascoe FP, Robertshaw NS (2008) PEDS: developmental milestones - an accurate brief tool for surveillance and screening. Clin Pediatr 47(3):271–279

Brown TE (2006) Executive functions and attention deficit hyperactivity disorder: implications of two conflicting views. Int J Disabil Dev Educ 53(1):35–46

Burden V, Stott CM, Forge J et al (1996) The Cambridge Language and Speech Project (CLASP). 1. Detection of language difficulties at 36 to 39 months. Dev Med Child Neurol 38(7):613–631

Burris C, Vorperian HK, Fourakis M et al (2014) Quantitative and descriptive comparison of four acoustic analysis systems: vowel measurements. J Speech Lang Hear Res 57(1):26–45

Bushnell EW, Boudreau JP (1991) The development of haptic perception during infancy. In: Heller MA, Schiff W (eds) The psychology of touch. Erlbaum, Hillsdale, pp 139–161

Carlson ML, Neff BA, Link MJ et al (2015) Magnetic resonance imaging with cochlear implant magnet in place: safety and imaging quality. Otol Neurotol 36(6):965–971

Carson DK, Klee T, Perry CK et al (1998) Comparisons of children with delayed and normal language at 24 months of age on measures of behavioral difficulties, social and cognitive development. Infant Ment Health J 19(1):59–75

Case-Smith J, Butcher L, Reed D (1998) Parent's report of sensory responsiveness and temperament in preterm infants. Am J Occup Ther 52(7):547–555

CHADD (2017) Rating scales and checklists. Available via http://www.chadd.org/Understanding-AD(H)D/For-Professionals/For-Healthcare-Professionals/Clinical-Practice-Tools/Rating-Scales-and-Checklists.aspx. Accessed 15 Feb 2017

Cheung PSP, Ng A, To CKS (2006) Hong Kong Cantonese articulation test. Language Information Sciences Research Centre, City University of Hong Kong, Hong Kong

CHILDES (2014) Child language data exchange system. Available via http://childes.talkbank.org/. Accessed 1 June 2014

Clahsen H (1986) Die Profilanalyse. Ein linguistisches Verfahren für die Sprachdiagnose im Vorschulalter. Marhold, Berlin

Cohen NJ, Farnia F, Im-Bolter N (2013) Higher order language competence and adolescent mental health. J Child Psychol Psychiatry 54(7):733–744

Conners CK (2004) Conners' CPT II continuous performance test II. Multi Health Systems, North Tonawanda

Conti-Ramsden G, Botting N (2008) Emotional health in adolescents with and without a history of specific language impairment (SLI). J Child Psychol Psychiatry 49(5):516–525

Coplan J, Gleason JR (1988) Unclear speech: recognition and significance of unintelligible speech in preschool children. Pediatrics 82(3):447–452

Culicchia G, Nobilia M, Asturi M et al (2016) Cross-cultural adaptation and validation of the Jebsen-Taylor Hand Function Test in an Italian population. Rehabil Res Pract 2016:8970917. https://doi.org/10.1155/2016/8970917. Epub 2016 Jul 18

Dale PS (1991) The validity of a parent report measure of vocabulary and syntax at 24 months. J Speech Hear Res 34(3):565–571

DaParma A, Geffner D, Martin N (2011) Prevalence and nature of language impairment in children with attention deficit/hyperactivity disorder. Contemp Issues Commun Sci Disord 38:119–125

Debuschewitz A, Winkler U, Günther T et al (2004) Die Bedeutung der taktil-kinästhetischen Wahrnehmung bei Kindern mit Aussprachestörungen. Sprache-Stimme-Gehör 28(4):171–177

Dilling H, Mombour W, Schmidt MH (2008) Internationale Klassifikation psychischer Störungen, 6th edn. Hans Huber, Bern

Dodd B (2005) Differential diagnosis and treatment of children with speech disorder, 2nd edn. Whurr, London

Dodd B (2014) Differential diagnosis of pediatric speech sound disorder. Curr Dev Disord Rep 1(3):189–196

Dodd B, Hua Z, Crosbie S et al. (2002) Diagnostic evaluation of articulation and phonology (DEAP). Psychology Corporation. Pearson Education, London (UK edition)

Dodd B, Hua Z, Crosbie S et al (2006) Diagnostic evaluation of articulation and phonology (DEAP). Psychology Corporation. Pearson Education, London (US edition)

Duffy JR (2016) Functional speech disorders: clinical manifestations, diagnosis, and management. Handb Clin Neurol 139:379–388

Dunn W, Griffith JW, Sabata D et al (2015) Measuring change in somatosensation across the lifespan. Am J Occup Ther 69(3):6903290020p1–6903290020p9. https://doi.org/10.5014/ajot.2015.014845

Durkin K, Conti-Ramsden G (2010) Young people with specific language impairment: a review of social and emotional functioning in adolescence. Child Lang Teach Ther 26(2):107–123

Ebejer JL, Medland SE, van der Werf J et al (2012) Attention deficit hyperactivity disorder in Australian adults: prevalence, persistence, conduct problems and disadvantage. PLoS One 7(10):e47404

Ege P, Acarlar F, Turan F (2004) Ankara Artikülasyon Testi. Key Tasarim, Ankara

Engle RW, Tuholski SW, Laughlin JE et al (1999) Working memory, short-term memory, and general fluid intelligence: a latent-variable approach. J Exp Psychol 128(3):309–331

Fenichel GM (2009) Clinical pediatric neurology. A signs and symptoms approach, 6th edn. Elsevier, New York

Fenson L, Marchman VA, Thal DJ et al (2007) MacArthur-Bates communicative development inventories: user's guide and technical manual, 2nd edn. Paul H. Brookes Publishing, Baltimore

Flipsen P Jr, Ogiela DA (2015) Psychometric characteristics of single-word tests of children's speech sound production. Lang Speech Hear Serv Sch 46(2):166–178

Folio R, Fewell RR (2000) The Peabody Developmental Motor Scales, 2nd edn (PDMS-2). PRO-ED, Austin

Folker JE, Murdoch BE, Cahill LM et al (2010) Differentiating impairment levels in temporal versus spatial aspects of linguopalatal contacts in Friedreich's ataxia. Motor Control 14(4):490–508

Folker JE, Murdoch BE, Cahill LM et al (2011) Articulatory kinematics in the dysarthria associated with Friedreich's ataxia. Motor Control 15(3):376–389

Fox AV (2006) Kindliche Aussprachestörungen. Phonologischer Erwerb – Differenzialdiagnostik – Therapie. Schulz-Kirchner Verlag, Idstein

Fox AV, Dodd BJ (1999) Der Erwerb des phonologischen Systems in der deutschen Sprache. Sprache - Stimme - Gehör 23:183–191

Fox-Boyer A (2014) Psycholinguistische Analyse kindlicher Aussprachestörungen (PLAKKS-II) (revised edition of PLAKKS, 2002). Pearson Assessment, Frankfurt

Fox-Boyer A, Salgert K, Clausen MC (2016) Diagnostik von kindlichen Aussprachestörungen unklarer Genese. Sprache Stimme Gehör 40(02):61–67

Francis DO, Chinnadurai S, Morad A et al (2015) Treatments for ankyloglossia and ankyloglossia with concomitant lip-tie. Rockville: Agency for Healthcare Research and Quality (US). Comparative Effectiveness Reviews, No. 149. Available via https://www.effectivehealthcare.ahrq.gov/ehc/products/558/2074/ankyloglossia-report-150504.pdf. Accessed 7 May 2017

Gardner JT (2010) Ultrasonographic investigation of clarinet multiple articulation. D.M.A. thesis, Graduate College, Arizona State University, Tempe. Available via http://gradworks.umi.com/34/10/3410697.html. Accessed 8 April 2016

Gardner JT, Stone M (2010) A comparison of midsagittal tongue shapes during clarinet performance and vowel production using ultrasound. Poster presented at Ultrafest V, Haskins Labs, New Haven, 26 March 2010. Available via http://www.haskins.yale.edu/conferences/UltrafestV/abstracts/Gardner_Stone_Poster_UltrafestV.pdf. Accessed 8 April 2016

Gerken L (1994) Child Phonology. In: Gernsbacher MA (ed) Handbook of psychology. Academic, San Diego, pp 781–820

Gibbon FE, Lee A (2016) Electropalatographic (EPG) evidence of covert contrasts in disordered speech. Clin Linguist Phon 31(1):4–20

Glascoe FP (1999) Using parents' concerns to detect and address developmental and behavioral problems. J Soc Pediatr Nurs 4(1):24–35

Glascoe FP, Dworkin PH (1995) The role of parents in the detection of developmental and behavioral problems. Pediatrics 95(6):829–836

Glaspey AM, Stoel-Gammon C (2007) A dynamic approach to phonological assessment. Adv Speech Lang Pathol 9(4):286–296

Goddard S (2005) Reflexes, learning and behavior: A window into the child's mind. Fern Ridge Press, Eugene

Goldstein B, Iglesias A (2006) CPACS: contextual probes of articulation competence: Spanish. Super Duper, Greenville

Götze B, Kiese-Himmel C, Hasselhorn M (2001) Haptische Wahrnehmungs- und Sprachentwicklungsleistungen bei Kindergarten- und Vorschulkindern. Prax Kinderpsychol Kinderpsychiatr 50(8):640–648

Grech H, Dodd B, Franklin S (2011) Maltese-English Speech Assessment (MESA). University of Malta, Guardamangia

Grunwald M (ed) (2008) Human haptic perception. Basics and applications. Birkhäuser, Basel

Grunwald M, Beyer L (eds) (2001) Grundlagen und Anwendungen zur haptischen Wahrnehmung. Birkhäuser, Basel

Grunwell P (1993) Analysing cleft palate speech. Whurr Publishers, London

Guerreiro MM, Hage SR, Guimaraes CA et al (2002) Developmental language disorder associated with polymicrogyria. Neurology 59(2):245–250

de Guibert C, Maumet C, Jannin P et al (2011) Abnormal functional lateralization and activity of language brain areas in typical specific language impairment (developmental dysphasia). Brain 134(10):3044–3058. https://doi.org/10.1093/brain/awr141

Hardcastle WJ (2006) Electromyography. In: Hardcastle WJ, Hewlett N (eds) Coarticulation: theory, data and techniques. Cambridge University Press, Cambridge, pp 270–283

Hatch F, Maietta L (1991) The role of kinesthesia in pre- and perinatal bonding. J Prenat Perinat Psychol Health 5(3):253–270

Head H (1905) The afferent nervous system from a new aspect. Brain 28(2):99–115

Healey DM, Rucklidge JJ (2008) The relationship between AD(H)D and creativity. The AD(H)D report. The Guilford, New York, pp 1–5

Hendrickson K, Mitsven S, Poulin-Dubois D et al (2015) Looking and touching: what extant approaches reveal about the structure of early word knowledge. Dev Sci 18(5):723–735

Henry JD, Beatty WW (2006) Verbal fluency deficits in multiple sclerosis. Neuropsychologia 44(7):1166–1174

Heyne M, Derrick D (2014) Some initial findings regarding first language influence on playing brass instruments. In: Proceedings of the 15th Australasian international conference on speech science and technology, Christchurch, 2014, pp 180–183. Available via http://ir.canterbury.ac.nz/xmlui/handle/10092/10656. Accessed 22 April 2016

Heyne M, Derrick D (2015) The influence of tongue position on trombone sound: a likely area of language influence, Christchurch. Available via http://ir.canterbury.ac.nz/handle/10092/11122. Accessed 22 April 2016

Hickok G, Poeppel D (2015) Neural basis of speech perception. Handb Clin Neurol 129:149–160. https://doi.org/10.1016/B978-0-444-62630-1.00008-1

Hirschfeld G, Zernikow B, Krämer N et al (2012) Development of somatosensory perception in children: a longitudinal QST-study. Neuropediatrics 43(1):10–16

Hodson B, Paden E (1991) Targeting intelligible speech: a phonological approach to remediation, 2nd edn. Pro-Ed/College Hill, Austin

Hollo A, Wehby JH, Oliver RM (2014) Unidentified language deficits in children with emotional and behavioral disorders: a meta-analysis. Except Child 80(2):169–186

Im-Bolter N, Cohen NJ, Farnia F (2013) I thought we were good: social cognition, figurative language, and adolescent psychopathology. J Child Psychol Psychiatry 54(7):724–732

International Expert Panel on Multilingual Children's Speech (2012) Multilingual children with speech sound disorders: position paper. Available via http://www.csu.edu.au/research/multilingual-speech/position-paper. Accessed 28 May 2016

International Phonetic Association (IPA) (1999) Handbook of the International Phonetic Association: a guide to the use of the International Phonetic Alphabet. Cambridge University Press, Cambridge

IPA Chart. http://www.internationalphoneticassociation.org/content/ipa-chart, available under a Creative Commons Attribution-Sharealike 3.0 Unported License. Copyright © 2015 International Phonetic Association

Itabashi R, Nishio Y, Kataoka Y et al (2016) Damage to the left precentral gyrus is associated with apraxia of speech in acute stroke. Stroke 47(1):31–36. https://doi.org/10.1161/strokeaha.115.010402

Jebsen RH, Taylor N, Trieschmann RB et al (1969) An objective and standardized test of hand function. Arch Phys Med Rehabil 50(6):311–319

Jones D (1972) An outline of English phonetics, 9th edn. W. Heffer & Sons, Cambridge

Jones LA, Lederman SJ (2006) Human hand function. Oxford University Press, Oxford

Kalisch T, Kattenstroth JC, Kowalewski R et al (2012) Cognitive and tactile factors affecting human haptic performance in later life. PLoS One 7(1):e30420. https://doi.org/10.1371/journal.pone.0030420

Karmiloff K, Karmiloff-Smith A (2001) Pathways to language. From fetus to adolescent. Harvard University Press, Cambridge

Kaufman AS, Kaufman NL (1983) Kaufman Assessment Battery for Children. American Guidance Service, Circle Pines MN

Kaufman AS, Kaufman NL (2004) Kaufman-Assessment Battery for Children, 2nd edn (KABC-II). AGS Publications, Circle Pines MN

Kauschke C (1999) Der Erwerb des frühkindlichen Lexikons – eine empirische Studie zur Entwicklung des Wortschatzes im Deutschen. Narr, Tübingen

Kauschke C, Siegmüller J (2009) Patholinguistische Diagnostik bei Sprachentwicklungsstörungen (PDSS), 2nd edn. Elsevier, Amsterdam

Kavanagh G, O'Hanrahan S, Hughes G et al (2014) Review of clinical guidelines for children and adolescents with attention deficit hyperactivity disorder and their application to an Irish context. Ir J Psychol Med 1(3):1–11

Kell CA, Neumann K, von Kriegstein K et al (2009) How the brain repairs stuttering. Brain 132(Pt 10):2747–2760. https://doi.org/10.1093/brain/awp185

Keller T (2014) ROC-Analysen. Available via http://www.acomed-statistik.de/roc-kurve.html. Accessed 1 June 2014

Kelsey CA, Minifie FD, Hixon TJ (1969) Applications of ultrasound in speech research. J Speech Hear Res 12(3):564–575

Kent RD (2000) Research on speech motor control and its disorders: a review and prospective. J Commun Disord 33(5):391–428

Kent RD (2015) Nonspeech oral movements and oral motor disorders: a narrative review. Am J Speech Lang Pathol 24(4):763–789

Kiese-Himmel C (unter Mitarbeit von Kiefer S) (2000) Diagnostischer Elternfragebogen zur taktil-kinästhetischen Responsivität im frühen Kindesalter (DEF-TK). Beltz, Göttingen

Kiese-Himmel C (2003) Göttinger Entwicklungstest der TAktil-KInästhetischen WAhrnehmung (TAKIWA). Beltz, Göttingen

Kiese-Himmel C (2005) Taktil-Kinästhetik - eine funktionale Grundlage der Sprachentwicklung? L.O.G.O.S. Interdisziplinär. Fachzeitschrift für Logopädie und andere kommunikationstherapeutische und benachbarte Gebiete 13:202–211

Kiese-Himmel C (2006) Wahrnehmung taktiler Reize. In: Funke J, Frensch PA (eds) Handbuch der Psychologie. Bd: Allgemeine Psychologie: Kognition und Handlung. Hogrefe, Göttingen, pp 147–151

Kiese-Himmel C (2007) Die Bedeutung der taktil-kinästhetischen Sinnesmodalität für die Sprachentwicklung. Forum Logopädie 21:26–29

Kiese-Himmel C (2008) Haptic perception in infancy and first acquisition of object words: developmental and clinical approach. In: Grunwald M (ed) Human haptic perception. Basics and applications. Birkhäuser, Basel, pp 321–334

Kiese-Himmel C, Kruse E (1998) Höhere taktil-kinästhetische Funktionen ehemalig sprachentwicklungsgestörter Kinder im Grundschulalter - eine neuropsychologische Studie. Folia Phoniatr Logop 50(4):195–120

Kiese-Himmel C, Schiebusch-Reiter U (1999) Haptische Formdiskrimination: Gruppenvergleich von sprachunauffälligen und ehemals sprachentwicklungsgestörten Kindern. HNO 47(1):45–50

Kiese-Himmel C, Witte C, von Steinbüchel N (2015) Graphästhesie und Sprachleistungen bei 3- bis 6-Jährigen mit Migrationshintergrund. Praxis Sprache 60(3):148–154

Kim Y, Shin M (2004) Urimal Test of Articulation and Phonology (U-TAP). Hakjisa Publisher, Seoul

Kim M, Pae S, Bak C (2007) Assessment of Phonology and Articulation for Children (APAC). Human Brain Research and Consulting Company, Inchon

Kirk C, Vigeland L (2014) A psychometric review of norm-referenced tests used to assess phonological error patterns. Lang Speech Hear Serv Sch 45(4):365–377

Klajman S, Huber W, Neumann H (1988) Ultrasonographische Unterstützung der Artikulationsanbahnung bei gehörlosen Kindern. Sprache-Stimme-Gehör 12:117–120

Kliegman RM, Stanton BF, St. Geme JW et al (eds) (2011) Nelson textbook of pediatrics, 19th edn. Elsevier, Philadelphia

Kunnari S, Savinainen-Makkonen T, Saaristo-Helin K (2012) Fonologiatesti. Niilo Mäki Instituutti, Jyväskylä

Ladefoged P (2006) A course in phonetics, 5th edn. Thomson Wadsworth, Boston

Laing GJ, Law J, Levin A et al (2002) Evaluation of a structured test and a parent led method for screening for speech and language problems: prospective population based study. BMJ 325(7373):1152–1154

de Langen-Müller U, Kauschke C, Kiesel-Himmel C et al (eds. in equal authorship) (2011) Diagnostik von Sprachentwicklungsstörungen (SES), unter Berücksichtigung umschriebener Sprachentwicklungsstörungen (USES) (Synonym: Spezifische Sprachentwicklungsstörungen (SSES)) Interdisziplinäre S2k-Leitlinie. Register-Nr: 049/006. Available via: http://www.awmf.org/uploads/tx_szleitlinien/049-006l_S2k_Sprachentwicklungsstoerungen_Diagnostik_2013-06-abgelaufen_01.pdf. Accessed 11 April 2018

de Langen-Müller U, Kiese-Himmel C, Neumann K et al (equal authorship) (2012) Diagnostik von (umschriebenen) Sprachentwicklungsstörungen, 1st edn. Peter Lang, Frankfurt am Main

de Langen-Müller U, Kauschke C, Kiese-Himmel C et al (eds in equal authorship) (2013) Diagnostik von Sprachentwicklungsstörungen (SES), unter Berücksichtigung umschriebener Sprachentwicklungsstörungen (USES). [Diagnostics of developmental disorders of speech and language with special attention to specific developmental disorders of speech and language.] Guidelines of the Deutsche Gesellschaft für Phoniatrie und Pädaudiologie e.V. (DGPP) and Deutsche Gesellschaft für Kinder- und Jugendpsychiatrie, Psychosomatik und Psychotherapie (DGKJP). Arbeitsgemeinschaft der Wissenschaftlichen Medizinischen Fachgesellschaften e.V. (AWMF). Register-Nr. 049/006. Available via http://www.awmf.org/uploads/tx_szleitlinien/049-006l_S2k_Sprachentwicklungsstoerungen_Diagnostik_2013-06_01.pdf. Accessed 13 Nov 2016

Largo RH, Molinari L, Comenale PL et al (1986) Language development of term and preterm children during the first five years of life. Dev Med Child Neurol 28(3):333–350

Law J, Boyle J, Harris F et al (2000) The feasibility of universal screening for primary speech and language delay: findings from a systematic review of the literature. Dev Med Child Neurol 42(3):190–200

Lederman SJ, Klatzky RL (1987) Hand movements: a window into haptic object recognition. Cogn Psychol 19(3):342–368

Lejeune F, Berne-Audéoud F, Marcus L et al (2014) The effect of postnatal age on the early tactile manual abilities of preterm infants. Early Hum Dev 90(5):259–264

Leonard MA, Milich R, Lorch P (2011) The role of pragmatic language use in mediating the relation between hyperactivity and inattention and social skills problems. J Speech Lang Hear Res 54(2):567–579

Li M, Kambhamettu C, Stone M (2005) Automatic contour tracking in ultrasound images. Clin Linguist Phon 19(6-7):545–554

Liégeois FJ, Morgan AT (2012) Neural bases of childhood speech disorders: lateralization and plasticity for speech functions during development. Neurosci Biobehav Rev 36(1):439–458

Liégeois F, Mayes A, Morgan A (2014) Neural correlates of developmental speech and language disorders: evidence from neuroimaging. Curr Dev Disord Rep 1(3):215–227. https://doi.org/10.1007/s40474-014-0019-1

Lietz R (1996) Klinisch-neurologische Untersuchung im Kindesalter. Deutscher Ärzte Verlag, Köln

Lin E, Hornibrook J, Ormond T (2012) Evaluating iPhone recordings for acoustic voice assessment. Folia Phoniatr Logop 64(3):122–130

Lindner C, Angerstein W, Aurich V et al (2007) An algorithm for pseudo-3D representation of the contour of the tongue while playing the didgeridoo. In: Agulló J, Barjau A (eds) International symposium on musical acoustics (ISMA). Program and Abstracts, Barcelona, 9–12 Sept 2007, pp 40–48. ISBN: 84-934142-0-4. Available via http://www.uniklinik-duesseldorf.de/fileadmin/Datenpool/einrichtungen/phoniatrie_und_paedaudiologie_id495/dateien/paper_barcelona.pdf. Accessed 8 April 2016

Logan GD (1994) On the ability to inhibit thought and action: a users' guide to the stop signal paradigm. In: Dagenbach D, Carr TH (eds) Inhibitory processes in attention, memory, and language. Academic, San Diego, pp 189–239

Lohmander A, Borell E, Henningsson G et al (2005) SVANTE- Svenskt artikulations- och Nasalittets Test: Pedagogisk Design. Skivarp, Sweden

Loonstra AS, Tarlow AR, Sellers AH (2001) COWAT metanorms across age, education, and gender. Appl Neuropsychol 8(3):161–167

Lopez C (2016) The vestibular system: balancing more than just the body. Curr Opin Neurol 29(1):74–83

Luiz D, Barnard A, Knosen N et al (2006) Griffiths Mental Development Scales - extended revised: 2 to 8 years (GMDS-ER 2-8). Administration and Analysis Manual. Available via http://www.hogrefe.co.uk/clinical-and-educational/child-development/gmds-er-2-8.html. Accessed 15 Nov 2016

Maassen BAM, Terband HR (2015) Process-oriented diagnosis of childhood and adult apraxia of speech (CAS and AOS). In: Redford MA (ed) The handbook of speech production, 1st edn. Wiley, Hoboken, pp 331–350

Maassen B, Thoonen G, Boers I (1997) Quantitative assessment of dysarthria and developmental apraxia of speech. In: Hulstijn W et al (eds) Speech production: motor control, brain research and fluency disorders. Elsevier Science BV, Amsterdam, pp 611–619

MacWhinney B (1995) The CHILDES project: tools for analyzing talk, 2nd edn. Erlbaum, Mahwah

Mandelli ML, Caverzasi E, Binney RJ et al (2014) Frontal white matter tracts sustaining speech production in primary progressive aphasia. J Neurosci 34(29):9754–9767

Manfredi C, Lebacq J, Cantarella G et al (2016) Smartphones offer new opportunities in clinical voice research. J Voice 31(1):111.e1–111.e7. https://doi.org/10.1016/j.jvoice.2015.12.020

Massy-Westropp NM, Gill TK, Taylor AW et al (2011) Hand grip strength: age and gender stratified normative data in a population-based study. BMC Res Notes 4:127. https://doi.org/10.1186/1756-0500-4-127

Mazurkiewicz-Bełdzińska M (2017) Neurological evaluation – from newborns to teenagers. In: Steinborn B (ed) Neurology of development age, 1st edn. PZWL, Waszawa, pp 68–84

McCauley RJ, Strand EA (2008) A review of standardized tests of nonverbal oral and speech motor performance in children. Am J Speech Lang Pathol 17(1):81–91

McGrath LM, Hutaff-Lee C, Scott A et al (2008) Children with comorbid speech sound disorder and specific language impairment are at increased risk for attention-deficit/hyperactivity disorder. J Abnorm Child Psychol 36(2):151–163

McGregor KK, Waxman SR (1998) Object naming at multiple hierarchical levels: A comparison of preschoolers with and without wordfinding deficits. J Child Lang 25(2):419–430

McGregor KK, Friedman RM, Reilly RM et al (2002) Semantic representation and naming in young children. Speech Lang Hear Res 45(2):332–346

McGrew KS (2005) The Cattell-Horn-Carroll theory of cognitive abilities: past, present, and future. In: Flanagan DP, Harrison PL (eds) Contemporary intellectual assessment: theories, tests, and issues, 2nd edn. Guilford, New York, pp 136–181

McIntosh B, Dodd B (2011) Toddler Phonology Test (TPT). Pearson Education, London

McLeod S (2012a) Multilingual children's speech. Available via http://www.csu.edu.au/research/multilingual-speech/. Accessed 28 May 2016

McLeod S (2012b) Summary of 250 cross-linguistic studies of speech acquisition. Available via http://www.csu.edu.au/research/multilingual-speech/speech-acquisition. Accessed 28 May 2016

McLeod S (2012c) Multilingual speech assessments. Available via http://www.csu.edu.au/research/multilingual-speech/speech-assessments. Accessed 28 May 2016

McLeod S (2015) Intelligibility in context scale: a parent-report screening tool translated into 60 languages. J Clin Pract Speech Lang Pathol 17(1):7–12

McLeod S, Verdon S (2014) A review of 30 speech assessments in 19 languages other than English. Am J Speech Lang Pathol 23(4):708–723

McLeod S, Harrison LJ, McCormack J (2012a) Intelligibility in context scale. Available via http://www.csu.edu.au/research/multilingual-speech/ics. Accessed 4 Sept 2016

McLeod S, Harrison LJ, McCormack J (2012b) Intelligibility in context scale: validity and reliability of a subjective rating measure. J Speech Lang Hear Res 55(2):648–656

McLeod S, Verdon S, Bowen C (2013) International aspirations for speech-language pathologists' practice with multilingual children with speech sound disorders: development of a position paper. J Commun Disord 46(4):375–387

McLeod S, Crowe K, Shahaeian A (2015) Intelligibility in Context Scale: normative and validation data for English-speaking preschoolers. Lang Speech Hear Serv Sch 46(3):266–276

Melchers P, Melchers M (2015) Kaufman Assessment Battery for Children-II (deutschsprachige Fassung der Originalversion von Kaufman AS, NL Kaufman (eds)). Pearson Assessment, Frankfurt/Main

Menyuk P, Liebergott JW, Schultz MC (1995) Early language development in full-term and premature infants. Erlbaum, Hillsdale

Michaelis R (2004) Das Grenzsteinprinzip als Orientierungshilfe für die pädiatrische Entwicklungsbetrachtung. In: Schlack HG (ed) Entwicklungspädiatrie. Marseille, München, pp 123–129

Michelson DJ, Shu SK (2012) Cognitive and motor regression. In: Swaiman KF et al (eds) Pediatric neurology: principles and practice, 5th edn. Mosby Elsevier, Philadelphia

Miller J, Andriacchi K, Nockerts A (2011) Assessing language production using SALT software: a clinician's guide to language sample analysis. SALT Software LLC, Middleton

Minifie FD, Kelsey CA, Zagzebski JA et al (1971) Ultrasonic scans of the dorsal surface of the tongue. J Acoust Soc Am 49(6):1857–1860

Montague A (1995) Körperkontakt. Die Bedeutung der Haut für die Entwicklung des Menschen, 8th edn. Klett, Stuttgart

Morgan AT, Liegeois F, Occomore L (2007) Electropalatography treatment for articulation impairment in children with dysarthria post-traumatic brain injury. Brain Inj 21(11):1183–1193

Morgan AT, Masterton R, Pigdon L et al (2013) Functional magnetic resonance imaging of chronic dysarthric speech after childhood brain injury: reliance on a left-hemisphere compensatory network. Brain 136(2):646–657

Morgan AT, Bonthrone A, Liégeois FJ (2016) Brain basis of childhood speech and language disorders: are we closer to clinically meaningful MRI markers? Curr Opin Pediatr 28(6):725–730. https://doi.org/10.1097/mop.0000000000000420

Mueller KL, Tomblin JB (2012) Examining the comorbidity of language disorders and AD(H)D. Top Lang Disord 32(3):228–246

Müürsepp I, Aibast H, Pääsuke M (2011) Motor performance and haptic perception in preschool boys with specific impairment of expressive language. Acta Paediatr 100(7):1038–1042

Namasivayam AK, Pukonen M, Goshulak D et al (2013) Relationship between speech motor control and speech intelligibility in children with speech sound disorders. J Commun Disord 46(3):264–280

Neumann K, Euler HA (2013) Kann ein Sprachstandsscreening zwischen Sprachförder- und Sprachtherapiebedarf trennen? In: Redder A, Weinert S (eds) Sprachförderung und Sprachdiagnostik - interdisziplinäre Perspektiven. Waxmann, Münster, pp 297–321

Neumann K, Keilmann A, Rosenfeld J et al (2009) Leitlinien der Deutschen Gesellschaft für Phoniatrie und Pädaudiologie zu Sprachentwicklungsstörungen bei Kindern (gekürzte Fassung). Kindh Entwickl 18(4):222–231

Neumann K, Holler-Zittlau I, van Minnen S et al (2011) Katzengoldstandards in der Sprachstandserfassung. Sensitivität-Spezifität des Kindersprachscreenings (KiSS). HNO 59(1):97–109

Neuschaefer-Rube C, Matern G, Ballero Flores V et al (1999) Einsatz des Ultraschalls zur Untersuchung artikulatorischer Zungenbewegungen am Beispiel des spanischen Multivibranten [rr]. Sprachtypol Univ Forsch (STUF) 52(3–4):397–406

New AB, Robin DA, Parkinson AL et al (2015) Altered resting-state network connectivity in stroke patients with and without apraxia of speech. Neuroimage Clin 8:429–439. https://doi.org/10.1016/j.nicl.2015.03.013

NICE (2008) Attention deficit hyperactivity disorder: diagnosis and management of AD(H)D in children, young people and adults. NICE Clinical Guideline 72. Available via www.nice.org.uk/CG72. Accessed 23 Jan 2017

Nicolosi L, Harryman E, Kresheck J (2003) Terminology of communication disorders. Speech-language-hearing, 5th edn. Lippincott Williams & Wilkins, Philadelphia

Novik TS, Hervas A, Ralston SJ et al (2006) Influence of gender on attention-deficit/hyperactivity disorder in Europe - ADORE. Eur Child Adolesc Psychiatry 15(suppl 1):15–24

Oller KD, Eilers RE, Neal AR et al (1999) Precursors to speech in infancy: the prediction of speech and language disorders. J Commun Disord 32(4):223–247

Panhellenic Association of Logopedists (PAL) [Πανελλήνιο" Συλλογο"Λ ογοπεδικwvn (ΠISL)] [Panellinios Syllogos Logopedikon] (1995) Dokimasía Φwnntikή" & 8wnologikή" Exélixn". Author, Athens

Papoušek M, Papoušek H (1989) Stimmliche Kommunikation im frühen Säuglingsalter als Wegbereiter der Sprachentwicklung. In: Keller H (ed) Handbuch der Kleinkindforschung. Huber, Bern, pp 466–489

Parthasarathy V, Stone M, Prince JL (2005) Spatiotemporal visualization of the tongue surface using ultrasound and kriging (SURFACES). Clin Linguist Phon 19(6–7):529–544

Peña ED, Gutiérrez-Clellen VF, Iglesias A et al (2014) BESA: Bilingual English-Spanish Assessment. AR-Clinical Publications, San Rafael

Penner Z (2000) Phonologische Entwicklung. Eine Übersicht. In: Grimm H (ed) Sprachentwicklung. Enzyklopädie der Psychologie, Themenbereich C, Serie III, Bd, vol 3. Hogrefe, Göttingen, pp 105–139

Penner Z, Kölliker-Funk M (1998) Therapie und Diagnose von Grammatikerwerbsstörungen. Ein Arbeitsbuch. Edition SZH, Luzern

Petermann F, Macha T (2005) Psychologische Tests für Kinderärzte. Hogrefe, Göttingen

Petermann F, Macha T (2013) Entwicklungstest sechs Monate bis sechs Jahre - Revision (ET 6-6-R). Pearson Assessment, Frankfurt, Main

Plante E, Vance R (1994) Selection of preschool language tests: a data-based approach. Lang Speech Hear Serv Sch 25(1):15–24

Polanczyk G, de Lima MS, Horta BL et al (2007) The worldwide prevalence of AD(H)D: a systematic review and metaregression analysis. Am J Psychiatry 164(6):942–948

Poole ML, Brodtmann A, Darby D et al (2017) Motor speech phenotypes of frontotemporal dementia, primary progressive aphasia, and progressive apraxia of speech. J Speech Lang Hear Res 60(4):897–911

Posner MI, Peterson SE (1990) The attention system of the human brain. Annu Rev Neurosci 13:24–42

Powell TW (2008) An integrated evaluation of non-speech oral motor treatments. Lang Speech Hear Serv Sch 39:422–227

Purves D, Augustine GJ, Fitzpatrick D et al (eds) (2004) Chapter 8: The somatic sensory system. In: Neuroscience, 3rd edn. Sinauer Associates, Inc. Sunderland, Massachusetts, USA, pp 189–208

Raven J, Raven JC, Court JH (2004) Manual for Raven's progressive matrices and vocabulary scales. Updated. Harcourt Assessment, San Antonio, TX

Redmond SM (2016) Language impairment in the attention-deficit/hyperactivity disorder context. J Speech Lang Hear Res 59(1):133–142

Reichmuth K (2018) Kommunikationsorientierte-sprachspezifische Therapie nach Reichmuth [German]. In: Wachtlin B, Bohnert A (eds) Kindliche Hörstörungen in der Logopädie. Thieme, Stuttgart

Rescorla L (1989) The language development survey: A screening tool for delayed language in toddlers. J Speech Hear Disord 54(4):587–599

Rice ML, Smolik F, Perpich D et al (2010) Mean length of utterance levels in 6-month intervals for children 3

to 9 years with and without language impairments. J Speech Lang Hear Res 53(2):333–349

Roberts HC, Denison HJ, Martin HJ et al (2011) A review of the measurement of grip strength in clinical and epidemiological studies: towards a standardised approach. Age Ageing 40(4):423–429

Rosenbaum S, Simon S (eds) (2016) Speech and language disorders in children: implications for the social security administration's supplemental security income program. National Academies of Sciences, Engineering, and Medicine. The National Academies Press, Washington, DC

Rothweiler M (1999) Der Erwerb von Nebensätzen im Deutschen. Niemeyer, Tübingen

Rothweiler M (2002) Spracherwerb. In: Meibauer J et al (eds) Einführung in die Germanistische Linguistik. Metzler, Stuttgart, pp 251–293

Royeen CB, Fortune JC (1990) Touch inventory for elementary-school-aged children. Am J Occup Ther 44(2):155–159

SALT Software (2014) Computerized language sample analysis. Available via http://www.saltsoftware.com/. Accessed 1 June 2014

Schäfer B, Fox AV (2006) Der Erwerb konsequenter Wortproduktion deutschsprachiger Zweijähriger. Sprache - Stimme - Gehör 30:186–192

Schöler H, Scheib K (2004) Desiderate und Thesen zur Diagnostik bei Sprachentwicklungsstörungen [Desiderata and theses for a diagnosis and differential diagnosis of developmental language impairment]. Sprache - Stimme - Gehör 28(1):37–41

Schönweiler R (1993) Diagnostik und Therapie kindlicher Sprachstörungen. DMW 118:707–711

Schönweiler R (2004) Mittelohrschwerhörigkeit und Sprachentwicklung: Korrelation. Kausalität und Konsequenzen Laryngo-Rhino-Otologie 83:1–2

Sciberras E, Mueller K, Efron D et al (2014) Language problems in children with AD(H)D: a community-based study. Pediatrics 133(5):793–800

Shawker TH, Sonies BC (1984) Tongue movement during speech: a real-time ultrasound evaluation. J Clin Ultrasound 12(3):125–133

Shawker TH, Sonies BC (1985) Ultrasound biofeedback for speech training. Instrumentation and preliminary results. Invest Radiol 20(1):90–93

Shellikeri S, Green JR, Kulkarni M et al (2016) Speech movement measures as markers of bulbar disease in amyotrophic lateral sclerosis. J Speech Lang Hear Res 59(5):887–899

Shimokata H, Kuzuya F (1995) Two-point discrimination test of the skin as an index of sensory aging. Gerontology 41(5):267–272

Snijders JT, Tellegen PJ, Laros JA (1989) Snijders-Oomen Non-Verbal Intelligence Test: SON-R 5.5-17. Manual and research report. Wolters-Noordhoff, Groningen

So LKH, Jing Z (2000) Putonghua Segmental PhonologyTest (PSPT). Nanjing Normal University Press, Nanjing

Soreni N, Crosbie J, Ickowicz A et al (2009) Stop signal and Conners' continuous performance tasks. Test-retest reliability of two inhibition measures in AD(H)D children. J Atten Disord 13(2):137–143

Soriano-Mas C, Pujol J, Ortiz H et al (2009) Age-related brain structural alterations in children with specific language impairment. Hum Brain Mapp 30(5):1626–1636

Squires J, Twombly E, Bricker D et al (2009) ASQ-3 user's guide, 3rd edn. Brookes, Baltimore

Stackhouse J, Wells BW (1997) Children's speech and literacy difficulties. A Psycholinguistic Model. Whurr, London

Steinhausen HC, Nøvik TS, Baldursson G et al (2006) Co-existing psychiatric problems in AD(H)D in the ADORE cohort. Eur Child Adolesc Psychiatry 15(suppl 1):i25–i29

Stepp CE (2012) Surface electromyography for speech and swallowing systems: measurement, analysis, and interpretation. J Speech Lang Hear Res 55(4):1232–1246. https://doi.org/10.1044/1092-4388(2011/11-0214)

Stevenson J, McCann D, Law CM et al (2011) The effect of early confirmation of hearing loss on the behaviour in middle childhood of children with bilateral hearing impairment. Dev Med Child Neurol 53(3):269–274

Stone M (2005) A guide to analyzing tongue motion from ultrasound images. Clin Linguist Phon 19(6-7):455–501

Stone M, Lundberg A (1996) Three-dimensional tongue surface shapes of English consonants and vowels. J Acoust Soc Am 99(6):3728–3737

Stone M, Morrish KA, Sonies BC et al (1987) Tongue curvature: a model of shape during vowel production. Folia Phoniatr 39(6):302–315

Stow C, Pert S (2006) BiSSS: bilingual speech sound screen: Pakistani heritage languages. Speechmark, Winslow

Strand EA, McCauley RJ (2008) Differential diagnosis of severe speech impairment in young children. AHSA Leader 13:10–13

von Suchodoletz W (2009) Wie wirksam ist Sprachtherapie? Kindh Entwickl 18(4):213–221

Suzuki A (2011) Wind instrument tonguing: comparison of tongue shape during performance and speaking. University of Aizu, Graduation Thesis, March 2011. Available via https://clrlab1.u-aizu.ac.jp/libraries/2011-thesis-01.pdf. Accessed 11 April 2016

Svec JG, Granqvist S (2010) Guidelines for selecting microphones for human voice production research. Am J Speech Lang Pathol 19(4):356–368. https://doi.org/10.1044/1058-0360(2010/09-0091)

Svensson P (1990) Ultraljudsobservationer av tungrörlighet hos normala och dysartriska individer under tal och sväljning/Ultrasound observations of tongue movements in normal and dysarthric speakers. Nord Tidskrift Logop Foniatr/Sand J Log Phon 15:5–11

Svensson P (1991) Tongue dynamics during speech and swallowing in laryngectomees - an ultrasound demonstration. Sand J Log Phon 16(1-2):25–28

Swaiman KF (2012) Neurologic examination of the older child. In: Swaiman KF et al (eds) Pediatric neurology. Principles and practice, 5th edn. Mosby Elsevier, Philadelphia

Szagun G, Steinbrink C (2004) Typikalität und Variabilität in der frühkindlichen Sprachentwicklung: Eine Studie mit einem Elternfragebogen. Sprache - Stimme - Gehör 28:137–145

Tannock R, Purvis L, Schachar RJ (1993) Narrative abilities in children with attention deficit hyperactivity disorder and normal peers. J Abnorm Child Psychol 21(1):103–117

Taylor E, Döpfner M, Sergeant J et al (2004) European clinical guidelines for hyperkinetic disorder - first upgrade. Eur Child Adolesc Psychiatry 13(suppl 1):i7–i30

Taylor S, McLean B, Falkmer T et al (2016) Does somatosensation change with age in children and adolescents? A systematic review. Child Care Health Dev 42(6):809–824

Tellegen P, Laros J (1993) The construction and validation of a nonverbal test of intelligence: the revision of the Snijders-Oomen test. Eur J Psychol Assess 9(2):147–157

Tellegen PJ, Laros JA (2005) Fair assessment for children from cultural minorities: a description of the SON-R non-verbal intelligence tests. In: Kopcanová D (ed) Quality education for children from socially disadvantaged settings. Commission of UNESCO, Bratislava, pp 50–73

Tellegen PJ, Winkel M, Wijnberg-Williams BJ et al (1998) Snijders-Oomen Non-Verbal Intelligence Test. SON-R 2.5-7. Manual and research report. Swets Test Publishers, Lisse

Tellegen PJ, Winkel M, Wijnberg-Williams BJ et al (2009) Snijders-Oomen Non-Verbal Intelligence Test. SON-R 2.5-7. Manual and research report. Hogrefe, Göttingen

Terband H, Maassen B, van Lieshout P et al (2011) Stability and composition of functional synergies for speech movements in children with developmental speech disorders. J Commun Disord 44(1):59–74. https://doi.org/10.1016/j.jcomdis.2010.07.003

The ASEBA Approach (2017) Achenbach system of empirically based assessment ASEBA. Available via https://aseba.org/preschool/. Accessed April 23, 2019

Thoonen G (1998) Developmental apraxia of speech in children. Quantitative assessment of speech characteristics. Dissertation, University of Nijmegen, The Netherlands

Thoonen G, Maassen B, Gabreëls F et al (1994) Feature analysis of singleton consonant errors in developmental verbal dyspraxia (DVD). J Speech Hear Res 37(6):1424–1440

Tomasello M (2000) Acquiring syntax is not what you think. In: Bishop DVM, Leonard LB (eds) Speech and language impairments in children: causes, characteristics, intervention and outcome. Psychology Press, Hove, pp 1–16

Topbaş S (2004/2005) Türkçe Sesletim-Sesbilgisi Testi (SST). TC Milli Eğitim Yayınevi, Ankara, p 4. Akşam Sanat Okulu Matbaası. Test Bataryası

Trochim WMK (2006) The research methods knowledge base, 2nd edn. Available via http://www.socialresearchmethods.net/kb/. Accessed 23 July 2016

Trochim WMK, Donnelly JP (2007) The research methods knowledge base, 3rd edn. Custom Solutions/Cengage Inc., Houston

Tsanas A, Zañartu M, Little MA et al (2014) Robust fundamental frequency estimation in sustained vowels: detailed algorithmic comparisons and information fusion with adaptive Kalman filtering. J Acoust Soc Am 135(5):2885–2901. https://doi.org/10.1121/1.4870484

Tsugawa L (2002) Spanish Preschool Articulation Test: SPAT. Lexicon Press, Billings

Unser M, Stone M (1992) Automated detection of the tongue surface in sequences of ultrasound images. J Acoust Soc Am 91(5):3001–3007

Urban PP (2013) Speech motor deficits in cerebellar infarctions. Brain Lang 127(3):323–326. https://doi.org/10.1016/j.bandl.2013.10.001

Vannorsdall TD, Maroof DA, Gordon B et al (2012) Ideational fluency as a domain of human cognition. Neuropsychology 6(3):400–405

Verhoeven JS, Rommel N, Prodi E et al (2012) Is there a common neuroanatomical substrate of language deficit between autism spectrum disorder and specific language impairment? Cereb Cortex 22(10):2263–2271. https://doi.org/10.1093/cercor/bhr292

Vieregge WH, Maassen B (1999) ExtIPA transcriptions of consonants and vowels spoken by dyspractic children: agreement and validity. In: Maassen B, Groenen P (eds) Pathologies of speech and language: advances in clinical phonetics and linguistics. Whurr Publishers, London, pp 275–284

Vogel AP, Fletcher J, Maruff P (2010) Acoustic analysis of the effects of sustained wakefulness on speech. J Acoust Soc Am 128(6):3747–3756. https://doi.org/10.1121/1.3506349

Vogel AP, Maruff P (2008) Comparison of voice acquisition methodologies in speech research. Behav Res Methods 40(4):982–987

Vogel AP, Maruff P (2014) Monitoring change requires a rethink of assessment practices in voice and speech. Logoped Phoniatr Vocol 39(2):56–61. https://doi.org/10.3109/14015439.2013.775332

Vogel AP, Morgan AT (2009) Factors affecting the quality of sound recording for speech and voice analysis. Int J Speech Lang Pathol 11(6):431–437

Vogel AP, Fletcher J, Snyder PJ et al (2011) Reliability, stability, and sensitivity to change and impairment in acoustic measures of timing and frequency. J Voice 25(2):137–149. https://doi.org/10.1016/j.jvoice.2009.09.003

Vogel AP, Shirbin C, Churchyard AJ et al (2012) Speech acoustic markers of early stage and prodromal Huntington's disease: a marker of disease onset? Neuropsychology 50(14):3273–3278. https://doi.org/10.1016/j.neuropsychologia.2012.09.011

Vogel AP, Rosen KM, Morgan AT et al (2014) Comparability of modern recording devices for speech analysis: smartphone, landline, laptop, and hard disc recorder. Folia Phoniatr Logop 66(6):244–250

Vogel AP, Wardrop MI, Folker JE et al (2017) Voice in Friedreich ataxia. J Voice 31(2):243.e9–243.e19. https://doi.org/10.1016/j.jvoice.2016.04.015. Epub 2016 Aug 5

Watkin KL, Rubin JM (1989) Pseudo-three-dimensional reconstruction of ultrasonic images of the tongue. J Acoust Soc Am 85(1):496–499

Wechsler D (2003) The Wechsler Intelligence Scale for children, 4th edn. The Psychological Corporation, San Antonio, TX

Wechsler D (2011) Wechsler Intelligence Scale for Children. 4th edn. (WISC-IV, ehemalig HAWIK-IV). Pearson Assessment, Frankfurt/Main (German Version: Petermann F, Petermann U (eds))

Wechsler D (2012) Wechsler Preschool and Primary Scale of Intelligence–IV (WPPSI-IV). The Psychological Corporation, San Antonio, TX (German version; Petermann F, Daseking M, 2018)

Wechsler D (2014) Wechsler Intelligence Scale for Children, 5th edn (WISC-V). Pearson, Bloomington, MN (German version: Petermann F, 2017)

Wein B (1990) Ein neues Verfahren zur 3D-Rekonstruktion der Zungenoberfläche aus Ultraschallbildern. Ultraschall Med 11(6):306–310

Wein B, Alzen G, Tolxdorff T et al (1988) Computersonographische Darstellung der Zungenmotilität mittels Pseudo-3D-Rekonstruktion. Ultraschall Med 9(2):95–97

Wein B, Böckler R, Huber W et al (1990a) Computersonographische Darstellung von Zungenformen bei der Bildung der langen Vokale des Deutschen. Ultraschall Med 11(2):100–103

Wein B, Drobnitzky M, Klajman S (1990b) Magnetresonanztomographie und Sonographie bei der Lautbildung. Fortschr Röntgenstr 153(10):408–412

Wein B, Böckler R, Meixner R et al (1991) Ultraschalluntersuchungen der Zunge bei der Artikulation. Sprachheilarbeit 36:24–27

Wein B, Angerstein W, Klajman S (1993) Suchbewegungen der Zunge bei einer Sprechapraxie: Darstellung mittels Ultraschall und Pseudo-3D-Abbildung. Nervenarzt 64:143–145

Weinberger S (2015) Speech accent archive. George Mason University. Available via http://accent.gmu.edu. Accessed 28 May 2016

Weinstein S (1968) Neuropsychological studies of the phantom. In: Benton AL (ed) Contributions to clinical neuropsychology. Aldine Publishing, Chicago, pp 73–106

Weissenborn J (2000) Erwerb von Morphologie und Syntax. In: Grimm H (ed) Sprachentwicklung.

Enzyklopädie der Psychologie. Themenbereich C, Serie III, Bd. 3. Hogrefe, Göttingen, pp 141–169

Willcutt EG (2012) The prevalence of DSM-IV attention-deficit/hyperactivity disorder: a meta-analytic review. Neurotherapeutics 9(3):490–499

Willcutt EG, Pennington BF, Chhabildas NA et al (1999) Psychiatric comorbidity associated with DSM-IV ADHD in nonreferred sample of twins. J Am Acad Child Adolesc Psychiatry 38(11):1355–1362

Willcutt EG, Doyle AE, Nigg JT et al (2005) Validity of the executive function theory of attention-deficit/ hyperactivity disorders: a meta-analytic review. Biol Psychiatry 57(11):1336–1346

World Health Organization (1993) The ICD-10 classification of mental and behavioural disorders: diagnostic criteria for research. World Health Organization, Geneva

World Health Organization (2011) International statistical classification of diseases and related health problems, 10th revision, edition 2010. Available via http://www. who.int/classifications/icd/en/. Accessed 1 June 2014

World Health Organization (WHO) (2007) International classification of disability and functioning. Children and youth version (ICF-CY). Available via http://apps.who.int/iris/bitstr eam/10665/43737/1/9789241547321_eng.pdf. Accessed 28 May 2016

Yew SGK, O'Kearney R (2013) Emotional and behavioural outcomes later in childhood and adolescence for children with specific language impairments: meta-analyses of controlled prospective studies. J Child Psychol Psychiatry 54(5):516–524

Zafeiriou DI (2004) Primitive reflexes and postural reactions in the neurodevelopmental examination. Pediatr Neurol 31(1):1–8

Zielke A, Angerstein W, Schwarze S et al (2010) Échographie de la langue et motricité du visage et du cou chez les instrumentistes à vent. Médecine des arts 71:2–10

Zielke A, Muth T, Massing T et al (2012) Zungenbewegungen und Gesichts-Hals-Motorik beim Spielen von Blasinstrumenten. Musikphysiol Musikermed 19(3): 189–195

Zimmer R (2012) Handbuch der Sinneswahrnehmung. Herder, Freiburg im Breisgau

Zollinger B (2004) Die Entdeckung der Sprache, 6th edn. Haupt Verlag, Bern

Zolotas K, Bird S (2010) An ultrasound investigation of didgeridoo articulations. Can Acoust 38(3):198–199

Mona Hegazi, Katrin Neumann, and Jochen Rosenfeld

12.1 Early Identification of Developmental Disorders of Speech and Language

Jochen Rosenfeld

12.1.1 Why Is Early Identification of Developmental Disorders of Speech and Language Desirable?

The early identification of developmental disorders of speech and language (DDSL; synonym: language impairment, LI) is a measure of secondary prevention, i.e. it aims at detecting and addressing an existing DDSL before the full appearance of symptoms.

So far, no universal screening procedure has been implemented nationwide on a legal basis

M. Hegazi
ENT Department, Ain Shams University,
Cairo, Egypt

K. Neumann
Department of Phoniatrics and Pediatric Audiology,
ENT Clinic, St. Elisabeth Hospital, University of
Bochum, Bochum, Germany
e-mail: Katrin.neumann@rub.de

J. Rosenfeld
Abteilung Gehör-, Sprach- u. Stimmheilkunde,
Kantonsspital St.Gallen, St. Gallen, Switzerland
e-mail: jochen.rosenfeld@kssg.ch

in any European country, and three evidence-based criteria in particular may be the cause of this: (1) lack of evidence that early intervention leads to long-term benefit, (2) nonexistence of valid, reliable tests for confirmatory diagnostics of language impairment and (3) lack of valid language screening instruments for identification of children with a specific developmental disorder of speech and language (SDDSL) (e.g. Institute for Quality and Efficiency in Health Care IQWiG 2009).

Against these difficulties, two causes are mainly discussed that favour early identification of DDSL: child-centred social and economic ones. As DDSL may lead to the negative long-term effects described above, early identification and intervention offer the possibility of enhancing developmental opportunities of a child, even if complete healing might be difficult. Considering the economic aspect, there is the question if early identification and intervention save costs in comparison with the consequential costs of language impairment that has not been treated.

Social Reasons for Favouring Early Identification of Developmental Disorders of Speech and Language DDSL usually have negative long-term sequelae for the cognitive, social and emotional development of a child until adulthood, such as an impaired perception or production of complex linguistic structures; difficulties in acquisition of spelling and reading; academic achievements that lie below what would be expected from the intellectual and social background, with the consequent decreased chances of education and career; and behavioural disorders with the risk of psychic disorders, decreased social competence and reduced independence (Felsenfeld et al. 1992, 1994; Snowling et al. 2001). Children have a much better prognosis for their future if the symptoms of DDSL have disappeared before entry into school (Law et al. 2004). This underscores why early identification and a timely start of intervention programmes are important for these children.

Economic Reasons for Favouring Early Identification of Developmental Disorders of Speech and Language In order to estimate the resource use and economic benefit of early identification and intervention in comparison with developmental disorders that have not been treated appropriately, cost-effectiveness analyses have been performed for both alternatives. Heckman (2008; see also Heckman et al. 2006) analysed the economic benefit of various early intervention programmes for disadvantaged children in general in comparison with consequential

costs without intervention (e.g. special schooling, social benefit payments, arrangement of placement, etc.) on the basis of long-term observational studies in which children with and without early intervention programmes were observed until adulthood. It has been shown that early intervention in particular is efficient and that the cost-effectiveness ratio is better than for intervention at any later time (Fig. 12.1).

12.1.2 Requirements

Instruments for assessing language skills may be either language screening, which determines a categorial aspect (ill vs. healthy or normal developmental language status vs. abnormal developmental language status), or language tests, which assess a dimensional aspect (degree of language proficiency). It is a prerequisite for early identification of DDSL that there are instruments available that permit a reliable conclusion concerning a child's language level (evidence-based diagnostics). The quality of a screening or a diagnostic instrument has to be shown by its fulfilment of the usual test-constructive quality criteria.

Fig. 12.1 Rates of return to human capital investment. With kind permission from Prof. James J. Heckman (Heckman 2008)

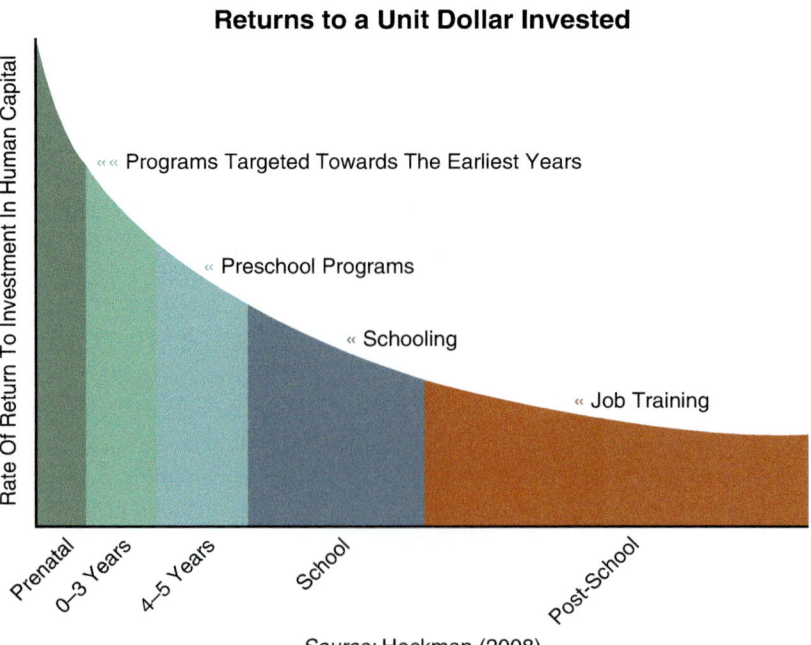

Returns to a Unit Dollar Invested

Rate Of Return To Investment In Human Capital

«« Programs Targeted Towards The Earliest Years

« Preschool Programs

« Schooling

« Job Training

Prenatal 0–3 Years 4–5 Years School Post-School

Source: Heckman (2008)

These primary quality criteria of objectivity (standardised procedure across examiners, absence of examiner bias), reliability (grade of accuracy of a measurement with respect to repeated measurements) and validity (grade of accuracy of the test result with respect to the parameter that it is supposed to measure) are essential preconditions for determining reliably a child's level of language development. Most important during the construction or evaluation of a screening or diagnostic test is the calculation of its concurrent validity by determining its concordance with another method (reference test, gold standard, external criterion). Normative data that are regularly updated are obligatory requirements for tests assessing a child's language skills for comparison with the range of variation among its peers. As secondary quality criteria, economic aspects and feasibility are especially important. A summary of psychometric criteria and design features for the assessment of instruments for early identification of linguistic skills in the German language is described in Rosenfeld and Kiese-Himmel (2011) and in Kiese-Himmel and Rosenfeld (2012). Section 11.3 provides tables of English and German language screening methods and tests, together with the quality criteria they fulfil, as well as an instruction on how to interpret the results of language testing and screening.

Because the application of each screening/test instrument for early language evaluation also results in a categorical decision (at risk of being language impaired—typically developing—borderline or unclear, control needed), cut-off criteria for the test scores need to be determined that enable an examiner to make this decision. Furthermore, information about the predictive validity, which demonstrates the extent to which a test score predicts scores from some criterion measurement that is collected at a later time, is desirable.

The most important criteria of diagnostic accuracy are sensitivity, specificity and positive or negative predictive values (Klee 2008). These criteria are not fixed parameters but depend on the population investigated and case definitions both for the analysed and reference tests. By convention and for practical reasons, sensitivity and specificity values of about 80% for each have been proposed as acceptable for screening for DDSL (Plante and Vance 1994). Higher sensitivity values are desirable but are hardly obtainable owing to the high variability of language development, the lack of objective tests and construction difficulties of language screening. For the evaluation of diagnostic accuracy of language tests, a generally accepted definition of SDDSL that determines the cut-off discrepancy between a child's achieved language status and the average language status of typically developed peers is lacking to date. Therefore, an SDDSL definition proposed for the ICD-11, the upcoming International Classification of Diseases by the World Health Organization, contains the following sentence:

> The individual's ability to understand, produce or use language is markedly below what would be expected given the individual's age and level of intellectual functioning (by convention and according to prevalence rates about 1.5 to 2 standard deviations below the age-related normative values in standardised and normed speech-language tests).
>
> Neumann (2017)

12.1.3 Risks

In addition to the expected benefit of early identification of language impairment, its potential risks have also to be considered. Possible downsides include the concern of parents, the wasted resources incurred by erroneous classification, stigmatisation by the social environment and a disordered familial interaction.

Currently the instruments used for early identification of language impairment often show relatively high rates of false-positive and false-negative results. These cause children to be classified as potentially language impaired although they are not (false positive). Through this, on the one hand, parents may be made to feel insecure, and on the other, financial and time resources could be wasted on an unnecessary intervention. Even more crucial, parents of children falsely classified as negative are misleadingly appeased and would have probably sought intervention for their child much earlier without screening. Hence, early screening for language risks appears reasonable provided that it fulfils high-quality standards and that appropriate diagnostic and intervention methods are available so that the benefit outweighs potential risks.

12.1.4 Methods

Generally, two basic approaches can be distinguished for the early identification of language abnormalities or DDSL: (1) direct evaluation of a child's linguistic skills during examination and (2) indirect evaluation of language development by means of parent questionnaires.

For direct evaluation of a child, methods such as the analysis of spontaneous speech, informal (non-standardised) techniques and standardised, normed language tests are used (see Sect. 11.3). It is often discussed that non-structured, informal and non-standardised methods approximate more a non-artificial communicative situation and thus describe a child's linguistic skills best. On the other hand, this approach is limited by the uniqueness of the investigation, dependence on the specific test situation and by the subjectivity of the examiner. Quality criteria such as objectiveness and reliability are usually poor, and standardised procedures are difficult to apply. On the contrary, standardised language tests are quite often time-consuming and costly in resource use and normally require specific linguistically or psychologically trained personnel.

Parent questionnaires, in particular those that focus on the assessment of the vocabulary of a child, have been proven as both reliable and economic diagnostic instruments for the early identification of impaired language development. Parents, as 'experts' who know their child in his or her daily environment, in various situations and over a long period, estimate the linguistic level of their child by standardised questionnaires that do not require special knowledge. Short instruments with a careful choice of items in particular reduce the dread of filling in lengthy questionnaires and provide comparable reliability to longer ones. Examples for suitable questionnaires are the SBE-2-KT (German: von Suchodoletz et al.

2009), the SBE-3-KT (German: von Suchodoletz and Sachse 2009), the PLS-5 (Zimmerman et al. 2011a) and the PLS-5 ST (Zimmerman et al. 2011b). The SBE-2-KT has been translated into 33 languages and is freely accessible on the Internet. For more examples see Sect. 11.3.

12.1.5 Implications

Both the diagnostic accuracy and the prognostic power (prognostic validity) are decisive for early identification methods of developmental language abnormalities or disorders. Only if these are given are early identification procedures useful.

Until the end of the first year of life, early identification of developmental language disorders is quite unreliable and causes more uncertainty for parents that would trigger intervention. Hence, this approach cannot be recommended. For the end of second year of life, there are valid and reliable instruments available, especially parent questionnaires that have been proven to be of value in practice. Even if their prognostic validity is limited in identifying children who will be language impaired at a later age, they detect quite reliably children at risk of developing later developmental disorders of speech and language. As a consequence, these children can be offered an early intervention. For language screening from the end of the third year of life on, there are a few valid instruments available that offer the option of a timely intervention, as shown in Sect. 11.3.

12.2 Stimulation of Child Language Development

Mona Hegazi and Katrin Neumann

12.2.1 Introduction

Children acquire language inherently by a strong genetically determined motivation, given that their biological conditions and social environment are not extremely adverse (child illness or neglect, absence of social bonds). The extent and quality to which they develop language, however, depend both on environmental input—from parent-child interaction, early literacy, a language-stimulating familial and social surrounding—and genome-environment interplay. The parental input style is correlated with the child language development in several respects, which seem to reflect the influence of the input style on a child's language proficiency. However, as, for example, shown in a recent large twin study, there are also child-to-parent effects that make an interpretation based on parent-to-child effects alone inadequate. Moreover, both parental language input factors and child language have been shown to be moderately heritable. The fact that parent and child share genes produces in itself a correlation between parent-language input style and child-language acquisition. Thus, social influences on a child's language acquisition may not be overestimated, considering the effects of shared gene variants on parent and child, the partially inherited parental input style and child-to-parent effects. Nevertheless, parental language stimulation is important, and interventions can be effective. This section deals with evidence-based, culturally appropriate interventions that support child language development, parenting skills and language-related child-parent (caregiver) interaction.

12.2.2 Biological and Environmental Stimulation of Language Development

Language acquisition of children is driven by genome-environment interplay. Genetic factors are the motor of language development. Children have a strong inherent motivation to develop oral language, most probably caused by their genetic endowment and an evolutionary 'necessity' for functioning in a human social context (Pinker 2002; Berwick et al. 2013). Apart from a frequently uttered public opinion, they need not be taught explicitly in language but develop it inherently by themselves, given that some physiological preconditions are fulfilled, such as the absence of severely impaired hearing or cognitive abilities, and that they grow up in a social environment that is neither neglecting nor language-suppressing (e.g. lacking social bonds). However, the extent and level to which children develop language depend, among other causes, on the input they receive, in particular at early ages when brain development is very dynamic. During early child development, the home environment, in particular the parent-child interactions, establishes a major component of the environmental factors. Parents play an effective role with regard to the rate and quality of a child's language acquisition. A language-stimulating environment entails talking empathetically to a child, sufficiently frequently and with an appropriate quality, responding to the child's utterances, repeating and expanding them and making talk time as enjoyable as possible. Later on, around the age of 3 years in community settings, peers increasingly overtake parts of the language-directing influences, together with caregivers and other adults or adolescents. Language proficiency, as well as school readiness and educational success, increases with the amount of early literacy a child experiences, i.e. the extent to which dealing with written and spoken language, such as the presence and use of scripts, books or narratives, plays a role in the family or social environment of a child (e.g. Navsaria and Sanders 2015).

Much research has been performed on the characteristics of speech that is directed to young children or produced in interaction with them during early stages of language acquisition (e.g. Hoff 2006; Rowe 2012). To what extent this kind of child-directed speech predicts a child's language development is of great interest. In particular, the quantity of input is related to the rate of language development but with wide variations with respect to the vocabulary of children. Additionally, qualitative factors have been shown to predict child language proficiency, usually with weak-to-moderate effect sizes (Dale et al. 2015). Qualitative factors concern all subdomains of language, i.e. phonology, lexicon, syntax, semantics and pragmatics, and comprise, among others, vocabulary diversity, age-appropriate mean length of utterance, repetition, exaggerated prosody, promotion of joint attention, proportion of conversation-eliciting speech as opposed to behaviour regulation, semantic contingency, decontextualized language use such as narratives and 'grammatical tutorials' such as sentence recasts and expansions (Dale et al. 2015; Hoff 2006; Rowe 2012).

The influence of specific aspects of child-directed speech differs with age and the developmental status of a child. During early child development, promotion of joint attention and use of exaggerated intonation play an important role, followed by vocabulary diversity and use of sentence recasts at later ages. The quantity of parental input has been shown to be most important during the second year of life, while diversity of parental vocabulary is more important in the third year, and the use of decontextualized language such as narratives and explanations is most important in the fourth year (Dale et al. 2015; Rowe 2012).

The majority of child-directed speech domains that facilitate a child's language development are intercorrelated. Moreover, they correlate with the parents' socio-economic status—corresponding to their educational level—that in itself encompasses a variety of parental behaviour. In addition, a variety of more proximate environmental factors contribute significantly to a child's language acquisition and are reflected in specific features of child-directed speech (e.g. Rowe 2012). They include, among others, prenatal care and nutrition, exposure to toxins and disease, caregiver education and mental health, type and quality of childcare and multilingual versus monolingual context (Dale et al. 2015).

A recent large twin study including more than 8000 twin pairs showed that both language stimulation by the parents and subdomains of the child language itself were moderately heritable (Dale et al. 2015). Moreover, a child-to-parent effect also influences the way parents talk to their child. Hence, a substantial portion of the parental language input to child language represents the effect of shared genes on both parent and child.

Sometimes parents need to be made aware that it is important for their child to be exposed to a stimulating language environment in order to enhance his or her language skills and motivation to speak. This becomes particularly important in the case of developmental language delays (late talkers). For example, short and highly struc-tured parent-based language intervention group programmes have been reported in a randomised controlled trial to be effective in overcoming specific expressive language delays (Buschmann et al. 2009).

In any population, a considerable number of children are at risk of experiencing developmental language abnormalities. Among these abnormalities, developmental disorders of speech and language (DDSL; synonym: language impairment, LI) have to be discerned from sociogenically caused language abnormalities, due to a socially weak environment with poor language stimulation or when multilingual children face difficulties in acquiring the common language. All these groups of children would benefit from more and high-quality language input. However, for developmental speech-language disorders, a sole improvement of input is not sufficient; speech and language treatment together with an optimised language input is required (de Langen-Müller et al. 2012).

12.2.3 Risk Factors for Delayed Language Development

In addition to comorbid diseases that are frequently associated with developmental speech-language disorders, such as hearing loss or neurological diseases, certain risk factors for language impairment are known. They include:

- Family history of language impairment
- Male sex
- Perinatal risk factors, such as prematurity (Nelson et al. 2006)

Other risk factors are reported with less consistency, such as childhood illnesses (Brookhouser et al. 1979; Singer et al. 2001), being born late in the family birth order (Tomblin et al. 1991), family size (Choudhury and Benasich 2006), older parents (Choudhury and Benasich 2006) or a younger mother (Tomblin et al. 1997) at birth, parental psychiatric disorders (Weindrich et al. 2000), low socio-economic status of the family or being of a minority race (Singer et al. 2001).

Recurrent otitis media and related hearing loss has been suspected as a risk factor for developmental speech-language disorders (e.g. Roberts et al. 2002). However, the results of meta-analyses do not reveal a clear indication for such a risk (Casby 2001; Roberts et al. 2004). Nevertheless, there are indications for a negative impact of even mild conductive hearing loss on phonological, lexical, grammatical and pragmatic development, at least at younger ages (Schönweiler 2002). Typically, however, children seem to make up for these language affections at school age, and the home environment of a child seems to be a stronger predictor of language skills than recurrent otitis media (Roberts et al. 2002). Thus, the inclusion of more complex parameters, such as assessment of speech-in-noise and binaural hearing, and appropriate, 'softer' outcomes is recommended to be considered in further studies.

12.2.4 Other Potentially Adverse Factors That May Influence Child Language Development

Common beliefs of parents and the public concern factors of a contemporary lifestyle or behaviour as hindering the language development of children, such as background noise in homes, nurseries or other social contexts, long TV exposure, busy parents, reflecting workload and habits, little talking among family members, lack of shared familial meals or lack of parental interaction with their children, but only some of these beliefs are supported by high-quality studies. Other studies point to potential risk factors, but do not provide evidence for a causal role in language acquisition. For example, several electrophysiological experiments have demonstrated that background noise distracts children and may hamper their speech processing (e.g. White-Schwoch et al. 2015). However, the impact of such noise on language acquisition is supported only by some studies (e.g. Wright et al. 1997) not by others (e.g. Alston and James-Roberts 2005).

A considerable proportion of children have TV or video exposures for more than 2 h per day (Chandra et al. 2016; Zimmerman and Christakis 2005). It has been shown that exten-

sive TV watching in childhood and adolescence is associated with adverse health indicators such as obesity, poor fitness, sleep disturbances, musculoskeletal disorders, smoking and raised cholesterol (Chandra et al. 2016; Zimmerman and Christakis 2005). Television viewing before the age of 3 years has also some moderate but significant negative effects on the cognitive development of children (Hancox et al. 2004), makes both children and parents less attentive and shortens toy play time of young children (Schmidt et al. 2008). Nevertheless, there is no strong evidence that extensive TV watching has a negative impact on language development. A few studies have found such a negative impact (Chonchaiya and Pruksananonda 2008, Tomopoulos et al. 2010; Zimmerman et al. 2007), but others have not (e.g. Ruangdaraganon et al. 2009). The results of Zimmerman et al. (2007) were not confirmed by a reanalysis (Ferguson and Donnellan 2014), and scientific debates on this topic continue. Positive or negative effects of television viewing also differ among distinct sociocultural populations and are content and screen time dependent. Indirect effects have to be expected, in that long screen times withhold children from more creative or energy expending activities (Hancox et al. 2004).

12.2.5 Language-Stimulating Family Interventions

Family intervention strategies usually follow one of two approaches that can be used by parents to stimulate their children's language skills—a child-centred approach and a hybrid approach.

There is no conclusive evidence to guide selection of the most effective approach for children with varying types of delays and disabilities (McCauley and Fey 2006).

12.2.5.1 Child-Centred Approaches

Child-centred strategies are indirect approaches where the parent follows the child's lead and adds language to each activity performed by the child. The adult chooses the materials but does not direct the activity. Rather he or she follows the child's lead, providing follow-up on a child's utterance with his or her own language that is appropriate to the context and the child's level of understanding. No specifications are prescribed, as the focus is on general communication (Fey 1986; Wolery and Sainato 1996).

The following are some examples of parent-specific language strategies in this approach:

- Naturalistic
  Example: Wait for the child to show interest, get down to the child's linguistic level and initiate communication.
- Interaction-promoting strategies
  Example: Encourage the child to take turns in a conversation. Ask questions and wait for a response.
- Language-modelling strategies
  Example: Label objects and actions, expand utterances and extend topics.

12.2.5.2 Hybrid Approaches

The hybrid approach encompasses a combination of a child-centred approach and structured training. This procedure requires a child to learn specific 'lessons', i.e. small and informal practices, or complete specific tasks as directed by the adult. In structured training, artificial reinforcers are basically used for language intervention.

Two examples of hybrid approaches:

- Responsive Interaction Technique
  In order to elicit verbal utterances, this technique prompts the child to make a response. The parent is taught to use target words (while avoiding directly prompting the child), to keep using the word within the context of situation and to encourage, but not insist on, the child to produce an utterance. For example, in a play situation, involving bathing a doll, the parent emphasises words such as baby and bath in a focused way at least five times (Yoder and Warren 2001).
- Prelinguistic Milieu Teaching
  When a child shows an interest in an object or an activity, the parent will ask the child about its name 'What is this?' or ask 'What do you want?' Then the parent will continue asking the child questions about it (Alpert and Kaiser 1992).

12.2.6 Efficacy of Home Intervention by Families

As shown in a meta-analysis by Roberts and Kaiser (2011), parents can be taught and may learn successfully how to promote their child's communication in the case of a developmental speech-language disorder with or without an intellectual disability. The authors concluded that parents play a key role in the intervention process and allow this process to be an ongoing one. Parents are powerful role models and reinforcers of desirable behaviour. Children made good progress when their parents learned to use specific techniques designed to improve the childrens' communication skills. The trained parents were sometimes more effective than speech-language pathologists in supporting the child. The earlier parents get involved in intervention programmes for their children, the better the outcome (Rosetti 2001).

The Hanen Program (*It Takes Two to Talk*) is a well-established family-centred non-structured intervention programme considering the child as part of a dynamic social system and the family as the most important element in a child's life (Girolametto and Weitzman 2006; Weitzman et al. 2017). This programme is led by a certified Hanen speech-language pathologist. It is supported by user-friendly resources, such as a parent guidebook (Pepper and Weitzman 2004), available in English, French, Spanish, Dutch and Danish and on DVD.

12.2.7 Tips for Parents or Caregivers when Talking to a Child

Sometimes parents are not aware that communication skills are the basis for future personal-social and academic success. Parents may regard language development as a natural process that occurs without the need for their active role. There is a partial truth in this statement because children are biologically programmed to acquire language, without direct teaching, provided basic requirements are met, such as being surrounded by language from birth and being exposed to "normal" social

Table 12.1 Examples of advice that can be given to parents (American Speech-Language-Hearing Association 1997, Weitzman and Greenberg 2010, Peterson 2004, Manolson 1995, Rosetti 2001, Wittmer and Petersen 2010)

- Talk a lot to your baby or young child whenever you are together. Try to build a language-rich environment for the child. Wherever you are, make the world come alive; point to birds in the garden, and chat about which fruit to buy and which picture to colour.
- Talk during all activities such as eating, washing, dressing and at bath time about what is going on. Children learn by repetition. Comment on what is in the context and what the child sees or does in the different situations.
- Listen and respond to babbles or any sound or words produced by the child or repeat them.
- Don't be embarrassed to talk 'motherese' (high-pitched 'baby-talk' with exaggerated prosody) to your baby. It is the optimal language input for babies and strengthens attachment.
- Try to make the talk time as enjoyable as possible by, e.g. playing games. Smile, laugh, encourage and praise the verbal productions of the child.
- Find time to spend with your children and have a shared focus. The one-to-one time will benefit the child.
- Minimise the time a child is put in front of the TV, because TV is passive entertainment and does not encourage any interaction. Choose TV productions with high quality with respect to child education.
- Minimise solitary activities that don't foster dialogue among the family members.
- You do not need any special toys or equipment to develop your child's communication skills. You only need time to talk and respond to the child's attempts to communicate while sharing and enjoying everyday's experiences together.
- Know that pretend (or symbolic) play, music, rhythm and songs are important for language development.
- Your child's age guides the level of the complexity of the language you use with the child. Do not use too complex sentences. If the child doesn't understand, then you may use key words, use more stress, or use gesture as you say the words.
- Avoid continually asking your child to name various items. Talk more than you ask questions. When you ask, give the child enough time to respond.
- Allow your child time to ask questions and be patient while doing so. By responding to them, your child experiences that you are attentive.
- Get and maintain your child's attention, for example, by varying pitch and intonation of your voice and putting emphasis on the key words in a sentence. Repeat when needed.

Table 12.1 (continued)

- Try to notice what interests your child and then comment on it (child-directed speech).
- Use parallel talk, a technique where the adult talks about what a child is doing.
- Take a step back during play and let your child take the lead.
- Always continue to build vocabulary. Introduce, for example, spatial relationships and opposites. Add new words to your child's utterances in order to promote longer ones (extended feedback).
- Use the correct pronunciation of the words and the correct sentence structure (corrective feedback).
- Read to your child. Do it in a narrative and dialoging way. Sometimes 'reading' is simply describing the pictures in a book without following the written words. As the child grows, sequential events are introduced. Story telling is a good way of stimulating the syntactic rules of the child's speech as well as pragmatics.

communication and interaction. However, language skills are generally improved by increased and high-quality language input, and, in particular in at-risk populations as described above, intensive exposure to a stimulating environment is beneficial for children. The examples given in Table 12.1 of advice that can be given to parents to promote their children's language skills are taken from the scientific literature (American Speech-Language-Hearing Association 1997; Weitzman and Greenberg 2010; Peterson 2004; Manolson 1995; Rosetti 2001; Wittmer and Petersen 2010). All or most of these recommendations usually come naturally to the parent of a healthy child. A piece of general advice thus is to listen to one's heart rather than listen to recommendations which are given in mass media and which vary as do fashions.

12.3 Genetic Counselling

See Part I, Chap. 3, Sect. 3.2.

12.4 Diagnostics of Hearing Impairments

See Part IV, Chap. 16, Sects. 16.1–16.25.

References

Alpert C, Kaiser A (1992) Training parents as milieu language teachers. J Early Interv 16(1):31–52

Alston E, James-Roberts IS (2005) Home environments of 10-month-old infants selected by the WILSTAAR screen for pre-language difficulties. Int J Lang Commun Disord 40(2):123–136

American Speech-Language-Hearing Association (1997) Activities to encourage speech and language development. http://www.asha.org/public/speech/development/parent-stim-activities.htm. Accessed 8 Jan 2017

Berwick RC, Friederici AD, Chomsky N et al (2013) Evolution, brain, and the nature of language. Trends Cogn Sci 17(2):89–98

Brookhouser PE, Hixson PK, Matkin ND (1979) Early childhood language delay: the otolaryngologist's perspective. Laryngoscope 89(12):1898-1913

Buschmann A, Jooss B, Rupp A et al (2009) Parent based language intervention for 2-year-old children with specific expressive language delay: a randomised controlled trial. Arch Dis Child 94(2):110–116

Casby MW (2001) Otitis media and language development: a meta-analysis. Am J Speech Lang Pathol 10(3 Pt 1):65–80

Chandra M, Jalaludin B, Woolfenden S et al (2016) Screen time of infants in Sydney, Australia: a birth cohort study. BMJ Open 6(10):e012342. https://doi.org/10.1136/bmjopen-2016-012342

Chonchaiya W, Pruksananonda C (2008) Television viewing associates with delayed language development. Acta Paediatr 97(7):977–982

Choudhury N, Benasich AA (2006) A family aggregation study: the influence of family history and other risk factors on language development. J Speech Lang Hear Res 46(2):261–272

Dale PS, Tosto MG, Hayiou-Thomas ME et al (2015) Why does parental language input style predict child language development? A twin study of gene-environment correlation. J Commun Disord 57:106–117

de Langen-Müller U, Kiese-Himmel C, Neumann K et al (2012) Diagnostik von (umschriebenen) Sprachentwicklungsstörungen. [Diagnostics of (specific) developmental disorders of speech and language.] [German]. Peter Lang, Frankfurt am Main

Felsenfeld S, Broen PA, McGue M (1992) A 28-year follow-up of adults with a history of moderate phonological disorder: linguistic and personality results. J Speech Hear Res 35(5):1114–1125

Felsenfeld S, Broen PA, McGue M (1994) A 28-year follow-up of adults with a history of moderate phonological disorder: educational and occupational results. J Speech Hear Res 37(6):1341–1353

Ferguson CJ, Donnellan MB (2014) Is the association between children's baby video viewing and poor language development robust? A reanalysis of Zimmerman, Christakis, and Meltzoff (2007). Dev Psychol 50(1):129–137

Fey M (1986) Language intervention with young children. College-Hill, San Diego, CA

Girolametto L, Weitzman E (2006) It takes two to talk - the Hanen Program® for parents: early language intervention through caregiver training. In: McCauley R, Fey M (eds) Treatment of language disorders in children. Brookes Publishing, New York, pp 77–103

Hancox RJ, Milne BJ, Poulton R (2004) Association between child and adolescent television viewing and adult health: a longitudinal birth cohort study. Lancet 364(9430):257–262

Heckman JJ, Stixrud J, Urzua J (2006) The effects of cognitive and noncognitive abilities on labor market: outcomes and social behavior. J Labor Econ 24(3):411–482

Heckman JJ (2008) Schools, skills and synapses. Econ Inq 46(3):289–324

Hoff E (2006) How social contexts support and shape language development. Develop Rev 26(1):55–88

Institut für Qualität und Wirtschaftlichkeit im Gesundheitswesen (Institute for Quality and Efficiency in Health Care IQWiG) (2009) Früherkennungsuntersuchung auf umschriebene Entwicklungsstörungen des Sprechens und der Sprache. Abschlussbericht S06–01. Köln: IQWiG Juni. https://www.iqwig.de/download/S06-01_Abschlussbericht_Frueherkennung_umschriebener_Stoerungen_des_Sprechens_und_der_Sprache.pdf. Accessed 24 Apr 2017

Kiese-Himmel C, Rosenfeld J (2012) Analyse aktueller Untersuchungsinstrumente zur Früherkennung von Auffälligkeiten in Sprechen und Sprache in der pädiatrischen Vorsorgeuntersuchung U8 (Evaluation of current assessment tools in early detection of developmental deviations in speech and language in the German Preventive Paediatric Examination U8) (Kindervorsorgeuntersuchung U8) (Preventive Paediatric Examination U8). Georg Thieme, Stuttgart, NY

Klee T (2008) Considerations for appraising diagnostic studies of communication disorders. Evid Based Commun Assess Interv 2(1):34–45

Law J, Garrett Z, Nye C (2004) The efficacy of treatment for children with developmental speech and language delay/disorder: a meta-analysis. J Speech Lang Hear Res 47(4):924–943

Manolson A (1995) You make the difference in helping your child to learn. Hanen Early Language Programme. Hanen Centre, Toronto, ON, Canada

McCauley R, Fey M (2006) Treatment of language disorders in children. Brookes, Baltimore, MA

Navsaria D, Sanders LM (2015) Early literacy promotion in the digital age. Pediatr Clin N Am 62(5): 1273–1295

Nelson HD, Nygren P, Walker M et al (2006) Screening for speech and language delay in preschool children: evidence synthesis no. 41. Rockville, Md.: Agency for Healthcare Research and Quality. http://www.ahrq.gov/downloads/pub/prevent/pdfser/speechsyn.pdf. Accessed 13 June 2006

Neumann K (2017) Content enhancement proposal "Specific developmental speech-language disorder" for ICD-11. http://apps.who.int/classifications/icd11/browse/proposals/l-m/en#/http://id.who.int/icd/entity/862918022?readOnly=true&action=ContentEnhancementProposal&stableProposalGroupId=329ceabe-8745-4ea4-869a-fdfd7b0c0859. Accessed 8 Apr 2017

Pepper J, Weitzman E (2004) It Takes Two to Talk: a practical guide for parents of children with language delays, 4th edn. The Hanen Centre, Toronto, Canada

Peterson P (2004) Naturalistic language teaching procedures for children at risk for language delays. Behav Anal Today 5(4):404–424

Pinker S (2002) The blank slate. Allen Lane, London

Plante E, Vance R (1994) Selection of preschool language tests: a data-based approach. Lang Speech Hear Serv Sch 25(1):15–24

Roberts JE, Burchinal MR, Zeisel SA (2002) Otitis media in early childhood in relation to children's school-age language and academic skills. Pediatrics 110(4):696–706

Roberts JE, Rosenfeld RM, Zeisel SA (2004) Otitis media and speech and language. A meta-analysis of prospective studies. Pediatrics 113(3 Pt 1):e238–e248

Roberts M, Kaiser A (2011) The effectiveness of parent-implemented language intervention: a meta-analysis. Am J Speech Lang Pathol 20(3):180–199

Rosenfeld J, Kiese-Himmel C (2011) Evaluation of current assessment tools in the early detection of language retardation in the German preventive paediatric examinations (Kindervorsorgeuntersuchung U7/U7A). Gesundheitswesen 73(10):668–679

Rosetti LM (2001) Communication intervention—birth to three, 2nd edn. Singular Thomson Learning, Independence, KY

Rowe ML (2012) A longitudinal investigation of the role of quantity and quality of child-directed speech in vocabulary development. Child Develop 83(5):1762–1774

Ruangdaraganon N, Chuthapisith J, Mo-suwan L et al (2009) Television viewing in Thai infants and toddlers: impacts to language development and parental perceptions. BMC Pediatr 9:34

Schmidt ME, Pempek TA, Kirkorian HL et al (2008) The effects of background television on the toy play behavior of very young children. Child Dev 79(4):1137–1151

Schönweiler R (2002) Ergebnisse zur Ätiologie kindlicher Spracherwerbsstörungen.[Findings on the etiology of developmental disorders of speech and language in children]. [German]. Hör-Bericht 71

Singer LT, Siegel AC, Lewis B et al (2001) Preschool language outcomes of children with history of bronchopulmonary dysplasia and very low birth weight. J Dev Behav Pediatr 22(1):19–26

Snowling MJ, Adams JW, Bishop DVM et al (2001) Educational attainments of school leavers with a pre-school history of speech-language impairments. Int J Lang Commun Disord 36(2):173–183

Tomblin JB, Hardy JC, Hein HA (1991) Predicting poor-communication status in preschool children using risk factors present at birth. J Speech Hear Res 34(5):1096–1105

Tomblin JB, Smith E, Zhang X (1997) Epidemiology of specific language impairment: prenatal and perinatal risk factors. J Commun Disord 30(4):325–344

Tomopoulos S, Dreyer BP, Berkule S et al (2010) Infant media exposure and toddler development. Arch Pediatr Adolesc Med 164(12):1105–1111

von Suchodoletz W, Kademann S, Tippelt S (2009) Sprachbeurteilung durch Eltern, Kurztest für die U7a (SBE-3-KT). http://www.kjp.med.uni-muenchen.de/download/SBE-3-KT.pdf. Accessed 24 Jan 2017

von Suchodoletz W, Sachse S (2009) Sprachbeurteilung durch Eltern, Kurztest für die U7 (SBE-2-KT), non-normalized translation in 33 languages. http://www.kjp.med.uni-muenchen.de/sprachstoerungen/sbe2kt_fremd.php. Accessed 24 Jan 2017

Weindrich D, Jennen-Steinmetz C, Laucht M et al (2000) Epidemiology and prognosis of specific disorders of language and scholastic skills. Eur Child Adolesc Psychiatry 9(3):186–194

Weitzman E, Greenberg J (2010) ABC and beyond: building emergent literacy in early childhood settings. The Hanen Centre, Toronto

Weitzman E, Girolametto L, Drake L (2017) Hanen Programs® for parents: parent implemented early language intervention. In: McCauley RJ, Fey ME, Gillam RB (eds) Treatment of language disorders in children, 2nd edn. Paul H. Brookes Publishing, Baltimore, MA, pp 27–56

White-Schwoch T, Davies EC, Thompson EC et al (2015) Auditory-neurophysiological responses to speech during early childhood: effects of background noise. Hear Res 328:34–47

Wittmer DS, Petersen SH (2010) Strategies to encourage language learning, strategies to support language development and learning. Pearson Allyn Bacon Prentice Hall. http://www.education.com/reference/article/strategies-language-learning/. Accessed 8 Jan 2017

Wolery M, Sainato D (1996) General curriculum and intervention strategies. In: Odom SL, McLean ME (eds) Early intervention/early childhood special education: recommended practices. Pro-Ed, Austin, TX, pp 125–158

Wright BA, Lombardino LJ, King WM (1997) Deficits in auditory temporal and spectral resolution in language-impaired children. Nature 387(6629):176–178

Yoder P, Warren S (2001) Relative treatment effects of two prelinguistic communication interventions on language development in toddlers with language delays vary by maternal characteristics. J Speech Lang Hear Res 44(1):224–237

Zimmerman FJ, Christakis DA (2005) Children's television viewing and cognitive outcomes: a longitudinal analysis of national data. Arch Pediatr Adolesc Med 159(7):619–625

Zimmerman FJ, Christakis DA, Meltzoff AN (2007) Associations between media viewing and language development in children under age 2 years. J Pediatr 151(4):364–368

Zimmerman IL, Steiner VG, Pond RE (2011a) PLS-5 preschool language scales, 5th edn. Pearson, San Antonio, TX

Zimmerman IL, Steiner VG, Pond RE (2011b) Preschool language scale-5 screening test (PLS-5 Screening Test), 5th edn. Pearson, San Antonio, TX

Rehabilitation and Prognosis of Developmental Disorders of Speech and Language

13

Karina Dancza, Dirk Deuster, Mona Hegazi,
Christiane Kiese-Himmel, Claudia Koch-Günnewig,
Katrin Neumann, Karen Reichmuth,
Amélie Elisabeth Tillmanns, and Sharon Tuppeny

13.1 Basics of Speech and Language Therapy in Children

See Part I, Chap. 1, Sect. 1.14.

K. Dancza
Singapore Institute of Technology, Health and Social
Sciences Cluster, Singapore, Singapore
e-mail: Karina.Dancza@singaporetech.edu.sg

S. Tuppeny
Royal College of Occupational Therapists,
London, UK
e-mail: sharon@mgaconsulting.org.uk

D. Deuster · K. Reichmuth · A. E. Tillmanns
Clinic of Phoniatrics and Pedaudiology,
University Hospital Münster, Münster, Germany
e-mail: deusted@uni-muenster.de;
karen.reichmuth@ukmuenster.de;
AmelieElisabeth.Tillmanns@ukmuenster.de

M. Hegazi
ENT Department, Ain Shams University,
Cairo, Egypt

C. Kiese-Himmel
Phoniatrics/Pediatric Audiological Psychology,
University Medical Center Göttingen,
Göttingen, Germany
e-mail: ckiese@med.uni-goettingen.de

C. Koch-Günnewig
Physiotherapy Practice for Children, Münster, Germany

K. Neumann
Department of Phoniatrics and Pediatric Audiology,
ENT Clinic, St. Elisabeth Hospital, University of
Bochum, Bochum, Germany
e-mail: Katrin.neumann@rub.de

13.2 Role of the Phoniatrician in the Intervention of Developmental Disorders of Speech and Language

Katrin Neumann, Mona Hegazi,
Amélie Elisabeth Tillmanns, and Dirk Deuster

13.2.1 Predispositions

The proper management of developmental disorders of speech and language (DDSL) belongs to the main duties of a phoniatrician. In order to accomplish this task, several preconditions need to be fulfilled:

- Profound knowledge and continuous education of the phoniatrician on the nature, causes, epidemiology, symptoms, co-morbidities, differential diagnostics, valid screening and diagnostic tools, treatment and rehabilitation methods of DDSL including behavioural, drug, physio- and psycho-therapy, as well as augmentative and alternative communication (AAC) and special education.
- An interdisciplinary working team including staff of one or more of the following medical specialties: logopaedists/speech and language therapists (SLPs), special pedagogues, psychologists, nurses or other healthcare professionals and optional audiologists/audiometrists or engineers/physicists.

© Springer-Verlag GmbH Germany, part of Springer Nature 2020
A. am Zehnhoff-Dinnesen et al. (eds.), *Phoniatrics I*, European Manual of Medicine,
https://doi.org/10.1007/978-3-662-46780-0_13

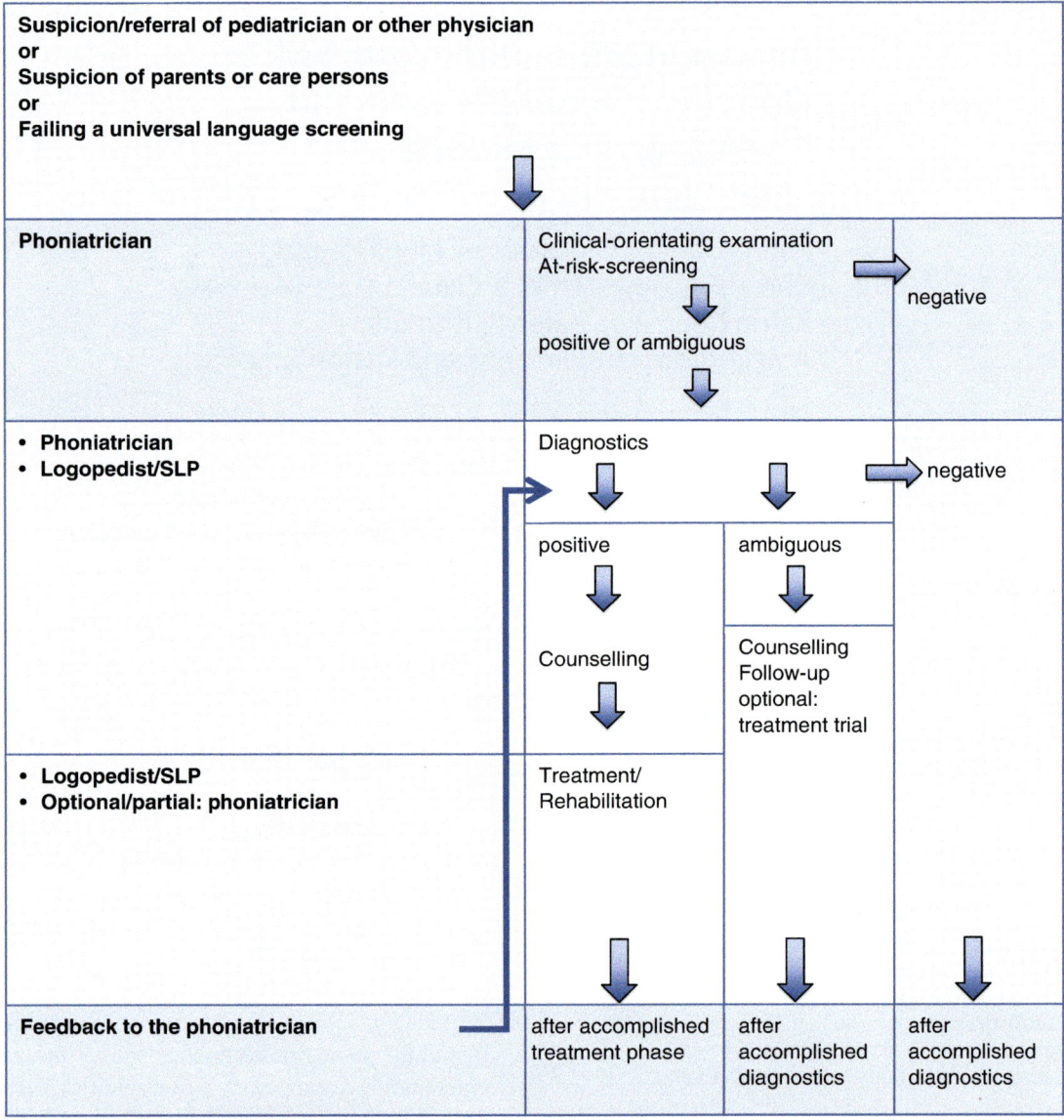

Fig. 13.1 Algorithm for phoniatric management of identification, diagnostics, treatment/rehabilitation, therapy supervision and outcome control of DDSL (modified from Neumann et al. 2016)

- A regular interdisciplinary exchange with other professionals in the field, including physicians such as (neuro)paediatricians, geneticists, ophthalmologists, radiologists, otorhinolaryngologists, oral and maxillofacial surgeons, orthodontists and psychiatricians, logopaedists/SLPs, psychologists, psychotherapists, teachers and special pedagogues, nursery nurses, and employees of health insurances or administrative bodies.

- Involvement in the training and education of logopaedists/SLPs.

13.2.2 Phoniatric Management of Developmental Disorders of Speech and Language

An appropriate phoniatric management of DDSL involves:

- A first identification process by medical history, orientating examination or screening.
- Professional diagnostics by valid assessment tools.
- Making or excluding the diagnosis of a DDSL.
- Counselling the parents or care persons.
- Setting up a treatment or rehabilitation plan together with the parents/care persons and the initiation/prescription of treatment/rehabilitation.
- Optional: the execution of parts of the treatment/rehabilitation by the phoniatrician her- or himself.
- A supervision of the treatment/rehabilitation and a regular outcome control of its effects.

The whole process is depicted in Fig. 13.1. In the following subsections, the named duties are described more in detail.

13.2.2.1 First Identification

Parents usually consult a phoniatrician if they or other related persons/caregivers, relatives, nursery nurses, physicians or other health professionals suspect a developmental language abnormality of a child. Often children are referred by a paediatrician or another physician to a phoniatrician. In some regions, universal screenings for speech and language are implemented and may lead to a referral of children who fail the screening to a phoniatric institution. Initially, the phoniatrician should identify whether there is a risk for an individual child to have a DDSL owing to sensory, physical, cognitive or behavioural factors such as permanent hearing loss; recurrent otitis media with effusion; DDSL history of siblings, parents or other close relatives; autism spectrum disorder and other pervasive developmental disorders; syndromes or craniofacial disorders that may impair cognitive or speech and language development; cleft palate or developmental disorders. For this, she or he will ask the parents about the medical and language developmental history of the child and will probably get a first impression by an orientating examination of the child's spontaneous or elicited language. Parent questionnaires, informal tests and at-risk screenings may be helpful in this process (see Sects. 11.1–11.3 and 12.1).

13.2.2.2 Diagnostics

The diagnostics is performed either by the phoniatrician himself and by his co-workers according to the algorithm depicted in Sect. 11.3. At first a hearing loss and other co-morbidities of a DDSL have to be excluded by an appropriate audiological and supplementary diagnostics. If a hearing loss is present, it should be treated before a DSSL intervention starts. If other co-morbidities are present, such as intellectual disability, autism or multiple needs, they have to be considered during the set-up of an intervention plan. The phoniatrician has to manage the whole diagnostic procedure including the involvement of other expertise, e.g. from (neuro)paediatric, genetic, radiological, ophthalmological, maxillo-facial-surgical, orthodontic or psychological specialties. Central to the diagnostics of DDSL are language tests, either embedded in language-covering general developmental tests or as general developmental language tests, or as specific language tests examining distinct areas of linguistic competence (see Sect. 11.3). The phoniatrician needs to know about the validity of the applied screenings and diagnostic tests, to ensure that they are up to date and provide proper performance and analysis, according to the test manuals, and to confirm the correct documentation of the results, either by her- or himself or by co-workers. The phoniatrician has to ensure the precise documentation of the test results in the medical record including the measurement conditions (such as 'good co-operation', 'tired child', or 'no compliance'). If there remains an ambiguity, she or he has to organise repeated measurements in order to obtain a diagnosis by 'dynamic assessment'. The phoniatrician has an important regulatory role in the analysis of the diagnostic results, not only for referring children with DDSL to an appropriate treatment but also to align the proportion of children who undergo a therapy with the prevalence expected for DDSL. For example, given that about 10% of children suffer from a DDSL (including children with language-relevant co-morbidities) and 5–8% from a specific DDSL (SDDSL; see Sect. 9.6), there is an imbalance compared with the numbers of children who undergo therapy (for example, in

Germany 24% of all boys and 17% of all girls at age of 6 years received a language therapy in 2014 according to the report of the largest German health insurance (Waltersbacher and Scientific Institute of AOK 2015)). Such an inappropriateness has to be prevented by the phoniatrician, who should initiate and finish interventions according to evidence-based best practices (see Sect. 2.3).

13.2.2.3 Making a Diagnosis

The identification and diagnostic process is completed by a clear diagnosis, which needs to be documented by the phoniatrician. It is not sufficient to describe findings only. If there is an ambiguity with respect to the diagnosis, a planned follow-up needs to be documented in the medical record and the physician's letters.

13.2.2.4 Counselling of Parents

Parents or caregivers need to be counselled by the phoniatrician in a quiet, sensitive and empathic atmosphere about the nature, treatment options and prognosis of the language disorder of their child/ward. Here, it is indispensable that the phoniatrician has a thorough and up-to-date knowledge about the state of the art of evidence-based interventions for DDSL according to scientific guidelines, systematic reviews, meta-analyses and randomised controlled trials (RCTs) (see Sect. 2.3). Even if she or he prefers one treatment method over others, it is necessary to inform the parents about the alternatives. The options for particular settings such as extensive treatments in logopaedic/SLP practices, intensive treatments courses, single or group therapies, out-patient or in-patient treatments need to be discussed with the parents/caregivers. The perspective of a child and her family with respect to the criteria of the International classification of functioning, disability, and health: children and youth version (ICF-CY; World Health Organization 2007) needs to be considered as well as the resources of a family (e.g. financial, time, driving distance, workload, knowledge of the common language, number of siblings). Furthermore, the phoniatrician needs to find out the expectations of the parents/caregivers with respect to the treatment

goals. The end of this process should be an informed consent, i.e. parents/caregivers should agree to the initiation of a distinct treatment from the perspective of well-informed decision makers in terms of the best interest of the child (Engelhardt 1996).

13.2.2.5 Set-Up of the Treatment/ Rehabilitation Plan and Initiation/Prescription of the Treatment

The duties of a phoniatrician include setting up a treatment plan, or at least to be involved in its elaboration. Here, precise treatment goals and a timeline have to be determined. It may, for example, be necessary to arouse enjoyment of speaking of a child before dealing with linguistic issues. If a treatment does not show an effect within a certain period (e.g. for stuttering within 3 months according to the German evidence-based guidelines on fluency disorders, Neumann et al. 2016), the treatment method should be reconsidered and changed or adapted.

13.2.2.6 Performance of Treatment/ Rehabilitation by the Phoniatrician

There is a long tradition of phoniatrics in language therapy. The profession of logopaedists has been founded and further developed by an initiative and under leadership of phoniatricians such as Emil Froeschels and Hermann Gutzmann. Language therapies have been developed in particular by Hermann Gutzmann, one of the pioneers of phoniatrics, who has earned much merit in the field of language therapy (e.g. Gutzmann 1912). Hence, a phoniatrician needs to know the principles of language therapy and should be able to perform at least parts of it by her- or himself. In particular, she or he may be actively involved if instrument-based procedures are applied, such as computer-feedback or tele-training.

13.2.2.7 Treatment Supervision and Outcome Control

One of the more important duties of a phoniatrician is the supervision and outcome control of a

DDSL treatment. This requires treatment reports of the therapists and repeated measures combining objective and subjective assessment methods (tests and parent reports or questionnaires, respectively) that evaluate social participation and interaction, and the quality of life of a child. Again, good medical practice requires a change of the therapy approach if a treatment is not successful within a defined period (Neumann et al. 2016). The phoniatrician has a key role in the further application, adaptation or finalisation of an intervention. In order to fulfill these tasks, regular monitoring of a child and a trustful and honest communication between phoniatrician and therapist are inevitable.

13.2.3 Integrated Approach

In order to achieve the highest benefit for a child from a treatment or rehabilitation in the case of a DDSL, a highly interdisciplinary approach is necessary. This needs a strong collaboration among all participants of the interdisciplinary network described in Sect. 13.2.1. The phoniatrician has to organise, manage and supervise this collaborative work by organising or participating in interdisciplinary case conferences for severe cases of DDSL or for children with multiple needs. She or he needs to communicate with nurseries, schools, special schools and health insurances in order to enable a child with DDSL the full integration in its familial and social environment, and participation in social activities according to the principles of the ICF-CY.

An important task of phoniatricians is their involvement in the education and training of therapists for DDSL. It is recommended that they be involved in giving lectures and providing regular practical traineeships of upcoming therapists in phoniatric institutions. Frequently, theses for bachelor, master and doctoral degrees are supervised by phoniatricians. Furthermore, phoniatricians are involved in basic and clinical research on the improvement of the quality of identification, assessment and intervention programmes, and on the implementation of evidenced-based procedures in the field of developmental language disorders.

13.3 Physiotherapy for Children with Neuromotor or Neurodevelopmental Diseases and Associated Communication Disorders

Claudia Koch-Günnewig

13.3.1 Introduction

Physiotherapy is a medical profession that assesses, diagnoses, treats and works to prevent diseases and disabilities through physical means for people of all ages. Physiotherapists support patients affected by injury, illness or disability through movement and exercise, manual therapy, education and advice. They are experts in movement and function. They work in partnership with their patients, assisting them to overcome movement disorders, which may have been present from birth, acquired through accident or injury or are the result of ageing or life-changing events.

In paediatric physiotherapy, it is important to consider several aspects that may influence the execution and the success of the treatment. The therapist needs to focus not only on the child but also on the parents and the familial background in general. Each long-term therapeutic intervention has an impact on the child's life and of the family's routine. Therefore, individual concepts with daily exercises need to be established in accordance with the family or caregivers of a child. Parents need to take on the function of a co-therapist during the treatment process. They need to be trained and guided through therapeutic measures and aids. In addition, the motivation and compliance of both parties need to be ensured and promoted without overtaxing the child or the parents. During the recent years, increasing attention has been paid to the role of the family in the child's life, and the term 'family-centred services' has been introduced to improve the care for children with special needs and their families. Systematic analyses suggest two recent trends:

> from child-focused to family-focused orientation and from professionally directed guidance to coaching based on equal partnership
> Dirks and Hadders-Algra (2011)

of both therapists and parents

Furthermore, and differing from that in adults, physiotherapy in children has to consider that diseases or injuries in children do not only affect their somatic state but also other developmental aspects of their neurological and sensorimotor systems. This may cause a deceleration, interruption or even cessation of the sensorimotor, cognitive, perceptual, social and emotional development of the child. The general aim of paediatric physiotherapy is to promote the normal development of the postural and movement apparatus. Therefore, the therapist needs detailed knowledge about the process of growth and maturation in the early stages of child development. Paediatric physiotherapy involves assessing the needs of a child and providing neurological rehabilitation in order to improve the child's participation and function.

Moreover, common goals should be established and consented to in an interdisciplinary approach. Paediatric physiotherapists work together with physicians, occupational therapists, nurses, speech therapists and orthopaedic technicians to support both child and parents. The primary goal should be to enable children with disabilities to achieve the highest possible level of independence throughout all stages of therapy. However, one should be aware that even with therapy not every child will achieve a healthy, normal state of life. In the following, four basic treatment methods in paediatric physiotherapy are introduced.

13.3.2 Vojta Therapy in Children

The Vojta Therapy is a concept of early assessment and treatment that focuses on the integrated treatment of disturbances of the posture and movement apparatus and of somatosensory perception disorders. It is based on reflex locomotion. The brain is stimulated in order to activate innate, stored movement patterns (International Vojta Society: http://www.vojta.com/en/organisation/international-vojta-society). The treatment generates involuntary muscular activity that patients with impairments of the central nervous system, which affect the posture and movement

apparatus, are unable to perform voluntarily, regardless of their age.

An activation of movement patterns can be obtained through the precise positioning of the child (prone position, supine position, lying on the side) as well as using predefined stimuli and specific pressure points on distinct body parts (stimulation zones). The combination of positioning, stimuli and pressure elicits coordinated movement patterns involving the muscles of the trunk and extremities. Visceral muscles and muscles of the face are also involved. These movement patterns occur 'reflex-like' and are called 'reflex creeping' and 'reflex rolling'—the two main movement complexes of the Vojta Therapy. Both movement complexes include fundamental components of locomotion such as postural regulation, standing up against gravity and phasic mobility of extremities.

Repeated activation of the reflex-like movement patterns (preferably four activation intervals per day) is assumed to induce a reorganisation of nerve and central nervous system functioning (brain and spinal cord). Dr. Václav Vojta has postulated that these pathways may be blocked in newborns. Vojta Therapy neither trains nor teaches functions such as grasping, rolling or crawling but activates innate skills (extension of the spine; muscle function differentiation of arms, legs and trunk; inducement of swallowing; increase of breathing depth; activation of visceral muscles). The treatment usually increases the quality of spontaneous posture and movement and also aims to improve somatosensory perception and the ability to initiate contact and to communicate. These effects can be observed over the entire day, in case reflex locomotion is activated regularly. The treatment focuses on replacing substitute and abnormal movement patterns used by the affected child.

Parents take on the role as co-therapist and therefore have to be instructed in the basic application of Vojta Therapy. One considerable aspect in their guidance is to explain that crying during the treatment is not caused by pain but rather expresses exhaustion and unfamiliar activation. Premature infants should be treated with Vojta Therapy as early as possible, because the central nervous system is still malleable, abnormal substitute patterns have not been established yet and growth and maturation processes may be supported by the treatment.

Although the Vojta Therapy is a popular approach, it is criticised because evidence for its effectiveness has not been clearly established on the basis of well-controlled trials as it has, for example, been shown in the literature and systematic reviews on children with cerebral palsy (Franki et al. 2012; Patel 2005). Furthermore, it is a child-oriented but not family-orientated approach, and the latter is favoured according to more recent treatment trends (Dirks and Hadders-Algra 2011).

13.3.3 Bobath Therapy in Children

The Bobath Therapy is a worldwide used neurophysiological assessment and treatment concept for patients with motor disorders caused by disturbed neurological functions, as developed by Berta and Dr. Karel Bobath (1984). It is applied in patients of all ages, but mainly in infants and children, with congenital or early-in-life acquired cerebral motor disorders, developmental delays of unknown origin, sensorimotor difficulties and other neurological and neuromuscular diseases. The neurophysiologically and neurodevelopmentally based concept focuses on both the:

> inhibition or suppression of abnormal tonic reflex activity responsible for patterns of hypertonia, and the facilitation of normal reactions and highly integrated postural control and balance in their own sequence of development, progressing to specialised activities.
>
> Hirata and Santos (2012)

It is an interdisciplinary, active hands-on therapy used to treat patients with an impairment of the central nervous system caused by lesions. Locomotor, sensorimotor, cognitive, perceptual, social and emotional development is assumed to be positively influenced by the Bobath Therapy. The treatment is performed by physiotherapists, occupational therapists, logopaedists, nursing staff and physicians such as phoniatricians and paediatricians.

For children, the paediatric physiotherapist applies a resource-orientated, problem-solving approach in order to access the individual's activity and participation. Therefore, special therapeutic handling techniques are used and taught to the parents during each intervention. Furthermore, customised equipment (specialised seating, orthotics) supports the effects of the Bobath Therapy. In case of sensory deficits or damaged processing of sensory information, the tactile and proprioceptive input is increased in order to support the child with his or her own body exploration (The Bobath Centre: http://www.bobath.org.uk). To achieve optimal sensorimotor processing and task performance, mutual dynamic interaction between the child and the paediatric physiotherapist is essential. Parents take on the role of a co-therapist and are guided in the correct use of therapeutic aids and the thorough application of basic, play-centred physiotherapeutic techniques. During each intervention, the main objective is to enable the child to participate in daily life by influencing and regulating the abnormal postural tone to more normal coordination patterns. Improved postural alignment is assumed to increase the efficiency of the child's movements and activities. The aim of the therapy is to lead the child towards developing and enhancing new functional skills and to involve the child further in active participation in everyday life activities with gradual reduction in assistance.

13.3.4 Castillo Morales Therapy in Children

The Castillo Morales Therapy, known as 'orofacial regulation therapy' (Castillo Morales Vereinigung e.V http://www.castillomoralesvereinigung.de/index_e.html), is a treatment concept developed by Dr. Castillo Morales (1999). This integrative therapeutic approach addresses children with orofacial, communicative and sensorimotor disorders. Dr. Castillo Morales discovered the interdependence of posture and movement of head, neck and jaw positions. This interdependence further influences the mimic, oral and pharyngeal muscles. Children with neurological or anatomical dysfunctions often face challenges in coordination of differentiated sensorimotor performance of the orofacial muscular system. These difficulties frequently cause problems in the ability to communicate (mimic expression and articulation) and to eat, drink and swallow. The Castillo Morales Therapy aims to support and improve the ability to communicate and strives towards enabling the children to participate in normal day activities, such as eating and drinking.

The Castillo Morales concept focuses on function and not only the movement itself, addressing each part of the oral complex and turning all of them into a dynamic system through coordinated activities (Hirata and Santos 2012; Morales 1999). It uses functional jaw orthopaedics through the palatine plate.

The paediatric physiotherapist applies manual vibration and pressing and pulling techniques to give proprioceptive experience to the orofacial system. Beyond orofacial functions, these techniques are assumed to activate also the hands, feet and trunk. The activation aims at positively re-influencing the muscular system of the whole orofacial region.

Patients with muscular hypotonia; sensorimotor impairment, e.g. in cerebral palsy; and special sensorimotor defects in the region of the face, throat and mouth may particularly benefit from Castillo Morales Therapy. It is also applied in premature infants with difficulties in ingestion, children with hypotonia (e.g. Down syndrome) and children with congenital, anatomically based malformations in the oral region. Positive short-term and long-term effects of the therapy in children with Down syndrome have been shown in several studies (e.g. Korbmacher et al. 2006).

13.3.5 Psychomotor Therapy in Children

Psychomotor therapy aims to facilitate the appropriate and age-relevant development of children with perception and movement disorders. It focuses on the improvement of perception, balance, coordination and strength. This integrated therapy approach includes play, rest and relaxation, perception, graphomotor, painting and movement exercises, as well as consulting parents. The training is organised in small groups of three to five children. Sensory integration and interpersonal relations are key elements of psychomotor therapy. A close collaboration between therapist, parents and family is essential. A supporting environment empowers the child to gain new sensory, motor, social and emotional experiences. Psychomotor therapy should enable the child to bring together, organise and assess information and stimuli in order to ensure self-controlled movement patterns.

13.4 Occupational Therapy

Karina Dancza and Sharon Tuppeny

13.4.1 Introduction

Occupational therapists are experts in occupations. Occupations refer to everything that people do in the course of their everyday life. Occupations for children and young people may include self-care (e.g. getting ready to go out, eating a meal, using the toilet), being productive (e.g. going to nursery, school or work or volunteering) and leisure (e.g. playing with friends or doing hobbies). Occupational therapists work not only with children but with people of all ages who have complex needs or circumstances, which means that they require expert advice and guidance. The role of occupational therapists with children and young people with developmental disorders of speech and language is to enable participation in everyday life and promote independence. Through doing activities that are meaningful to the child/young person, it is believed that there will be a positive impact on his/her health and wellbeing.

Children and young people with developmental language disorders are likely to experience challenges when engaging in aspects of their day-to-day life such as playing with friends, doing their schoolwork, interacting with their family, etc. Language disorders are also a feature of other developmental disorders, and as such the impact on functioning may not be solely related to their language issues.

13.4.2 Occupational Therapy Assessment and In-Context Observations

The starting point of an occupational therapy assessment is to understand the child/young person and the family's priorities in terms of the occupations they want to, need to, or are expected to do. On the basis of these priority areas, an occupational therapist will assess and analyse multiple elements that have an impact on a child/young person's ability to carry out the occupations, which extend beyond the diagnosis. This would likely involve an observation of the child/young person doing the priority activity (ideally in context) and if necessary additional standardised or nonstandardised assessments to illuminate the strengths, needs, barriers and enablers of participation.

With respect to the International Classification of Functioning, Disability and Health (ICF, World Health Organization 2001), occupational therapists will consider person factors and body functions (e.g. values, roles, habits and physical/cognitive/communication/emotional functions), demands of the occupation (e.g. required steps/timing, space, tools, actions), and environmental context (e.g. characteristics of the physical space/materials, social context). In addition, consideration should be given to how these elements are influenced by societal and cultural expectations

(Fisher 2009). The integral nature of these factors on the ability of the child/young person to do his/her occupation (e.g. playing, doing schoolwork, organising themselves, etc.) is shown in Fig. 13.2.

Benefits of in-context observations for a child/young person with a developmental disorder of speech and language are that the impact of the environment on the ability to participate successfully in a given task can be considered and the assessment would thus not rely on the child/young person's understanding of assessment instructions.

13.4.3 Intervention Approaches

Intervention approaches will depend on the reasons for the challenges, as identified from the assessment. Collaboration with the child/young person, family and school (if relevant) is essential. The focus could be on the exploration of alternative ways of doing activities, making changes to the environment or developing skills or strategies to enable successful participation. Some occupational therapists may focus on the development or remediation of underlying body functions (such as motor skills, sensory skills, perceptual skills, etc.), although increasingly the evidence within the profession highlights the benefit of practicing the actual activity rather than focusing at a body function and structure level (Law and Darrah 2014).

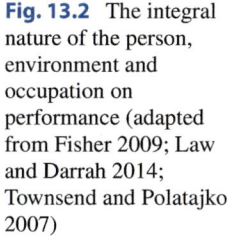

Fig. 13.2 The integral nature of the person, environment and occupation on performance (adapted from Fisher 2009; Law and Darrah 2014; Townsend and Polatajko 2007)

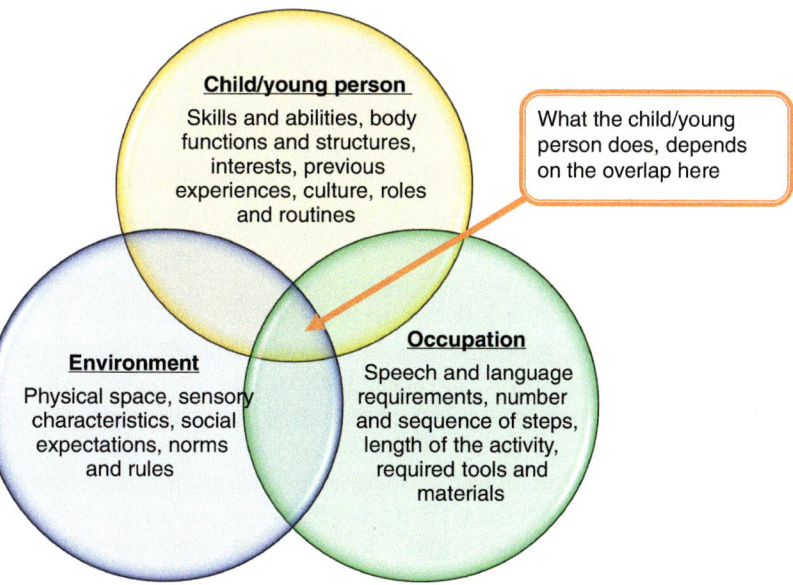

Child/young person
Skills and abilities, body functions and structures, interests, previous experiences, culture, roles and routines

What the child/young person does, depends on the overlap here

Environment
Physical space, sensory characteristics, social expectations, norms and rules

Occupation
Speech and language requirements, number and sequence of steps, length of the activity, required tools and materials

For example, if a priority occupation for a child is to ride his or her bike, then practicing the actual task of riding (at a level that is challenging yet achievable) may be more effective than undertaking activities not associated with riding a bike but are designed to improve balance or sensory processing. Moreover, utilising the motivation of the child/young person and family through collaborative goal setting and focusing on their priorities also demonstrates effective results (Graham et al. 2013; Locke and Latham 2002). Interventions are thus likely to be contextual to the situation and specific to the child/young person. The effectiveness is measured by the change they make to the child/young person's ability to engage and participate in their daily life tasks.

Case Study 13.1

Viktor is an 8-year-old student identified by his teachers as having challenges relating to his schoolwork tasks and associated speech, language and communication difficulties. The priority occupations identified by Viktor's teacher, his parent and Viktor are related to completing tabletop activities such as drawing and writing. The occupational therapist observed Viktor during the classroom routine of the children's receiving instructions whilst they were sitting on the carpet and then going to their desks and undertaking a writing and drawing activity. A School Version of the Assessment of Motor and Process Skills (School AMPS; Fisher et al. 2007) was undertaken. According to the School AMPS, Viktor was observed to have some mild clumsiness and increase in effort as he did his writing and drawing (percentile rank 50). On the School AMPS process scale, Viktor was observed to be markedly inefficient in his use of time, space and objects during the writing and drawing task (percentile rank <1). This appeared to be influenced by four main factors: (1) Viktor not remembering how to spell the words he wanted to write, (2) Viktor looking around and becoming distracted, (3) long verbal instructions being given by the teacher, and (4) a cluttered desk.

The results were clustered and documented as a baseline. A goal was developed that focused on what Viktor would like to achieve following intervention (i.e. what success would look like). For example, 'By the end of term (4 weeks), Viktor will write his English story within the time allocated within the lesson'.

Interventions were collaboratively determined and included Viktor having a dictionary of commonly used words on his desk so that he could recall how to spell what he wanted to write. In addition, environmental modifications were made such as reducing the clutter in the class so Viktor was less distracted during the task, the teacher giving all instructions to students verbally and in writing and organising Viktor's desk.

The interventions were trialled and evaluated, where the goal was reviewed and the School AMPS was re-administered. Viktor (and many other children in the class) was reported to have benefited from the interventions and the goal was achieved. Viktor's school motor measure remained stable (percentile rank 50), and his school process measure was significantly improved (percentile rank 10).

13.5 Principles of Augmentative Communication Methods

Karen Reichmuth

13.5.1 Introduction

Augmentative and alternative communication (AAC) interventions are methods and technologies used to compensate for an individual's reduced communicative competence (see Branson and Demchak 2009 for review). Following the broader definition of the American Speech-Language-Hearing Association (ASHA 2005):

AAC refers to an area of research, clinical, and educational practice. AAC involves attempts to study and when necessary compensate for temporary or permanent impairments, activity limitations, and participation restrictions of individuals with severe disorders of speech-language production and/or comprehension, including spoken and written modes of communication.

13.5.2 When Is AAC Indicated in Children with Developmental Disorders of Speech and Language (DDSL) and Hearing Disorders?

The following classification of three target groups for AAC interventions introduced by von Tetzchner and Martinsen (1992) is commonly used (see review Branson and Demchak 2009):

- The expressive language group: individuals understanding others' spoken language but having difficulty in expressing themselves
- The supportive language group:
  - Subgroup A: children who temporarily use AAC in order to facilitate their comprehension of spoken language, as well as to express themselves
  - Subgroup B: children who speak but who have difficulty being understood
- The alternative language group: individuals who use AAC as a permanent means of receptive and expressive communication

The children this section focuses on may belong to any of these three groups. Children at any age are reliant upon AAC if their speech is inadequate to meet their communicative goals and if they are at risk of a profound impairment of their expressive communication (Cress and Marvin 2003). Children, especially those showing or expected to show a general or mental developmental delay or impairment (e.g. children with Down syndrome or other syndromes, with cognitive impairment, with multiple disabilities, with autism) and who exhibit special or even complex needs, meet these criteria for AAC, often from birth on (Cress and Marvin 2003; Light and Drager 2007; Wilkinson and Hennig 2007; Sevcik et al. 2008).

More than 40% of children with sensorineural hearing impairment show additional impairments or will develop them during their life (Meinzen-Derr et al. 2011). These children are also at high risk of developing insufficient communicative competence via oral language, even if they have received hearing devices (hearing aids or cochlear implants) early in life (Meinzen-Derr et al. 2013; Kim et al. 2010; Boons et al. 2012).

If the continuous monitoring of communication and language development in the children named above confirms a considerable retardation, intervention should include AAC and advice to parents in using AAC in daily communication at home as early as possible (Cress and Marvin 2003; Meinzen-Derr et al. 2013; Branson and Demchak 2009).

13.5.3 Classification of AAC Modes

AAC includes a large variety of communication forms and can be categorised as 'unaided' and 'aided' modes (see Branson and Demchak 2009 and von Loeper and ISAAC 2012 for overview):

- Unaided AAC modes are all the body's own modes and therefore need no external devices: e.g. natural gestures, manual signs (e.g. Makaton®, see Fig. 13.3), gestural cueing systems, vocalisation and speech and eye gaze body language.

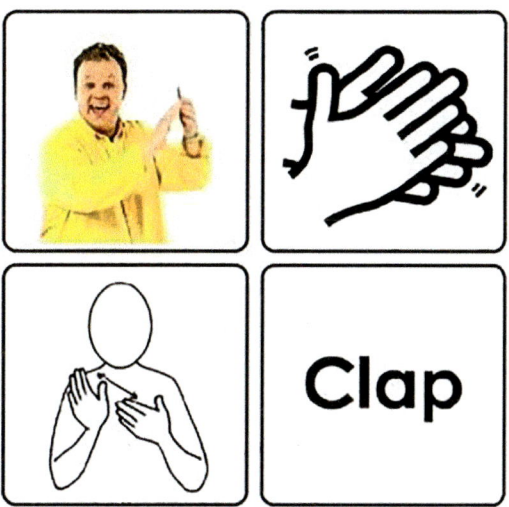

Fig. 13.3 *Makaton®* is a multimodal language programme using signs and symbols to help children to communicate. It is available in several languages. Reprinted from http://helloautismresources.weebly.com/home/free-makaton-resources-and-signs

- Aided AAC modes require an external device to display and store symbols or pictures, photos and objects or letters. These external aids can be:
  - Non-electronic, e.g. miniature objects, pictures, photos, communication boards and binders (e.g. see Fig. 13.4a, b), individual diaries/communication books
  - Electronic, that range from light-technology components without or with voice output (e.g. switches, see Fig. 13.5) to highly sophisticated speech-generating devices (VOCA, electronic device with voice output communication) (e.g. see Figs. 13.6, 13.7, and 13.8).

An AAC intervention aiming at successful communication should generally include an individualised multimodal combination of different communication forms (Sevcik et al. 2008). The selection depends on the user's individual motor, visual, cognitive, language and communication strengths and weaknesses.

13.5.4 Evidence of ACC Intervention

AAC does not hinder speech production. Available research indicates that AAC actually facilitates vocal communication by increasing interaction

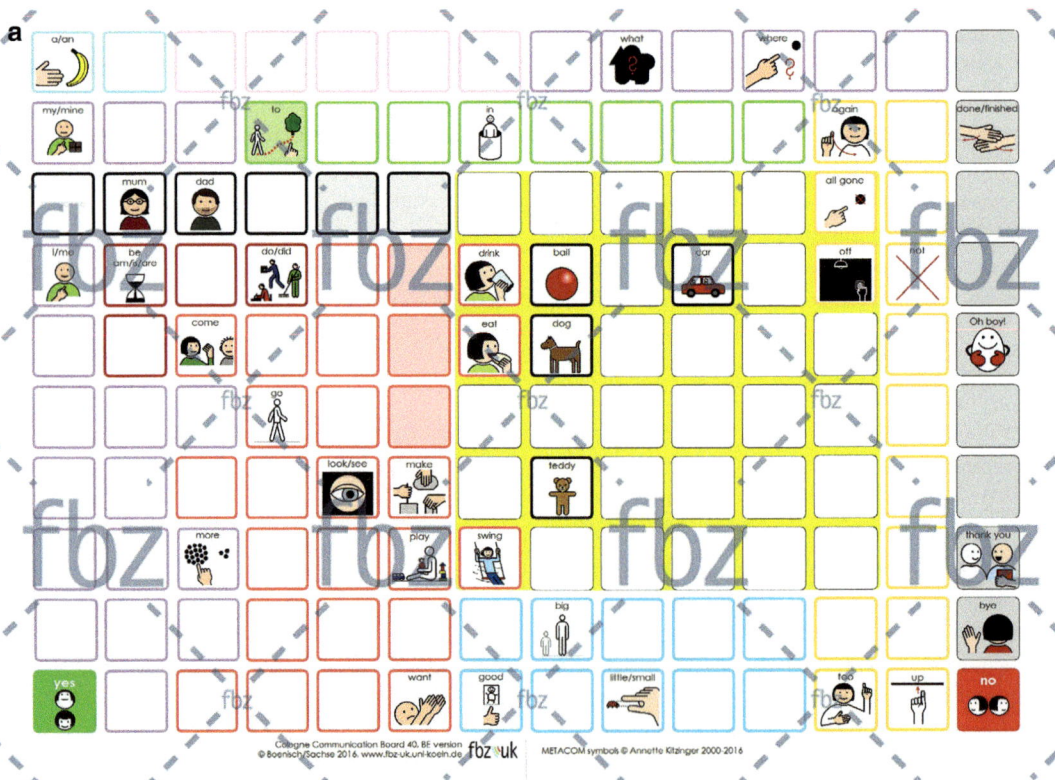

Fig. 13.4 (**a**) *Cologne Communication Board®*; Version 3.0. Reprinted from www.fbz-uk.uni-koeln.de with kind permission of © Boenisch and Sachse (2017). Reprinted with *METACOM* symbols with kind permission of © Kitzinger (2011–2015). The depicted board has a size of DIN A3 with 140 symbol fields (100 fields as a static frame for core vocabulary in white and a flexible block of 6 × 5 fields for fringe vocabulary in yellow). Here a reduced vocabulary is used, which can individually be expanded (*Cologne Vocabulary*). The board supports language learning via symbol-based communication combined with procedural memory learning. (**b**) *Cologne*

Communication Binder®; Version 3.0. Reprinted from www.fbz-uk.uni-koeln.de with kind permission of © Boenisch and Sachse (2017). Reprinted with *METACOM* symbols with kind permission of ©Kitzinger (2011–2015). The binder has a static frame for core vocabulary and a flexible block for fringe vocabulary of several topics with approx. 450 words (*Cologne Vocabulary*). Montessori colour coding is used for word forms. The binder supports language learning via symbol-based communication combined with procedural memory learning. The binder is available in English and German

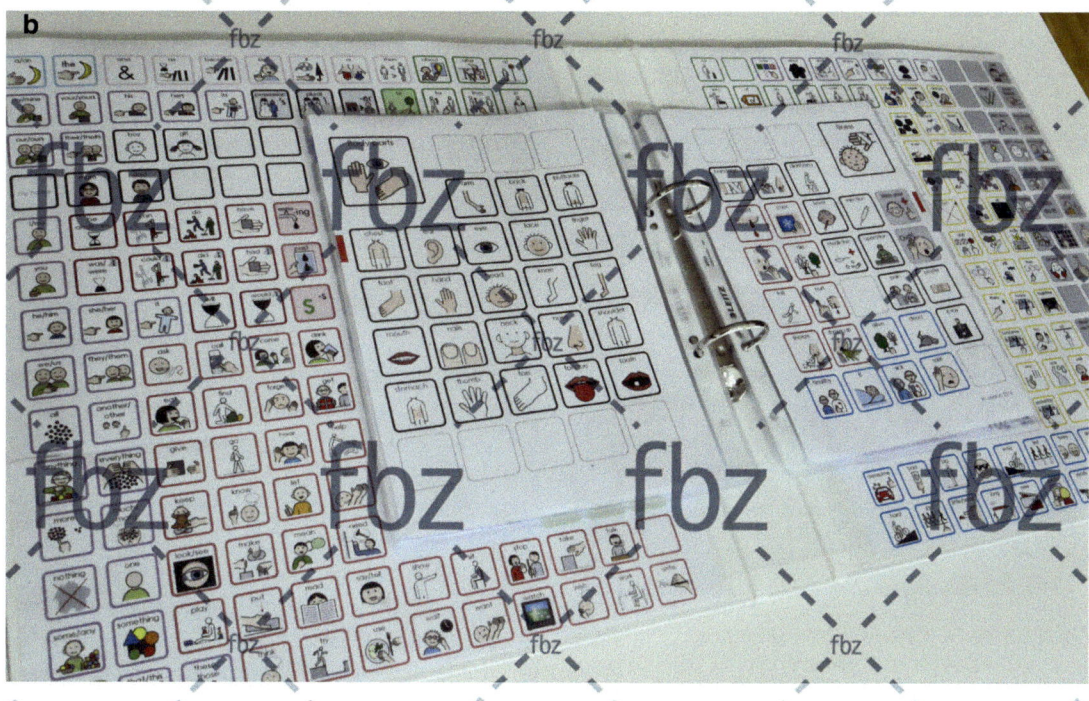

Fig. 13.4 (continued)

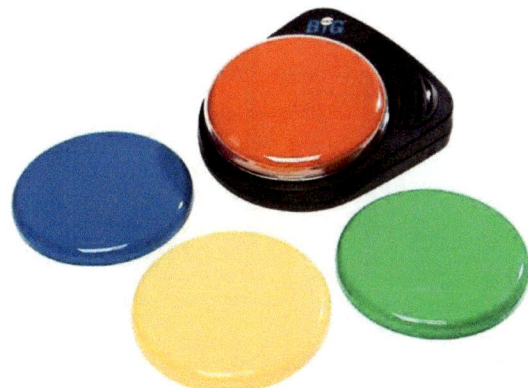

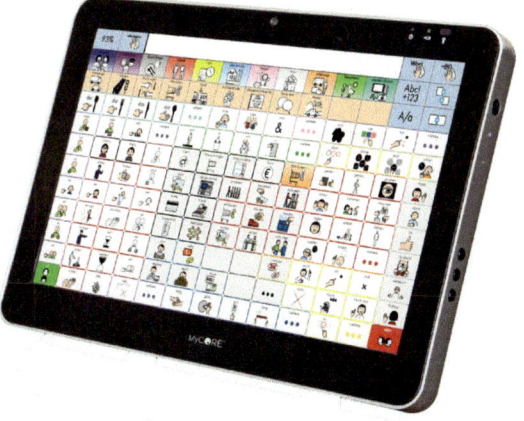

Fig. 13.5 *BIGmack®* (light-tech communication kit, size 17 cm). Reprinted from www.rehamedia.de. With kind permission of © AbleNet (2016). The *BIGmack®* is one of several switches suitable for initiating communication with voice. Utterances (e.g. intentions or wishes) can be recorded for up to 2 min in a loop and played back in an interaction with the child who presses the switch. So the child can manipulate the interaction himself or herself actively (e.g. recorded wish for more blowing of bubbles may be composed of a core vocabulary suitable for several play activities: 'More' or 'Again' or 'Do it again!'). The uses of at least two *BIGmacks®* with different coloured buttons are recommended for providing the possibility for decision-making or alternative wishes. Additionally, transparent buttons allow for fixing a symbol under them

Fig. 13.6 *MyCore13®*. Reprinted from www.rehamedia. de. With kind permission of © MyCore (2017). It is a VOCA (here with touch screen) with 2000 words. Vocabulary selection and organisation are based on the *Cologne Vocabulary*. The high-frequency words (core vocabulary) are statically provided as a frame around the topic pages with changing fringe vocabulary (raster of 6 × 5 in grey as a dynamic block). *MyCore13®* is available in English and German

and language skills and by providing a voice output model for speech (Cress and Marvin 2003). A meta-analysis of Millar et al. (2006) shows that none of the individuals treated with AAC had a decrease in speech production, but on the contrary, the majority (89%) had increased speech production as a result of AAC intervention. Regardless of a child's diagnosis, AAC systems have been provided to very young children, with positive gains in receptive and expressive language and communication skills (Sevcik et al. 2008). The existing literature suggests that AAC may provide strategies and systems to compensate for impairments and disabilities of individuals with severe communication disorders. AAC may also support literacy learning in children with special educational or complex needs (see Hetzroni 2004 and Koppenhaver and Williams 2010 for review).

Early intervention with AAC for young children at risk of expressive communication impairments is successful and recommended (Cress and Marvin 2003; Walker and Snell 2013). Access to AAC systems serves as a means to acquire some of the necessary prelinguistic and cognitive skills that are essential for language development (for overview, see Cress and Marvin 2003).

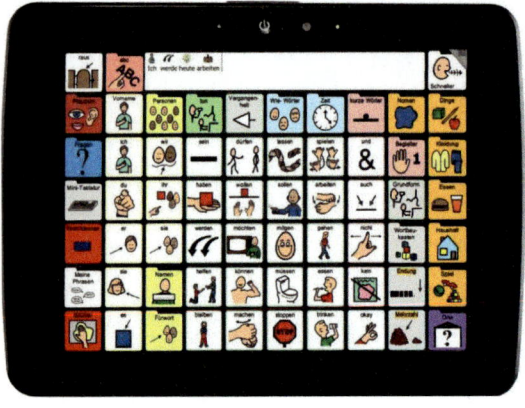

Fig. 13.7 *Tobii Dynavox T10®*. Reprinted from www.rehamedia.de. With kind permission of © Tobii Dynavox (2016). It is a very light tablet-based VOCA (here with touchscreen)

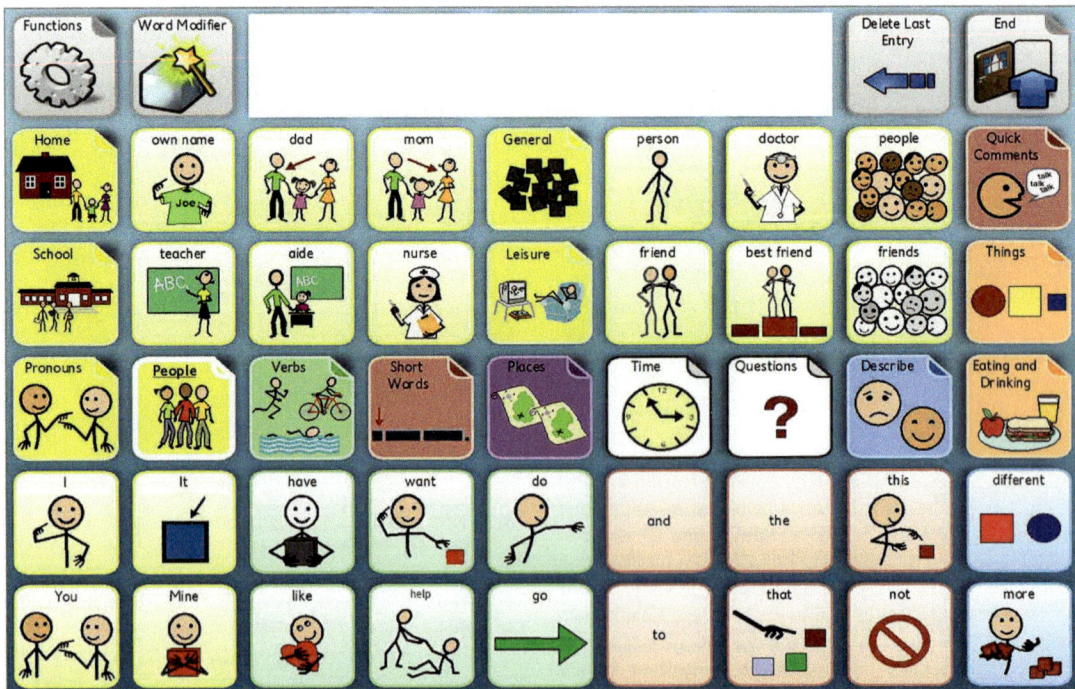

Fig. 13.8 *Tobii Sono Lexis®*. Reprinted from www.tobii-dynavox.de/sono-lexis/. With kind permission of © Tobii Dynavox (2016). Sono Lexis is a symbol-based communication software for VOCAs of Tobii Dynavox. It offers both a core and fringe vocabulary with static architecture and supports language learning via symbol-based communication combined with procedural memory learning. It uses the Fitzgerald Key colour coding. *Sono Lexis®* is available in English, German and other languages

As an example, a child who cannot independently hit a switch or who is not yet an intentional communicator might not be referred for AAC services if practitioners do not recognize that learning these skills is part of AAC service delivery, not a prerequisite to being qualified for AAC.

Cress and Marvin (2003)

The research for evidence of AAC intervention is demanding, because of the large heterogeneity of the population of children who need AAC and the large variety of AAC modes and the fast growth of innovative approaches (Costantino and Bonati 2014). A meta-analysis by Walker and Snell (2013) showed that AAC intervention is equally effective across a broad spectrum of participants and interventions. But it is even more effective in younger children than in older children or adults. Limitations of efficacy of AAC intervention are reviewed by Costantino and Bonati (2014). The number of AAC intervention studies with randomised controlled trials is still limited, and they are often of low quality. Hence, important intervention studies with higher methodological quality are required.

There are still some myths, already debunked, that may prevent clinicians from recommending AAC for intervention in children with delay in communication development. Table 13.1 shows the common myths and the evidence against them collected by Sevcik et al. (2008).

It is important to differentiate between sign languages primarily used by deaf people or in the deaf community and signs used in AAC as a means of intervention. In linguistic terms, sign languages include the fundamental properties that exist in all languages, executed in the visual-manual mode including a spatial grammar (Sandler and Lillo-Martin 2006). Signs used in AAC (e.g. Makaton®, see Fig. 13.3) are manual communication systems/programmes and artificially generated collections of signs, often borrowed from sign languages, to support the development of using language and communication in children with communication disorders. The Makaton® language programme, for example, has been effectively used with individuals who have cognitive impairments, autism, Down syndrome or multisensory impairment

Table 13.1 Myths regarding AAC and evidence against them

Myths	Evidence against myth
AAC is (only useful as) a last resort in speech and language intervention	AAC is in the speech-language pathologist's practice[a]
AAC hinders or stops further speech development	AAC approaches do not hinder speech development. In fact, data from young children show that it facilitates speech
Children must have certain skills to benefit from AAC	There are no prerequisites for using an AAC system. There is a continuum of [applicable] systems
Speech-generating devices are only for children with intact cognition	There are many types of speech-generating devices from simple to sophisticated available to choose from
Children have to be at a certain age to benefit from AAC	Children of all ages can learn to use AAC
There is a representational hierarchy from objects to printed words	Children can learn and use a variety of symbols

Table cited from Sevcik et al. (2008) with kind permission from Thieme Medical Publishers

[a]Complementary note from the author: certified training courses that fulfil the requirements of ISAAC (International Society for Augmentative and Alternative Communication) are recommended (www.isaac-online.org)

that negatively affect the ability to communicate (Beukelman and Mirenda 2005). Makaton® is a multimodal language programme using signs and symbols to help people to communicate. It was developed by MAgaret Walker, KAthy Johnston and TONy Conforth (Walker and Armfield 1981).

13.5.5 Selection and Organisation of a Vocabulary for AAC Intervention

Besides the decision on which AAC device suits the toddler's or child's needs and abilities best, the identification of suitable and age-appropriate vocabularies is challenging (Banajee et al. 2003).

To determine vocabulary for AAC intervention in children, there are three main approaches:

developmental, environmental and functional (for overview, see Banajee et al. 2003):

- Developmental: the use of developmental vocabulary lists, knowledge of the development of different word forms (e.g. nouns, verbs) and the number of words that children typically use at a certain age or the developmental level is used to determine vocabulary for AAC systems.
- Environmental: following an ecological inventory process, in which words appropriate for specific communication environments (i.e. fringe vocabulary) are identified for AAC.
- Functional: following functional communication needs by focusing on the pragmatic aspect of language. Vocabularies are chosen on the basis of expressed communication functions such as requesting, commenting, greeting and protesting.

The identification of vocabularies for toddlers involves aspects of all three approaches. As practice shows, the different focuses of these approaches lead to a large diversity of vocabulary lists recommended for ACC intervention without always matching the needs of children relying on AAC for language development. Resent research findings on vocabulary selection for ACC users underline the importance of distinguishing between core and fringe vocabularies (see, e.g. Beukelman et al. 1991; Balandin and Iacono 1999; Banajee et al. 2003; Boenisch 2014; Boenisch and Soto 2015). The core vocabulary research in AAC users of Beukelman and colleagues dates back to the 1980s (Beukelman et al. 1991) and is based on the idea of investigating the frequency and commonality of word occurrence in functional communication.

> Core vocabularies are small in size and do not change across environments or between individuals. Common words used across all communication environments comprise core vocabulary lists, which [especially] include structure words (e.g., want, more) that provide a framework for functional language use.
>
> Banajee et al. (2003)

Whereas core vocabulary especially includes structure words such as pronouns, auxiliary verbs, adverbs, prepositions, articles, conjunctions and some content words (nouns, verbs and adjectives) (Boenisch 2014), fringe vocabulary especially includes content words (nouns, verbs, adjectives) that change depending on topic and environment. A growing body of studies performed in various languages and populations (subjects differ, e.g. by age, cognition status, academic skills) on core vocabulary underlines the finding that the 50 most frequently used words (top 50) represent 50% of daily communication and that the 250 most frequently used words (top 250) represent 85% (for overview, see Boenisch 2014).

Applying these findings to vocabulary selection and organisation in AAC intervention, and on AAC devices, leads to the following conclusions and recommendations:

- Both core and fringe vocabularies are important for communication purposes and language development (Banajee et al. 2003).
- The selection and organisation of vocabulary in AAC have to account for the fact that children use core vocabulary more frequently than fringe vocabulary.
- Individual, developmental and environmental aspects have to be considered by selecting an AAC vocabulary for a child.
- AAC interventions aiming to support language development should follow a common underlying educational and therapeutic concept for vocabulary selection and organisation independent from the AAC modes and devices.

How are these findings implemented in ACC materials for intervention for children with DDSL? There are different approaches for applying these findings to practice:

- *Makaton®*: The multimodal language programme Makaton® (see Fig. 13.3) focuses on teaching core vocabulary as the base for communication. The signs and symbols are used with speech in spoken word order. Starting with the core vocabulary is recommended (core vocabulary sign book). The programme is available in several languages (www.makaton.org).

- *Cologne Communication Board and Binder®* (see Fig. 13.4a, b): Here, Boenisch and colleagues apply research data from a range of studies on core and fringe vocabulary in German (e.g. Boenisch and Sachse 2007) and English (e.g. Boenisch and Soto 2015) to their *Cologne Communication Boards and Binders®* and to the VOCA *MyCore®* (see Fig. 13.6). In all these AAC materials and devices of the Cologne group, a static visible and accessible raster for core vocabulary frames a flexible and dynamic adaptable raster for fringe words (Fig. 13.9). In practice the communication partner gives feedback to the child by correcting and expanding his or her communication attempts: he or she touches the symbols or guides the child's hand with accompanying talk. When she or he talks to the child, the boards or binders are also used in parallel (modelling). By this, children experience and learn the use of language. The frequent recurring of simple motoric procedures by touching the static symbols for utterances with core vocabulary supports children's language use and comprehension (procedural memory learning), even if the complexity of the device increases. The use of the vocabulary and expanding it is supported by the so-called focus-word approach of Sachse and Willke (2011). Enhancing grammar skills is possible to correct expressive grammar use with the *MyCore®*. The Cologne AAC material constitutes a comprehensive multimodal approach to support language development based on current research findings.

- *Minspeak®*: This is an internationally widely used coding strategy for VOCAs only. It is a word strategy that uses semantic coding, developed by Baker in the 1980s. It uses multi-meaning icons associated with a single picture. The use of core vocabulary is also supported by *Minspeak®* (Baker et al. 2000). It uses rules and patterns for organising and coding vocabulary. Simple pictures represent a category of words, such as *Mr. Action Man* for

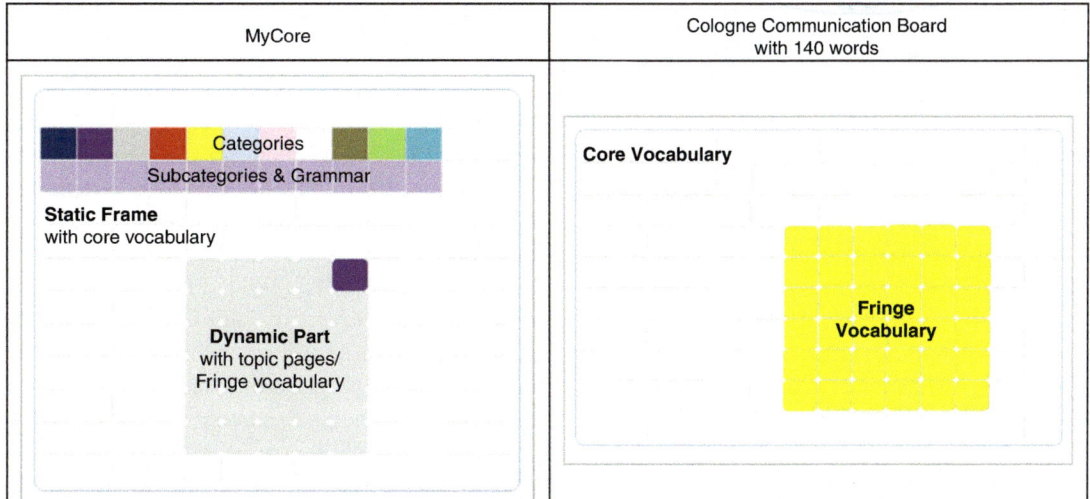

Fig. 13.9 Scheme of organisation of core and fringe vocabulary for the *Cologne Vocabulary* on the *Cologne Communication Board®*, (right, see also Fig. 13.4b) and its application on the VOCA *MyCore®* (left, see also Fig. 13.6). Reprinted from www.fbz-uk.uni-koeln.de/36720. With kind permission of © Boenisch and Sachse (2017)

verbs, *Mother Hubbard* for nouns and *Paintbrush* for adjectives. The person using *Minspeak®* has to learn a small set of pictures—usually less than 100—and then learns the rules for combining those icons to short icon sequences. *Minspeak®* icons are combined in two- or three-part sequences (e.g. by combining the pictures *cube* and *paintbrush*, a child says the word 'little') *(http://www.minspeak.com/).* Expanding the vocabulary and enhancing grammar skills are possible to correct expressive grammar use. The memory requirements for icon sequences are high for a user. *Minspeak®* strategy is used on the following VOCAs with dynamic display: *Accent®* or *Nova chat®* (© Prentke Romich, www.minspeak.com).

13.5.6 Aims of AAC Intervention

AAC interventions use a flexible and child-and-family-centred approach that focuses on early enhancing the communicative competence of a child and his or her successful participation in social life (Granlund et al. 2008; WHO 2007). Via ACC intervention the expansion of vocabulary and an enhancement of grammar and literacy skills should be individually supported as well as possible within the cognitive and communicative resources of the child. The speech and language therapy should implement a multimodal approach in order to enhance effective communication that is (pre)linguistically appropriate and aims at facilitating the quality of life of a child (ASHA 2005; WHO 2007).

13.6 Principles of Computerised Rehabilitation

Karen Reichmuth

13.6.1 Introduction

Despite the enormous influence digital media have on daily life, fundamental research on computer-based learning and its effects on child development in general are still limited. The impact that computer-based learning may have on language and literacy development in children with related disorders is currently of particular interest. The advantages of digital media for the rehabilitation of developmental language, literacy and hearing disorders seem obvious. Digital media have a highly stimulative nature, enable higher training frequency at home and may reduce costs of rehabilitation. The following report on the efficacy of computerised training on developmental language, literacy and hearing disorders is based on an electronic search of the *MEDLINE* database and manual search for reviews and meta-analyses since the year 2000. The reviews were based on intervention studies published in peer-reviewed journals.

13.6.2 'Fast ForWord'® (FFW)

Most reviews found addressed the language intervention programme *Fast ForWord®* (developed by Scientific Learning Corporation, 1999; www.scilearnglobal.com), which is commonly used in English-speaking countries (Sisson 2009; Cirrin and Gillam 2008; Loo et al. 2010; Strong et al. 2011).

Fast ForWord® (FFW) consists of a sample of computer-based intervention programmes designed to advance language and literacy skills in children with language-learning difficulties who are from 4 to 14 years of age. It was developed on the basis of the *rapid auditory processing deficit* theory of Tallal (1980, 2013), which states that impaired perception and discrimination of auditory stimuli negatively influence the typical development of language and reading. FFW uses acoustically modified non-speech and speech sounds. The developers of FFW claim that appropriate training may lead to lasting improvements in the neural systems that underlay the learning of language and, as a consequence, to better language and reading skills. Results of intervention studies with FFW by Merzenich et al. (1996) and Tallal (2013) supported the theory. However, the *rapid auditory processing deficit* theory is not universally accepted as an exclusive explanation for specific language and reading disorders. A large corpus of studies can be found that reflects the very controversial discussion on the efficacy of FFW (for an overview, see Strong et al. 2011; Loo et al. 2010). The meta-analytical review by Strong et al. (2011) revealed that:

> there is no evidence from the analysis carried out that 'Fast ForWord'-Program is effective as a treatment for children's oral language or reading difficulties.

These results support the conclusions drawn by Sisson (2009), Cirrin and Gillam (2008) and Loo et al. (2010) that there is a gap in the body of evidence supporting the efficacy of FFW. Despite this, Tallal (2013), the developer of the theory on which FFW is based, still describes FFW as a 'neurocognitive training revolution.' But following the conclusion of an evidential gap reported in the reviews cited here, FFW cannot be recommended uncritically for the computerised rehabilitation of developmental language and literacy disorders.

13.6.3 'My Sentence Builder'© (MSB) to Train Expressive Grammar

The computer-assisted treatment programme 'My Sentence Builder'© (MSB) (Washington and Warr-Leeper 2006) was developed to train expressive grammar in preschool children with specific developmental disorders of speech and language (SDDSL; synonym: specific language impairment, SLI). The development of the programme was based on the theory that verbal memory deficits in children with SDDSL lead to

> slow processing of rapid successive and unstressed elements in the spoken language stream (Washington et al. 2011)

especially for grammatical morphemes. In consequence, this

> inability to process the auditory elements hinders the abstraction of underlying rules and thus results in agrammatical productions (Washington et al. 2011)

in children with SDDSL. The MSB therefore provides additional visual support by the use of pictures and colour codes to visualise different sentence elements, syntactics and grammatical morphemes. The authors themselves conducted an intervention study with a randomised, controlled procedure to test the efficacy of MSB (Washington et al. 2011). The study compared the outcomes of treatment of preschool children with SDDSL by MSB, an alternative noncomputerised grammar treatment, and 'just waiting' without treatment (the control group). The results showed significant treatment benefits for both treatment groups compared with the control group, but no significant difference between MSB and the alternative conventional noncomputerised treatment. The authors themselves concluded that the MSB is

> viable, but not necessarily a better treatment option (Washington et al. 2011)

for expressive grammar deficits in preschool children with SDDSL. From the design of the study, the effects found are of good evidential standard, but the researchers were themselves the distributor of MSB and therefore had conflicts of interest. Further independent research, including reviews and meta-analyses, are needed to prove the efficacy of MSB that Washington et al. (2011) found.

13.6.4 'Earobics'® and Other Auditory Training Programmes

A review by Loo et al. (2010) reports the evidence for different computer-based auditory training programmes in children with language, reading and related learning difficulties. Studies with different commercial programmes, such as FFW and 'Earobics'® (http://www.earobics.com/), and noncommercial programmes focusing on phonological awareness, non-speech and simple speech sound training were analysed. 'Earobics' comprises a suite of computer-based programmes to improve phonological awareness and auditory-language processing as well as reading and spelling skills. Very few studies have been conducted with this programme on children with problems in language and reading development. In summarising the results, Loo et al. (2010) pointed out that

'Earobics' seems to have a positive impact on phonological awareness but not on reading or spelling skills.

Loo et al. (2010) also reported various non-commercial computer-based training studies for children with developmental language and reading disorders. The training activities included non-speech and simple speech sounds, such as phonemes or consonant-vowel syllables. The results demonstrated that there was an effect on reading skill but only if the training delivered a combination of audio-visual methods. None of the studies reviewed included language measures, so nothing can be reported about the effect the programmes may have on receptive or expressive language development (see Loo et al. 2010 for an overview).

13.6.5 'Cogmed Working Memory Training' (CWMT)

Because verbal working memory is a basic neuropsychological skill that plays a key role in language processing, reviews reporting 'Cogmed working-memory training' (CWMT) (http://www.cogmed.com/) are included here. CWMT is designed to improve visuospatial and verbal working memory as well as attention (Shinaver et al. 2014). CWMT has been evaluated for different target groups, but not for children with developmental disorder of speech and language and literacy difficulties (Shinaver et al. 2014). Controversial discussion around the efficacy of CWMT can be found in various reviews (for overview, see Shinaver et al. 2014). CWMT has been used in a pilot study for children with a severe or profound bilateral hearing loss from birth, after receiving cochlear implants (CI; Kronenberger et al. 2011). This study performed a within-group comparison with only a 2–5-week waiting period after a first assessment as control condition, a subsequent training period with CWMT and a 6-month follow-up period. Working memory skills improved during the training period, but there were rather weak or no long-term effects, except for the ability of sentence repetition which improved later on. Although the training effect found was of low evidential standard (no correction for typical improvement by age was made), the authors pointed to the importance of conducting a large-scale, randomised clinical trial with this population. In sum, Shinaver et al. (2014) rate the CWMT programme positively but suggest the need for further research, which seems worthwhile, especially for children with developmental language, literacy and hearing disorders.

13.6.6 Résumé and Perspectives

To summarise, research on the use of computerised intervention programmes in the rehabilitation of developmental language, literacy and hearing disorders has so far been very limited. The reviews and meta-analyses found in the literature since the year 2000 reveal no convincing efficacy for the widespread language intervention programme FFW. To treat expressive grammar in preschool children with SDDSL, the programme 'My Sentence Builder' seems to be effective but no better than common behavioural language treatment without a computer. Independent research on the MSB is necessary. A low level of efficacy has been shown for auditory training to improve phonological awareness, for example, by using 'Earobics'. The use of specific noncommercial programmes can also be beneficial for reading skills, as long as training delivers a combination of audio-visual methods. Studies on other linguistic skills are still lacking. There are some promising findings on computer-based training for working memory as an important underlying skill for children in the target groups focused on here, e.g. for sentence repetition in children fitted with CI. Further research following the principles of high-quality, evidence-based practice is necessary.

13.7 Prognosis

Christiane Kiese-Himmel

13.7.1 Introduction

The prognosis for a particular child with a developmental disorder of speech and language (DDSL) depends on a variety of factors. In general, a trend for improvement of DDSL can be observed over time. Difficulties in language functioning (residual symptoms), however, persist—carrying into mid-childhood, adolescence and adulthood—even when the disorder appears to be resolved after treatment (see Johnson et al. 2010). Moreover, children, adolescents and adults may also suffer from lifelong consequences in terms of communication disorders, psychosocial disturbances, academic deficits and behaviour problems. Nevertheless, substantial individual differences in outcome can be found. Primarily, the prognosis of a DDSL depends on the type of language disorder, severity in the symptom domains of the language disorder, associated disorders (co-morbidities), multilevel risk factors such as concomitant problems in the family environment (e.g. poverty and its associated factors, socio-economic disadvantage, unstimulating environment) and other individual conditions (e.g. preterm born, poor health, history of recurrent or chronic otitis media). Children who receive early and appropriate therapy are more likely to have a better outcome.

The following passages depict some disorders from the spectrum of DDSL listed in Sect. 9.1 as examples.

13.7.2 Late Talking/Developmental Language Delay in the Absence of Other Developmental Problems

Late talkers may show uneven profiles of language outcome. Developmental language delay can change for the better or even remit without intervention ('late bloomers'), but this is not necessarily the case though catch-up development may be expected (see Rescorla and Dale 2013). As a rough estimate, 35–60% (e.g. Dale et al. 2003; 56% reported for Germany, Sachse and von Suchodoletz 2013) improve until the age of 3–4 years and reach language abilities within the normal range. However, on average they obtain significantly lower scores in the outcome measures compared with children with typical language history (Rescorla 2011). In the remainder, late talker status may be a precursor of specific language impairment by 3 or 4 years of age (e.g. Dale et al. 2003).

13.7.3 Specific Developmental Disorders of Speech and Language (SDDSL)

SDDSL is also called 'primary language impairment' or 'specific language impairment' (SLI). The prognosis depends on the type (receptive or expressive) and severity of the SLI. Children with a history of SLI often have deficits in literacy skills and school attainment. Findings provide strong evidence that children with DDSL demonstrate persisting difficulties with oral narrative skills in mid-childhood; continued deficits in verbal short-term memory, phonological processing and reading; and a weakness in language-related skills into adolescence, sometimes even in adulthood. A family history of specific reading disorders is a sensitive predictor of specific reading or spelling disorders at primary school ages. In addition, various negative psychological outcomes have been reported (poor psychosocial adjustment, affective disturbance, abnormalities in interpersonal relationships and emotional and behavioural disorders, attention deficit disorders with or without hyperactivity). However, the relationship between language impairment and difficulties in mid-childhood and later childhood as well as in adolescence remains unclear. Expressive language deficits are often associated with internalising problems and social withdrawal. Receptive language deficits involve substantial social adaption difficulties and carry the greatest risk of childhood psychopathology and psychiatric disorder in adult life.

13.7.4 Childhood Dysphasia with Landau-Kleffner Syndrome

Language improves over time by speech language therapy, but language deficits tend to persist in most children (Duran et al. 2009). The older a child is at onset of the auditory processing/receptive and expressive language disorder, the better seems to be the prognosis for language development.

13.7.5 Other Developmental Disorders of Speech and Language

These include lisping or DDSL associated with co-morbidities, for example:

- Hearing loss

    Children with early-identified permanent hearing loss without additional disabilities in a beneficial living environment, who received early adequate assisting hearing devices (before 6 months of age) and were enrolled in auditory-verbal rehabilitation, may reach performances in speech and language tests within the normal range. Outcomes in communication skills and quality of life are usually improved. This is also true for children with severe or profound bilateral sensorineural hearing loss. A low educational level of the mother is a negative factor. Compared with children who are hard of hearing from birth on, children who loose their hearing post-lingually, which means after oral language acquisition, have less impaired language development.
- Pervasive developmental disorders such as autism spectrum disorders

    Language development in children may vary considerably as a result of cognitive functioning and social development but rarely reach a normal level. Longitudinal research has found a relationship between joint attention abilities (i.e. shared attention between social partners in relation to objects or events including gaze following and pointing), interactive play behaviour and imitation abilities in typically developing young children and their later language skills. Thus, such non-verbal communication skills at age 2–3 years, especially the frequency of joint attention, are strong predictors of expressive language outcome in autistic children. Additionally, early language ability and social communication skills in children with autism are associated with later academic achievement. Even though variability in language increases over time, children tend also to experience continued deficits in reading skills, especially in reading comprehension skills.

In summary, children with less severe DDSL will show a greater improvement than those with more or with severe problems who need special treatment and education. In general, the younger the child at the onset of therapy, the better the prognosis except for childhood dysphasia with Landau-Kleffner Syndrome, here the opposite is true. Evidence demonstrates a positive effect of an optimal early age- and grade-appropriate language intervention (including parental advice, parent-directed programmes and positive family support), particularly for children with expressive-only DDSL.

References

American Speech-Language-Hearing Association (2005) Roles and responsibilities of speech-language pathologists with respect to augmentative and alternative communication: position statement. Available via www.asha.org/policy. Accessed 3 May 2018

Baker B, Hill K, Devylder R (2000) Core vocabulary is the same across environments. Paper presented at a meeting of the technology and persons with disabilities conference at California State University, Northridge, Los Angeles, CA

Balandin S, Iacono T (1999) Crews, Wusses, and Whoppas: core and fringe vocabularies of Australian meal-break conversations in the workplace. Augment Altern Commun 15(2):95–109

Banajee M, Dicarlo C, Buras Stricklin S (2003) Core vocabulary determination for toddlers. Augment Altern Commun 19(2):67–73

Beukelman D, Mirenda P (2005) Symbols and rate enhancement. Augmentative alternative communication: supporting children and adults with complex communication need. Paul H. Brookes Pub. Co., Baltimore, pp 65–67

Beukelman D, McGinnis J, Morrow D (1991) Vocabulary selection in augmentative and alternative communication. Augment Altern Commun 7(3):171–185

Bobath K (1984) Uma base neurofisiológica para o tratamento da paralisia cerebral, 2nd edn. Manole, São Paulo

Boenisch J (2014) Kern-Vokabular im Kindes- und Jugendalter: Vergleichsstudie zum Sprachgebrauch von Schülerinnen und Schülern mit und ohne geistige Behinderung und Konsequenzen für die UK. UK & Forschung 3:4–23. Sonderbeilage Unterstützte Kommunikation 1/2014

Boenisch J, Sachse S (2007) Diagnostik und Beratung in der Unterstützten Kommunikation. Theorie, Forschung, Praxis. Von Loeper Literaturverlag, Karlsruhe

Boenisch J, Soto G (2015) The oral core vocabulary of typically developing English-speaking school-aged children. Augment Altern Commun 31(1): 77–84

Boons T, Brokx JP, Dhooge I et al (2012) Predictors of spoken language development following pediatric cochlear implantation. Ear Hear 33(5):617–639

Branson D, Demchak M (2009) The use of augmentative and alternative communication methods with infants and toddlers with disabilities: a research review. Augment Altern Commun 25(4):274–286

Cirrin FM, Gillam RB (2008) Language intervention practices for school-age children with spoken language disorders: a systematic review. Lang Speech Hear Serv Sch 39:110–137

Costantino MA, Bonati M (2014) A scoping review of interventions to supplement spoken communication for children with limited speech or language skills. PLoS One 9(3):e90744. https://doi.org/10.1371/journal.pone.0090744

Cress CJ, Marvin CA (2003) Common questions about AAC services in early intervention. Augment Altern Commun 19(4):264–272

Dale PS, Price TS, Bishop DV et al (2003) Outcomes of early language delay: I. Predicting persistent and transient language difficulties at 3 and 4 years. J Speech Lang Hear Res 46(3):544–560

Dirks T, Hadders-Algra M (2011) The role of the family in intervention of infants at high risk of cerebral palsy: a systematic analysis. Dev Med Child Neurol 53(Suppl 4):62–67

Duran MH, Guimaraes CA, Medeiros LL, Guerreiro MM (2009) Landau-Kleffner syndrome: long-term follow-up. Brain Dev 31(1):58–63

Engelhardt HT (1996) The foundations of bioethics. Oxford University Press, New York

Fisher AG (2009) Occupational therapy intervention process model: a model for planning and implementing top-down, client centred, and occupation-based interventions. Three Star Press, Fort Collins

Fisher AG, Bryze K, Hume V et al (2007) School assessment of motor and process skills, 2nd edn. Three Star Press, Fort Collins

Franki I, Desloovere K, De Cat J et al (2012) The evidence-base for conceptual approaches and additional therapies targeting lower limb function in children with cerebral palsy: a systematic review using the ICF as a framework. J Rehabil Med 44(5):396–405

Graham F, Rodger S, Ziviani J (2013) Effectiveness of occupational performance coaching in improving children's and mothers' performance and mothers' self-competence. Am J Occup Ther 67(1):10–18

Granlund M, Björck-Akesson E, Wilder J et al (2008) Interventions for children in a family environment: implementing evidence in practice. Augment Altern Commun 24(3):207–219

Gutzmann H (1912) Sprachheilkunde. Vorlesungen über die Störungen der Sprache mit besonderer Berücksichtigung der Therapie. Fischer's medicinische Buchhandlung, H. Kornfeld, Berlin

Hetzroni OE (2004) AAC and literacy. Review. Disabil Rehabil 26(21–22):1305–1312

Hirata GC, Santos RS (2012) Rehabilitation of oropharyngeal dysphagia in children with cerebral palsy: a systematic review of the speech therapy approach. Int Arch Otorhinolaryngol 16(3):396–399

Johnson CJ, Beitchman JH, Brownlie EB (2010) Twenty-year follow-up of children with and without speech-language impairments: family, educational, occupational, and quality of life outcomes. Am J Speech Lang Pathol 19(1):51–65

Kim LS, Jeong SW, Lee YM et al (2010) Cochlear implantation in children. Auris Nasus Larynx 37(1):6–17

Koppenhaver D, Williams A (2010) A conceptual review of writing research in augmentative and alternative communication. Augment Altern Commun 26(3):158–176. https://doi.org/10.3109/07434618.2010.505608

Korbmacher HM, Limbrock JG, Kahl-Nieke B (2006) Long-term evaluation of orofacial function in children with Down syndrome after treatment with a stimulating plate according to Castillo Morales. J Clin Pediatr Dent 30(4):325–328

Kronenberger WG, Henning SC, Colson BG et al (2011) Working memory training for children with cochlear implants: a pilot study. J Speech Lang Hear Res 54(4):1182–1196

Law M, Darrah J (2014) Emerging therapy approaches: an emphasis on function. J Child Neurol 29(8):1101–1107

Light J, Drager K (2007) AAC technologies for young children with complex communication needs: state of the science and future research directions. Augment Altern Commun 23(3):204–216

Locke EA, Latham GP (2002) Building a practically useful theory of goal setting and task motivation: a 35-year odyssey. Am Psychol 57(9):705–717

Loo JH, Bamiou DE, Campbell N et al (2010) Computer-based auditory training (CBAT): benefits for children with language- and reading-related learning difficulties. Review. Dev Med Child Neurol 52(8):708–717

Meinzen-Derr J, Wiley S, Grether S et al (2011) Children with Cochlea implants and developmental disabilities: a language skills study with developmentally matched hearing peers. Res Dev Disabil 32(2):757–767

Meinzen-Derr J, Wiley S, Grether S et al (2013) Functional performance among children with cochlear implants and additional disabilities. Cochlear Implants Int 14(4):181–189. https://doi.org/10.1179/17547628 12Y.0000000019. Epub 2013 Feb 9

Merzenich MM, Jenkins WM, Johnston P et al (1996) Temporal processing deficits of language-learning impaired children ameliorated by training. Science 271(5245):77–81

Millar DC, Light JC, Schlosser RW (2006) The impact of augmentative and alternative communication intervention on the speech production of individuals with developmental disabilities: a research review. J Speech Lang Hear Res 49(2):248–264

Morales RC (1999) Terapia de regulação orofacial: Conceito RCM. Memnon, São Paulo

Neumann K, Euler HA, Bosshardt HG et al (2016) Pathogenese, Diagnostik und Behandlung von Redeflussstörungen. Evidenz- und konsensbasierte S3-Leitlinie, AWMF-Registernummer 049-013, Version 1. 2016. Im Auftrag der Leitliniengruppe [Pathogenesis, diagnostics, and treatment of fluency disorders. Evidence and consensus-based S3-guideline, AWMF-registry number 049-013, version 1. 2016. On behalf of the consensus group]. Available via http://www.awmf.org/leitlinien/detail/ll/049-013.html. Accessed 5 Oct 2016

Patel DR (2005) Therapeutic interventions in cerebral palsy. Indian J Pediatr 72(11):979–983

Rescorla LA (2011) Late talkers: do good predictors of outcome exist? Dev Disabil Res Rev 17(2):141–150

Rescorla LA, Dale PS (2013) Late talkers: language development, interventions, and outcomes. Paul H Brookes Publishing, Baltimore

Sachse S, von Suchodoletz W (2013) Sprachentwicklung von der U7 bis zur U7a bei Kindern mit und ohne Sprachentwicklungsverzögerungen. Klin Pediatr 225(4):194–200

Sachse S, Willke M (2011) Fokuswörter in der Unterstützten Kommunikation. Ein Konzept zum sukzessiven Wortschatzaufbau. In: Bollmeyer H et al (eds) UK inklusive—Teilhabe durch Unterstützte Kommunikation. Von Loeper Literaturverlag, Karlsruhe

Sandler W, Lillo-Martin D (2006) Sign language and linguistic universals. Cambridge University Press, Cambridge

Sevcik RA, Barton-Hulsey A, Romski M (2008) Early intervention, AAC, and transition to school for young children with significant spoken communication disorders and their families. Semin Speech Lang 29(2):92–100

Shinaver CS, Entwistle PC, Söderqvist S (2014) Cogmed WM training: reviewing the reviews. Appl Neuropsychol Child 3(3):163–172

Sisson CB (2009) A meta-analytic investigation into the efficacy of Fast ForWord intervention on improving academic performance. Doctoral dissertation, Regent University. Diss Abstr Int, Section A: Humanities and Social Sciences 69(12-A):4633

Strong GK, Torgerson CJ, Torgerson D et al (2011) A systematic meta-analytic review of evidence for the effectiveness of the 'Fast ForWord' language intervention program. J Child Psychol Psychiatry 52(3):224–235

Tallal P (1980) Auditory temporal perception, phonics, and reading disabilities in children. Brain Lang 9(2):182–198

Tallal P (2013) Fast ForWord®: the birth of the neurocognitive training revolution. Prog Brain Res 207:175–207

Townsend E, Polatajko HJ (2007) Enabling occupation II: advancing an occupational therapy vision for health, well-being and justice through occupation. Canadian Association of Occupational Therapists, Ottawa

von Loeper Literaturverlag, isaac—Gesellschaft für Unterstützte Kommunikation e. V. (eds) (2012) Handbuch der Unterstützten Kommunikation, vol 1–2. Von Loeper Literaturverlag, Karlsruhe

von Tetzchner S, Martinsen H (1992) Introduction to symbolic and augmentative communication. Whurr/Wiley, London

Walker M, Armfield A (1981) What is the Makaton vocabulary? Spec Educ Forward Trends 8(3):19–20

Walker VL, Snell ME (2013) Effects of augmentative and alternative communication on challenging behavior: a meta-analysis. Review. Augment Altern Commun 29(2):117–131

Waltersbacher A, Wissenschaftliches Institut der AOK (WIdO) (2015) Heilmittelbericht 2015. [Scientific Institute of the AOK (WIdO). Remedy report 2015]. Available via http://www.wido.de/fileadmin/wido/downloads/pdf_heil_hilfsmittel/wido_hei_hmb2015_1512.pdf. Accessed 11 Sept 2016

Washington KN, Warr-Leeper GA (2006) A collaborative approach to computer-assisted treatment of preschool children with specific language impairment. OSLA Connect J 2(2):10–11

Washington KN, Warr-Leeper G, Thomas-Stonell N (2011) Exploring the outcomes of a novel computer-assisted treatment program targeting expressive-grammar deficits in preschoolers with SLI. J Commun Dis 44(3):315–330

Wilkinson KM, Hennig S (2007) The state of research and practice in augmentative and alternative communication for children with developmental/intellectual disabilities. Ment Retard Dev Disabil Res Rev 13(1):58–69

World Health Organization (2001) International classification of functioning, disability and health: ICF. World Health Organization, Geneva

World Health Organization (2007) International classification of functioning, disability, and health: children and youth version: ICF-CY. WHO Press, Geneva. Available via http://apps.who.int/iris/bitstream/10665/43737/1/9789241547321_eng.pdf. Accessed 31 Aug 2014

Part IV

Disorders of Hearing Development

Editor: Antoinette am Zehnhoff-Dinnesen

Lectors: Manfred Gross,
Antoinette am Zehnhoff-Dinnesen,
Ross Parfitt

Basics of Disorders of Hearing Development

14

Antoinette am Zehnhoff-Dinnesen,
Wendy Albuquerque, Hanno J. Bolz,
Steffi Johanna Brockmeier, Thorsten Langer,
Radha Narayan, Ross Parfitt,
Simona Poisson-Markova, Ewa Raglan,
Sabrina Regele, Rainer Schönweiler,
Pavel Seeman, Eva Seemanova,
Amélie Elisabeth Tillmanns, and Oliver Zolk

A. am Zehnhoff-Dinnesen · R. Parfitt · S. Regele
A. E. Tillmanns
Clinic of Phoniatrics and Pedaudiology, University
Hospital Münster, Münster, Germany
e-mail: am.zehnhoff@uni-muenster.de;
ross.parfitt@ukmuenster.de;
sabrina.regele@ukmuenster.de;
AmelieElisabeth.Tillmanns@ukmuenster.de

W. Albuquerque
Department of ENT and Audiovestibular Medicine,
St Georges Healthcare NHS Trust, London, UK
e-mail: Wendy.albuquerque@stgeorges.nhs.uk

H. J. Bolz
Senckenberg Centre for Human Genetics,
Frankfurt am Main, Germany
e-mail: h.bolz@senckenberg-humangenetik.de

S. J. Brockmeier
ENT Clinic, Audiology, Phoniatrics, Neuro-Otology,
Kantonsspital Aarau AG, Aarau, Switzerland
e-mail: hanna.brockmeier@ksa.ch

T. Langer
Department of Pediatric Oncology and Hematology,
University Hospital Schleswig-Holstein, Campus
Lübeck, Lübeck, Germany
e-mail: thorsten.langer@uksh.de

R. Narayan
The Whittington Hospital, London, UK
e-mail: radha.narayan@nhs.net

S. Poisson-Markova · P. Seeman · E. Seemanova
Department of Child Neurology, 2nd Medical School
of Charles University Prague,
Prague, Czech Republic
e-mail: s.markova@lfmotol.cuni.cz;
Pavel.seeman@lfmotol.cuni.cz;
Eva.seemanova@lfmotol.cuni.cz

E. Raglan
Department of Audiology and Audiovestibular
Medicine, Great Ormond Street Hospital for Children
NHS Foundation Trust, London, UK
e-mail: eraglan@doctors.org.uk

R. Schönweiler
Department of Phoniatrics and Pediatric Audiology,
University Clinic of Schleswig-Holstein, Campus
Lübeck, Lübeck, Germany
e-mail: rainer.schoenweiler@phoniatrie.uni-luebeck.de

O. Zolk
Institute of Pharmacology of Natural Products and
Clinical Pharmacology, University Hospital Ulm,
Ulm, Germany
e-mail: oliver.zolk@uni-ulm.de

© Springer-Verlag GmbH Germany, part of Springer Nature 2020
A. am Zehnhoff-Dinnesen et al. (eds.), *Phoniatrics I*, European Manual of Medicine,
https://doi.org/10.1007/978-3-662-46780-0_14

14.1 Definition of Hearing Loss and Audiological Grading Scales

Antoinette am Zehnhoff-Dinnesen

> Hearing loss, hearing impairment, or deafness is a partial or total inability to hear.
> Encyclopaedia Britannica Online (2011)

Diseases of the outer or middle ear cause conductive hearing loss, impairment of inner ear structures/auditory nerves evokes sensorineural hearing loss, and damage to the central auditory system generates central hearing loss. Combinations are possible, called mixed hearing loss, when conductive and sensorineural hearing loss are collated. Hearing impairment is the most frequent sensory deficit (Mathers et al. 2003). The focus of Part IV is the development of hearing and its disorders. Hearing loss in childhood impedes speech and language acquisition, leading to reduced communication ability, adverse psychosocial effects and academic disadvantages. Audiological classifications with different aims and complexity have been developed for reporting the incidence and severity of hearing loss, e.g. the Common Terminology Criteria for Adverse Events (CTCAE) v4.0 considers functional aspects (National Institutes of Health NIH and National Cancer Institute NCI 2010), and the Münster Classification (Schmidt et al. 2007) includes slight hearing changes and tinnitus for early detection of hearing loss. The WHO defines the degrees slight, moderate, severe and profound (Mathers et al. 2003; World Health Organization 2013). Some grading systems are shown in Table 14.1; some are presented and discussed in detail, e.g. in Stevens et al. (2011), Lafay-Cousin et al. (2013), Landier et al. (2014) and Knight et al. (2016). Hearing loss can affect one or both ears and different frequencies to different extents. Types and time courses of hearing loss are presented in detail in Sect. 15.1.

14.2 Epidemiology of Hearing Disorders in Children

Ross Parfitt and Amélie Elisabeth Tillmanns

14.2.1 Introduction

Epidemiology is

> the study of the distribution and determinants of disease frequency in [the] human population.
> Davis et al. (2004)

The distribution of hearing disorders is usually reported by *prevalence*, which is

> the proportion of individuals with a defined type of hearing impairment in a specified population cohort.
> Sancho et al. (1998), cited in Davis et al. (2004)

This is typically expressed as a percentage of that population or the number of affected individuals per thousand of the population. The term *incidence* means the number of new cases within a defined time period.

Various figures for the prevalence of hearing disorders in children have been reported, such as 1.3 per 1000 (Fortnum and Davis 1997), 5.6 per 1000 (Watkin et al. 1990) and 1.4% (Stevens et al. 2013). Faced with such differing prevalence values, we need to know the details behind each study. When factors such as differences in the study populations and definitions of hearing impairment are taken into account, the prevalence emerging from these studies is more clearly comparable, resulting in the figures 1.3 per 1000 (Fortnum and Davis 1997), 2.1 per 1000 (Watkin et al. 1990) and 4.0 per 1000 (Stevens et al. 2013). The following section goes into greater detail about these and other examples.

Table 14.1 Audiological grading scales

Grade	ASHA Guidelines (1994)	BIAP (1996)[a]	WHO Global Burden of Disease 2000 (Mathers et al. 2003)[a]	Münster classification (Schmidt et al. 2007)	CTCAE v.4.0 NIH NCI (2010)	Chang Practical Grading System (Chang and Chinosornvatana 2010)	SIOP Boston Ototoxicity Scale (Brock et al. 2012)	WHO Global Burden of Disease (2013)[a]
0		I. Normal or subnormal: <20 dB	0: No impairment: ≤25 dB HL	0: No impairment: ≤10 dB HL at all frequencies		0: ≤20 dB HL at 1, 2 and 4 kHz	0: ≤20 dB HL at all frequencies	
1	(A) 20 dB or greater decrease in pure-tone threshold at any test frequency	II. Mild: 21–40 dB	1: Slight impairment: 26–40 dB HL	1: Onset of impairment: >10 and ≤20 dB HL at one or more frequencies, or tinnitus	1: Mild; asymptomatic or mild symptoms; clinical or diagnostic observations only; intervention not indicated: In adults 15–25 dB HL at two contiguous frequencies/subjective change; in children >20 dB HL at 8 kHz	1a: ≥40 dB HL at any frequency 6–12 kHz 1b: >20 and <40 dB HL at 4 kHz	1: >20 dB HL above 4 kHz	Mild: 20–34 dB HL
2	(B) 10 dB or greater decrease at two adjacent test frequencies	III. Moderate: 1st degree: 41–55 dB 2nd degree: 56–70 dB IV. Severe: 1st degree: 71–80 dB 2nd degree: 81–90 dB	2: Moderate impairment: 41–60 dB HL	2: Moderate impairment: >20 dB HL at 4 kHz and above 2a: >20 to ≤40 dB HL 2b: >40 to ≤60 dB HL 2c: >60 dB HL	2: Moderate; minimal intervention indicated: In adults >25 dB HL at two contiguous frequencies/limiting instrumental ADL; in children >20 dB HL at 4 kHz and above	2a: ≥40 dB HL at 4 kHz and above 2b: >20 dB HL and <40 dB at any freq below 4 kHz	2: >20 dB HL at 4 kHz and above	Moderate: 35–49 dB HL Moderately severe: 50–64 dB HL

(continued)

Table 14.1 (continued)

Grade	ASHA Guidelines (1994)	BIAP (1996)[a]	WHO Global Burden of Disease 2000 (Mathers et al. 2003)[a]	Münster classification (Schmidt et al. 2007)	CTCAE v.4.0 NIH NCI (2010)	Chang Practical Grading System (Chang and Chinosornvatana 2010)	SIOP Boston Ototoxicity Scale (Brock et al. 2012)	WHO Global Burden of Disease (2013)[a]
3	(C) Loss of response at three consecutive test frequencies where responses were previously obtained	V. Very severe: 1st degree: 91–100 dB 2nd degree: 101–110 dB 3rd degree: 111–119 dB	3: Severe impairment: 61–80 dB HL	3: Considerable impairment, rehabilitation with hearing aids indicated: >20 dB HL at <4 kHz 3a: >20 to ≤40 dB HL 3b: >40 to ≤60 dB HL 3c: >60 dB HL	3: Severe or medically significant; disabling: In adults >25 dB HL at three contiguous frequencies/ therapeutic intervention indicated/limiting self-care ADL; in children >20 dB HL at 3 kHz and above	3: ≥40 dB HL at 2 or 3 kHz	3: >20 dB HL at 2 or 3 kHz and above	Severe: 65–79 dB HL Profound: 80–94 dB HL
4		VI. Total hearing loss: >120 dB	4: Profound impairment including deafness: ≥81 dB HL	4: Loss of function, cochlear implant indicated: ≥80 dB HL at <4 kHz	4: Life-threatening consequences; urgent intervention indicated: In adults >80 dB HL at 2 kHz and above; in children cochlear implant indicated	4: ≥40 dB HL at 1 kHz and above	4: >40 dB HL at 2 kHz and above	Complete: ≥95 dB HL

All except ASHA (1994), BIAP (1996) and WHO (2013) use the numbering scheme 0–4 or 1–4, but each audiological grading scale defines these intervals differently.

Abbreviations: ASHA American Speech-Language-Hearing Association, ADL Activities of Daily Living, BIAP Bureau International d'Audiophonologie, CTCAE Common Terminology Criteria for Adverse Events, NCI National Cancer Institute, NIH National Institutes of Health, SIOP International Society of Paediatric Oncology, WHO World Health Organization

[a]The grades described by BIAP, WHO 2000 and WHO 2013 reflect average hearing thresholds across 0.5, 1, 2 and 4 KHz

14.2.2 Prevalence of Childhood Hearing Loss and Case Definition

Fortnum and Davis (1997) reported the prevalence of permanent childhood hearing impairment as 1.3 per 1000. The population sampled was all children born and resident within a defined regional health authority within the UK between 1985 and 1993 (552,558 live births). Hearing loss in this study was defined as a permanent hearing threshold of $\geq$40 dB HL in the better ear, averaged across 0.5, 1, 2 and 4 kHz, including sensorineural, permanent conductive and mixed impairments. 0.73 per 1000 were moderate hearing losses (40–69 dB HL), 0.28 were severe (70–94 dB HL) and 0.31 were profound ($\geq$95 dB HL).

Watkin et al. (1990) studied the population of children born between 1973 and 1988 in a different UK regional health authority and reported a prevalence of 5.6 per 1000. In this case, hearing loss was defined as permanent bilateral thresholds >21 dB HL averaged in the better ear or unilateral hearing loss >55 dB HL in the affected ear. 1.3 per 1000 had mild hearing loss (21–40 dB HL), 0.8 moderate (41–70 dB HL), 0.4 severe (71–95 dB HL) and 0.7 profound (>95 dB HL). Unilateral hearing losses accounted for 2.4 per 1000. Once the unilateral and mild bilateral hearing losses were removed, the prevalence rate was reduced to 2.1 per 1000.

In 2013, the World Health Organization's Global Burden of Disease Hearing Loss Expert Group reported the global prevalence of hearing impairment in children aged 5–14 years old as 1.4%, which equates to 16 million children, based on a meta-review of 42 studies across 29 countries (Stevens et al. 2013). Prevalence was lowest in high-income countries (Western Europe, Australia and the USA) at 0.4% and highest in South Asia at 2.2%. 'Hearing impairment' was defined here as an average hearing threshold of $\geq$35 dB HL in the better ear calculated across 0.5, 1, 2 and 4 kHz. Data were taken only from studies that reported their methodology in detail, had adequate sample sizes, had response rates $\geq$80% and where study samples were representative of the target population. All contributing studies had to report detailed audiological data (thresholds and frequencies tested) and include audiological test techniques of sufficient quality (e.g. specific minimum background noise levels), but no distinction between temporary and permanent hearing loss was made.

The differences between the three examples cited above are largely removed once the definitions of hearing loss used in each case and the sample populations are considered. Watkin's results are comparable to Fortnum and Davis when mild and unilateral hearing impairments are excluded (2.1 per 1000 and 1.4 per thousand, respectively). When focusing on high-income countries, the WHO figures are reduced to 4.0 per 1000. The remaining difference of 1.9–2.6 per thousand between the WHO and the two UK-based studies may be accounted for by the lower threshold used by the WHO to define hearing loss (35 dB HL rather than 40 dB HL) and inclusion of temporary hearing impairments.

Other factors may also contribute to such differences as discussed above. Age range, for example, is crucial, as highlighted by Morton and Nance (2006) who reported increasing prevalence of hearing loss within the US increasing from 1.86 per 1000 at birth to approx. 2.7 per 1000 by 5 years old and 3.5 per 1000 during adolescence (hearing loss here defined as bilateral or unilateral sensorineural loss of >35 dB HL). All of these prevalence figures are legitimate but their specific contexts must be understood.

Two relatively recent studies analyse changes in the prevalence of hearing loss over time. Shargorodsky et al. (2010) compared the data gathered on teenagers between 1988–1994 and 2005–2006. The authors found a 77% increase in the prevalence of uni- and bilateral hearing loss $\geq$25 dB HL (air-conduction thresholds averaged across frequencies) over this time period (from 3.2 to 5.3% of the US teen population). Van Naarden Braun et al. (2015) used data on 8-year-old children during each of the years 1991–2010, finding an average prevalence of 1.4 per 1000 (bilateral thresholds $\geq$40 dB HL averaged over 500–2000 Hz) with no significant change across the 20-year time period. Comparing WHO data from 1985 to 2011, the prevalence of hearing disability has risen about eightfold, partly because of the inclusion of lower hearing loss grades in the definition but also due to—among others—increasing presbyacusis, earlier detection of hearing loss and increasing use of ototoxic medication (Olusanya et al. 2014).

14.2.3 Normal Hearing in Children

Normal-hearing in adults, which has been set as 0 dB HL for purposes of audiometric measurement, is defined as the average of the lowest distinguishable sound pressure level measurable in young adults. This level has been studied and revised several times over the years (International Organization for Standardization (2010) 8253-1), so when comparing auditory thresholds described in the literature, the fact that the baseline may not always be the same has to be taken into account.

In children there is no clear definition of normal-hearing threshold in tone audiometry because hearing sensitivity changes with age and results from different hearing test methods of differing sensitivity and considerable variation (especially in subjective tests) also change with age. In general, children and adolescents often show lower hearing thresholds than the audiometric zero. For example, one study found that 75% of children aged from 5 to 14 years had hearing threshold levels better than audiometric zero (calibration according to the American standard specification for audiometers for general diagnostic purposes Z24.5-1951) (Eagles et al. 1963). Two other studies found that over 50% of children and adolescents showed lower threshold results than the 1951 ASA audiometric zero (Roberts and Ahuja 1975; Roberts and Huber 1970), but when compared with the audiometric zero from ANSI 1969, a substantially lower percentage showed results under zero (Roberts and Ahuja 1975).

Another problem that has to be considered is differences in children's sensitivity or responsiveness to different stimuli, with pure tones, warble tones, narrowband noise and FRESH noise (frequency-specific hearing assessment noise, a narrowband noise with steep filter slopes (see Moore and Violetto (2016)) being the most commonly used nowadays). Greatest sensitivity/responsiveness has been found in response to warble tones (Orchik and Rintelmann 1978; Walker et al. 1984). Close agreement between warble tone and pure-tone thresholds has been found in adults (Dockum and Robinson 1975) with equally high test-retest reliability for both types of stimuli (Staab and Rintelmann 1972).

Behavioural observation audiometry is the most common subjective hearing test used in babies, with visual reinforcement audiometry (VRA) being the standard from about 8 months of age and play audiometry from approximately 2.5 years of age. These different methods are described in Sect. 16.4.

Babies and young children generally show auditory responses at higher levels than adult hearing thresholds, and this is reflected in the common use of the term 'minimal response level' instead of 'threshold'. Increasing hearing sensitivity can be seen with increasing age. This can be explained by the greater test sensitivity and compliance with age but also by maturation of the auditory pathway after birth (Talero-Gutierrez et al. 2008) and by changes in the anatomy of the middle and external ear (Schneider et al. 1980).

Various studies have reported measurable hearing thresholds in babies younger than 1 year of age, down to 6 dB HL at some frequencies (e.g. Olsho et al. 1988), by using VRA with two observers, usually more than one reward, and measurements at more than one time point in some cases. According to Olsho et al. (1988), pure-tone thresholds improve most in high frequencies between 3 and 6 months of age, while an improvement in low-frequency sensitivity is observed at some later time between 6 months of age and adulthood. Over the age of 5 years, when ear-specific and frequency-specific testing is used regularly, most but not all studies still describe increasing sensitivity with age (Eagles et al. 1963; Roberts and Ahuja 1975; Roberts and Huber 1970; Orchik and Rintelmann 1978; Holmes et al. 2004; Haapaniemi 1996).

According to Eagles et al. (1963), girls' hearing is most sensitive at age 11–12 and boys' hearing 1 year later. From age 12 years and onwards, no further trend towards changes in hearing sensitivity was found (Eagles et al. 1963; Roberts and Ahuja 1975; Holmes et al. 2004). School-aged girls have been found to have lower hearing thresholds than boys, especially at higher frequencies, but not all studies support this difference (Roberts and Ahuja 1975; Roberts and Huber 1970; Holmes et al. 2004; Shepard et al. 1981; Costa et al. 1988). Many studies also show slightly different hearing levels in the left and right ears, but these results are also often contradictory (Eagles et al. 1963; Roberts and Ahuja 1975; Roberts and Huber 1970; Karma et al. 1989; Pirila et al. 1992). Table 14.2 gives a detailed overview of studies of normal-hearing thresholds/minimal response levels in children of different ages and lists methodological differences and key details of each study.

14.3 Normal Development Stages of Hearing and Auditory Processing

Rainer Schönweiler

Hearing develops continuously but it is often classified in stages (Table 14.3).

It is interesting that hearing begins long before birth when the hair cells are fully developed and connected to the central nervous system. Normally, this is the case at a gestational age of around 19 weeks (Hepper and Shahidullah 1994). From that time on, the foetus uses hearing intensively, so far as we can judge by reports from pregnant women experiencing foetal movements in reaction to loud sounds, music and shouting.

These sounds are transmitted to the foetal cochleae via bone conduction. Testing of prenatal behavioural bone conduction seems to be feasible in utero and might be a promising method for the detection of hearing impairment—once a standard testing procedure and normative values for such a prenatal 'diagnostic test' have been made available. Other interesting observations are foetal auditory-evoked potentials (Cook et al. 1987). In animal studies with lambs, these have been detected at a gestational age of 117 days (from a total 144 days until birth). Human auditory-evoked potentials can be detected immediately before birth (Staley et al. 1990; Woods and Plessinger 1985) by the use ECG monitoring electrodes and clicks delivered by a loudspeaker, which has been used as an alternative to the conventional newborn hearing screening. In fact, much of the auditory abilities measured in newborns and infants are present long before birth. But this is true only for healthy children without congenital hearing loss and genetic hearing disorders. In contrast, children with genetic hearing loss have never been able to hear until they have been fitted with hearing aids or cochlear implants.

The next developmental stage of hearing begins after birth. In this neonatal state, the newborn uses prenatal experience (Table 14.3). Within the first 2 to 3 days after birth, the newborn still hears sounds from the outside via bone conduction, although less damped. By the end of the third day, provided that the newborn is healthy and able to drink, the remaining amniotic fluid will have left the middle ear cavities during swallowing. From that time on, the newborn hears sounds from the outside via air conduction and much louder than before. This is normally the moment in time when the newborn hearing screening test is done. With normal hearing and evoked potential thresholds around 20 dB, the newborn shows reactions at 80 dB in a behavioural hearing test (Table 14.4) (Northern and Downs 2014).

With air conduction, owing to experience from the foetal stage, the newborn is able to recognise a presented female voice as belonging to his or her mother (DeCasper and Fifer 1980).

In the postnatal stage, infants develop reactions to sounds of lower intensities and begin to localise sounds by turning their heads to the sound source (Table 14.4) (Northern and Downs 2014). Sound localisation requires two hearing ears and binaural interaction in the auditory pathway of the central nervous system.

Table 14.2 Overview of studies of normal-hearing thresholds in childhood

Group	Age	Stimulus, calibration	Method	Criteria for patient selection	Results (special remarks, explanation for given thresholds) Mean threshold (standard deviation)	Normal-hearing thresholds/minimal response levels (dB HL/dB SPL where given) at frequency (Hz) (std. deviation)										Source
						125	250	500	1000	2000	3000	4000	6000	8000	10,000	
USA, $n = 132$	6 months	250 ms tones, Earphones	Tone burst VRA, go/no-go	Normal and healthy upon paediatric examination				23		20				19		Berg and Smith (1983)
	10 months							27		17				23		
	10 months	Sound field						20		18				21		
	14 months							19		20				21		
	18 months							19		18				21		
USA, $n = 22$	8 months	30-s Pure tones, sound field	Behavioural observation, 2 observers, ascending method of limits	Screened to eliminate "high-risk" babies and considered to be developmentally normal				45				50				Hoversten and Moncur (1969)
Sweden, $n = 120$	3 months to 1 year	Pure tones	VRA mean monaural sound field thresholds/conditioned orientation reflex audiometry-mean binaural thresholds	Reported normal hearing, clinical exam	Estimated threshold from figures		29	31	30	33		33				Liden and Kankkunen (1969)
	1–2 years						29/33	29/33	34/34	29/34		32/40				
	2–3 years						24/31	21/31	20/32	21/34		23/40				
	3–4 years						14/30	14/33	13/31	15/34		18/40				
	4–5 years						12/26	12/26	10/26	10/27		12/29				
	5–6 years						12/22	9/19	7/24	7/23		8/23				

Population	Age	Stimulus	Condition				Reference
USA, n = 39	8–24 months	Warble tone	Negative otological history, normal acoustic immittance, normal development, good health	29.0		28.0	McDermott and Hodgson (1982)
	25–36 months			29.0		27.8	
	37–48 months			23.9		25.0	
	8–24 months	Narrow band noise		22.0		25.0	
	25–36 months			25.9		24.4	
	37–48 months			22.9		23.6	
USA, n = 9	6–7 months	2-s, 5% warbled tones	Supra-aural headphones	38	25	23	Moore and Wilson (1978)
n = 10	12–13 months			31	27	25	
n = 9	6–7 months		Sound field	18	18	18	
n = 10	12–13 months			21	16	14	
USA, screened n = 11	6 months	500-ms pure tones	If screened: Tympanometry pressure peak >−100 daPa H₂O Supra aural headphone VRA, go/no-go Mean threshold (Standard Deviation)	21 (5.72)		16 (4.2)	Nozza and Wilson (1984)
n = 17 unscreened				23 (7.3)		20 (10.00)	
n = 12 screened	12 months			18 (3.62)		14 (6.10)	
n = 17 unscreened				22 (9.4)		15 (6.75)	

(continued)

Table 14.2 (continued)

Group	Age	Stimulus, calibration	Method	Criteria for patient selection	Results (special remarks, explanation for given thresholds) Mean threshold (standard deviation)	Normal-hearing thresholds/minimal response levels (dB HL/dB SPL where given) at frequency (Hz) (std. deviation) 125	250	500	1000	2000	3000	4000	6000	8000	10,000	Source
USA, $n = 11$	8–11 months	1 s pure tones	Insert earphones, left ear, operant head turn with VRA, yes/no, infants with >25% false-positive rate on two occasions were excluded from the study	Tympanometric screening					12.6 (3.7)							Nozza (1995)
USA, $n = 10-28$	3 months	Pure tone	VRA, observer-based psychoacoustic procedure	Full-term birth, no complications, normal postnatal development, never diagnosed hearing loss, no colds, no middle ear infection <3 weeks before testing, no >2 prior ear infection, no family history of congenital hearing loss	Estimated values from Fig. 4 in reference		47	41	30	26		23		36		Olsho et al. (1988)
$n = 10-22$	6 months						47	30	21	12		14		16		
$n = 10-11$	12 months						43	32	22	10		13		21		
UK, $n = 46$	8–11 months	Warble tones	Insert earphone VRA, 2 testers, 1–2 visits	Screening passed, tympanometry, TEOAE, development questionnaire	Mean minimal response levels			16.4	13.3	7.1		6.4				Parry et al. (2003)

Country, n	Stimuli	Age	Method	Condition	Notes	Data 1	Data 2	Data 3	Data 4	Data 5	Data 6	Data 7	Data 8	Data 9	Reference
Canada, n = 23–31 per freq./age	Half-octave bands	6 months	Refined VRA, free-field, 2 speakers 45° right/left from baby	–	19,000 Hz: 6 months: 41 dB; 12/18 months: 38 dB; 24 months: 31 dB	24									Schneider et al. (1980)
		12, 18 months				22									
		24 months				19									
USA, n = 11–16	1-s wave tones, sound field	7–11 months	VRA, go/no-go operant head-turning technique	Appeared in good health on test days		37.7	30.3	31.2	36.1	34.3					Sinnott et al. (1983)
n = 2–7	0.5-s wave tones, sound field					33.6	35.0	36.5	31.2	25.0					
Canada, n = 89	Octave-band noise	6 months	VRA modification with 2 speakers in 45°	Free of cold		200 Hz: 38	400 Hz: 33	25	28	23	18				Trehub et al. (1980)
n = 74		12 months				27	25	18	16	17	10				
n = 76		18 months				31	24	19	20	14	19				
Brazil, n = 50	Instrumental sounds	6–12 months	VRA	Absence of risk indicators for hearing loss, presence of bilateral otoacoustic emissions, type A tympanometric curve	Average	32.24	27.07	26.72	27.41						Vieira and Azevedo (2007)
		13–24 months				27.5	22.14	20.71	21.79						
		24–34 months				24.29	21.43	21.43	21.43						
USA, n = 2078	Octave band	5 years	Earphones, hand raising/play technique	Representative cross selection of Pittsburg school children, otoscopy	Increasing sensitivity with age, girls more sensitive than boys	11.8	11.4	9.6	6.9	5.1	9.4	12.6			Eagles et al. (1963)
		7 years				6.6	8.5	6.1	4.5	2.9	7.7	8.8			
		10 years				6.2	7.3	5.7	5.1	2.8	7.9	8.7			
		14 years				6.2	7.0	6.0	5.5	4.4	9.2	9.3			
Finland, n = 471	Pure tones, earphones	7 years	Pure tone audiometry with bracketing method	Healthy tympanic membrane, normal objective acoustic immittance tympanometry and acoustic reflex measures		10.2	6.9	3.7	0.8	0.7	1.2	1.6	6.1	5.8	Haapaniemi (1996)
		10 years				5.9	2.7	0.1	-1.2	-5.1	-0.8	-0.7	3.3	2.6	
		14 years				5.2	2.6	-0.7	-1.5	-1.8	-1.4	-0.5	4.8	2.1	

(continued)

Table 14.2 (continued)

Group	Age	Stimulus, calibration	Method	Criteria for patient selection	Results (special remarks, explanation for given thresholds) Mean threshold (standard deviation)	125	250	500	1000	2000	3000	4000	6000	8000	10,000	Source
USA, n = 6166	6–11 years	ANSI S3.6-1969		Screening questionnaire	AC, average left/right ear, male:female			7.2:7.1	5.3:5.5	4.0:3.6	5.7:5.2	5.3:5.0	8.9:9.5	11.7:11.7		Holmes et al. (2004)
	12–19 years							6.2:6.0	4.8:4.4	3.4:3.2	6.5:4.2	5.8:3.9	10.1:10.4	9.3:8.9		
Finland, n = 420	5 years	Pure tone, cal. ISO 389 std.	Air/bone conduction thresholds	No otological selection	AC, average left/right ear, male:female	18.3:15.7	13.1:11.2	10.5:9.5	8.1:7.9	7.1:7.4		8.0:7.6	12.7:11.2	14.3:13.6		Karma et al. (1989)
USA, n = 20	3.5 years	Pure tone, warble tone, narrowband	Earphone 3.5/4.5 years: conditioned play audiometry 5.5/6.5 years: raising hand when sound was heard	Normally-hearing = passing a pure-tone screening test at the 20 dB hearing threshold level (re ANSI, 1969)	Estimated threshold from Fig. 1 in reference. Thresholds for the three test stimuli (pure tone, warble tone and narrow-band noise) are combined			25	16	15						Orchik and Rintelmann (1978)
	4.5 years							24	14	13						
	5.5 years						36	21	12	9		15				
	6.5 years						33	18	10	10.5		13				
Denmark, n = 46	10–12 years	2 s pure tones	Quasi free-field, stimulus from a point source	Normal medical history, hearing anamnesis (no noise exposure, middle ear dysfunction), otoscopy, impedance								4.02		25.33	28.75	Osterhammel (1978)
Korea, n = 15,606	12–19 years	Pure tones, GSI SA-203 audiometer	Air cond., earphones, modified Hughson-Westlake procedure	Normal tympanic membrane and no history of regular or occupational noise exposure	Better ear, average 12–19 years, male:female			7.2:6.9	2.0:1.9	1.7:2.1	1.9:1.6	1.9:2.0	9.0:10.6			Park et al. (2016)

Normal-hearing thresholds/minimal response levels (dB HL/dB SPL where given) at frequency (Hz) (std. deviation)

Study	Age	Pure tone	Method	Exclusion	Hearing loss in better ear	Estimated 50th percentile								Reference
						9.0	9.5	6.0	4.0		3.0		6.0	
UK, n = 11370 n = 12406	7 years	Pure tone	Air conduction audiometry locally done	No exclusion	Hearing loss in better ear	9.5	9.5	5.0	2.5		1.5		3.0	
	11 years													Richardson et al. (1976)
USA, n = 7119	6 years	Pure tone, 1951 American Standard	Air-conduction earphones	Non-institutionalised children, no otological selection	Median hearing levels of the better ears, male:female	−7.8:−7.7	−7.3:−7.6	−7.0:−7.2	−8.1:−8.7		−4.1:−4.8	−2.6:−3.0	−4.7:−6.6	Roberts and Huber (1970)
	7 years					−8.7:−8.3	−7.6:−8.0	−7.2:−7.8	−8.8:−8.8		−4.7:−4.9	−2.8:−2.7	−6.4:−5.9	
	8 years					−10.2:−10.1	−9.3:−9.9	−7.8:−8.6	−9.4:−9.8		−5.5:−5.7	−3.5:−4.0	−6.9:−7.9	
	9 years					−11.1:−9.6	−10.0:−9.4	−8.9:−8.3	−10.1:−10.1		−5.9:−5.2	−3.8:−3.5	−7.6:−7.4	
	10 years					−11.5:−10.8	−10.5:−11.1	−9.2:−9.8	−9.6:−10.4		−5.6:−6.4	−3.0:4.0	−7.7:−7.5	
	11 years					−11.9:−11.2	−11.2:−10.8	−10.0:−10.3	−9.9:−10.5		−6.0:−5.9	−3.1:−3.4	−7.2:−7.8	
USA, n = 7119	7 years	Pure tone	Modified Hughson-Westlake method	Without reported hearing trouble	Average of better ear	8.0	7.9	4.7	1.5	5.5	6.5	10.1	8.9	Roberts and Federico (1972)
USA, n = 6768	10 years	Pure tones, ASA 1951/ANSI-1969	Modif. Hughson-Westlake method, 40 locations in the USA	Probability sample of the non-institutionalised youths 12–17 years in the USA	Mean threshold of better ear vs. audiometric 0 ANSI 1969	5.9	5.1	2.6	0.7	4.3	5.3	8.9	7.6	Roberts and Ahuja (1975)
	12 years					9.2	6.4	2.0	1.1	5.2	8.0	10.2	7.0	
	13 years					9.4	6.2	1.8	1.1	5.6	8.4	11.0	7.2	
	14 years					8.8	5.8	1.6	1.1	5.2	7.7	10.9	6.5	
	15 years					9.0	6.0	1.5	1.2	5.6	8.0	11.4	6.8	
	16 years					9.0	5.5	1.4	1.0	5.2	8.0	12.2	6.2	
	17 years					9.4	5.4	1.2	1.0	5.0	8.0	11.4	6.4	
Taiwan, n = 1411	7 years	Pure tone, ANSI S3.1-1991 std.		Normal otoscopy and tympanometry	Mean threshold AC, male:female		15.7:14.7	13.2:11.6	11.5:10.2		10.4:9.7			Yang et al. (2011)
	10 years						13.8:13.1	12.4:10.6	11.4:10.4		9.5:8.7			
	14 years						14.2:12.4	12.4:9.5	11.5:9.2		10.6:7.6			
	16 years						14.2:12.6	12.7:10.1	11.4:9.1		10.5:7.4			

Table 14.3 Developmental stages of hearing and auditory processing (Northern and Downs 2014)

Development stage	Age	Developmental steps
Foetal stage	Conceptional age 26 weeks to birth	Hearing of maternal sounds and speech as well as damped external sounds and speech via bone conduction
Neonatal stage	First days after birth	Loss of amniotic fluid from the middle ear; hearing of external sounds and speech switches from bone conduction to air conduction
Postnatal stage	First year	Lowering of reaction thresholds and development of sound localisation (see Table 14.4); acceleration of auditory brainstem responses (auditory maturation (see Table 14.5)); use of hearing to control crying, babbling and first words
Infantile stage	1 to ~16 years	Development of auditory processing abilities; speech and language development

Data from Chapter 3. Auditory and Speech-Language Development in Hearing in Children, Sixth Edition by J.L. Northern and M.P. Downs. Copyright © 2014 by Plural Publishing, Inc. Used with permission. Modification with permission from the author.

Table 14.4 Development of auditory behaviour in children (Northern and Downs 2014)

Age	Behavioural threshold (dB) as deviation from behavioural thresholds in adults (nHL)	Sound localisation
Newborn	80	No localisation but arousal from sleep
3 months	60	Rudimentary head turn in the horizontal plane
6 months	50	Slow localisation to side
9 months	45	Slow localisation to side and below
12 months	40	Slow localisation to side, below and above
18 months	30	Rapid localisation to side, below and above
2 years	20	Rapid localisation in all directions
4 years	10	Rapid localisation in all directions
6 years	5	Rapid localisation in all directions

Data from Chapter 3. Auditory and Speech-Language Development in Hearing in Children, Sixth Edition by J.L. Northern and M.P. Downs. Copyright © 2014 by Plural Publishing, Inc. Used with permission. Modification with permission from the author.

Table 14.5 Indicators of auditory maturation, observed in auditory brainstem evoked potential Jewett V (Eggermont and Salamy 1988; Picton et al. 2012)

Conceptional age (weeks)	Deviation from the latency of adults (ms)	Deviation from the threshold of adults (dB nHL)
25	+4	
30	+2	
35	+1.5	
40	+1	+20
50	+0.75	+10
100	+0.5	+0
200	+0.25	
300	+0.1	

If a baby fails the newborn hearing screening test, it has to undergo further diagnostic tests. Measurement of auditory evoked potentials involves estimation of both latencies and thresholds with respect to the individual gestational age (Table 14.5) (Eggermont and Salamy 1988).

For instance, if a 3-month-old infant born at term presents a behavioural threshold around 90 dB (Table 14.4) and a threshold in the auditory brainstem response of around 40 dB (Table 14.5), then the estimated 'true' threshold is around 30 dB. Assuming a conceptional age of 50 weeks for this example, the calculation is as follows: 90 − 60 = 30 (Table 14.4) and 40 − 10 = 30 (Table 14.5).

In the postnatal stage, infants develop abilities that allow for auditory feedback in the control of vocalisations and speech-sound production. It has been shown that at the age of 4 months, infants are able to imitate the vowels /a/, /i/ and /u/ selectively (Kuhl and Meltzoff 1996); at the age of 4 to 9 months, normal-hearing infants are able to control prosodic patterns of crying by using auditory feedback, while infants with so far unaided profound hearing loss are not (Möller and Schönweiler 1999). These abilities cannot be perceived by untrained listeners but can be discovered by acoustic analyses and linguistic transcripts (Kuhl and Meltzoff 1996; Möller and Schönweiler 1999). Finally, at the age of 8–10 months, untrained listeners can perceive reduplicated babbling in infants with normal hearing. In children with unaided profound hearing loss, reduplicated babbling cannot be observed (Northern and Downs 2014).

In the infantile stage, children develop abilities of auditory processing and auditory perception that allow for speech understanding in noisy environments, speech-sound discrimination, dichotic listening, auditory memory and phonological awareness. For many of these abilities, a number of test procedures have been developed that permit comparison with age-dependent normative data. If a child presents typical symptoms of auditory processing disorders (APD), the diagnosis can be confirmed

from age 7 on. These issues will be discussed in the sections on auditory processing disorders (Sects. 15.2 and 16.8).

14.4 Normal Development of Behavioural Responses to Sound in Children

Wendy Albuquerque

In a study by Hepper and Shahidullah (1994), one foetus had been observed to move in response to sound as early as at 19 weeks of gestational age, and babies are born with basically functioning hearing. In those incredible early months after birth, babies grow and learn, demonstrating behavioural responses to sound that change as they mature.

In Table 14.6 an attempt is made to summarise the different types of behavioural

Table 14.6 Different types of behavioural responses to sound that develop in normal children

Approximate age (months)	Behavioural responses to sound (Northern and Downs 2014; American Speech-Language-Hearing Association 2005; Lewis et al. 2006; First Years 2011; Center for Early Intervention on Deafness 2016; Centers for Disease Control and Prevention 2016)
0–2	Arousal from sleep; eye widening; change in sucking patterns during feeding; limbs move or slow down; change in breathing pattern; quietens, cries, startles to sudden loud sounds; may be soothed by certain songs or music
2–4	Eye widening or searching; stilling or quietens to sounds; crying/smiling or other change in facial expression; limb extension; rudimentary head turn; turn taking cooing; vocalises to get attention
4–6	Localisation of sound to side; looks puzzled when hears something new or unexpected; turns quickly to mother's voice across room; begins to imitate vocalisations of adults
6–9	Localisation of sound to side and directly below; able to make a full head turn to the sound; increasingly interested in its own voice and sounds; sways/bounces to music; begins to copy rhythm and actions of rhymes/songs; begins to make bisyllabic babble, practising the sequence of the same sounds
9–12	Localises to side and below; answers to/recognises its own name; responds to keywords in play; understands the meaning associated with some environmental sounds (e.g. telephone ringing)
12–15	Localises to side, below and immediately above; immediately turns to its own name; points to pictures in a book when item named; finds an object when asked to
15–18	Localises to side, below and above; follows simple spoken commands; begins to fill in a familiar missing word when an adult leaves a pause in rhymes and story books; increasing quality of prosody in vocalisations; increasing 'word-like' babble; emergence of single words
18–24	Recognises and names environmental sounds; understands when called from another room; follows a conversation on a known topic
24–36	Understands most of a direct conversation; enjoys listening to longer stories; answers questions about familiar topics
36–48	Hears television at same level of loudness as others; listens closely and retells stories; accurately repeats predictable sentences
48–60	Understands most of what is said in school and at home; can follow more complex instructions; can identify rhyming or non-rhyming words from small sets

responses to sound that develop in normal children.

There are important concepts to remember:

- There is a great variability as to when different babies reach different milestones.
- Babies do not consistently respond to sound until they are around 7–9 months of age when they sit up and turn their head; one cannot rely solely upon the observation of development of behavioural hearing responses to exclude deafness.
- Very young babies do not respond to the quietest sounds that they can hear but only to supra-threshold sounds that they can hear (Williamson 2002).
- In most babies born with significant hearing loss, this impairment is invisible. In a baby with a syndrome (e.g. Down syndrome), professionals are more easily alerted to the possibility of hearing loss.

14.5 Speech and Language Development of Normal-Hearing and Hearing-Impaired Children

Steffi Johanna Brockmeier

14.5.1 Language Acquisition

Language acquisition is the most complex task humans have to accomplish in their early development. Hearing, cognitive, motor as well as social development must work hand in hand to promote this process. However, no explicit instruction is necessary to achieve this. During the sensitive period for language acquisition, adequate language input of the environment is sufficient. Discrimination of phonemic contrasts for all language is an inborn ability, and the base for the production of vowel-like sounds typically starts at 3 months of age. During the first year of life, foreign language-specific perception abilities decline as native language perception is enhanced. Speech production starts with a universal phase in which the production of non-speech sounds is followed by vowel-like sounds

and canonical babbling. Around 10 months of age, language-specific speech production starts, and first words are expected at age 1 year. Generally speaking, children have acquired the full phonemic repertoire of their specific language, as well as most grammatical structures and a wide range of vocabulary, from the ages 4 to 5.

There is a slight variation in the acquisition of sounds depending on the language of a child. However, generally the phonemes first acquired are bilabial sounds, followed by first and second articulation zone sounds and succeeded around 2.5 years by the third articulation zone sounds. By 3 years the first complicated consonant combinations are present. At age 4 all phonemes of the mother tongue have been learned, though difficult consonant combinations and sibilant sounds might still be imperfect. In a normally developing child, perfection is achieved by age 6 (O'Hare and Bremner 2015).

The first words are nouns that are connected with the environment of the child and therefore depend on where and how the child lives. By age 2 around 50 words are known and the first verbs and adjectives appear. In the period from 2 to 4 years, active and passive vocabulary multiplies, and when school starts, the vocabulary should be from 2000 to 3000 active words. Acquisition of vocabulary never stops and adult vocabulary consists of 20,000–250,000 words (O'Hare and Bremner 2015).

One-word utterances around the age 1 consist of nouns. At age 2 most children use two- to three-word utterances and ask first questions by changing intonation. Sentences are grammatically still incorrect. Children start to use interrogatives at approximately age 3, and short sentences are grammatically accurate, subordinate clauses appear. Around age 4 sentences get longer and grammatical constructions more complex. Grammar is usually correct at age 6, and children are able to express their thoughts in different time forms as well as re-narrate events and stories (O'Hare and Bremner 2015).

14.5.2 Sign Language

If an auditory-oral approach is not possible, or signed language may be helpful as an additional communication mode, or the child is born to deaf parents and sign language is preferred, characteristics of signed language have to be considered. Signed languages such as British Sign Language (BSL) or German Sign Language (DGS) are natural languages with the same structures as spoken languages, and learning these is a task as complex as learning spoken languages. Caregivers adapt their sign language to the need of the child as is done for spoken language, and the child develops speech the same way as children do in spoken language, starting with 'sign babble', simple signs and one-word utterances (Morgan 2014). As for spoken language, competent role models are needed to facilitate normal sign language development. As less than 5% of prelingually deaf children have signing deaf parents, early acquisition of sign language for a child in a hearing family has to be supported by bringing a natural signing adult into the child's environment.

14.5.3 Conductive Hearing Loss

Conductive hearing loss is the most prevalent type of hearing loss in childhood, commonly due to otitis media with effusion. Although this condition is the most frequent, little consistency is found regarding its long-term consequence on speech and hearing. This is partly because there are hardly any studies available covering the most sensitive period of these developmental processes, which lies between birth and age 2. Furthermore, most reports are retrospective, and the chosen methodology and the age at test may not be suitable for the detection of the consequences of early disease (see Zumach et al. 2009 for discussion).

Studies have shown a greater signal-to-noise ratio in children of age 7 (Zumach et al. 2009) than 4 (Gravel and Wallace 1992). This is a relevant finding, as hearing in noise is the normal condition in everyday life. In the Zumach study, correlations were not found between socio-economic status and cognitive development but with the frequency and level of hearing loss due to middle ear effusion.

Another study has shown that when long lasting, otitis media with effusion is prone to lead to auditory deprivation and can result in deterioration of listening and language performance as well as central auditory processing deficits (Klausen et al. 2007).

On basis of auditory event-related potentials, Haapala et al. (2015) studied neural mechanisms of involuntary attention in 22–26-month-old children with repetitive middle ear infections and healthy controls. The analysis of auditory P3a showed an atypical neural organisation, the late negativity LN a longer latency in children with recurrent middle ear problems suggesting long-term effects on the developing central auditory system.

In conclusion, although a direct correlation between otitis media and long-term effects on speech and language development cannot be proven at present, children having problems in language acquisition need to be considered at risk of further deterioration of their condition by an additional conductive hearing loss due to effusion. Therefore, they should be treated straight away, not only taking conservative but also surgical options into consideration.

14.5.4 Speech and Language Development in Subgroups of Sensorineural Hearing Loss

Bilateral Sensorineural Hearing Loss If pancochlear bilateral sensorineural hearing loss exceeds 40 dB, deficits in speech perception have to be expected. The individual extent of deviation from the norm varies a lot, ranging from a simple delay to a complete inability to acquire spoken language. Generally speaking, a higher degree of hearing loss leads to more abnormalities. Deficits can be seen in all linguistic fields.

Articulation of vowels and consonants may be problematic with substitutions, distortions and omissions. For affected children it may be difficult to differentiate between different vowels and voiced and voiceless consonant sounds. Phonological development is considerably slowed (Dobie and Van Hemel 2004); speech intelligibility is reduced.

Vocabulary acquisition is slowed and might plateau early. Nonliteral and abstract words are especially difficult to integrate in the lexicon (Briscoe et al. 2001; Jerger et al. 2002). Grammatical knowledge is impaired with sentences being shorter, of more simple structure, and passive voice is rarely seen (Dobie and Van Hemel 2004). As language proficiency is a prerequisite for reading achievement, literacy skills are often impaired in school age children with hearing loss (Carney and Moeller 1998).

This statement is still true with today's hearing aid technology and timely rehabilitation (Eisenberg 2007; Tomblin et al. 2015).

Bilateral High-Frequency Sensorineural Hearing Loss Bilateral high-frequency hearing loss is known to cause problems with phoneme acquisition for fricatives. It is important to remember that high-frequency hearing loss cannot be detected by the measurement of TEOAE (transient evoked otoacoustic emissions), which is the most common method applied for newborn hearing screening in Europe. So children with deficits in the pronunciations of these sounds have to be tested differently, since the deficits might have been missed in early testing. Behavioural testing, DPOAE (distortion product evoked OAE) and frequency-specific evoked response audiometry have to be applied.

Mid-frequency Sensorineural Hearing Loss Mid-frequency hearing loss up to a maximum of 50 dB may not cause significant symptoms during early stages of language acquisition. However, those children, if not detected by newborn hearing screening or preschool hearing test, often are presented at school age with listening problems in the classroom environment.

Low-Frequency Sensorineural Hearing Loss There is no literature on isolated low-frequency hearing loss and speech development. The low frequency loss seldom exceeds 50 dB and is a relatively rare condition. As these children are usually only presented for doctor's advice at school age, one can assume that their speech development is not grossly disabled. Late

diagnosis is possible as for cases with unilateral or mild hearing impairment (Feder et al. 2017).

Unilateral and Mild Sensorineural Hearing Loss Mild and unilateral hearing loss primarily result in difficulties understanding speech in noisy situations and impaired localisation abilities (Bess et al. 1986, 1998).

About 30% of children with mild or unilateral hearing loss are found to have delayed speech development if not supplied with an amplifying hearing device (Yoshinaga-Itano et al. 2009). Difficulties arise in the fields of use of language, vocabulary, articulation and phonological discrimination (Tharpe 2008). Lower performance in reading and spelling is possible (Winiger et al. 2016). Nevertheless this kind of hearing loss may be unnoticed and late-diagnosed (Feder et al. 2017).

Auditory Processing Disorder The influence of auditory processing disorders on speech development is discussed controversially, and there is limited literature on direct correlations between particular deficits in auditory processing and specific features of speech development. This is partly because there is little knowledge about norms in many fields of auditory perception and little agreement on what auditory processing really is. However, children with delay in speech development often have pathological scores in auditory memory tests. A defined subset of dyslexic children has difficulties with the discrimination of phonemes. Though, the most common reason for dyslexia is a deficient phoneme grapheme assignment (McArthur et al. 2013).

Auditory Dyssynchrony The group of children with auditory dyssynchrony is very heterogeneous with many subjects suffering from additional neurological and intellectual handicaps that impact on speech development. Children suffering from this condition, but who are cognitively within the normal range, show variable outcomes in respect to speech development, ranging from near normal to severely retarded or disturbed (Uhler et al. 2012; Nikolopoulos 2014).

14.5.5 Outcomes After Interventions for Sensorineural Hearing Loss

In general, it is agreed that intervention for sensorineural hearing loss should be as early as possible. In the age of universal newborn hearing screening, the goal therefore is that children are diagnosed and get their hearing aids by the age of 6 months. For all other children, intervention should start immediately after diagnosis of hearing loss (Silverman 1983).

Hearing Aids Little prospective, controlled design research has been undertaken to study formally the impact of hearing aids and hearing aid fitting on the hearing and speech development of children with hearing impairment. Clinical experience shows that acquisition of language is facilitated by hearing aids. However, there are vast differences in the progress between children who suffer from a similar hearing loss. Apart from the degree of hearing loss, the following contributing factors have been assessed retrospectively to reveal a positive impact on speech development: early use of hearing aids, highly educated mothers, reliance on spoken language, integration and structured teaching individually (Yoshinaga-Itano et al. 1998; Tomblin et al. 2015).

Cochlear Implantation For the profoundly hearing-impaired, cochlear implantation is a valuable way to gain more auditory access to speech. Owing to the success of this rehabilitation method, inclusion criteria for cochlear implantation have been broadened towards more residual hearing.

Today if young children receive cochlear implants of high technological standard, acceleration of speech development is observed. However, Nittrouer showed that for implant recipients who received their first implants at an average age of 20 months, at age 80 months, speech measures (utterance length in morphemes, number of conjunctions, personal pronouns, bound morphemes, different words) were at least one standard deviation or more below those of the normal-hearing group (Nittrouer et al. 2014). We expect that bilateral implantation at an even earlier age will bring additional improvements. According to Levine et al. (2016), it is crucial to experience a language model in the first year of life. But still further studies are needed concerning the acquisition of complex language, vocabulary and literacy skills for the population of children who were implanted early and profited from newer technologies.

Intelligibility of speech, which in the hearing aid area had always been a major concern for the population with profound hearing loss, has improved dramatically through cochlear implantation, both in quality and in the time needed to achieve it (see review Flipsen 2008).

Factors with an impact on speech development in early implanted children are new coding strategies, implantation at younger age, more residual hearing preimplantation, (re)habilitation emphasising auditory perception and speech development (Geers 2006).

14.6 Psychomotor and Cognitive Stages of Normal Children of Different Ages

See Part III Sect. 9.2.

14.7 Aetiology of Hearing Disorders and the Likelihood of Involvement of Other Systems

Radha Narayan and Ewa Raglan

14.7.1 Risk Factors for Permanent Childhood Hearing Impairment

Thirty to 50% of cases of hearing loss are of unknown aetiology (Fortnum and Davis 1997; Parving 1984; Davis and Wood 1992; Newton 1985). Where the aetiology is known, at least half are genetic (Smith et al. 1993), and approximately

30% of this group is syndromal (Davis et al. 2004). Fortnum and Davis state that 10% of hearing loss cases in their study had pre- or perinatal aetiologies and 6% had postnatal aetiologies. Postnatally acquired and late-onset cases account for 7.5–25% of permanent childhood hearing impairment (Fortnum 2003; Weichbold et al. 2006). By far the most common childhood hearing loss is the typically temporary, conductive hearing loss caused by Otitis Media (OM) which, in its various forms, has a prevalence of 1.41 per 1000 in high-income North America and as high a prevalence as 97 per 1000 in South Asia (with hearing loss defined as auditory thresholds >25 dB HL in the better ear) (Monasta et al. 2012).

Various expert lists of risk factors for permanent childhood hearing impairment (PCHI) have been compiled. According to the Year 2007 Position Statement: Principles and Guidelines for Early Hearing Detection and Intervention Programs by the Joint Committee on Infant Hearing (2007), risk indicators associated with permanent congenital, delayed-onset or progressive PCHI are:

- Caregiver concern§ regarding hearing, speech, language or developmental delay.
- Family history§ of permanent childhood hearing loss.
- Neonatal intensive care of more than 5 days or any of the following regardless of length of stay: ECMO§, assisted ventilation, exposure to ototoxic medications (gentamicin and tobramycin) or loop diuretics (furosemide) and hyperbilirubinemia that requires exchange transfusion.
- In utero infections, such as CMV§, herpes, rubella, syphilis and toxoplasmosis.
- Craniofacial anomalies, including those that involve the pinna, ear canal, ear tags, ear pits and temporal bone anomalies.
- Physical findings, such as white forelock, that are associated with a syndrome known to include a sensorineural or permanent conductive hearing loss.
- Syndromes associated with hearing loss or progressive or late-onset hearing loss§, such

as neurofibromatosis, osteopetrosis and Usher syndrome; other frequently identified syndromes include Waardenburg, Alport, Pendred and Jervell and Lange-Nielsen.
- Neurodegenerative disorders§, such as Hunter syndrome, or sensory motor neuropathies, such as Friedreich ataxia and Charcot-Marie-Tooth syndrome.
- Culture-positive postnatal infections associated with sensorineural hearing loss, § including confirmed bacterial and viral (especially herpes viruses and varicella) meningitis.
- Head trauma, especially basal skull/temporal bone fracture§ that requires hospitalisation.
- Chemotherapy§.

Risk indicators that are marked with a "§" are of greater concern for delayed-onset hearing loss.

The US Preventive Services Task Force (2008) lists the following risk factors: NICU admission for ≥2 days, family history of hereditary childhood sensorineural hearing loss, craniofacial abnormalities, certain congenital syndromes (such as Usher or Waardenburg) and infections (e.g. toxoplasmosis, bacterial meningitis, syphilis, rubella, *Cytomegalovirus*, *Herpes virus*).

A retrospective study conducted by Connolly et al. (2005) found that 1 of 75 infants with such risk factors had a hearing loss, but only 1 of 811 infants without risk factors did. The National Institutes of Health (NIH) (1993) reported that of all babies born with hearing loss each year, approximately 50% were discharged from the well-baby clinic with no known risk factors for hearing loss. Universal newborn hearing screening programmes, which are already implemented in many countries, are therefore of crucial importance.

Detailed information on the aetiology of childhood hearing loss will be given in the Sect. 14.8 Infection with Neurotropic Viruses, Sect. 14.9 Ototoxicity in Children, Sect. 14.10 Genetics of Hearing Loss and Sect. 14.11 Syndromes Associated with Hearing Impairment. Aetiological aspects of special kinds of hearing loss are presented in the Sect. 15.1 Types and Time Courses of Hearing Loss, Sect. 15.2

Auditory Processing Disorders, Sect. 15.3 Hyperacusis, Sect. 15.4 Tinnitus and Sect. 15.5 Nonorganic (Functional) Hearing Loss.

14.7.2 Additional Disabilities

Prevalence data concerning additional disabilities vary in the literature from approximately 20–40% of children born with hearing loss. For example, the 2007–2008 Annual Survey of Deaf and Hard of Hearing Children in the USA shows 39.3% of children with educationally relevant conditions; the study of Cupples et al. (2014) reported 26.4% of hearing-impaired children with additional handicaps. In spite of such differences—possibly due to different methodological approaches and demographical distinctions— mental retardation and learning disability are more frequent than visual impairment, cerebral palsy or autism spectrum disorder (Cupples et al. 2014) (for further details, see Sect. 16.23).

To identify the cause of hearing loss and to detect possible coexisting medical conditions, the following overview presents a pathway for medical investigations offering the chance to avoid progression of hearing impairment and to prevent complications. Further details can be found in Sect. 16.20.

14.7.3 Medical Investigations for Clarification of Aetiology

Since the introduction of the newborn hearing screening programme (NHSP), permanent childhood hearing impairment (PCHI) is being identified at an earlier age. Parents and families are being provided with a wealth of medical information and intervention within days of having a new baby. Investigating hearing loss in a timely manner has a direct impact on understanding the cause of hearing loss in the child and importantly on the acceptance of the diagnosis by the family, although it is recognised that sometimes it may affect bonding between child and a parent. Medical investigations must be initiated by a pro-

fessional with training and understanding of the complexities associated with a diagnosis of hearing loss.

Historically, congenital PCHI has been classified as either hereditary or acquired. Investigations aim to identify the cause of hearing loss, identify coexisting medical conditions (e.g. renal pathology in Branchio-Oto-Renal syndrome) and prevent progression in hearing loss in those children identified with widened vestibular aqueduct (WVA) or congenital *cytomegalovirus* infection (CMV). In addition, investigations may help us understand genetic hearing loss and secure genetic counselling. Investigations may help identify and prevent complications in some children with profound sensorineural hearing loss (SNHL) and cardiac conduction defects (Jervell and Lange-Nielsen syndrome). Children identified with mitochondrial m.1555A > G mutation will be given advice regarding development of progressive hearing loss associated with aminoglycoside medications, thereby preventing further deterioration in hearing by avoiding exposure to those medicines.

The objectives of performing investigations are therefore to provide the best clinical and audiological outcomes in a child with PCHI. A robust and systematic pathway for investigations by a suitably trained professional is essential for the success of the process.

14.7.4 Timing of Investigations

Investigations should be offered as soon as possible so as to maximise the chance of arriving at a diagnosis (BAAP 2015a, b, c) with consideration given to parental readiness and the general health of the baby.

Investigations should be considered as an active process as new data emerge as the child grows; therefore a review of the diagnosis at each clinical encounter is extremely useful. One positive investigation does not automatically exclude other conditions, as varied aetiology providing diagnostic clues may be present in an individual child.

Some treatable viral infections that may improve clinical outcomes benefit from early identification. Other investigations can be delayed in a family where there are difficulties with acceptance of the diagnosis.

14.7.5 History

General History The aetiology can be traced by careful history-taking and should include the details of pregnancy (possible maternal intrauterine infections in the first trimester, exposure to drugs and alcohol during pregnancy, ABO incompatibility, rhesus disease and maternal diabetes/hypothyroidism), birth and postnatal period.

Perinatal events including hypoxia, hyperbilirubinaemia, sepsis and the potential exposure to ototoxic medication and the need for mechanical ventilation should be asked for.

Postnatal history should cover history of meningitis (neonatal meningitis is a well-known risk factor for hearing loss), noise exposure including incubator noise, ototoxic medication/radiotherapy, history of falls and accidents leading to head injuries, viral illnesses of childhood such as mumps, measles and rubella and immunisation status (Bamiou et al. 2000) (see Sect. 16.1).

Family History A detailed family history of hearing loss or risk factors associated with hearing loss in at least three generations should be recorded wherever possible (BAAP 2015a, b, c). Any consanguinity between parents must be noted. A pedigree chart can indicate modes of inheritance such as Mendelian dominant, recessive, X-linked or mitochondrial (see Sect. 16.1).

14.7.6 Clinical Examination

It is imperative to carry out a complete physical examination after undressing the child. Height, weight and head circumference should be measured and plotted on an appropriate growth chart recording centiles for comparison. Particular note must be made of the ocular region, ears, nose, midface and neck. Otoscopy and examination of the palate are essential. Further, examination of the skin for pigmentation, limbs and digits, spine, cardiovascular system and cranial nerves is important (BAAP 2015a, b, c) (see Sect. 16.1).

14.7.7 Family Audiograms

All first- and second- (if possible) degree relatives should have formal audiometric assessment whether or not they report hearing difficulties. It is recommended that each Paediatric Audiology Department has a robust policy for performing family audiograms with the necessary referrals should a hearing loss be identified (see Sect. 17.4).

14.7.8 Consultative Examinations

Ophthalmology It is estimated that 40% of children with PCHI may in addition have an ophthalmological condition (Guy et al. 2003). Vision and the development of communication are closely linked (Laffan 1993). Children with deafness are more reliant on their vision for their communication as they may use Picture Exchange Communication System (PECS) and lip reading to aid their communication.

The Royal College of Ophthalmologists recommends targeted clinical surveillance of certain groups at high risk of eye disorders, including children with a sensorineural deafness. It recommends the inclusion of a full orthoptic examination, cycloplegic refraction and a fundus examination (NDCS and Sense 2014).

In some children with SNHL, the eye examination may help make the diagnosis such as CHARGE association, Usher syndrome or congenital CMV.

Electrocardiography (ECG) All children with bilateral profound SNHL must be offered an ECG to examine the possibility of a long QT interval. Jervell Lange-Nielsen Syndrome (JLNS) is an extremely rare condition with a long QT interval and profound SNHL but associated risk of sudden death, preventable if identified early.

An immediate referral to a Paediatric Cardiologist is recommended.

Genetic Investigation Examinations for connexin 26 and 30 mutations, mitochondrial mutation m.1555A > G where there is history of hearing loss through maternal inheritance or hearing loss following application of the aminoglycosides, Pendrin gene testing in children with bilateral widened vestibular aqueduct (WVA) and Mondini anomaly (Bogazzi et al. 2004) are currently recommended.

Families can also be referred to a geneticist if there are dysmorphic features, developmental delay, multiple unexplained pathologies or on parental request. The geneticist may be able to suggest additional investigations that are not routinely available. Parents must be given a thorough explanation of the advantages and disadvantages of those tests and must be assisted in making an informed decision regarding whether or not they would like to have their child investigated (see Sect. 16.22).

14.7.9 Serological Investigations

Testing for Congenital Infections Congenital *cytomegalovirus* (cCMV) accounts for 20% of all childhood sensorineural hearing loss (SNHL) but is not routinely tested for at birth. Valganciclovir has been shown to prevent hearing deterioration and improve neurocognitive outcomes if started in the first month of life (Kadambari et al. 2015a).

In babies less than 1 year old, urinary or salivary CMV DNA PCR on two separate occasions should be performed. In babies less than 3 weeks of age, a positive test confirms congenital CMV. In children greater than 1 year of age, CMV IgG antibody testing with or without urinary CMV DNA PCR should be performed. In both groups a positive result must be confirmed with neonatal dried blood spot testing for CMV DNA. At any age maternal CMV IgG antibody testing can be performed; a negative result rules out congenital CMV.

Serology for rubella, toxoplasma, syphilis and HIV can also be carried out where clinically indicated.

Thyroid Function Tests These should be carried out in families with history of thyroid disease or goitre. They should be considered in children with WVA or Mondini deformity; as the thyroid dysfunction in Pendred syndrome tends to occur in late childhood, testing should be timed accordingly.

Urine Examination Dipstick studies for the presence of blood and protein should be carried out in order to exclude Alport syndrome.

Autoimmune Tests These should be reserved for children with progressive hearing loss or where there is evidence of systemic involvement. Tests may include antinuclear antibodies, antineutrophil cytoplasmic antibodies, dsDNA, RA factor, antiphospholipid, anticardiolipin, antithyroid antibody, antibodies to Sm, ESR, CRP and others as indicated (BAAP 2015a, b, c).

14.7.10 Imaging

Magnetic resonance imaging (MRI) of the inner ears and internal auditory meatuses (IAMs) is the first-line radiological investigation in children (BAAP 2015a, b, c). This investigation will show structural anomalies of the ear (soft tissue) apart from details of the ossicular chain. The computed tomography (CT) scan of the petrous temporal bone in children with permanent conductive hearing loss and craniofacial anomalies will show the bony structures (see Sect. 16.21).

14.7.11 Vestibular Investigations

These investigations should be considered when motor milestones are delayed or there are reported problems with balance or complaints of dizziness. Children presenting with imbalance, motor developmental delay and hearing impairment of various degrees should be suspected of having vestibular dysfunction. This discovery will help the establishment of the diagnosis in a child presenting with hearing impairment but also will allow for treatment and possible avoidance of life-threatening circumstances in the future.

Reported prevalence of vestibular disorders in the deaf population of children is 30–40% (Moller 2002) (see Sect. 16.15).

At times, despite thorough medical investigations, no cause of hearing impairment can be established. These children require periodic review of their investigations, concurrently with reassessment of their medical and audiological status.

14.8 Infection with Neurotropic Viruses

Antoinette am Zehnhoff-Dinnesen, Sabrina Regele, and Ross Parfitt

14.8.1 Definition and Classification

Neurotropic viruses have a predilection for nervous tissue and may be neuroinvasive (entering or infecting tissue) and neurovirulent (causing disease). Viruses may enter the nervous system via blood when infected immune cells carry the virus to nervous tissue or when blood capillaries are crossed by free viruses or in leukocytes (Nath and Berger 2003). Viruses can also travel along the axons of nerves, thus escaping the immune system (Wright et al. 2008). Once viruses are inside neurons, they can survive for the host's lifetime and cause damage to the nervous system (Nath and Berger 2003).

Hotta (1997) classified neurotropic viruses according to the course of the infection:

- Acute infection possible by: Japanese encephalitis, *Venezuelan equine encephalitis and California encephalitis viruses, tick-borne encephalitis virus (TBEV)*, polio, coxsackie, echo, mumps, measles, influenza, rabies viruses, members of the family *Herpesviridae* such as *herpes simplex, varicella-zoster, cytomegalo, HHV-6 and Epstein-Barr viruses*

- Latent infection possible by: *herpes simplex and varicella-zoster viruses*
- Slow virus infection possible by: *measles, rubella and John Cunningham (JC) viruses*, retroviruses such as *human T-lymphotropic virus 1* and *human immunodeficiency virus*

Neurotropic viruses are typically classified as DNA, RNA or retroviruses (RNA viruses that replicate through a DNA intermediate).

According to Jackson (2013), the following viruses may also cause damage to the human nervous system: *enterovirus, West Nile virus, chikungunya virus, Nipah virus and viral haemorrhagic fever (VHF) agents.*

Hearing impairment may be caused by viral-induced labyrinthitis, by neuritis of the vestibulo-cochlear nerve or by meningitis/encephalitis, with the subtypes sensorineural hearing loss (SNHL), central hearing loss or a combination of both. Inner ear structures may be damaged by infection or by inflammatory responses (Newton and Vallely 2006). Harris et al. (1984) found strong immunologic responses within the inner ear, with the production of a fibro-osseous matrix being responsible for nonreversible cochlear injury. Ječmenica and Opančina (2015) stated that retrocochlear damage in children with purulent meningitis, or who were born with a rubella virus or CMV infection, was detectable on auditory-brainstem response (ABR) testing.

14.8.1.1 DNA Viruses, Family *Herpesviridae*

Human Cytomegalovirus (CMV) Infection CMV belongs to the beta-herpes virus subfamily and is transmitted by saliva, blood, organ transplantations, genital secretions, urine or breast milk. In the USA, nearly 90% of the population is infected by the eighth decade of life (Swanson and Schleiss 2013). CMV may persistently infect the inner ear (Sugiura et al. 2004), may be reactivated and may cause congenital infection (Cook 2007).

Congenital CMV (cCMV) is caused by new infections or reactivated latent infection in the mother. The greatest risk of symptomatic disease caused by CMV is found during the first trimester. There is also a high risk of symptomatic disease in infants if the infection occurred in the mother around the time of conception. The highest risk for foetal infection is in the third trimester. However infection in the third trimester shows a low risk of symptomatic disease (Enders et al. 2011).

According to Choo and Meinzen-Derr (2010), almost 1% of newborns are infected with CMV. 11–13% of neonates with CMV are symptomatic, with petechiae, jaundice, hepatosplenomegaly, microcephaly, seizures, chorioretinitis, SNHL and small size for gestational age being common symptoms. 40–58% of symptomatic CMV children develop long-term sequelae, such as SNHL, visual impairment, intracranial calcifications (especially in the germinal matrix and periventricular), seizure disorder, cerebral palsy and intellectual or physical disabilities.

13.5% of children who are asymptomatic at birth may develop neurological impairment, most often hearing loss (Swanson and Schleiss 2013). CMV is the main cause of nonhereditary congenital hearing loss, and without any doubt cytomegalovirus infections are underdiagnosed dramatically in childhood hearing loss.

In a longitudinal study, Dahle et al. (2000) found unilateral hearing loss in 40%, bilateral hearing loss in 60% and progressive hearing loss in 54% of cases. Fowler (2013) suggests the possibility of late-onset hearing loss and fluctuating hearing loss. Bilavsky et al. (2016) diagnosed hearing impairment in 36.2% of infants with symptomatic congenital cytomegalovirus. Unilateral hearing impairment occurred in 57.4% of these cases and bilateral hearing impairment in 42.6%. Monitoring of auditory function is therefore urgently needed in these children (Foulon et al. 2008; Fowler 2013). Follow-up investigations over at least 6 years are recommended (Goderis et al. 2014).

Qiao et al. (2011) found fibrous degeneration of the scala media and the cochlear duct and thickening of Reissner's membrane in animals infected with CMV, and Teissier et al. (2011) found extensive damage of the stria vascularis and non-sensory epithelia in the inner ear of human foetuses with cCMV infection. The severity of the inner ear infection correlated with the extent of CNS lesions. High risk of hearing loss has been found in clinical studies in children with cerebral involvement, a failure to thrive, petechiae or disseminated affectation (Smets et al. 2006; Grosse et al. 2008; Rosenthal et al. 2009).

It is important to detect congenital CMV infections in the first 2–3 weeks after birth in order to differentiate them from postnatal CMV infections (de Vries et al. 2012). CMV DNA can be found in saliva and urine (Ross et al. 2015). It is also possible to detect CMV DNA in dried blood spotted on filter paper, which is used for the metabolic screening of newborns (Koontz et al. 2015). A positive result here will identify congenital CMV infection. A negative result however does not exclude a congenital CMV infection (Boppana et al. 2010).

Nigro et al. (2005) treated pregnant women who had CMV or CMV DNA in their amniotic fluid with intravenous CMV hyperimmune globulin, which significantly reduced the incidence of CMV disease in their infants from 50% in the untreated control group to 3.2%. The intravenous application of Ganciclovir was found to prevent hearing loss in infants with symptomatic CMV infection (Kimberlin et al. 2003), and neutropenia was controllable. Initial intravenous and subsequent oral application of Ganciclovir/Valganciclovir (which after oral administration is rapidly converted into Ganciclovir) was also found to be effective in preventing hearing loss (Amir et al. 2010). Significantly less developmental delay was apparent in infants with symptomatic congenital CMV infection, including cerebral involvement, after preventive intravenous therapy with Ganciclovir (Oliver et al. 2009). Valganciclovir has been shown to prevent hearing deterioration and improve neurocognitive outcomes if started in the first month of life (Kadambari et al. 2015b). For symptomatic congenital CMV, Kimberlin et al. (2015) showed that long-term hearing and neurodevelopmental outcomes are better following 6 months of treatment with oral Valganciclovir than just 6 weeks. Bilavsky et al. (2016) treated infants with symptomatic congenital cytomegalovirus for 1 year with Ganciclovir/Valganciclovir. Hearing impairment improved in 64.8% of cases. Improvement in hearing sensitivity was more common in infants born with mild or moderate hearing loss than with severe hearing impairment.

In infants with asymptomatic CMV infection, SNHL has also been shown to be prevented (Lackner et al. 2009) or improved (Çiftdoğan and Vardar 2011) by Ganciclovir/Valganciclovir treatment. In cases of resistance to Ganciclovir, Cidofovir may be used (White et al. 2006).

Different immunisation strategies are being tested in clinical trials (Swanson and Schleiss 2013), and implications for vaccine design are discussed in Wang and Fu (2014).

Until a vaccine is licensed in different countries, and vaccination is routinely performed, strategies aimed at reducing CMV transmission have to be defined (Swanson and Schleiss 2013).

Stowell et al. (2012) found that CMV survives for 6 h on rubber, cloth and crackers, 3 h on glass and plastic and 1 h on wood and metal. To reduce the risk of infection, pregnant women are advised to wash their hands frequently, avoid intimate contact with children and not to share towels or food (Picone et al. 2009). Cordier et al. (2012a, b) recommend education programmes for pregnant women and further training for healthcare providers. Kadambari et al. (2013) postulate the combination of screening for cCMV with the Neonatal Hearing Screening to improve early detection/prevention of SNHL, especially in infants with cCMV who are asymptomatic at birth, and to enhance aetiological clarification. Consensus recommendations for prevention, diagnosis and management of congenital CMV infection are presented in (Rawlinson et al. 2017; Luck et al. 2017).

Herpes Simplex Virus (HSV) Infection *HSV-1* (labial herpes) and *HSV2* (genital herpes) are both encapsulated, double-stranded DNA viruses of the herpesvirus family (Cohen et al. 2014).

Neonatal infection with HSV affects 1 in 2000 to 1 in 8000 live births in the USA (Muller et al. 2010). The highest transmission rate of infected neonates takes place during the peripartum period.

Only 5% of cases are believed to be in utero infections (Kimberlin 2004).

It is therefore important to prevent the genital HSV infection near term. The infection rate can be reduced by Caesarean delivery (Brown et al. 2003).

HSV infection causes a wide spectrum of clinical diseases: skin, mucous membrane and eye infections, encephalitis and multi-organ disease (Muller et al. 2010).

After a systematic review of the literature, Westerberg et al. (2008) stated that SNHL in children with exposure to HSV is rare. Following intrauterine infection, other clinical sequelae of HSV infection and comorbid conditions may themselves be causative or contributory factors to the development of SNHL in neonates. The authors conclude that there is at present no advantage from routine serological screening for HSV infection in addition to newborn hearing screening in otherwise healthy neonates. In neonates with clinical or serological findings of HSV infection, newborn hearing screening and hearing evaluation before the age of 30 months should be performed. There is currently no knowledge about HSV as a risk factor for delayed-onset SNHL.

Cohen et al. (2014) demonstrated in another review that hearing loss is bilateral and severe when caused by HSV1 infection after infancy associated with meningitis or encephalitis.

Hearing loss associated with HSV-1 or HSV-2 infections is treated with antiherpetic agents and steroids.

In connection with cochlear implantation of children with idiopathic SNHL, Noorbakhsh et al. (2011) found HSV DNA in the perilymph of 1 out of 18 children investigated, but these findings were not supported by Sugiura et al. (2004).

Human Herpes Virus (HHV6) Infection *HHV-6* belongs to the beta-herpes virus subfamily. *HHV-6* is present in ~1 in every 101 births (Caserta et al. 2014). According to Sugiura et al. (2004), *HHV-6* is transmitted with high prevalence during early infancy. *HHV-6* causes a febrile disease with rash and may provoke illnesses of the CNS, the gastrointestinal and respiratory tracts and blood cells. The relationship between *HHV-6* and SNHL, for example, the appearance of a sudden hearing loss, is still unclear. Little is known about neurodevelopmental deficits, including SNHL, by congenital HHV-6 infection (Hall et al. 2010).

Caserta et al. (2014) examined children with HHV-6 congenital infection. Information on newborn hearing was collected, and an audiological evaluation was performed between 12 and 24 months of age. No child had an abnormal newborn screening or any identifiable hearing loss at the evaluation. However, the children showed cognitive impairment at 12 months of age, as defined by the Mental Development Index (MDI) of the Bayley Scales of Infant Development II (Steiner 2013).

14.8.1.2 RNA Viruses, Paramyxoviruses

Measles According to the Advisory Committee on Immunization Practices (ACIP) (McLean et al. 2013), measles, which is caused by *Morbillivirus* (the family of the Paramyxoviruses), is highly contagious and transmitted by airborne respiratory droplets. The incubation period lasts 10–12 days, and sufferers are infectious from 4 days before rash onset until 4 days afterwards. Reports from before the introduction of vaccination suggested that 5–10 % of profound bilateral sensorineural hearing loss was caused by measles (McKenna 1997) but measles had been nearly eliminated by vaccination. However, infection from people who decline vaccination still occurs. By the age of 6 months, the infant is no longer protected by maternal antibodies if vaccination is not completed. If infants aged 6 to 11 months are exposed to the virus, immunoglobulin products should be applied (McLean et al. 2013). One measles patient per 1000 suffers from encephalitis with a risk of developing SNHL but reliable recent estimates of the role of the measles virus in SNHL are lacking (Rima 2006). Seven percent of patients suffer from otitis media, and this prevalence increases to 30% in cases with severe respiratory involvement (Rima 2006). Measles may play a role in

the development of otosclerosis (Niedermeyer and Arnold 2008).

Mumps Mumps is caused by *Rubulavirus* from the Paramyxoviruses family (McLean et al. 2013). The incubation period lasts 16–18 days, and the symptoms are fever and inflammation of the salivary glands. Encephalitis occurs in 1 out of 6000 cases. In the pre-vaccine era, mumps was a major cause of hearing loss in children and adolescents (mostly permanent, unilateral impairment, though bilateral and reversible cases are reported), even after asymptomatic infections (Wright 2006). Incidence of mumps-related hearing loss varies considerably, from as low as 1 out of 30,000 to as high as 3 out of 100, depending on levels of vaccination in different communities (Cohen et al. 2014). El-Badry et al. (2015) reported unilateral peripheral vestibular dysfunction in 58% of mumps patients with profound unilateral SNHL. Initial transmission of the virus is via respiratory secretions and routes of infection of the inner ear include blood, CSF/perilymph and (rarely) the eighth cranial nerve (Wright 2006). In the USA, outbreaks are still observed, for example, in clusters of unvaccinated people, such as religious communities or on university campuses (McLean et al. 2013). Vaccination is effective and safe ((SNHL following the live measles, mumps and rubella vaccine is reported as 1 out of 6,000,000–8,000,000 doses (Asatryan et al. 2008)) but is still not available in all parts of the world (Wright 2006).

14.8.1.3 RNA Viruses, Togaviruses

Rubella Rubella is caused by *Rubivirus*, which belongs to the Togavirus family, and is transmitted by nasopharyngeal secretions. The symptoms consist of rash, low-grade fever, lymphadenopathy and malaise. Encephalitis is reported in 1 out of 6000 cases, with adults being the most affected (McLean et al. 2013). Bilateral SNHL is the most common consequence of congenital rubella (Cohen et al. 2014). Infection during the first trimester of pregnancy leads to congenital rubella syndrome (CRS), characterised by cataracts, hearing loss, intellectual disability and heart defects. In the USA, rubella has been nearly eliminated by vaccination; rare cases are related to importation. Muscat et al. (2012) report a median rubella incidence of 0.3 in 1 million inhabitants in Europe in 2008. Hamdan et al. (2011) measured a rubella prevalence of 65.3% in a sample of 231 pregnant women in western Sudan.

Salt-and-pepper retinopathy is crucially suggestive of rubella-induced deafness (see Tamayo et al. 2013, who recommended a thorough ophthalmologic examination in all cases of hearing impairment). Dewan and Gupta (2012) reported ophthalmic signs of CRS in 29% of 374 deaf school children in southern India.

Since rubella vaccine is scarce in Nigeria, Onakewhor and Chiwuzie (2011) recommend the immunisation of children and women of child-bearing age. The worldwide eradication of rubella has still not been successful, and its contribution to congenital hearing loss and childhood disability has still to be taken into account (Tookey 2006).

14.8.1.4 RNA Viruses, Flaviviruses

Tick-Borne Encephalitis (TBE) The causative virus belongs to the family of flaviviruses, of which more than 10,000 cases are reported annually worldwide (Marsala et al. 2014). Schuler et al. (2014) reported an average annual incidence of tick-borne encephalitis/meningitis of two cases per 100,000 in Switzerland. According to Marsala et al. (2014), the tick bite goes unnoticed in about a third of patients. A third of patients develop disease, of whom two-thirds experience an initial incubation period of 4–28 days, followed by the first stage of illness with fever, headache and body pain (2–10 days); then a symptom-free interval of 1–21 days occurs before the start of the second phase, which features a febrile syndrome and possible complications, such as meningitis/encephalitis/myelitis and consecutive neurological symptoms including balance disorders (Kaiser 2012) and hearing loss. The outcome is worse after infection with Siberian and Far Eastern virus subtypes than with the European subtype. Increasing age is a risk factor for a worse clinical course. Genetic factors also have to be considered (Bogovic and Strle 2015). In case of a combined infection with *Borrelia burgdorferi*, the course of disease is more severe (Marsala et al. 2014). TBE vaccination coverage is still low, even in endemic regions. Efforts to promote vaccination should be intensified.

14.8.1.5 Retroviruses

Human Immune Deficiency Virus (HIV)/ Acquired Immunodeficiency Syndrome (AIDS) The number of HIV-infected children worldwide is estimated to be 3.4 million, of whom approximately 28% have access to antiretroviral therapy (Laughton et al. 2013). Opportunistic infections, ototoxic drugs and the virus itself may cause hearing loss in HIV-/AIDS-positive children. The type of hearing loss may be sensorineural, conductive or mixed (da Silva Araújo et al. 2012).

Various international studies have found hearing loss in 13–39% of HIV-positive children: Makar et al. (2012) observed approximately equal numbers of sensorineural versus conductive hearing losses, Ndoleriire et al. (2013) sensorineural hearing loss in 64% and Chao et al. (2012) predominantly conductive hearing loss. Torre et al. (2012) additionally reported a correlation between the incidence of hearing loss and the severity of the HIV illness. Hrapcak et al. (2016) found hearing loss in 24% of 380 HIV-infected children (82% conductive, 14% sensorineural and 4% mixed). The authors observed the following risk factors: frequent ear infections, ear drainage, tuberculosis, severe HIV disease and low BMI.

Harris et al. (2012) emphasise the necessity of considering ototoxic drugs in HIV-positive patients, especially ototoxic tuberculosis drugs. Highly active antiretroviral therapy (HAAT) seems to damage outer hair cell mitochondria, especially in combination with noise exposure.

HIV-/AIDS-positive children should have routine screening for hearing impairment and periodic otorhinolaryngological/pedaudiological assessment.

14.8.2 Diagnostics/Audiological Monitoring

Diagnostics should be performed in cooperation with a paediatrician/neuropaediatrician. Possible diagnostic techniques for viral brain diseases include neuroimaging by CT and MRI scans, lumbar puncture, analysis of cerebrospinal fluid (CSF), real-time polymerase chain reaction (PCR) assays from the CSF in the first days of infection, and serology with determination of acute and convalescent viral antibody titres (at onset and 1 month and 3 months later) (Wilson and Gulya 1993).

Because of possible progression, fluctuation, reversibility or late-onset of hearing loss caused by neurotropic viruses, regular pedaudiological controls and long-term follow-up are essential. Possible additional effects of ototoxic drugs should be considered.

14.8.3 Therapy/Rehabilitation

Specific paediatric/neuropaediatric intervention is necessary, possibly including active and passive immunisation strategies.

Rehabilitative pedaudiological provisions may include hearing aid supply, FM system supply (Frequency Modulation System, a wireless transmitter system, e.g. transmitting sound from the teacher's microphone to the pupil's hearing aid), cochlear implantation, advice regarding preferential classroom seating, absorption of background noise in classrooms, information to parents/teachers and advice against noise exposure.

14.8.4 Prevention

In cases of an existing vaccine, the vaccination coverage should be increased worldwide to reduce avoidable virus-induced hearing loss in infants and children and its consecutive sequelae for language acquisition, psychosocial development, literacy acquisition and academic chances. Long-lasting immunity is provided by mumps, measles and rubella vaccination (McLean et al.

2013). Immunity following TBE vaccination extends up to at least 3 years. The necessity for revaccination has to be considered. Bochennek et al. (2014) underline that a significant number of paediatric tumour patients lose their pre-existing humoral immunity against measles, mumps and rubella after the end of chemotherapy. This risk is higher in children with acute lymphatic leukaemia and in younger children. Post-chemotherapy revaccination is necessary.

In cases of as-yet non-existent vaccination, efforts to develop a vaccine and to promote licensing in different countries and utilisation by the population should be intensified.

14.9 Ototoxicity in Children

Antoinette am Zehnhoff-Dinnesen, Thorsten Langer, and Oliver Zolk

More than 700 drugs are known to be ototoxic. Ototoxic drugs can act on the cochlea, the vestibular system or both, potentially resulting in tinnitus, sensorineural hearing loss, disequilibrium or nausea. Data on the incidence of drug-induced disequilibrium, nausea and tinnitus in paediatric patients are sparse, although more information is available about drug-induced hearing loss, which is the focus of this chapter.

14.9.1 Anticancer Drugs

Among the anticancer drugs, platinum compounds pose the highest risk of damage to the inner ear (Langer et al. 2013; Stöhr et al. 2005). Cisplatin and carboplatin are effective antineoplastic agents widely used for the treatment of a variety of paediatric cancers. Ototoxic side effects are common and occur in up to 90% of patients receiving cisplatin, and these effects are dose-dependent. The incidence of cisplatin-related ototoxicity increases by an average of 5–7% per additional 100 mg/m^2 cumulative dose of cisplatin. Moreover, younger age, prior irradiation, concomitant ototoxic drugs and renal dysfunction individually contribute to the severity of hearing deficits at any given cisplatin dose (Langer et al. 2013). Carboplatin is less ototoxic, with incidence rates of up to 50%; however, the incidence markedly increases when the brain disposition of carboplatin is enhanced by transient osmotic opening of the blood-brain barrier for treatment of brain tumours or brain metastases (Brock et al. 2012).

Platinum drugs induce apoptosis of the outer hair cells and degeneration of the stria vascularis and spiral ganglion cells via formation of DNA adducts, which activate the inflammatory cascade and generate oxidative stress in the cells (Waissbluth and Daniel 2013). Platinum ototoxicity usually manifests as bilateral, symmetrical, sensorineural hearing loss and is often accompanied by tinnitus and vertigo. Platinum drug-induced hearing loss initially affects the higher frequencies ($\geq$4 kHz) but can progress to encompass the speech frequencies (<3.5 kHz) (Knight et al. 2005). High-frequency hearing loss renders certain consonants (e.g. sibilant sounds) inaudible and may compromise speech recognition and comprehension, especially in the presence of noise. This complication renders affected children vulnerable to underachievement in school and has debilitating effects on the patients' quality of life (Langer et al. 2013). Hearing loss is especially problematic in infants and young children in the phase of language development. In addition, these ototoxic symptoms can progress even further after therapy.

Even after controlling for established clinical risk factors, interindividual variation in susceptibility to platinum ototoxicity remains high (Langer et al. 2013). This variation has prompted the search for genetic markers, such as single nucleotide polymorphisms in hereditary deafness genes, in genes involved in the transport, metabolism and detoxification of cisplatin, as well as in the nucleotide excision repair pathway, to be utilised for risk stratification (Langer et al. 2013). As a result, information on the association of polymorphisms in the thiopurine *S*-methyltransferase gene with cisplatin-induced hearing loss has been included in the Food and Drug Administration (FDA) drug label for cisplatin. Nevertheless, markers with sufficient predictive value to be used in routine clinical practice in identifying susceptible individuals before commencement of platinum drug treatment are still lacking.

Among anticancer drugs, etoposide and vinca alkaloids have also been documented to cause sensorineural hearing loss, although at a much lower frequency than the platinum compounds.

14.9.2 Anti-infective Agents

Aminoglycoside antibiotics (e.g. amikacin, gentamicin, tobramycin and neomycin), although oto- and nephrotoxic, are essential for the treatment of serious bacterial infections. Their adverse effects on auditory functions may be related to the dosage and dosing interval (i.e. drug levels in the plasma) and the duration of therapy. Changing dosing regimens of aminoglycosides from multiple times per day to a once-daily regime, however, reduces the resultant nephrotoxicity but not the ototoxicity. Aminoglycosides accumulate in the inner ear fluid from which these molecules are slowly eliminated. The subsequent degeneration of hair cells and neurons causes high-frequency hearing loss that is usually irreversible, bilateral and progressive and which extends to lower frequencies with prolonged treatment. Cochleotoxic effects may also manifest as tinnitus. Moreover, aminoglycosides can be vestibulotoxic, causing transient nystagmus and imbalance (Mudd et al. 2012). Ototoxicity of aminoglycosides is regarded highest in neomycin, followed by gentamicin, kanamycin and tobramycin, with least toxicity in amikacin and netilmicin. Cochleotoxicity is considered to be predominant in amikacin and neomycin and vestibulotoxicity in gentamicin (Schacht et al. 2012).

The incidence of aminoglycoside-induced ototoxicity, which can reach 60%, depends on the compound, the dose, the duration of treatment and the patient age group. Inflammation seems to boost the uptake of aminoglycosides into the inner ear (Koo et al. 2015). Incidences are generally underestimated because long-term follow-up is rare and specific high-frequency audiometry is not always performed (So 2009). While some children do not develop noticeable hearing loss despite high exposure to aminoglycosides, others may experience irreversible, profound hearing loss after very low exposure. This interindividual variability is, in part, related to a familial predisposition, which has been attributed to mutations in the mitochondrial genome and in particular to the m.1555A > G polymorphism (rs267606617) in the mitochondrially encoded 12S RNA (Bitner-Glindzicz and Rahman 2007).

Other potentially ototoxic anti-infective agents include the macrolide antibiotics vancomycin, teicoplanin and minocycline; the antifungal drug amphotericin B; the antiprotozoal drug chloroquine; and the antiviral drug Ganciclovir. Combination therapy of anti-infective drugs with ototoxic potential, as for the treatment of serious infections, may potentiate auditory adverse reactions. Unfortunately, limited information on the possible ototoxicity of anti-retroviral therapy is available, and, thus, discrimination between the effects of the therapy and the direct effects of HIV on auditory function from the viral neurotropism is quite difficult.

Both reversible and irreversible sensorineural hearing loss and tinnitus are well-known side effects of the quinolone-type antiprotozoal drugs (e.g. quinine, chloroquine and mefloquine) that are used for treatment of malaria (Bitner-Glindzicz and Rahman 2007; Bortoli and Santiago 2007). Malaria is a disease of high prevalence worldwide and affects mostly children less than 15 years old. Therefore ototoxic side effects may cause a significant individual and societal burden. Unlike that for quinolines, ototoxicity has not been reported with the use of other antimalarials, such as atovaquone/proguanil and artemeter/lumefantrine (Gürkov et al. 2008).

14.9.3 Loop Diuretics

Although generally safe, a side effect of loop diuretics (e.g. furosemide, bumetanide and ethacrynic acid) is ototoxicity, which has been related to the blood level of the drug. Rapid infusion and drug accumulation following use of large parenteral doses for renal failure increase toxicity. These drugs can cause either a temporary or in some cases a permanent loss of hearing. Less common are tinnitus and disequilibrium, which rarely occur in the absence of hearing loss. Animal experiments show that these drugs act on the stria vascularis, producing oedema of these tissues and resulting in a decrease of the endocochlear potential. Ototoxicity seems to be less frequent following the use of bumetanide than furosemide, whereas irreversible hearing loss seems to be much more common with ethacrynic acid use (Greenberg 2000; So 2009). As a consequence of immature drug elimination capabilities, preterm infants exhibit a prolonged plasma half-life of furosemide and thus may be at increased risk of ototoxicity (Peterson et al. 1980), although an increased frequency of acute hearing loss in these patients has not been confirmed (Rais-Bahrami et al. 2004; de Hoog et al. 2003).

14.9.4 Ototopical Medications

As the debate between studies arguing for and against ototoxicity by topical otic antibiotics has not come to an end up to now (Crowson et al. 2016), in case of perforation of the tympanic membrane, grommets, mastoid cavity with open middle ear and, in case of pre-existing sensorineural hearing loss, non-ototoxic antibiotic preparations, such as the fluoroquinolone ofloxacin, should be used (Mudd et al. 2012; Haynes et al. 2007). For the treatment of otitis media, the effect of intratympanic injection of ciprofloxacin hydrogel providing sustained release of the drug to the middle ear was superior to conventional ototopical application in an animal study (Wang et al. 2014).

A combination of Colistin (polymyxin E), bacitracin (polypeptide antibiotic, orally nephrotoxic) and hydrocortisone was applicated topically in children with acute otorrhoea after insertion of ventilation tubes and was found to be superior to oral amoxicillin–clavulanate suspension (van Dongen et al. 2014). While in 21% of the children in the group with topical therapy ear drops were aggravating or painful, in the group with systemic therapy 23% had gastrointestinal trouble.

If potentially ototoxic ear drops are urgently needed for open middle ear, a pre-therapeutic audiogram should be performed (Mudd et al. 2012), informed permission of parents/patients should be obtained, advice concerning possible ototoxic reactions should be provided and aminoglycosides and long-term therapy should be avoided (Haynes et al. 2007).

The antiseptics Vosol (acetic acid otic solution), gentian violet, povidone-iodine and chlorhexidine have ototoxic potential (Haynes et al. 2007), whereas, at least in animal studies, Ciclopirox (antimycotic) (Baylancicek et al. 2008), Burow's solution (aluminium acetate; antibacterial, anti-oedematous) (Serin et al. 2007), mitomycin C (against granulation/scar tissue) (Babu et al. 2005) and the adhesive octylcyanoacrylate (Maw et al. 2000) do not cause a reduction in the auditory brainstem response (ABR) threshold when applied topically to the middle ear.

14.9.5 Audiological Diagnostics

The hearing anamnesis should comprise familial risk, pre-therapeutic hearing loss and competing causes (e.g. acoustic trauma, noise, infections, dose and duration of previous ototoxic medication). Details of cranial irradiation should be documented (time interval, dose, path of rays). A pre-therapeutic baseline audiogram is indispensable. Tinnitus, as a first sign of ototoxicity, should be documented and characterised with respect to quality (e.g. ringing and humming), ear side, frequencies, loudness and course. To rule out conductive hearing loss by a middle ear problem, ear microscopy and impedance audiometry are necessary. In addition, pure-tone audiometry (PTA), beginning at the age of 3 years, should be carried out via air (0.25–10 kHz) and bone conduction (up to 6 kHz). Incorrect earphone placement may induce an artificial high-frequency hearing loss because of standing waves in the ear canal producing sound pressure changes (Beahan et al. 2012). Free field audiometry (visual reinforcement audiometry and conditioned play audiometry, 0.25–8 kHz) in children younger than 3 years

is not reliable but may hint at high-frequency hearing loss. For speech audiometry, age-specific tests are selectable from the age of 2 years. Speech audiometry in noise in patients of at least 5 years (Fig. 14.1a, b) is of major significance in high-frequency hearing loss diagnosis, especially to document the reduced speech discrimination in the context of school.

Extended high-frequency audiometry (EHF) measuring frequencies higher than 8 kHz and up to 16 kHz provides reliable results in patients who are at least 7 years old (Beahan et al. 2012). Special high-frequency headphones are recommended (Gordon et al. 2005).

14.9.6 Audiological Monitoring

Early detection of ototoxic damage enables therapeutic modifications and protective strategies. To diagnose early changes in auditory function, EHF (Knight et al. 2007) and objective measurements of distortion product otoacoustic emissions (DPOAE) are recommended (Knight et al. 2007). Jacobs et al. (2012) presented the portable audiometer OtoID for high-frequency screening in homes and clinics. The extrapolation of DPOAE input/output function can be used to estimate pure-tone thresholds up to 8 kHz (Stavroulaki et al. 2001).

Experimental studies have been performed to explore high-frequency ABR (Mitchell et al. 2004), high-frequency auditory steady state response (ASSR) (Tlumak et al. 2007) and high-frequency click-evoked otoacoustic emissions (Keefe et al. 2011). For high frequency ABR special high frequency stimuli (e.g. 8000 Hz tone bursts) and high frequency earphones are needed (Hall 2013). Rosner et al. (2011) have described a combination of DPOAE and ASSR recordings. Goodman (2011) presented technical solutions for the clinical application of high-frequency transient-evoked otoacoustic emissions (TEOAEs) in ototoxicity monitoring. Dreisbach et al. (2018) showed repeatable measurements of high-frequency DPOAE.

Audiological monitoring of patients receiving platinum drugs should not be performed immediately after the platinum cycle because

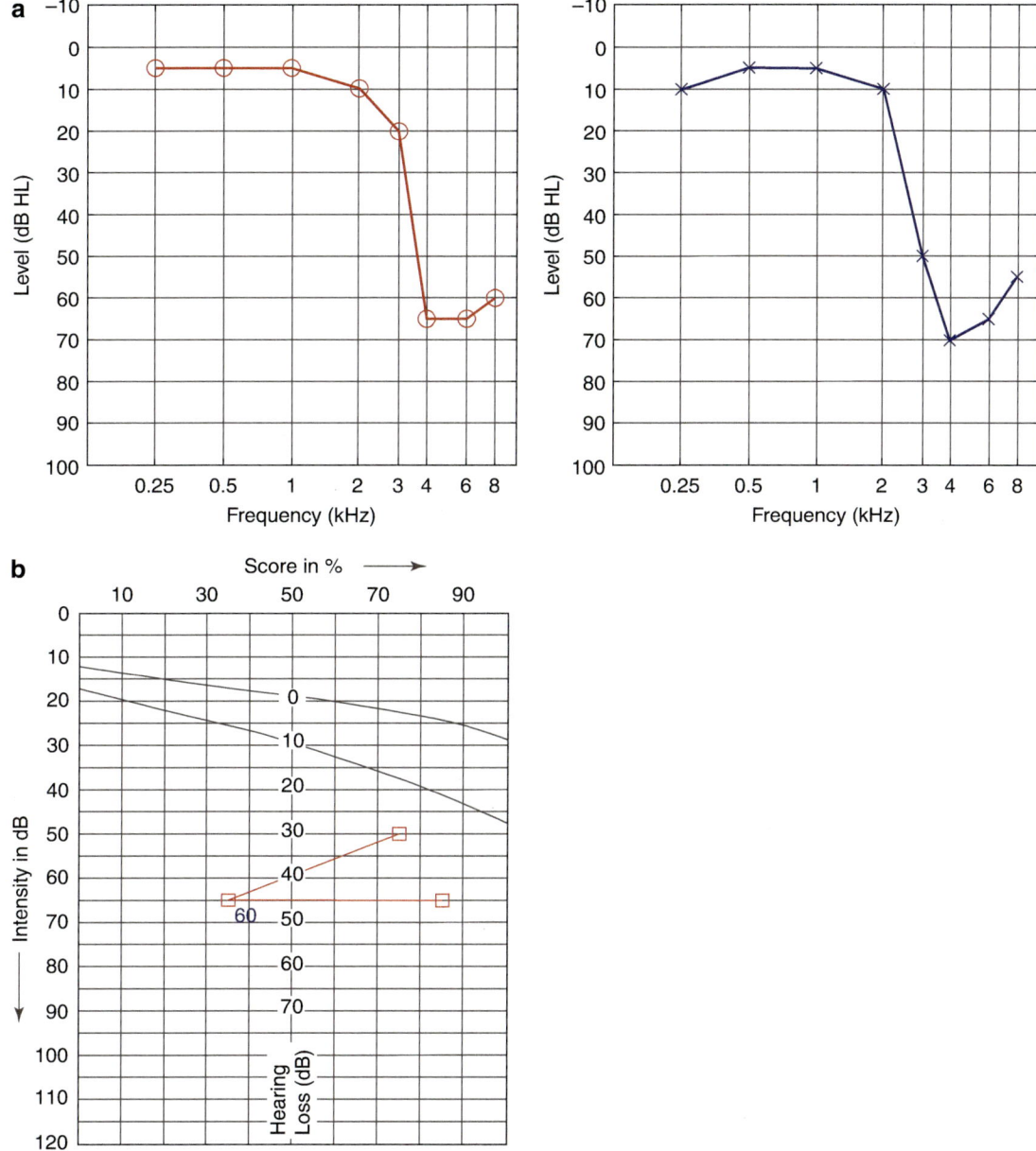

Fig. 14.1 (**a**) Audiogram showing platinum-induced high-frequency hearing loss in both ears. (**b**) Speech audiogram showing unaided (i.e. without hearing aids) binaural speech discrimination score of 75% at 50 dB speech level, 85% at 65 dB speech level and 35% in noise at 65 dB speech level with 60 dB noise level

chemotherapy-related fatigue and transient hearing impairment may produce unreliable results (Knight et al. 2007). Monitoring evaluations within the 24 h before platinum chemotherapy cycles is recommended (Knight et al. 2007). In addition to the degree of hearing loss, the time course of hearing impairment during platinum chemotherapy should also be recorded and evaluated. Detection of early variations may be important in predicting final hearing toxicity

(Schmücker et al. 2009). In fact, Lafay-Cousin et al. (2013) showed that patients with earlier cisplatin-induced ototoxicity (i.e. the presence of a ≥Münster grade 1 hearing loss; >10 to ≤20 dB) after only the second cisplatin cycle had a five times greater risk of permanent hearing loss and of ultimately requiring hearing support.

14.9.7 Audiological Post-therapeutic Follow-Up

Because of possible hearing loss progression even after the end of the cisplatin therapy, Weissenstein et al. (2012) recommend post-therapeutic audiological evaluation every 6 months in the first 2 years and then annually for at least 5 years. In the case of hearing loss progression, the audiological evaluation period should be extended (Weissenstein et al. 2012). Even in previously unaffected children, post-therapeutic progressive hearing loss is seemingly possible (Knight et al. 2005), supporting the requirement for at least one audiological evaluation after 6 months. Additional cranial irradiation necessitates close monitoring (Warrier et al. 2012), and because of the possible late-onset adverse effects, a longer follow-up period after irradiation is needed (Gurney and Bass 2012). In children with retinoblastoma, a late onset of hearing loss, which is considered to be 3 years after the last dose of carboplatin, has been observed, supporting long-term follow-up of these patients for at least 5 years (Jehanne et al. 2009a, b). After application of aminoglycosides, which have a long half-life, patients should be monitored for cochleotoxic and vestibulotoxic damages for as many as 6 months after cessation of the treatment, and these patients should avoid noise for at least this time span.

14.9.8 Therapy and Prevention

In the cases of high-risk patients and those where signs of ototoxic damage necessitate intervention, modification of therapeutic strategies, including a reduction of dose, switching to a less ototoxic treatment, or application of otoprotective substances, is useful. The latter were tested in recent studies to reduce Platinum- or aminoglycoside-induced hearing loss. The antioxidants sodium thiosulfate (Brock et al. 2018; Freyer et al. 2017, 2018) and N-acetylcysteine (Kranzer et al. 2015) have received FDA orphan drug designation as otoprotective drugs (US Food and Drug Administration 2011, 2012) and trans-tympanic administration (Riga et al. 2011), e. g. as a gel (Berglin et al. 2011), seems to be promising (Schroeder et al. 2018).

Patients should be advised to avoid noise exposure. Hearing aid availability should not be protracted, in order to facilitate optimal circumstances for language development and school performance. Because isolated acoustic amplification of high frequencies with conventional hearing aids is technically difficult, and background noise may be simultaneously enhanced, in school a wireless personal frequency-modulated (FM) communication system should be utilised (see Sect. 18.11). In addition, special hearing aid solutions for high-frequency hearing loss such as frequency compression, frequency transposition (Alnahwi and AlQudehy 2015) and frequency composition (Kuriger and Lesimple 2012) should be considered as should electric-acoustic stimulation (see Sect. 18.7). In conjunction with preferential classroom seating, an educational audiologist should provide the necessary advice on the absorption of background noise, e.g. via reduction of reverberation time. Additional caution should be exercised in cases of family history of ototoxicity or in case of pre-existing hearing impairment or decreased renal or hepatic function.

For treatment with aminoglycosides, it should be considered that the risk of ototoxicity depends on the compound, the dose, the duration of treatment and the patient's age. Genetic tests may identify patients at risk (Bitner-Glindzicz and Rahman 2007). In a tissue culture with auditory hair cells, Bodmer et al. could show the prevention of gentamicin-induced oxidative stress and apoptosis by the peroxisome proliferator-activated receptor-gamma and peroxisome proliferator-activated receptor-alpha agonist pioglitazone (published in Bausch 2016).

In general, the lowest effective dose of an ototoxic drug should be chosen, and drug levels, renal function and hearing thresholds should be monitored. Extended duration of therapy, application of ototoxic agents in parallel, and exposure to noise should be avoided.

14.10 Genetics of Hearing Loss

Pavel Seeman, Simona Poisson-Markova, Eva Seemanova, and Hanno J. Bolz

Hearing loss is the most common sensory deficit. Hearing loss which starts before speech development is termed 'prelingual hearing loss'. Prelingual hearing loss may cause speech impairment and cognitive delay if insufficiently treated. The population prevalence of severe, early-onset hearing loss in different countries ranges from 1:500 to 1:1000 (Fortnum and Davis 1997; Morton 1991; Morton and Nance 2006; Fortnum et al. 2001). Approximately 60% of these cases are genetic.

The proportion of hearing loss of genetic origin is increasing because acquired hearing loss following infections (e.g. cytomegalovirus, measles or toxoplasmosis), perinatal trauma, CNS bleeding or ototoxic drugs has become more rare, owing to improved general health and perinatal care.

The most common type of genetic hearing loss is non-syndromic (accompanied by no other symptoms), accounting for approximately 70% of cases. Syndromic hearing loss (accompanied by symptoms affecting other organs) occurs in about 30% of cases (Welch et al. 2007; Schrijver 2004).

Genetic hearing impairment is extremely heterogeneous. More than 70 genes have been identified as potential causes of non-syndromic hearing loss. More than 400 genetic syndromes feature hearing loss.

Genetic hearing loss may follow any Mendelian inheritance mode (autosomal recessive-AR, autosomal dominant-AD and X-linked), but responsible genes can also be located in the mitochondrial DNA (Van Camp and Smith 2016; Toriello and Smith 2013; Kozlova et al. 1996).

In non-syndromic hearing loss (NSHL), the AR mode of inheritance is by far the most common (approximately 80%). AD inheritance occurs in approximately 15% of cases, and X-linked and mitochondrial types are rare (representing less than 2%).

An ARNSHL hearing loss generally shows early, usually prelingual, onset and may be moderate to severe. Mutations in *GJB2* are responsible for HL in up to 50% of cases (Snoeckx et al. 2005). ADNSHL hearing losses are generally of later onset than ARNSHL forms (but may still often manifest in childhood), mild to moderate and progressive.

A systematic classification of all known syndromic genes associated with HL, based on the mode of inheritance, is available via 'http://hereditaryhearingloss.org'. ARNSHL loci are classified by the term 'DFNB', and to date DFNB1–DFNB108 have been classified. ADNSHL loci are classified as DFNA1–DFNA73 and X-linked as DFNX1–DFNX6 (Van Camp and Smith 2016).

Several syndromic hearing losses are AD-determined, for example, Stickler syndrome with skeletal dysplasia, Waardenburg syndrome with pigmentation defects, Treacher Collins syndrome with mandibulofacial dysostosis, Townes-Brocks syndrome with skeletal defects, branchio-otorenal (BOR) syndrome with renal disorder and facioscapulohumeral muscular dystrophy.

Other syndromic hearing impairments are AR inherited, for example, Usher syndrome with retinitis pigmentosa, of which at least 11 genetic types are known, Pendred syndrome with thyreopathy, Alström syndrome with obesity, type 2 diabetes mellitus, cardiomyopathy and retinopathy Alport syndrome with nephropathy and Fabry disease, a lysosomal storage disease causing a wide range of systemic dysfunctions (e.g. angiokeratoma, kidney and ocular involvement, cardiac manifestations, neuropathy).

Syndromic hearing impairment can also have a chromosomal aetiology. For example, hearing loss is common in Wolf-Hirschhorn syndrome, resulting from a deletion of the short arm of chromosome 4. Hearing loss can also be a symptom of DiGeorge syndrome, a result of microdeletion of the long arm of chromosome 22, and of Schinzel-Giedion syndrome, with mutations in the *SETBP1* gene. Numerical chromosomal aberrations can manifest as hearing impairment, for example, when due to trisomy of chromosome 21 in Down syndrome or due to trisomy of chromosome 18 in Edwards syndrome. Recurrent risk in chromosomal aberrations is low in the majority of cases because of de novo mutations.

The rarest mode of inheritance of syndromic genetic hearing loss is X-linked recessive. Only hemizygous males are affected; females are asymptomatic carriers.

The risk of genetic recurrence in AR hearing loss is 25% for siblings. AD forms have a 50% risk of recurrence (for offspring of affected persons) if the mutation is inherited. However, in both AD and X-linked hearing losses, it is necessary to differentiate inherited from de novo mutations in order to determine the true recurrence risk.

14.11 Syndromes Associated with Hearing Impairment

Antoinette am Zehnhoff-Dinnesen,
Pavel Seeman, Simona Poisson-Markova,
Eva Seemanova, and Hanno J. Bolz

More than 400 hearing loss syndromes have been described. The following Tables 14.7, 14.8, 14.9, 14.10, 14.11, 14.12, 14.13 and 14.14 list the most important and well-defined syndromes, classified on the basis of:

- Numerical chromosomal aberrations
- Structural chromosomal aberrations
- Mode of inheritance (autosomal dominant, autosomal recessive, X-linked, mitochondrial)

In addition, examples of two non-genetic syndromes are given.

In the tables, the names of the syndromes with synonyms, the phenotype OMIM number (underlined), affected genes/chromosomal regions, prevalence/incidence, clinical manifestations possibly relevant for hearing function, ear-specific anomalies, type of hearing impairment, cognitive function and other clinical manifestations are considered. Clinical manifestations of potential relevance for hearing include immuno deficiencies causing middle ear infections, autoimmune diseases involving the inner ear and muscular hypotonia or palatal anomalies affecting Eustachian tube function. Ear-specific anomalies are malformations/deformities that may affect the outer, middle or inner ear, the auditory nerve or the internal auditory canal.

In most syndromes, severity and combination of symptoms are variable. The presumably main clinical manifestations are underlined.

The tables are not exhaustive. They closely refer to the descriptions given in Orphanet (http://www.orpha.net/consor/cgi-bin/index.php) and in the OMIM database (Online Mendelian Inheritance in Man®, http://omim.org/) and list the most important characteristics given there. The incidence and prevalence are given as reported but can, for rare syndromes, at best represent estimates and vary significantly depending on the population/ethnic background. Because there may be different modes of inheritance for a syndrome or mutations in a gene, more than one inheritance mode may be listed.

Some syndromes are also listed in Sect. 9.10 (Syndromes Associated with Language Impairment).

Further information on syndromes with hearing impairment may be found on the Hereditary Hearing Loss Homepage (Van Camp and Smith 2015). For more detailed descriptions of hereditary hearing loss syndromes, we recommend, e.g. Toriello and Smith (2013) and Smith et al. (1999).

Table 14.7 Numerical chromosomal aberrations

Name of syndrome, synonyms, phenotype MIM numbers	Karyotype	Incidence/ prevalence	Clinical manifestations possibly relevant for hearing, ear-specific clinical manifestations and hearing	Cognitive ability	Clinical manifestations
Down syndrome, Trisomy 21 190685	47, XX + 21 or 47, XY + 21 free trisomy (95%; 2–3% in mosaic status), translocation trisomy (5%)	Increasing with maternal age	– Muscular hypotonia – Autoimmune pathology – Small ear canals, impacted wax – Early degeneration of hair cells – Conductive hearing loss, sensorineural hearing loss or both (Austeng et al. 2013)	Intellectual disability	**Dysmorphic Signs and Malformations** – Characteristic facies with upslanting palpebral fissures, epicanthus, short neck, round face, broad nasal bridge – Bilateral single palmar crease, polydactyly – Short stature **Organ/Systemic Manifestations** – Heart defects, particularly atrioventricular septal defect – Intestinal malformations (duodenal stenosis/atresia, imperforate anus, Hirschsprung disease) – Muscular hypotonia, joint laxity – Leukaemia reactions – Endocrine pathologies (hypothyroidism, diabetes mellitus) – Premature ageing, Alzheimer disease, seizures

Orphanet (2014a), OMIM (2015a)

788

Table 14.7 (continued)

Name of syndrome, synonyms, phenotype MIM numbers	Karyotype	Incidence/ prevalence	Clinical manifestations possibly relevant for hearing, ear-specific clinical manifestations and hearing	Cognitive ability	Clinical manifestations
Turner syndrome 45,X syndrome 45,X/46,XX syndrome 300082	Xq monosomy of the X chromosome (45,X), throughout or in mosaicism; can also be due to an abnormal X chromosome (deletion, ring chromosome X, dicentric chromosome)	1/2,500 female live births (prevalence)	– Low-set ears – Hearing impairment by middle ear infections/middle ear effusions during infancy, sensorineural hearing loss in adolescence (Alves and Silva Oliveira 2014) – Possibly cholesteatoma, craniofacial abnormalities, low-set ears, narrow and/or high-arched palate, micrognathia (Bergamaschi et al. 2008)	Normal intelligence, Turner syndrome-associated cognitive profile with impaired visuospatial/perceptual abilities possible Hong et al. (2009) OMIM (2000)	**Dysmorphic Signs and Malformations** – Growth retardation, short stature, broad, shield-like chest – High-arched palate, low-set ears, pterygium colli, low hairline **Organ/Systemic Manifestations** – Gonadal dysgenesis, hypogenitalism – Congenital lymphoedema – Cardiovascular anomalies (aortic coarctation) – Gastrointestinal anomalies – Kidney anomalies – Hypothyroidism – Immune system disease

Orphanet (2007a), OMIM (2005)

Table 14.8 Structural chromosomal aberrations (microdeletion/microduplication syndromes; contiguous gene syndromes)

Name of syndrome and synonyms	Microdeletion	Microduplication	Inheritance incidence/prevalence	Clinical manifestations possibly relevant for hearing function, ear-specific clinical manifestations and hearing	Cognitive ability	Clinical manifestations
DiGeorge syndrome, Velocardiofacial syndrome, CATCH22 Microdeletion 22q11.2, Monosomy 22q11 Sedlackova syndrome Shprintzen syndrome 602054	Long arm of chromosome 22		Autosomal dominant 1/2000–1/4000 live births (incidence)	– Immune deficiency/ autoimmune disease – Palatal anomalies – Conductive hearing loss, sensorineural hearing loss or mixed HL (Zarchi et al. 2011)	Normal to moderately impaired (Woodin et al. 2001; Furniss et al. 2011), learning disability	**Dysmorphic Signs and Malformations** – Palatal anomalies (overt/ submucous cleft), typical facies with hypertelorism, epicanthal folds, prominent nasal root, dental anomalies, eye anomalies, ptosis **Organ/Systemic Manifestations** – Cardiac anomalies – Gastrointestinal/renal anomalies – Immune deficiency (thymic aplasia/hypoplasia) autoimmune disease
Orphanet (2012a), OMIM (2013a)						
Goldenhar syndrome Facioauriculovertebral dysplasia Oculoauriculovertebral dysplasia, OAV Oculoauriculovertebral syndrome, OAVS 164210	1p22.2–p31.1 5q13.2 5p15 12p13.33 14q31.1–q31.3 15q24.1 22qter 22q11.2	10p14–p15 14q23.1 22q11.1–q11.21	Indications for autosomal dominant, autosomal recessive and multifactorial inheritance 1/5600 (incidence)	– Orofacial clefts – Ear anomalies (pre-auricular tags or pits, auricle dysplasia, anotia, microtia, atresia of external auditory canal, middle ear anomalies) (Chetcuti et al. 2014) – Anomalies of inner ear structures (Scholtz et al. 2001) – Conductive and/or sensorineural hearing loss	Normal	**Dysmorphic Signs and Malformations** – Hemifacial microsomia, facial asymmetry, orofacial clefts, ocular defects, coloboma of upper eye lid – Growth retardation **Organ/Systemic Manifestations** – Heart malformation – Genitourinary malformation – Cerebrum malformation – Vertebral anomalies – Epibulbar dermoid cyst
Orphanet (2014b), OMIM (2016a)						

(continued)

Table 14.8 (continued)

Name of syndrome and synonyms	Microdeletion	Microduplication	Inheritance incidence/prevalence	Clinical manifestations possibly relevant for hearing function, ear-specific clinical manifestations and hearing	Cognitive ability	Clinical manifestations
Langer-Giedion syndrome Deletion 8q24.1, Monosomy 8q24.1Trichorhinophalangeal syndrome type 2 <u>150230</u>	8q23.3-q24.13, leading to the loss of at least two genes: *TRPS1* and *EXT1*		Autosomal dominant, often de novo mutations <1/1,000,000 (prevalence)	– Frequent respiratory infections in infancy – Hypotonia – <u>Large anteverted ears</u> – Conductive hearing loss or sensorineural hearing loss	Mild-to-severe intellectual deficit, normal in about 25%	**Dysmorphic Signs and Malformations** – Bulbous nose, wide prominent philtrum, thin upper lip, small mandible, enophthalmos, malocclusion, dental anomaly, <u>sparse scalp hair</u> – <u>Redundant skin</u> – <u>Cartilaginous exostoses</u>, cone-shaped phalangeal epiphyses, <u>winged scapulae</u>, narrow ribs, growth retardation – Microcephaly **Organ/Systemic Manifestations** – Hypotonia – Frequent respiratory infections in infancy

Orphanet (2016), National Organization for Rare Disorders (2005), OMIM (2013b)

| Wolf–Hirschhorn syndrome 4p-syndrome Distal deletion 4p Distal monosomy 4p Telomeric deletion 4p 194190 | 4p16.3 microdeletion, affecting *LETM1* and *WHSC1* | Autosomal dominant 1/50,000 births (prevalence) | Moderate to severe impairment in most cases | – Hypotonia – Cleft palate – Otitis – Malformation of outer (poorly formed ears with pits/tags), middle and inner ear (Ulualp et al. 2004) | **Dysmorphic Signs and Malformations** – Cleft palate, characteristic facies with broad nasal bridge, prominent glabella, ("Greek warrior helmet appearance"), hypertelorism, epicanthus, high-arched eyebrows, protruding eyes, divergent strabismus, short philtrum, mouth with downturned corners, micrognathia, dental anomalies, microcephaly – Malformed vertebral bodies, accessory/fused ribs, clubfeet, split hands, severe growth deficiency **Organ/Systemic Manifestations** – Heart anomalies – Urogenital anomalies – Seizure disorder – Hypotonia |

Orphanet (2012b), OMIM (2015b)

Table 14.9 Autosomal dominant disorders

Name of syndrome and synonyms	Gene, chromosomal regions	Inheritance incidence/prevalence	Clinical manifestations possibly relevant for hearing function, ear-specific clinical manifestations and hearing	Cognitive ability	Clinical manifestations
BOR syndrome Branchiootorenal syndrome 113650 Orphanet (2007b), OMIM (2012a)	EYA1 (8q13.3) SIX1 (14q23.1) SIX5 (19q13.32)	Autosomal dominant 1/40,000 (prevalence)	– Malformations of outer, middle or inner ear, pre-auricular pits – Conductive, sensorineural or mixed hearing loss	Mostly normal	**Dysmorphic Signs and Malformations** – Branchial clefts, fistulae, cysts, stenosis/aplasia of lacrimal ducts **Organ/Systemic Manifestations** – Renal abnormalities (renal hypoplasia/agenesis, renal cysts), anomalies of urinary tract
Camurati-Engelmann disease Progressive diaphyseal dysplasia 131300	Camurati-Engelmann disease TGFB1 (19q13.2)	Autosomal dominant with reduced penetrance >300 cases reported	Camurati-Engelmann disease – Progressive hyperostosis, sclerosis – Conductive or sensorineural hearing loss or both in <20% of patients, progressive, internal auditory canal may be involved (Tibesar et al. 2004)	Normal	Camurati-Engelmann disease **Dysmorphic Signs and Malformations** – Progressive hyperostosis of long bones, sclerotic changes at the skull base – Limb pain, waddling gait, joint contractures, muscle weakness – Easy fatigability – Marfanoid body habitus – Possibly frontal bossing, enlarged mandible, facial paralysis, delayed dentition, extensive dental caries – Lumbar lordosis, kyphosis, scoliosis, coxa valga, genu valgum, flat feet – If involvement of the orbit proptosis, papilloedema, epiphora, glaucoma, subluxation of the globe **Organ/Systemic Manifestations** – Anaemia, leukocytopenia – Hepatosplenomegaly – Undernutrition, anorexia – Decreased subcutaneous tissue, hyperhidrosis – Delayed puberty, hypogonadism – Bladder incontinence – Possibly slurred speech, dysphagia, cerebellar ataxia
Camurati-Engelmann Disease Type II Progressive diaphyseal dysplasia with striations of the bones 606631 Orphanet (2013a), OMIM (2002a, 2006a)	Camurati-Engelmann Disease Type II no mutation in TGFB1	Camurati-Engelmann Disease Type II possibly autosomal dominant rare cases (IOF 2015)			Camurati-Engelmann Disease Type II **Dysmorphic Signs and Malformations** – Similar phenotype – Usually asymptomatic or mild limb pains

Syndrome	Gene / Inheritance	Hearing / ear findings	Mental status	Dysmorphic Signs and Malformations / Organ-Systemic Manifestations
CHARGE syndrome C: Coloboma H: Heart defects A: Atresia (choanal-) R: Retarded growth and development G: Genital abnormalities E: Ear anomalies 214800	CHD7 (8q12.2) SEMA3E (7q21.11) Mostly sporadic due to de novo mutation Autosomal dominant 1/15,000–1/17,000 (prevalence)	– Frequent chest infections – Mild-to-severe T-cell deficiency – Cleft lip or palate or both, unilateral or bilateral choanal atresia/stenosis, low-set lop or cup-shaped outer ear with deficient cartilage of the outer pinna (unusually shaped, asymmetrical pinnae, floppy), triangular concha, stenotic ear canal, middle ear ossicle malformations, dysplasia/aplasia of cochlea, semicircular canals, abnormality of auditory nerve – Eustachian tube dysfunction, chronic serous otitis media – Conductive hearing impairment/sensorineural hearing loss (Thelin and Krivenki 2008)	Normal to serve mental retardation	**Dysmorphic Signs and Malformations** – Choanal atresia/stenosis, cleft lip or palate or both, – Broad prominent forehead, prominent nasal bridge/columnella, flat midface, protruding jaw, overbite, unilateral or bilateral facial palsy, unilateral or bilateral coloboma of the iris – Hypoplastic nails, clinodactyly, polydactyly, brachydactyly, joint hyperflexibility, contractures, short stature **Organ/Systemic Manifestations** – Heart defects (tetralogy of Fallot, perimembranous ventricular septal defect, double-outlet right ventricle, AV canal defects) – Retina-choroid – Genitourinary and renal abnormalities – Laryngo-tracheomalacia, oesophageal atresia/tracheoesophageal fistula – Endocrine abnormalities – T-cell deficiency – Cerebral anomalies (corpus callosum agenesis), anomalies of the olfactory tracts, bulbs – Dysphagia – Developmental retardation – Autism spectrum disorder, anxiety disorder – Numerous chest infections

Orphanet (2015a), Thelin and Krivenki (2008), OMIM (2016b)

Syndrome	Gene / Inheritance	Hearing / ear findings	Mental status	Dysmorphic Signs and Malformations / Organ-Systemic Manifestations
Cleidocranial dysplasia Cleidocranial dysostosis 119600	RUNX2 (6p21.1) Autosomal dominant 1/1,000,000 (prevalence, regionally higher owing to a founder mutation)	– Recurrent infections of the upper respiratory tract – Predominantly middle ear conduction problem, structural abnormalities of the ossicles – Sometimes cochlear or eighth nerve problem dense sclerosis of the temporal bone (Candamourty et al. 2013)	Normal	**Dysmorphic Signs and Malformations** – Aplasia/hypoplasia of clavicles, dysplastic scapulae – Persistence of wide-open skull sutures, fontanels – Multiple dental abnormalities, hyperdontia, broad flat forehead, hypertelorism, midface hypoplasia, pointed jaw – Brachydactyly, tapering fingers, short, broad thumbs – Short stature, scoliosis, vertebral malformation, genu valgum, coxa vara, pes planus, wide pubic symphysis **Organ/Systemic Manifestations** – Frequent infections of the upper respiratory tract

Orphanet (2013b), MalaCards: The Human Disease Database (2016), OMIM (2013c)

(continued)

Table 14.9 (continued)

Name of syndrome and synonyms	Gene, chromosomal regions	Inheritance incidence/ prevalence	Clinical manifestations possibly relevant for hearing function, ear-specific clinical manifestations and hearing	Cognitive ability	Clinical manifestations
Crouzon disease Crouzon craniofacial dysostosis 123500	Crouzon disease *FGFR2* (10q25.3-q26) 80% IgIII domain 20% IgI-IgII domains	Crouzon disease autosomal dominant 0.9/100,000 (prevalence)	Crouzon disease - High palate - Posteriorly angulated ears, rarely external auditory canal atresia, ossicular fixation, serous otitis media - Conductive hearing loss/ sensorineural hearing loss/mixed hearing loss (Orvidas et al. 1999)	Intellectual disability uncommon	Crouzon disease **Dysmorphic Signs and Malformations** - Premature synostosis of cranial sutures, craniosynostosis, facial hypoplasia, hypertelorism, beaked nose, hypoplastic maxilla, mandibular prognathism, high palate, exophthalmos, palpebral malocclusion, strabismus **Organ/Systemic Manifestations** - Blindness - Hydrocephaly, descent of the cerebellar tonsils, anomalies in jugular venous drainage, intracranial hypertension
Crouzon syndrome— acanthosis nigricans 612247	Crouzon syndrome— acanthosis nigricans *FGFR3* (4p16.3)	Crouzon syndrome— acanthosis nigricans autosomal dominant, sporadic <70 cases up to now	Crouzon syndrome—acanthosis nigricans - In addition cleft palate, choanal atresia/stenosis		Crouzon syndrome —acanthosis nigricans **Dysmorphic Signs and Malformations** - Additional acanthosis nigricans, hyperpigmented skin, warty acanthomas, melanocytic nevi - Vertebra anomalies - Choanal atresia/stenosis, cleft palate, dental malocclusion, cementomas of the jaw **Organ/Systemic Manifestations** - Kidney affection
Crouzon-like syndrome	Crouzon-like syndrome *ERF* (19q13.2) *IL11RA* (9p21.1-p13.2) (Keupp et al. 2013)	Crouzon-like syndrome autosomal recessive			Crouzon-like-syndrome Dysmorphic Signs and Malformations - Multiple suture synostosis, exophthalmos, prominent forehead, no prognathism, no beaked nose

Orphanet (2013c, 2014c), OMIM (2016c, 2008)

Facioscapulo-humeral muscular dystrophy FSHD1 158900 FSHD2 158901	FSHD1 *DUX4* (4q35) FSHD2 *MCHD1* (18p11.32)	Autosomal dominant 1/20,000 (prevalence)	- Sensorineural hearing loss of cochlear origin, characteristic in cases with large 4q35 deletion (Trevisan et al. 2008)	Dependent on molecular defect normal or reduced	**Dysmorphic Signs and Malformations** - Degenerative myopathy primarily of facial and upper girdle muscles **Organ/systemic manifestations** - Cardiac signs - Neurological involvement - Anomaly of retinal vessels

Orphanet (2014d), OMIM (2013d)

Hypoparathyroidism, sensorineural hearing loss and renal dysplasia syndrome HDR HDRS Barakat syndrome nephrosis, nerve deafness and hypoparathyroidism 146255 Orphanet (2008a), OMIM (2011a)	Haploinsufficiency of *GATA3* (important for inner ear development) (10p14)	Autosomal dominant <1/1,000,000 (prevalence)	– Bilateral, symmetric, downsloping sensorineural hearing loss – Early-onset during childhood, cochlear origin in patients with *GATA3* mutations (Chien et al. 2014)	Mild mental retardation possible (Yesiltepe Mutlu et al. 2015)	**Organ/Systemic Manifestations** – Progressive renal disease, nephrotic syndrome, cystic kidney, renal dysplasia/hypoplasia/aplasia, renal scarring, vesicoureteral reflux, pelvicalyceal deformity – Hypoparathyroidism, hypocalcaemia, tetany, afebrile convulsions
Marshall syndrome 154780	*COL11A1* (1p21.1)	Autosomal dominant <1/1,000,000 (prevalence)	– Sensorineural or mixed hearing impairment, slight to severe, damage of auditory nerve	Intellectual functioning disability not described	**Dysmorphic Signs and Malformations** – Hypertelorism, anteverted nares, severe hypoplasia of the nasal bones, abnormal frontal sinuses, flat/retracted midface, prominent eyes, thick calvaria short stature, spondyloepiphyseal dysplasia **Organ/Systemic Manifestations** – Severe myopia, cataract, further eye anomalies – Intracranial calcifications – Early-onset osteoarthritis – Anhidrotic ectodermal anomalies – Hypogenitalism

Orphanet (2015b), National Organization for Rare Disorders (2015), OMIM (2012b)

Muckle-Wells syndrome Neutrophilic urticaria 191900	*Intermediate form of cryopyrin-associated periodic syndrome (CAPS)* NLRP3 (1q44)	Autosomal dominant about 140 cases known	– Progressive sensorineural hearing loss, cochlear origin, chronic inflammation as possible cause	Cognitive impairment	**Dysmorphic Signs and Malformations** – Episodic urticaria-like skin rash – Erythematous band over the hands, clubbed fingers – Conjunctivitis, uveitis, episcleritis **Organ/Systemic Manifestations** – Recurrent fever – Myalgia, arthralgia – Headache, chronic meningitis – Thoracic/abdominal pain – Fatigue – Oral aphthosis – Lymphadenopathy – Papillar oedema, optic atrophy – Secondary amyloidosis (causing renal disease) – Sterility in men

Orphanet (2014e), OMIM (2012c)

(continued)

Table 14.9 (continued)

Name of syndrome and synonyms	Gene, chromosomal regions	Inheritance incidence/prevalence	Clinical manifestations possibly relevant for hearing function, ear-specific clinical manifestations and hearing	Cognitive ability	Clinical manifestations
Muenke syndrome *FGFR3*-associated coronal synostosis 602849	*FGFR3* (4p16.3)	Autosomal dominant 1/15,000 births (incidence)	– Low-frequency sensorineural hearing loss, abnormal differentiation of organ of Corti supposed by animal study (Mansour et al. 2009) – Hearing loss by affection of sensory nerves	Developmental delay possible	**Dysmorphic Signs and Malformations** – Coronal craniosynostosis: bilateral—small antero-posterior diameter of skull (brachycephaly), decrease in the depth of the orbits, hypoplasia of the maxillae, unilateral—flattening of the orbit (plagiocephaly) – Thimble-shaped middle phalanges, carpal-tarsal fusion, brachydactyly, carpal bone malsegregation – Coned epiphyses
Orphanet (2017), Mercy Clinic Kids Plastic Surgery (2016), OMIM (2012d)					
Neurofibromatosis type 2 NF2 101000	*NF2* (22q12.2) in >50% new mutations in one third mosaicism	Autosomal dominant around 1/60,000 (prevalence)	– Auditory nerve affection: tinnitus, hearing loss, deafness, unilateral – Vestibular nerve affection: dizziness, imbalance nausea, vomiting, vertigo	Normal	**Organ/Systemic Manifestations** – Tumours of the eighth cranial nerve, schwannomas of cranial, spinal, peripheral nerves, intracranial meningiomas (incl. optic nerve) – Cataract – Ependymomas – Skin tumours
Orphanet (2009a), OMIM (2012e)					
Noonan syndrome 163950	*PTPN11* (12q24.1) (50%) *SOS1* (2p22.1) (13%) *RAF1* and *RIT1* each in 5%, *KRAS* <5% Various less frequent: see Allanson and Roberts (2016)	Autosomal dominant 1/1000–1/2500 live births (incidence)	– High-arched palate, low-set posteriorly rotated ears, thickened helix, anomalies of ossicular chain – Otitis media – Conductive hearing loss, sensorineural hearing loss, unilateral, bilateral (Scheiber et al. 2009)	Mild deficit, mental retardation possible	**Dysmorphic Signs and Malformations** – Short stature, spine deformity, cubitus valgus broad forehead, hypertelorism, ptosis, down-slanting palpebral fissures, high-arched palate, webbed neck **Organ/Systemic Manifestations** – Heart defects, cardiomyopathy, pulmonic stenosis – Thorax anomaly (pectus carinatum, infundibular thorax) – Cryptorchidism – Bleeding tendency – Lymphatic dysplasia
Orphanet (2008b), OMIM (2015c)					

Oculodentodigital syndrome Oculodentodigital dysplasia Oculodento-osseous dysplasia Oculodentodigital syndrome Oculodento-osseous dysplasia ODD syndrome ODDD ODOD Osseous-oculo-dental dysplasia 164200	*GJA1* (6q22.31)	*Mostly dominant, rarely recessive <1000 people worldwide (incidence unknown)*	Disability possible	**Dysmorphic Signs and Malformations** – Narrow pinched nose, hypoplastic alae nasi, anteverted nares, prominent columella, narrow nasal bridge, epicanthic folds, cleft palate, microphthalmia, microcornea, small or missing teeth, dysplastic enamel – Syndactyly of fingers, camptodactyly, syndactyly of toes – Brittle nails, palmoplantar keratoderma – Microcephaly **Organ/Systemic Manifestations** – Eye abnormalities, vision loss – Webbing of the skin, hypotrichosis – Lack of bladder or bowel control – Ataxia, spasticity, dysarthria
			– Cleft palate – Conductive hearing loss	

Genetics Home Reference (2016c), OMIM (2014a)

PAX6-related disorders) 607108	*PAX6* (11p13), encoding transcription regulator protein essential for eye and neural development	Autosomal dominant Aniridia in 1/64,000–1/96,000 live births (incidence)	Impact on academic performance possible	**Organ/Systemic Manifestations** – Ocular maldevelopment, aniridia – Structural brain anomalies, absent/hypoplastic anterior commissure, hypoplastic corpus callosum
			– Case study with congenital aniridia, auditory processing disorder, deficits in auditory and verbal working memory, normal brain MRI (Bamiou et al. 2007)	

Orphanet (2012c), OMIM (2017a)

Schinzel-Giedion syndrome SGS 269150	*SETBP1* (18q21.3) mostly sporadic due to de novo mutations	Autosomal dominant <1/1,000.000 (prevalence)	Severe mental retardation	**Dysmorphic Signs and Malformations** – Midface retraction, prominent forehead, short upturned nose, macroglossia, choanal stenosis – Short limbs, valgus or varus foot deformity, mesomelic brachymelia – Hypoplastic/hyperconvex nails, single palmar creases of the hands **Organ/Systemic Manifestations** – Visceral anomalies – Hypertrichosis – Cardiac abnormalities – Renal malformations – Genitourinary abnormalities – Hypotonia – Seizures – Visual impairment – Neuroepithelial tumours
			– Hypotonia – Choanal stenosis, low-set ears, posteriorly rotated, ear malformation – Sensorineural hearing loss	

Orphanet (2014f), Genetic Testing Registry (2016), OMIM (2014b)

(continued)

Table 14.9 (continued)

Name of syndrome and synonyms	Gene, chromosomal regions	Inheritance incidence/ prevalence	Clinical manifestations possibly relevant for hearing function, ear-specific clinical manifestations and hearing	Cognitive ability	Clinical manifestations
Stickler syndrome Hereditary progressive arthro-ophthalmopathy 108300	Stickler syndrome type 1 *COL2A1* (12q13.11-q13.2) Stickler syndrome type 2 *COL11A1* (1p21.1) Stickler syndrome type 3 (without ocular signs) *COL11A2* (6p21.32) Stickler syndrome type 4: *COL9A1* (6q12-q14) Stickler syndrome type 5: *COL9A2* (1p34.2)	Autosomal dominant forms: Stickler syndrome type 1, 2, 3 Autosomal recessive forms: Stickler syndrome type 4, 5 1/7500 births (incidence)	– Palatal defect, hypermobility of tympanic membrane – Sensorineural hearing loss more often than mixed, mixed more often than conductive hearing loss, hearing loss more often in Stickler syndrome type 2 and 3 than in 1 (Acke et al. 2012), in non-ocular type 3 hearing loss of cochlear origin (van Beelen et al. 2012)	Usually normal	**Dysmorphic Signs and Malformations** – Flat midface, Pierre Robin sequence (small lower jaw, glossoptosis, difficulty breathing), palatal defect, bifid uvula – Juvenile cataract, strabismus – Mild platyspondyly, abnormal epiphyses, juvenile joint laxity **Organ/Systemic Manifestations** – Myopia, vitreoretinal or chorioretinal degeneration, retinal detachment, chronic uveitis Type 1 membranous vitreous Type 2 beaded vitreous Type 3 non-ocular type Type 4 vitreous degeneration and liquefaction Type 5 same clinical symptoms as types 1 and 2 early osteoarthritis

Orphanet (2008c), OMIM (2013e)

| Townes-Brocks syndrome
TBS
Townes syndrome
107480 | About 50% *SALL1* (16q12.1) de novo mutations, sometimes *SALL4* (20q13.2) | Autosomal dominant about 1/250,000 (prevalence) | – Dysplastic ear helices
– Sensorineural/conductive/mixed hearing impairment | 10% intellectual deficit | **Dysmorphic Signs and Malformations**
– Thumb malformations (triphalangeal thumbs, preaxial polydactyly, absent bones), foot malformations, fusion of metatarsals
– Rib/vertebral anomalies, growth retardation
Organ/Systemic Manifestations
– Anomalies of kidneys
– Heart anomalies
– Imperforate anus
– Genitourinary malformations
– Ophthalmological malformations
– Gastrointestinal anomalies
– CNS anomalies (Type I Arnold-Chiari malformation)
– Congenital hypothyroidism |

Orphanet (2013d), OMIM (2011b)

Syndrome	Gene/Locus	Inheritance/Frequency	Intelligence	Hearing/ENT	Dysmorphic Signs and Malformations
Treacher Collins syndrome Mandibulofacial dysostosis 154500	Most common Type I *TCOF1* (5q32-q33) Less common Type II *POLR1D* (13q12.2) Type III *POLR1C* (6p21.1)	Autosomal dominant: Type I, II Autosomal recessive: Type III 1/50,000 (incidence)	Normal	– Narrow airways, high palate, cleft palate, microtia, malformed auricles, atresia of the external auditory canals, anomalies of ossicular chain, less common pretragal fistula – Bilateral conductive hearing loss	**Dysmorphic Signs and Malformations** – Malar/mandibular hypoplasia, retrognathia/micrognathia, retrogenia, dental malocclusion, anterior open bite, macrostomia, widely spaced teeth, ogival palate, cleft palate, hypoplasia of the zygomatic complex, abnormalities in the temporo-mandibular joint, limited mouth opening, antimongoloid slant of the eyes, palpebral fissures, inferolateral orbital cleft, coloboma of eyelids, partial absence of lid lashes – Narrow airways – Microcephaly – Spinal anomalies, enchondromas **Organ/Systemic Manifestations** – Heart defects
Waardenburg syndrome 4 types, most common WS1, WS2 WS4 Waardenburg-Shah syndrome 193500	WS1, WS3 *PAX3* (2q36.1) WS2 *MITF* (3p14-p13)/ *TYR* mutation/ homozygous deletions *SNAI2* (8q11.21) WS2, WS4 *SOX10* (22q13.1) WS4 *EDNRB* (13q22.3) *EDN3* (20q13.32)	Mostly autosomal dominant Autosomal recessive: WS4 1/20,000–1/40,000 (prevalence)	Average	– Sensorineural hearing loss of varying degree WS1 60% affected, congenital, mostly bilateral, profound (Milunsky 2001)	**Dysmorphic Signs and Malformations** – Pigmentation anomalies of eyes, hair (white forelock), skin, partial albinism, congenital leukoderma, heterochromic irides – Synophrys/medial eyebrow flare, broad/high nasal root, prominent columella, hypoplastic alae nasi WS1 with dystopia canthorum WS2 without dystopia canthorum WS3 with dystopia canthorum and upper limb anomalies **Organ/Systemic Manifestations** WS4 with M. Hirschsprung

Orphanet (2014g), OMIM (2016d)

Orphanet (2015c), OMIM (2016e))

Table 14.10 Autosomal recessive disorders

Name of syndrome and synonyms	Gene, chromosomal regions	Inheritance incidence/ prevalence	Clinical manifestations possibly relevant for hearing function, ear-specific clinical manifestations and hearing	Cognitive ability	Clinical manifestations
Alström syndrome 203800	*ALMS1* (2p13.1)	Autosomal recessive probably underestima-ted *ALMS1* mutations are a predominant cause for apparently isolated Leber congenital amaurosis (LCA) 1–9/1,000,000 (prevalence)	– Chronic respiratory illness – Mild-to-moderate slowly progressive bilateral sensorineural hearing loss, cochlear origin (Bahmad et al. 2014)	Often normal, developmental delay possible	**Dysmorphic Signs and Malformations** – Deep-set eyes, rounded face – Short fingers/toes **Organ/Systemic Manifestations** – Congenital progressive cone-rod retinal degeneration (LCA) – Cardiomyopathy – Childhood obesity, insulin resistance, hyperinsulinemia, type 2 diabetes mellitus – Liver dysfunction, steatosis, cirrhosis – Hypertriglyceridaemia – Hypogonadism in males/hyperandrogenism in females – Chronic respiratory illness – Progressive renal failure

Orphanet (2014h), OMIM (2016f)

	Genes	Inheritance/prevalence	Hearing	Cognitive outcome	Dysmorphic Signs and Malformations / Organ/Systemic Manifestations
Bardet-Biedl syndrome BBS 209900	At least 19 different genes *BBS1* *BBS2* *ARL6* (BBS3) *BBS4* *BBS5* *MKKS* (BBS6) *BBS7* *TTC8* (BBS8) *BBS9* *BBS10* *TRIM32* (BBS11) *BBS12* *MKS1* (BBS13) *CEP290* (BBS14) *WDPCP* (BBS15) *SDCCAG8* (BBS16) *LZTFL1* (BBS17) *BBIP1* (BBS18) *IFT27* (BBS19) (Forsythe and Beales 2015)	Autosomal recessive 1/125,000–1/175,000 in Europe (prevalence)	– Otitis media, glue ear – Conductive/sensorineural hearing loss	Normal cognitive outcome possible (Nikkel and Hunter 2013), behavioural dysfunction	**Dysmorphic Signs and Malformations** – Post-axial polydactyly **Organ/Systemic Manifestations** – Retinal degeneration – Polycystic kidneys – Hypogonadism hypogenitalism – Diabetes, obesity – Cardiovascular anomalies – Hirschsprung disease
Orphanet (2008d), Nikkel and Hunter (2013), OMIM (2017b)					
Biotinidase Deficiency BTD deficiency Juvenile-onset multiple carboxylase deficiency Late-onset multiple carboxylase deficiency 253260	*BTD* (3p25.1)	Autosomal recessive 1/61,000 (prevalence)	– Sensorineural hearing loss (Sivri et al. 2007)	Developmental delay	**Organ/Systemic Manifestations** – Metabolic inability to recycle biotin, ketolactic acidosis, organic aciduria, hyperammonaemia – Cutaneous abnormalities, eczematoid rash, alopecia – Fungal infections – Breathing problems (tachy-/apnoea) – Hepato-/splenomegalie – Optic atrophy – Neurologic abnormalities, cerebral atrophy, seizures, ataxia – Hypotonia
Orphanet (2011a), OMIM (2009a)					

(continued)

Table 14.10 (continued)

Name of syndrome and synonyms	Gene, chromosomal regions	Inheritance incidence/ prevalence	Clinical manifestations possibly relevant for hearing function, ear-specific clinical manifestations and hearing	Cognitive ability	Clinical manifestations
Cockayne syndrome 216400	*ERCC6* (*CSB*; 10q11) *ERCC8* (*CSA*; 5q12.1)	Autosomal recessive 1/200,000 (incidence in Europe)	– Large ears, possibly malformed – Sensorineural hearing loss like prebyacusis (Shemen et al. 1984)	Intellectual disability	**Dysmorphic Signs and Malformations** – Slow growth, "cachectic dwarfism" – Microcephaly, thin nose, enophthalmia, cataracts, dental caries – Premature ageing (progeria), thin, dry hair and skin – Long limbs, large hands and feet, contractures of joints **Organ/Systemic Manifestations** – Progressive retinal degeneration – Risk of malignancy (skin and other) – Subcutaneous lipoatrophy – Cerebellar ataxia, spasticity, peripheral demyelinating neuropathy – Serious reaction to metronidazole with liver failure Type1: symptoms in first year of life Type 2: more severe than type 1, congenital Type 3: later onset, milder symptoms

				Dysmorphic Signs and Malformations
Xeroderma pigmentosum—Cockayne syndrome complex (Orphanet 2014i) 278730 278760 278780 610651	*ERCC3* (2q21) or *ERCC2* (19q13.3) or *ERCC5* (13q22-q34)	Autosomal recessive about 40 cases known (Natale and Raquer 2017)	– Progressive hearing loss	<u>Cognitive deficit</u>	**Dysmorphic Signs and Malformations** – <u>Microcephaly, hydrocephalus</u> – Cachexia – Premature aging – <u>Dwarfism</u> **Organ/Systemic Manifestations** – <u>UV-sensitive skin lesions causing skin cancer, skin atrophy</u> – Spasticity, ataxia – Pigmentary retinopathy, optic atrophy – Arteriosclerosis
Orphanet (2009b), OMIM (2012f)					
Diastrophic dwarfism Diastrophic dysplasia 222600	*SLC26A2* (5q31-q34)	Autosomal recessive manner 1–1.3/100,000 (prevalence)	– Cleft palate, cysts on the external ear, <u>malformation of pinnae with cartilage calcification</u> – Middle ear disease – Conductive hearing loss/sensorineural hearing loss (Tunkel et al. 2012)	Normal	**Dysmorphic Signs and Malformations** – Short stature, short extremities, malformations and contractures of joints, mainly of shoulders, elbows, interphalangeal joints, hips, hyperlaxity of joints, bilateral clubfoot, short limb deformation of the wrists, <u>abducted thumbs ("hitchhiker thumb"), scoliosis</u>, premature calcification of costal cartilages – Cleft palate, mandible hypoplasia
Orphanet (2008e), OMIM (2010a)					
Jervell and Lange-Nielsen syndrome Long QT interval-deafness syndrome 220400	*KCNQ1* (*LQT1*; 11p15.5) or *KCNE1* (*LQT5*; 21q22.1-q22.2)	Autosomal recessive 1/200,000–1/1,000,000 (prevalence)	– <u>Congenital profound bilateral sensorineural hearing loss</u>	Pecularities not described	**Organ/Systemic Manifestations** – <u>Prolonged QT interval on electrocardiogram, risk of ventricular tachyarrhythmias, syncopal attacks, sudden death</u>
Orphanet (2009c), OMIM (2006b)					

(continued)

Table 14.10 (continued)

Name of syndrome and synonyms	Gene, chromosomal regions	Inheritance incidence/prevalence	Clinical manifestations possibly relevant for hearing function, ear-specific clinical manifestations and hearing	Cognitive ability	Clinical manifestations
Kartagener syndrome Primary ciliary dyskinesia Dextrocardia-bronchiectasis-sinusitis syndrome Immotile cilia syndrome Kartagener type Siewert syndrome 244400	*DNAH5* 15–21% *CCDC39* 2–10% *DNAI1* 2–9% *CCDC40* 1–8% *DNAH11* 6% *DNAAF1* 4–5% *LRRC6* 3% *DNAI2* 2% *DNAAF2* <2% a third of patients did not have mutations in these genes (Orphanet 2014j)	Autosomal dominant or autosomal recessiveor X-linked dominant 1/15,000–1/30,000 live births (incidence)	– Chronic upper and lower respiratory tract infection, rhinitis, sinusitis – Chronic otitis media – Temporary or permanent conductive hearing loss – Risk of tympanic perforation after grommet (Prulière-Escabasse et al. 2010)	Very rarely X-linked PCD associated with intellectual deficiency	**Dysmorphic Signs and Malformations** – Pectus excavatum, scoliosis **Organ/Systemic Manifestations** – Chronic upper/lower respiratory tract infection, rhinitis, sinusitis, chronic cough, bronchiectasis – Situs inversus (in half of patients) – Congenital heart disease – Reduced fertility in women, ectopic pregnancies, abnormal motility of spermatozoa – Very rarely X-linked PCD with retinitis pigmentosa

Orphanet (2014j), OMIM (2009b)

Maternal phenylketonuria Hyperphenlyalaninemic embryopathy Maternal PKU Maternal hyperphenyl-alaninemia Phenylketonuric embryopathy 261600	Mutations in the *PAH* gene (12q22-q24.2)	Autosomal recessive 1/10,000 (incidence)	– Dysplastic ear helices, high palate	Severe to profound intellectual disability	**Dysmorphic Signs and Malformations** – Growth retardation – Receding forehead, fused eyes, strabismus, underdeveloped philtrum, anteverted nostrils, flat nasal bridge, deviated nasal septum, micrognathia, ptosis, high palate – Hypopigmentation, eczema, rashes – "Mousy" musty body odour by phenylacetic acid – Microcephaly **Organ/Systemic Manifestations** – Congenital heart disease – Seizures – Autistic-like behaviour – Early diagnosis essential, treatable by diet

Orphanet (2015d), OMIM (2015d), American Academy of Pediatrics (2008)

(continued)

Table 14.10 (continued)

Name of syndrome and synonyms	Gene, chromosomal regions	Inheritance incidence/prevalence	Clinical manifestations possibly relevant for hearing function, ear-specific clinical manifestations and hearing	Cognitive ability	Clinical manifestations
Mucopolysaccharidosis Hurler disease MPSIH Mucopolysaccharidosis type IH 607014	Hurler disease *IDUA* (4p16.3)	Hurler disease autosomal recessive 1/200,000 in Europe (prevalence)	MPS – Damage of auditory nerve secondary to skeletal deformations – Otitis media, acute, chronic or with effusion Hurler disease – Nasal secretion, hyperplastic adenoids – Middle ear problem – Sensorineural hearing loss, reduced number of hair cells (Kariya et al. 2012)	Hurler disease progressive cognitive/sensorial deterio-ration	Hurler disease **Dysmorphic Signs and Malformations** – Short stature, dysostosis multiplex, thoracic-lumbar kyphosis – Progressively large head, bulging frontal bones, coarse face, depressed nasal bridge, broad nasal tip, anteverted nostrils, nasal secretion, full cheeks, enlarged lips, corneal opacity **Organ/Systemic Manifestations** – Cardiomyopathy, valvular abnormalities – Hyperplastic tonsils/adenoids – Hydrocephaly – Hepatosplenomegaly, hernias, hirsutism

Mucopolysaccharidosis type II Hunter syndrome Iduronate 2-sulfatase deficiency MPS2 MPSII 309900	Hunter syndrome *IDS* (Xq28)	Hunter syndrome X-linked recessive 1/166,000 (prevalence at birth in Europe)	Hunter syndrome – Respiratory tract infections – Acute/chronic otitis media – Conductive hearing loss – Sensorineural hearing loss (Keilmann et al. 2012)	Hunter syndrome MPS2, severe form, early psycho-motor regression MPS2, attenuated form, without cognitive involvement	Hunter syndrome **Dysmorphic Signs and Malformations** – Prominent lips, enlarged nostrils, protruding tongue – Macrocephaly, skeletal deformities – Skin lesions like orange peel (on the shoulder, back, thighs) **Organ/Systemic Manifestations** – Airway obstruction, respiratory tract infections – Cardiomyopathy – Umbilical/inguinal hernia – Intractable diarrhoea – Hepatosplenomegaly – Neurological deterioration
Sanfilippo disease MPS3 MPSIII Mucopolysaccharidosis type III 252900	Sanfilippo disease *MPS IIIA* (17q25) *MPS IIIB* (17q21) *MPS IIIC* (pericentromeric region chromosome 8) *MPS IIID* (12q14)	Sanfilippo disease autosomal recessive 1–9/1,000,000 (prevalence)	Sanfilippo disease Type A: – Ear infections – Sensorineural hearing loss (Buhrman et al. 2013)	Sanfilippo disease severe, rapid intellectual deterioration	Sanfilippo disease **Dysmorphic Signs and Malformations** – Slight coarse facial dysmorphism, macrocephaly – Short stature, joint stiffness, slight dysostosis multiplex **Organ/Systemic Manifestations** – Severe neurological degeneration, affection of brain, spinal cord – Hyperkinesia, aggressiveness, sleep disorders, seizures – Mild hepatomegaly – Umbilical/inguinal hernia

(continued)

Table 14.10 (continued)

Name of syndrome and synonyms	Gene, chromosomal regions	Inheritance incidence/prevalence	Clinical manifestations possibly relevant for hearing function, ear-specific clinical manifestations and hearing	Cognitive ability	Clinical manifestations
Morquio disease MPS4 MPSIV Mucopolysaccharidosis type IV 253010	Morquio disease *MPS IVA, MPS IVBGALNS* (16q24) *GLB1* (3p22.3)	Morquio disease autosomal recessive MPS IVA 1/250,000 MPS IVB rarer	Morquio disease – Frequent infections of upper respiratory tract – Middle ear disease – Conductive/sensorineural/mixed hearing loss, frequently progressive, rarely worse than moderate (Pauli 2009)	Morquio disease normal intelligence	Morquio diseaseMPS IVA, MPS IVB **Dysmorphic Signs and Malformations** – Mildly coarse facies, corneal clouding – Short-trunked dwarfism, spondylo-epiphyso-metaphyseal dysplasia, platyspondyly, kyphosis, scoliosis, pectus carinatum, genu valgum, long bone deformities, joint hyperlaxity **Organ/Systemic Manifestations** – Osteoporosis – Damages of nervous system secondary to skeletal deformations – Instability of first two cervical vertebra by hypoplasia of odontoid vertebra/joint hyperlaxity, intubation difficulties – Mild hepatomegaly – Valvular heart disease – Cervical myelopathy – Frequent infections of upper respiratory tract

Maroteaux-Lamy disease RSB deficiency ASB deficiency Arylsulfatase B deficiency MPS6 MPSVI Mucopolysaccharidosis type VI N-acetylgalactosamine 4-sulfatase deficiency 253200	Maroteaux-Lamy disease *ARSB* (5q13-5q14)	Maroteaux-Lamy disease autosomal recessive 1/43,261–1/1,505,160 live births (prevalence)	Maroteaux-Lamy disease - Sinusitis - Otitis media - Damage of inner ear, damage of nerve - Conductive/sensorineural/mixed hearing loss	Maroteaux-Lamy disease intellectual deficit generally absent	Maroteaux-Lamy disease **Dysmorphic Signs and Malformations** - Chubby face, thickened lips due to gingival hypertrophy, prominent forehead, broad, flattened bridge of the nose, macroglossia, short, stiff neck, corneal clouding - Short stature, dysostosis multiplex, degenerative joint disease with stiff joints - Hirsutism **Organ/Systemic Manifestations** - Inguinal/umbilical hernia - Cardiac valve disease - Pulmonary function affected, sinusitis - Hepatosplenomegaly - Sleep apnoea - Optic nerve atrophy, blindness - Cervical spinal instability causing cervical cord compression, meningeal thickening, bony stenosis with damage of neurological structures, hydrocephalus

(continued)

Table 14.10 (continued)

Name of syndrome and synonyms	Gene, chromosomal regions	Inheritance incidence/ prevalence	Clinical manifestations possibly relevant for hearing function, ear-specific clinical manifestations and hearing	Cognitive ability	Clinical manifestations
Scheie syndrome MPS1S MPSIS Mucopolysaccharidosis type 1S Mucopolysaccharidosis type IS 607016	Scheie syndrome *IDUA* (4p16.3)	Scheie syndrome autosomal recessive 1/500,000 (prevalence)	Scheie syndrome – Nasal secretion – Middle ear infection conductive hearing loss – Sensorineural hearing loss	Scheie syndrome little if any intellectual deficiency	Scheie syndrome **Dysmorphic Signs and Malformations** – Corneal opacification, large mouth, thick lips, nasal secretion – Stiff joints, mild skeletal changes **Organ/Systemic Manifestations** – Glaucoma – Aortic valve disease with aortic regurgitation – Spastic paresis by glycosaminoglycan infiltration of the dura with compression of the cervical spinal cord

Orphanet (2007c, 2007d, 2010, 2011b, 2013e, 2014k), Genetics Home Reference (2016d), National Organization for Rare Disorders (2014), OMIM (2002b, 2007a, 2015e, 2016g, 2016h, 2016i)

Name of syndrome and synonyms	Gene, chromosomal regions	Inheritance incidence/ prevalence	Clinical manifestations possibly relevant for hearing function, ear-specific clinical manifestations and hearing	Cognitive ability	Clinical manifestations
Pendred syndrome (PDS) Goitre-deafness syndrome 274600	Biallelic *SLC26A4* (7q22.3) or double heterozygous mutations in *SLC26A4* and *FOXI1* (5q34) or in *SLC26A4* and *KCNJ10* (1q23.2)	Autosomal recessive 1–9/100,000 (prevalence)	– Enlargement of the vestibular aqueduct (EVA), cochlear hypoplasia – Congenital sensorineural hearing loss, possibly progressive, fluctuating	Peculiarities not described	**Organ/Systemic Manifestations** – Euthyroid goitre, hypothyroidism if low nutritional iodide intake, thyroid carcinoma possible

Orphanet (2013f), OMIM (2012g)

Syndrome (OMIM)	Gene (locus)	Inheritance (prevalence)	Hearing loss	Other	Dysmorphic Signs and Malformations / Organ/Systemic Manifestations
Refsum syndrome 266500	90% *PHYH* (10p13) 10% *PEX7* (6q21-q22.2)	Autosomal recessive 1/1,000,000 in the UK (prevalence)	– Progressive symmetric mild-to-profound sensorineural hearing loss	Mental retardation in infantile Refsum disease	**Dysmorphic Signs and Malformations** – Cataract, nystagmus – Skeletal abnormalities, epiphyseal dysplasia, short metacarpals/metatarsals **Organ/Systemic Manifestations** – Accumulation of phytanic acid in plasma/tissues – Peripheral neuropathy, cerebellar ataxia, anosmia – Early-onset retinal degeneration – Cardiomyopathy – Autism spectrum disorder, attention deficit-hyperactivity disorder – Early diagnosis essential, treatable by diet

Orphanet (2015e), OMIM (2009c)

Syndrome (OMIM)	Gene (locus)	Inheritance (prevalence)	Hearing loss	Other	Organ/Systemic Manifestations
Usher syndrome 601067	Type 1: *MYO7A, USH1C, CDH23, PCDH15, USH1G* Type 2: *USH2A, ADGRV1, WHRN, PDZD7* (digenic, *USH2A* modifier) Type 3: *CLRN1*	Autosomal recessive, rarely digenic; up to 1/6000 (prevalence)	Type 1: – Congenital hearing loss, profound Type 2: – Prelingual moderate to severe, slowly progressive Type 3: – Early progressive hearing loss	Normal	**Organ/Systemic Manifestations** Type 1 (35%): – Vestibular dysfunction, early retinal degeneration Type 2 (>60%): – Normal vestibular function, retinal degeneration from puberty on Type 3 (<3% of cases, more frequent in the Finnish and Ashkenazi Jewish populations): – 50% with vestibular dysfunction, retinal degeneration; variable: may clinically correspond to type 1 or 2

Orphanet (2009d), OMIM (2012h)

Table 14.11 Disorders with X-Linked Inheritance

Name of syndrome and synonyms	Gene, chromosomal regions	Inheritance incidence/ prevalence	Clinical manifestations possibly relevant for hearing function, ear-specific clinical manifestations and hearing	Cognitive ability	Clinical manifestations
Alport syndrome Alport deafness-nephropathy 301050	COL4A5 (Xq22) COL4A3 (2q36-q37) COL4A4 (2q35-q37) COL4A3 (2q36-q37) COL4A4 (2q35-q37)	Mostly X-linked dominant COL4A5 15% autosomal recessive COL4A3, COL4A4 Rarely autosomal dominant COL4A3, COL4A4 1/50,000 (prevalence)	– Sensorineural hearing loss, cochlear	Normal	**Dysmorphic Signs and Malformations** – Ocular; anterior lenticonus, corneal lesions **Organ/Systemic Manifestations** – Glomerular nephropathy with progressive renal failure – Thrombopenia – Leiomyomatosis
Orphanet (2007e), OMIM (2015f)					
FG syndrome FGS Keller syndrome FGS2 300321 FGS3 300406 FGS4 300422 FGS5 300581 FGS6 300298 FGS7 300553	FG syndrome FGS FGS2 FLNA (Xq28.2) FGS3 (Xp22.3), candidate gene MID1 FGS4 CASK (Xp11.4) FGS5 (Xq22.3) FGS6 UPF3B (Xq25-26) FGS7 BRWD3 (Xq21.1)	FG syndrome FGS incompletely recessive X-linked disorder 1/500 (prevalence)	FG syndrome FGS – Hypotonia – Cleft palate – Recurrent otitis – Conductive hearing loss – Sensorineural hearing loss	FG syndrome FGS intellectual deficit, delayed development of sensory integration	FG syndrome FGS **Dysmorphic Signs and Malformations** – Relative shortness compared to large head – dysmorphic facies, cleft palate, squint – Limb defects **Organ/Systemic Manifestations** – Laryngeal cleft – Intestinal atresia, anal anomalies, constipation, hernia – Gastro-oesophageal involvement, reflux – Sleep apnoea – Hypospadia, hydrocele – Congenital hypotonia – Attention deficit disorder, behavioural disturbances, fascination with mechanical toys/objects – Partial agenesis of corpus callosum, Chiari I malformation – Congenital heart defects FGS2 – Typical periventricular nodular heterotopia on MRI

Opitz G/BBB syndrome (OS) ADOS Autosomal dominant Opitz BBB/G syndrome Autosomal dominant Opitz syndrome Hypertelorism-oesophageal abnormality-hypospadias syndrome Hypospadias-dysphagia syndrome Hypospadias-hypertelorism syndrome Opitz syndrome Opitz-Frias syndrome 300000	Opitz G/BBB syndrome G/BBB syndrome (XLOS) *MID1* (Xp22.2) G/BBB syndrome (ADOS) 22q11.2 deletion Opitz G/BBB syndrome X-linked G/BBB XLOS 1/50,000–1/100,000 (prevalence) Autosomal dominant G/BBB ADOS Prevalence unknown	Opitz G/BBB syndrome – Cleft lip/palate – Conductive hearing loss	Opitz G/BBB syndrome intellectual deficit with short attention span, learning difficulties	Opitz G/BBB syndrome **Dysmorphic Signs and Malformations** – Prominent forehead, hypertelorism, telecanthus, broad nasal bridge, cleft lip/palate, anteverted nares – Syndactyly **Organ/Systemic Manifestations** – Hypospadia, cryptorchidism, hypoplastic/bifid scrotum – Laryngo–tracheo–esophageal (LTE) abnormalities – Imperforate/ectopic anus – Cardiac defects – Renal malformations – Corpus callosum agenesis, cerebellar vermis agenesis/hypoplasia – Mostly only hypertelorism in female carriers
Opitz-Kaveggia/FG syndrome FGS1 305450	Opitz-Kaveggia/FG syndrome *MED12* (Xq13.1) Opitz-Kaveggia/FG syndrome X-linked recessive Prevalence unknown	Opitz-Kaveggia/FG syndrome – Hypotonia in childhood – Small external ears – Conductive hearing loss – Sensorineural hearing loss	Opitz-Kaveggia/FG syndrome learning disability, mental retardation (Risheg et al. 2007)	Opitz-Kaveggia/FG syndrome **Dysmorphic Signs and Malformations** – Joint laxity/contractures – Relative macrocephaly, high broad forehead with upsweep of the frontal hairline (cow's lick), hypertelorism, downslanted palpebral fissures – Broad thumbs, broad halluces, great toes, short stature **Organ/Systemic Manifestations** – Imperforate anus or severe constipation – Reduced or lax muscle tone in childhood, increased tone in adulthood – Congenital heart defect – Partial agenesis of corpus callosum – Seizures, hyperactivity, tantrums

Orphanet (2009e, 2012d), Contact a Family (2016), OMIM (2006c, 2007b, 2009d, 2010b, 2012i), Santoro and Hedlund (2008)

(continued)

Table 14.11 (continued)

Name of syndrome and synonyms	Gene, chromosomal regions	Inheritance incidence/ prevalence	Clinical manifestations possibly relevant for hearing function, ear-specific clinical manifestations and hearing	Cognitive ability	Clinical manifestations
Mohr–Tranebjaerg syndrome DDON syndrome Deafness-dystonia-optic neuronopathy syndrome 304700	*TIMM8A* (Xq22) encoding a translocase polypeptide of the inner mitochondrial membrane or *CGS* (Xq22)	X-linked recessive >90 cases known	– Recurrent infections – Early childhood onset hearing loss, progressive loss of cochlear neuronal cells and vestibular neurons, auditory neuropathy (Bahmad et al. 2007)	Slowly progressive dementia from the fourth decade on	**Organ/Systemic Manifestations** – From early adulthood decreasing visual acuity, photophobia, acquired colour vision defect, central scotoma, cortical blindness – Progressive dystonia from adolescence on, ataxia – Personality changes, paranoia – Resistance to limb movement – Agile tendon reflexes, ankle clonus, extensor–plantar responses, fractures – Recurrent infections
Orphanet (2013g), OMIM (2016j) Otopalatodigital syndrome type I OPD I syndrome Taybi syndrome 311300	*FLNA* (Xq28)	X-linked dominant >100 cases known	– Cleft palate – Malformed auditory ossicles – Conductive hearing loss	Mild intellectual disability	**Dysmorphic Signs and Malformations** – Frontal bossing with prominent supraorbital ridges, flat nasal bridge, hypertelorism, microstomia, dental abnormalities, occipital prominence, cleft palate – Mild skeletal anomalies, camptodactyly, "tree frog" hands and feet, pectus carinatum, mild campomelia, slight femoral bowing, limitation of joint movement

Orphanet (2015f), OMIM (2009e)

Disease	Gene/Mechanism	Inheritance	Auditory	Neurological	Organ/Systemic Manifestations
X-linked adrenoleukodystrophy X-ALD Addison disease and cerebral sclerosis melanodermic leukodystrophy Schilder-Addison Complex Schilder disease Siemerling-Creutzfeldt disease 300100	ABCD1 (Xq28) Demyelination, associated with deficient beta-oxidation of very long chain fatty acids	X-linked 1/20,000–1/50,000 (prevalence)	– Auditory processing disorder in a case study, on brain MRI involvement of the auditory pathway at the level of the trapezoid body/posterior corpus callosum (Bamiou et al. 2004)	In childhood cerebral form learning problems, aggressive behaviour In adreno-myeloneuropathy type changes in behaviour and thinking ability	– Progressive neurodegeneration Childhood cerebral form **Organ/Systemic Manifestations** – Vision problems – Swallowing difficulty – Poor coordination – Disturbed adrenal gland function Adrenomyeloneuropathy type **Organ/Systemic Manifestations** – Progressive stiffness, weakness in legs (paraparesis) – Urinary/genital tract disorders – Adrenocortical insufficiency Addison disease **Organ/Systemic Manifestations** – Adrenocortical insufficiency

Genetics Home Reference (2016b), OMIM (2013f)

Disease	Gene/Mechanism	Inheritance	Auditory	Neurological	Organ/Systemic Manifestations
X-linked agammaglobulinaemia XLA Agammaglobulinaemia Bruton's agammaglobulinaemia congenital agammaglobulinaemia hypogammaglobulinaemia 300755	BTK (Xq22.1)	X-linked recessive or not applicable 1–9/1,000,000 (prevalence)	– Recurrent otitis in spite of antibiotics – Conductive hearing loss – Viral infections – Cochlear or retro-cochlear hearing loss (Berlucchi et al. 2008)	Normal	**Organ/Systemic Manifestations** – Frequent infections (pneumonia, bronchitis, otitis, conjunctivitis, sinusitis, chronic diarrhoea), serious or fatal course possible

Genetics Home Reference (2016a), Orphanet (2013h), OMIM (2010c)

Table 14.12 Postzygotic mutation with effect on sex development

Name of syndrome and synonyms	Gene, chromosomal regions	Inheritance incidence/ prevalence	Clinical manifestations possibly relevant for hearing function, ear-specific clinical manifestations and hearing	Cognitive ability	Clinical manifestations
McCune–Albright syndrome Gonadotrophin-independent female-limited sexual precocity Polyostotic fibrous dysplasia 174800	Somatic mutations of *GNAS1* (20q13.1-13.2) in very early development, mosaicism, effects on development of sex	Inheritance not applicable 1/100,000–1/1,000,000 (prevalence)	– Abnormal bone growth in the skull – Secondary hearing loss	Normal	**Dysmorphic Signs and Malformations** – Polyostotic fibrous dysplasia – Abnormal skull bone growth – Café-au-lait skin pigmentation **Organ/Systemic Manifestations** – Rarely malignant transformation of fibrous dysplasia of bone, pathological fractures – Blindness – Precocious puberty – Endocrinological anomalies (hyperthyroidism, growth hormone excess, Cushing syndrome) – Renal phosphate wasting, renal disease

Orphanet (2008f), University of Maryland Medical Center (2014), WebMD Magazine (2007), OMIM (2011c)

Table 14.13 Mitochondrial mutations associated with syndromic hearing impairment

Name of syndrome and synonyms	Anomalies of mitochondrial DNA (mtDNA)	Incidence/prevalence	Clinical manifestations possibly relevant for hearing function, ear-specific clinical manifestations and hearing	Cognitive ability	Clinical manifestations
Kearns-Sayre syndrome KSS 530000	Sporadic several large deletions of mtDNA heteroplasmic (single cell can harbour deleted and normal DNA, symptoms depend on proportion of abnormal DNA)	1/125,000 (prevalence)	– Progressive sensorineural hearing loss (Zwirner and Wilichowski 2001)	Intellectual deficit	**Dysmorphic Signs and Malformations** – Ptosis, weakness of facial muscles – Small stature **Organ/Systemic Manifestations** – Retinal degeneration, progressive external ophthalmoplegia – Cardiomyopathy, cardiac conduction defect – Weakness of pharyngeal muscles, skeletal muscle myopathy – Intestinal disorders – Endocrine disorders – Renal disease – Cerebellar ataxia – Dysarthria

Orphanet (2014l), Hereditary Hearing Loss Homepage (2016), OMIM (2016k)

Maternally inherited diabetes and deafness MIDD Mitochondrial diabetes 520000	*MTTL1* m.3243A > G *MTTK* m.8296A > G *MTTE* m.14709T > C Several large deletions/duplications of mtDNA	Unknown	– Progressive sensorineural hearing loss, more profound at higher frequencies	Mental retardation (Chen et al. 2004)	**Dysmorphic Signs and Malformations** – Ptosis **Organ/Systemic Manifestations** – Diabetes – Diabetic retinopathy – Muscle pain, myopathy – Cardiomyopathy – Gastrointestinal tract symptoms – Renal disease – Neuropsychiatric symptoms

Orphanet (2009f), Hereditary Hearing Loss Homepage (2016), OMIM (2012j)

(continued)

Table 14.13 (continued)

Name of syndrome and synonyms	Anomalies of mitochondrial DNA (mtDNA)	Incidence/prevalence	Clinical manifestations possibly relevant for hearing function, ear-specific clinical manifestations and hearing	Cognitive ability	Clinical manifestations
Mitochondrial encephalopathy, lactic acidosis and stroke-like episodes MELAS Mitochondrial myopathy, encephalopathy, lactic acidosis and stroke-like episodes 540000	*MTTL1* *MTTQ* *MTTH* *MTTK* *MTTC* *MTTS1* *MTND1* *MTND5* *MTND6* *MTTS2* most common: m.3243A-G transition in *MTTL1*	1–9/1,000,000 (prevalence)	– Progressive sensorineural hearing loss (Chen et al. 1998; Zwirner and Wilichowski 2001)	Dementia	**Dysmorphic Signs and Malformations** – Short stature **Organ/Systemic Manifestations** – Myopathy, proximal limb weakness – Lactic acidosis, episodic vomiting – Encephalopathy, hemiparesis, stroke-like episodes, hemianopsia, cortical blindness – Psychiatric manifestations – Endocrinopathy – Diabetes – Heart disease

Orphanet (2015g), Hereditary Hearing Loss Homepage (2016), OMIM (2016l)

Name of syndrome and synonyms	Anomalies of mitochondrial DNA (mtDNA)	Incidence/prevalence	Clinical manifestations possibly relevant for hearing function, ear-specific clinical manifestations and hearing	Cognitive ability	Clinical manifestations
Myoclonus epilepsy associated with ragged-red fibres MERRF Fukuhara syndrome 545000	*MTTK* *MTTL1* *MTTH* *MTTS1* *MTTS2* *MTTF* most common: m.8344A > G in *MTTK* heteroplasmy in cells	0.9/100,000 in Europe (prevalence)	– Sensorineural hearing loss	Dementia	**Dysmorphic Signs and Malformations** – Short stature **Organ/Systemic Manifestations** – Myoclonic epilepsy – Retinal degeneration, optic atrophy, ophthalmoparesis – Peripheral neuropathy, pyramidal signs, ataxia, spasticity – Myopathy, muscle weakness, ragged-red muscle fibres – Cardiomyopathy – Lipomatosis

Orphanet (2006), Hereditary Hearing Loss Homepage (2016), OMIM (2014c)

Table 14.14 Non-genetic syndromes with hearing loss

Name of syndrome and synonyms	Caused by	Incidence/prevalence	Clinical manifestations possibly relevant for hearing function, ear-specific clinical manifestations and hearing	Cognitive ability	Clinical manifestations
Foetal alcohol syndrome FAS	Alcohol abuse by mother during pregnancy	At least 2–7/1000 children in the USA in difficult socio-economic populations 2–5% **Foetal Alcohol Spectrum Disorders (FASD)** in the USA	– Cleft lip/palate – Conductive hearing loss, sensorineural hearing loss, central hearing loss (Katbamna 2010)	Learning disabilities, mental retardation possible	**Dysmorphic Signs and Malformations** – Facial anomalies with small eye size, skin folds at the corner of the eye, low nasal bridge, short upturned nose, indistinct philtrum, thin upper lip, retrognathism, hypoplastic maxilla, cleft lip/palate, microcephaly – Growth retardation **Organ/Systemic Manifestations** – Behavioural abnormalities **FASD** Partial foetal alcohol syndrome (pFAS) with subtypes alcohol-related neurodevelopmental disorder (ARND) and alcohol-related birth defects (ARBD)
Katbamna (2010), Medscape (2016) Foetal Hydantoin syndrome Foetal dihydantoin syndrome Phenytoin embryo-foetopathy	Anticonvulsant drug phenytoin applied by mother during pregnancy	Unknown 5–10% of exposed children develop embryo-foeto-pathy	– Cleft lip/palate, malformed and low-set ears – Conductive hearing loss	Cognitive deficits, motor developmental delay	**Dysmorphic Signs and Malformations** – Short neck, short nose, deep nasal bridge, hypertelorism, epicanthal folds, cleft lip/palate, microcephaly, ocular defects – Hypoplastic distal phalanges, hypoplastic nails of fingers/toes, growth deficiency **Organ/Systemic Manifestations** – Cardiac anomalies – Neurological impairment – Umbilical/inguinal hernias – Hypospadias

Orphanet (2015h), National Organization for Rare Disorders (1993)

References

Acke FRE, Dhooge IJM, Malfait F et al (2012) Hearing impairment in Stickler syndrome: a systematic review. Orphanet J Rare Dis 7:84. https://doi.org/10.1186/1750-1172-7-84

Allanson JE, Roberts AE (2016) Noonan syndrome. In: Pagon RA et al (ed) GeneReviews® [Internet]. Available via https://www.ncbi.nlm.nih.gov/books/NBK1124. Accessed 3 June 2017

Alnahwi M, AlQudehy ZA (2015) Comparison between frequency transposition and frequency compression hearing aids. Egypt J Otolaryngol 31(1):10–18

Alves C, Silva Oliveira C (2014) Hearing loss among patients with Turner's syndrome: literature review. Braz J Otorhinolaryngol 80(3):257–263

American Academy of Pediatrics Committee on Genetics (2008) Maternal Phenylketonuria Committee on Genetics Policy Statement. Available via http://pediatrics.aappublications.org/content/pediatrics/122/2/445.full.pdf. Accessed 1 May 2017

American Speech-Language-Hearing Association (2005) How does your child hear and talk? Available via http://www.asha.org/public/speech/development/chart/. Accessed 14 July 2017

American Speech-Language-Hearing Association ASHA (1994) Audiologic management of individuals receiving cochleotoxic drug therapy. https://doi.org/10.1044/policy.GL1994-00003. Accessed 30 Dec 2016

Amir J, Wolf DG, Levy I (2010) Treatment of symptomatic congenital cytomegalovirus infection with intravenous ganciclovir followed by long-term oral valganciclovir. Eur J Pediatr 169(9):1061–1067

Asatryan A, Pool V, Chen RT et al (2008) Immunization Safety Office, Office of the Chief Science Officer, Centers for Disease Control and Prevention, Atlanta, GA, USA, The VAERS Team. Live attenuated measles and mumps viral strain containing vaccines and hearing loss: Vaccine Adverse Event Reporting System (VAERS), United States, 1990-2003. Vaccine 26(9):1166–1172

Austeng ME, Akre H, Falkenberg ES et al (2013) Hearing level in children with Down Syndrome at the age of eight. Res Dev Disabil 34(7):2251–2256

BAAP (2015a) Guidelines for aetiological investigation into unilateral permanent childhood hearing impairment. Available via http://www.baap.org.uk/Portals/0/Guidelines%20for%20aetiological%20investigation%20into%20unilateral%20permanent%20childhood%20hearing%20impairment.pdf. Accessed 17 May 2017

BAAP (2015b) Guidelines for aetiological investigation into severe to profound bilateral permanent childhood hearing impairment. Available via http://www.baap.org.uk/Portals/0/Guidelines%20for%20aetiological%20investigation%20into%20severe%20to%20profound%20bilateral%20permanent%20childhood%20hearing%20impairment.pdf. Accessed 17 May 2017

BAAP (2015c) Guidelines for aetiological investigation into mild to moderate bilateral permanent childhood hearing impairment. Available via http://www.baap.org.uk/Portals/0/Guidelines%20for%20aetiological%20investigation%20into%20mild%20to%20moderate%20bilateral%20permanent%20childhood%20hearing%20impairment.pdf. Accessed 17 May 2017

Babu SC, Kartush JM, Patni A (2005) Otologic effects of topical mitomycin C: phase I-evaluation of ototoxicity. Otol Neurotol 26(2):140–144

Bahmad F Jr, Merchant SN, Nadol JB et al (2007) Otopathology in Mohr-Tranebjaerg syndrome. Laryngoscope 117(7):1202–1208

Bahmad F Jr, Costa CS, Teixeira MS et al (2014) Familial Alström syndrome: a rare cause of bilateral progressive hearing loss. Braz J Otorhinolaryngol 80(2):99–104

Bamiou DE, MacArdle B, Bitner-Glindzicz M et al (2000) Aetiological investigations of hearing loss in childhood. A review (98 references). Clin Otolaryngol Allied Sci 25(2):98–106

Bamiou DE, Davies R, Jones S et al (2004) An unusual case of X-linked adrenoleukodystrophy with auditory processing difficulties as the first and sole clinical manifestation. J Am Acad Audiol 15(2):152–160

Bamiou DE, Campbell NG, Musiek FE et al (2007) Auditory and verbal working memory deficits in a child with congenital aniridia due to a PAX6 mutation. Int J Audiol 46(4):196–202

Bausch A (2016) Strekin AG announces the presentation of key STR001 data at the conference on molecular biology of hearing and deafness, Cambridge UK. Available via http://www.prnewswire.com/news-releases/strekin-ag-announces-the-presentation-of-key-str001-data-at-the-conference-on-molecular-biology-of-hearing-and-deafness-cambridge-uk-585189461.html. Accessed 15 Apr 2017

Baylancicek S, Serin GM, Ciprut A et al (2008) Ototoxic effect of topical ciclopirox as an antimycotic preparation. Otol Neurotol 29(7):910–913

Beahan N, Kei J, Driscoll C et al (2012) High-frequency pure-tone audiometry in children: a test-retest reliability study relative to ototoxic criteria. Ear Hear 33(1):104–111

Berg KM, Smith MC (1983) Behavioral thresholds for tones during infancy. J Exp Child Psychol 35(3):409–425

Bergamaschi C, Bergonzoni L, Mazzanti E et al (2008) Hearing loss in Turner syndrome: results of a multicentric study. J Endocrinol Invest 31(9):779–783

Berglin CE, Pierre PV, Bramer T et al (2011) Prevention of cisplatin-induced hearing loss by administration of a thiosulfate-containing gel to the middle ear in a guinea pig model. Cancer Chemother Pharmacol 68(6):1547–1556

Berlucchi M, Soresina A, Redaelli De Zinis LO et al (2008) Sensorineural hearing loss in primary antibody deficiency disorders. J Pediatr 153(2):293–296

Bess FH, Tharpe AM, Gibler AM (1986) Auditory performance of children with unilateral sensorineural hearing loss. Ear Hear 7(1):20–26

Bess FH, Dodd-Murphy J, Parker RA (1998) Children with minimal sensorineural hearing loss: prevalence, educational performance, and functional status. Ear Hear 19(5):339–354

BIAP (1996) Audiometric classification of hearing impairments. Available via https://www.biap.org/en/recommandation/recommendations-pdf/ct-02-classification-des-deficiences-auditives-1/55-02-1-audiometric-classification-of-hearing-impairments. Accessed 4 May 2017

Bilavsky E, Shahar-Nissan K, Pardo J et al (2016) Hearing outcome of infants with congenital cytomegalovirus and hearing impairment. Arch Dis Child 101(5):433–438

Bitner-Glindzicz M, Rahman S (2007) Ototoxicity caused by aminoglycosides. BMJ 335(7624):784–785

Bochennek K, Allwinn R, Langer R et al (2014) Differential loss of humoral immunity against measles, mumps, rubella and varicella-zoster virus in children treated for cancer. Vaccine 32(27):3357–3361

Bogazzi F, Russo D, Raggi F et al (2004) Mutations in the SLC26A4 (pendrin) gene in patients with sensorineural deafness and enlarged vestibular aqueduct. J Endocrinol Invest 27(5):430–435

Bogovic P, Strle F (2015) Tick-borne encephalitis: a review of epidemiology, clinical characteristics, and management. World J Clin Cases 3(5):430–441

Boppana SB, Ross SA, Novak Z et al (2010) Dried blood spot real-time polymerase chain reaction assays to screen newborns for congenital cytomegalovirus infection. JAMA 303(14):1375–1382

Bortoli R, Santiago M (2007) Chloroquine ototoxicity. Clin Rheumatol 26(11):1809–1810

Briscoe J, Bishop DV, Norbury CF (2001) Phonological processing, language, and literacy: a comparison of children with mild-to-moderate sensorineural hearing loss and those with specific language impairment. J Child Psychol Psychiatry 42(3):329–340

Brock PR, Knight KR, Freyer DR et al (2012) Platinum-induced ototoxicity in children: a consensus review on mechanisms, predisposition, and protection, including a new International Society of Pediatric Oncology Boston ototoxicity scale. J Clin Oncol 30(19):2408–2417

Brock PR, Maibach R, Childs M et al (2018) Sodium thiosulfate for protection from cisplatin-induced hearing loss. N Engl J Med 378(25):2376–2385

Brown ZA, Wald A, Morrow RA et al (2003) Effect of serologic status and cesarean delivery on transmission rates of herpes simplex virus from mother to infant. JAMA 289(2):203–209

Buhrman D, Thakkar K, Poe M et al (2013) Natural history of Sanfilippo syndrome type A. J Inherit Metab Dis 37(3):431–437. https://doi.org/10.1007/s10545-013-9661-8

Candamourty R, Venkatachalam S, Yuvaraj V et al (2013) Cleidocranial dysplasia with hearing loss. J Nat Sci Biol Med 4(1):245–249. https://doi.org/10.4103/0976-9668.107318

Carney AE, Moeller MP (1998) Treatment efficacy: hearing loss in children. J Speech Lang Hear Res 41(1):S61–S84

Caserta MT, Hall CB, Canfield RL et al (2014) Early developmental outcomes of children with congenital HHV-6 infection. Pediatrics 134(6):1111–1118

Center for Early Intervention on Deafness (2016) Stages of early development: birth through three years of age. Available via http://ceid.org/wp-content/uploads/2014/06/Stages_of_auditory_development.pdf. Accessed 14 July 2017

Centers for Disease Control and Prevention (2016) Learn the signs: developmental milestones. Available via https://www.cdc.gov/ncbddd/actearly/milestones/index.html. Accessed 14 July 2017

Chang KW, Chinosornvatana N (2010) Practical grading system for evaluating cisplatin ototoxicity in children. J Clin Oncol 28(10):1788–1795

Chao CK, Czechowicz JA, Messner AH et al (2012) High prevalence of hearing impairment in HIV-infected peruvian children. Otolaryngol Head Neck Surg 146(2):259–265

Chen JN, Ho KY, Juan KH (1998) Sensorineural hearing loss in MELAS syndrome—case report. Kaohsiung J Med Sci 14(8):519–523

Chen YN, Liou CW, Huang CC et al (2004) Maternally inherited diabetes and deafness (MIDD) syndrome: a clinical and molecular genetic study of a Taiwanese family. Chang Gung Med J 27(1):66–73

Chetcuti K, Abernethy LJ, Bruce C (2014) An 8-year-old girl with congenital deafness and musculoskeletal abnormalities. Arch Dis Child 99(7):665. https://doi.org/10.1136/archdischild-2013-305836

Chien W, Leiding JW, Hsu AP et al (2014) Auditory and vestibular phenotypes associated with GATA3 mutation. Otol Neurotol 35(4):577–581. https://doi.org/10.1097/MAO.0000000000000238

Choo D, Meinzen-Derr J (2010) Universal newborn hearing screening in 2010. Curr Opin Otolaryngol Head Neck Surg 18(5):399–404. https://doi.org/10.1097/MOO.0b013e32833d475d

Çiftdoğan DY, Vardar F (2011) Effect on hearing of oral valganciclovir for asymptomatic congenital cytomegalovirus infection. J Trop Pediatr 57(2):132–134

Cohen BE, Durstenfeld A, Roehm PC (2014) Viral causes of hearing loss: a review for hearing health professionals. Trends Hear 18:1–17

Connolly JL, Carron JD, Roark SD (2005) Universal newborn hearing screening: are we achieving the Joint Committee on Infant Hearing (JCIH) objectives? Laryngoscope 115(2):232–236

Contact a Family (2016) Opitz-Kaveggia/FG syndrome. Available via http://www.cafamily.org.uk/medical-information/conditions/o/opitz-kaveggiafg-syndrome-keller-syndrome-opitz-fg-syndrome-opitz-kaveggia-syndrome/. Accessed 2 Aug 2016

Cook C (2007) Cytomegalovirus reactivation in "immunocompetent" patients: a call for scientific prophylaxis. J Infect Dis 196(9):1273–1275

Cook CJ, Williams C, Gluckman PD (1987) Brainstem auditory evoked potentials in the fetal sheep, in utero. J Dev Physiol 9(5):429–439

Cordier AG, Guitton S, Vauloup-Fellous C et al (2012a) Awareness of cytomegalovirus infection among pregnant women in France. J Clin Virol 53(4): 332–337

Cordier AG, Guitton S, Vauloup-Fellous C et al (2012b) Awareness and knowledge of congenital cytomegalovirus infection among health care providers in France. J Clin Virol 55(2):158–163

Costa OA, Axelsson A, Aniansson G (1988) Hearing loss at age 7, 10 and 13—an audiometric follow-up study. Scand Audiol Suppl 30:25–32

Crowson M, Schulz K, Tucci D (2016) National utilization and forecasting of ototopical antibiotics: Medicaid Data versus "Dr. Google". Otol Neurotol 37(8):1049–1054

Cupples L, Ching TYC, Crowe K et al (2014) Outcomes of 3-year-old children with hearing loss and different types of additional disabilities. Deaf Stud Deaf Educ 19(1):20–39

da Silva Araújo E, Zucki F, Corteletti LCBJ et al (2012) Hearing loss and acquired immune deficiency syndrome: systematic review. J Soc Bras Fonoaudiol 24(2):188–192

Dahle AJ, Fowler KB, Wright JD et al (2000) Longitudinal investigation of hearing disorders in children with congenital cytomegalovirus. J Am Acad Audiol 11(5):283–290

Davis A, Wood S (1992) The epidemiology of childhood hearing impairment: factor relevant to planning of services. Brit J Audiol 26(2):77–90

Davis A, Mencher G, Moorjani P (2004) An epidemiological perspective on childhood hearing impairment. In: McCormick B (ed) Paediatric audiology 0-5 years, 3rd edn. Whurr Publishers, London, pp 1–40

de Hoog M, van Zanten BA, Hop WC et al (2003) Newborn hearing screening: tobramycin and vancomycin are not risk factors for hearing loss. J Pediatr 142(1):41–46

de Vries JJ, Barbi M, Binda S et al (2012) Extraction of DNA from dried blood in the diagnosis of congenital CMV infection. Methods Mol Biol 903: 169–175

DeCasper AJ, Fifer WP (1980) Of human bonding: newborns prefer their mothers' voices. Science 208(4448):1174–1176

Dewan P, Gupta P (2012) Burden of congenital Rubella syndrome (CRS) in India: a systematic review. Indian Pediatr 49(5):377–399

Dobie RA, Van Hemel S (2004) Hearing loss: determining eligibility for social security benefits, Chapter 7 hearing loss in children. National Academies Press, Washington, DC, p 180–223. Available via https://www.ncbi.nlm.nih.gov/books/NBK207837/. Accessed 12 Feb 2017

Dockum GD, Robinson DO (1975) Warble tone as an audiometric stimulus. J Speech Hear Disord 40(3):351–356

Dreisbach L, Zettner E, Chang LM et al (2018) High-frequency distortion-product otoacoustic emission repeatability in a patient population. Ear Hear 39(1):85–100

Eagles EL, Wishik SM, Doerfler LG et al (1963) Hearing sensitivity and related factors in children. University of Pittsburgh, Graduate School of Public Health, Pittsburgh, 1st edn. Laryngoscope, St. Louis

Eggermont JJ, Salamy A (1988) Maturational time course for the ABR in preterm and full term infants. Hear Res 33(1):35–47

Eisenberg LS (2007) Current state of knowledge: speech recognition and production in children with hearing impairment. Ear Hear 28(6):766–772

El-Badry MM, Abousetta A, Kader RMA (2015) Vestibular dysfunction in patients with post-mumps sensorineural hearing loss. J Laryngol Otol 129(4):337–341

Encyclopædia Britannica Online (2011) Deafness. Encyclopædia Britannica Inc. Accessed 22 Feb 2012

Enders G, Daiminger A, Bader U et al (2011) Intrauterine transmission and clinical outcome of 248 pregnancies with primary cytomegalovirus infection in relation to gestational age. J Clin Virol 52(3):244–246

Feder KP, Michaud D, McNamee J et al (2017) Prevalence of hearing loss among a representative sample of Canadian Children and adolescents, 2 to 19 years of age. Ear Hear 38(1):7–20

First Years (2011) Developmental milestones, birth to 8 years. Available via http://firstyears.org/miles/chart.htm. Accessed 14 July 2017

Flipsen P (2008) Intelligibility of spontaneous conversational speech produced by children with cochlear implants: a review. Int J Pediatr Otorhinolaryngol 72(5):559–564

Forsythe E, Beales PL (2015) Bardet-Biedl syndrome. In: Pagon RA et al (ed) GeneReviews® [Internet]. University of Washington, Seattle, Seattle

Fortnum H (2003) Epidemiology of permanent childhood hearing impairment: implications for neonatal hearing screening. Audiol Med 1(3):155–164

Fortnum H, Davis A (1997) Epidemiology of permanent childhood hearing impairment in Trent Region, 1985-1993. Br J Audiol 31(6):409–446. Available via http://www.ncbi.nlm.nih.gov/pubmed/9478287. Accessed 11 May 2018

Fortnum HM, Summerfield AQ, Marshall DH et al (2001) Prevalence of permanent childhood hearing impairment in the United Kingdom and implications for universal neonatal hearing screening: questionnaire based ascertainment study. BMJ 323(7312):536–540. https://doi.org/10.1136/bmj.323.7312.536

Foulon I, Naessens A, Foulon W et al (2008) A 10-year prospective study of sensorineural hearing loss in children with congenital cytomegalovirus infection. J Pediatr 153(1):84158

Fowler KB (2013) Congenital cytomegalovirus infection: audiologic outcome. Clin Infect Dis 57(Suppl 4):S182–S184

Freyer DR, Chen L, Krailo MD et al (2017) Effects of sodium thiosulfate versus observation on development of cisplatin-induced hearing loss in children with cancer (ACCL0431): a multicentre, randomised, controlled, open-label, phase 3 trial. Lancet Oncol 18(1):63–74

Freyer DR, Frazier AL, Sung L (2018) Sodium thiosulfate and cisplatin-induced hearing loss. N Engl J Med 379(12):1180–1181

Furniss F, Biswas AB, Gumber R et al (2011) Cognitive phenotype of velocardiofacial syndrome: a review. Res Dev Disabil 32(6):2206–2213

Geers AE (2006) Factors influencing spoken language outcomes in children following early cochlear implantation. In: Moller AR (ed) Cochlear and brainstem implants. Adv Otorhinolaryngol. Karger, Basel, pp 50–65

Genetic Testing Registry (2016) Schinzel-Giedion syndrome. Available via https://www.ncbi.nlm.nih.gov/gtr/conditions/C1849294/. Accessed 27 July 2016

Genetics Home Reference (2016a) X-linked agammaglobulinemia. Available via https://ghr.nlm.nih.gov/condition/x-linked-agammaglobulinemia#synonyms. Accessed 4 Sept 2016

Genetics Home Reference (2016b) X-linked adrenoleukodystrophy. Available via https://ghr.nlm.nih.gov/condition/x-linked-adrenoleukodystrophy. Accessed 4 Sept 2016

Genetics Home Reference (2016c) Oculodentodigital dysplasia. Available via https://ghr.nlm.nih.gov/condition/oculodentodigital-dysplasia#definition. Accessed 30 July 2016

Genetics Home Reference (2016d) Mucopolysacch aridosis type III. Available via https://ghr.nlm.nih.gov/condition/mucopolysaccharidosis-type-iii. Accessed 31 July 2016

Goderis J, De Leenheer E, Smets K et al (2014) Hearing loss and congenital CMV infection: a systematic review. Pediatrics 134(5):972–982

Goodman S (2011) Comparison of high-frequency TEOAEs and DPOAEs for monitoring ototoxicity in pediatric cancer patients. Lecture presented at Illinois Speech-Language-Hearing Association 2011. Available via https://clas.uiowa.edu/sites/clas.uiowa.edu.comsci/files/groups/arl/pubs/goodman_isha_2011.pdf. Accessed 21 Jan 2017

Gordon JS, Phillips DS, Helt WJ et al (2005) Evaluation of insert earphones for high-frequency bedside ototoxicity monitoring. J Rehabil Res Dev 42(3):353–361

Gravel JS, Wallace IF (1992) Listening and language at 4 years of age: effects of early otitis media. J Speech Hear Res 35(3):588–595

Greenberg A (2000) Diuretic complications. Am J Med Sci 319(1):10–24

Grosse SD, Rossa DS, Dollard SC (2008) Congenital cytomegalovirus (CMV) infection as a cause of permanent bilateral hearing loss: a quantitative assessment. J Clin Virol 41(2):57–62

Gürkov R, Eshetu T, Miranda IB et al (2008) Ototoxicity of artemether/lumefantrine in the treatment of falciparum malaria: a randomized trial. Malar J 7:179

Gurney JG, Bass JK (2012) New International Society of Pediatric Oncology Boston Ototoxicity Grading Scale for pediatric oncology: still room for improvement. J Clin Oncol 30(19):2303–2306

Guy R, Nicholson J, Pannu SS et al (2003) A clinical evaluation of ophthalmic assessment in children with sensorineural deafness. Child Care Health Dev 29(5):377–384

Haapala S, Niemitalo-Haapola E, Raappana A et al (2015) Long-term influence of recurrent acute otitis media on neural involuntary attention switching in 2-year-old children. Behav Brain Funct 12:1

Haapaniemi JJ (1996) The hearing threshold levels of children at school age. Ear Hear 17(6):469–477

Hall C, Caserta M, Schnabel K et al (2010) Transplacental congenital human herpesvirus 6 infection caused by maternal chromosomally integrated virus. J Infect Dis 201(4):505–507. https://doi.org/10.1086/650495

Hall JW III (2013) Should Tone Burst ABR be Performed at 8000 Hz for Infant Hearing Assessment? https://www.audiologyonline.com/ask-the-experts/should-tone-burst-abr-performed-11941. Accessed 25 April 2019

Hamdan HZ, Abdelbagi IE, Nasser NM et al (2011) Seroprevalence of cytomegalovirus and rubella among pregnant women in western Sudan. Virol J 8:217

Harris JP, Woolf NK, Ryan AF et al (1984) Immunologic and electrophysiological response to cytomegaloviral inner ear infection in the guinea pig. J Infect Dis 150(4):523–530

Harris T, Peer S, Fagan JJ (2012) Audiological monitoring for ototoxic tuberculosis, human immunodeficiency virus and cancer therapies in a developing world setting. J Laryngol Otol 126(6):548–551

Haynes DS, Rutka J, Hawke M et al (2007) Ototoxicity of ototopical drops—an update. Otolaryngol Clin North Am 40(3):669–683

Hepper PG, Shahidullah BS (1994) Development of fetal hearing. Arch Dis Child Fetal Neonatal Ed 71(2):F81–F87

Hereditary Hearing Loss Homepage (2016) Mitochondrial mutations associated with syndromic hearing impairment. Available via http://hereditaryhearingloss.org/main.aspx?c=.HHH&n=86517&ct=78933&e=234541. Accessed 2 Aug 2016

Holmes AE, Niskar AS, Kieszak SM et al (2004) Mean and median hearing thresholds among children 6 to 19 years of age: the Third National Health And Nutrition Examination Survey, 1988 to 1994, United States. Ear Hear 25(4):397–402

Hong D, Kent JS, Kesler S (2009) Cognitive profile of Turner syndrome. Dev Disabil Res Rev 15(4):270–278. https://doi.org/10.1002/ddrr.79

Hotta H (1997) Neurotropic viruses: classification, structure and characteristics. Nihon Rinsho 55(4):777–782

Hoversten GH, Moncur JP (1969) Stimuli and intensity factors in testing infants. J Speech Hear Res 12(4):677–686

Hrapcak S, Kuper H, Bartlett P et al (2016) Hearing loss in HIV-infected children in Lilongwe, Malawi. PLoS One 11(8):e0161421. https://doi.org/10.1371/journal.pone.0161421. Accessed 8 Jan 2017

International Organization for Standardization (2010) 8253-1: Acoustics—audiometric test methods, part 1: pure tone air and bone conduction audiometry. Available via https://www.iso.org/standard/43601.html. Accessed 2 Apr 2017

International Osteoporosis Foundation (IOF) (2015) Camurati-Engelmanndiseasetype 2. Available via https://www.iofbonehealth.org/osteoporosis-musculoskeletal-disorders/skeletal-rare-disorders/camurati-engelmann-disease-type-2. Accessed 6 Mar 2017

Jackson AC (ed) (2013) Viral infections of the human nervous system. Springer, Basel

Jacobs P, Silaski G, Wilmington D et al (2012) Development and evaluation of a portable audiometer for high frequency screening of hearing loss from ototoxicity in homes/clinics. IEEE Trans Biomed Eng 59(11):3097–3103

Ječmenica JR, Opančina AAB (2015) Characteristics of brain stem auditory evoked potentials in children with hearing impairment due to infectious diseases. J Child Neurol 30(6):683–689

Jehanne M, Lumbroso-Le Rouic L, Savignoni A et al (2009a) Analysis of ototoxicity in young children receiving carboplatin in the context of conservative management of unilateral or bilateral retinoblastoma. Pediatr Blood Cancer 52(5):637–643

Jehanne M, Mercier G, Doz F (2009b) Monitoring of ototoxicity in young children receiving carboplatin for retinoblastoma. Pediatr Blood Cancer 53(6):1162

Jerger S, Lai L, Marchman VA (2002) Picture naming by children with hearing loss: I. Effect of semantically related auditory distracters. J Am Acad Audiol 13(9):463–477

Joint Committee on Infant Hearing (2007) Year 2007 position statement: principles and guidelines for early hearing detection and intervention programs. Pediatrics 120(4):898–921

Kadambari S, Luck S, Davis A et al (2013) Clinically targeted screening for congenital CMV—potential for integration into the National Hearing Screening Programme. Acta Paediatr 102(10):928–933

Kadambari S, Luck S, Davis A et al (2015a) Evaluating the feasibility of integrating salivary testing for congenital CMV into the Newborn Hearing Screening Programme in the UK. Eur J Pediatr 174(8):1117–1121

Kadambari S, Walter S, Stimson L et al (2015b) Integration rapid diagnostic testing for congenital CMV into the Newborn Hearing Screening Programme: the audio-vestibular physician's perspective. Arch Dis Child Fetal Neonatal Ed 100(5):F466–F467. https://doi.org/10.1136/archdischild-2015-308884

Kaiser R (2012) Tick-borne encephalitis: clinical findings and prognosis in adults. Wien Med Wochenschr 162(11–12):239–243

Kariya S, Schachern PA, Nishizaki K et al (2012) Inner ear changes in mucopolysaccharidosis type I/Hurler syndrome. Otol Neurotol 33(8):1323–1327. https://doi.org/10.1097/MAO.0b013e3182659cc3

Karma P, Sipila M, Rahko T (1989) Hearing and hearing loss in 5-year-old children. Pure-tone thresholds and the effect of acute otitis media. Scand Audiol 18(4):199–203

Katbamna B (2010). fetal alcohol syndrome: effects on the auditory system. Available via http://www.audiologyonline.com/articles/fetal-alcohol-syndrome-effects-on-845. Accessed 4 Sept 2016

Keefe DH, Goodman SS, Ellison JC et al (2011) Detecting high-frequency hearing loss with click-evoked otoacoustic emissions. J Acoust Soc Am 129(1):245–261

Keilmann A, Nakarat T, Bruce IA et al (2012) Hearing loss in patients with mucopolysaccharidosis II: data from HOS—the Hunter Outcome Survey. J Inherit Metab Dis 35(2):343–353. https://doi.org/10.1007/s10545-011-9378-5

Keupp K, Li Y, Vargel I et al (2013) Mutations in the interleukin receptor *IL11RA* cause autosomal recessive Crouzon-like craniosynostosis. Mol Genet Genomic Med 1(4):223–237. https://doi.org/10.1002/mgg3.28

Kimberlin DW (2004) Neonatal herpes simplex infection. Clin Microbiol Rev 17(1):1–13

Kimberlin DW, Lin CY, Sánchez PJ et al (2003) Effect of ganciclovir therapy on hearing in symptomatic congenital cytomegalovirus disease involving the central nervous system: a randomized, controlled trial. J Pediatr 143(1):16–25

Kimberlin DW, Jester PM, Sanchez PJ et al (2015) Valganciclovir for symptomatic congenital cytomegalovirus disease. N Engl J Med 372(10):933–943

Klausen O, Moller P, Holjefjord A et al (2007) Lasting effects of otitis media with effusion on language skills and listening performance. Acta Otolaryngol Suppl 543:73–76

Knight KR, Kraemer DF, Neuwelt EA (2005) Ototoxicity in children receiving platinum chemotherapy: underestimating a commonly occurring toxicity that may influence academic and social development. J Clin Oncol 23(34):8588–8596

Knight KR, Kraemer DF, Winter C et al (2007) Early changes in auditory function as a result of platinum chemotherapy: use of extended high-frequency audiometry and evoked distortion product otoacoustic emissions. J Clin Oncol 25(10):1190–1195

Knight K, Chen L, Freyer D et al (2016) Group-wide, prospective study of ototoxicity assessment in children receiving cisplatin chemotherapy (ACCL05C1): a report from the Children's Oncology Group. J Clin Oncol 2016:JCO2016692319. Epub ahead of print

Koo J-W, Quintanilla-Dieck L, Jiang M et al (2015) Endotoxemia-mediated inflammation potentiates aminoglycoside-induced ototoxicity. Sci Transl Med 7(298):298ra118. https://doi.org/10.1126/scitranslmed.aac5546

Koontz D, Baecher K, Amin M et al (2015) Evaluation of DNA extraction methods for the detection of cytomegalovirus in dried blood spots. J Clin Virol 66:95–99

Kozlova SN, Demikova NS, Seemanova E et al (1996) Nasledstvennie sindromy i mediko-genetičeckoe konsultirovanie [Inherited syndromes and medical—genetic consultancy]. Praktika, Moscow, p 470

Kranzer K, Elamin WF, Cox H et al (2015) A systematic review and meta-analysis of the efficacy and safety of N-acetylcysteine in preventing aminoglycoside-induced ototoxicity: implications for the treatment of multidrug-resistant TB. Thorax 70:1070–1077

Kuhl PK, Meltzoff AN (1996) Infant vocalizations in response to speech: vocal imitation and developmental change. J Acoust Soc Am 100(4 pt 1):2425–2438

Kuriger M, Lesimple C (2012) Frequency Composition™: a new approach to frequency lowering. Available via http://prof.bernafon.ca/downloads/~/media/pdf/english/global/bernafon/whitepaper/bf_wp_frequency_composition_uk.ashx. Accessed 29 Apr 2017

Lackner A, Acham A, Alborno T et al (2009) Effect on hearing of ganciclovir therapy for asymptomatic congenital cytomegalovirus infection: four to 10 year follow up. J Laryngol Otol 123(4):391–396

Lafay-Cousin L, Purdy E, Huang A et al (2013) Early cisplatin ototoxicity profile may predict the need for hearing support in children with medulloblastoma. Pediatr Blood Cancer 60(2):287–292

Laffan C (1993) Vision in communication. Talking Sense 39(4)

Landier W, Knight K, Wong FL et al (2014) Ototoxicity in children with high-risk neuroblastoma: prevalence, risk factors, and concordance of grading scales—a report from the Children's Oncology Group. J Clin Oncol 32(6):527–534

Langer T, am Zehnhoff-Dinnesen A, Radtke S et al (2013) Understanding platinum-induced ototoxicity. Trends Pharmacol Sci 34(8):458–469

Laughton B, Cornell M, Boivin M et al (2013) Neurodevelopment in perinatally HIV-infected children: a concern for adolescence. J Int AIDS Soc 16(1):18603

Levine D, Strother-Garcia K, Golinkoff R et al (2016) Language development in the first year of life: what deaf children might me missing before cochlear implantation. Otol Neurotol 37(2):e56–e62. https://doi.org/10.1097/MAO.0000000000000908. Nashville CI Papers

Lewis S, Moralee M, Skipp A et al (2006) The Early Support Monitoring protocol for deaf babies and children. Available via DfES Publications. http://www.batod.org.uk/content/resources/nhsp/useMP.pdf. Accessed 3 Apr 2016

Liden G, Kankkunen A (1969) Visual reinforcement audiometry. Acta Otolaryngol 67(2):281–292

Luck SE, Wieringa JW, Blázques-Gamero D et al (2017) Congenital cytomegalovirus: a European expert consensus statement on diagnosis and management. Pediatr Infect Dis J 36(12):1205–1213

Makar SK, Dhara S, Sinha AK et al (2012) Nature and onset of communication disorder in pediatrics with HIV. Int J Pediatr Otorhinolaryngol 76(7):1065–1066

MalaCards: The human disease database (2016) Cleidocranial dysplasia recessive form. Available via http://www.malacards.org/card/cleidocranial_dysplasia_recessive_form#related_genes. Accessed 31 July 2016

Mansour SL, Twigg SRF, Freeland RM et al (2009) Hearing loss in a mouse model of Muenke syndrome. Hum Mol Genet 18(1):43–50. https://doi.org/10.1093/hmg/ddn311

Marsala SZ, Pistacchi M, Gioulis M et al (2014) Neurological complications of tick borne encephalitis: the experience of 89 patients studied and literature review. Neurol Sci 35(1):15–21

Mathers C, Smith A, Concha M (2003) Global burden of hearing loss in the year 2000 (2003). Global Burden of Disease World Health Organization, Geneva, pp 1–30. Available via http://www.who.int/healthinfo/statistics/bod_hearingloss.pdf. Accessed 2 Nov 2016

Maw JL, Kartush JM, Bouchard K et al (2000) Octylcyanoacrylate: a new medical-grade adhesive for otologic surgery. Am J Otol 21(3):310–314

McArthur G, Kohnen S, Larsen L et al (2013) Getting to grips with the heterogeneity of developmental dyslexia. Cogn Neuropsychol 30(1):1–24

McDermott JC, Hodgson WR (1982) Auditory thresholds in children for narrow-band noise and warble tones in sound field. Brit J Audiol 16(4):221–225

McKenna MJ (1997) Measles, mumps, and sensorineural hearing loss. Ann N Y Acad Sci 830:291–298

McLean HQ, Fiebelkorn AP, Temte JL et al (2013) Prevention of measles, rubella, congenital rubella syndrome, and mumps, 2013: summary recommendations of the Advisory Committee on Immunization Practices (ACIP). MMWR Recomm Rep 62(42013):1–34

Medscape (2016) Fetal alcohol syndrome. Available via http://emedicine.medscape.com/article/974016-overview. Accessed 3 June 2017

Mercy Clinic Kids Plastic Surgery (2016) Muenke syndrome treatment. Available via https://www.mercy.net/practice/mercy-clinic-kids-plastic-surgery/muenke-syndrome-treatment. Accessed 30 July 2016

Milunsky JM (2001) Waardenburg syndrome type I. In: Pagon RA et al (eds) Gene reviews. University of Washington, Seattle

Mitchell CR, Ellingson RM, Henry JA et al (2004) Use of auditory brainstem responses for the early detection of ototoxicity from aminoglycosides or chemotherapeutic drugs. J Rehabil Res Dev 41(3A):373–382

Moller C (2002) Balance disorders. In: Newton VE (ed) Paediatric audiological medicine. Whurr Publishers, London

Möller S, Schönweiler R (1999) Analysis of infant cries for the early detection of hearing impairment. Speech Comm 28(3):175–193

Monasta L, Ronfani L, Marchetti F et al (2012) Burden of disease caused by otitis media: systematic review and global estimates. PLoS One 7(4):e36226

Moore K, Violetto D (2016) FRESH noise—a fresh approach to pediatric testing. AudiologyOnline, Article 17035. Available via http://www.audiology-online.com/articles/fresh-noise-approach-to-pediatric-17035. Accessed 3 Apr 2017

Moore JM, Wilson W (1978) Visual reinforcement audiometry (VRA) with infants. In: Gerber SE et al (eds)

Early diagnosis of hearing loss. Grune & Stretten, New York

Morgan G (2014) On language acquisition in speech and sign: development of combinatorial structure in both modalities. Front Psychol 5:1217

Morton NE (1991) Genetic epidemiology of hearing impairment. Ann N Y Acad Sci 630:16–31

Morton CC, Nance WE (2006) Newborn hearing screening—a silent revolution. N Engl J Med 354(20):2151–2164. https://doi.org/10.1056/NEJMra050700

Mudd PA, Edmunds AL, Glatz FR et al (2012) Ototoxicity. Medscape. Available via http://emedicine.medscape.com/article/857679-overview. Accessed 9 Sept 2016

Muller WJ, Jones CA, Koelle DM (2010) Immunobiology of herpes simplex virus and cytomegalovirus infections of the fetus and newborn. Curr Immunol Rev 6(1):38–55

Muscat M, Zimmerman L, Bacci S et al (2012) Toward rubella elimination in Europe: an epidemiological assessment. Vaccine 30(11):1999–2007

Natale V, Raquer H (2017) Xeroderma pigmentosum-Cockayne syndrome complex. Orphanet J Rare Dis 12(1):65

Nath A, Berger JR (2003) Clinical neurovirology: neurological disease and therapy. CRC Press, Boca Raton

National Institutes of Health (1993) Early identification of hearing impairment in infants and young children. NIH Consensus Statement Online 1993. 11(1):1–24. Available via https://consensus.nih.gov/1993/1993hearinginfantschildren092html.htm. Accessed 5 May 2017

National Institutes of Health NIH, National Cancer Institute NCI (2010) Common Terminology Criteria for Adverse Events (CTCAE) Version 4.0. Available via http://evs.nci.nih.gov/ftp1/CTCAE/About.html. Accessed 5 June 2014

National Organization for Rare Disorders (1993) Fetal hydantoin syndrome. Available via https://rarediseases.org/rare-diseases/fetal-hydantoin-syndrome/. Accessed 3 June 2017

National Organization for Rare Disorders (2005) Trichorhinophalangeal syndrome type II. Available via http://rarediseases.org/rare-diseases/trichorhinophalangeal-syndrome-type-ii/. Accessed 27 July 2016

National Organization for Rare Disorders (2014) Maroteaux Lamy syndrome. Available via http://rarediseases.org/rare-diseases/maroteaux-lamy-syndrome/. Accessed 1 Aug 2016

National Organization for Rare Disorders (2015) Marshall syndrome. Available via https://rarediseases.org/rare-diseases/marshall-syndrome/. Accessed 28 July 2016

NDCS and Sense (2014) Vision care for your deaf child. Available via https://www.sense.org.uk/sites/default/files/Vision_care_for_your_deaf_child_v2.pdf. Accessed 16 May 2016

Ndoleriire C, Turitwenka E, Bakeera-Kitaaka S et al (2013) The prevalence of hearing impairment in the 6 months – 5 years HIV/AIDS-positive patients attending paediatric infectious disease clinic at Mulago Hospital. Int J Pediatr Otorhinolaryngol 77(2):262–265

Newton VE (1985) Aetiology of bilateral sensori-neural hearing loss in young children. J Laryngol Otol Suppl 10:1–57

Newton EN, Vallely PJ (eds) (2006) Infection and hearing impairment. Whurr, Chichester

Niedermeyer HP, Arnold W (2008) Otosclerosis and measles virus—association or causation? ORL J Otorhinolaryngol Relat Spec 70(1):63–69

Nigro G, Adler SP, La Torre R et al (2005) Passive immunization during pregnancy for congenital cytomegalovirus infection. N Engl J Med 353(13):1350–1362

Nikkel SM, Hunter AG (2013) Normal intelligence and features of Bardet-Biedl syndrome in a family with a duplication of chromosome 20p13-p12.1. Genetics, Children's Hospital of Eastern Ontario, Ottawa, ON, Canada. Available via www.ashg.org/2013meeting/abstracts/fulltext/f130120786.htm. Accessed 2 Aug 2016

Nikolopoulos TP (2014) Auditory dyssynchrony or auditory neuropathy: understanding the pathophysiology and exploring methods of treatment. Int J Pediatr Otorhinolaryngol 78(2):171–173

Nittrouer S, Sansom E, Low K et al (2014) Language structures used by kindergartners with cochlear implants: relationship to phonological awareness, lexical knowledge and hearing loss. Ear Hear 35(5):506–518

Noorbakhsh S, Farhadi M, Daneshi A et al (2011) Viral infections detected by serology and PCR of perilymphatic fluid in children with idiopathic sensorineural hearing loss. World Health Organization Institutional Repository for Information Sharing. Available via http://apps.who.int/iris/bitstream/10665/118200/1/17_11_2011_0868_0871.pdf?ua=1. Accessed 31 Dec 2016

Northern JL, Downs MP (2014) Hearing in children, 6th edn. Plural Publishing Inc, San Diego

Nozza RJ (1995) Estimating the contribution of non-sensory factors to infant-adult differences in behavioral thresholds. Hear Res 91(1–2):72–78

Nozza RJ, Wilson WR (1984) Masked and unmasked pure-tone thresholds of infants and adults: development of auditory frequency selectivity and sensitivity. J Speech Hear Res 27(4):613–622

O'Hare A, Bremner L (2015) Management of developmental speech and language disorders. Arch Dis Child 101:272–277. https://doi.org/10.1136/archdischild-2014-307394

Oliver SE, Cloud GA, Sánchez PJ et al (2009) Neurodevelopmental outcomes following ganciclovir therapy in symptomatic congenital cytomegalovirus infections involving the central nervous system. J Clin Virol 46(4):S22–S26

Olsho LW, Koch EG, Carter EA et al (1988) Pure-tone sensitivity of human infants. J Acoust Soc Am 84(4):1316–1324

Olusanya BO, Neumann KJ, Saunders JE (2014) The global burden of disabling hearing impairment: a call to action. Bull World Health Organ 92(5):367–373

OMIM (2000) Turner syndrome-associated neurocognitive phenotype. Available via https://www.omim.

org/entry/313000?search=turner%20syndrome%20 patients&highlight=syndromic%20turner%20 patient%20syndrome. Accessed 23 Mar 2017

OMIM (2002a) Camurati-Engelmann disease, type 2. Available via https://www.omim.org/entry/606631. Accessed 3 June 2017

OMIM (2002b) Scheie syndrome. Available via https:// www.omim.org/entry/607016. Accessed 23 May 2017

OMIM (2005) Cognitive function 1, social; CGF1. Available via https://www.omim.org/entry/300082. Accessed 3 June 2017

OMIM (2006a) Camurati-Engelmann disease. Available via https://www.omim.org/entry/131300?search=camurati-engelmann%20disease&highlight=camurati%20camuratiengelmann%20disease%20engelmann. Accessed 11 May 2018

OMIM (2006b) Jervell and Lange-Nielsen syndrome 1. Available via https://www.omim.org/entry/220400. Accessed 23 May 2017

OMIM (2006c) Opitz Gbbb syndrome, type I. Available via https://www.omim.org/entry/300000. Accessed 23 May 2017

OMIM (2007a) Mucopolysaccharidosis, type IVB. Available via https://www.omim.org/entry/253010. Accessed 23 May 2017

OMIM (2007b) FG syndrome 3. Available via https:// www.omim.org/entry/300406. Accessed 23 May 2017

OMIM (2008) Crouzon syndrome with acanthosis nigricans. Available via https://www.omim.org/entry/612247. Accessed 3 June 2017

OMIM (2009a) Biotinidase deficiency. Available via https://omim.org/entry/253260. Accessed 23 May 2017

OMIM (2009b) Ciliary dyskinesia, primary, 1, with or without situs inversus. Avalaible via https://www.omim.org/entry/244400. Accessed 3 June 2017

OMIM (2009c) Refsum disease, classic. Available via https://www.omim.org/entry/266500. Accessed 23 May 2017

OMIM (2009d) FG syndrome 2. Available via https:// www.omim.org/entry/300321. Accessed 23 May 2017

OMIM (2009e) Otopalatodigital syndrome, type I. Available via https://www.omim.org/entry/311300. Accessed 23 May 2017

OMIM (2010a) Diastrophic dysplasia. Available via https://www.omim.org/entry/222600. Accessed 23 May 2017

OMIM (2010b) Opitz-Kaveggia syndrome. Available via https://www.omim.org/entry/305450. Accessed 23 May 2017

OMIM (2010c) Agammaglobulinemia, X-Linked. Available via https://www.omim.org/entry/300755. Accessed 23 May 2017

OMIM (2011a) Hypoparathyroidism, sensorineural deafness, and renal dysplasia. Available via https://www.omim.org/entry/146255. Accessed 3 June 2017

OMIM (2011b) Townes-Brocks syndrome 1. Available via https://www.omim.org/entry/107480. Accessed 23 May 2017

OMIM (2011c) McCune-Albright Syndrome. Available via https://www.omim.org/entry/174800. Accessed 23 May 2017

OMIM (2012a) Branchiootorenal syndrome 1; BOR1. Available via https://www.omim.org/entry/113650. Accessed 1 May 2017

OMIM (2012b) Marshall syndrome. Available via https:// www.omim.org/entry/154780. Accessed 23 May 2017

OMIM (2012c) Muckle-Wells syndrome. Available via https://www.omim.org/entry/191900. Accessed 3 June 2017

OMIM (2012d) Muenke syndrome. Available via https:// www.omim.org/entry/602849. Accessed 23 May 2017

OMIM (2012e) Neurofibromatosis, type II. Available via https://www.omim.org/entry/101000. Accessed 23 May 2017

OMIM (2012f) Cockayne syndrome A. Available via https://www.omim.org/entry/216400?search=Cockayne%20syndrome&highlight=syndromic%20cockayne%20syndrome. Accessed 23 May 2017

OMIM (2012g) Pendred syndrome. Available via https:// www.omim.org/entry/274600. Accessed 23 May 2017

OMIM (2012h) Usher syndrome, type ID. Available via https://www.omim.org/entry/601067. Accessed 23 May 2017

OMIM (2012i) FG syndrome 4. Available via https:// www.omim.org/entry/300422. Accessed 23 May 2017

OMIM (2012j) Diabetes and deafness, maternally inherited. Available via https://www.omim.org/entry/520000. Accessed 23 May 2017

OMIM (2013a) Velocardiofacial syndrome. Available via https://www.omim.org/entry/192430?search=Velocardiofacial%20syndrome%2C&highlight=syndromic%20syndrome%20velocardiofacial. Accessed 3 June 2017

OMIM (2013b) Langer-Giedion syndrome; LGS; chromosome 8q24.1 deletion syndrome. Available via https://www.omim.org/entry/150230?search=Langer-Giedion%20syndrome&highlight=giedion%20syndromic%20langer%20syndrome%20langergiedion. Accessed 3 June 2017

OMIM (2013c) Cleidocranial dysplasia; CCD. Available via https://www.omim.org/entry/119600. Accessed 3 June 2017

OMIM (2013d) Facioscapulohumeral muscular dystrophy 1. Available via https://www.omim.org/entry/158900?search=facioscapulohumeral%20muscular%20dystrophy&highlight=facioscapulohumeral%20dystrophy%20muscular. Accessed 1 May 2017

OMIM (2013e) Stickler syndrome, type I. Available via https://www.omim.org/entry/108300. Accessed 23 May 2017

OMIM (2013f) Adrenoleukodystrophy. Available via https://www.omim.org/entry/300100. Accessed 3 June 2017

OMIM (2014a) Oculodentodigital dysplasia. Available via https://www.omim.org/entry/164200. Accessed 23 May 2017

OMIM (2014b) Schinzel-Giedion midface retraction syndrome. Available via http://www.orpha.net/consor/cgi-bin/Disease_Search.php?lng=EN&data_id=2807&Disease_Disease_Search_diseaseGroup=Schinzel-Giedion-syndrome&Disease_Disease_Search_diseaseType=Pat&Disease(s)/group of diseases=Schinzel-Giedion-syndrome&title=Schinzel-Giedion-syndrome&search=Disease_Search_Simple. Accessed 23 May 2017

OMIM (2014c) Myoclonic epilepsy associated with ragged-red fibers. Available via https://www.omim.org/entry/545000. Accessed 23 May 2017

OMIM (2015a) Down syndrome. Available via https://www.omim.org/entry/190685?search=Morbus%20Down&highlight=down%20morbus. Accessed 3 June 2017

OMIM (2015b) Wolf-Hirschhorn syndrome; WHS. Available via https://www.omim.org/entry/194190?search=wolf-hirschhorn%20syndrome&highlight=wolfhirschhorn%20wolf%20hirschhorn%20syndrome%20syndromic. Accessed 3 June 2017

OMIM (2015c) Noonan syndrome 1. Available via https://www.omim.org/entry/163950. Accessed 23 May 2017

OMIM (2015d) Phenylketonuria. Available via https://www.omim.org/entry/261600. Accessed May 23rd, 2017

OMIM (2015e) Mucopolysaccharidosis, type IIIA. Available via https://www.omim.org/entry/252900. Accessed 23 May 2017

OMIM (2015f) Alport syndrome, X-Linked. Available via https://www.omim.org/entry/301050. Accessed 23 May 2017

OMIM (2016a) Hemifacial microsomia; HFM. Available via https://www.omim.org/entry/164210. Accessed 3 June 2017

OMIM (2016b) Charge syndrome. Available via https://www.omim.org/entry/214800. Accessed 3 June 2017

OMIM (2016c) Crouzon syndrome. Available via https://www.omim.org/entry/123500. Accessed 3 June 2017

OMIM (2016d) Treacher Collins syndrome 1. Available via www.omim.org/entry/154500. Accessed 23 May 2017

OMIM (2016e) Waardenburg syndrome, type 1. Available via https://www.omim.org/entry/193500. Accessed 23 May 2017

OMIM (2016f) Alstrom syndrome. Available via https://www.omim.org/entry/203800. Accessed 23 May 2017

OMIM (2016g) Mucopolysaccharidosis, type II. Available via https://www.omim.org/entry/309900. Accessed 23 May 2017

OMIM (2016h) Mucopolysaccharidosis type VI. Available via https://www.omim.org/entry/253200. Accessed 23 May 2017

OMIM (2016i) Hurler syndrome. Available via https://www.omim.org/entry/607014. Accessed 23 May 2017

OMIM (2016j) Mohr-Tranebjaerg syndrome. Available via https://www.omim.org/entry/304700. Accessed 23 May 2017

OMIM (2016k) Kearns-Sayre syndrome. Available via https://www.omim.org/entry/530000. Accessed 23 May 2017

OMIM (2016l) Mitochondrial myopathy, encephalopathy, lactic acidosis, and stroke-like episodes. Available via https://www.omim.org/entry/540000. Accessed 23 May 2017

OMIM (2017a) Paired box gene 6. Available via https://www.omim.org/entry/607108. Accessed 1 May 2017

OMIM (2017b) Bardet-Biedl syndrome 1. Available via https://www.omim.org/entry/209900. Accessed 23 May 2017

Onakewhor JU, Chiwuzie J (2011) Seroprevalence survey of rubella infection in pregnancy at the University of Benin Teaching Hospital, Benin City, Nigeria. Niger J Clin Pract 14(2):140–145

Orchik DJ, Rintelmann WF (1978) Comparison of puretone, warble-tone and narrow-band noise thresholds of young normal-hearing children. J Am Audiol Soc 3(5):214–220

Orphanet (2006) MERRF. Available via http://www.orpha.net/consor/cgi-bin/Disease_Search.php?lng=EN&data_id=64&Disease_Disease_Search_diseaseGroup=MERRF&Disease_Disease_Search_diseaseType=Pat&Disease(s)/group of diseases=MERRF&title=MERRF&search=Disease_Search_Simple. Accessed 2 Aug 2016

Orphanet (2007a) Turner syndrome. Available via http://www.orpha.net/consor/cgi-bin/Disease_Search.php?lng=EN&data_id=44&Disease_Disease_Search_diseaseGroup=Turner-Syndrome&Disease_Disease_Search_diseaseType=Pat&Disease(s)/group%20of%20diseases=Turner-syndrome&title=Turner-syndrome&search=Disease_Search_Simple. Accessed 27 July 2016

Orphanet (2007b) BOR syndrome. Available via http://www.orpha.net/consor/cgi-bin/Disease_Search.php?lng=EN&data_id=237&Disease_Disease_Search_diseaseGroup=Branchiootorenal-syndrome&Disease_Disease_Search_diseaseType=Pat&Disease(s)/group of diseases=BOR-syndrome&title=BOR-syndrome&search=Disease_Search_Simple. Accessed 4 Aug 2016

Orphanet (2007c) Mucopolysaccharidosis type 4. Available via http://www.orpha.net/consor/cgi-bin/Disease_Search.php?lng=EN&data_id=872&Disease_Disease_Search_diseaseGroup=Morquio-disease&Disease_Disease_Search_diseaseType=Pat&Disease(s)/group of diseases=Mucopolysaccharidosis-type-4&title=Mucopolysaccharidosis-type-4&search=Disease_Search_Simple. Accessed 31 July 2016

Orphanet (2007d) Mucopolysaccharidosis type 3. Available via http://www.orpha.net/consor/cgi-bin/Disease_Search.php?lng=EN&data_id=653&Disease_Disease_Search_diseaseGroup=Sanfilippo-disease&Disease_Disease_Search_diseaseType=Pat&Disease(s)/group of diseases=Mucopolysaccharidosis-type-3&title=Mucopolysaccharidosis-type-

3&search=Disease_Search_Simple. Accessed 31 July 2016

Orphanet (2007e) Alport syndrome. Available via http://www.orpha.net/consor/cgi-bin/Disease_Search.php?lng=EN&data_id=630&Disease_Disease_Search_diseaseGroup=Alport-syndrome&Disease_Disease_Search_diseaseType=Pat&Disease(s)/group of diseases=Alport-syndrome&title=Alport-syndrome&search=Disease_Search_Simple. Accessed 4 Aug 2016

Orphanet (2008a) Hypoparathyroidism-deafness-renal disease syndrome. Available via http://www.orpha.net/consor/cgi-bin/Disease_Search.php?lng=EN&data_id=2110&Disease_Disease_Search_diseaseGroup=hdr&Disease_Disease_Search_diseaseType=Pat&Disease(s)/group%20of%20diseases=Hypoparathyroidism-deafness-renal-disease-syndrome&title=Hypoparathyroidism-deafness-renal-disease-syndrome&search=Disease_Search_Simple. Accessed 4 Sept 2016

Orphanet (2008b) Noonan syndrome. Available via http://www.orpha.net/consor/cgi-bin/Disease_Search.php?lng=EN&data_id=206&Disease_Disease_Search_diseaseGroup=Noonan-syndrome&Disease_Disease_Search_diseaseType=Pat&Disease(s)/group of diseases=Noonan-syndrome&title=Noonan-syndrome&search=Disease_Search_Simple. Accessed 29 July 2016

Orphanet (2008c) Stickler syndrome. Available via http://www.orpha.net/consor/cgi-bin/Disease_Search.php?lng=EN&data_id=824&Disease_Disease_Search_diseaseGroup=Stickler-syndrome&Disease_Disease_Search_diseaseType=Pat&Disease(s)/group of diseases=Stickler-syndrome&title=Stickler-syndrome&search=Disease_Search_Simple. Accessed 28 July 2016

Orphanet (2008d) Bardet-Biedl syndrome. Available via http://www.orpha.net/consor/cgi-bin/Disease_Search.php?lng=EN&data_id=3244&Disease_Disease_Search_diseaseGroup=Bardet-Biedl-syndrome&Disease_Disease_Search_diseaseType=Pat&Disease(s)/group%20of%20diseases=Bardet-Biedl-syndrome&title=Bardet-Biedl-syndrome&search=Disease_Search_Simple. Accessed 1 Aug 2016

Orphanet (2008e) Diastrophic dwarfism. Available via http://www.orpha.net/consor/cgi-bin/Disease_Search.php?lng=EN&data_id=209&Disease_Disease_Search_diseaseGroup=Diastrophic-dysplasia&Disease_Disease_Search_diseaseType=Pat&Disease(s)/group%20of%20diseases=Diastrophic-dwarfism&title=Diastrophic-dwarfism&search=Disease_Search_Simple. Accessed 1 Aug 2016

Orphanet (2008f) McCune-Albright syndrome. Available via http://www.orpha.net/consor/cgi-bin/Disease_Search.php?lng=EN&data_id=279&Disease_Disease_Search_diseaseGroup=McCune-Albright-syndrome&Disease_Disease_Search_diseaseType=Pat&Disease(s)/group of diseases=McCune-Albright-syndrome&title=McCune-Albright-syndrome&search=Disease_Search_Simple. Accessed 2 Aug 2016

Orphanet (2009a) Neurofibromatosis type 2. Available via http://www.orpha.net/consor/cgi-bin/Disease_Search.php?lng=EN&data_id=183&Disease_Disease_Search_diseaseGroup=Neurofibromatosis-type-2&Disease_Disease_Search_diseaseType=Pat&Disease(s)/group of diseases=Neurofibromatosis-type-2&title=Neurofibromatosis-type-2&search=Disease_Search_Simple. Accessed 4 Aug 2016

Orphanet (2009b) Cockayne syndrome. Available via http://www.orpha.net/consor/cgi-bin/Disease_Search.php?lng=EN&data_id=638&Disease_Disease_Search_diseaseGroup=Cockayne-syndrome&Disease_Disease_Search_diseaseType=Pat&Disease(s)/group of diseases=Cockayne-syndrome&title=Cockayne-syndrome&search=Disease_Search_Simple. Accessed 31 July 2016

Orphanet (2009c) Jervell and Lange-Nielsen syndrome. Available via http://www.orpha.net/consor/cgi-bin/Disease_Search.php?lng=EN&data_id=12056&Disease_Disease_Search_diseaseGroup=Jervell-Lange-Nielsen-syndrome&Disease_Disease_Search_diseaseType=Pat&Disease(s)/group of diseases=Jervell-and-Lange-Nielsen-syndrome&title=Jervell-and-Lange-Nielsen-syndrome&search=Disease_Search_Simple. Accessed 4 Aug 2016

Orphanet (2009d) Usher syndrome. Available via http://www.orpha.net/consor/cgi-bin/Disease_Search.php?lng=EN&data_id=662&Disease_Disease_Search_diseaseGroup=Usher-syndrome&Disease_Disease_Search_diseaseType=Pat&Disease(s)/group of diseases=Usher-syndrome&title=Usher-syndrome&search=Disease_Search_Simple. Accessed 31 July 2016

Orphanet (2009e) FG syndrome phenotypic spectrum. Available via http://www.orpha.net/consor/cgi-bin/Disease_Search.php?lng=EN&data_id=1053&Disease_Disease_Search_diseaseGroup=FG-syndrome&Disease_Disease_Search_diseaseType=Pat&Disease(s)/group of diseases=FG-syndrome&title=FG-syndrome&search=Disease_Search_Simple. Accessed 2 Aug 2016

Orphanet (2009f) Maternally-inherited diabetes and deafness. Available via http://www.orpha.net/consor/cgi-bin/Disease_Search.php?lng=EN&data_id=7037&Disease_Disease_Search_diseaseGroup=Maternally-inherited-diabetes-and-deafness-&Disease_Disease_Search_diseaseType=Pat&Disease(s)/group of diseases=Maternally-inherited-diabetes-and-deafness&title=Maternally-inherited-diabetes-and-deafness&search=Disease_Search_Simple. Accessed 2 Aug 2016

Orphanet (2010) Mucopolysaccharidosis type 6. Available via http://www.orpha.net/consor/cgi-bin/Disease_Search. php?lng=EN&data_id=24&Disease_Disease_Search_ diseaseGroup=Maroteaux-Lamy-syndrome&Disease_ Disease_Search_diseaseType=Pat&Disease(s)/ group%20of%20diseases=Mucopolysaccharidosis-type-6&title=Mucopolysaccharidosis-type-6&search=Disease_Search_Simple. Accessed 1 Aug 2016

Orphanet (2011a) Biotinidase deficiency. Available via http://www.orpha.net/consor/cgi-bin/Disease_Search. php?lng=EN&data_id=11267&Disease_Disease_ Search_diseaseGroup=Biotinidase-deficiency&Disease_Disease_Search_ diseaseType=Pat&Disease(s)/group of diseases= Biotinidase-deficiency&title=Biotinidase-deficiency&search=Disease_Search_Simple. Accessed 4 Aug 2016

Orphanet (2011b) Scheie syndrome. Available via http:// www.orpha.net/consor/cgi-bin/Disease_Search. php?lng=EN&data_id=12382&Disease_Disease_ Search_diseaseGroup=mucopolysaccharidosis&Disease_Disease_Search_diseaseType=Pat&Disease(s)/ group%20of%20diseases=Scheie-syndrome&title=Scheie-syndrome&search=Disease_ Search_Simple. Accessed 1 Aug 2016

Orphanet (2012a) 22q11.2 deletion syndrome. Available via http://www.orpha.net/consor/ cgi-bin/Disease_Search.php?lng=EN&data_ id=126&Disease_Disease_Search_ diseaseGroup=Di-George-syndrome&Disease_ Disease_Search_diseaseType=Pat&Disease(s)/ group%20of%20diseases=22q11-2-dele-tion-syndrome&title=22q11-2-deletion-syndrome&search=Disease_Search_Simple. Accessed 27 July 2016

Orphanet (2012b) Wolf-Hirschhorn syndrome. Available via http://www.orpha.net/consor/cgi-bin/Disease_ Search.php?lng=EN&data_id=147&Disease_ Disease_Search_diseaseGroup=Wolf-Hirschhorn-syndrome&Disease_Disease_Search_ diseaseType=Pat&Disease(s)/group%20of%20 diseases=Wolf-Hirschhorn-syndrome&title=Wolf-Hirschhorn-syndrome&search=Disease_Search_ Simple. Accessed 27 July 2016

Orphanet (2012c) Aniridia. Available via http:// www.orpha.net/consor/cgi-bin/Disease_Search. php?lng=EN&data_id=6018&Disease_Disease_ Search_diseaseGroup=aniridia&Disease_ Disease_Search_diseaseType=Pat&Disease(s)/ group%20of%20diseases=Aniridia&title=Aniridia&search=Disease_Search_Simple. Accessed 4 Mar 2017

Orphanet (2012d) Opitz G/BBB syndrome. Available via http://www.orpha.net/consor/cgi-bin/Disease_Search. php?lng=EN&data_id=3423&Disease_Disease_ Search_diseaseGroup=BBB-G-syndrome&Disease_ Disease_Search_diseaseType=Pat&Disease(s)/ group%20of%20diseases=Opitz-G-BBB-syndrome&title=Opitz-G-BBB-

syndrome&search=Disease_Search_Simple. Accessed 2 Aug 2016

Orphanet (2013a) Camurati-Engelmann disease. Available via http://www.orpha.net/consor/cgi-bin/Disease_ Search.php?lng=EN&data_id=1551&Disease_ Disease_Search_diseaseGroup=Camurati-Engelmann-disease&Disease_Disease_ Search_diseaseType=Pat&Disease(s)/ group of diseases=Camurati-Engelmann-disease&title=Camurati-Engelmann-disease&search=Disease_Search_Simple. Accessed 29 July 2016

Orphanet (2013b) Cleidocranial dysplasia. Available via http://www.orpha.net/consor/ cgi-bin/Disease_Search.php?lng=EN&data_ id=443&Disease_Disease_Search_ diseaseGroup=Cleidocranial-dysplasia&Disease_ Disease_Search_diseaseType=Pat&Disease(s)/ group of diseases=Cleidocranial-dysplasia&title =Cleidocranial-dysplasia&search=Disease_Search_ Simple. Accessed 31 July 2016

Orphanet (2013c) Crouzon disease. Available via http:// www.orpha.net/consor/cgi-bin/Disease_Search. php?lng=EN&data_id=244&Disease_Disease_ Search_diseaseGroup=Crouzon-disease&Disease_ Disease_Search_diseaseType=Pat&Disease(s)/ group of diseases=Crouzon-disease&title=Crouzon-disease&search=Disease_Search_Simple. Accessed 30 July 2016

Orphanet (2013d) Townes-Brocks syndrome. Available via http://www.orpha.net/consor/cgi-bin/Disease_Search. php?lng=EN&data_id=218&Disease_Disease_ Search_diseaseGroup=Townes-Brocks-syndrome&Disease_Disease_Search_ diseaseType=Pat&Disease(s)/group of diseases=Townes-Brocks-syndrome&title=Townes-Brocks-syndrome&search=Disease_Search_Simple. Accessed 29 July 2016

Orphanet (2013e) Mucopolysaccharidosis type 2. Available via http://www.orpha.net/consor/ cgi-bin/Disease_Search.php?lng=EN&data_ id=131&Disease_Disease_Search_diseaseGro up=Mucopolysaccharidosis-type-2&Disease_ Disease_Search_diseaseType=Pat&Disease(s)/ group of diseases=Mucopolysaccharidosis-type-2&title=Mucopolysaccharidosis-type-2&search=Disease_Search_Simple. Accessed 2 Aug 2016

Orphanet (2013f) Pendred syndrome. Available via http://www.orpha.net/consor/cgi-bin/Disease_Search. php?lng=EN&data_id=558&Disease_Disease_ Search_diseaseGroup=Pendred-syndrome&Disease_ Disease_Search_diseaseType=Pat&Disease(s)/group of diseases=Pendred-syndrome&title=Pendred-syndrome&search=Disease_Search_Simple. Accessed 4 Aug 2016

Orphanet (2013g) Mohr-Tranebjaerg syndrome. Available via http://www.orpha.net/consor/cgi-bin/Disease_ Search.php?lng=EN&data_id=10691&Disease_ Disease_Search_diseaseGroup=Mohr-Tranebjaerg-syndrome&Disease_Disease_Search_ diseaseType=Pat&Disease(s)/group of diseases=Mohr-Tranebjaerg-syndrome&title=Mohr-Tranebjaerg-syndrome&search=Disease_Search_ Simple. Accessed 4 Aug 2016

Orphanet (2013h) X-linked agammaglobulin-emia. Available via http://www.orpha.net/ consor/cgi-bin/Disease_Search.php?lng=EN&data_ id=142&Disease_Disease_Search_diseaseGroup=X-linked-agammaglobulinemia&Disease_ Disease_Search_diseaseType=Pat&Disease(s)/ group%20of%20diseases=X-linked-agammaglobulinemia&title=X-linked-agam-maglobulinemia&search=Disease_Search_Simple. Accessed 4 Mar 2017

Orphanet (2014a) Down syndrome. Available via http:// www.orpha.net/consor/cgi-bin/Disease_Search. php?lng=EN&data_id=116&Disease_Disease_ Search_diseaseGroup=M%2D%2DDown&Disea se_Disease_Search_diseaseType=Pat&Disease(s)/ group%20of%20diseases=Down-syndrome&title=Down-syndrome&search=Disease_ Search_Simple. Accessed 27 July 2016

Orphanet (2014b) Goldenhar syndrome. Available via http://www.orpha.net/consor/ cgi-bin/Disease_Search.php?lng=EN&data_ id=499&Disease_Disease_Search_ diseaseGroup=Goldenhar-syndrome&Disease_ Disease_Search_diseaseType=Pat&Disease(s)/group of diseases=Goldenhar-syndrome&title=Goldenhar-syndrome&search=Disease_Search_Simple. Accessed 28 July 2016

Orphanet (2014c) Crouzon syndrome-acanthosis nigricans syndrome. Available via http://www. orpha.net/consor/cgi-bin/Disease_Search. php?lng=EN&data_id=12205&Disease_Disease_ Search_diseaseGroup=Crouzon-syndrome-acan-thosis-nigricans-syndrome&Disease_Disease_ Search_diseaseType=Pat&Disease(s)/group of diseases=Crouzon-syndrome-acanthosis-nigricans-syndrome&title=Crouzon-syndrome-acanthosis-nigricans-syndrome&search=Disease_Search_ Simple. Accessed 30 July 2016

Orphanet (2014d) Facioscapulohumeral dys-trophy. Available via http://www.orpha. net/consor/cgi-bin/Disease_Search. php?lng=EN&data_id=62&Disease_Disease_ Search_diseaseGroup=Facioscapulohumeral-muscular-dystrophy&Disease_Disease_Search_ diseaseType=Pat&Disease(s)/group%20 of%20diseases=Facioscapulohumeral-dystrophy&title=Facioscapulohumeral-dystrophy&search=Disease_Search_Simple. Accessed 1 May 2017

Orphanet (2014e) Muckle-Wells syndrome. Available via http://www.orpha.net/consor/cgi-bin/OC_Exp. php?Lng=GB&Expert=575. Accessed 1 May 2017

Orphanet (2014f) Schinzel-Giedion syndrome. Available via http://www.orpha.net/consor/cgi-bin/Disease_ Search.php?lng=EN&data_id=2807&Disease_

Disease_Search_diseaseGroup=Schinzel-Giedion-syndrome&Disease_Disease_ Search_diseaseType=Pat&Disease(s)/group of diseases=Schinzel-Giedion-syndrome&title=Schinzel-Giedion-syndrome&search=Disease_Search_Simple. Accessed 27 July 2016

Orphanet (2014g) Treacher-Collins syndrome. Available via http://www.orpha.net/consor/ cgi-bin/Disease_Search.php?lng=EN&data_ id=293&Disease_Disease_Search_ diseaseGroup=Treacher-Collins-&Disease_Disease_ Search_diseaseType=Pat&Disease(s)/group of diseases=Treacher-Collins-syndrome&title=Treacher-Collins-syndrome&search=Disease_Search_Simple. Accessed 29 July 2016

Orphanet (2014h) Alström syndrome. Available via http://www.orpha.net/consor/cgi-bin/Disease_Search. php?lng=EN&data_id=1328&Disease_Disease_ Search_diseaseGroup=Alstrom-syndrome&Disease_ Disease_Search_diseaseType=Pat&Disease(s)/group of diseases=Alstrom-syndrome&title=Alstrom-syndrome&search=Disease_Search_Simple. Accessed 1 Aug 2016

Orphanet (2014i) Xeroderma pigmentosum-Cockayne syndrome complex. Available via http://www. orpha.net/consor/cgi-bin/Disease_Search. php?lng=EN&data_id=18903&Disease_Disease_ Search_diseaseType=ORPHA&Disease_Disease_ Search_diseaseGroup=220295&Disease(s)/ group%20of%20diseases=XP-CS-complex&title=XP-CS-complex&search=Disease_ Search_Simple. Accessed 1 May 2017

Orphanet (2014j) Primary ciliary dyskinesia. Available via http://www.orpha.net/consor/cgi-bin/Disease_Search. php?lng=EN&data_id=665&Disease_Disease_ Search_diseaseGroup=Primary-Ciliary-Dyskinesia&Disease_Disease_Search_ diseaseType=Pat&Disease(s)/group%20of%20 diseases=Primary-ciliary-dyskinesia&title=Primary-ciliary-dyskinesia&search=Disease_Search_Simple. Accessed 1 Aug 2016

Orphanet (2014k) Hurler syndrome. Available via http:// www.orpha.net/consor/cgi-bin/Disease_Search. php?lng=EN&data_id=12381&Disease_Disease_ Search_diseaseGroup=Mucopolysaccharidosis&Dis ease_Disease_Search_diseaseType=Pat&Disease(s)/ group of diseases=Hurler-syndrome&title=Hurler-syndrome&search=Disease_Search_Simple. Accessed 31 July 2016

Orphanet (2014l) Kearns-Sayre syndrome. Available via http://www.orpha.net/consor/cgi-bin/Disease_Search. php?lng=EN&data_id=61&Disease_Disease_ Search_diseaseGroup=Kearns-Sayre-Syndrome-&Disease_Disease_Search_ diseaseType=Pat&Disease(s)/group of diseases= Kearns-Sayre-syndrome&title=Kearns-Sayre-syndrome&search=Disease_Search_Simple. Accessed 2 Aug 2016

Orphanet (2015a) CHARGE syndrome. Available via http://www.orpha.net/consor/

832

cgi-bin/Disease_Search.php?lng=EN&data_
id=110&Disease_Disease_Search_
diseaseGroup=CHARGE-syndrome&Disease_
Disease_Search_diseaseType=Pat&Disease(s)/group
of diseases=CHARGE-syndrome&title=CHARGE-
syndrome&search=Disease_Search_Simple.
Accessed 28 July 2016

Orphanet (2015b) Marshall syndrome. Available via
http://www.orpha.net/consor/cgi-bin/Disease_Search.
php?lng=EN&data_id=540&Disease_Disease_Sea
rch_diseaseGroup=Marshall-syndrome&Disease_
Disease_Search_diseaseType=Pat&Disease(s)/group
of diseases=Marshall-syndrome&title=Marshall-
syndrome&search=Disease_Search_Simple.
Accessed 28 July 2016

Orphanet (2015c) Waardenburg syndrome.
Available via http://www.orpha.net/consor/
cgi-bin/Disease_Search.php?lng=EN&data_
id=663&Disease_Disease_Search_
diseaseGroup=Waardenburg-syndrome&Disease_
Disease_Search_diseaseType=Pat&Disease(s)/group of
diseases=Waardenburg-syndrome&title=Waardenburg-
syndrome&search=Disease_Search_Simple. Accessed
29 July 2016

Orphanet (2015d) Maternal phenylketonuria. Available via
http://www.orpha.net/consor/www/cgi-bin/OC_Exp.
php?lng=EN&Expert=2209. Accessed 3 June 2017

Orphanet (2015e) Refsum disease. Available via http://
www.orpha.net/consor/cgi-bin/Disease_Search.
php?lng=EN&data_id=381&Disease_Disease_
Search_diseaseGroup=Refsum-disease&Disease_
Disease_Search_diseaseType=Pat&Disease(s)/
group of diseases=Refsum-disease&title=Refsum-
disease&search=Disease_Search_Simple. Accessed 4
Aug 2016

Orphanet (2015f) Otopalatodigital syndrome type 1.
Available via http://www.orpha.net/consor/cgi-bin/
Disease_Search.php?lng=EN&data_id=12059&Disease_
Disease_Search_diseaseGroup=Otopalatodigital-
syndrome-type-1&Disease_Disease_Search_
diseaseType=Pat&Disease(s)/group of diseases=
Otopalatodigital-syndrome-type-
1&title=Otopalatodigital-syndrome-type-
1&search=Disease_Search_Simple. Accessed 2
Aug 2016

Orphanet (2015g) MELAS. Available via http://
www.orpha.net/consor/cgi-bin/Disease_Search.
php?lng=EN&data_id=63&Disease_Disease_
Search_diseaseGroup=MELAS&Disease_Disease_
Search_diseaseType=Pat&Disease(s)/group of disease
s=MELAS&title=MELAS&search=Disease_Search_
Simple. Accessed 2 Aug 2016

Orphanet (2015h) Fetal hydantoin syndrome. Available via
http://www.orpha.net/consor/cgi-bin/Disease_Search.
php?lng=EN&data_id=1875&Disease_Disease_
Search_diseaseGroup=Fetal-Hydantoin-
Syndrome&Disease_Disease_Search_
diseaseType=Pat&Disease(s)/group%20of%20
diseases=Fetal-hydantoin-syndrome&title=Fetal-
hydantoin-syndrome&search=Disease_Search_
Simple. Accessed 4 Sept 2016

Orphanet (2016) Langer-Giedion syndrome. Available via
http://www.orpha.net/consor/cgi-bin/Disease_Search.
php?lng=EN&data_id=526&Disease_Disease_
Search_diseaseGroup=Langer-Giedion-
syndrome&Disease_Disease_Search_
diseaseType=Pat&Disease(s)/group of diseases=
Langer-Giedion-syndrome&title=Langer-Giedion-
syndrome&search=Disease_Search_Simple.
Accessed 27 July 2016

Orphanet (2017) Muenke syndrome. Available via http://
www.orpha.net/consor/cgi-bin/Disease_Search.
php?lng=EN&data_id=10716&Disease_Disease_
Search_diseaseGroup=Muenke-syndrome&Disease_
Disease_Search_diseaseType=Pat&Disease(s)/group
of diseases=Muenke-syndrome&title=Muenke-
syndrome&search=Disease_Search_Simple.
Accessed 30 July 2016

Orvidas LJ, Fabry LB, Diacova S et al (1999) Hearing and
otopathology in Crouzon syndrome. Laryngoscope
109(9):1372–1375

Osterhammel D (1978) High-frequency thresholds
using a quasi-free-field technique. Scand Audiol
7(1):27–30

Park YH, Shin SH, Byun SW et al (2016) Age- and
gender-related mean hearing threshold in a highly-
screened population: The Korean National Health and
Nutrition Examination Survey 2010-2012. PLoS One
11(3):e0150783

Parry G, Hacking C, Bamford J et al (2003) Minimal
response levels for visual reinforcement audiometry in
infants. Int J Audiol 42(7):413–417

Parving A (1984) Aetiological diagnosis in hearing-
impaired children—clinical value and application
of a modern examination programme. Int J Pediatr
Otorhinolaryngol 7(1):29–38

Pauli RM (2009) Morquio Syndrome Natural History.
Available via http://www.lpaonline.org/assets/docu-
ments/NH%20Morquio%20Syndrome.pdf. Accessed
1 Aug 2016

Peterson RG, Simmons MA, Rumack BH et al (1980)
Pharmacology of furosemide in the premature newborn infant. J Pediatr 97(1):139–143

Picone O, Vauloup-Fellous C, Cordier AG et al
(2009) A 2-year study on cytomegalovirus infection during pregnancy in a French hospital. BJOG
116(6):818–823

Picton TW, Taylor MJ, Durieux-Smith A (2012) Chapter
25—Brainstem auditory evoked potentials in infants
and children. In: Aminoff MJ (ed) Electrodiagnosis
in clinical neurology, 6th edn. Elsevier Saunders,
Philadelphia, pp 553–579

Pirila T, Jounio-Ervasti K, Sorri M (1992) Left-right
asymmetries in hearing threshold levels in three age
groups of a random population. Audiology 31(3):
150–161

Prulière-Escabasse V, Coste A, Chauvin P et al (2010)
Otologic features in children with primary cili-

ary dyskinesia. Arch Otolaryngol Head Neck Surg 136(11):1121–1126. https://doi.org/10.1001/archoto.2010.183. PMCID: PMC3307375

Qiao Y, Meng L, Wang J et al (2011) Effect of Ganciclovir on murine cytomegalovirus-induced hearing loss in a mouse model. Cell Biochem Biophys 61(2):407–412

Rais-Bahrami K, Majd M, Veszelovszky E et al (2004) Use of furosemide and hearing loss in neonatal intensive care survivors. Am J Perinatol 21(6):329–332

Rawlinson WD, Boppana SB, Fowler KB et al (2017) Congenital cytomegalovirus infection in pregnancy and the neonate: consensus recommendations for prevention, diagnosis, and therapy. Lancet Infect Dis 17(6):e177–e188

Richardson K, Peckham CS, Goldstein H (1976) Hearing levels of children tested at 7 and 11 years: a national study. Brit J Audiol 10(4):117–121

Riga MG, Chelis L, Kakolyris S et al (2011) Transtympanic injections of N-acetylcysteine for the prevention of cisplatin-induced ototoxicity: a feasible method with promising efficacy. Am J Clin Oncol 36(1):1–6

Rima B (2006) Measles. In: Newton EN, Vallely PJ (eds) Infection and hearing impairment. Whurr, Chichester

Risheg H, Graham J Jr, Clark RD et al (2007) A recurrent mutation in MED12 leading to R961W causes Opitz-Kaveggia syndrome. Nat Genet 39(4):451–453. https://doi.org/10.1038/ng1992

Roberts J, Ahuja EM (1975) Hearing levels of US youths 12-17 years. Vital and Health Statistics. Series 11. Data from the National Health Survey 145(145):1–84

Roberts J, Federico JV (1972) Hearing sensitivity and related medical findings among children. Vital and Health Statistics. Series 11. Data from the National Health Survey 114(114):1–72

Roberts J, Huber P (1970) Hearing levels of children by age and sex: United States. Vital and health statistics. Series 11. Data from the National Health Survey 102(102):1–51

Rosenthal LS, Fowler KB, Boppana SB et al (2009) Cytomegalovirus shedding and delayed sensorineural hearing loss: results from longitudinal follow-up of children with congenital infection. Pediatr Infect Dis J 28(6):515–520

Rosner T, Kandzia F, Oswald JA et al (2011) Hearing threshold estimation using concurrent measurement of distortion product otoacoustic emissions and auditory steady-state responses. J Acoust Soc Am 129(2):840–851

Ross SA, Ahmed A, Palmer AL et al (2015) Urine collection method for the diagnosis of congenital cytomegalovirus infection. Pediatr Infect Dis J 34(8):903–905

Santoro L, Hedlund G (2008) FG Syndrome (FGS) FG Syndrome (FGS). European Course on Clinical Dysmorphology Rome, Italy March 28 March 28 - 29, 2008. 40 -Year Retrospective Year Retrospective. Available via http://istituti.unicatt.it/genetica-medica-John_Opitz.pdf. Accessed 23 May 2017

Schacht J, Talaska AE, Rybak LP (2012) Cisplatin and aminoglycoside antibiotics: hearing loss and its prevention. Anat Rec (Hoboken) 295(11):1837–1850

Scheiber C, Hirschfelder S, Gräbel S et al (2009) Bilateral cochlear implantation in children with Noonan syndrome. Int J Pediatr Otorhinolaryngol 73(6):889–894

Schmidt CM, Bartholomaus E, Deuster D et al (2007) Die "Münsteraner Klassifikation": Eine neue Einteilung der Hochtonschwerhörigkeit nach Cisplatingabe. [The "Muenster classification" of high frequency hearing loss following cisplatin chemotherapy]. HNO 55:299–306

Schmücker M, Deuster D, Lanvers-Kaminsky C et al (2009) Dosisabhängigkeit der Cisplatin-Ototoxizität. In: Gross M, Am Zehnhoff-Dinnesen A (eds) Aktuelle phoniatrisch-pädaudiologische Aspekte 2009, vol 17. Rheinware Verlag, Mönchengladbach, pp 11–12

Schneider B, Trehub SE, Bull D (1980) High-frequency sensitivity in infants. Science (New York, NY) 207(4434):1003–1004

Scholtz AW, Fish JH 3rd, Kammen-Jolly K et al (2001) Goldenhar's syndrome: congenital hearing deficit of conductive or sensorineural origin? Temporal bone histopathologic study. Otol Neurotol 22(4):501–505

Schrijver I (2004) Hereditary non-syndromic sensorineural hearing loss: transforming silence to sound. J Mol Diagn 6(4):275824. https://doi.org/10.1016/S1525-1578(10)60522-3

Schroeder RJ 2nd, Audlin J, Luo J et al (2018) Pharmacokinetics of sodium thiosulfate in Guinea pig perilymph following middle ear application. J Otol 13(2):54–55

Schuler M, Zimmermann H, Altpeter E et al (2014) Epidemiology of tick-borne encephalitis in Switzerland, 2005 to 2011. Euro Surveill 19(13): pii: 20756

Serin GM, Ciprut A, Baylancicek S et al (2007) Ototoxic effect of Burow solution applied to the guinea pig middle ear. Otol Neurotol 28(5):605–608

Shargorodsky J, Curhan SG, Curhan GC et al (2010) Change in prevalence of hearing loss in US adolescents. JAMA 304(7):772–778. https://doi.org/10.1001/jama.2010.1124

Shemen LJ, Mitchell DP, Farkashidy J (1984) Cockayne syndrome-an audiologic and temporal bone analysis. Am J Otol 5(4):300–307

Shepard NT, Davis JM, Gorga MP et al (1981) Characteristics of hearing-impaired children in the public schools: part I—demographic data. J Speech Hear Disord 46(2):123–129

Silverman SR (1983) Speech training then and now: a critical review. In: Hochberg I et al (eds) Speech of the hearing impaired: research, training, and personnel preparation. University Park Press, Baltimore, pp 1–20

Sinnott JM, Pisoni DB, Aslin RN (1983) A comparison of pure tone auditory thresholds in human infants and adults. Infant Behav Dev 6(1):3–17

Sivri HS, Genç GA, Tokatli A et al (2007) Hearing loss in biotinidase deficiency: genotype-phenotype correlation. J Pediatr 150(4):439–442

834

Smets K, De Coen K, Dhooge I et al (2006) Selecting neonates with congenital cytomegalovirus infection for ganciclovir therapy. Eur J Pediatr 165(12):885–890

Smith RJH, Shearer AE, Hildebrand MS et al (1993) updated 2014. Deafness and hereditary hearing loss overview. In: Pagon RA et al (eds) GeneReviews(R). University of Washington, Seattle. Available via https://www.ncbi.nlm.nih.gov/books/NBK1434/. Accessed 31 Mar 2017

Smith RJH, Shearer AE, Hildebrand MS (1999) Deafness and hereditary hearing loss overview. In: Pagon RA et al (eds) GeneReviews® [Internet]. University of Washington, Seattle. Available via https://www.ncbi.nlm.nih.gov/books/NBK1434/. Accessed 3 June 2017

Snoeckx RL, Huygen PLM, Feldmann D et al (2005) GJB2 mutations and degree of hearing loss: a multicenter study. Am J Hum Genet 77(6):945–957. https://doi.org/10.1086/497996

So TY (2009) Use of ototoxic medications in neonates-the need for follow-up hearing test. J Pediatr Pharmacol Ther 14(4):200–203

Staab WJ, Rintelmann WF (1972) Status of warble-tone in audiometers. Audiology 11(3):244–255

Staley K, Iragui V, Spitz M (1990) The human fetal auditory evoked potential. Electroencephalogr Clin Neurophysiol 77(1):1–5

Stavroulaki P, Apostolopoulos N, Segas J et al (2001) Evoked otoacoustic emissions—an approach for monitoring cisplatin induced ototoxicity in children. Int J Pediatr Otorhinolaryngol 59(1):47–57

Steiner A (2013) Bayley scales of infants development-II. In: Volkmar FR (ed) Encyclopedia of autism spectrum disorders. Springer, New York, pp 399–400

Stevens G, Flaxman S, Brunskill E et al (2011) Global and regional hearing impairment prevalence: an analysis of 42 studies in 29 countries. Eur J Public Health 23(1):146–152

Stevens G, Flaxman S, Brunskill E et al (2013) Global and regional hearing impairment prevalence: an analysis of 42 studies in 29 countries. Eur J Public Health 23(1):146–152

Stöhr W, Langer T, Kremers A, Bielack S et al (2005) Cisplatin-induced ototoxicity in osteosarcoma patients: a report from the late effects surveillance system. Cancer Invest 23(3):201–207

Stowell JD, Forlin-Passoni D, Din E et al (2012) Cytomegalovirus survival on common environmental surfaces: opportunities for viral transmission. J Infect Dis 205(2):211–214

Sugiura S, Yoshikawa T, Nishiyama Y et al (2004) Detection of herpesvirus DNAs in perilymph obtained from patients with sensorineural hearing loss by real-time polymerase chain reaction. Laryngoscope 114(12):2235–2238

Swanson EC, Schleiss MR (2013) Congenital cytomegalovirus infection: new prospects for prevention and therapy. Pediatr Clin North Am 60(2):335–349

Talero-Gutierrez C, Carvajalino-Monje I, Samper BS et al (2008) Delayed auditory pathway maturation in the differential diagnosis of hypoacusis in young children. Int J Pediatr Otorhinolaryngol 72(4):519–527

Tamayo ML, García N, Bermúdez Rey MC et al (2013) The importance of fundus eye testing in rubella-induced deafness. Int J Pediatr Otorhinolaryngol 77(9):1536–1540

Teissier N, Delezoide AL, Mas AE et al (2011) Inner ear lesions in congenital cytomegalovirus infection of human fetuses. Acta Neuropathol 122(6):763–774

Tharpe AM (2008) Unilateral hearing loss in children: past and current perspectives. Trends Amplif 12(1):7–15

Thelin JW, Krivenki SE (2008) Audiologic issues in CHARGE syndrome. Available via http://www.asha.org/Articles/Audiologic-Issues-in-CHARGE-Syndrome/. Accessed 11 Jan 2017

Tibesar RJ, Brissett AE, Shallop JK et al (2004) Internal auditory canal decompression and cochlear implantation in Camurati-Engelmann disease. Otolaryngol Head Neck Surg 131(6):1004–1006

Tlumak AI, Durrant JD, Collet L (2007) 80 Hz auditory steady-state responses (ASSR) at 250 Hz and 12,000 Hz. Int J Audiol 46(1):26–30

Tomblin JB, Harrison M, Ambrose SE et al (2015) Language outcomes in young children with mild to severe hearing loss. Ear Hear 36(Suppl 1):76S–91S

Tookey PA (2006) Rubella. In: Newton EN, Vallely PJ (eds) Infection and hearing impairment. Whurr, Chichester

Toriello HV, Smith SD (2013) Hereditary hearing loss and its syndromes, 3rd edn. Oxford University Press, Oxford

Torre P III, Zeldow B, Hoffman HJ et al (2012) Hearing loss in perinatally HIV-infected and HIV-exposed but uninfected children and adolescents. Pediatr Infect Dis J 31(8):835–841

Trehub SE, Schneider BA, Endman M (1980) Developmental changes in infants' sensitivity to octave-band noises. J Exp Child Psychol 29(2):282–293

Trevisan CP, Pastorello E, Tomelleri GL et al (2008) Facioscapulohumeral muscular dystrophy: hearing loss and other atypical features of patients with large 4q35 deletions. Eur J Neurol 15(12):1353–1358

Tunkel D, Alade Y, Kerbavaz R et al (2012) Hearing loss in skeletal dysplasia patients. Am J Med Genet 158A(7):1551–1555. https://doi.org/10.1002/ajmg.a.35373

Uhler K, Heringer A, Thompson N et al (2012) A tutorial on auditory neuropathy/dyssynchrony for the speech-language pathologist and audiologist. Semin Speech Lang 33(4):354–366

Ulualp SO, Wright CG, Pawlowski KS et al (2004) Histopathological basis of hearing impairment in Wolf-Hirschhorn syndrome. Laryngoscope 114(8):1426–1430

University of Maryland, Medical Center (2014) McCune-Albright syndrome. Available via https://umm.edu/health/medical/ency/articles/mccunealbright-syndrome. Accessed 2 Aug 2016

US Food and Drug Administration (2011) Orphan drug designations and approvals, sodium thiosulfate. Available via http://www.accessdata.fda.gov/scripts/opdlisting/oopd/OOPD_Results_2.cfm?Index_Number=353311. Accessed 23 June 2014

US Food and Drug Administration (2012) Orphan drug designations and approvals, N-acetylcysteine. Available via http://www.accessdata.fda.gov/scripts/opdlisting/oopd/OOPD_Results_2.cfm?Index_Number=370012. Accessed 23 June 2014

US Preventive Services Task Force (2008) Universal screening for hearing loss in newborns: US Preventive Services Task Force recommendation statement. Pediatrics 122(1):143–148

van Beelen E, Leijendeckers JM, Huygen PL et al (2012) Audiometric characteristics of two Dutch families with non-ocular Stickler syndrome (COL11A2). Hear Res 291(1–2):15–23

Van Camp G, Smith R (2015) Hereditary hearing loss homepage. Available via http://hereditaryhearingloss.org/. Accessed 3 June 2017

Van Camp G, Smith RJH (2016) Hereditary hearing loss homepage. Available via http://hereditaryhearingloss.org. Accessed 7 June 2016

van Dongen TM, van der Heijden GJ, Venekamp RP et al (2014) A trial of treatment for acute otorrhea in children with tympanostomy tubes. N Engl J Med 370:723–733

Van Naarden Braun K, Christensen D, Doernberg N et al (2015) Trends in the prevalence of autism spectrum disorder, cerebral palsy, hearing loss, intellectual disability, and vision impairment, metropolitan Atlanta, 1991-2010. PLoS One 10(4):e0124120

Vieira EP, Azevedo MF (2007) Audiometria de reforço visual com diferentes estímulos sonorous em crianças. (Visual reinforcement audiometry with different sound stimuli in children). Pro Fono 19(2):185–194

Waissbluth S, Daniel SJ (2013) Cisplatin-induced ototoxicity: transporters playing a role in cisplatin toxicity. Hear Res 299:37–45

Walker G, Dillon H, Byrne D (1984) Sound field audiometry: recommended stimuli and procedures. Ear Hear 5(1):13–21

Wang D, Fu TM (2014) Progress on human cytomegalovirus vaccines for prevention of congenital infection and disease. Curr Opin Virol 6:13–23

Wang X, Fernandez R, Tsivkovskaia N et al (2014) OTO-201: nonclinical assessment of a sustained-release ciprofloxacin hydrogel for the treatment of otitis media. Otol Neurotol 35(3):459–469

Warrier R, Chauhan A, Davluri M et al (2012) Cisplatin and cranial irradiation-related hearing loss in children. Ochsner J 12(3):191–196

Watkin PM, Baldwin M, Laoide S (1990) Parental suspicion and identification of hearing impairment. Arch Dis Child 65(8):846–850

WebMD Magazine (2007) McCune Albright syndrome. Available via http://www.webmd.com/children/mccune-albright-syndrome. Accessed 2 Aug 2016

Weichbold V, Nekahm-Heis D, Welzl-Muller K (2006) Universal newborn hearing screening and postnatal hearing loss. Pediatrics 117(4):631–636

Weissenstein A, Deuster D, Knief A et al (2012) Progressive hearing loss after completion of cisplatin chemotherapy is common and more pronounced in children without spontaneous otoacoustic emissions before chemotherapy. Int J Pediatr Otorhinolaryngol 76(1):131–136

Welch KO, Marin RS, Pandya A et al (2007) Compound heterozygosity for dominant and recessive GJB2 mutations: effect on phenotype and review of the literature. Am J Med Genet A 143A(14):1567–1573. https://doi.org/10.1002/ajmg.a.31701

Westerberg BD, Atashband S, Kozak FK (2008) A systematic review of the incidence of sensorineural hearing loss in neonates exposed to Herpes simplex virus (HSV). Int J Pediatr Otorhinolaryngol 72(7):931–937

White DR, Choo DI, Stroup G et al (2006) The effect of cidofovir on cytomegalovirus-induced hearing loss in a guinea pig model. Arch Otolaryngol Head Neck Surg 132(6):608–615

WHO (2013) WHO methods and data sources for global burden of disease estimates 2000-2011. Available via http://www.who.int/healthinfo/statistics/GlobalDALYmethods_2000_2011.pdf. Accessed 4 May 2017

Williamson T (2002) Neonatal hearing screening and assessment behavioural observation audiometry. A recommended test protocol. Available via http://hearing.screening.nhs.uk/audiology. Accessed 19 Sept 2014

Wilson WR, Gulya AJ (1993) Sudden sensorineural hearing loss. In: Cummings CW, Fredrickson JF, Harker LA et al (eds) Otolaryngology: head and neck surgery, vol 4, 2nd edn. Mosby-Year Book Inc, St. Louis

Winiger AM, Alexander JM, Diefendorf AO (2016) Minimal hearing loss: from a failure-based approach to evidence-based practice. Am J Audiol 25(3):232–245

Woodin M, Wang PP, Aleman D et al (2001) Neuropsychological profile of children and adolescents with the 22q11.2 microdeletion. Genet Med 3(1):34–39. https://doi.org/10.1097/00125817-200101000-00008

Woods JR, Plessinger MA (1985) The fetal auditory brain stem response: serial measurements at two stimulus intensities. Otolaryngol Head Neck Surg 93(6):759–764

World Health Organization (2013) WHO methods and data sources for global burden of disease estimates 2000-2011. WHO, Geneva. Available via http://www.who.int/healthinfo/statistics/GlobalDALYmethods_2000_2011.pdf. Accessed 4 Jan 2017

Wright KE (2006) Mumps. In: Newton EN, Vallely PJ (eds) Infection and hearing impairment. Whurr, Chichester

Wright E, Brew B, Wesselingh S (2008) Pathogenesis and diagnosis of viral infections of the nervous system. Neurol Clin 26(3):617–733

Yang TH, Wu CS, Liao WH et al (2011) Mean hearing thresholds among school children in Taiwan. Ear Hear 32(2):258–265

Yesiltepe Mutlu G, Kirmizibekmez H, Nakamura A et al (2015) Novel de novo GATA binding protein 3 mutation in a Turkish boy with hypoparathyroidism, deafness, and renal dysplasia syndrome. J Clin Res Pediatr Endocrinol 7(4):344–348. https://doi.org/10.4274/jcrpe.2249

Yoshinaga-Itano C, AL S, Coulter DK et al (1998) Language of early- and later-identified children with hearing loss. Pediatrics 102(5):1161–1171

Yoshinaga-Itano C, Johnson CD, Carpenter K et al (2009) Outcomes of children with mild bilateral hearing loss and unilateral hearing loss. Sem Hear 29(2):196–211

Zarchi O, Attias J, Raveh E et al (2011) A comparative study of hearing loss in two microdeletion syndromes: velocardiofacial (22q11.2 deletion) and Williams (7q11.23 deletion) syndromes. J Pediatr 158(2):301–306. https://doi.org/10.1016/j.jpeds.2010.07.056. Epub 2010 Sep 16

Zumach A, Gerrits E, Chenault MN et al (2009) Otitis media and speech-in-noise recognition in school-aged children. Audiol Neurootol 14(2):121–129

Zwirner P, Wilichowski E (2001) Progressive sensorineural hearing loss in children with mitochondrial encephalomyopathies. Laryngoscope 111(3):515–521

Special Kinds of Disorders of Hearing Development

15

Antoinette am Zehnhoff-Dinnesen,
Doris-Eva Bamiou, Nicole G. Campbell,
David R. Moore, Haldun Oguz, Ross Parfitt,
Mustafa Asim Safak, Claus-Michael Schmidt,
Tony Sirimanna, Amélie Elisabeth Tillmanns,
and Dorothe Veraguth

15.1 Types and Time Courses of Hearing Loss

Dorothe Veraguth and
Amélie Elisabeth Tillmanns

15.1.1 Introduction

Hearing loss is present at birth or could appear at any time of life. Congenital hearing impairment includes hereditary hearing impairment or hearing loss due to other factors present either in utero (prenatal) or at the time of birth. Acquired hearing loss is a result of a disease, a condition or an injury.

The prevalence of hearing impairment among newborns and infants is estimated to be 1.5 to 6 per 1000 live births. The estimate 1–2/1000 is based on the number of children with a profound bilateral hearing loss and does not account for infants with a mild or moderate to severe hearing loss or for babies with a single-side hearing impairment (Ardle and Bitner-Glindzicz 2010; Gifford et al. 2009; Gregg et al. 2004). The prevalence may differ from country to country. Most children with congenital hearing impairment are identifiable by newborn hearing screening.

A. am Zehnhoff-Dinnesen · R. Parfitt
A. E. Tillmanns
Clinic of Phoniatrics and Pedaudiology,
University Hospital Münster, Münster, Germany
e-mail: am.zehnhoff@uni-muenster.de;
ross.parfitt@ukmuenster.de;
AmelieElisabeth.Tillmanns@ukmuenster.de

D.-E. Bamiou
National Hospital for Neurology and Neurosurgery,
London, UK
e-mail: d.bamiou@ucl.ac.uk

N. G. Campbell
Auditory Implant Service,
University of Southampton, Southampton, UK
e-mail: N.G.Campbell@soton.ac.uk

D. R. Moore
Communication Sciences Research Center,
Cincinnati Children's Hospital, Cincinnati, OH, USA
e-mail: david.r.moore@cchmc.org

H. Oguz
Fonomer, Ankara, Turkey

M. A. Safak
Department of Otolaryngology, Near East University,
Lefkosa, Turkey

C.-M. Schmidt
Gemeinschaftspraxis im Vitalcenter,
Münster, Germany
e-mail: michael.schmidt@pp-hno.de

T. Sirimanna
Audiological Medicine and Cochlear Implant
Department, Great Ormond Street Hospital,
London, UK
e-mail: Tony.Sirimanna@gosh.nhs.uk

D. Veraguth
Clinic of ENT, Head- and Neck-Surgery,
University Hospital Zurich, Zurich, Switzerland
e-mail: dorothe.veraguth@usz.ch

© Springer-Verlag GmbH Germany, part of Springer Nature 2020
A. am Zehnhoff-Dinnesen et al. (eds.), *Phoniatrics I*, European Manual of Medicine,
https://doi.org/10.1007/978-3-662-46780-0_15

Hearing loss also can be acquired during infancy or childhood for various reasons. Infectious diseases, especially meningitis, are a leading cause of acquired hearing loss. Trauma to the nervous system, damaging noise levels and ototoxic drugs can all place a child at risk of developing acquired hearing loss. Otitis media is a common cause of usually reversible hearing loss. Certain physical findings, historical events and developmental conditions may indicate a potential hearing problem. These conditions include, but are not limited to, anomalies of the ear and other craniofacial structures, significant perinatal events and global developmental or speech-language delays (Bachmann and Arvedson 1998; Joint Committee on Infant Hearing 2000).

Many epidemiological studies suggest that at least one third of all cases of hearing impairment are hereditary. Seventy percent of genetic-based congenital HL appears to be non-syndromic, and the other 30% is syndromic. One third of cases are acquired hearing loss with identifiable reasons, and the remaining one third is not clearly hereditary and not obviously correlated with a specific causative factor (Gregg et al. 2004).

15.1.2 Conductive Hearing Loss

Conductive hearing loss varies widely in degree and may be congenital or acquired.

The degree of conductive hearing loss can vary between 20 and 60 dB HL, depending on the cause. Further, many causes of conductive hearing losses are medically or surgically treatable. At pre-school age the most common cause is an otitis media with effusion.

Additional to the audiological tests, a radiological examination with computed tomography is often important for planning an adequate therapy for a permanent conductive hearing loss. Because the outer ear canal and the middle ear of the infant are small and growth is final at school age, surgical treatment with reconstruction of the middle ear is often meaningful for adolescents. In addition to the surgery, treatment with hearing aids is often mandatory for young children with conductive hearing loss. In some cases fitting hearing aids behind the ear is not possible because of the anatomy of the ear canal and the concha. Bone-anchored hearing aids are helpful, and bone conduction hearing devices can also be fixed with a headband for babies and infants (Janssen et al. 2012). An active middle ear implant (Vibrant Soundbridge®) is often more successful for hearing than a surgical reconstruction of the outer ear canal and the middle ear structures (Cremers et al. 2010).

In the following paragraphs, the most important causes of conductive hearing loss in children are presented.

Microtia and Aural Atresia The most developmental deformities of the external ear canal (Cremers et al. 2010) are associated with findings of middle ear and inner ear abnormalities and consequent hearing loss. In microtia a smaller than normal and probably misshapen auricle is a typical finding. The external canal is likely to be absent (see Fig. 15.1), and there are often abnormalities of the ossicular chain. The prevalence is 1–2/1,000,000 newborns, and 25% of cases are bilateral and 75% unilateral. Three types exist, graded according to severity (Luquetti et al. 2012). Assessment with CT scan is needed before surgery is discussed. Implantable hearing aids are today a good alternative option, especially bone-anchored hearing aids or active middle ear implants (see Sect. 18.5).

Clefts and Craniofacial Malformations Children with cleft lip and palate or cleft palate

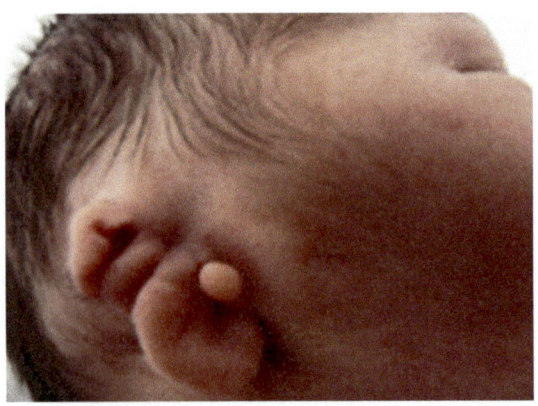

Fig. 15.1 Microtia and aural atresia

only or other craniofacial malformations have a high incidence of conductive hearing loss from otitis media with effusion (Swibel Rosenthal et al. 2012). The majority of children develop normal hearing by school age with palatoplasty and routine tube insertion. Hearing improves significantly from childhood to adolescence in patients with cleft lip and palate and cleft palate only.

Syndromal Conductive Hearing Impairment This type includes various ossicular chain malformations and abnormalities in combination with hearing loss from otitis media with effusion. In many syndromes the auricle is also dysplastic, and the fitting of normal behind-the-ear hearing aids is impossible. The children need bone-anchored hearing aids fixed by a softband for babies and infants. The most common syndromes are Goldenhar syndrome, Treacher Collins syndrome, Pierre Robin syndrome and craniofacial dysostoses (Apert syndrome, Pfeiffer syndrome, Crouzon disease) (Swibel Rosenthal et al. 2012) (see Sect. 14.11).

Abnormalities of the Tympanic Membrane and the Middle Ear Audiological abnormalities may include the following audiometry: air-bone gap <60 dB, depending on the degree of abnormality of the ossicular transmission, flattened tympanogram, and absence of stapedius reflexes. The most common causes are infections of the middle ear in different stages:

Acute Otitis Media Acute infections of the middle ear are frequently associated with upper respiratory infections; the typical pathogenic agent is *Pneumococcus*, *Haemophilus influenza* or *Moraxella*. In the literature different evidence-based recommendations exist, particularly those of the current American guidelines for medical treatment (Venekamp et al. 2013).

Chronic Otitis Media A variety of pathologies can be seen: chronic perforation of the tympanic membrane (see Fig. 15.2a), ossicular chain abnormalities, tympanosclerosis and cholesteatoma (see Fig. 15.2b). The therapy is often surgical, and secondarily hearing aids are an option if a conductive hearing loss persists.

Otitis Media with Effusion Otitis media with effusion (see Fig. 15.3) is the most common cause of conductive hearing loss with the presence of fluid in the middle ear or a bluish discolouration of the tympanic membrane and lack of compliance of the ear drum. Otitis media with effusion is associated with allergies, adenoid hypertrophy or craniofacial abnormalities, especially cleft palate. The therapy includes decongestants, myringotomy and insertion of ventilation tubes, according to the different guidelines of treatment of otitis media with effusion (Rosenfeld et al. 2013). Also anti-allergic medication may be an option. Hearing aids

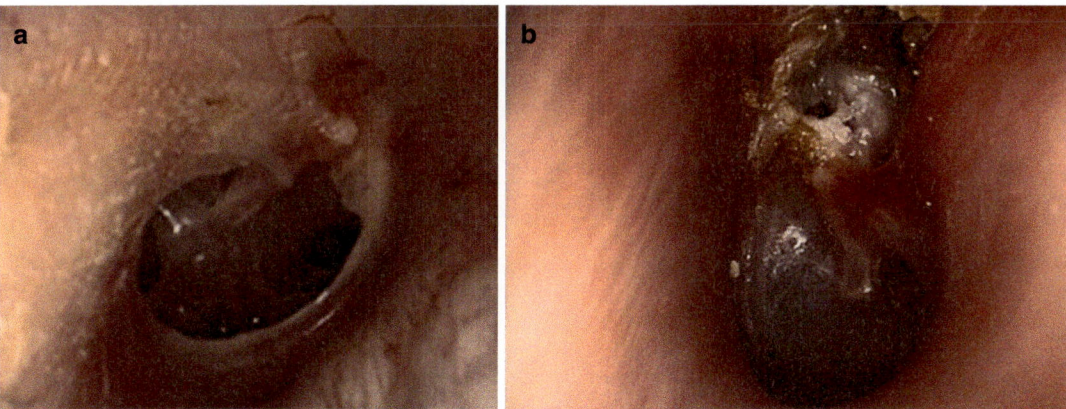

Fig. 15.2 (**a**) Chronic Otitis media with subtotal perforation of tympanic membrane. (**b**) Cholesteatoma with epitympanal perforation

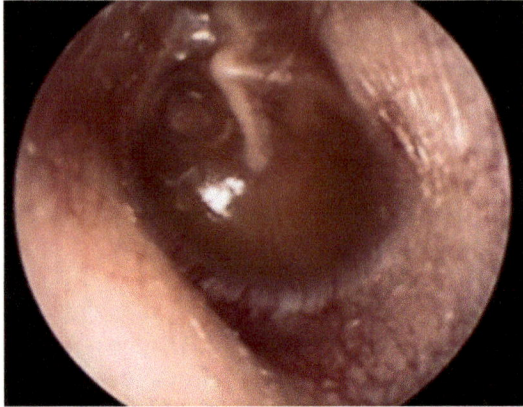

Fig. 15.3 Otitis media with effusion

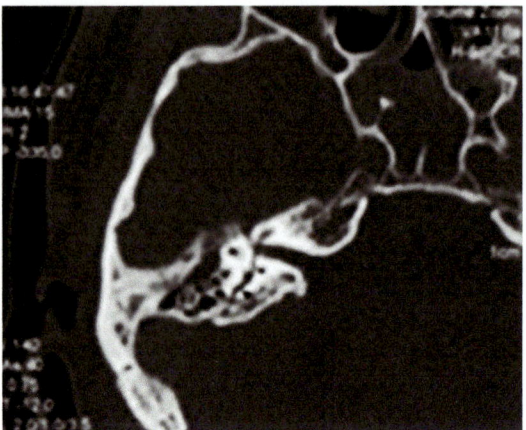

Fig. 15.4 Fracture of the petrous temporal bone

for children with recurrent otitis media with effusions can be evaluated, especially if ventilation tube insertion is difficult or not successful (e.g. children with Down syndrome, Kartagener syndrome, mucoviscidosis, immunodeficiency disorders).

Otosclerosis and Tympanosclerosis In children otosclerosis is rarely reported. Typically a conductive hearing loss is seen early with a reduced air-bone gap at 2 kHz; later a sensorineural hearing loss may be seen as well. In this age group, the diagnosis is usually suggested by a positive family history of otosclerosis but must be distinguished from more frequent aetiologies of stapes ankylosis with a normal tympanic membrane, such as tympanosclerosis of the oval window or minor aplasia (Lescanne et al. 2008).

Trauma Longitudinal fractures of the petrous temporal bone are associated with perforation of the tympanic membrane and possible dislocation of the ossicular chain (see Fig. 15.4). A total sensorineural hearing loss is suggestive of a transverse fracture of the petrous temporal bone.

15.1.3 Sensorineural Hearing Loss

A sensorineural hearing loss affects the inner ear (cochlea) or auditory nerve (eighth cranial nerve). Most sensorineural hearing losses are sensory and restricted to the cochlea and do not result from an abnormality of the auditory nerve.

Routine audiometric testing does not differentiate between a sensory loss and a neural loss. Electrophysiological measures (auditory brainstem response, ABR; Cochlear Microphonics, CM) and otoacoustic emissions (OAE) reveal the difference between sensory and neural causes (Gifford et al. 2009; Gregg et al. 2004; Harlor and Bower 2009). Imaging studies by MRI (magnetic resonance imaging) and CT (computed tomography) show congenital malformations of the inner ear: cochlear hypoplasia, incomplete partition, common cavity or enlarged vestibular aqueduct (Huang et al. 2012). In 1987 Jackler published a classification system for congenital malformation of the inner ear (Jackler et al. 1987). Sensorineural hearing loss ranges from mild to profound degree and needs early fitting with hearing aids or cochlear implants, according to audiological test results. In addition, infants with congenital hearing loss benefit from special education with training for speech and language development.

The most important causes of sensorineural hearing impairment are as follows:

- Genetic hearing impairment (see Sect. 14.10)
- Chromosomal abnormalities: Down syndrome and Turner's syndrome (see Sect. 14.11)
- Pre-/perinatal factors: low birth weight, hypoxia, hyperbilirubinaemia (see Sect. 14.7)
- Prenatal infections: rubella, cytomegalovirus infection, toxoplasmosis, lues, herpes simplex (see Sects. 14.7 and 14.8)

- Postnatal infections: meningitis, encephalitis, mumps, measles, chicken pox, influenza (see Sects. 14.7 and 14.8)
- The most common major sequela of meningitis is hearing loss to different degrees with overall worldwide prevalence among meningitis patients of 20%, in Europe 9%. Twenty percent of all patients have multiple impairments: hearing loss, seizures, hydrocephalus, spasticity/paresis, cranial nerve palsies and visual impairment (Edmond et al. 2010). The prevalence of bilateral hearing loss of at least 70 dB HL after pneumococcal meningitis with the risk of ossification of the labyrinth system in high-income countries is 8%, and for hearing loss of at least 30 dB HL in one ear, the prevalence increases to 26% (Jit 2010). In the literature it is also reported that the risk of sequelae in children aged less than 5 years is twice as high as for older people (Edmond et al. 2010).
- Ototoxicity: aminoglycosides affect the cochlear and vestibular systems; cisplatin has a cochleotoxic effect (see Sect. 14.9).
- Noise exposure: the threshold pattern results in a notch-type audiogram configuration. Initially temporary threshold shifts are observed. With repeated exposure the threshold shift can progress to permanent noise-induced hearing loss in the high frequencies. Loud sounds often occur in modern music machines used with ear phones, in different toys and in explosives (pyrotechnics).
- Head injury: a dull head injury can lead to isolated damage of the inner ear (cochlear labyrinthine concussion) or damage of the otolith organ due to a bone conduction pressure. A typical sign is a high-frequency sensorineural hearing loss in form of a c5-dip (Brusis 2011) (at frequency 4000 Hz). In case of a unilateral skull base fracture, a contralateral labyrinthine concussion is also possible. Many cases also show an accompanying tinnitus.

15.1.4 Combined Sensorineural and Conductive Hearing Loss

Mixed hearing loss occurs when an individual has a conductive hearing loss overlying a sensori-neural hearing loss. The air conduction threshold exceeds the bone conduction threshold by more than 10 dB, and the bone conduction thresholds are outside the normal range. With a mixed hearing loss, abnormalities are identified in the outer or middle ear as well as the inner ear. Mixed hearing loss varies in degree. In some cases, the conductive component of the mixed hearing loss can be medically or surgically treated. Ventilation tubes are especially helpful in infants with otitis media with effusion and a permanent sensorineural hearing loss.

15.1.5 Auditory Neuropathy/ Auditory Dyssynchrony/ Auditory Neuropathy Spectrum Disorder

In rare instances, a sensorineural hearing loss can be neural, i.e. the deficit is at the level of the auditory nerve. These types typically are labelled as auditory neuropathy (AN), auditory dyssynchrony (AD) or auditory neuropathy spectrum disorder (ANSD). In addition, children who have an auditory neuropathy generally do not respond well to traditional forms of audiological management, such as hearing aids. Preliminary case reports indicate positive outcomes with cochlear implants if the damage is located perisynaptically. Auditory neuropathy can be congenital or acquired.

Since the introduction of newborn hearing screening, there has been increasing recognition of children who present with normal outer hair cell (sensory) function but absent or abnormal auditory nerve function. Thus, when screened with otoacoustic emissions (OAEs), these babies will show a clear response on newborn hearing screening, because their outer hair cells are initially functioning but lack waves in the auditory brainstem response (ABR) (Gregg et al. 2004; Walker et al. 2016). Round window electrococh-leography (RWECochG) and electric auditory brainstem responses (EABR) may be useful tools that will help with deciding on management (e. g. Cochlea Implantation) (Gibson and Sanli 2007) but are restricted to specialised audiologists and need a high degree of compliance.

Aetiologically, this is a very heterogeneous group of children who have a variety of clinical histories and no single identifiable pathology (see below). This group of children can present with impaired speech perception and have difficulty with processing rapidly changing acoustic signals. The audiometric thresholds may range from mild to severe to profound hearing loss patterns. It has recently been suggested that this group should be described as having an auditory neuropathy spectrum disorder. The true prevalence of auditory neuropathy is unknown, and it is estimated that about 10% of all infants with hearing disorders show symptoms of ANSD.

Potential aetiologies for this group are (Ardle and Bitner-Glindzicz 2010):

- Genetic conditions: non-syndromic, such as mutations in the otoferlin (*OTOF*) gene or pejvakin gene (*PJVK*). Syndromic, such as hereditary motor and sensory neuropathies (e.g. Charcot-Marie-Tooth), Friedreich ataxia, Mohr-Tranebjaerg syndrome, some mitochondrial mutations or other generalised neuropathies
- Aplasia or hypoplasia of the vestibulocochlear nerve
- Perinatal events: hyperbilirubinaemia, hypoxia, extremely low birth weight, complicated perinatal course

15.1.6 Central Hearing Disorders

Central hearing disorders are a consequence of a disruption in processing at varying levels of the hearing pathway, from the auditory nerve to inferior colliculus to the auditory cortex. They often present in a similar way as problems in auditory pathway development and can be manifested in a huge variety of ways that usually do not affect peripheral hearing or exhibit discrepancies between peripheral hearing and speech discrimination or other auditory functions, such as noise localisation, suppression of disturbing noise, binaural hearing or auditory memory. Children with central auditory disorders mostly present as easily distractible, having difficulties in remembering orally given tasks or to understand speech in noisy backgrounds. However, even more differentiated tasks, such as music perception, differentiation of pitch levels and recognition of emotional prosody or animal sounds can be affected (Peretz et al. 2001; Taniwaki et al. 2000; Griffiths et al. 1997; Yuvaraj et al. 2015; Bisiach et al. 1984; Hattiangadi et al. 2005). Generally, clinical differentiation from behavioural problems such as hyperactivity, learning disorders, attentiveness disorders or memory problems can be challenging. Specific testing of central auditory functions, and often psychological or developmental testing, is needed for differentiation, and an audiological follow-up is essential.

If a discrepancy between a pure-tone audiogram and a speech audiogram with or without background noise appears, more diagnostic steps have to be taken to assess central hearing. When a newly appearing central hearing disorder is suspected, cranial imaging with magnetic resonance tomography or computed tomography should be considered. For audiological diagnosis, measures of acoustically evoked potentials are crucial, if possible auditory brainstem responses, middle latency response and cortical evoked response audiometry, to detect disturbances of all parts of the auditory pathway. The diagnosis is completed by measuring OAE, contralateral OAE suppression, stapedius reflexes and acoustic reflex decay.

Central hearing disorders can be the first symptom of a beginning central pathology. As an example, this was the case in a 9-year-old boy who presented first with a subjective unilateral hearing loss without vertigo or tinnitus but had a normal pure-tone audiogram. When the hearing loss got subjectively worse, further pedaudiological testing was performed, showing reduced hearing in background noise, so an auditory processing disorder was suspected. After 6 more months of waiting, he developed a unilateral slight sensorineural hearing loss and following this was diagnosed with a benign brainstem tumour of the cerebellopontine angle after the course of 2 years of diagnosis. In the literature, a similar case of word deafness due to compression of the inferior colliculus has been described as being reversible after radiation (Joswig et al. 2015).

A very common reason for neural hearing loss is a benign tumour of the inner ear canal, such as acoustic neurinomas, in children most commonly neurinomas in neurofibromatosis or meningiomas, mostly presenting with unilateral hearing loss, tinnitus and vertigo. In most acoustic neurinomas, latencies of early brainstem potentials are prolonged or lacking (Selters and Brackmann 1977; Hoth 1991), OAE can be present or absent, depending on whether the inner ear is affected. Central hearing disorders can also be due to central inflammatory or vascular processes, tumours, trauma or other brain lesions, as well as neurodegenerative diseases, asphyxia during birth and other reasons, and grades of possible reversibility differ (Griffiths et al. 1997; Yuvaraj et al. 2015; Bisiach et al. 1984; Hattiangadi et al. 2005; Kihara et al. 2012; Zhu et al. 2010; Tabuchi et al. 2007; Iizuka et al. 2007; Hoistad and Hain 2003; Wakabayashi et al. 1999). In the case of central hyperbilirubinaemia, severity can range from slight reversible hearing loss to deafness (Nickisch et al. 2009). Auditory agnosia describes cases in which patients show clinical deafness in spite of normal or slightly reduced peripheral hearing, for example, after stroke, inflammatory processes or trauma, mostly in bilateral temporal lobes (Hattiangadi et al. 2005; Mendez 2001; Kaga et al. 2000a, b, 2003, 2015; Brody et al. 2013).

15.1.7 Progressive, Fluctuating and Sudden Hearing Loss

The clinical presentation of immune-mediated inner-ear disorders is very variable. The symptom most commonly associated with immune-mediated inner-ear disorders is a progressive or fluctuating sensorineural hearing loss (Agrup 2008). This is partially because auditory symptoms are the most studied inner-ear symptom, whereas vestibular symptoms can be overlooked, even though the two symptoms often develop together. Progressive hearing loss of late-onset type is typical in eye disorders, nervous system disorders and endocrine or metabolic diseases. Fluctuating patterns are common with immune-mediated inner-ear disorders (Gregg et al. 2004). However, sudden hearing loss or sudden vestibular loss also occurs. High-frequency hearing loss has been associated with patho-aetiological mechanisms involving vasculitis.

Sudden sensorineural hearing loss appears to be less frequent in the paediatric population than in adults. The definition of sudden hearing loss is a unilateral or bilateral hearing loss of 30 dB or more in three contiguous frequencies developing within a period of a few days. Several possible patho-aetiologies have been suggested with isolated sudden sensorineural hearing loss including viral/bacterial infections and vascular disorders. Hearing loss, especially when unilateral, may be missed in children because younger children are unable to express the complaint or parents are unable to recognise the loss of function. A progressive sensorineural hearing loss is present in 2–6% of all hearing-impaired children aged 8–13 years (Parving 1988). Progression in hearing loss is most frequent in early childhood and was found in more than 40% of participants in a study with 688 patients in the first years of infancy/childhood. Only 6% of children have progression defined as >15 dB for the averaged thresholds 0.5–4 kHz at age exceeding 4 years. The higher frequencies 2 and 4 kHz seem to be the most vulnerable (Johansen et al. 2004).

The cause of a hearing loss often remains unknown. Because of progression or fluctuation, the need for frequent surveillance of the hearing loss in infants and children before school age and repeated testing seems mandatory (Joint Committee on Infant Hearing 2000; Muse et al. 2013).

15.2 Auditory Processing Disorders

David R. Moore, Nicole G. Campbell, Doris-Eva Bamiou and Tony Sirimanna

Definition and History There are many definitions of auditory processing disorder (APD; Vermiglio 2014), but 'listening difficulty despite normal auditory sensitivity' is a simple and mostly inclusive one. 'Listening' is the process by which people actively engage with their auditory environment. It is synonymous with 'auditory perception' and includes both the sensory and cognitive aspects of hearing. Although the primary functional consequence of APD is difficulty in hearing speech, especially in challenging auditory environments, APD has historically been distinguished from a primary language or intellectual impairment. The importance of auditory perception, distinct from auditory sensitivity, was first recognised more than 60 years ago (Jerger 2009), although the interchangeable terms 'APD' and 'central APD' (CAPD; AAA 2010) are more recent (Keith 1977; Willeford 1974). APD may be 'developmental' (in children), 'acquired' (stroke, trauma or ageing brain) or 'secondary' to hearing loss (BSA 2011; Moore et al. 2013).

Demographics APD is diagnosed primarily in children (7–17 years old) of both sexes, but adults of any age (Humes et al. 2012) and younger children are also affected (Emanuel et al. 2011; Lucker 2012). Among children, boys are more commonly referred and diagnosed than girls. Retention of developmental APD into adulthood has recently been found (Del Zoppo et al. 2015). Prevalence among the general population is not known with any precision, but rationalised estimates from one service suggested 0.5–1.0% (Hind et al. 2011). In three studies, 22% (Moore and Hunter 2013), 34% (Tomlin et al. 2015) and 46% (Ludwig et al. 2014) of children with normal auditory sensitivity referred to audiology were diagnosed with APD.

Mechanisms Because APD does not involve a loss of auditory sensitivity, it has long been assumed to be a disorder of the central auditory nervous system (CANS; Fig. 15.5) with most definitions specifying impaired 'neural' (BSA 2011) or 'central' (AAA 2010) function. However, this assumption has recently been challenged by clear evidence that both specific pathology within the cochlea (Bharadwaj et al. 2014; Kujawa and Liberman 2009) and modulation of CANS function by higher-level cortical

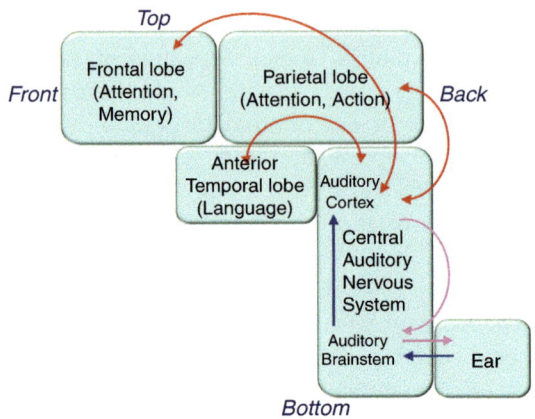

Fig. 15.5 The 'real' auditory system

processes (Atiani et al. 2014; Nelken et al. 2014) may contribute to the clinical symptoms of APD without affecting the audiogram. In fact, it is increasingly unclear exactly where the CANS begins or ends. In the cochlea (Fig. 15.6: Moser et al. 2013), malfunction or loss of inner hair cell 'ribbon' synapses or the distal processes of afferent auditory nerve fibres during ageing or following noise damage can degrade temporal coding in the brain. In the cortex, auditory stimulation can directly excite neurons in the anterior temporal, frontal and parietal lobes, well beyond the classical CANS (Moore 2012). Finally, descending efferent pathways from the cortex influence function throughout the CANS and ear (Fig. 15.5). Lesions in various parts of the CANS result in impaired hearing (Bamiou et al. 2012), but the relation of these lesions and impairments to developmental or secondary APD is unclear.

Identification and Referral Speech and language delays and inconsistent responses to sounds are often the first signs to caregivers that a young child may need help. Cross-referrals between community nurses, speech-language professionals and audiologists are common through the pre-school years (UK study; Hind et al. 2011). For older children, poor progress in school may be found, and family doctors, nurses and paediatricians often refer these cases. A US survey (Emanuel et al. 2011) found that audiologists measured pure-tone thresholds (100%), tympanometry (97%), speech

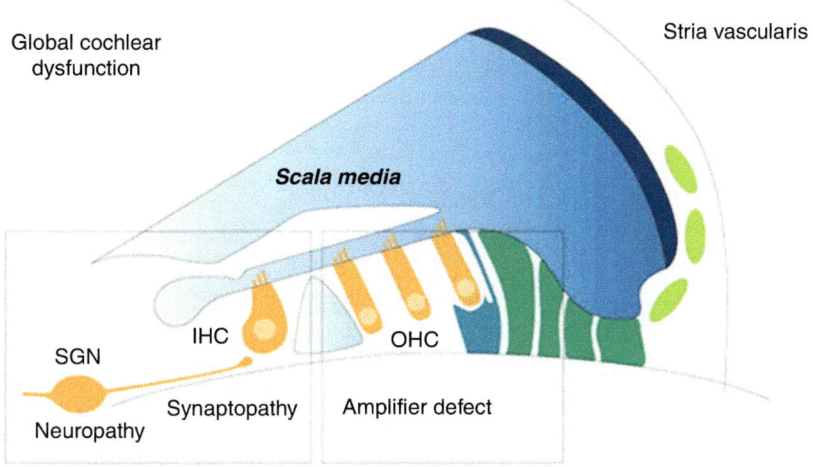

Fig. 15.6 Pathology in the cochlea (Moser et al. 2013). *SGN* spiral ganglion neuron, *IHC* inner hair cell, *OHC* outer hair cells. Image copyright and with permission from Wolters Kluwer Health, Inc.

recognition in quiet (92%), acoustic reflexes (69%), otoacoustic emissions (58%) and words in noise (54%) upon referral. Questionnaires were also usually given to parents or teachers. Referred children and adults with normal audiology nevertheless reported a variety of difficulties, including speech recognition and discrimination in challenging environments, spatial hearing, music/song perception and reproduction as well as auditory attention and memory. Children additionally can have delayed auditory and academic developmental milestones (Campbell et al. 2012).

Diagnosis There is no universally agreed diagnostic procedure for APD. For example, in Germany APD is called 'auditory processing and perception disorder' (APPD) (German: auditive Verarbeitungs- und Wahrnehmungsstörung (AVWS)) to include impaired short-term memory and attention that are primarily in the auditory domain, as well as phoneme listening and the range of auditory perceptual problems recognised by ASHA (2005). In each case, APPD is diagnosed with the appropriate qualifier by using a multidisciplinary approach (GSPPA 2014). In one study, deficits in three such audiological tests resulted in a diagnosis of APD (Ludwig et al. 2014). In a multicentre UK study, performance below the recommended clinical cut-off on one or more subtests of the SCAN-C (Keith 2000), which is widely used as a screening test for auditory processing disorders, plus failure in one or

more additional tests (random gaps, pitch pattern, duration pattern) was used (Dawes et al. 2009; Emanuel et al. 2011; Moore and Hunter 2013).

Intervention Three management strategies (environmental, remediation, compensatory) were examined in a survey of nearly 200 US audiology services (Emanuel et al. 2011). Environmental modification was delivered by almost all services polled and included preferential seating, directing attention and wireless listening devices (e.g. Bluetooth). 'Remediation' was used by the majority of services, which consisted of training exercises, either computer-delivered or conventional. Compensatory strategies, including listening and metamemory, were also widely used. There is now considerable, high-quality evidence for the efficacy of wireless devices to improve listening, both during and following use of the devices (Hornickel et al. 2012; Keith and Purdy 2014). Computer-based training has received both positive (Kraus 2012; Moore et al. 2005) and negative (Stanford Center on Longevity 2014; Halliday et al. 2012) reviews, but in general, training benefit currently appears to be limited to skills closely related to those trained. Simple advice is low-cost and may be efficacious if actively promoted, but limited training and compliance monitoring have precluded critical evaluation.

Summary APD is currently diagnosed following reports of listening difficulties, normal audiometry and poor performance in additional tests of auditory and cognitive function. Listening difficulties may derive either from top-down cognitive processing or control dysfunction or from suprathreshold sensory temporal processing dysfunction in the cochlea or brainstem. The most effective treatment strategies appear to be advice on listening and use of a communication device.

15.3 Hyperacusis

Ross Parfitt, Mustafa Asim Safak, Haldun Oguz and Antoinette am Zehnhoff-Dinnesen

15.3.1 Definition and Epidemiology

Hyperacusis is a symptom defined as an

> experience of inordinate loudness of sound that most people tolerate well, associated with a component of distress… this experience has a physiologic basis… but it also has a psychological component.
>
> Baguley and Andersson (2007)

Other related terms include *phonophobia*, which literally means fear of sound but is often used clinically to describe an aversion to sound in general (e.g. in migraine); *misophonia*, which means dislike of particular soft sounds (e.g. the sound of somebody chewing); and *decreased sound tolerance* to refer to any of the above (Hall 2013). *Loudness recruitment*, in which a small increase in sound intensity is perceived as a large increase (as is typically found in sensorineural hearing loss), should not be confused with hyperacusis. There is a lack of clarity and consistency in the definitions and terminology used in the literature, so such distinctions are important to note.

Hyperacusis is reported to affect 9–16% of the general population (Andersson et al. 2002; Skarzyński et al. 2000) and is severe in 2% (Baguley and McFerran 2011). It is closely associated with tinnitus: hyperacusis is reported in 40% of patients whose primary concern is tinnitus (Jastreboff et al. 1996), and tinnitus is reported in 86% of those whose primary concern is hyperacusis (Anari et al. 1999).

15.3.2 Mechanisms

Various peripheral and central mechanisms for hyperacusis have been proposed. These mechanisms may combine to different degrees in different patients.

Stapedial reflex dysfunction is one such potential peripheral mechanism. This proposal originated in the observation that decreased sound sensitivity is a common symptom of several conditions with accompanying facial palsy (e.g. Bell's palsy) or stapedial muscle dysfunction (e.g. following stapedectomy) (Baguley and McFerran 2011). Dysfunction of the medial or lateral efferent auditory systems, which innervate the outer and inner hair cells (OHCs/IHCs) of the cochlea, respectively, has also been proposed (e.g. Herráiz and Diges 2011): disinhibition of the OHCs or increased glutamate release at the base of the IHCs may lead to constant overstimulation of the IHCs.

Given the high rates of various forms of loudness intolerance reported in disorders known to be influenced by serotonin dysregulation (such as Williams syndrome, depression, migraine and post-traumatic stress disorder), it is believed that serotonin may play a significant role. There is, however, some dispute about whether true hyperacusis is found in these latter cases or whether it is in fact a general intolerance of sound, in which case other mechanisms may be involved (e.g. Blomberg et al. 2006).

Change in central auditory gain is a normal consequence of change in the peripheral auditory system, but where dysregulated it may be a significant factor in hyperacusis. For example, Formby et al. (2003) demonstrated in normal-hearing listeners that auditory deprivation by means of earplugs worn continuously for 2 weeks leads to increased central auditory gain, observed as hearing threshold shifts on pure-tone audiometry and on loudness scaling measures once the earplugs have been removed. The reverse, 2 weeks of constant low-level noise through in-the-ear wearable devices, leads to decreased central auditory gain (i.e. decreased loudness perception and increased sound tolerance). Sun et al. (2012) demonstrated in rats that the sensory deafferentation that follows cochlear hearing loss induced by noise exposure also leads to an increase in central auditory gain. These and other studies imply that central auditory gain is adaptable and can be affected by changes in levels of peripheral auditory stimulation, that such change affects loudness judgements and that dysregulated central auditory gain may therefore play a significant role in the pathophysiology of hyperacusis. Sun et al. (2014) proposed that even temporary hearing loss at an early age may affect tolerance of sound during development.

Involvement of the amygdala, limbic and autonomic systems, perhaps triggered by this abnormal auditory gain, has also been postulated (e.g. Jastreboff and Hazell 1993; Herráiz et al. 2006). Activation of these systems in association with sound gives rise to emotional responses such as anxiety, fear and depression. Baguley and Andersson (2007) have developed a fear-avoidance model of hyperacusis, in which fear of the experience of loud sound leads to increased awareness of the presence of sound and more frequent (unconscious) avoidance activities and possibly phobic reactions.

One limitation of the above-described mechanisms is that many patients with hyperacusis do not have abnormal peripheral function (Baguley and McFerran 2011), so any alteration in central auditory gain may be modulated by other factors.

15.3.3 Assessment

Hyperacusis is a subjective symptom, and no objective diagnostic assessment is currently possible. Diagnosis is based chiefly on the symptom report. The following assessment methods do, however, provide useful information to help exclude underlying pathology and enable successful, individually tailored treatment and counselling steps.

Baguley and Andersson (2007) proposed that an appropriate clinical history should include asking the patient or their parent/carer about their sound sensitivity (onset, development over time, types of sounds, reaction), its impact on their life,

avoidance activities (including the use of hearing protection), other diagnoses (e.g. depression, migraine or Williams syndrome) and other sensory sensitivities. A clinical examination of the ears and cranial nerve function is also recommended.

Audiometric Assessment Audiometric assessment is essential but should be undertaken with a level of caution, bearing in mind the risk of triggering or exacerbating the very problem for which the patient is seeking help. Hall (2013) recommends reminding the patient that they can stop the tests at any time. Pure-tone audiometry (including the extended high-frequency range) and tympanometry are beneficial in order to identify any underlying hearing loss. Presentation of the initial audiometric stimuli at a lower level than usual may help avoid triggering the patient's symptoms. Uncomfortable loudness level (ULL) testing, which measures the level at which a sound becomes uncomfortably loud, is often performed in order to investigate the severity of the problem and provide a baseline against which therapeutic benefit can be measured. Categorical loudness scaling tests such as Würzburger Hörfeld (Goebel and Günther 2014) or Oldenburger Hörfeld (Lehnhardt and Laszig 2009) can deliver even more detailed information than ULL testing (see Sect. 4.3.3 for further detail (pure-tone audiometry)).

Acoustic reflex testing may seem beneficial in order to test stapedial reflex function but risks exacerbating hyperacusis symptoms and, for this reason, is strongly advised against by various authors (e.g. Hall 2013; Baguley and McFerran 2011). If acoustic reflex testing is undertaken, consider using broadband noise stimuli for which the normal reflex threshold is ca. 20 dB lower than for pure tones (Margolis 1993), and avoid a screening approach that automatically tests at ca. 85 dB SPL and above. Outer hair cell function can be investigated by using otoacoustic emission (OAE) testing. Large amplitude responses on transient-evoked or distortion-product OAEs may indicate hyperexcitability (Hesse et al. 1999).

Self-report questionnaires, such as the Mini-HQ9 in Goebel and Günther (2014) (in German), which is based on questionnaires by Khalfa et al. (2002) (in English) and Nelting and Finlayson (2004) (in German), can be beneficial in indicating the severity of hyperacusis and associated distress. Such questionnaires can also be used as tools for monitoring progress during treatment.

Some centres perform additional tests such as speech audiometry in noise to investigate whether an associated auditory processing component is present.

The absence of abnormal audiological findings should not be taken to imply that hyperacusis is not present. The most common outcome of audiometric assessment in cases of hyperacusis is essentially normal-hearing sensitivity (Hall 2013).

15.3.4 Treatment

A range of treatment approaches has been proposed, including various forms of counselling and sound therapy. A multidisciplinary management approach is recommended, given the complexity of this disorder.

Counselling for hyperacusis should involve giving clear, individual-appropriate information, including a description of normal peripheral and central auditory system function, a clear explanation of hyperacusis, the involvement of the limbic and autonomic systems in regulating emotional responses and anxiety, and reasons (specific to the individual) why hyperacusis could occur (Baguley and Andersson 2007). Such discussion may not be possible with a younger patient, in which case counselling of their parents/carers is crucial. It is particularly valuable to encourage the continued exposure of their child to sound in a controlled way and with a great deal of positive reinforcement throughout. The involvement of clinical psychologists pursuing a structured approach such as cognitive behavioural therapy would be very beneficial in more extreme cases (Andersson 2013).

Sound therapy approaches follow the principle that increased peripheral auditory stimulation leads to a reduction in central auditory gain,

thereby reducing the perception of moderate sounds as distressingly loud. Sound therapy must be performed in a controlled manner, for example, by listening daily to a broadband sound generator in an otherwise quiet environment and gradually increasing the sound level over time. Open-fit hearing aids set to provide a level of gain in quiet situations but no gain at higher levels can be a useful alternative to a separate sound generator. Sound therapy can also function as a tool of desensitisation to perceived loud sounds or even to specific sounds with a distressing emotional association. Hall (2013) recommends the patient/parent make audio recordings of specifically troublesome sounds, to which the patient should then listen daily. Such an approach should be carried out in combination with counselling.

The use of hearing protection (e.g. headphones or earplugs) is contrary to the sound therapy approach. Long-term use of hearing protection has the effect of increasing central auditory gain (Formby et al. 2003) (therefore increasing the likelihood that when a moderately loud sound is heard it is perceived as too loud). However, short-term use of hearing protection in cases where the individual has become extremely handicapped by their hyperacusis may allow them to continue their normal life, for example, to attend school. Where hearing protection is judged necessary, hearing aids with a full silicone mould and active compression of moderate-high level input could be beneficial in the short term. Hearing aids have the advantage over other hearing protection in that they allow the finely controlled adjustment of gain over time. Their therapy must, however, encourage the gradual weaning of the hearing protection so that the above risks do not become overly ingrained.

Tinnitus retraining therapy (TRT) is a well-accepted treatment approach for hyperacusis that combines counselling and sound therapy (Jastreboff and Jastreboff 2000). Tinnitus and hyperacusis are very closely linked, and controlled desensitisation to the distressing sound is a key principle of treatment for both. The structure of TRT can therefore also be applied to individuals whose main complaint is hyperacusis. Jastreboff and Jastreboff (2000) reported that at least 75% of 163 hyperacusis patients who started TRT obtained significant improvement. Madeira et al. (2007) found TRT to be effective in improving hyperacusis symptoms in 75–88.5% of patients.

The use of medication for hyperacusis is rare. Antidepressants or anxiolytics are sometimes used to manage psychological side-effects. Evidence supporting the possible role of serotonin may open new avenues of treatment (Herráiz et al. 2006). Zazzio (2010) noted benefits following treatment with lasers projected down the outer ear canal in combination with pulsed electromagnetic field therapy/repetitive transcranial magnetic stimulation applied near the mastoid and the control of reactive oxygen species by various antioxidants. Silverstein et al. (2016) saw benefit in six adult patients with severe hyperacusis who had not responded to other therapy by reinforcing the round and oval window with temporalis fascia or tragal perichondrium. The benefit of this new therapeutic approach has to be investigated by further studies.

Other potential therapies abound but are not widely supported or used in clinical practice.

Case Study 15.1
Harry suffered from recurrent middle ear diseases in early childhood. His parents brought him to the clinic for phoniatrics and pedaudiology when he was 12 years old because of hyperacusis alongside severe difficulties at school, problematic social behaviour and poor social functioning. He had been given a psychotropic drug which caused several side-effects (tiredness among others). Harry filled in the Mini-HQ9: noise aggravated him, diminished his concentration and made communication difficult. He was angry about noises; he avoided them and immediately withdrew from them. He believed that he could not manage his daily life if the hyperacusis remained to the same extent. His ENT examination was without pathological findings. The audiological examination showed:

- Mild, combined, conductive/sensorineural hearing loss.
- ULLs at 60 dB HL in both ears.

- Normal speech audiogram, normal speech audiogram in noise.
- Categorical loudness scaling (Oldenburger Hörfeld) was abnormal at 500 Hz, 1, 2 and 4 kHz.
- Slightly flattened tympanograms.
- Abnormally high amplitudes of TEOAE.

His tinnitus could not be characterised in detail during the test sessions.

Harry was supplied with open-fit hearing aids set to provide a level of gain in quiet situations but no gain at higher levels. When tested with his hearing aids, ULLs were measured at levels of 90 dB HL. He found the hearing aids helpful at school, but it became necessary to change his school placement to a special school for hearing and communication with small and quiet classes. Tinnitus retraining therapy and psychological therapy were finally discussed.

15.4 Tinnitus

Mustafa Asim Safak, Haldun Oguz, and Ross Parfitt

Introduction Tinnitus can be described as the perception of a sound in the absence of an external acoustic stimulus. Tinnitus is a symptom, rather than a disease, and can arise as a result of dysfunction at any point in the auditory pathway.

Objective tinnitus (also called somatic tinnitus (Hazell et al. 1995)) can be distinguished from subjective (or neurophysiological (Hazell et al. 1995)) tinnitus. Objective tinnitus refers to sounds generated in bodily structures and conducted to the ear. These sounds can often be heard by the clinician. Common causes of objective tinnitus include blood vessels near the ear (often reported as sounding pulsatile), palatal myoclonus and stapedius muscle dystonia, all of which warrant medical attention (Elziere et al. 2007; Fritsch et al. 2001). The vast majority of cases of tinnitus are, however, subjective, and the term 'tinnitus' is often taken to refer solely to this type. Subjective tinnitus reflects non-pathological dysfunction of normal auditory processes and cannot be heard by anyone except for the person with tinnitus. As such, the main concerns regarding subjective tinnitus are the psychological impact it can have on the patient (such as distress and reduced quality of life) and tinnitus as a possible indicator of hearing loss or other dysfunction.

Epidemiology Ten percent of adults experience prolonged tinnitus, which is reported as moderately-severely annoying in 5% and has a severe effect on quality of life in 1% (Davis and Rafaie 2000). Tinnitus is a primary complaint in 0.5–3.8% of children seen in audiology clinics (Baguley et al. 2013). In normal-hearing children, the prevalence of tinnitus has been reported to be from 6 to 40% (Aksoy et al. 2007; Juul et al. 2012; Mills et al. 1986; Nodar 1972; Savastano et al. 2009). The prevalence of tinnitus increases up to 66% in children with increasing age or greater degree of hearing impairment (Shetye and Kennedy 2009). Tinnitus is reported in 38% of children with cochlear implants, most commonly in the implanted ear when the implant is not in use (Chadha et al. 2009).

Symptoms/Percept The tinnitus percept differs between individuals and is often described as a buzzing, ringing, roaring or clicking sound. It is heard continuously in some people and intermittently in others. Its subjective localisation is not always clear to the patient but is generally described as being in one ear, both ears or in the head. Acoustic hallucinations and pseudo-hallucinations are sometimes mistakenly considered to be forms of tinnitus; their characteristics are explained in an overview by Bernard and Quante (2011) and by Cope and Baguley (2009).

By matching the level of an externally generated sound to the loudness of the tinnitus percept, studies on loudness matching suggested that tinnitus is often surprisingly quiet even when patients describe it as being distressing (see review by Henry and Meikle 2000). There is, however, no correlation between the properties of

the tinnitus percept (including loudness, type, quality and pitch) and its subjective severity (e.g. Meikle et al. 1984).

Effects/Impact Many researchers suggest that the link between tinnitus and distress stems not from the loudness of the tinnitus percept but from associated psychological factors (Holmes and Padgham 2009), with anxiety, depression, sleep disturbance and reduced attention/concentration being experienced by many.

Tinnitus may cause concentration/attention difficulties in children and can bring about behavioural problems such as irritation, nervousness, deterioration in linguistic capacity, learning and writing difficulties (Kentish et al. 2000).

Tinnitus can be related to permanent hearing impairment (HI) or temporary hearing threshold shift (TTS) (Juul et al. 2012). Approx. 90% of people with tinnitus have some form of hearing loss (Davis and Rafaie 2000). Many tinnitus patients also report increased sensitivity to loud sound (hyperacusis) (see Sect. 15.3).

Significant differences between children with and without tinnitus were found on measurement of self-perception of hearing loss, dizziness, headache and concern about obesity (Kim et al. 2012). Trait anxiety in particular was found to be strongly associated with tinnitus.

Pathogenesis/Mechanism The pathophysiology of subjective tinnitus is much more complex than that of objective tinnitus. In the past, scientific opinion regarding underlying mechanisms was based on an analogy between tinnitus and intractable pain; both were believed to be caused by deafferentation of neural fibres (Tonndorf 1987). Recent studies suggest various neural changes occurring in the auditory pathways relating to the deafferentation of central auditory structures following cochlear injury (e.g. Brozoski et al. 2012). These include tonotopic map reorganisations in auditory cortical and thalamic structures; hyperactivity in these structures (but typically not in auditory nerve fibres) increased burst firing in subcortical auditory nuclei and increased synchronous neural activity, particularly in tonotopic regions affected by hearing loss where tinnitus perception is also localised (Noreña et al. 2006). The limbic system is also involved in the chronic perception of tinnitus (Lockwood et al. 1998; Leaver et al. 2011) and is a key part of Jastreboff and Hazell's influential neurophysiological model of tinnitus (1993), which describes a complex interaction between sensory and emotional systems.

Aetiology The aetiology of tinnitus is idiopathic in most children. Probable aetiological factors include a wide variety of infections, metabolic or vascular diseases, haemodynamic changes, tumours, allergies, ototoxic medication, neurological disorders, dietary changes, depression or anxiety, stress, craniomandibular disorders or traumatic events such as acoustic trauma, barotrauma or head and neck trauma (Bösel et al. 2008; Elziere et al. 2007; Nicolas-Puel et al. 2006; Rodriguez-Casero et al. 2006; Aust 2002). Relevant pathology usually relates to the ear, head and neck area. Tinnitus can occur with or without prior noise exposure (noise-induced tinnitus (NIT) and spontaneous tinnitus (ST), respectively).

15.5 Non-organic (Functional) Hearing Loss

Claus-Michael Schmidt

Introduction 'Non-organic hearing loss' (NOHL) (pseudohypacusis, functional or psychogenic hearing loss) is described as accounting for from 1 to 3% of all cases of hearing loss in children. It is characterised by a discrepancy between elevated pure-tone audiometry thresholds and normal speech discrimination. In adults, elevated pure-tone thresholds are often found with conscious intentions and gains: malingering means faking or worsening a hearing loss in order to achieve premature retirement or get out of military service. In children, NOHL is regarded as more or less unconscious (Austen and Lynch 2004).

Clinics Non-organic (functional) hearing loss in children is characterised by a hearing loss without a detectable corresponding pathology in the auditory system. Schmidt et al. (2013) have reviewed the current literature. Mean age at diagnosis was 11.3 years. Girls were twice as often affected as boys. Mean pure-tone threshold was 40–50 dB (often air and bone conduction). Most of the patients had no problems understanding oral instruction. Speech audiometry (additionally speech in noise) often showed normal results. A brainstem audiometry with threshold estimation and latency interpretation should confirm the diagnosis. Middle ear pathologies should be ruled out by ear microscopy, tympanometry and stapedial reflex measurement. Cochlear function is additionally investigated with otoacoustic emissions. Single-sided NOHL can be ruled out with the Stenger test.

Differential Diagnosis Table 15.1 includes mild sensorineural hearing loss, auditory processing disorder, auditory neuropathy and elevated thresholds in mental retardation.

Biographic History The child's history frequently shows school and education problems or family conflicts. A discrepancy between parental expectations and school performance is discussed as a risk factor (Aplin and Rowson 1990). The typical onset between 10 and 12 years and the increased frequency during periods of intense performance assessments are discussed as an indication of educational and emotional stress. Children, especially those with low average intelligence, having managed primary school without, or with little, difficulty, may develop NOHL after transfer to secondary school. Severe psychic trauma such as neglect and abuse is also described. Pre-existing organic hearing loss can be worsened by non-organic causes. Prognosis seems to be dependent on the severity of the patient's school or personal problems.

Management and Counselling The clinical follow-up in children with NOHL should include auditory brainstem response measurement and repetition of subjective audiometry. The biographical

Table 15.1 Differential diagnosis of NOHL (modified from Schmidt et al. 2013)

	Age at diagnosis	Pure-tone audiometry thresholds	Speech audiometry	Speech in noise	ABR
NOHL	End of primary school/secondary school	Often >40 dB	Mostly normal	Normal or mild impairment	Normal thresholds and latencies
Mild sensorineural hearing loss	Before primary school	≤30–40 dB	Normal or mild impairment	Impaired	Click threshold nearly normal
Auditory processing disorder	Primary school	Normal	Normal	Impaired	Normal thresholds and latencies
Auditory neuropathy	Infant/toddler	0–100 dB	Worse than pure-tone audiometry	Impaired	Pathological
Mental retardation	Infant/toddler	Difficult to estimate	Different, difficult to estimate	Often not possible to perform	Normal thresholds, often prolonged latencies

history is essential. An intelligence test, preferably in the context of a psychological investigation as a first step, and a child psychiatrist consultation as a second step, can be generally recommended. If serious developmental disorders are suspected, a child neurologist should be consulted. A history of speech or reading problems should lead to speech and language evaluation. Teachers should be involved, especially in cases of school- and learning-based problems. Additionally, consultation of external pedagogues can be considered.

References

AAA (2010) Guidelines for the diagnosis, treatment, and management of children and adults with central auditory processing disorder. http://www.audiology.org/publications-resources/document-library/central-auditory-processing-disorder. Accessed 10 Oct 2016

Agrup C (2008) Immune-mediated audiovestibular disorders in the paediatric population: a review. Int J Audiol 47(9):560–565

Aksoy S, Akdogan O, Gedikli Y et al (2007) The extent and levels of tinnitus in children of central Ankara. Int J Pediatr Otorhinolaryngol 71(2):263–268

Anari M, Axelsson A, Eliasson A et al (1999) Hypersensitivity to sound—questionnaire data, audiometry and classification. Scand Audiol 28(4):219–230

Andersson G, Lindvall N, Hursti T et al (2002) Hypersensitivity to sound (hyperacusis): a prevalence study conducted via the Internet and post. Int J Audiol 41(8):545–554

Andersson G (2013) The treatment of hyperacusis with cognitive behavioral therapy. ENT Audiol News 21:86–87

Aplin DY, Rowson VJ (1990) Psychological characteristics of children with functional hearing loss. Br J Audiol 24(2):77–87

Ardle BM, Bitner-Glindzicz M (2010) Investigation of the child with permanent hearing impairment. Arch Dis Child Educ Pract 95(1):14–23

ASHA (2005) (Central) auditory processing disorders: the role of the audiologist. http://www.asha.org/docs/html/tr2005-00043.html. Accessed Sept 2013

Atiani S, David SV, Elgueda D et al (2014) Emergent selectivity for task-relevant stimuli in higher-order auditory cortex. Neuron 82(2):486–499. https://doi.org/10.1016/j.neuron.2014.02.029

Aust G (2002) Tinnitus in childhood. Int Tinnitus J 8(1):20–26

Austen S, Lynch C (2004) Non-organic hearing loss redefined: understanding, categorizing and managing non-organic behaviour. Int J Audiol 43(8):449–457

Bachmann KR, Arvedson JC (1998) Early identification and intervention for children who are hearing impaired. Pediatr Rev 19(5):155–165

Baguley DM, Andersson G (2007) Hyperacusis: mechanisms, diagnosis, and therapies. Plural Publishing, San Diego

Baguley DM, McFerran DJ (2011) Hyperacusis and disorders of loudness perception. In: Møller M et al (eds) Textbook of tinnitus. Springer, New York, pp 13–23

Baguley DM, Bartnik G, Kleinjung T et al (2013) Troublesome tinnitus in childhood and adolescence: data from expert centres. Int J Pediatr Otorhinolaryngol 77(2):248–251

Bamiou DE, Werring D, Cox K et al (2012) Patient-reported auditory functions after stroke of the central auditory pathway. Stroke 43(5):1285–1289. https://doi.org/10.1161/strokeaha.111.644039

Bernard F, Quante A (2011) Akustische Halluzinationen und Pseudohalluzinationen bei erworbener Schwerhörigkeit (Acoustic hallucinations and pseudo-hallucinations in acquired deafness). HNO 59(5):519–521. https://doi.org/10.1007/s00106-010-2249-9

Bharadwaj HM, Verhulst S, Shaheen L et al (2014) Cochlear neuropathy and the coding of supra-threshold sound. Front Syst Neurosci 8:26. https://doi.org/10.3389/fnsys.2014.00026

Bisiach E, Cornacchia L, Sterzi R et al (1984) Disorders of perceived auditory lateralization after lesions of the right hemisphere. Brain 107.(Pt 1:37–52

Blomberg S, Rosander M, Andersson G (2006) Fears, hyperacusis and musicality in Williams syndrome. Res Dev Disabil 27(6):668–680

Bösel C, Mazurek B, Haupt H et al (2008) Chronischer Tinnitus und kraniomandibuläre Dysfunktionen (Chronic tinnitus and craniomandibular disorders. Effectiveness of functional therapy on perceived tinnitus distress). HNO 56(7):707–713

Brody RM, Nicholas BD, Wolf MJ et al (2013) Cortical deafness: a case report and review of the literature. Otol Neurotol 34(7):1226–1229

Brozoski T, Odintsov B, Bauer C (2012) Gamma-aminobutyric acid and glutamic acid levels in the auditory pathway of rats with chronic tinnitus: a direct determination using high resolution point-resolved proton magnetic resonance spectroscopy (1H-MRS). Front Syst Neurosci 6:9. https://doi.org/10.3389/fnsys.2012.00009

Brusis T (2011) Innenohrschwerhörigkeit nach stumpfem Schädelhirntrauma bzw. Kopfpralltrauma (Sensorineural hearing loss after dull head injury or concussion trauma). Laryngo-Rhino-Otologie 90(2):73–80

BSA (2011) Position statement: auditory processing disorder (APD). http://www.thebsa.org.uk/wp-content/uploads/2014/04/BSA_APD_PositionPaper_31March11_FINAL.pdf. Accessed 29 Dec 2014

Campbell NG, Bamiou DE, Sirimanna T (2012) Current progress in auditory processing disorder. ENT Audiol News 21(2):86–90

Chadha NK, Gordon KA, James AL et al (2009) Tinnitus is prevalent in children with cochlear implants. Int J Pediatr Otorhinolaryngol 73(5):671–675

Cope TE, Baguley DM (2009) Is musical hallucination an otological phenomenon? a review of the literature. Clin Otolaryngol 34(5):423–430. https://doi.org/10.1111/j.1749-4486.2009.02013.x

Cremers CW, O'Connor AF, Helms J et al (2010) International consensus on Vibrant Soundbridge® implantation in children and adolescents. Int J Pediatr Otorhinolaryngol 74(11):1267–1269

Davis A, El Rafaie A (2000) Epidemiology of tinnitus. In: Tyler RS (ed) Tinnitus handbook. Singular, San Diego, CA

Dawes P, Sirimanna T, Burton M et al (2009) Temporal auditory and visual motion processing of children diagnosed with auditory processing disorder and dyslexia. Ear Hear 30(6):675–686. https://doi.org/10.1097/AUD.0b013e3181b34cc5

Del Zoppo C, Sanchez L, Lind C (2015) A long-term follow-up of children and adolescents referred for assessment of auditory processing disorder. Int J Audiol 54(6):368–375

Edmond K, Clark A, Korczak VS et al (2010) Global and regional risk of disabling sequelae from bacterial meningitis: a systematic review and meta-analysis. Lancet Infect Dis 10(5):317–328

Elziere M, Roman S, Nicollas R et al (2007) Objective tinnitus associated with essential palatal myoclonus: report in a child. Int Tinnitus J 13(2):157–158

Emanuel DC, Ficca KN, Korczak P (2011) Survey of the diagnosis and management of auditory processing disorder. Am J Audiol 20(1):48–60. https://doi.org/10.1044/1059-0889(2011/10-0019

Formby C, Sherlock LP, Gold SL (2003) Adaptive plasticity of loudness induced by chronic attenuation and enhancement of the acoustic background. J Acoust Soc Am 114(1):55–58

Fritsch MH, Wynne MK, Matt BH et al (2001) Objective tinnitus in children. Otol Neurotol 22(5):644–649

Gibson WP, Sanli H (2007) Auditory neuropathy: an update. Ear Hear 28(2 Suppl):102S–106S

Gifford KA, Holmes MG, Bernstein HH (2009) Hearing loss in children. Pediatr Rev 30(6):207–215

Goebel G, Günther S (2014) Nachweis der Geräuschüberempfindlichkeit (Hyperakusis) mit überschwelliger Audiometrie: evaluation eines neuen Verfahrens auf Basis der kategorialen Hörfeldaudiometrie (Würzburger Hörfeld) zur Klassifizierung des Hyperakusis-Schweregrades (Assessment of decreased sound tolerance (hyperacusis) with suprathreshold audiometry: evaluation of a new method based on categorial loudness scaling (Würzburger Hörfeld) to classify the severity of hyperacusis). Z Audiol 53(3):98–109

Gregg R, Wiorek L, Arvedson J (2004) Pediatric audiology: a review. Pediatr Rev 25(7):224–234

Griffiths TD, Rees A, Witton C et al (1997) Spatial and temporal auditory processing deficits following right hemisphere infarction. A psychophysical study. Brain 120(Pt 5):785–794

GSPPA (2014) Auditory processing and perception disorders: definition. Professional guidelines. German Society of Phoniatrics and Pediatric Audiology

Hall JW (2013) What can be done for patients with hyperacusis and other forms of decreased sound tolerance. Available via Audiology Online, Article #11679. http://www.audiologyonline.com/articles/20q-what-can-done-for-11679. Accessed 16 Nov 2016

Halliday LF, Taylor JL, Millward KE et al (2012) Lack of generalization of auditory learning in typically developing children. J Speech Lang Hear Res 55(1):168–181. https://doi.org/10.1044/1092-4388(2011/09-0213

Harlor AD, Bower C (2009) Hearing assessment in infants and children: recommendations beyond neonatal screening. Committee on Practice and Ambulatory Medicine; Section on Otolaryngology-Head and Neck Surgery. Pediatrics 124(4):1252–1263

Hattiangadi N, Pillion JP, Slomine B et al (2005) Characteristics of auditory agnosia in a child with severe traumatic brain injury: a case report. Brain Lang 92(1):12–25

Hazell JW, McKinney CJ, Aleksy W (1995) Mechanisms of tinnitus in profound deafness. Ann Otol Rhinol Laryngol Suppl 166:418–420

Henry JA, Meikle MB (2000) Psychoacoustic measures of tinnitus. J Am Acad Audiol 11(3):138–155

Herráiz C, Plaza G, Aparicio JM (2006) Mechanisms and management of hyperacusis (decreased sound tolerance). Acta Otorrinolaringol Esp 57(8):373–377

Herráiz C, Diges I (2011) Tinnitus and Hyperacusis/Phonophobia. In: Møller M et al (eds) Textbook of Tinnitus. Springer, New York, pp 455–461

Hesse G, Masri S, Nelting M et al (1999) Hypermotility of outer hair cells: DPOAE findings with hyperacusis patients. In: Hazell J (ed) Proceedings of the sixth international tinnitus seminar. Tinnitus and Hyperacusis Center, London, pp 342–344

Hind SE, Haines-Bazrafshan R, Benton CL et al (2011) Prevalence of clinical referrals having hearing thresholds within normal limits. Int J Audiol 50(10):708–716. https://doi.org/10.3109/14992027.2011.582049

Hoistad DL, Hain TC (2003) Central hearing loss with a bilateral inferior colliculus lesion. Audiol Neurootol 8(2):111–113

Holmes S, Padgham ND (2009) Review paper: more than ringing in the ears: a review of tinnitus and its psychosocial impact. J Clin Nurs 18(21):2927–2937

Hornickel J, Zecker SG, Bradlow AR et al (2012) Assistive listening devices drive neuroplasticity in children with dyslexia. Proc Natl Acad Sci U S A 109(41):16731–16736. https://doi.org/10.1073/pnas.1206628109

Hoth S (1991) Veränderungen der frühen akustisch evozierten Potentiale bei Akustikusneurinom (Changes in early auditory evoked potentials in acoustic neuroma). HNO 39(9):343–355

Huang BY, Zdanski C, Castillo M (2012) Pediatric sensorineural hearing loss, part 1: practical aspects for neuroradiologists. AJNR Am J Neuroradiol 33(2):211–217

Humes LE, Dubno JR, Gordon-Salant S et al (2012) Central presbycusis: a review and evaluation of the evidence. J Am Acad Audiol 23(8):635–666

Iizuka O, Suzuki K, Endo K et al (2007) Pure word deafness and pure anarthria in a patient with frontotemporal dementia. Eur J Neur 14(4):473–475

Jackler RK, Luxford WM, House WF (1987) Congenital malformations of the inner ear: a classification based on embryogenesis. Laryngoscope 97(3 Pt 2 Suppl 40):2–14

Janssen RM, Hong P, Chadha NK (2012) Bilateral bone-anchored hearing aids for bilateral permanent conduc-

tive hearing loss: a systematic review. Otolaryngol Head Neck Surg 147(3):412–422

Jastreboff PJ, Hazell JW (1993) A neurophysiological approach to tinnitus: clinical implications. Br J Audiol 27(1):7–17

Jastreboff PJ, Gray WC, Gold SL (1996) Neurophysiological approach to tinnitus patients. Am J Otol 17(2):236–240

Jastreboff PJ, Jastreboff MM (2000) Tinnitus retraining therapy (TRT) as a method for treatment of tinnitus and hyperacusis patients. J Am Acad Audiol 11(3):162–177

Jerger J (2009) The concept of auditory processing disorder: a brief history. In: McFarland ATCDJ (ed) Controversies in central auditory processing disorder. Plural Publishing, San Diego, CA, pp 1–13

Jit M (2010) The risk of sequelae due to pneumococcal meningitis in high-income countries: a systematic review and meta-analysis. J Infect 61(2):114–124

Johansen IR, Hauch AB, Christensen B et al (2004) Longitudinal study of hearing impairment in children. Int J Pediatr Otorhinolaryngol 68(9):1157–1165

Joint Committee on Infant Hearing (2000) Year 2000 position statement: principles and guidelines for early hearing detection and intervention programs. Am J Audiol 9(1):9–29

Joswig H, Schonenberger U, Brugge D et al (2015) Reversible pure word deafness due to inferior colliculi compression by a pineal germinoma in a young adult. Clin Neur Neurosurg 139:62–65

Juul J, Barrenäs ML, Holgers KM (2012) Tinnitus and hearing in 7-year-old children. Arch Dis Child 97(1):28–30

Kaga M, Shindo M, Kaga K (2000a) Long-term follow-up of auditory agnosia as a sequel of herpes encephalitis in a child. J Child Neur 15(9):626–629

Kaga K, Shindo M, Tanaka Y et al (2000b) Neuropathology of auditory agnosia following bilateral temporal lobe lesions: a case study. Acta Otolaryngol 120(2):259–262

Kaga K, Kaga M, Tamai F et al (2003) Auditory agnosia in children after herpes encephalitis. Acta Otolaryngol 123(2):232–235

Kaga K, Shinjo Y, Enomoto C et al (2015) A case of cortical deafness and loss of vestibular and somatosensory sensations caused by cerebrovascular lesions in bilateral primary auditory cortices, auditory radiations, and postcentral gyruses—complete loss of hearing despite normal DPOAE and ABR. Acta Otolaryngol 135(4):389–394

Keith RW (ed) (1977) Central auditory dysfunction. Grune & Stratton, New York

Keith RW (2000) Development and standardization of SCAN-C test for auditory processing disorders in children. J Am Acad Audiol 11(8):438–445

Keith WJ, Purdy SC (2014) Assistive and therapeutic effects of amplification for auditory processing disorder. Semin Hear 35(01):27–38

Kentish RC, Crocker SR, McKenna L (2000) Children's experience of tinnitus: a preliminary survey of children presenting to a psychology department. Br J Audiol 34(6):335–340

Khalfa S, Dubal S, Veuillet E et al (2002) Psychometric normalization of a hyperacusis questionnaire. ORL J Otorhinolaryngol Relat Spec 64(6):436–442

Kihara M, de Haan M, Were EO et al (2012) Cognitive deficits following exposure to pneumococcal meningitis: an event-related potential study. BMC Infect Dis 12:79

Kim YH, Jung HJ, Kang SI et al (2012) Tinnitus in children: association with stress and trait anxiety. Laryngoscope 122(10):2279–2284

Kraus N (2012) Biological impact of music and software-based auditory training. J Commun Disord 45(6):403–410. https://doi.org/10.1016/j.jcomdis.2012.06.005

Kujawa SG, Liberman MC (2009) Adding insult to injury: cochlear nerve degeneration after "temporary" noise-induced hearing loss. J Neurosci 29(45):14077–14085. https://doi.org/10.1523/jneurosci.2845-09.2009

Leaver AM, Renier L, Chevillet MA et al (2011) Dysregulation of limbic and auditory networks in tinnitus. Neuron 69(1):33–43

Lehnhardt E, Laszig R (eds) (2009) Praxis der audiometrie. Thieme, Stuttgart, p 140

Lescanne EB, Bakhos D, Metais JP et al (2008) Otosclerosis in children and adolescents: a clinical and CT-scan survey with review of the literature. Int J Pediatr Otorhinolaryngol 72(2):147–152

Lockwood AH, Salvi RJ, Coad ML et al (1998) The functional neuroanatomy of tinnitus: evidence for limbic system links and neural plasticity. Neurology 50(1):114–120

Lucker JR (2012) What school psychologists need to understand about auditory processing disorders. School Psych 66(2):9–18

Ludwig AA, Fuchs M, Kruse E et al (2014) Auditory processing disorders with and without central auditory discrimination deficits. J Assoc Res Otolaryngol 15(3):441–464. https://doi.org/10.1007/s10162-014-0450-3

Luquetti DV, Heike CL, Hing AV et al (2012) Microtia: epidemiology and genetics. Am J Med Genet A 158A(1):124–139

Madeira G, Ch M, Decat M et al (2007) TRT: efficacité après un an de traitement (TRT: results after one year treatment). Rev Laryngol Otol Rhinol (Bord) 128(3):145–148

Margolis RH (1993) Detection of hearing impairment with the acoustic stapedius reflex. Ear Hear 14(1):3–10

Meikle MB, Vernon J, Johnson RM (1984) The perceived severity of tinnitus. Some observations concerning a large population of tinnitus clinic patients. Otolaryngol Head Neck Surg 92(6):689–696

Mendez MF (2001) Generalized auditory agnosia with spared music recognition in a left-hander. Analysis of a case with a right temporal stroke. Cortex 37(1):139–150

Mills RP, Albert DM, Brain CE (1986) Tinnitus in childhood. Clin Otolaryngol Allied Sci 11(6):431–434

Moore DR, Rosenberg JF, Coleman JS (2005) Discrimination training of phonemic contrasts enhances phonological processing in mainstream school children. Brain Lang 94(1):72–85. https://doi.org/10.1016/j.bandl.2004.11.009

Moore DR (2012) Listening difficulties in children: bottom-up and top-down contributions. J Commun Disord 45(6):411–418. https://doi.org/10.1016/j.jcomdis.2012.06.006

Moore DR, Rosen S, Bamiou DE et al (2013) Evolving concepts of developmental auditory processing disorder (APD): a British Society of Audiology APD special interest group 'white paper'. Int J Audiol 52(1):3–13. https://doi.org/10.3109/14992027.2012.723143

Moore DR, Hunter LL (2013) Auditory processing disorder (APD) in children: a marker of neurodevelopmental syndrome. Hearing Balance Commun 11(3):160–167

Moser T, Predoehl F, Starr A (2013) Review of hair cell synapse defects in sensorineural hearing impairment. Otol Neurotol 34(6):995–1004

Muse C, Harrison J, Yoshinaga-Itano C et al (2013) Supplement to the JCIH 2007 position statement: principles and guidelines for early intervention after confirmation that a child is deaf or hard of hearing. Joint Committee on Infant Hearing of the American Academy of Pediatrics. Pediatrics 131(4):e1324–e1349

Nelken I, Bizley J, Shamma SA et al (2014) Auditory cortical processing in real-world listening: the auditory system going real. J Neurosci 34(46):15135–15138. https://doi.org/10.1523/jneurosci.2989-14.2014

Nelting M, Finlayson NK (2004) GÜF Geräuschüberempfindlichkeits-Fragebogen. Manual. Hogrefe Verlag, Göttingen

Nickisch A, Massinger C, Ertl-Wagner B et al (2009) Pedaudiologic findings after severe neonatal hyperbilirubinemia. Eur Arch Otorhinolaryngol 266(2):207–212

Nicolas-Puel C, Akbaraly T, Lloyd R et al (2006) Characteristics of tinnitus in a population of 555 patients: specificities of tinnitus induced by noise trauma. Int Tinnitus J 12(1):64–70

Nodar RH (1972) Tinnitus aurium in school age children. J Audit Res 12:133–135

Noreña AJ, Gourévitch B, Aizawa N et al (2006) Spectrally enhanced acoustic environment disrupts frequency representation in cat auditory cortex. Nat Neurosci 9(7):932–939

Parving A (1988) Longitudinal study of hearing-disabled children. A follow-up investigation. Int J Pediatr Otorhinolaryngol 15(3):233–244

Peretz I, Blood AJ, Penhune V et al (2001) Cortical deafness to dissonance. Brain 124(Pt 5):928–940

Rodriguez-Casero MV, Mandelstam S, Kornberg AJ et al (2006) Acute tinnitus and hearing loss as the initial symptom of multiple sclerosis in a child. Int J Pediatr Otorhinolaryngol 69(1):123–126

Rosenfeld RM, Schwartz SR, Pynnonen MA et al (2013) Clinical practice guideline: tympanostomy tubes in children. Otolaryngol Head Neck Surg 149(1 Suppl):S1–S35

Savastano M, Marioni G, de Filippis C (2009) Tinnitus in children without hearing impairment. Int J Pediatr Otorhinolaryngol 73(Suppl 1):13–15

Schmidt CM, am Zehnhoff-Dinnesen A, Deuster D (2013) Nonorganic (functional) hearing loss in children. (Nichtorganische (funktionelle) Hörstörungen bei Kindern). HNO 61(2):136–141

Selters WA, Brackmann DE (1977) Acoustic tumor detection with brain stem electric response audiometry. Arch Otolaryngol (Chicago, Ill: 1960) 103(4):181–187

Shetye A, Kennedy V (2009) Tinnitus in children: an uncommon symptom? Arch Dis Child 95(8):645–648

Silverstein H, Ojo R, Daugherty J et al (2016) Minimally invasive surgery for the treatment of hyperacusis. Otol Neurotol 37(10):1482–1488

Skarzyński H, Rogowski M, Bartnik G et al (2000) Organization of tinnitus management in Poland. Acta Otolaryngol 120(2):225–226

Stanford Center on Longevity (2014) Redesigning Long Life. A consensus on the brain training industry from the scientific community. http://longevity3.stanford.edu/blog/2014/10/15/the-consensus-on-the-brain-training-industry-from-the-scientific-community/. Accessed 10 Mar 2015

Sun Fu Q, Zhang C et al (2014) Loudness perception affected by early age hearing loss. Hear Res 313:18–25. http://www.sciencedirect.com/science/article/pii/S0378595514000471

Sun W, Deng A, Jayaram A et al (2012) Noise exposure enhances auditory cortex responses related to hyperacusis behavior. Brain Res 1485:108–116

Swibel Rosenthal LH, Caballero N, Drake AF (2012) Otolaryngologic manifestations of craniofacial syndromes. Otolaryngol Clin N Am 45(3):557–577

Tabuchi S, Kadowaki M, Watanabe T (2007) Reversible cortical auditory dysfunction caused by cerebral vasospasm after ruptured aneurysmal subarachnoid hemorrhage and evaluated by perfusion magnetic resonance imaging. Case report. J Neurosurg 107(1):161–164

Taniwaki T, Tagawa K, Sato F et al (2000) Auditory agnosia restricted to environmental sounds following cortical deafness and generalized auditory agnosia. Clin Neur Neurosurg 102(3):156–162

Tomlin D, Dillon H, Sharma M et al (2015) The impact of auditory processing and cognitive abilities in children. Ear Hear 36(5):527–542

Tonndorf J (1987) The analogy between tinnitus and pain: a suggestion for a physiological basis of chronic tinnitus. Hear Res 28(2–3):271–275

Venekamp RP, Sanders S, Glasziou PP et al (2013) Antibiotics for acute otitis media in children. Otolaryngol Clin N Am 31(1):557–577. Cochrane Database Syst Rev 31(1):CD000219

Vermiglio AJ (2014) On the clinical entity in audiology: (central) auditory processing and speech recognition in noise disorders. J Am Acad Audiol 25(9):904–917. https://doi.org/10.3766/jaaa.25.9.11

Wakabayashi Y, Nakano T, Isono M et al (1999) Cortical deafness due to bilateral temporal subcortical hemorrhages associated with moyamoya disease: report of a case. No shinkei geka. Neurol Surg 27(10):915–919

Walker EA, McCreery RW, Spratford M et al (2016) Children with ANSD fitted with hearing aids applying the AAA pediatric amplification guideline: current practice and outcomes. J Am Acad Audiol 27(3):204–218. https://doi.org/10.3766/jaaa.15050

Willeford J (1974) Central auditory function in children with learning disabilities. Paper presented at the American Speech-Language-Hearing Association Annual Convention, 1974, Las Vegas

Yuvaraj P, Jayaram M, Abubacker R et al (2015) Auditory neuropathy spectrum disorder in hypomyelinating leukodystrophy—a case study. Int J Pediatr Otorhinolaryngol 79(12):2479–2483

Zazzio M (2010) Pain threshold improvement for chronic hyperacusis patients in a prospective clinical study. Photomed Laser Surg 28(3):371–317

Zhu RJ, Lv ZS, Shan CL et al (2010) Pure word deafness associated with extrapontine myelinolysis. J Zhejiang Univ Sci B 11(11):842–847

Diagnosis and Differential Diagnosis of Disorders of Hearing Development

16

Ahmet Atas, Songul Aksoy,
Antoinette am Zehnhoff-Dinnesen,
Doris-Eva Bamiou, Sylva Bartel-Friedrich,
Claire Benton, Hanno J. Bolz, Nicole G. Campbell,
Frans Coninx, Martine de Smit, Jakub Dršata,
Mona Hegazi, Armagan Incesulu, Kristin Kerkhofs,
Arne Knief, Sabrina Kösling, Jill Massey,
Peter Matulat, David R. Moore, Dirk Mürbe,
Katrin Neumann, Haldun Oguz,
Levent N. Ozluoglu, Waheeda Pagarkar,
Ross Parfitt, Simona Poisson-Markova,
Ewa Raglan, Charlotte Rogers,
Mustafa Asim Safak, Pavel Seeman,
Eva Seemanova, Tony Sirimanna, Piotr Swidzinski,
Monika Tigges, and Thomas Wiesner

Electronic Supplementary Material The online version of this chapter (https://doi.org/10.1007/978-3-662-46780-0_16) contains supplementary material, which is available to authorized users.

A. Atas
Department of Audiology, Faculty of Health Science, Istanbul University Cerrahpasa, İstanbul, Turkey

Department of ENT—Audiology and Speech Pathology, Faculty of Medicine, Istanbul University Cerrahpasa, İstanbul, Turkey

S. Aksoy
Department of Audiology, Hacettepe University, Sıhhiye-Ankara, Turkey

A. am Zehnhoff-Dinnesen · A. Knief · P. Matulat
R. Parfitt
Clinic of Phoniatrics and Pedaudiology,
University Hospital Münster, Münster,
Germany
e-mail: am.zehnhoff@uni-muenster.de;
knief@uni-muenster.de; matulat@uni-muenster.de;
ross.parfitt@ukmuenster.de

D.-E. Bamiou
National Hospital for Neurology and Neurosurgery,
London, UK
e-mail: d.bamiou@ucl.ac.uk

S. Bartel-Friedrich
Department of Otorhinolaryngology—Head and Neck Surgery, University Hospital Martin Luther University Halle-Wittenberg, Halle (Saale), Germany
e-mail: sylva.bartel-friedrich@uk-halle.de

C. Benton
Nottingham Audiology Services, Ropewalk House,
Nottingham, UK
e-mail: claire.benton@nuh.nhs.uk

C. Rogers
Leicester School of Allied Health Sciences,
De Montfort University, Hawthorn Building,
Leicester, UK
e-mail: charlotte.rogers@dmu.ac.uk

H. J. Bolz
Senckenberg Centre for Human Genetics,
Frankfurt am Main, Germany
e-mail: h.bolz@senckenberg-humangenetik.de

N. G. Campbell
Auditory Implant Service,
University of Southampton,
Southampton, UK
e-mail: N.G.Campbell@soton.ac.uk

F. Coninx
Institut für Audiopädagogik, University of Cologne,
Solingen-Ohligs, Germany
e-mail: f.coninx@ifap.info

M. de Smit
Artevelde University College, Ghent, Belgium
e-mail: martine.desmit@arteveldehs.be

J. Dršata
Department of Otorhinolaryngology and Head and
Neck Surgery, University Hospital Hradec Kralove,
Hradec Kralove, Czech Republic
e-mail: drsata@fnhk.cz

M. Hegazi
ENT Department, Ain Shams University, Cairo, Egypt

A. Incesulu
Faculty of Medicine, Department of Otolaryngology-
Head and Neck Surgery, Eskisehir Osmangazi
University, Eskişehir, Turkey
e-mail: saincesulu@ogu.edu.tr

K. Kerkhofs
Rehabilitationcentre De Poolster, Brussels, Belgium
e-mail: Kristin.kerkhofs@vgc.be

S. Kösling
Department of Diagnostic Radiology, Martin-Luther
University Halle-Wittenberg, Halle (Saale), Germany
e-mail: sabrina.kosling@medizin.uni-halle.de

J. Massey
Evelina London Children's Hospital, Guys and
St Thomas' NHS Foundation Trust, London, UK

D. R. Moore
Communication Sciences Research Center,
Cincinnati Children's Hospital, Cincinnati, OH, USA
e-mail: david.r.moore@cchmc.org

D. Mürbe
Department of Audiology and Phoniatrics, Charité—
University Medicine Berlin, Berlin, Germany
e-mail: dirk.muerbe@charite.de

K. Neumann
Department of Phoniatrics and Pediatric Audiology,
ENT Clinic, St. Elisabeth Hospital, University of
Bochum, Bochum, Germany
e-mail: Katrin.neumann@rub.de

H. Oguz
Fonomer, Ankara, Turkey

L. N. Ozluoglu
Department of Otolaryngology, Baskent University,
Etimesgut/Ankara, Turkey
e-mail: leventozluoglu@baskent-ank.edu.tr

W. Pagarkar
Royal National Throat Nose & Ear Hospital, Nuffield
Hearing and Speech Centre, London, UK
e-mail: wpagarkar@nhs.net

E. Raglan
Department of Audiology and Audiovestibular
Medicine, Great Ormond Street Hospital for Children
NHS Foundation Trust, London, UK
e-mail: eraglan@doctors.org.uk

S. Poisson-Markova · P. Seeman · E. Seemanova
Department of Child Neurology, 2nd Medical School of
Charles University Prague, Prague, Czech Republic
e-mail: Pavel.seeman@lfmotol.cuni.cz;
Eva.seemanova@lfmotol.cuni.cz

M. A. Safak
Department of Otolaryngology, Near East University,
Lefkosa, Turkey

T. Sirimanna
Audiological Medicine and Cochlear Implant
Department, Great Ormond Street Hospital, London, UK
e-mail: Tony.Sirimanna@gosh.nhs.uk

P. Swidzinski
Department of Phoniatrics and Audiology,
Poznan University of Medical Sciences, Poznan,
Poland

M. Tigges
Städt. Klinikum Karlsruhe GmbH, ENT Clinic,
Phoniatrics and Pedaudiology,
Karlsruhe, Germany
e-mail: monika.tigges@klinikum-karlsruhe.de

T. Wiesner
Department of Phoniatrics and Pediatric Audiology,
Werner Otto Institut gGmbH, Hamburg, Germany
e-mail: twiesner@werner-otto-institut.de

16.1 Diagnostic Interview, Recording of Family Tree and Clinical Examination

Monika Tigges

16.1.1 Diagnostic Interview

The evaluation of a suspected hearing disorder begins with a detailed medical anamnesis. The history is usually obtained from the parents or caregivers. Clinical signs of hearing disorders are often unspecific. The purpose of the history is to obtain information regarding the onset, duration and degree of the hearing disorder, possible risk factors and cause of the disease.

The child should also be spoken to in an age-appropriate manner. In this way, information regarding the speech development of the child can be obtained, and a basis of trust can be established for the subsequent physical examination. Observing the child is also important. A thorough history is essential for a fruitful relationship between the physician and the child/family, and it additionally affects the choice and specification of further tests.

The history should include the following topics:

Reactions to Sound The interview begins with questions regarding the child's reactions to acoustic signals. Reactions should be appropriate to their age (being startled by very loud noises, attentive listening for low noises, reactions to speech and music). Results of previous hearing tests and possible newborn hearing screening should be requested. Relevant information regarding speech development, including the age at which first words were spoken, the number of words spoken, the length of sentences, the child's understanding of speech and bilingualism, should be gathered.

Risk Factors In the following paragraphs, risk factors are presented.

Questions regarding risk factors during the pre- and perinatal periods should include:

- Prematurity
- Low birth weight
- Complications of delivery
- Perinatal distress, delivery by Caesarean section and the indications for this
- Asphyxia
- Treatment in a neonatal intensive care unit
- Hyperbilirubinaemia, ABO and rhesus incompatibility
- Sepsis
- Maternal endocrine disorders (diabetes, hyperthyroidism)
- Maternal infections (CMV, rubella, toxoplasmosis, syphilis, HIV)
- Maternal drug abuse

The following postnatal risk factors should be assessed:

- Meningitis
- Viral infection (rubella, mumps, CMV)
- Ototoxic drugs
- Recurrent otitis media

- Head injury
- Noise exposure

General Development In order to establish a picture of general developmental progress, the dates of the main milestones of motor development should be asked for (crawling, ability to walk, gross motor skills, fine motor skills, interest in play). Bear in mind that behavioural disorders may occur as a result of a hearing problem.

Vestibular Symptoms Vestibular involvement can lead to delay in milestones. Direct questions regarding possible tinnitus or vertigo can be asked of older children, in order to indicate a possible vestibular problem.

Illnesses Possibly Connected with Hearing Problems Disorders of the kidneys, heart and eyes, among many others, may be linked to certain diseases or syndromes with associated hearing abnormalities.

16.1.2 Family History and Recording of Family Tree

The family history may suggest a hearing disorder of genetic origin. As genetic factors are a major cause of hearing disorders, a family history of possible hearing loss and speech disorders should be taken. Number, gender, ages and state of health of siblings should be provided. In families with hearing disorders, a family tree of at least three generations should be constructed. The possibility of consanguinity should be inquired into, as the risk for an autosomal recessive hearing disorder is higher in these cases.

An example of a family with an autosomal recessive hearing disorder is given in Fig. 16.1.

16.1.3 Clinical Examination

During the examination neonates and smaller children will usually sit on the lap of the caregiver. Older children may sit alone on the examination chair.

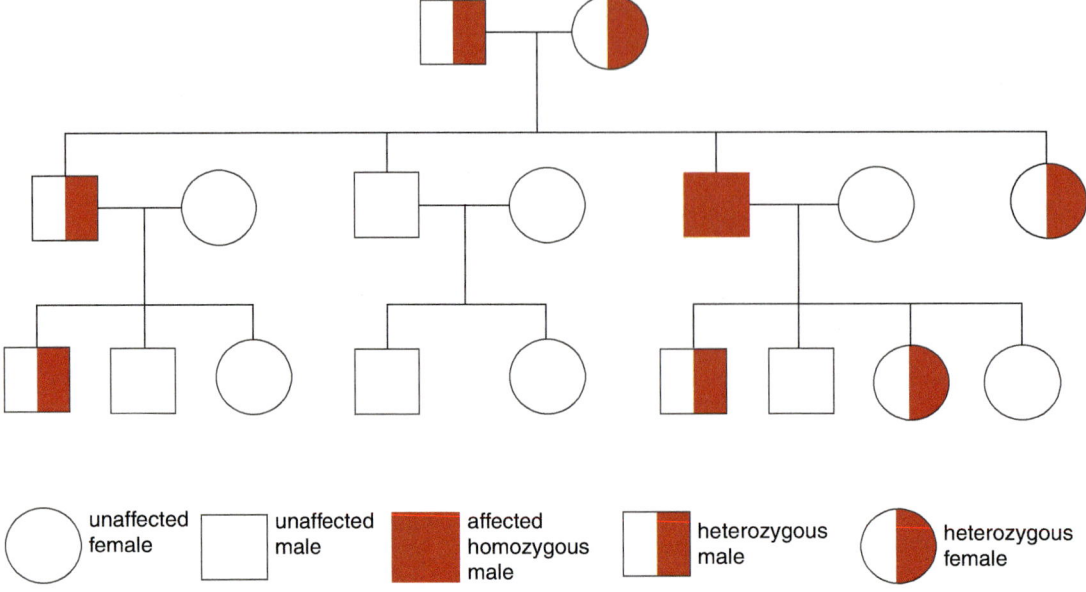

Fig. 16.1 Family tree of an autosomal recessive hearing disorder

Examination begins with an assessment of the head and neck. Any craniofacial abnormality is to be regarded as suspicious when found in relation with a hearing disorder. For example, heterochromia of the iris and a patch of white hair are observed in Waardenburg syndrome. An enlarged thyroid gland may be a sign of hypothyroidism (Pendred syndrome). Microgenia is related to Pierre Robin sequence. Malformations of the jaw occur in syndromes such as Franceschetti or Goldenhar. Branchiogene developmental disorders such as cervical cysts or fistulas may be related to hearing disorders as well.

The pinnae and their surrounding area should be examined for malformations such as pre-auricular pits or pre-auricular tags, atresia or microtia.

Pre-auricular pits may be connected with a fistula and an epidermal cyst at its end. Some authors recommend surgery before superinfection (Shoman et al. 2014).

Microtia is classified in Grades I–IV:

- I: malformation of the external ear with identifiable structures and a small but present external ear canal
- II: partially developed ear with a closed or stenotic external ear canal

- III: absence of the external ear with a small tissue structure, absence of the external ear canal
- IV: absence of the total ear

These abnormalities may be associated with middle ear malformation and congenital or progressive hearing loss (Germiller 2007).

A binocular inspection with the microscope is essential to assess the ear canal and the tympanic membrane. The width or possible atresia of the external canal should be examined. Cerumen should be removed until at least a part of the tympanic membrane is visible—if tolerated.

The tympanic membrane is judged for decline, translucency, colour, integrity and morphology of manubrium of malleus. The most common pathological findings are effusions and acute or chronic otitis media.

By inspection of the nose and nasopharynx, mucosal swelling, erythema and secretion may give hints to allergies, inflammation or reflux (Alexiades and Hoffmann 2008).

A nasal pit may be associated with a fistula and an epidermal cyst at its end extending into the nasal cavity or even intracranially. Because of the risk of infection, surgery should be performed; preoperative MRI is strongly recommended (Rizzi and Dunham 2014).

The size of the adenoids should be assessed. Choanal opening can be judged indirectly by strained expiration through the nose on a Link mirror. If necessary flexible or rigid endoscopes can be used. Examination of the oral area should include the teeth, tongue and tonsils. Additional attention should be paid to the soft and hard palate (high palate, short velum, cleft palate). Cleft or bifid uvula may hint to submucous cleft palate. Palpation and inspection of the velum during phonation are useful to exclude submucous cleft palate. Submucous cleft palate may affect the soft or the bony palate.

If a hearing disorder has been diagnosed, a full clinical examination is recommended to look for signs of syndromal disease, for example, café au lait spots in neurofibromatosis (Ruben 2001; Potsic and Lando 2012; Gibbin 2007).

During the examination every care should be taken to ensure that the child remains as comfortable as possible. In this way the cooperation of the child is maintained for the further audiological evaluations.

16.2 Basics of Technical Standards and Calibration

Arne Knief

In clinical audiometry there are many sources of error. The patient may vary in his or her answers and may not be cooperative; the audiometric technician may misinterpret the responses of the patient. Therefore it is important to reduce errors with well-maintained equipment. The standards provide good instructions for purchasing and assuring error-free operation. A huge spectrum is covered from the properties of microphones for calibration to word lists for speech audiometry as well as service for hearing aids. A rough list of standards is shown in Table 16.1.

More about standards are on the worldwide web:

Table 16.1 Selection of standards important in audiometry

ISO 266	Preferred frequencies
ISO 389	Standard reference zero for the calibration of audiometric equipment (all kinds of signals and sound sources)
ISO 7029	Statistical distribution of hearing thresholds as a function of age
ISO 8253	Audiometric test methods (pure tones, narrowband tones, frequency-modulated tones with air and bone conduction and one or more loudspeakers; minimum requirements of precision and comparability between different test procedures; basic methods of speech recognition tests and requirements for the composition, validation and evaluation (not the content) of speech material; noise for masking and as competing sound)
EN 15927	Services offered by hearing aid professionals
ISO 16832	Loudness scaling by means of categories
EN 60118	Hearing aids
EN 60318	Simulators of human head and ear (ear simulator for the measurement of earphones, acoustic coupler for the calibration of earphones, occluded-ear simulators, coupler for the measurement of hearing aids and earphones coupled to the ear by means of ear inserts, mechanical coupler for the measurement of bone vibrators, head and torso simulator for the measurement of hearing aids)
EN 60645	Equipment for audiometry: pure-tone audiometry, speech audiometry, test signals, high-frequency audiometry (8–16 kHz), instruments for the measurement of aural acoustic impedance/admittance, otoacoustic emissions and auditory brainstem responses
EN 60942	Sound calibrators
EN 61094	Specification for measurement microphones
EN 62489	Audio-frequency induction loop systems for assisted hearing

- European Committee for Standardization www.cen.eu.
- International Organization for Standardization www.iso.org.
- Sound and Vibration Standards acoustic-standards.co.uk/index.htm.
- Freestd Standards Worldwide www.freestd.us.

For detailed overview see Wilber (2002). It is important to implement good calibration practice into the daily performance of audiometry. Various guidelines and protocols for audiometry mention calibration as part of essential practice (e.g. British Society of Audiology 2011a).

16.3 Pure-Tone Audiometry

Piotr Swidzinski and Ross Parfitt

16.3.1 Introduction

Pure-tone audiometry (PTA) is the most common test within audiology, apart from newborn hearing screening tests, and forms the backbone of audiological diagnosis and management. PTA is a behavioural test (i.e. responses require the conscious cooperation of the patient) of the threshold of hearing (the lowest level of an acoustic signal that the patient can hear). It is appropriate for patients of approximately 3–5 years of developmental age and older.

Various protocols and guidelines for PTA have been created by different international organisations, such as the American Speech-Language-Hearing Association (1978), British Society of Audiology (2011a), US National Health and Nutrition Examination Survey (National Centre for Health Statistics 2003), Ireland's Health and Safety Authority (2007) and World Health Organization (2013). A well-structured PTA protocol, if correctly followed, has high test-retest reliability (Stuart et al. 1991), and intra-subject deviation of less than 10 dB is expected in >94% of subjects (Schmuziger et al. 2004). This article gives an overview of the core concepts of PTA which underlie most modern pure-tone audiometry protocols.

16.3.2 Resources

PTA is performed with an audiometer (which generates the sound stimuli), transducers (which deliver the stimuli to the patient) and a patient response button (which the patient presses to indicate that they have heard the sound stimulus). Audiometers can be stand-alone devices but are these days often attached to conventional computers and controlled by software, allowing results to be digitally recorded and connected with patient medical systems.

Air-conduction transducers include supra-aural headphones, typically Telephonics TDH 39 or Beyerdynamic DT 48 (Fig. 16.2), and (occasionally) insert earphones, such as Etymotics ER-3C (Fig. 16.3). Bone-conduction signals are delivered through a dedicated transducer such as Radioear B71 (Fig. 16.4).

Calibration of each audiometer (together with its dedicated transducers) must be performed at least annually (Stage B calibration, defined in ISO 8253-1 (2010)) in order to ensure the accuracy of the stimuli delivered to the patient. Simple checks (also known as Stage A checks) ought to be performed before each session of use to flag any technical issues or drift in the calibration.

PTA is typically performed within a sound-treated room, which reduces both background noise from outside the room and resonance within it. Soundfield audiometry is not covered in this article (see Sect. 16.4 for more details).

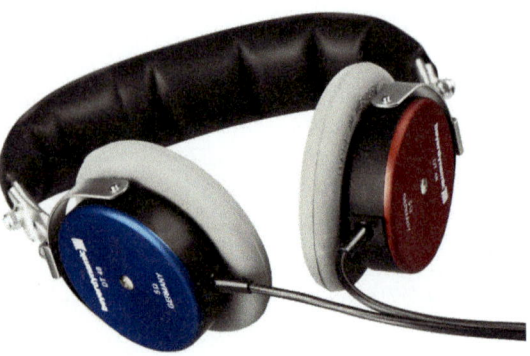

Fig. 16.2 Beyerdynamic DT 48 headphones. Image copyright and with permission from Beyerdynamic

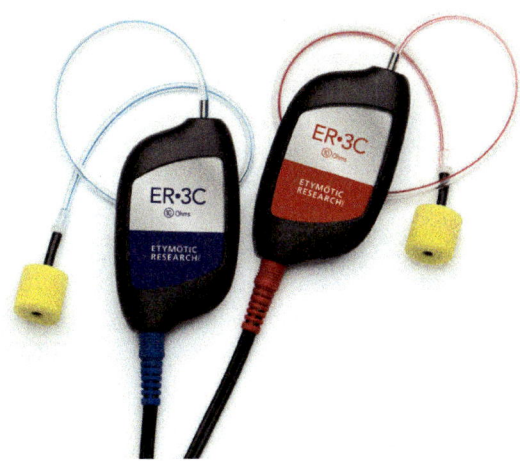

Fig. 16.3 Etymotics ER-3C insert earphone. Image copyright and with permission from Etymotic Research, Inc.

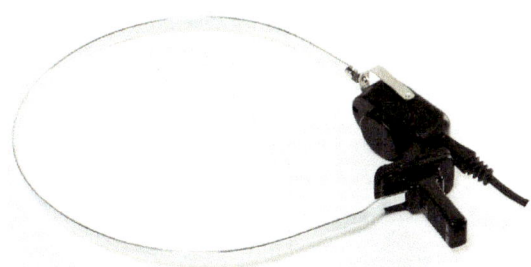

Fig. 16.4 Radioear B71 bone-conduction transducer. Image copyright and with permission from Radioear

16.3.3 Key Principles of PTA

Stimulus Type The stimuli (also known as 'signals' or 'tones') used in PTA are pure tones (i.e. sine waves) (see Sect. 1.4), which are the most frequency-specific stimuli possible.

Frequency and Level of Stimulus PTA is typically performed over the frequency range 250 Hz to 8 kHz and includes frequencies at each octave (250, 500, 1000, 2000, 4000 and 8000 Hz). Additional testing at intermediate frequencies, such as 1.5, 3 and 6 kHz, is sometimes done for specific purposes, such as to enable the gain of hearing aids to be set more accurately. Air-conduction testing can be performed at all of the above standard frequencies and is occasionally performed at higher frequencies (known as extended high-frequency audiometry), for example, in younger patients at risk of sensorineural hearing loss, such as those receiving ototoxic medication. Specific headphones are required for high-frequency audiometry, such as the Sennheiser HDA 200.

Bone-conduction testing is typically only performed between 500 Hz and 4 kHz, though some centres test up to 6 kHz. Bone-conduction signals can lead to vibrotactile sensation at lower frequencies (Boothroyd and Cawkwell 1970) and be airborne at higher frequencies (Lightfoot 1979) because of poor distortion performance of bone-conduction transducers at both low and high frequencies (Lightfoot 2000; Lightfoot and Hughes 1993). For this reason, precautions should be taken when using bone conduction above 2 kHz, such as covering the test ear with a supra-aural headphone (BSA 2011a). Both air- and bone-conduction stimulations are limited in their maximum output levels (air conduction is limited to approx. 120–130 dB HL output and bone conduction to approx. 60 dB HL output (both varying at different frequencies and dependent on audiometer manufacturer).

16.3.4 Test Procedure

Before Testing Otoscopy before PTA is recommended. PTA is not advised in cases of obstructed ear canal (owing to a risk of falsely raised air-conduction thresholds) or ear infection (owing to a risk of discomfort and cross infection). See more detailed protocols, such as those named in the introduction, for other specific contraindications.

The patient should be clearly instructed to press the response button every time he hears a sound, even if the sound is very quiet. Other responses, such as the patient's raising their hand or saying 'yes', are reasonable if the patient is physically unable to push the button. Adaptations for patients who do not understand their task (e.g. younger children or people with cognitive difficulties) are covered in Sects. 16.4 and 16.24.

Care should be taken to position the transducers accurately in order to avoid artificially lowering the level of the signal delivered to the ear.

Supra-aural headphones should rest on the pinnae with the centre of each headphone-loudspeaker in line with the auditory meatus. The bone-conduction transducer should be placed on the mastoid behind the 'test' ear (i.e. the ear which is being tested at the time), not touching any part of the ear and with as little hair between the transducer and the skin as possible.

Test Protocol Most PTA test protocols are based on the modified Hughson-Westlake procedure (Carhart and Jerger 1959), which establishes the 'ascending' psychometric threshold by presenting a stimulus to the test ear at a suprathreshold level and reducing the level in 10 or 20 dB steps until no response is present (i.e. the signal level is too low for the patient to hear). The level is then increased in 5 dB steps until a response is obtained (i.e. until the patient can again hear the signal). From this level the '10 down, 5 up' procedure is repeated until more than 50% of these ascending responses occur at the same level, with a minimum of two ascending trials. As soon as 2/2, 2/3, 3/5, etc., responses have been obtained at the same level, that level can be accepted as the threshold of hearing at that frequency (see, e.g. Fig. 16.5a–d). In practice, it is unwise to pursue individual thresholds for a great number of ascending trials because the patient can become tired and the reliability of their responses can suffer. If no threshold is identified within approx. 5 ascending trials, either start again at a clearly

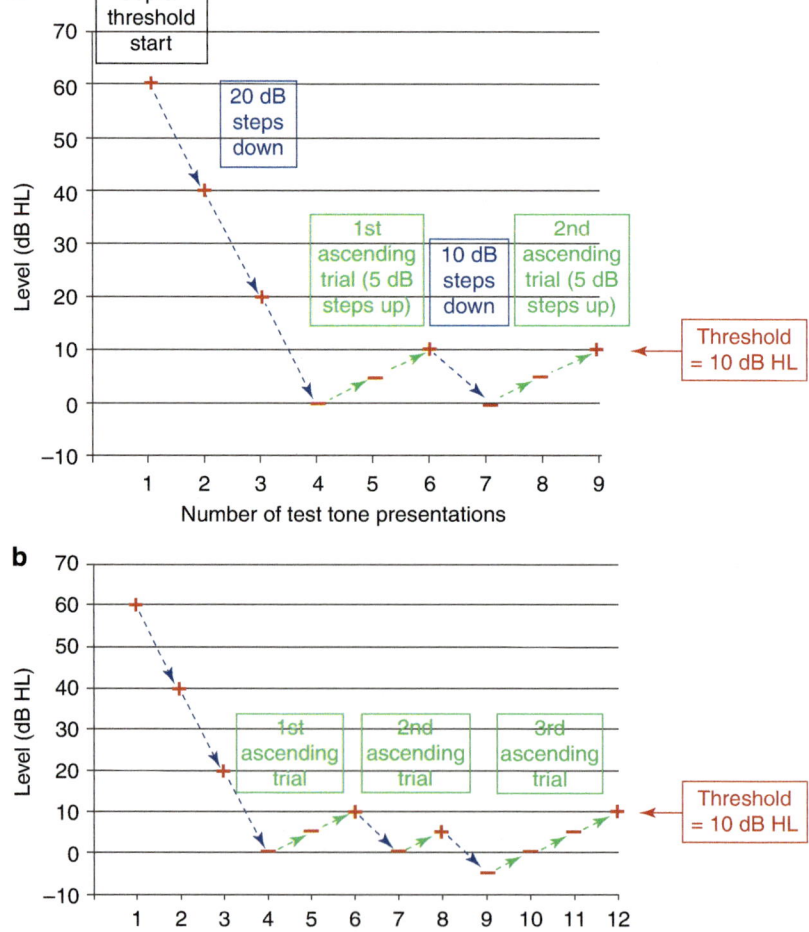

Fig. 16.5 (**a–d**) Four examples of tone presentations, ascending trials and responses in pure-tone audiometry, in the search for the auditory threshold, based on the modified Hughson-Westlake procedure (Carhart and Jerger 1959). The + symbol indicates a patient response; the − symbol indicates no patient response. (**a**) Two positive responses at 10 dB HL out of two ascending trials: threshold = 10 dB HL. (**b**) Two positive responses at 10 dB HL out of three ascending trials: threshold = 10 dB HL. (**c**) Two positive responses at 5 dB HL out of three ascending trials: threshold = 5 dB HL. (**d**) Three positive responses at 10 dB HL out of five ascending trials: threshold = 10 dB HL

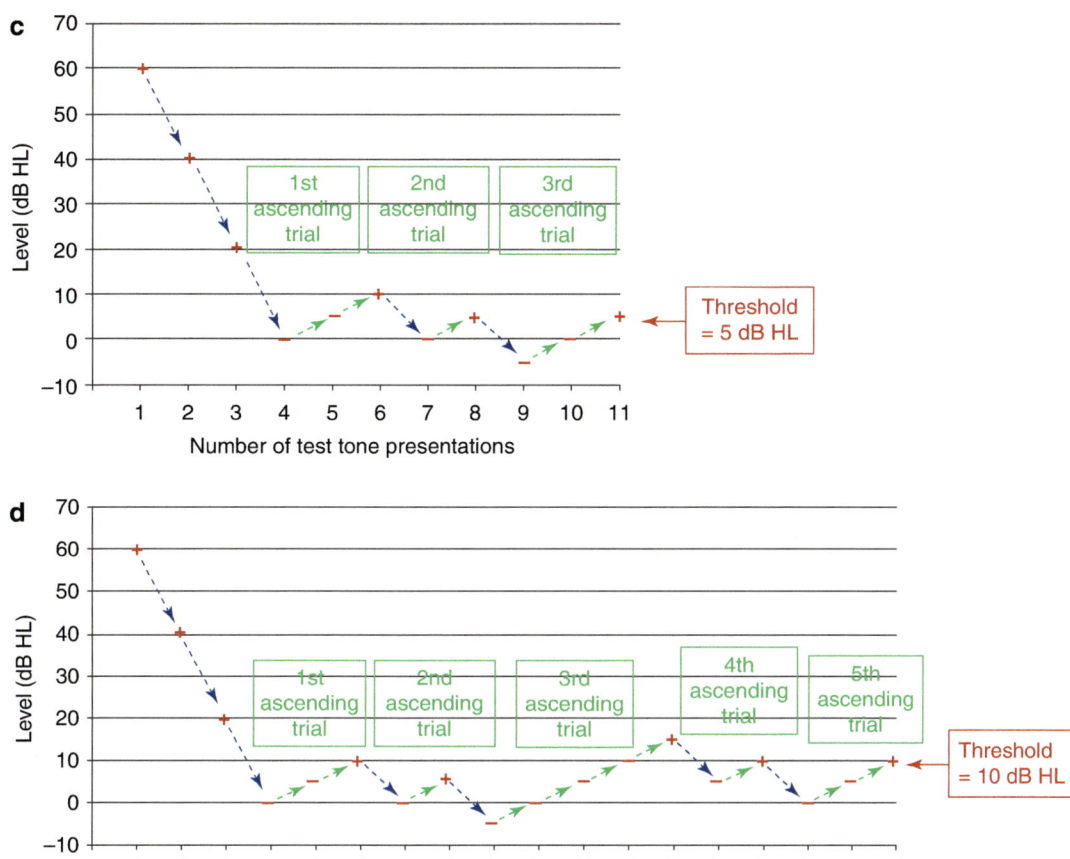

Fig. 16.5 (continued)

suprathreshold level, move on to another frequency and come back later or take a short break. Different protocols for measuring threshold exist, and results obtained will be slightly different for each one. Consistency of test protocol used is essential in order for results to be truly comparable (Franks 2001).

Presentation of the test tones should be arrhythmic with silences in between; otherwise the patient could (consciously or not) predict the presence of a tone which they cannot actually hear, thus resulting in falsely lowered thresholds. The tones should vary in length, and the patient should be instructed to hold the response button for as long as the sound is present, rather than just pressing it when they first hear the sound. This enables the tester to check the response to both

the onset and offset of the tone, thereby increasing the certainty of the response.

This procedure is typically carried out beginning with air-conduction stimuli (starting at 1 kHz) on the suspected better ear. All desired air-conduction frequencies are usually tested on the same ear and then moving to the other ear and then finally using bone conduction.

If air-conduction thresholds are within the normal range (usually accepted as <20–25 dB HL; see Sect. 1.4 and the 'Interpretation' subsection), bone-conduction testing is usually not clinically indicated.

Masking Munro and Agnew (1999) measured inter-aural attenuation levels (i.e. the level at which a signal played from a transducer to one ear could be 'cross-heard' by the other ear) of 40 dB for Telephonics TDH 39 supra-aural headphones and 55 dB for Etymotics ER-3A insert earphones. In clinical terms, this means that a large asymmetry in air-conduction thresholds between the two ears may mistakenly appear to be no greater than 40 dB (using supra-aural headphones) or 55 dB (using insert earphones). Masking is the essential process by which we can measure the 'true' threshold in these cases.

In masking, a noise (usually 1/3-octave narrowband noise, though white noise or others are used in some clinics) is played to the non-test ear at the 'effective masking level' (the lowest level of masking noise required to prevent the threshold-level pure-tone signal from being heard). The patient is asked to ignore the noise and only respond when they hear the pure-tone signals (played to the test ear). Using the common 'plateau' technique, the levels of noise and signal are increased to the point at which responses occur consistently at a particular signal level despite the noise level increasing further. This is taken as the true threshold.

Masking as part of bone-conduction testing is somewhat more problematic because the interaural attenuation of bone-conduction signals can be as low as 0 dB. Bone-conduction masking (in which a bone-conduction signal is masked by noise via an air-conduction transducer) is therefore essential in cases of asymmetrical air-conduction thresholds and where bone-conduction thresholds appear significantly better than air-conduction thresholds (the 'air-bone gap'). It is, however, clinically inefficient to mask all incidences of an air-bone gap because they are actually more likely than not to occur (Studebaker 1967). Small air-bone gaps should not necessarily be taken as evidence of middle ear pathology (Margolis 2015). The BSA protocol therefore recommends bone-conduction masking only where there is a ≥ 10 dB gap between the not-masked bone-conduction threshold and the air-conduction threshold of either ear (BSA 2011a).

The tester must be careful not to play uncomfortably loud sound into the non-test ear and must be aware of the risks of central masking and cross-masking. In central masking the patient is unable to identify a tone when masking noise is present. In cross-masking the masking noise is itself cross-heard, with the effect of masking the test ear. In cases such as this, masking to find the true threshold may not be possible.

A more comprehensive guideline for masking is beyond the scope of this article. See specific protocols (e.g. BSA 2011a) for further detail.

16.3.5 Recording the Results of PTA

The Audiogram The results of PTA are typically displayed on an audiogram (see Fig. 16.6), which is a graph showing auditory thresholds with frequency (Hz) on the X-axis and level (dB HL) on the Y-axis. Different countries and clinics use different symbols, though the circle and cross (representing right- and left-sided air-conduction thresholds, respectively), the use of red and blue (for right and left sides) and results for the right side being displayed on the left side of the page, and vice versa, are universal. Not-masked bone-conduction thresholds are represented by triangles in Fig. 16.6 and masked bone-conduction thresholds by square brackets.

Interpretation of Normal Range of Hearing Various descriptions of the 'normal range' of hearing can be found (see Sect. 14.1) and are generally accepted as being hearing thresholds better than 20–25 dB HL.

Interpretation of Conductive Hearing Loss Where bone-conduction thresholds are within the normal range and air-conduction thresholds are outside of the normal range, a conductive hearing loss is indicated (see Fig. 16.7).

Interpretation of Sensorineural Hearing Loss Where air- and bone-conduction thresholds are outside of the normal range to the same degree, a sensorineural hearing loss is indicated (see Fig. 16.6, right ear).

Interpretation of Mixed Hearing Loss Where air- and bone-conduction thresholds are both outside of the normal range but there is a difference between them (an air-bone gap)

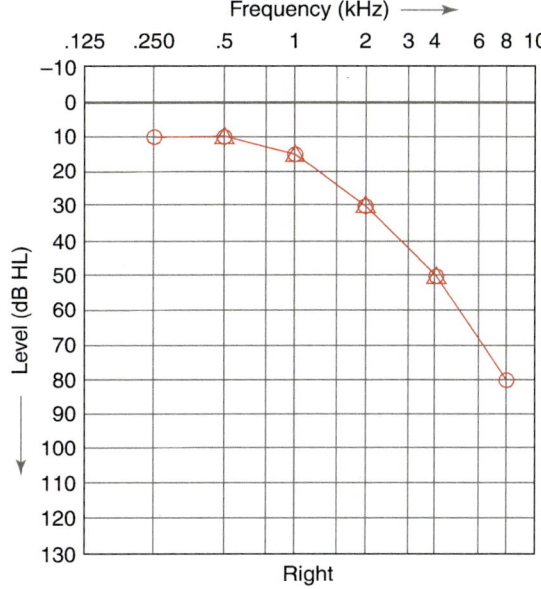

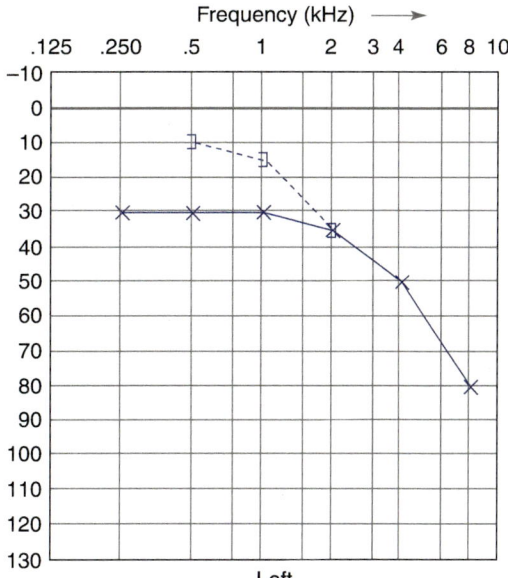

Fig. 16.6 An audiogram showing hearing thresholds for a hypothetical bilateral high-frequency sensorineural hearing loss with a low-frequency conductive component on the left. Results for the right ear are shown in red on the left side and results for the left ear in blue on the right side. The circles and crosses represent air-conduction thresholds; triangles represent not-masked bone-conduction thresholds; square brackets represent masked bone-conduction thresholds. These symbols are standard in the UK. Different symbols are used in different countries and clinics

and bone-conduction thresholds are better than air-conduction thresholds, a mixed hearing loss is indicated (see Fig. 16.8).

Different threshold levels are typically found at different frequencies. For example, otitis media with effusion is typically characterised by conductive hearing loss in the lower frequencies and normal thresholds in the higher frequencies (see Fig. 16.7). Presbyacusis (age-related sensorineural hearing loss) is characterised by normal or near-normal-hearing thresholds in the low frequencies and a sensorineural hearing loss affecting higher frequencies (see Fig. 16.6, right ear).

16.3.6   Limitations of PTA

As with all audiological tests, the cross-check principle (Jerger and Hayes 1976), which encourages the use of other tests (such as tympanometry; see Sect. 16.9) and the subjective impression

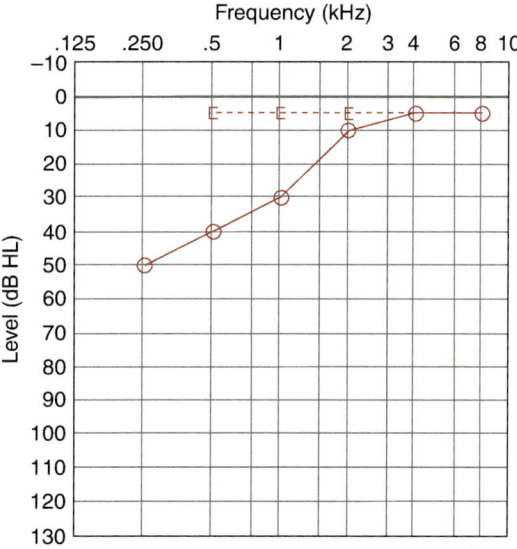

Fig. 16.7 Audiogram showing typical hearing thresholds found in conductive hearing loss caused by otitis media with effusion. This audiogram shows right-sided air-conduction thresholds (circles) and masked bone-conduction thresholds (square brackets)

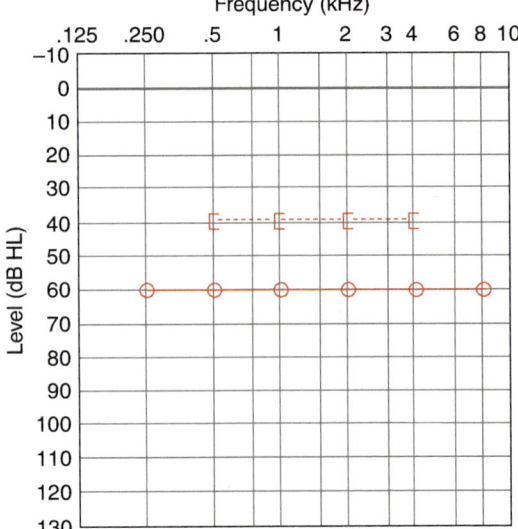

Fig. 16.8 Audiogram showing possible hearing thresholds found in mixed hearing loss. This audiogram shows right-sided air-conduction thresholds (circles) and masked bone-conduction thresholds (square brackets)

made by the patient to corroborate the result, is worth following. As the test results rely on behavioural responses, falsely raised thresholds (whether conscious or not) could be obtained. See Sect. 15.5 for insight into nonorganic hearing loss (NOHL) and Lightfoot and Kennedy (2006) on the use of cortical electric response audiometry (which measures the electrical response to auditory stimulation within the auditory cortex) as 'objective pure-tone audiometry'. Expectation bias can lead to inaccuracy during testing (Margolis et al. 2015), and there is a risk of responses being falsely interpreted by the tester (especially where time pressure and insufficient training are factors).

Classic pure-tone audiometry only tests the threshold of hearing in response to pure tones. Although this is sufficient for the diagnosis of many audiological conditions, it does not provide full evidence about the patient's functional hearing (e.g. his/her ability to process suprathreshold speech and other functional sounds or their tolerance of loud sound). See Sect. 16.7 for information on speech audiometry. Loudness investigations are outlined in the following subsection.

16.3.7 Loudness Tests

'Loudness' refers to the subjective perception of a sound, whereas 'sound level' is an objective measure (see Sects. 1.3 and 1.4). Uncomfortable loudness level (ULL) (also known as 'loudness discomfort level' (LDL)) testing measures the lowest level at which a sound becomes uncomfortable for the subject. This can be useful in providing additional accuracy regarding the patient's degree of loudness recruitment (in which a small increase in sound intensity is perceived as a large increase, as is typically found in sensorineural hearing loss) (see Sect. 1.4), thereby informing hearing aid gain settings, and is also often used in cases of suspected hyperacusis (see Sect. 15.3).

The basic procedure of ULL testing is to increase the level of a sound stimulus gradually until it just becomes uncomfortably loud for the patient (BSA 2011b). It is important to remember that the ULL is not the same as the threshold of pain. Agreeing an appropriate response method with the patient and issuing clear instructions are obviously crucial. ULLs are usually shown on the audiogram using the ⌐ and ⌐ symbols for right and left ears, respectively. Sherlock and Formby (2005) surveyed previous literature and proposed a normal ULL of around of 100 dB HL, but they noted considerable variance in normal ULLs reported between different studies across different signals, frequencies and transducers.

Loudness scaling seeks to investigate the subjective loudness of sound in more detail. Various scales exist, and most use verbal descriptors, e.g. very soft, soft, OK, loud, very loud and too loud (Loudness Growth in 1/2-Octave Bands, LGOB scale) (Allen et al. 1990), and specific test procedures to measure the subjective perception of loudness. The highly subjective and non-linear nature of (loudness) sensation can lead to potentially significant interindividual and inter-scale differences, e.g. Elberling (1999); however the international standard ISO 16832 (2006), based on Brand and Hohmann's Adaptive Categorical Loudness Scaling (ACALOS) (Brand and Hohmann 2002), has sought to increase reliability. The 'Würzburger Hörfeld' and 'Oldenburger Hörfeld' loudness scaling tests are well established within German clinics (Lehnhardt and Laszig 2009).

16.3.8 Dead-Region Testing

A cochlear dead region is an area of the cochlea in which the inner hair cells or auditory neurons are damaged to the extent that none are functional (Moore 2001). Given the tonotopic nature of the cochlea and the spread of acoustic sensation over the basilar membrane (see Sect. 1.4), stimulation of a cochlear dead region by using a signal of a frequency to which the non-functioning hair cells/neurons were tuned results in 'off-frequency listening', in which functional hair cells/neurons of a neighbouring region of the cochlea respond. Off-frequency listening is not detected on classic PTA, so specific tests are required. The threshold-equalising noise (TEN) test is one such test (Moore et al. 2000).

In the TEN test, a pure tone is played at the frequency of the suspected dead region, and a specifically designed TEN stimulus is played at 10 dB above the notional threshold of the suspected dead region. If the pure-tone threshold in the presence of TEN stimulus is <10 dB above the level of the TEN stimulus, then no dead region is judged to be present; if the pure-tone threshold is >10 dB above the level of the TEN stimulus, then a dead region is present. If a dead region is identified in a hearing aid user, the gain of the hearing aid could be adjusted to avoid stimulation at the affected frequencies, thus avoiding the distorted perceptual effects of off-frequency listening which can include impaired speech perception (Moore et al. 2000).

16.4 Paediatric Behavioural Audiometry (0–6 Years)

Kristin Kerkhofs and Martine de Smit

16.4.1 Introduction

Behavioural audiometry is an essential part of the diagnosis of hearing loss in very young children, even those younger than 6 months of age. Physiological measures (i.e. tympanometry, otoacoustic emissions, ABR and ASSR) should be complemented with behavioural measures to be able to determine the type and degree of hearing loss. The purpose of behavioural audiometry is to obtain air- and bone-conduction thresholds for the whole frequency range. Cross-checking of all measurements is needed before starting hearing aid fitting. This cross-check principle was described 40 years ago by Jerger and Hayes (1976) and is still up to date.

Behavioural audiometry needs well-experienced audiologists and is a time-consuming measurement that has to be done in optimal conditions. The test protocol will vary with the chronological age of the child. In case of retardation, it follows the developmental age of the child. Therefore you have to know the level of development and physical status (i.e. visual, motor abilities) before starting testing.

Testing can be done in a single or double soundproof booth. In a single soundproof booth, the examiner(s) and the child are in the same room. In a double soundproof booth, two examiners are needed, one with the child and one outside with the audiometer. The choice depends on personal preference. It may be useful to have both options.

General test strategy:

- To select the appropriate test method and setup, look into the *developmental status* of the child, especially in case of prematurity and mental or motor retardation.
- Try to *collect the results of all previous measurements*. This information helps you to find the optimal starting level.
- Always start with *bone conduction* if possible. It gives you the opportunity to use a vibrotactile stimulus (65 dBHL at 500 Hz or 45 dBHL at 250 Hz) (Cole and Flexer 2011), which you can use for conditioning the child when testing visual reinforcement audiometry (VRA) or conditioned play audiometry (CPA) (both outlined below). Even deaf children can feel these stimuli. At the same time, you obtain the result of the best inner ear, which you can compare with air-conduction results. Middle ear problems are very common in this age group. Moreover keep in mind that not every conductive hearing loss can be excluded with tympanometry.

- Continue with *air conduction*. Always try to obtain ear-specific thresholds. Insert earphones are recommended for this population to avoid a collapsed ear. A higher inter-aural attenuation makes masking less necessary. Using the child's earmould instead of the foam tip is even better.

- Use warble tones, narrowband noise or fresh noise (a more frequency-specific stimulus than typical narrowband noise (which usually has a 1/3-octave range)) instead of pure tones. Sometimes it will be necessary to find other more interesting frequency-specific stimuli to get the child's attention.

- Be very *flexible* during the test. The proposed flowcharts can be a support for those who are not used to working in this way. It will be important to maximise the child's attention span.

- Sometimes it will be necessary to *repeat* the test. Some children need more time, are not in the best condition or ask for a different way of working. Tests may need to be conducted over several sessions in order to obtain appropriate diagnostic information.

16.4.2 Behavioural Observation Audiometry (BOA): 0–5 Months

Leading-In Since universal hearing screening has been introduced in many countries, diagnosis will often happen before the age of 3 months. At this age behavioural observation audiometry can be an added value with the results of objective measurement, not only as an essential part of the cross-checking but also in counselling and supporting parents.

Although BOA is not generally accepted as an integral part of the paediatric audiometry test protocol, some paediatric audiologists provided evidence of BOA in this target group many years ago (e.g. Delaroche 2001; Delaroche et al. 2004, 2005; Madell and Flexer 2008).

BOA's purpose is to obtain air- and bone-conduction data as close as possible to the hearing threshold for a broader frequency range of at least 500–4000 Hz.

This can only be performed in optimal conditions and by following a strict protocol.

Developmental Milestones In the first 3 months of life, auditory reactions are unisensory and are based on reflexes. The most common reflexes are the cochleo-palpebral reflex, rudimentary head spin, changes in sucking, breathing, etc.

Between 3 and 5 months of age, unisensorial development becomes intersensory (i.e. the child becomes more able to combine input from more than one sensory system) (Piaget and Inhelder 1969). Most babies are already able to make a head turn to the sound, which can be reinforced by multimodal communication and personalised relationships. This has been described in the Delaroche protocol (Delaroche et al. 2011) as 'congratulating with smiles, signs, caresses and speech'.

In the following paragraphs, test equipment and setup are explained:

Conditions It is not the purpose of behavioural audiometry to search for strong reflexes as a reaction to loud sounds, but to look for minimal changes in behaviour as a reaction to soft sounds. These reactions are called the minimal response levels (MRLs). They can only be obtained in optimal conditions, as in a light sleep or while feeding or sucking (awake but peaceful). If the child is in a deep sleep, it will not respond, so its sleep state should be confirmed, by touching the eyelashes (the eyelids will move slightly when the child is not in a deep sleep).

When the child is hungry or does not feel comfortable, it may be too distracted to respond to the quietest sounds it can hear.

Testing has to be done in a soundproof booth with minimal distraction. Minimise tactile or visual impulses; no people other than the parents are allowed. When the mother is feeding, ideally the test can start from the moment the sucking becomes effortless and regular.

Transducers It is preferable to use the vibrator for bone conduction on an adapted diadem or softband. Air conduction with insert earphones gives ear-specific information with a great inter-aural difference. Therefore sound-field is not recommended. Furthermore, sound-field stimulation is less reactive (i.e. clear responses are more difficult to observe) and limited in loudness for finding the minimal response level (MRL) at this age.

Start with bone conduction to obtain the MRL of the better-functioning cochlea without influence of middle ear problems. The vibrator has to be placed only at the mastoid. The diadem of the vibrator has to be adjusted to the size of the child's head. Continue with insert earphones and be aware that the foam tip is not blocked with earwax (Fig. 16.9). In a later stage, one can use the customised earmould of the hearing aid instead of the foam tip.

Stimuli To obtain a proper response of the child, use warble tone, fresh noise or narrowband noise. At this age pure tones are not attractive enough. It may be necessary to change the nature of the stimulus while testing.

Procedure To obtain the minimal response level of the child, it is necessary to start below the expected threshold. A proper reaction can only be obtained when reaching the minimal response level for the first time for each frequency.

Start with *bone conduction*. Place the vibrator on the mastoid (Fig. 16.9 left), and observe the child's behaviour for a few minutes before presenting any sound in order to know the behaviour without auditory stimulation. If a bone-conduction hearing loss can be expected, start at the MRL of a normal-hearing child at this age, which will be 30–40 dBHL (Delaroche et al. 2011).

Follow the steps as indicated in the flowchart (Fig. 16.10).

Continue with *air conduction* using insert earphones (Fig. 16.9 right) on the basis of information from objective measurements, if available, or start from the bone-conduction thresholds you have just measured.

If click ABR testing was performed, start at 2 kHz, 20 dB below the ABR threshold level, and choose the better ear. Preferably it is necessary to obtain ear-specific information as soon as possible. Eventually binaural stimulation by insert phones can be used to have an initial idea about the type of hearing loss and the responsiveness of the better inner ear.

Follow the steps as indicated in the flowchart (Fig. 16.11).

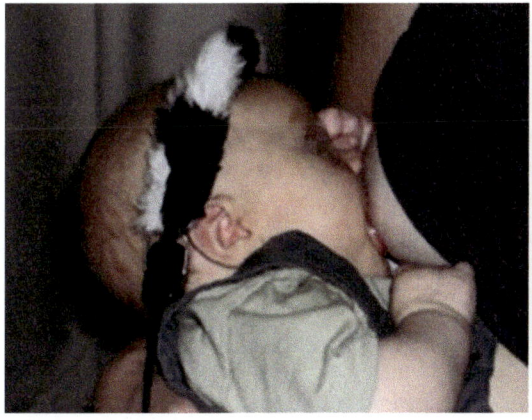 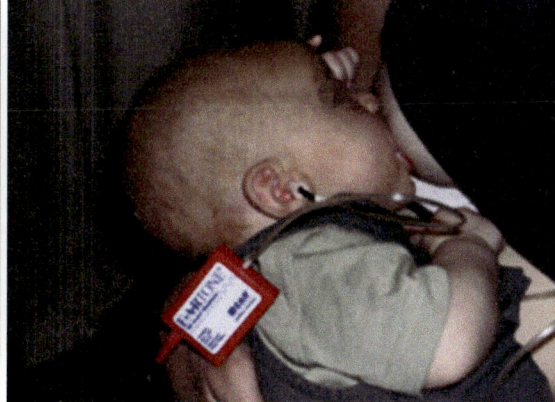

Fig. 16.9 BOA with vibrator (left) and insert earphones with foam tip (right). Photo with kind permission of the parents

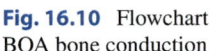

Fig. 16.10 Flowchart BOA bone conduction

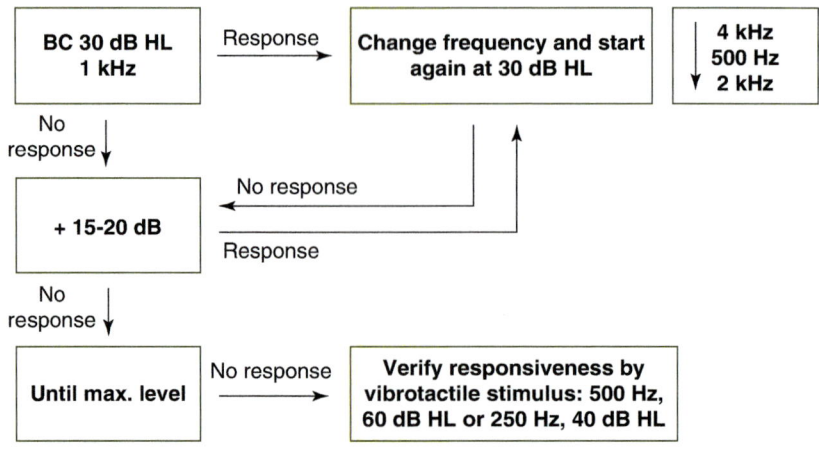

Fig. 16.11 Flowchart BOA air conduction

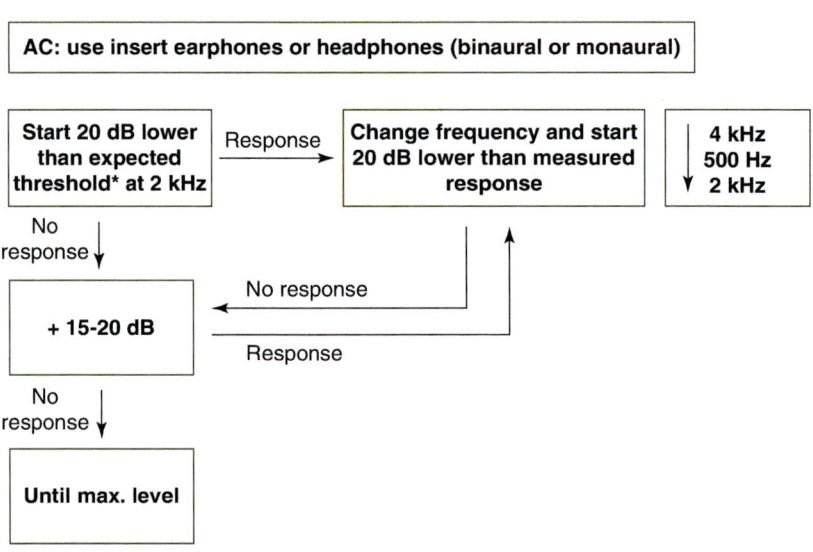

* Use information from BC or AC ABR threshold best ear

Characteristics of Responses Most common responses are opening eyes, moving eyelashes and starting or stopping sucking.

The stimulation and response delay are different for each child. Make sure that this delay remains the same for the same child.

The number of observable responses is limited because of the problem of habituation. With BOA it is not possible to confirm each response as with conditioned behavioural audiometry with older children.

Minimal Response Level (MRL) In threshold estimation with BOA, a clear distinction has to be made between neonates with normal hearing and neonates with a sensorineural hearing loss. While normal-hearing babies have higher response levels, hearing-impaired babies with a loss of 50 dBHL or more react closer to their real hearing threshold. These findings are well described by Delaroche (Delaroche et al. 2011). One possible cause is the phenomenon of recruitment, which results in faster loudness scaling in case of sensorineural hearing loss. Another cause is the effect of surprise, which makes babies with a hearing loss respond faster and clearer to a sound that is right on or just above their threshold level.

16.4.3 Visual Reinforcement Audiometry (VRA): 5–24 Months

Leading-In From the age of 5–6 months, most children can be conditioned to make a head turn response towards an auditory stimulus (Northern and Downs 2001). This will be the start of visual reinforcement audiometry (VRA) and conditioned orientation reflex audiometry (COR). In both cases a child's turning response is rewarded with a visual incentive. In VRA we use one reward. COR, using two rewards, requires adequate ability to localise a sound source. In this chapter we only discuss VRA.

Developmental Milestones In a normal developing child of 5–6 months of age, the intersensory phase is expanding rapidly. Every time an audible sound is presented, we use the natural strong interest in coloured and illuminated animation to condition the child to look at a visual reward as reinforcer.

This will not be possible in children with intersensory problems such as autism spectrum disorders.

Conditions VRA can be performed in a single or double soundproof booth where the lights can be dimmed. The younger the child, the more we prefer to work in a single booth. The test room should not be cluttered because, as in BOA testing, it is important to have fewer potential distractions. The examiner and test assistant keep the child attentive by being relatively quiet and not interfering while presenting the test stimuli. The presence of one parent, without interfering with the process of testing, can keep the child calm. The child needs to be seated in such a way that a head turn can easily be carried out in the direction of the visual reward.

Transducers All transducers can be used.

Stimuli Do not use pure tones but more reactive stimuli such as warble tone, frequency-specific fresh noise or narrowband noise. With hard-to-test children, it can be necessary to change the nature

of sound during the test or even use familiar sounds (i.e. barking dog, melody, crying baby, etc.).

Setup (Fig. 16.12)

Animation and Distractors A variety of visual animations and moving toys can be used as reinforcement. Moore et al. (1975) investigated in the effect of different kinds of visual animation. They demonstrated that auditory localisation behaviour of infants is influenced by the type of reinforcement. At the youngest age, three-dimensional animations are preferable, such as a flashing lamp and brightly illuminated mechanical toys (i.e. clown playing drums, dancing bear).

These toys have to be enclosed in a cloudy Lucite box so the child cannot easily see the animation until it is turned on. Older children, who are no longer interested in moving toys, can be reinforced with two-dimensional reinforcements such as a video or animation on a screen.

The test assistant keeps the child attentive, often by quietly playing with (interesting, but not fascinating) toys in front of the child. The tester and assistant should be relatively quiet, making

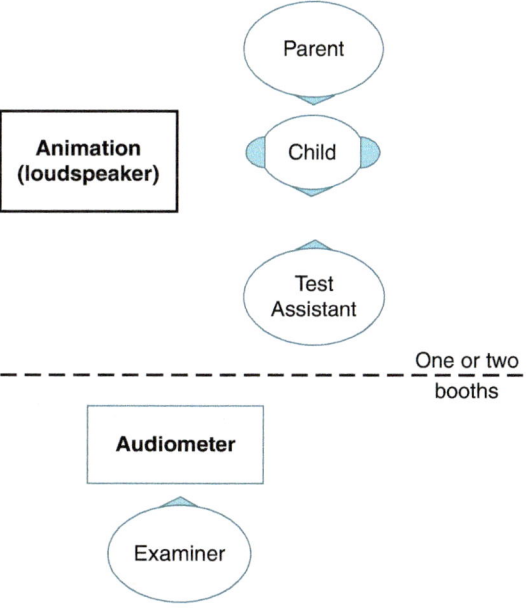

Fig. 16.12 The VRA test setup

sure not to interfere while the test stimuli are being presented. If the child finds the visual reinforcement very interesting, they might keep 'checking' (i.e. looking at the reinforcer even when there is no sound stimulus). In this case, the test assistant can help to distract the child from the visual animation, perhaps by temporarily increasing their level of play.

Procedure The test procedure consists of two phases: the conditioning and the testing. It is recommended to start with *bone conduction on a vibrotactile level (500 Hz at 65 dBHL or 250 Hz at 45 dBHL)* in order to condition the child to respond by consistently turning the head to the auditory stimulus and to determine the bone-conduction thresholds.

Continue with *insert earphones* or *headphones* to determine ear-specific and air-conduction thresholds.

Follow the steps as indicated in the flowchart (Fig. 16.13).

In case of uncooperative behaviour when the vibrator or headphones cannot be used, it is better to work in free field in the first contact. In a second stage, ear-specific information should be obtained.

Free-field measurements are also useful for looking for the functional gain with hearing aids or cochlear implants. Soundfield can also be necessary to give the parents insight into the level of hearing impairment.

In cases where any contact with a vibrator or headphones is refused, it will be necessary to start in a soundfield setting.

Follow the steps as indicated in the flowchart (Fig. 16.14).

Minimal Response Level Normal and hearing-impaired children can respond close to their hearing threshold at this age. Madell and Flexer

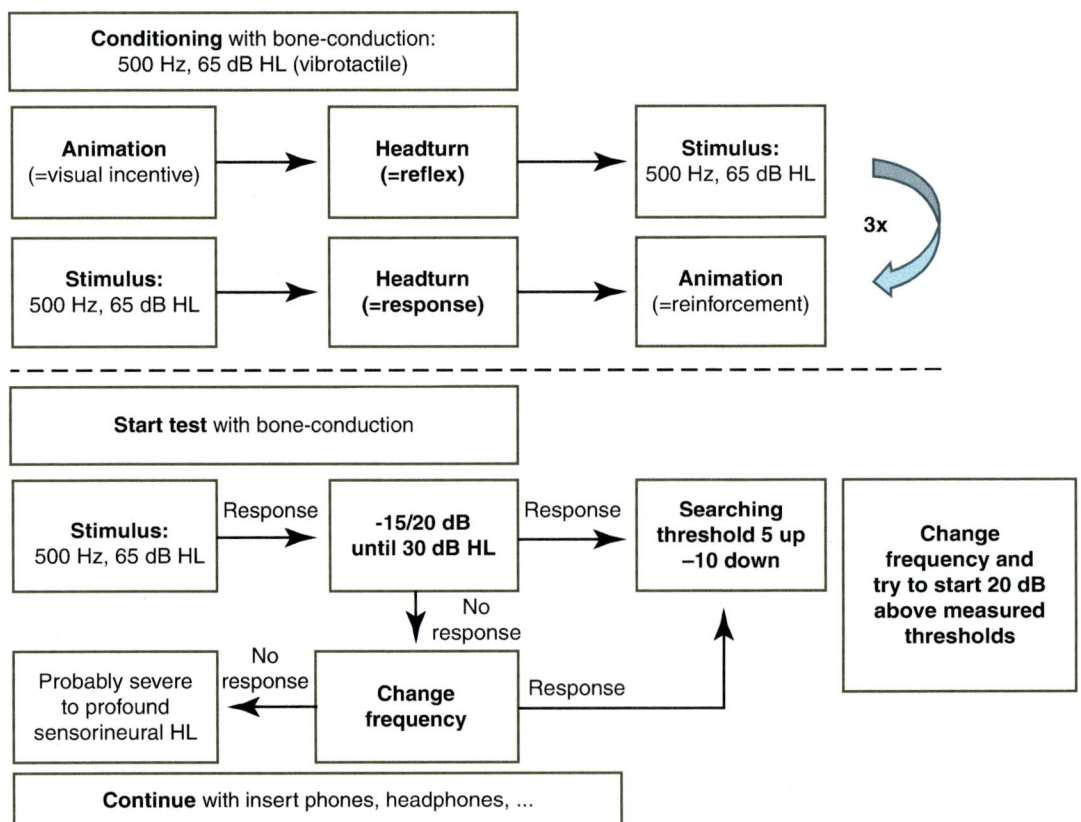

Fig. 16.13 Flowchart VRA starting with bone conduction

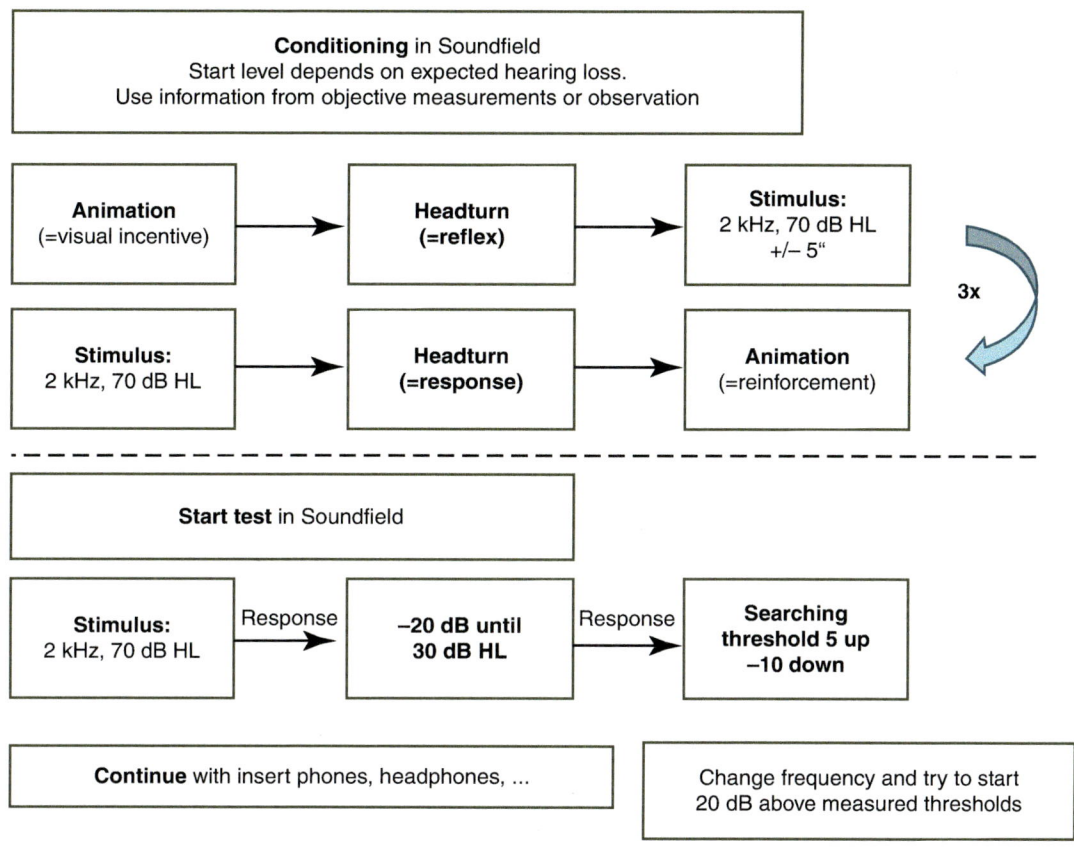

Fig. 16.14 Flowchart VRA starting in free field

(2008) refer to several studies that demonstrate that infants with normal hearing respond to sound no higher than 15–20 dBHL and children at the age of 1 respond at an adult level. But it is still advisable to consider MRL because of the variability between the children. The responses in normal-hearing infants should not be higher than 20 dBHL for all frequencies.

16.4.4   Conditioned Play Audiometry (CPA): 2–5 Years

Leading-In CPA demands the child's active cooperation by the need to perform an action after hearing an audible sound. This is a conditioned response. The 'listen and drop' task is the simplest level. The child may drop a block in a box or put a ring on a ring bar. The 'button-pushing response' to activate a rewarding

animation requires a higher cognitive level, so is reserved for older children. Nowadays an interesting PowerPoint programme can be used on a laptop that is controlled by a remote mouse operated by the audiologist. Madell (Madell and Flexer 2008) called this special technique a 'computer-assisted reinforcement' procedure.

Developmental Level Most normally developing children are near 2 or 2.5 years of age before they are able to participate in play audiometry. Children with hearing loss, who frequently have hearing tests, are able to learn the 'listen and drop' task earlier.

Infants at this age are not always cooperative. The paedaudiologist will have to be creative and flexible to obtain enough testing information. Good paedaudiologists should be able to swap quickly between a repertoire of games with different levels of engagement aimed at children with different attention and cooperation. More complex games can be reserved for older or more mature children. Similarly, different types and levels of reward are appropriate. Even CPA may need to be conducted over several sessions in order to obtain appropriate diagnostic information.

Conditions If one audiologist is performing the test, it will be necessary to work in a single soundproof booth. The test room should be orderly to avoid distraction. Parents can be involved during the training.

Transducer Air- and bone-conduction transducers can be used in order to determine the type and the degree of hearing loss.

Stimuli Use warble, fresh noise, speech sounds or familiar sounds.

Setup The infant can sit at a children's table or in a highchair.

There are several possible test setups for CPA (example in Fig. 16.15). The examiner, preferably, has to sit close (next or in front of) the child in order to control their play quickly and provide social reinforcement.

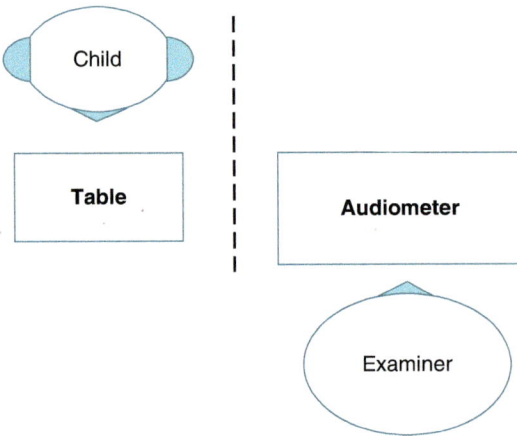

Fig. 16.15 An example of CPA test setup

Material A variety of toys is needed, according to the interest and developmental age of the child, to be able to maintain the child's attention.

The 'listen and drop' task is the simplest level.

When using 'computer-assisted reinforcement', the child uses a push button that is not actually connected to the computer. The button-pushing responses of the child will only be rewarded if there was a preceding stimulus. Even a simple PowerPoint presentation with popular characters can maintain the child's interest.

Procedure The test procedure consists of two phases: conditioning and testing. To start the conditioning session, it is important to use a test stimulus that the child is expected to hear. In case of doubt, bone conduction on a vibrotactile level (e.g. 500 Hz, 65 dBHL) can be used.

Conditioning

- Demonstrate the task: the audiologist and the child hold a toy to the ear to highlight the listening task. When sound (for at least 5 s) is presented, the audiologist clearly shows the presence of sound by dropping the toy. The child has to do the same. Parents can be involved as model in this process.
- After a few presentations, the child should hold the toy to the ear alone. When the sound is presented, the child must drop the toy on his/her own. Encouragement is important in this stage.
- When the child is able to do the task without assistance, the test can start.
- Remark: conditioning should be repeated at any point during the test if the child's responses seem to indicate that it is no longer cooperating.

Testing

- Rapidly decrease the level of the sound that you used for the conditioning task and continue with the '5-up-10-down method' (Hughson-Westlake method) to find the threshold.
- Change frequency and start approximately 20 dBHL above the measured response.

- If the child gets bored, the toys may need to be changed.
- When testing with insert earphones or headphones and the attention span seems to be very short, it may be necessary to change to the left or right ear after each frequency.

Response Behaviour At this age the child may respond at an adult level, so the term 'minimal response level' is no longer appropriate.

16.4.5 Hard-to-Test Populations

Testing children with special needs follows the same principles as testing children without additional problems. Some adaptations and specific knowledge may be necessary.

The test procedure should be chosen according to the developmental age of the child.

- For children with an intellectual disability, the response can be significantly delayed because of the time needed to recognise the sound. Therefore it can be necessary to hold the stimulus for a longer time.
- For children with motor problems, modifications of the child's position may be necessary in order to enable clearly visible responses (i.e. when a child does not have a good trunk control, an adapted chair is needed).
- Children with visual impairment can benefit from dimming the room light in order to make the reinforcers more visible.
- For blind children, tested with VRA, air-puff reinforcement can be used instead of a visible reinforcer.
- A special technique for this population is TROCA (tangible reinforced operant conditioning audiometry), where food or tokens are used as reinforcers instead of flashing lights or mechanical toys.

With disabled children, it will be important to keep the carers involved in behavioural tests to be able to choose the right procedure and material and interpret the child's responses.

16.5 Assessment of Tinnitus: A Specialist Otorhinolaryngology Perspective

Armagan Incesulu, Haldun Oguz, Mustafa Asim Safak, Ahmet Atas, Songul Aksoy, Levent N. Ozluoglu and Ross Parfitt

16.5.1 Introduction

Tinnitus evaluation may differ according to the time of onset (acute vs chronic), classification (objective vs subjective) and accompanying symptoms; however the following steps are important and performed for almost all cases.

16.5.2 Medical History

An adequate, detailed medical history should gather information about possible causes (such as hearing loss, use of ototoxic drugs including salicylates, quinine and aminoglycosides), otological diseases (sensation of aural fullness, sporadic rotatory vertigo lasting hours or temporarily reduced hearing may give a hint towards Meniére's disease), non-otological diseases (head trauma, noise exposure and the presence of metabolic diseases symptoms) and the tinnitus percept: date of onset (sudden or gradual), localisation (unilateral, bilateral, in the head), subjective loudness, type of sound (ringing, buzzing, hissing, pulsating), temporal aspects (continuous, intermittent), anything that improves or worsens the tinnitus and impact upon the patient (depression, anxiety, concentration, disrupted sleep). Questionnaires to evaluate the psychological influence of the tinnitus (e.g. the Tinnitus Handicap Inventory (Newman et al. 1996)) are useful.

16.5.3 Clinical Examination

Ear, nose, throat and neck examination is essential for each patient in order to investigate possible objective causes. During this assessment, a temporomandibular joint examination, evaluation of the cranial nerves as well as auscultation of the neck and pressure on the ipsilateral internal jugular vein are very important. If the tinnitus percept is reduced during these manoeuvres, venous aetiology may be indicated (Baguley et al. 2013). In a very small percentage of tinnitus patients, the vascular aetiology may be due to a serious underlying disease such as carotid artery dissection or aneurysm.

16.5.4 Audiological Examination

Audiological Tests Given that subjective tinnitus results primarily from dysfunction within the auditory system, an age-appropriate assessment of hearing thresholds and middle ear status may be worthwhile, both to investigate the aetiology and to guide later treatment. Such audiological investigation may include pure-tone audiometry, speech discrimination testing and tympanometry; however, uncomfortable loudness-level measurements and acoustic reflexes should be treated with caution as high-level sound may exacerbate the symptoms. Some evidence suggests that a causative auditory system change may not be detected by standard audiological tests (e.g. Fabijańska et al. 2012); therefore testing in an extended high-frequency range and the use of otoacoustic emissions may be useful. Electrocochleography (e.g. to diagnose Meniére's disease), auditory brainstem response audiometry (e.g. as one diagnostic element in detecting a cerebellopontine tumour) and videonystagmography (to find vestibular system dysfunction) (Jozefowicz-Korczynska et al. 2005) may be performed if needed.

Psychophysical and Other Tinnitus Assessment Procedures Audiological tests, such as pitch and loudness matching, are often performed in order to define the parameters of the tinnitus percept. Note that these tests can only be carried out when the patient's tinnitus is audible to them during testing.

The basic procedure of pitch matching involves presenting low-level pure tones or narrowband noise of various frequencies and asking the patient to indicate when the pitch is similar to that of their tinnitus. As tinnitus may be a spectrum of sounds, spectral matching is recommendable (Henry 2016).

Loudness matching involves increasing the level of the pitch-matched signal (usually in 1 dB steps) from threshold until the patient indicates that the loudness of the signal and tinnitus are equal. Both procedures should be performed separately for each affected ear if possible.

It is important that the patient understands the difference between pitch and loudness during these matching procedures and that they are informed that slightly inexact responses will not hinder their treatment. The matched frequency and level are often indicated by a 'T' sign on the audiogram.

Minimum masking level (MML) procedures are sometimes carried out with the aim of determining the patient's ability to suppress the tinnitus signal in the presence of competing noise. The level of white noise (a random broadband signal that includes energy at all audible frequencies) is gradually increased until the patient reports any change in the tinnitus (such as it becoming louder, softer or entirely suppressed). Tinnitus matching and MML testing are, however, much less simple than one might expect. For example, many different matching procedures have been tested since the 1940s, and this area is rife with methodological difficulties (see Henry and Meikle 2000).

Tinnitus can be inhibited for up to approx. 1 min in some patients following some types of auditory stimulation. This is known as residual inhibition. According to Henry (2016), studies should be performed to develop optimal stimuli for extending this effect as basis for a new therapeutic approach.

Given that parameters of the tinnitus percept, such as loudness, pitch and quality, do not correlate with the perceived severity of tinnitus (Meikle et al. 1984), tinnitus severity may be better assessed from questionnaires (such as the Tinnitus Handicap Inventory) which address the patient's perception of their tinnitus and its impact on their lives, rather than psychophysical investigation.

The Tinnitus Handicap Inventory (THI) (Newman et al. 1996) contains 25 self-reporting closed questions related to personal and social situations as well as feelings about tinnitus, designed to assess the severity of the patient's tinnitus (slight, mild, moderate, severe or catastrophic). Other tinnitus questionnaires exist, such as the Iowa Tinnitus Handicap Questionnaire (Kuk et al. 1990), the Tinnitus Reaction Questionnaire (Wilson et al. 1991) and the Tinnitus Functional Index (TFI) (Henry et al. 2014). But as to our knowledge, there are no standardised questionnaires for children (BSA 2014).

In patients with hearing impairment, the ten-item Tinnitus and Hearing Survey (THS) (Henry et al. 2015) separates complaints caused by hearing loss from self-perceived problems induced by tinnitus by two specific subscales.

Given the strong connection between tinnitus and anxiety/depression, some clinics also use tools such as the Hospital Anxiety and Depression Scale (Zigmond and Snaith 1983) to assess the psychological impact on the patient.

16.5.5 Other Investigations

If, e.g. chronic otitis media or otosclerosis is suspected, high-resolution computed tomography may be useful. Magnetic resonance imaging is usually the preferred method in patients with asymmetric hearing loss or asymmetric tinnitus to rule out a cerebellopontine angle tumour, such as vestibular schwannoma. Magnetic resonance angiography or venography may be necessary in cases with suspected cerebral ischemia, dural sinus thrombosis or neoplastic lesion (Sismanis 2011). Doppler ultrasonography may be useful for exploring the vascular structures in the neck. Blood tests for haemodynamic and metabolic diseases are also important.

16.6 Assessment of Tinnitus in Children and Teenagers: A Specialist Paediatric Audiology and Hearing Therapy Perspective[1]

Claire Benton and Charlotte Rogers

Prevalence figures for tinnitus in children in studies vary from 12 to 36% for normally hearing children and go up to 66% for children with known hearing loss (Shetye and Kennedy 2010). The impact of tinnitus in children is in many ways similar to that in adults, affecting sleep, concentration and listening skills (Kentish et al. 2000).

History A comprehensive history is necessary to get a full picture of the impact of a child's tinnitus, ensuring the child's views are fully included. The history should cover the following points:

- Description of tinnitus sounds: children can use very descriptive language to describe what they hear such as 'buzzing bees', 'swishing' and 'like a train'. Younger children may find it helpful to draw a picture of their tinnitus. Where possible details of onset, duration and how often it is heard are useful.
- Impact of tinnitus: there are currently no standardised tinnitus questionnaires for children. The impact and concerns of both the parents and the child should be investigated. Finding out about the effects of the tinnitus on school and home life is important. Standardised measures of anxiety and depression in children do exist and these can be helpful.
- Hearing difficulties and other audiovestibular symptoms: it is important to rule out any physiological reason for the tinnitus. Asking about their history of otitis media with effusion is also useful.
- Medical and neurological factors: any history of head trauma or noise trauma should be noted. Other general medical problems may also be relevant, for example, migraine can be associated with auditory sensitivity and tinnitus.
- Factors affecting their tinnitus: some children or families may have noticed factors that make the tinnitus better or worse, such as tiredness, school situations or stress. It is very important to find out about the child's whole life and potential areas of stress for him or her, such as bereavement or family breakdowns.

Clinical Assessment Children with tinnitus can find audiometry particularly stressful; they may have a history of being difficult to assess or have variable results on previous tests. The testing environment should be child-friendly and the children

---

[1] Article written on behalf of the British Society of Audiology Paediatric Tinnitus Working Party. Supported by the British Tinnitus Association.

given time to do the test at their own pace. It is important to establish accurate, ear-specific thresholds by using age-appropriate testing techniques. Observing the child closely throughout the test allows any signs of anxiety to be seen and reassurance given. Otoscopy and middle ear admittance measurements are always needed to rule out any pathology that requires further medical treatment. At the moment, loudness discomfort measures or any tinnitus-matching tests are not recommended, as there is very limited evidence for either the diagnostic or therapeutic benefit of such tests (see Henry and Meikle 2000 for a review of such psychoacoustic measures).

16.7 Speech Audiometry at the Phoneme and Word Level

Frans Coninx

16.7.1 Introduction

The assessment of auditory processing and recognition of speech in infants and children is important and complex: the child's performance in a speech recognition test does not only depend on the auditory skills themselves but also on factors such as language, cognition, articulation

and speech, visual cognition, attention and concentration. Typically, these factors are dynamic and changing over time.

On the basis of the Erber (1982) level scheme for auditory functions (see Table 16.2), auditory speech tasks may be at the detection, discrimination or identification/recognition level. Comprehension is not included here, as such tasks (certainly in an open-set format) depend not only on hearing but are also determined to a major extent by central linguistic and cognitive skills.

16.7.2 Phoneme/Syllable Level

The Ling 6 sound test contains the phonemes for [m], [ah], [oo], [ee], [sh] and [s], being familiar speech sounds that cover the relevant speech range from 250 to 8000 Hz (Ling 1989). It can be used with children who are conditioned for and familiar with this task, by professionals as well as by parents. The aim is to assess or verify the detection or identification of the six speech sounds. With the purpose of assessing detection thresholds, a Ling sounds-based PTA paradigm can be used. The 'Ling Audiogram' result (see Fig. 16.16) will show the six thresholds for detection-identification of Ling sounds and allows a quick and easy judgement of whether or not the six phonemes will be audible in normal running speech.

Table 16.2 Structured overview of auditory tests at four functional levels

Level	Phonemes/syllables	Words
Detection	• Ling 6 sound test • Ling sounds-based 'PTA' (pure-tone audiometry)	
Discrimination	• A§E (auditory speech sounds evaluation; Govaerts et al. 2006) • H-LAD (Heidelberger Lautdifferenzierungstest; Brunner et al. 1998) • WADT (Wepman auditory discrimination test; Ross 1979)	
Identification/ recognition		Pictures tasks • MTS (Monosyllable-Trochee-Spondee test; Erber and Alencewicz 1976) • AAST (adaptive auditory speech test; Coninx 2005)
Comprehension		

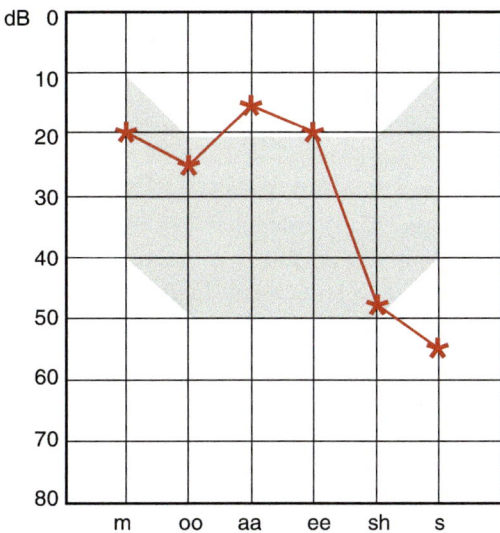

Fig. 16.16 The Ling Audiogram shows the detection thresholds of the six Ling sounds. In this example, the detection of the two fricatives is most likely not good enough for them to be heard in normal running speech

The Ling test uses isolated phonemes. A phoneme-based test, supplying useful information on the basic listening level, can also be based on a syllable form or even by using words.

As an example, in the A§E test (Govaerts et al. 2006), syllables are used to assess detection and discrimination skills in the child. For both skills, an operant conditioning protocol is used: visual reinforcement audiometry (VRA). The response of the child to the detection of a stimulus or the discrimination of a stimulus change has to be reliably observed by using paradigms that are adapted to the developmental level of the child. For the difficult-to-test younger children, VRA (Coninx and Moore 1997) might be the only successful procedure; for older children the usual techniques of play audiometry can be used. With the VRA paradigm, not only phoneme detection but also phoneme discrimination can be investigated. In case of discrimination testing, the visual reinforcer is presented in relation to a sudden change in a sequence of 'stable' phonemes or syllables (e.g. da-da-da…) to another sequence of 'stable' stimuli (e.g. ta-ta-ta…). A response of the child to the sudden phoneme change is visually reinforced.

For older children, easier and faster 'same-different'-based tasks can be used instead. The stimuli would be two isolated phonemes (/s/-/f/ or /a/-/e/), two consonant-vowel syllables (/sa/-/fa/ or /ba/-/be/) or a minimal word pair, differing only in the same phoneme contrast (seat-feet or ball-bell). Various responses from the child can be used: verbal feedback ('same' versus 'different') or pointing to a picture representing same or different. Isolated phonemes or consonant-vowel syllables are considered to be better than words, because the test result for word pairs might depend on the vocabulary of the child. This is caused by lexical neighbourhood processes (Janse and Newman 2013). Examples of word-pair tests are H-LAD (German, Brunner et al. 1998) and WADT (English, Ross 1979).

16.7.3 Word Level

The most frequently used form of speech audiometry in children is based on words. Children develop skills to identify or recognise words earlier than full sentences, as well as earlier than isolated phonemes (a subskill of phonological awareness). For test applications, the words have to be chosen carefully in order to be within the vocabulary of children in the target group age. The words can be presented as stimuli in a quiet or noisy environment. The response of the child can be different: repeating the spoken word or pointing (or comparable action) to a picture or object that represents the spoken word.

A well-known version of such a test is the MTS test (Erber and Alencewicz 1976). Each of the 12 words used as stimulus is in one of three prosodic categories: monosyllables, trochees and spondees. Within each of the categories, the child can identify the words only on phoneme-based information. A picture table is shown (see Fig. 16.17) and the child has to point; as a consequence, the MTP test is a closed-set test. Results can be analysed and differentiated at the prosodic and segmental levels. These closed-set tests are available in many languages.

Open-set tests are similar to many tests used for adult listeners. This choice has to be carefully

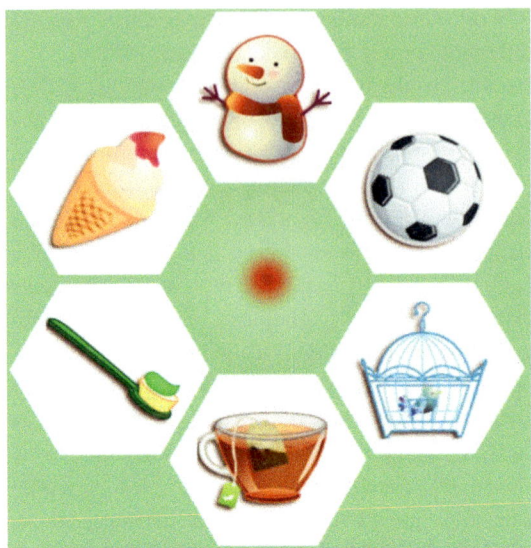

Fig. 16.17 The six spondee words of the AAST UK version. The red dot in the centre cell is a visual prompt during stimulus presentation

considered, as interference with the speech and articulation skills and the vocabulary of the child will interfere with the auditory skills as such. A gold standard for an open-set test—for English—is the PB-K test (Haskins 1949), which uses a phonetically balanced word list for children in kindergarten.

Closed tests as described above are used to assess a word recognition score at a selected fixed intensity, at 65 dB SPL or at the individually different most comfortable level (MC).

In order to find a speech recognition threshold (SRT), the test has to be repeated several times; alternatively, adaptive paradigms have to be used. A typical example is the adaptive auditory speech test (AAST) for children aged 3–4 years and above (Coninx 2005). Only six spondee words are used, requiring little vocabulary and minimised influence of working memory and visual cognition when the child is searching for the correct picture to click. When using touchscreen technology, even young children 3–4 years old can do the test and are highly motivated and concentrated. After typically 1–1.5 min, the SRT measurement is completed. The result of a test

has to be interpreted by taking the age-dependent normal values into account. An important advantage of AAST is the multi-lingual applicability with nearly language-independent normal values.

For tests in noise, steady-state noise can be used (more likely related to cochlear dysfunctions) (Smits et al. 2013) or fluctuating noises, such as the International Female Fluctuating Masker (IFFM, Holube et al. 2011). The thresholds in IFFM are more likely to be related to retrocochlear dysfunctions, i.e. auditory processing disorders.

Future development in speech audiometry for children will increasingly include modern technology with a touchscreen. This not only increases the level of motivation but also opens options for remote screening and testing.

16.8 Auditory Processing Tests

David R. Moore, Nicole G. Campbell, Doris-Eva Bamiou and Tony Sirimanna

16.8.1 Diagnosis

There is no universally agreed diagnostic procedure for auditory processing disorder (APD). Diagnostic recommendations have been made by the American Speech-Language-Hearing Association (ASHA 2005a, b) and by the American Academy of Audiology (AAA 2010) on the basis of several distinct forms of impaired auditory processing outlined below. These recommendations are a quasi-international standard, but in practice the recommendations are adhered to only loosely in the USA (Emanuel et al. 2011) and even less so in other countries (Hind et al. 2011). In Germany, the diagnosis of 'auditory processing and perception disorder' (APPD) (German: auditive Verarbeitungs- und Wahrnehmungsstörung (AVWS)) includes auditory-specific cognitive impairment as a designated form of APPD (GSPP 2014), but only if that impairment is judged not to be described by other, more widely accepted terms (e.g. attention deficit disorder, language impairment). Some countries have issued practice guidelines in recent years, rather than stipulating comprehensive diagnostic measures and criteria. For example, Australian Hearing has implemented standard procedures for the diagnosis, assessment and management of some aspects of APD (Hearing 2013), and the British Society of Audiology (BSA APD SIG 2011a, 2018) has provided an evidence-based commentary to guide practice.

An attempt to reach a consensus on APD definition, diagnosis and management was the principal aim of two ASHA Technical Reports (ASHA 1996, 2005b). Auditory processing was determined to be the neural mechanisms underlying auditory discrimination and pattern recognition; temporal, spatial and binaural aspects of hearing; and perception of competing and degraded auditory signals. APD was defined as a disorder of one or more of these processes, which were noted to be necessary for both non-verbal and verbal perception. Impairments should be diagnosed by using a variety of non-standard indices (e.g. case history, observation of behaviour, questionnaires) and standardised auditory measures that use both non-verbal and verbal stimuli. Electrophysiological testing (e.g. auditory brainstem response, cortical event-related potentials) was also suggested, but details were not provided. Performance of at least two standard deviations (s.d.) below the (standardised) mean on two auditory processing tests, or 3 s.d. on one test, is 'generally required for diagnosis'. However, both the ASHA Reports and the AAA (2010) Guidelines suggest that the number and specific type of tests used should depend on individual cases. There is no specification of the number of tests that are to be used, and the criteria, like those proposed by other groups, are arbitrary. Statistically, the more tests performed, the more likely an individual will fail two of them. Wilson and Arnott (2013) showed in a large sample of children ($n = 150$) that diagnosis rates of APD can range from 7 to 93% depending upon which criteria are applied, even using the same test battery.

16.8.2 Differential Diagnosis

Because APD typically presents as problems involving speech perception, most guidelines recommend verbal (speech-based) testing. For example, the commonly used SCAN test battery (Keith 2009) has four core tests that all use verbal stimuli. Verbal stimuli used in APD diagnosis vary from nonmeaningful phonemes (e.g. 'da') or vowel-consonant-vowel (VCV) syllables (e.g. 'ata') through commonly used short words (e.g. 'dog') to longer words and whole sentences. These stimuli all involve a lesser or greater degree of memory and linguistic processing that strong neurological evidence suggests occurs beyond the central auditory nervous system, primarily in the anterior temporal and frontal brain lobes. An ongoing debate concerns whether APD should be diagnosed when only 'unimodal' auditory deficits (i.e. deficits specific to hearing) are found (Cacace and McFarland 2013).

To segregate distinctly auditory deficits, non-verbal testing for APD diagnosis is also recommended. Non-verbal tests attempt to isolate those aspects of auditory processing, as listed above (discrimination, pattern recognition, etc.), that are the building blocks of everyday listening. However, there is scant evidence that either these tests or those involving verbal stimuli are very good predictors of the listening problems that people being assessed for APD typically report (Moore et al. 2010; Watson and Kidd 2009). The most common of those problems are, for children, academic difficulties and attentive listening to speech, especially in challenging environments (AAA 2010; Campbell et al. 2012). In addition, listening to both speech in everyday life, and to verbal or non-verbal tests in the clinic, necessarily accesses cognitive resources that are mostly 'supra-modal' (not specific to hearing). These resources include attention, memory, fluid intelligence, motivation and emotion. Professional guidelines urge the clinician to ensure that the person being tested is attentive, but clinicians cannot adequately control or measure cognitive influences on perception with current test procedures.

16.8.3 Occurrence of APD (not ADP!) with Other Learning Problems

Only a small proportion of children referred to audiology clinics are assessed for APD, and only a fraction of them receive a diagnosis of APD (Hind et al. 2011; Moore and Hunter 2013). However, around 20% of all children have speech, language, attention, behaviour, reading or intellectual difficulties. A substantial proportion of them perform poorly on tests of auditory processing (Amitay et al. 2002; Ferguson et al. 2011; Miller and Wagstaff 2011; Sharma et al. 2009) or have behaviour that overlaps extensively with that seen in children with APD (Chermak et al. 1999, 2002). Conversely, most children diagnosed with APD have multiple difficulties. Do those children all have APD? The relation between perception and cognition has been debated for well over 100 years, i.e. whether hearing or vision determines intelligence or vice versa (Spearman 1904). Surprisingly, this is still a current debate, for example, in the extensive literature on language and reading difficulties (Ziegler et al. 2005, 2009). The problem faced by hearing specialists is whether to diagnose APD, recognising the non-specific nature of the diagnosis, or to refer a child for a more broadly based assessment. In either case, identifying individual difficulties is the first step towards appropriate treatment.

16.8.4 How Should APD Be Diagnosed?

It has recently been suggested (Dillon et al. 2012) that specific treatment for APD may be an appropriate form of management for some children. These children may be identified by specific tests, for each of which there is a specific treatment, delivered in a hierarchical fashion. A scheme that builds on this model is shown in Fig. 16.18. The aim here is to provide a specific strategy for clinicians, so that a more rational and uniform approach to management may be delivered and the outcome may better describe a more specific problem that the child has.

16.8.5 Current Situation and Way Forward

Several groups around the world have now issued APD statements, guidelines or white papers, including the American Speech-Language-Hearing Association (ASHA 2005a, b), the American Academy of Audiology (AAA 2010), the British Society of Audiology (BSA APD SIG 2011a, b, 2018; Moore et al. 2013), the Canadian Interorganizational Steering Group for Speech-Language Pathology and Audiology (2012), the German Society of Phoniatrics and Paediatric Audiology (Nickisch et al. 2015), the Australian National Acoustics Laboratory (NAL 2015), the Dutch Position Statement (De Wit et al. 2017) and more recently a group in Europe which has published its perspective on APD (Iliadou et al. 2017). As outlined at the beginning of this section, there is no universally agreed diagnostic procedure for APD, but all of the above documents contribute to international debate and better understanding. High-calibre research, alongside international and interdisciplinary dialogue, is imperative for informing future evidence-based practice. The APD MESHGuide, a new evidence based online resource, offers practical guidance (Campbell et at. 2019).

Remediation is considered in Sect. 18.14.

Fig. 16.18 Draft hierarchical scheme for the diagnosis and rehabilitation of APD by using specific assessments that incorporate a problem-orientated approach and differential and adaptive testing (Moore 2012; Dillon et al. 2012). The scheme includes conventional (audiometry) and research procedures. A validated questionnaire (e.g. ECLiPS (Barry and Moore 2014, Barry et al. 2015)) assesses everyday listening skills which, if deficient, lead to further objective assessments. Electrophysiological testing (auditory brainstem and frequency-following response) determines ear and brainstem function objectively. Speech-in-noise testing (e.g. LiSN-S) and 'forced attention' dichotic CV syllables (Hugdahl et al. 2009) differentiate 'bottom-up' and 'top-down' processing difficulties

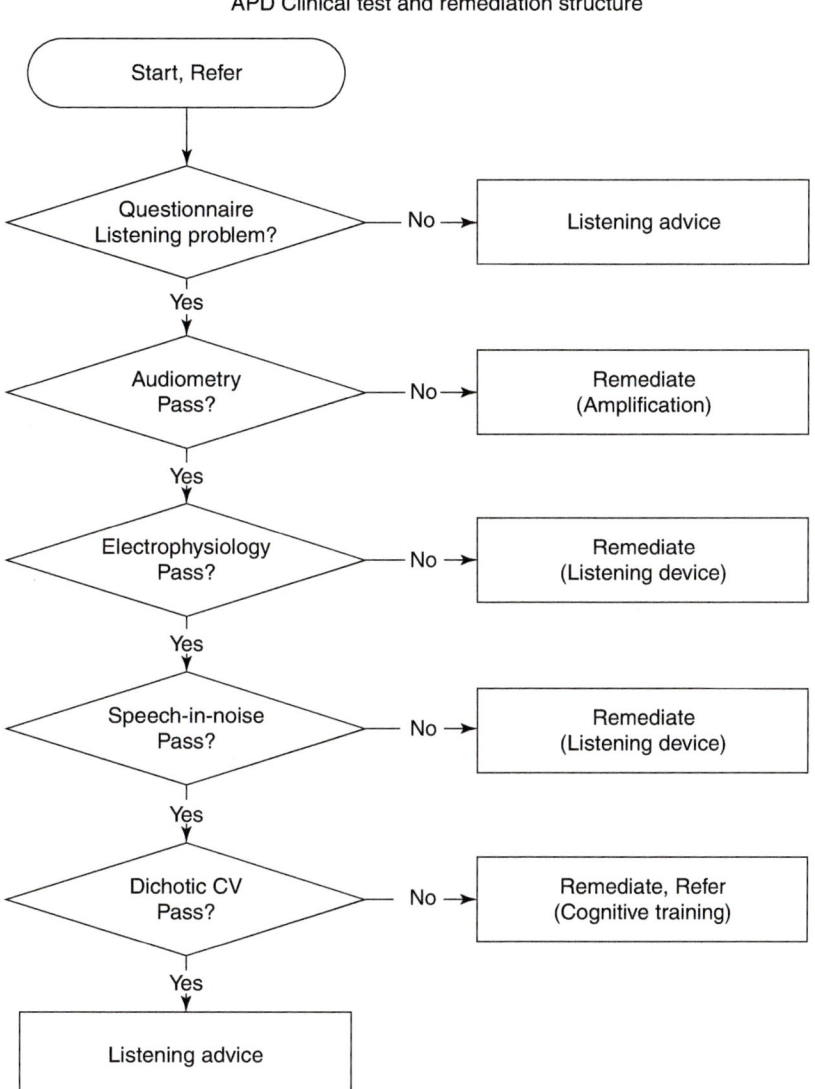

16.9 Acoustic Immittance Measurements

Piotr Świdziński and Ross Parfitt

16.9.1 Introduction

The ability of the tympanic membrane and ossicular chain to transfer sound waves from the outer ear canal through the middle ear is known by a variety of related terms that have specific techni-cal differences but are often used interchangeably in common practice: admittance, compliance, conductance, immittance and susceptance. The opposite (i.e. the ability of the mechanism to resist the transfer of sound) is typically known as impedance or reflectance.

The stiffer the tympanic membrane, the smaller the amount of sound energy admitted through it (low admittance) and the greater the amount of sound energy reflected by it (high impedance). Sound energy is optimally trans-ferred across the tympanic membrane when the air pressure within the middle ear is equal to that in the outer ear canal, which is typically an atmospheric pressure of 0 daPa (decapascals). Most common disorders of the middle ear, such as middle ear effusion or Eustachian tube dysfunction, affect the air pressure within it, thus stiffening the tympanic membrane.

Tympanometry measures admittance at various external air pressures in order to assess the presence of middle ear disorders. Acoustic reflex testing assesses the basic function of cochlear and retrocochlear structures involved in the acoustic reflex arc by measuring the lowest sound level that triggers contraction of the stapedius muscle (a response that stiffens the ossicular chain and tympanic membrane, resulting in measurably reduced admittance).

While tympanometry and acoustic reflex testing are not direct measures of hearing sensitivity, tympanometry especially plays a crucial role in audiological diagnostics, providing further information in cases of conductive hearing loss and functioning as a cross-check to support the findings of other tests. Other acoustic immittance tests exist (e.g. acoustic reflectometry and tests of Eustachian tube function) but are not common in clinical audiology and are not discussed in this article.

The patient does not need to respond actively during acoustic immittance tests and should ideally be still and quiet.

A tympanometer is used for both tympanometry and acoustic reflex testing. Modern tympanometers are often hand-held, wireless devices linked to a computer, but older, larger stand-alone models are still common. The core mechanism is a probe consisting of three tubes: one attached to an air pump, another to deliver a pure tone (the 'probe tone') generated by a miniature loudspeaker in the main body of the device and the third a microphone (Fig. 16.19). The probe is inserted into the outer ear canal with an appropriately sized disposable silicone tip to create an air-tight seal with the wall of the ear canal.

International standards for the calibration of tympanometers (ISO 60645-5 2005) must be adhered to.

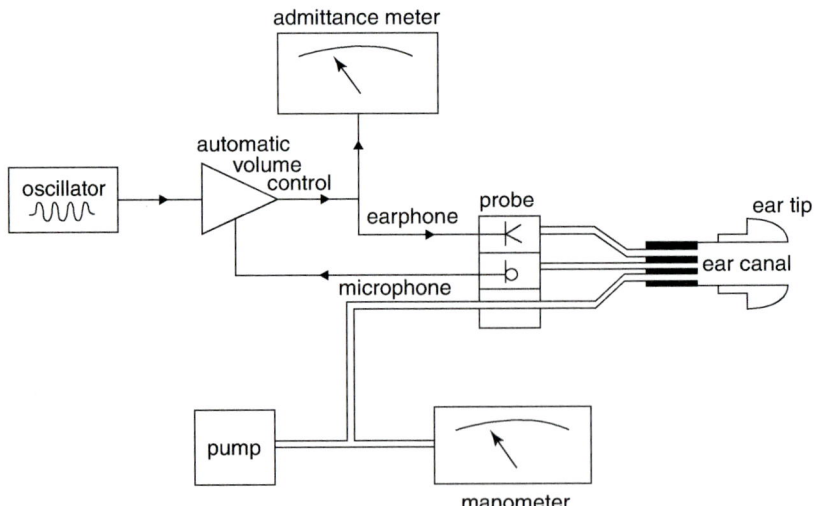

Fig. 16.19 Block diagram showing key components of an audiometer, the probe and ear tip and an air pump and manometer, to change and monitor air pressure in the outer ear canal; the probe tone is generated by the oscillator and conducted to the ear canal via the earphone; the microphone measures the level (dB SPL) of the probe tone in the opening of the outer ear canal and admittance is calculated. Image from Benton et al. (2004), with kind permission from Wiley © (2004)

16.9.2 Tympanometry

In tympanometry, the air pressure in the outer ear canal is varied over the course of a few seconds, usually from a positive pressure of approximately 200 daPa to a negative pressure of approximately −400 daPa at a rate of 50 daPa/s (e.g. British Society of Audiology (BSA) 2013). The rate and direction of pressure change can be varied in many tympanometers, but variations in these parameters play little role in typical clinical testing. During this pressure change, the probe tone (usually 226 Hz) is played constantly into the outer ear canal, and the sound that is reflected from the tympanic membrane is detected by the microphone.

Results and Interpretation A real-time trace of the inverse of the amount of reflected sound across the gradually changing air pressure is shown on the tympanometer display (admittance or compliance on the Y-axis and pressure on the X-axis) (Fig. 16.20). This graph is known as a tympanogram. The peak of the trace (i.e. the point at which compliance is highest) reflects the point at which air pressure is equal in the outer and middle ear. This can be compared

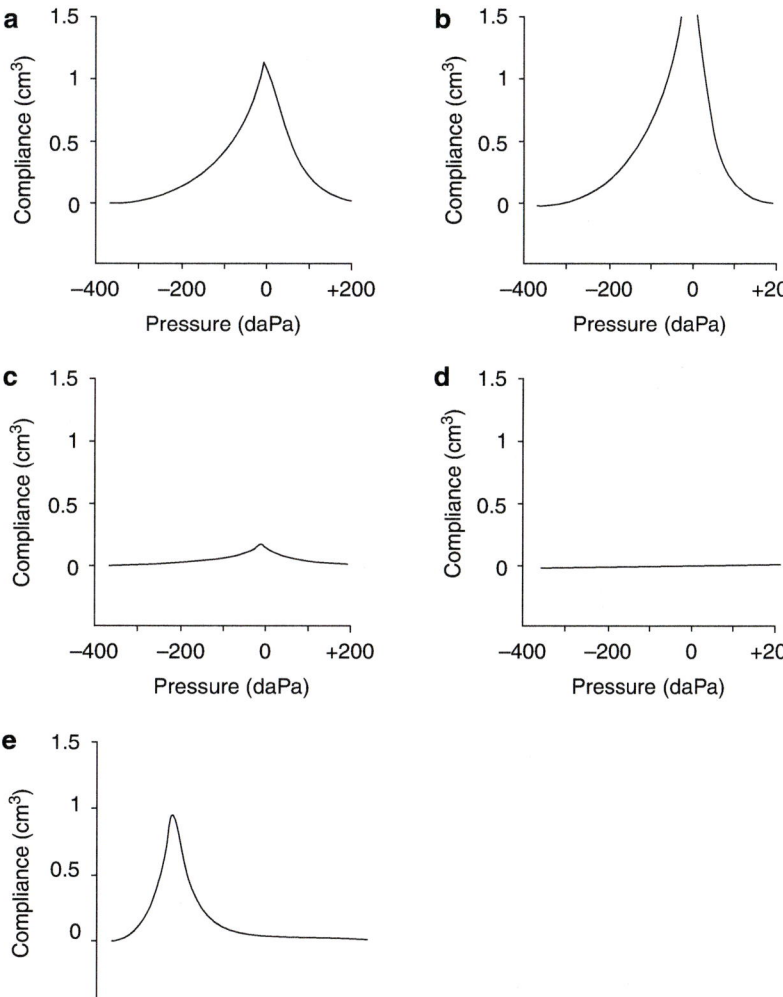

Fig. 16.20 Classic tympanogram shapes: (**a**) normal, (**b**) hypermobile, (**c**) reduced compliance, (**d**) flat, (**e**) negative

Table 16.3 Tympanogram interpretation when using a 226 Hz probe tone

Result				Description	
Peak compliance (mL, mmho/L or cm³)	Peak pressure (daPa)	Ear canal volume (cm³)	Interpretation	Commonly used term	Audiogram type (Jerger 1970)
Adults: 0.3–1.6 Children (6m–6y): ≥0.2 (BSA 2013)	Adults: −50 to +50 Children: −200 to +50 (BSA 2013)	Adults: 0.6–1.5 Children: 0.4–1.0 (BSA 2013)	Middle ear function within the normal range	Normal	A
Higher than normal range	Normal range	Normal range	Hypermobile tympanic membrane or ossicular discontinuity	Hypermobile	A_D
Lower than normal range	Normal range	Normal range	Reduced tympanic membrane mobility or ossicular fixation	Reduced compliance	A_S
Flat	Flat	Normal range	Middle ear effusion	Flat	B
Normal range	Higher than normal range	Normal range	Possible acute middle ear pathology	Positive	–
Normal range	Lower than normal range	Normal range	Eustachian tube dysfunction	Negative	C
Flat	Flat	Higher than normal range	Grommet in situ and patent or perforated tympanic membrane	Large ECV	–
Flat	Flat	Lower than normal range	Occluding wax or incorrectly placed probe	–	–

with established normal values (Table 16.3). The volume of air required to fill the ear canal (known as the equivalent ear canal volume (EECV) or just the ear canal volume) is also recorded and can be compared with norms (Table 16.3). The norms shown in Table 16.3 are from the British Society of Audiology (2013). Other norms exist but the principle of interpretation is the same.

A classification system is sometimes used when reporting tympanometric results (e.g. Jerger 1970, Table 16.3), but it is preferable to report the actual values obtained. Some commonly used terms for reporting audiogram shape are also indicated in Table 16.3 (Fig. 16.20a–e showing common results of tympanometry).

Many tympanometers also show gradient, which essentially reports the sharpness or roundedness of the peak, but different manufacturers use different algorithms to calculate this (BSA 2013) so interpretation is not always clear. Gradient does not play an important role in typical clinical interpretation guidelines.

Contraindications Tympanometry should be preceded by otoscopy or microscopy in order to check for occluding wax (which should be removed before testing), inflammation or infection of the outer ear (which would contraindicate the test owing to the risk of pain or cross infection) and to provide a visual check of the status of the tympanic membrane. Previous tympanic membrane surgery may contraindicate tympanometry because of the risk of the change in air pressure damaging the TM.

The change in air pressure should not be painful or uncomfortable for the patient in the absence of infection or inflammation. Subjects with pressure-related vertigo, such as that resulting from a perilymph fistula in the vestibular system, may feel some dizziness, but other patients typically do not.

Tympanometry can be performed on compliant patients of any age, with a small but crucial change in probe tone frequency for younger patients (see below).

Probe Tone Frequency For children younger than 6 months corrected age (BSA 2013) or with an ear canal volume less than 0.9 mL (Limberger et al. 2007), a probe tone frequency of 1000 Hz provides a better measure than the typical 226 Hz. This is because the walls of the infant ear canal are more flexible than those of older children and adults, and a large contribution to the tympanometry results can come from the compliance of the outer ear canal itself, rather than just the middle ear. This effect is reduced when using a higher-frequency probe tone.

Tympanogram interpretation is different when using the 1 kHz probe tone. The BSA recommends the following steps (see BSA 2013 for more details): first, drawing a straight line between the compliance levels at the positive and negative pressure endpoints of the trace (−400 and +200 daPa) and then determining if the peak is above this line ('positive peak'), when middle ear function is essentially normal, or below this line ('negative peak') or there is no peak, when ear function should be considered abnormal (Fig. 16.21).

Wideband Tympanometry Wideband tympanometry (also known as 3D or multi-frequency tympanometry) is a comparatively new development in the clinic. A broadband click is used instead of a single-frequency probe tone, allow-

ing the response of the middle ear at many frequencies (typically 226–8000 Hz) to be measured simultaneously. The results are plotted on a 3D tympanogram (Fig. 16.22). The main measure is no longer compliance or admittance (in mmho/L, mL or cm³) but absorption or absorbance, which is the percentage of the incoming sound energy absorbed by the middle ear (i.e. the percentage which is not reflected back to the probe microphone). Wideband tympanometry has potential benefits, such as measuring multiple different-frequency tympanograms simultaneously, the ability to measure without changing air pressure (therefore safer for postoperative ears) and potentially higher diagnostic power for specific pathologies such as otosclerosis (Shahnaz et al. 2009).

16.9.3   Acoustic Reflex Testing

Significantly suprathreshold acoustic stimulation triggers the acoustic reflex, by which the stapedius muscle contracts. The acoustic reflex arc involves acoustic stimulation of the inner hair cells of one cochlea, followed by afferent innervation of the vestibulocochlear (8th) nerve and the ventral cochlear nucleus, where it is sent to both superior olivary complexes and medial nuclei of the facial (7th) nerve, leading to bilat-

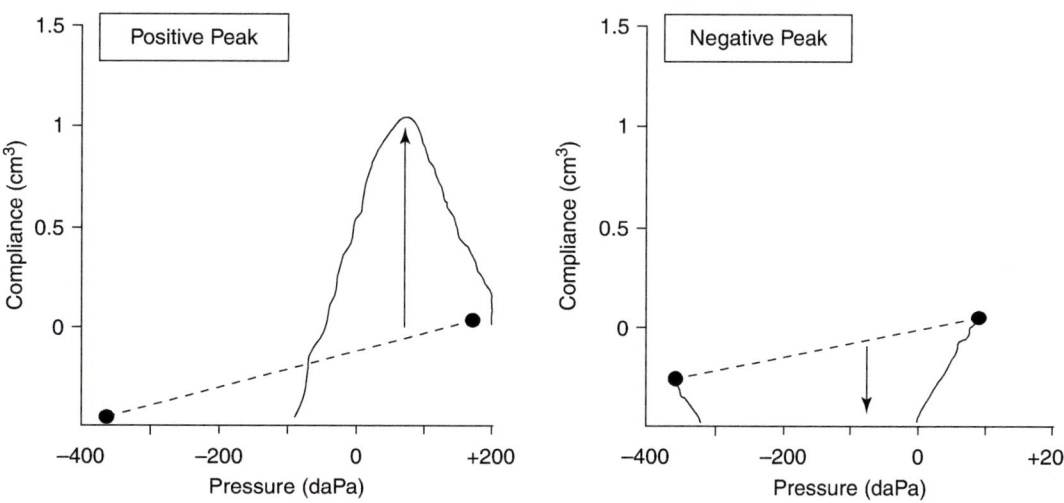

Fig. 16.21 Interpretation of tympanometry when using a 1 kHz probe tone. Image adapted with kind permission of the British Society of Audiology (2013)

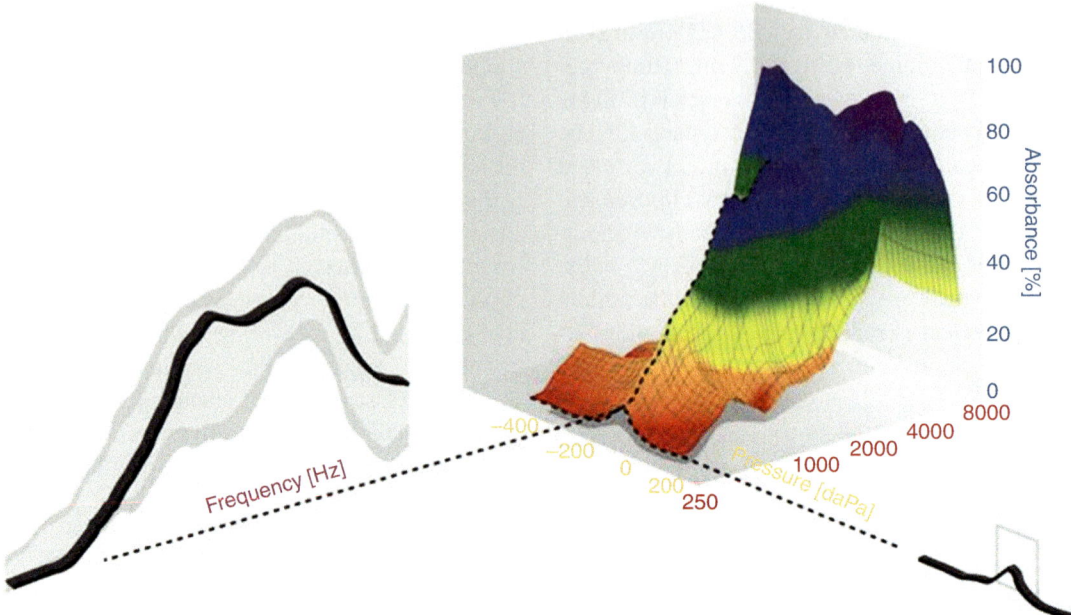

Fig. 16.22 A hypothetical 3D tympanogram on which frequency (in red), pressure (in orange) and absorbance (in blue) are shown. Image copyright and with kind permission of Interacoustics

Fig. 16.23 Schematic diagram of the acoustic reflex arc. *ME* middle ear; *SM* stapedius muscle; *VIII* vestibulocochlear (8th) nerve; *SOC* superior olivary complex; *VII MN* medial nucleus of 7th nerve; *VII* facial (7th) nerve

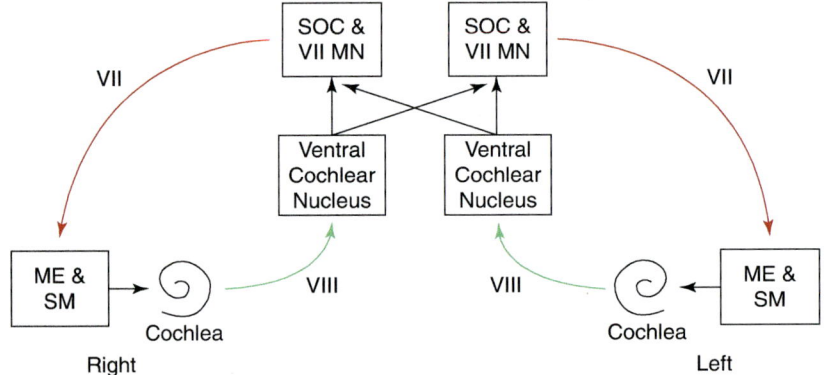

eral efferent innervation of the 7th nerve terminating at the stapedius muscles of both ears (Fig. 16.23). The contraction of these muscles stiffens the ossicular chain and therefore stiffens the tympanic membrane, a movement that is measurable using a tympanometer.

The acoustic reflex threshold (ART) is the lowest signal level (dB SPL) from which the acoustic reflex is triggered. This is usually performed at the pressure level of peak compliance for the individual subject, in order that the response obtained is as large as possible. Various stimuli can be used, typically pure tones (500, 1000, 2000 and 4000 Hz) and broadband noise. Normal values are 90–95 dB SPL for tones and 70–75 dB SPL for broadband noise (Margolis 1993). Pathology affecting any of the structures of the reflex arc can lead to an increase in the threshold or obliterate the response. The acoustic reflex can also be used as an objective measure of recruitment in sensorineural hearing loss (Metz recruitment) (e.g. Thomsen 1955).

Ipsilateral measurements involve stimulating and measuring the response in the same ear; contralateral measurements involve stimulating one ear and measuring the response in the other. Combining the results of ipsi- and contralateral measurements can help identify the site of lesion within the reflex arc (e.g. Emanuel 2009). Contralateral measures are also used to avoid test artefacts that can result from interference of the probe and stimulus tones on ipsilateral measurements (Benton et al. 2004).

Esser et al. (1987) proposed comparing acoustic reflex thresholds elicited by pure tones with those elicited by narrowband noises. They found a 10 dB higher pure-tone acoustic reflex threshold in children with auditory processing disorder (APD). Kunze et al. (2016) could not find such differences in children with or without APD. Another test paradigm in occasional use is the reflex decay. In this test, an acoustic reflex is evoked by a sound signal sustained over a longer duration, usually 10 s. The reflex decay is the amount of time during this acoustic stimulation by which the reflex is sustained at a level above 50%. The normal value is ≥ 5 s. A shorter duration (i.e. a quicker decay) may indicate retrocochlear or other central pathology, such as myasthenia gravis (e.g. Bischoff et al. 1989). This test is, however, not used very often these days because of the prevalence of imaging techniques such as MRI.

Acoustic reflex testing can be performed on patients of any age; however, given that high signal levels are required to evoke a response even in normal-hearing patients, caution should be used, especially in patients reporting sensitivity to loud sounds, such as suspected hyperacusis, patients with lowered uncomfortable loudness levels or patients with tinnitus. Contraindications are otherwise the same as for tympanometry.

16.10 Otoacoustic Emissions

Jakub Dršata and Ross Parfitt

16.10.1 Nature and History of Otoacoustic Emissions

Otoacoustic emissions (OAEs) are very low-level sounds that arise during active contraction of the outer hair cells in the organ of Corti. OAEs can emerge spontaneously or be evoked intentionally. The principle of OAE measurement is the detection of these sounds.

OAEs result from the active mechanism of cochlear amplification (see Sect. 1.4), a function that plays a significant role in the sensitivity and discrimination of hearing (Heinz et al. 2001). Detection of the OAE is therefore an important objective indicator of inner ear function. It does not, however, provide information about the general status of the auditory system.

The history of OAE measurement dates back to 1978, when David Kemp first demonstrated their existence and utility. Since then, several types of OAE, which can be used in the investigation of inner ear function, have been discovered. The most important clinical applications of OAEs are the transient-evoked OAE (TEOAE) and distortion product OAE (DPOAE). The most common use of TEOAEs these days is in newborn hearing screening programmes (see Sect. 17.1) and of DPOAEs is in audiological monitoring during therapy with ototoxic drugs (see Sect. 14.9).

16.10.2 Measurement of OAEs

All forms of OAE are based on the same principle: the detection of sounds produced by the cochlea by using a microphone placed in the outer ear canal. The difference between the various OAE methods lies essentially in the stimuli presented and the processing of results.

OAE measurements are widely used in audiological examination. Various pieces of OAE test equipment can be used, from basic screening devices to more sophisticated clinical equipment, depending on the purpose of the investigation. Screening devices are most common in routine practice and are typically user-friendly, to the extent that they can be operated by trained staff with a secondary school level of education. These devices report results simply as 'positive' (OAEs are present) or 'negative' (OAEs are absent and further audiological investigation is necessary) (Fig. 16.24).

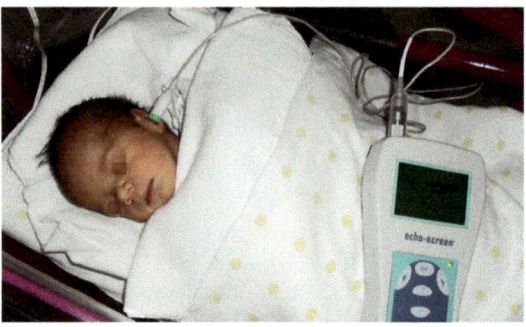

Fig. 16.24 Automated transient-evoked otoacoustic emission (TEOAE) testing in a neonate. Photograph with kind permission of the parents

In all OAE tests, the response must be distinguished from the presence of noise. Various strategies are used to aid this process, such as filtering of the response to focus only on the frequency range of interest. Averaging strategies work on the principle that the response occurs within a particular time window following the stimulus but that noise is essentially random. The results of repeated stimulation and measurement ('sweeps') can therefore be averaged to reduce the effects of noise. Artefact rejection is also employed in order to reject sweeps that feature recorded sound higher than a particular sound pressure level, thereby omitting transient background noise.

Measurement Conditions The main conditions for acquiring reliable OAE results are:

- Proper sealing of the probe in the outer ear canal (i.e. no gap between the probe and the ear canal, orientation of the probe towards the tympanic membrane, no blockage of the ear canal (e.g. by earwax)
- Use of fully functional equipment (appropriate calibration, probe patency)
- Minimal environmental/background noise and subject movement during testing
- Absence of middle ear pathology (see below)

Because OAEs are produced in the cochlea but measured by a microphone in the outer ear canal, the ability to measure them is hindered by the presence of any obstruction in the middle or outer ear. Such obstructions may include amniotic fluid and debris present in the ears of neonates on the first day of life, possibly until the second day of life.

OAEs do not measure the status of the entire auditory system: they may still be present in retrocochlear pathology (e.g. auditory neuropathy).

The reproducibility of OAEs decreases with age, and they are almost never present in any cochlear pathology. The correspondence of age-related 'normal' hearing with OAE presence in older age is, therefore, not reliable.

16.10.3 Spontaneous OAEs

Definition and Principle Spontaneous otoacoustic emissions (SOAEs) are typically stable pure tones that are measurable at low intensity (10–15 dB SPL) in the outer ear canal (Hall 1999) and that occur without external stimulation. Current models of SOAE genesis suggest that SOAEs arise as a consequence of a complex sustained motion of the outer hair cells in the organ of Corti (Kemp 2002).

Importance, Interpretation and Limitations SOAEs are measurable in 30–40% of healthy young people (Burns et al. 1992). SOAEs can occur at a broad range of frequencies, but the specific frequency measured is not particularly important, as it does not relate to the outer hair cell function at a particular tonotopic area of the cochlea. The detectability of the SOAE is critically dependent on the health of the cochlea; therefore the presence of an SOAE is a particularly sensitive indicator of the integrity of cochlear function. However, the absence of measurable SOAE should not necessarily be taken to indicate pathology or hearing loss.

16.10.4 Transient-Evoked OAEs

Definition and Principle Transient-evoked otoacoustic emissions (TEOAEs) are very brief sounds, emitted over a 0.5–4 kHz frequency range as a response to transient (i.e. very brief) acoustic stimuli (usually click stimuli) presented at intensities of 80–85 dB SPL. A series of transient stimuli with very short pauses in between is used during stimulation.

Importance and Limitations TEOAE testing is quick (usually lasting just a few seconds for each ear), non-invasive and technically simple and requires no active participation by the patient, and the result is very reliable. These features make TEOAE testing particularly useful for neonatal hearing screening, applied in an automated version.

The presence of amniotic fluid or debris in the ears of neonates may mean that the TEOAE cannot be recorded shortly after delivery.

Newborns at risk of retrocochlear pathology, such as auditory neuropathy, should not be tested solely with TEOAEs. Automated auditory brainstem response (AABR) audiometry should be used in these cases.

Interpretation High-level click stimuli reliably evoke a response if the hearing threshold is 20 dB HL or better across frequencies (Kemp 1978). TEOAEs can also be evoked (though less reliably) where mild sensorineural hearing loss is present (Robinette et al. 2007). The presence of TEOAE indicates healthy cochlear function (Kemp 2002) or, at worst, mild hearing loss (Ramos et al. 2013). A positive response is indicated where the signal-to-noise ratio (SNR) is 3–6 dB (i.e. the level of the response is 3–6 dB higher than that of the noise), depending on the protocol and equipment used. Modern screening devices typically include automated data analysis, with positive result (TEOAE present) indicated as 'pass' or similar. A negative response ('refer') indicates that normal hearing cannot be confirmed and the patient requires further investigation (such as rescreening or AABR testing if within a newborn hearing screening programme).

Clinical devices enable more detailed analysis of the test data for scientific and research purposes. First studies are performed in the clinical application of high-frequency TEOAEs (Goodman 2011).

16.10.5 Distortion Product OAEs

Definition and Principle DPOAEs are responses from non-linear elements in the cochlea to stimulation by the travelling wave of basilar membrane displacement that is the physical manifestation of sound as it moves through the cochlea. The stimulus is different from that used in TEOAE testing: instead of a click stimulus, two pure tones with closely related frequencies (f1, f2) and intensity characteristics (L1, L2) are presented simultaneously to the same ear. The intermodulation of these two tones results in predictable basilar membrane activity at various different relative frequencies (known as distortion products). Clinical DPOAE testing measures the amplitude of the response at one of these frequencies, usually 2f1-f2, which has the largest amplitude.

Importance, Interpretation and Limitations DPOAEs complement TEOAEs in clinical practice. DPOAEs seem to be less sensitive to minor and subclinical conditions of the hearing system (e.g. Kemp 2002). They allow the measurement of a wider frequency range than do TEOAEs (Kemp 2002). The response corresponds to the hearing threshold near the f2 frequency (Robinette and Glattke 2007). Furthermore, the DPOAE can be detected at higher frequencies (up to 8 or 10 kHz), and the measurement of DPOAE amplitudes seems to be a promising method for the early detection of high-frequency cochlear damage (e.g. ototoxicity, noise). DPOAEs can be detected up to a cochlear hearing loss of 50 dB HL, so they cannot be used to identify lower degree hearing impairments.

The examination is usually performed and interpreted for individually tested frequencies, though many OAE devices run through a standard battery of tested frequencies. The frequency-specific characteristic of DPOAEs means that manufacturers have been able to place on the market devices with DPOAE-based hearing threshold estimation (DP audiogram) capability. The extrapolation of DPOAE input/output function can be used to estimate pure-tone thresholds up to 8 kHz (Stavroulaki et al. 2001). The clinical importance of DPOAE is nonetheless a subject of further research.

16.10.6 Other Applications of OAEs

Sustained-frequency otoacoustic emissions are acoustic responses to the presentation of an ongoing tonal stimulus. The wide frequency range (0.5–8 kHz) of these emissions enables the study of inner ear function at specific frequencies, whereas TEOAEs and DPOAEs rely on the combined response or interaction of various areas of the basilar membrane. Because they are identifiable even in cases of severe hearing loss, sustained-frequency otoacoustic emissions may be useful as an objective tool for the quantification of hearing loss. Nevertheless, the method is still an object of study and is not routinely used in practice.

The bibliography includes some articles in which other applications of OAE have been studied, such as synchronised SOAE (Jedrzejczak et al. 2008), stimulus-frequency OAE (Ellison and Keefe 2008) and others. The utility of these methods is under study, and their clinical use in routine practice is currently marginal.

16.11 Evoked Response Audiometry

Arne Knief and Jakub Dršata

16.11.1 Impact of Evoked Response Audiometry on Objective Threshold Audiometry

The gold standard for hearing threshold assessment is pure-tone audiometry (PTA). This subjective examination requires active cooperation of the investigated subject. On the basis of this principle, a significant number of subjects (infants, psychically and mentally diseased persons, malingerers) cannot pass the examination. Objective threshold audiometry is aimed at covering this gap. Among

its methods, evoked response audiometry (ERA) plays a most prominent role in newborn hearing screening and in auditory diagnostics of children and their hearing rehabilitation (Dršata et al. 2015). Optimising these methods has been a subject of intensive research, the essential goal of which is finding a method with the best correlation to the behavioural threshold (Stapells 2011).

Different stages of the auditory pathways can be studied with ERA signals. Early latency responses originate from the brainstem (the auditory brainstem response, ABR). Auditory steady-state responses (ASSR) have generators in the brainstem as well as in more central areas (Picton et al. 2003). Middle latency responses come from the primary auditory cortex and long latency response from the non-primary cortex (cortical ERA, CERA).

The more centrally the source of activity can be found, the more the activity is dependent on the arousal of the patient. Nonetheless, we are in a favourable position to measure responses from the brainstem in sleep as well as in narcosis.

16.11.2 Broadband and Frequency-Specific ABR

There are two kinds of ABR measurements: one with broadband stimuli such as clicks, to test the integrity of the auditory pathway and to determine an overall hearing threshold, and the other with frequency-specific stimuli, to estimate the hearing thresholds at these frequencies.

Jewett (1970) and Jewett et al. (1970) first described evoked responses from the brainstem. Therefore, the potentials from the brainstem were named after him, Jewett waves, enumerated I to V or J1 to J5. The sources of these waves were analysed by dipole analysis of the EEG (Scherg 1991). Scherg (1991) showed that wave I is identical with the compound action potential of the auditory nerve. Wave II is generated at the opening of the internal acoustic meatus, the porus acusticus internus. Scherg (1991) found the source of wave III in the efferent part of the ventral cochlear nucleus, still in the ipsilateral hemisphere. Waves IV and V were thought to originate from the nucleus olivaris superior and lemniscus lateralis, on the ipsi- and contralateral sides, respectively.

Nevertheless, Picton (2011) argued:

> At any point in time after … 2.5 ms, activities in many different places in the pathway overlap.

The conventional click stimulus (Fig. 16.25) excites the whole cochlea, which results in a clear identification of Jewett's waves. The intensities used in air-conduction ERA reach from threshold up to 100 dB HL and above. A healthy auditory pathway is characterised by latencies of Jewett's waves that fall within standard ranges. These latency ranges are age-specific. Jewett's waves appear delayed and altered or can vanish in cases of conductive, sensorineural or retrocochlear neural hearing loss. An increase of the synchrony of neural activation is reached with the use of chirp stimuli (Fig. 16.25), which compensates for the frequency-dependent time delay of sensory perception in the cochlea (Dau et al. 2000; Elberling et al. 2007). The sound of a broadband chirp starts at low frequency and ascends to high frequency. These stimuli evoke higher amplitudes near threshold and therefore a higher signal-to-noise ratio than clicks.

Although the click and broadband chirp stimuli excite the whole cochlea and generate relatively well-synchronised neural responses, these stimuli are not frequency-specific, and so these methods cannot assess the hearing levels at individual frequencies.

Tone bursts (Fig. 16.25) compared with clicks are referred to as providing more frequency-specific results with good correlation with pure-tone behavioural thresholds (Gorga et al. 2006). In a clinical setting, the tone bursts are usually presented at 500, 1000, 2000 and 4000 Hz. To enhance the frequency specificity, the tonal stimuli are masked with notched-noise (so-called notched-noise ABR, Picton et al. 1979). The effect of masking is to prevent neighbouring regions of the cochlear from contributing to the response (Fig. 16.26, review: Stapells and Oates 1997).

Comparable to the application of broadband chirps for overall threshold ABR measurements, narrowband chirps can also be used for frequency specificity, for which a part of the whole chirp is cut out and covers, for example, only one octave (Wegner and Dau 2002). Especially at low frequency, this narrowband chirp is more efficient than tone bursts (Mühlenberg and Schade 2012). Narrowband chirps have been proven to generate a frequency-specific response, with a reduction in the test time in newborns (Ferm et al. 2013).

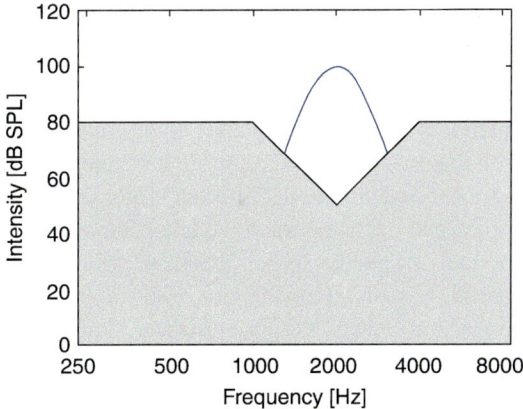

Fig. 16.26 Schematic spectrum of a frequency-specific notched-noise stimulus. The noise (in grey) is notched at the stimulus frequency and masks the possible side bands of the tone burst (blue line)

Fig. 16.25 Time courses of different stimuli are shown: left click, middle tone burst and right chirp stimulus

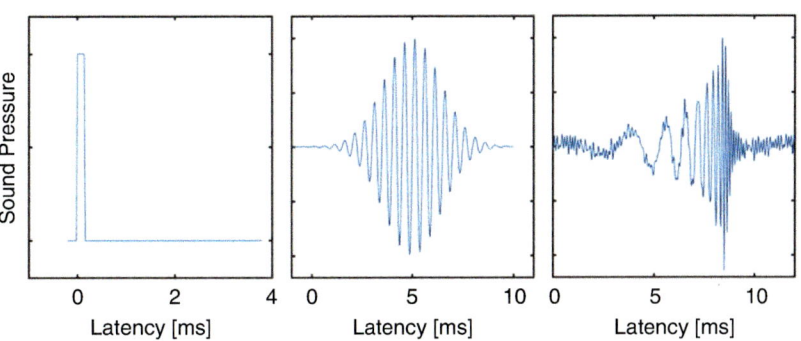

The reliability and technical mastering of the described methods have resulted in commercially available ABR systems that offer different kinds of stimulation.

16.11.3 Auditory Steady-State Responses

Auditory steady-state responses (ASSR; steady-state evoked potentials, SSEP; amplitude-modulation following response, AMFR) are auditory evoked potentials from the brainstem and more central structures (Beck et al. 2007). The stimuli are usually continuous pure tones, modulated mostly with modulation frequency around 80 Hz in the amplitude alone or both the amplitude and frequency domains (see Sect. 16.12).

16.11.4 Cortical ERA

Cortical ERA (CERA), also called measurement of late auditory evoked potentials (LAEP), is much less sensitive to muscle activity than ABR, with the drawback that it is more dependent upon vigilance and attention. Different kinds of stimuli come into consideration: clicks, tone bursts (frequency-specific with a length of ≥50 ms) or speech signals (consonant-vowel or vowel-consonant-vowel). The examination requires the patient's alertness or at the most video sedation.

The reliance of CERA on the patient's mental vigilance makes the method suitable mostly for calm but awake children and adults (Stapells 2002). The observed response pattern is in a time window between 50 ms and 1000 ms and in a frequency range from near 0 Hz up to 600 Hz.

The CERA has its diagnostic value in the examination of the auditory pathway beyond the brainstem up to the cortical areas. The clinical application of CERA is not widespread and is at its beginnings. It can be useful in questions of maturation (after hearing aid use or cochlear implant), auditory neuropathy, auditory processing disorders, psychogenic hearing disorders, autism, lesions of the central pathway or aggravation and simulation (Walger et al. 2014).

16.11.5 Specific Issues of ERA

Patient Preparation and Test Implementation For measurement of ERA—broadband and frequency-specific—the patient has to be relaxed and quiet. This means in the case of small children that they have at least to sleep. In the case of well-collaborating parents of children without neuropsychological disorders, the examination can be performed in a deep natural sleep following previous sleep deprivation. However, sedation or general anaesthesia is often to be considered for infants. Among sedatives and anaesthetics, different drugs are used (e.g. chloral hydrate, midazolam, ketamine and others), with variable pharmacokinetics, side effects and brain activity influences. Anaesthesia is accompanied by risks and a high logistic effort and therefore to be avoided if possible. The alternative is natural sleep. Sleep can be induced by oral administration of melatonin, a naturally produced hormone adjusting the circadian rhythm (Schmidt et al. 2007).

The measurement is comparable to that of electroencephalography. Four electrodes are fixed: at the vertex (or forehead), both mastoids and a ground electrode at the forehead, cheek, clavicle or neck (Fig. 16.27). The stimuli are presented via headphone, insert earphones or bone-conduction transducer (Fig. 16.28).

Frequency-specific ERA examination is carried out principally in an identical way as for conventional click-evoked ABR. Obviously, the estimation of hearing thresholds at individual frequencies takes a significantly longer time, and feeble responses to the specific stimuli are more sensitive to the ambient noise and measurement conditions than with a conventional click-evoked ABR.

Estimated Audiogram (EA) The ABR objective threshold audiometry is based on detection of the most prominent Jewett V wave. The key point for the correct hearing level estimation is a faultless identification of the Jewett's wave complex. An expert audiologist takes the pattern of waves, their latencies and intensities and the age of the patient and measurement condi-

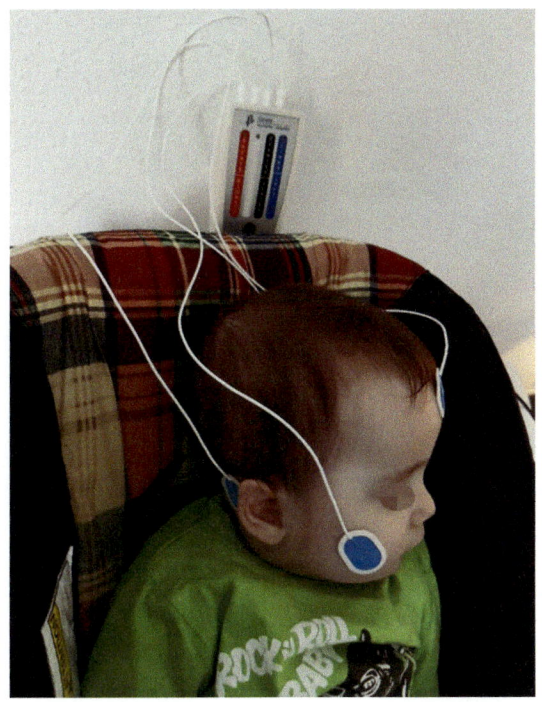

Fig. 16.27 Electrode positions are shown for ERA measurement. Photo from electrodes with kind permission from Ambu GmbH, photo from preamplifier of the BERA system Corona with kind permission from Pilot Blankenfelde medizinisch elektronische Geräte GmbH, photo of child with kind permission of the parents

tions into account when identifying Jewett waves and the thresholds. Evaluation algorithms specified by the manufacturers, based on automatic ERA analysis, may help to eliminate possible human errors. Nevertheless, the results of these algorithms have to be scrutinised critically, especially in nonoptimal measurement conditions.

ASSR measurements generally follow a complete automatic protocol. Thresholds at different frequencies as well as in both ears can be measured simultaneously (Korczak et al. 2012). This possibility leads to a shorter measurement time for a complete threshold estimation. Nevertheless, the major advantage of ABR (controlled by an audiologist) over ASSR remains the traceability of the results and the information about the auditory pathway given by the wave pattern above thresholds.

Level-Latency Curves With the correct identification of the Jewett waves, especially wave V and in addition wave I, information is gained for differential diagnosis. The latencies of the waves t_V and t_I are a function of stimulus intensity: they increase with decreasing intensity. The compari-

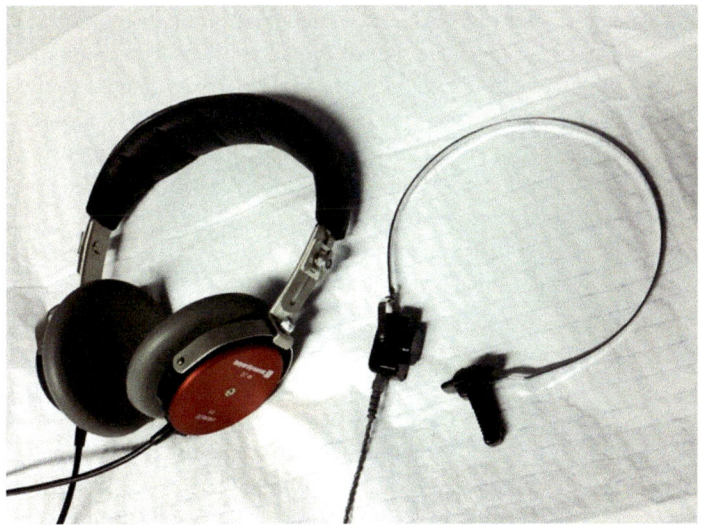
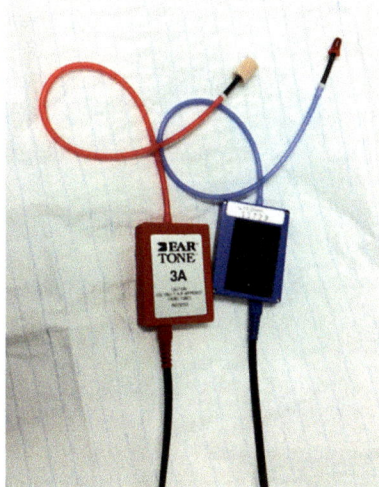

Fig. 16.28 For stimulation in ERA measurement, a headphone (left, type DT 48 with kind permission from Beyerdynamic), a transducer for bone-conduction ERA (middle, type B-71 with kind permission of Radioear) and

insert earphones (right, with kind permission from 3M) can be used. The earphones are shown with different ear tips for different sizes of the ear canal

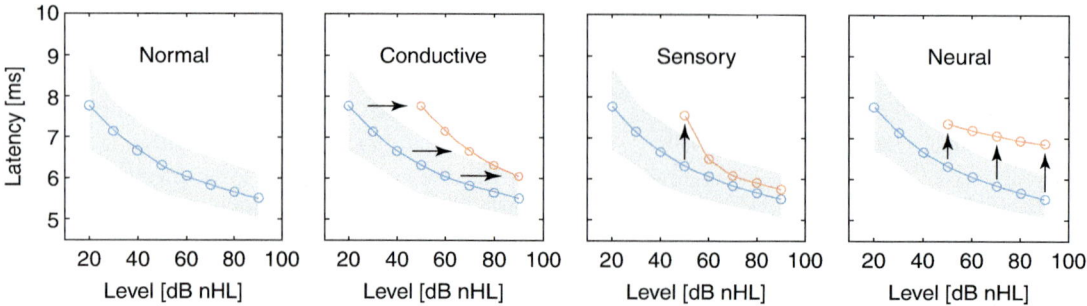

Fig. 16.29 Level-latency curves are shown for different pathologies. In grey is the normal range of latencies for wave V shown, in blue their mean. In red the divergent latencies for the noted pathologies are shown

son of these functions with normal ranges helps to identify different pathologies (Fig. 16.29). The latency difference $\Delta t = t_V - t_I$ is also taken into account.

In conductive hearing loss, the stimulus reaches the cochlea quieter than normal. Therefore, the curves are parallel but shifted to higher intensities. The difference Δt remains normal.

In sensory hearing loss, the curves at high levels are almost normal and prolonged only at levels near threshold. In the case of low-frequency loss, t_V can even be shortened because of the lacking later low-frequency portion of the signal. The curve shape conforms to a defect of the outer hair cells and normal neuronal processing.

In contrast, in retrocochlear hearing loss latency, t_I is normal but t_V is severely prolonged. The wave pattern can also be irregular, e.g. in auditory neuropathy (Schmidt et al. 2012).

The interpretation of the level-latency graphs provides important hints for diagnostics. But be aware: in infants it is more difficult because of maturation of the auditory pathway, so additional diagnostics should be taken into account.

Bone Conduction in ABR If conductive hearing loss is suspected, measurement of bone-conduction ABR is indicated. Unlike in (the normal) air-conduction ABR, the stimulus is presented by a transducer (Fig. 16.28) as similarly used for bone-conduction behavioural thresholds. The transducer ideally is held by an elastic band or clamp. The intensities used reach

a maximal of 50 dB, which is sufficient for diagnostics of conductive problems. A large early artefact may occur owing to the vibrating mass, but the ABR response to frequency-specific stimuli appears after that artefact (Stapells and Oates 1997). In cases of threshold differences between ears, masking comparable to that for behavioural measurement is necessary. To identify conductive or mixed hearing loss, ear microscopy, tympanometry, stapedius reflex measurement and otoacoustic emissions should be taken into account.

Hearing Rehabilitation Based on ERA Results The estimated audiogram is not identical to the behavioural threshold of hearing examined with PTA. The correlation of estimated audiogram and the behavioural threshold is strongly influenced by the chosen method and measurement conditions, individual hearing loss and condition (maturation) of the auditory pathways as well as experience of the audiologist. Nevertheless, in preschool children, infants and non-cooperating young patients, threshold estimation by physiological measurements is the best that can be achieved. In group means, the thresholds are within 10–15 dB of the behavioural threshold. In cases of steep hearing loss, the difference may be larger (~20 dB) in the range of the steep slope. The hearing loss is rather underestimated (Johnson and Brown 2005). The results of the electrophysiological measurements have to be checked for plausibility in synopsis with otoacoustic emissions, middle ear status, stapedius reflex measurements, sound field behavioural audiometry and language development of the child. The estimated thresholds are suitable for establishing the basal hearing aid settings. It is necessary to control the fitting, the development of hearing and language of the children regularly.

The results of objective threshold audiometry in the hearing rehabilitation process must be continually monitored, also with the help of behavioural methods, as soon as their achievement is possible.

16.12 Indication and Interpretation of Auditory Steady-State Responses

Piotr Swidzinski and Arne Knief

16.12.1 Characteristics of Auditory Steady-State Responses (ASSR)

Registration of the auditory evoked potentials (AEP) of specific frequencies, from the point of view of response correctness, has been and still is inconvenient (long time of stimulus duration—short time of response latency of auditory potentials). Towards the end of the twentieth century (1998), auditory steady-state responses (ASSR) were developed and introduced to the techniques of electrophysiological auditory investigations (Kuwada et al. 1986, Tlumak et al. 2012; review and tutorial: Korczak et al. 2012, Pruszewicz and Obrębowski 2010). The advantage of this method is the possibility of automatic assessment by statistical processing algorithms. Frequency specificity is obtained by the use of pure tones (sine waves) or 'chirp'-type auditory stimuli (Stürzebecher et al. 2006) as 'carrier signal' with frequencies of 500, 1000, 2000 and 4000 Hz, which are modulated by a signal with frequency around 80 Hz. It is possible to use multiple carriers in parallel by modulation with different frequencies around 80 Hz (Lins and Picton 1995; John et al.

1998). This enables time-saving acquisition setups. The sites where the potentials are generated are the brainstem and the thalamus—thus the test is a combination of two registrations: ABR (auditory brainstem responses) and MLR (middle latency responses). In the auditory system, a steady-state response is evoked at the frequency of the modulation. Names for this method are auditory steady-state response (ASSR) or amplitude-modulation following response (AMFR). Figure 16.30 presents a simple diagram of the ASSR production.

16.12.2 Aim of the ASSR Production

The ASSR test is aimed first at producing a simple objective measurement of hearing whose result correlates directly with the audiogram; it is an instrument complying with the principle of audiological diagnostics, the 'cross-check principle' according to Jerger and Hayes (1976), in particular in the diagnostics of young children. The automatic analysis of the ASSR is based on a transformation into frequency space, e.g. by a fast Fourier transform (FFT). In the next step, it is evaluated by statistical testing to determine if there is a response to the stimuli at the modulation frequency or not. The methods used can be the calculation of phase coherence values or the F-test (Dobie and Wilson 1996). Phase coherence is calculated if the measured signal has random phases: then there is no response; if in each repetition the phase is the same and related to the stimulus, there is a valid response. In the F-test the energy at the modulation frequency is compared with that of neighbouring frequencies. Different variations and flavours of these algorithms are possible (Picton et al. 2003). Each device manufacturer uses its own estimation algorithm, and usually they do not disclose their methods.

The result of the measurement is not demonstrated as a typical wave form with assessment of registered wave latency, but evaluated as a graph resembling an audiogram. An example of the ASSR test result is presented in Fig. 16.31.

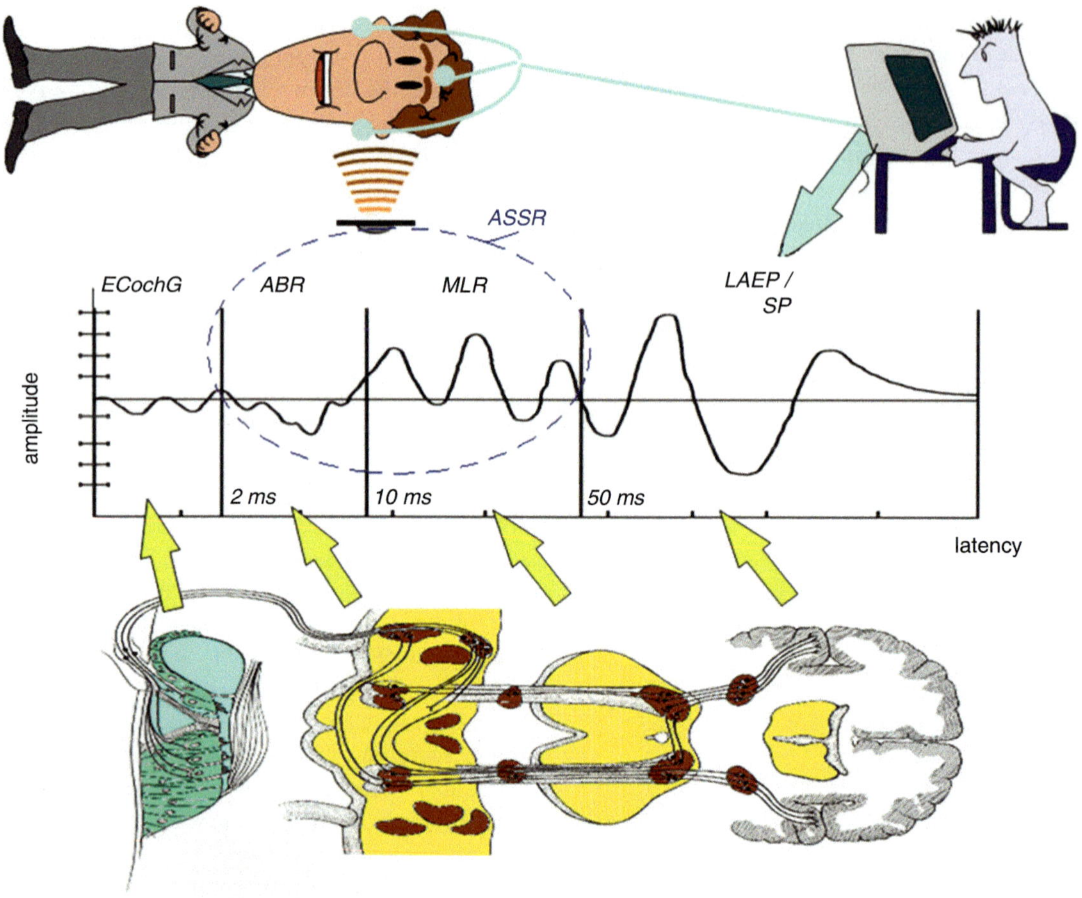

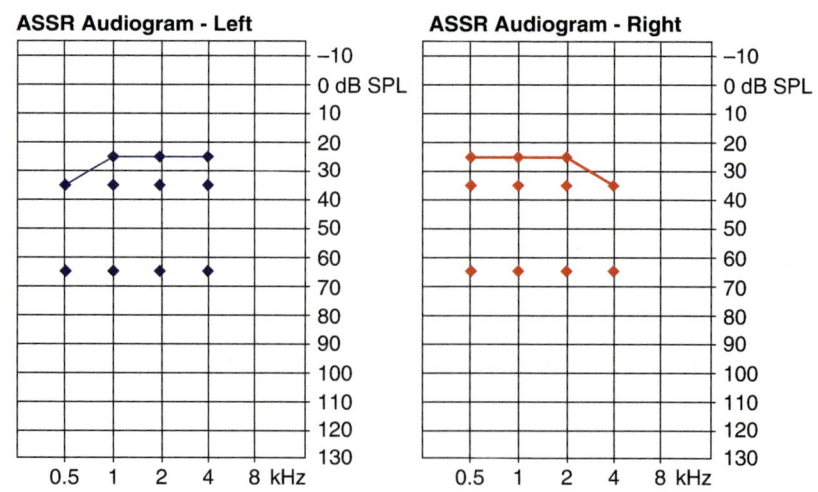

Fig. 16.30 The site of the ASSR response production (the author's own study based on the materials from the Department of Phoniatrics and Audiology, University of Medical Sciences in Poznań). *ECochG* electrocochleography; *ABR* auditory brainstem response; *MLR* middle latency response; *SP* sustained potential; *LAEP* late auditory evoked potential

Fig. 16.31 An example of the ASSR registration in an 11-year-old child (legend: X-axis, frequency in kHz; Y-axis, sound pressure level in dB)

ASSR Audiogram - Left

| | | | | | |
| −10 |
| 0 dB SPL |
| 10 |
| 20 |
| 30 |
| 40 |
| 50 |
| 60 |
| 70 |
| 80 |
| 90 |
| 100 |
| 110 |
| 120 |
| 130 |

0.5   1   2   4   8 kHz

ASSR Audiogram - Right

| | | | | | |
| −10 |
| 0 dB SPL |
| 10 |
| 20 |
| 30 |
| 40 |
| 50 |
| 60 |
| 70 |
| 80 |
| 90 |
| 100 |
| 110 |
| 120 |
| 130 |

0.5   1   2   4   8 kHz

16.12.3 Indication and Interpretation of ASSR

The indication for the ASSR test is the need to obtain an objective audiogram, besides its use in newborn hearing screening. As the ASSR method makes use of tonal, frequency-specific stimuli (similar to that in the audiometric test), the test result can be compared with the behaviourally obtained audiogram. It can be a perfect instrument for objective hearing tests in children and uncooperative patients through earphones and in a free acoustic field through loudspeakers. The problem of this method is the need for a correction to estimate the hearing threshold. In normal-hearing adults and older children, this correction is averaged at 11 dB for 2 kHz up to 17 dB for 500 Hz (Tlumak et al. 2007). In hearing-impaired adults, it varies from 8 to 14 dB. Despite this correction the method is considered to give a good estimate of hearing threshold. In children <6 years and infants, compared with ABR thresholds—which may lie 10 dB above behavioural thresholds—the ASSR for normal hearing is 17 dB, 13 dB, 13 dB and 9 dB worse than ABR in normal hearing and 9 dB, 9 dB, 9 dB and 6 dB worse in patients with hearing loss at 500 Hz, 1000 Hz, 2000 Hz and 4000 Hz, respectively (Van Maanen and Stapells 2010). These corrections vary in different publications (e.g. Chou et al. 2012; Luts et al. 2006; Rance et al. 2005) because of different study groups, stimuli, measurement time, noise floor and other parameters. Considerable variability in interpersonal and intrapersonal results is noticed. A large number of audiologists seem to indicate that so far the method represents poor diagnostic value (Pruszewicz and Obrębowski 2010; Tlumak et al. 2012). Owing to the good correlation of the ABR and ASSR thresholds, the method is quite usable. In commercial ASSR systems, an automatic correction is normally included; therefore the result of measurement is an estimated audiogram. The audiological assistant or semi-skilled examiner does not need to know much about the interpretation of the response, as in click or notched-noise ABR, as the measurement system delivers an audiogram. But this audiogram should be interpreted with caution depending on the degree of hearing loss, age and measurement conditions.

16.13 Promontory Test

Dirk Mürbe

Aim and Method The promontory test assesses whether external electrical stimulation at the cochlear promontory generates an auditory percept. The test was initially introduced to ascertain deaf patients' candidacy for cochlear implantation, since conductivity of the auditory nerve is an essential prerequisite for a successful outcome after implantation.

The subjective test aims to assess thresholds and dynamic ranges of hearing sensation and can be performed in an outpatient procedure, in which the patient is seated and the external ear canal is under local anaesthesia. Under microscopic control, a needle electrode is then transtympanically positioned at the cochlear promontory, via the external ear canal. Different stimulation paradigms have been introduced to determine whether a patient will benefit from electrical stimulation. Commonly used stimulation rates include 50, 100 and 200 Hz. During stimulus application, the patient is asked to describe the hearing sensation associated with the different stimuli. For each stimulation rate, the patient indicates if there is an increase in perceptual loudness as stimulant current is increased. Further, the discrimination between the different stimulation rates is assessed. Thresholds and dynamic ranges can then be documented for the different stimulation rates.

Alternatively, to avoid the application of a needle electrode, the promontory test can be modified, and a ball electrode can be positioned in the external ear canal in contact with the tympanic membrane.

Interpretation and Diagnostic Value In the early years of cochlear implantation, in which most patients scheduled for implantation suffered from complete deafness, the promontory test was an essential part of candidacy assessment. Since then, the indications for cochlear implantation have expanded to include patients with profound sensorineural hearing loss and residual hearing. In these cases, the promontory test is usually postponed, because reliable thresholds in pure-tone audiometry describe the basic conductivity of the auditory nerve. The promontory test has, however, been suggested to be a useful tool in predicting postoperative speech perception in patients at risk of poor auditory nerve functioning (neuropathies), especially in postinflammatory conditions such as meningitis, or after long auditory deprivation (Alfelasi et al. 2013).

16.14 Electro-audiometry

Arne Knief

In deaf or nearly deaf patients, the only possibility of evoking an impression of hearing is the electrical stimulation of the auditory system. Electrical stimulation can be used to measure the

capability of the auditory pathway, as does acoustic brainstem audiometry. This examination can provide information about the status of the auditory pathway as well as thresholds for electrical stimulation to be used in cochlear implants.

Electro-audiometry may be used before cochlear implantation to examine if the post-cochlear system is adequate for electrical stimulation via a cochlear implant. There are two possibilities of measurement: the patients report their subjective impression of the stimulation (the so-called promontory test; see Sect. 16.13), or, perhaps more reliable, the nerve response is recorded with synchronous averaging by auditory brainstem response acquisition equipment. Nevertheless, its predictive value is low and the method has disappeared from medical guidelines (Lesinski et al. 1997).

After cochlear implantation, the electrically evoked compound action potentials can be measured by using the implanted electrodes (Fig. 16.32).

The test is controlled by proprietary software of the implant producer. As result of the measurement, threshold values are obtained that can be used for adjusting the speech processor programme

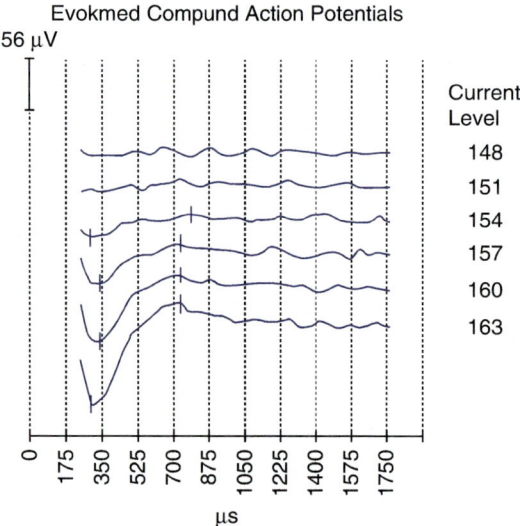

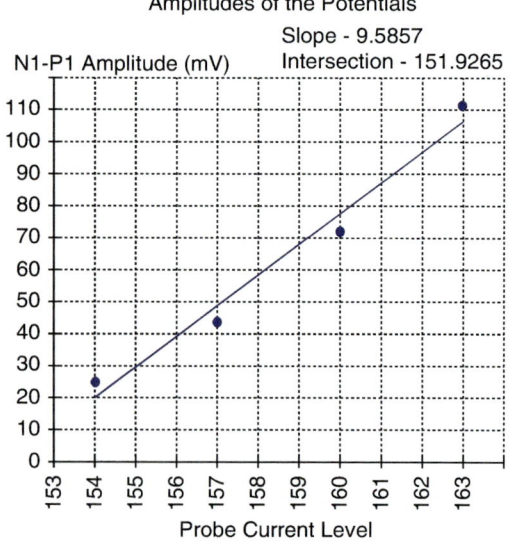

Fig. 16.32 Measurement of evoked compound action potentials with a cochlear implant (Software Custom Sound EP ver. 5.0, Cochlear Ltd., Australia). In the left panel, compound action potentials are shown for one electrode (no. 6) at increasing current levels (current levels are arbitrary units of the manufacturer and can be translated to currents in microampere range). In the middle panel, the amplitude differences of the marked positive and negative peaks are drawn over the current levels. The linearity of the amplitudes enables the extrapolation of a threshold. In the right panel, the extrapolated amplitude thresholds of the evoked compound action potentials are drawn for different electrodes. They generate a profile for speech processor fitting

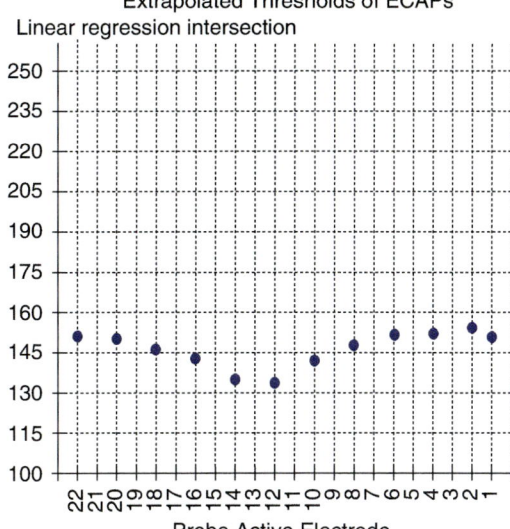

Extrapolated Thresholds of ECAPs
Linear regression intersection

Probe Active Electrode

Fig. 16.32 (continued)

of the implant recipient (Smoorenburg et al. 2002). This measurement is useful in non-cooperative patients such as small children, but it also enables adequate fitting of the speech processor in patients with intense tinnitus.

An electrically evoked brainstem response can also be measured in special cases, for example, if there is doubt that the auditory pathway is functioning well. The stimulation is executed with intra-cochlear electrodes and acquisition of the response with surface electrodes as in normal brainstem response measurement (Brown 2003).

16.15 Balance/Vestibular Assessment in Children

Waheeda Pagarkar and Ewa Raglan

16.15.1 Developmental Balance Assessment in Children: Development of Balance, History and Observation

Development of Balance Balance is a complex modality that develops with input from the visual, proprioceptive/somatosensory and vestibular systems. This sensory information is integrated and processed within the central nervous system and results in outputs that help stabilise our eyes and body in space through the vestibulo-ocular (VOR) and vestibulospinal (VSR) reflexes, respectively, and help in perception and awareness of our posture and movement in space through cortical connections. Development of balance depends on the development of each of these sensory systems and on the development of the integrating pathways.

The vestibular labyrinth and receptors are developed to an adultlike form by 32-week gestation. The vestibular nerve is the first cranial nerve to complete myelinisation. The slow (reflexive) component of VOR can be seen at birth, but the fast (saccadic or central) component is immature and continues to develop until the age of 2 years. Absence of the VOR by the age of 10 months is an abnormal finding (Eviatar and Eviatar 1979; Fife et al. 2000). Infants prefer visual inputs to maintain balance, whereas adults rely more on somatosensory information. Infants perform better under conditions of sensory loss [e.g. visual difficulties] than conditions of sensory conflict, indicating that the central vestibular integrative pathways are immature. The role of the vestibular system in postural control depends on these integrative pathways, and the ability to resolve intersensory conflict is mature approximately at the age of 15 years (Steindl et al. 2006; Shinjo et al. 2007).

Balance difficulties in children may present as delayed motor milestones, poor tone and floppy posture, frequent falls and unusual gait. They may be related to visual, neurological or vestibular pathology or psychological factors. Cardiac pathology and metabolic disturbances such as hypoglycaemia should also be considered. A comprehensive balance evaluation should include a clinical assessment of all the above conditions. The vestibular aspects of a child's balance can be assessed from history, examination and selected investigations.

History The onset and progress of the balance difficulty is often a pointer to its cause. In combination with deafness, poor tone and delayed walking in a neonate are likely to be due to a congenital vestibular hypofunction. Sudden vertigo, resolving in days, preceded by a viral infection and followed by fluctuating imbalance is likely to be related to vestibular neuritis. Associated conditions should be noted, as balance difficulties occur in Pendred's syndrome (with deafness and goitre), Usher syndrome (with deafness and retinitis pigmentosa), CHARGE syndrome (with deafness and dysmorphism) and migraine (often with headaches and vertigo). Family history is a pointer to inherited conditions (i.e. affected parents/siblings in branchio-oto-renal syndrome). Perinatal history is important, as deafness and cerebral palsy can be related to neonatal jaundice and perinatal hypoxia.

Observation and Examination The key to successful examination of balance in a child, particularly the young toddler, involves knowledge of normal development, a keen eye for observing the child during natural activity and the ability to engage children in play. The general examination must include looking for dysmorphism, otoscopy, examination of the nose and throat, looking for neurocutaneous markers and a complete systemic examination to look for associated conditions and syndromes. A detailed neurological examination is mandatory. Clinical vestibular examination includes assessing the VOR, the vestibulospinal reflex (from postural tests) and the developmental reflexes.

16.15.2 Tests for Posture/ Vestibulospinal Reflex

This can be started by simple observation of the child. How is their posture? Newborns with poor tone may have a frog-leg posture. Children with balance difficulties will often hold on to their parent or to the walls or banister for support. A broad-based gait is a pointer of poor balance. Unusual gaits can be observed in cerebral palsy, neuropathy and hemiparesis. Keeping a few obstacles in the path of a walking child or engaging them to kick a football and observing how they manoeuvre these will prove useful. A child who is running around, rolling on the floor and climbing chairs is unlikely to have a significant

balance problem! The principle of postural tests is to reduce the visual and proprioceptive inputs, thereby uncovering vestibular dysfunction (Valente 2011).

- Romberg's test: the child stands with feet together, and sway is noted with eyes both open and closed. A variation is the sharpened Romberg's test whereby this stability is evaluated in a heel-to-toe stance.
- Foam test: the child stands on foam with eyes open and closed and sway is noted.
- Unterberger's test: the child is asked to march on the spot with the eyes closed and the deviation is noted.
- Tandem gait: the child walks heel to toe and steadiness is noted.

The postural tests are limited by lack of specificity for vestibular dysfunction and paucity of normative data for children.

16.15.3 Tests for Eye Movements and VOR

The VOR in children is dependent on the attention and state of arousal of the child, unintended ocular fixation due to light leaks and difficulty with head stabilisation during testing. Examination of children is helped by using child-friendly visual targets (e.g. stickers, toys). Begin by looking for a squint and spontaneous nystagmus. The best way to look for vestibular nystagmus is by using Frenzel's or Video-Frenzel's glasses in the central, right and left gaze (angle of gaze should be <30°). Smooth pursuit is best checked with a toy and optokinetic nystagmus with a striped drum with child-friendly pictures.

Halmagyi's Head Thrust The child's head is gently rotated by approximately 30° in the yaw plane (about the vertical body axis) while asking the child to focus on the examiner's nose. A rapid head thrust is incorporated ensuring maintenance of visual fixation. A 'catch-up' saccade indicates loss of function of the ipsilateral lateral semicircular canal.

Head-Shaking Nystagmus The child's head is briskly rotated in the yaw plane with eyes closed for about 30 s. The eyes are then opened and examined preferably using Frenzel's/Video-Frenzel's glasses. Vestibular asymmetry causes nystagmus beating away from the side of the lesion.

Vibration-Induced Nystagmus This can be done with a vestibular vibrator applied to the mastoid process for approximately 10 s. The test also elicits vestibular asymmetry. The nystagmus begins when the vibration is applied and beats opposite to the direction of the lesioned side.

Dynamic Visual Acuity Children may be evaluated with modification of the Snellen eye chart using child-friendly characters. The child is asked to read this chart from a distance of 1.5 m with the head steady. A baseline visual acuity is obtained. The child's head is rotated in the yaw plane at approximately 1–2 Hz. A loss of three lines or more of visual acuity may indicate a VOR deficiency.

16.15.4 Tests for Neonatal Reflexes

In the article of O'Reilly et al. (2011), various approaches are presented.

Moro Reflex This is elicited by holding the child supine and allowing its head to drop by approximately 30° in relation to the trunk. There is extension and abduction of the arms with fanning out of the fingers followed by adduction of the arms at the shoulder and crying. This reflex normally disappears by the age of 5–6 months. Its presence before this age is indicative of vestibular function.

Farmers Rotation Test The baby is held at arm's length (facing the examiner) and rotated in one direction around the examiner. There is a deviation of the eyes and head in the direction of the rotation, in the presence of vestibular function. This response can be elicited up to the age of 6 weeks. At a later age, the nystagmus supersedes the eye deviation.

Parachute Reflex The child is held face down horizontally and moved downward suddenly. This causes an extension and abduction of the lower limbs and outstretched hands. A backward and sideward parachute reflex can also be elicited. This can occur beyond the age of 5 months and is indicative of vestibular function.

Head Righting Reflexes These develop by the age of 4–6 months. The child's trunk is held 30° from the vertical, and a normally responding infant will tilt its head so as to remain vertical. At about age 5 months, the child will also move the lower limbs away from the side to which they have been tilted.

16.15.5 Other Tests: Dix-Hallpike Positional Test

This involves rapidly taking the child from a seated to a lying back position with the head turned to one side (right or left). The eyes are observed for nystagmus. The child is then rapidly taken to the seated position and the eye observation is repeated. The presence of horizontal, rotatory, geotropic nystagmus with vertigo after a short latent period and fatigue on repeated testing occurs in benign paroxysmal positional vertigo (BPPV).

16.15.6 Vestibular Investigations

Adequate preparation for the tests is important. Vestibular sedatives are withheld for 24–48 h prior to testing, and it is important that the child eats only a light meal before the appointment.

Electronystagmography and Video-Oculography These are techniques used for recording eye movements during rotational chair testing. They can also be used for recording eye movements for gaze, smooth pursuit, saccades and optokinetic nystagmus. It is important to understand the differences between child and adult traces, and normative data should be collected. Testing in a dark room, the need for placing electrodes or goggles and the rotational chair stimulus itself make these tests challenging in children. Furthermore, inattention and alertness will influence responses.

Video Head Impulse Test (vHIT) could be used successfully to test dizzy children (Khater and Afifi 2016). This test provides vestibular ocular reflex analysis of high-frequency vestibular activity of the horizontal and vertical semicircular canals. It is based on Halmagyi's head thrust response. With the video head impulse test, eye movements can be recorded by a high-speed lightweight video camera and mini-gyroscopes fitted to eye glasses (MacDougall et al. 2009; Petrak et al. 2013).

Computerised Rotational Chair Testing The response to impulsive and sinusoidal rotation indicates the presence of vestibular function. The limitation is that this test assesses the overall vestibular function rather than for individual ears. The advantage is that children may sit on their mother's lap and this test is better tolerated than the caloric test. Using this method, young infants can be examined for VOR. The gain, phase and time constant of the nystagmus is calculated. In the event that recording of the nystagmus is difficult, simple observation with an infra-red camera is useful in detecting per-rotatory and post-rotatory nystagmus. VOR gain increases linearly as a function of age from 3 to 9 years (Casselbrant et al. 2010).

Bithermal Caloric Testing Warm and cool irrigation of water or air may be used. This test allows individual ear testing of vestibular function and, from the Jongkees formula, will give the canal paresis and directional preponderance. Studies of ice-cold caloric responses in infants indicate that nystagmus is observed by the age of 6 months in full-term infants (Eviatar and Eviatar 1979). Practically, children younger than 5 years of age may not tolerate this test well.

Computerised Dynamic Posturography The test can be used in children as young as 3–6 years

of age (Foudriat et al. 1993). The sensory organisation test (SOT) is the commonest subtest used. This test consists of six conditions of varying combinations of fixed and moving platforms and visual surroundings done with eyes open or closed. The child must try to maintain the best balance possible despite conflicting clues. Normative data should be obtained, although it has been shown that younger children perform worse than older ones (Valente 2007). Special adaptations should be made for testing children. Information may be gained regarding how well a patient integrates visual, vestibular and proprioceptive cues and whether there is an overdependence on one modality.

Vestibular Evoked Myogenic Potentials Test (VEMPs) Both cervical and ocular VEMPs (cVEMPs and oVEMPs) have been done in children to evaluate the integrity of the otolith system (Valente 2007; Wang et al. 2008; Lin et al. 2010). cVEMPs are commonly recorded from the sternocleidomastoid muscle and test the vestibulocollic reflex, whereas the oVEMPs assess the otolithic VOR. Rectification methods may be employed to correct for the difference in background muscle activity. Latency, threshold and asymmetry may be measured. VEMPs are well tolerated and can give information on individual ear otolith function. VEMPs have been demonstrated in neonates and children and the wave latencies may be shorter than in adults (Valente 2007).

Subjective Visual Vertical/Subjective Visual Horizontal (SVV/SVH) Test This test involves setting a linear marker to the vertical or horizontal in a dark room, in the absence of visual clues. The patient is asked to adjust the marker to his/her subjective vertical/horizontal. The degree of deviation is recorded. This can be done in older children but head restraint may be required to avoid the effect of head tilt. The values may be abnormal in acute unilateral vestibular lesions.

16.16 Evaluation of Speech Communication in Hearing-Impaired Children

Antoinette am Zehnhoff-Dinnesen
and Mona Hegazi

16.16.1 Introduction: Relation of Hearing, Language and Speech

According to Aslin and Smith (1988) and Carney (1996), basic sensory perception (sound detection) is followed by coding perceptual representations (phonetic discrimination) and cognitive/linguistic processing (word recognition). These levels are mirrored in speech production by primitive vocalisations, complex vocal utterances (babbling) and phonemic or syllabic speech patterns (Eisenberg et al. 2007). Hearing loss (HL) in early childhood impairs the development of speech recognition and speech production by hindering the generation of correct recognition categories, linguistic and motoric patterns. Recognition of word boundaries, of syllables, of prosodic elements of speech, of sound patterns in words is basically essential for language development in early infancy.

Results in speech recognition and production depend on the type and degree of hearing loss, onset of manifestation, age at detection and start of intervention, additional handicaps, kind and quality of hearing device supply, communication mode, support by parents and intensity of therapeutic training.

Typical findings in hearing-impaired children, dependent on the degree of hearing loss, may be:

- Prolonged phase of primitive vocalisations.
- Delay in onset of babbling and differences in babbling behaviour, less consonantal types.
- Delay in development of phonemic/syllabic speech patterns.
- Lagging behind in vowel and consonant production.
- More problems in recognising consonant than vowel contrasts.

- More problems in recognising consonant manner and rear place than consonant voicing and front place.
- Substitution particularly for fricatives and affricates.
- Mild to moderate hoarseness.
- Nasal resonance problems (Eisenberg et al. 2007).

Furthermore, school achievement and academic chances may be impaired by hearing loss-related disorders of speech and language development.

Evaluation of speech communication in hearing-impaired children will be presented in this section concerning:

- Communication mode (oral-aural, manual, combined, total).
- Nasality and voice function.
- Non-verbal communication.
- Receptive language/comprehension with/without lip reading, narrative and supralinguistic skills, expressive phonetic, phonological levels, semantic levels, working memory and word finding, morphological, syntactic levels, prosody, intelligibility, pragmatics.
- Auditory and visual perception.

For assessment of kinaesthetic and tactile perception see Sect. 11.10; oral motor examination protocol and assessment of speech sound development see Sects. 11.4 and 11.5; details of literacy (phonological awareness, reading, writing) see Volume 2, Part III.

In recent years, evaluation of speech and language development in hearing-impaired children has focused on testing oral language in children with cochlear implants in comparison with children with hearing aids and normal-hearing children. Often-used tests and exemplary results are presented.

The choice of test material may be motivated by the aim to evaluate signal processing strategies, the intention to identify perceptual processes or the purpose to detect individual promotive or hindering factors (Kirk et al. 2012). Only a selection of tests can be included in this article. For further reading, see e.g. the systematic review from da Silva et al. (2011) on Instruments to Assess the Oral Language of Children fitted with a Cochlear Implant, and the book on Clinical Management of Children with Cochlear Implants by Eisenberg (2016).

16.16.2 Evaluation of Communication Mode

In a first step, the communication mode used in the education of the child should be clarified. The most common types are:

Oral Communication The use of residual hearing to develop oral communication is emphasised.

- Auditory-Verbal: This method maximises the use of residual hearing to develop spoken language and restricts the use of visual cues, speech reading (lip reading) and signs.
- Auditory-Oral: This method maximises the use of both residual hearing and speech reading (lip reading) to develop spoken language.

Manual Communication This method refers to communication by using the hands without dependence on verbal communication:

- Sign Language: A visuospatial language that uses handshapes, movements and locations of the hands, facial expressions and other body movements; each sign in a sign language is like a word in a spoken language; sign language is a real language with its own grammar rules.
- Fingerspelling: Each letter in any language is represented by a sign and words are simply spelt letter-by-letter.
- Cued Speech: This method uses eight handshapes—none of which are derived from sign languages—to represent consonants and four hand placements around the face to represent vowels.

Simultaneous Communication 'Sim-Comm' Sign language and spoken language are simultaneously used.

Total Communication Any means of communication is utilised such as formal sign language, fingerspelling, natural gestures, speech, lip reading, listening with amplification, pictures and writing.

16.16.3 Evaluation of Nasality and Voice Function

Nasal Resonance Disorders in Hearing Loss Abnormal resonance in children with hearing loss (HL children) may be explained by an uncoordinated velopharyngeal function (Kim et al. 2012) due to the absence of complete auditory feedback. By auditory perceptual evaluation, the type of nasality may be defined:

- Hypernasality, typical in children with sensorineural hearing loss.
- Cul-de-sac resonance (typical in children with sensorineural hearing loss, caused by muffled airflow near the lower pharynx and incomplete velopharyngeal closure).
- Hyponasality, typical in children with conductive hearing loss.
- Mixed nasality, e.g. sensorineural hearing loss and adenoids, for details see Volume 2, Part I Speech Disorders (Dysglossia/Nasality/Velopharyngeal Insufficiency).

Henningsson et al. (2008) developed, as a working group, a set of five parameters with hypernasality, hyponasality, audible nasal air emission or nasal turbulence, consonant production errors and voice disorder, also considering speech understandability and speech acceptability. They presented guidelines for scoring procedures in relation to these parameters.

The Nasometer (Kay Elemetrics Corp.) is considered the most reliable tool for objectively evaluating resonance disorders (Van Lierde et al. 2005). The Nasometer (Kummer 2008) (Kay Elemetrics Corp.) is a computer system that measures the proportion of acoustic energy produced in the oral and nasal cavities during speech and calculates the proportion of nasal and oral resonance as a nasalance score: nasal acoustic energy divided by the (sum of nasal and oral energy) × 100 = nasalance percentage.

The MacKay-Kummer SNAP Test-R in the revised version from 2005 comprises a syllable-repetition subtest (oral + /a:/, oral + /i:/, nasal + /a:/, nasal + /i:/), a prolonged sounds subtest (/a:/, /i:/, /s:/, /m:/), a picture-cued subtest (sentences) and a paragraph (reading) subtest (https://www.researchgate.net/publication/282586585_SNAP_TEST_II_Score_Sheet_32505).

By such a test in combination with Nasometer measurements, nasalance scores for oral (bilabial, alveolar, velar and sibilant) and nasal phonemes may be obtained (Nguyen et al. 2008).

Kim et al. (2012), in addition to nasalance tests by nasometer, used the 'vertical focus of resonance' (VFR), for evaluation of perceptual rating, which focuses on the resonance energy in the frontal, throat, pharyngeal and nasal locations. Their results showed inappropriate coordination of velopharyngeal function in HL subjects and that the air flow and the resonance energy were not released from the resonance cavity in this group.

Baudonck et al. (2015) studied nasalance and nasality in 36 children with cochlear implants (CI children), 25 children with hearing aids (HA children) and 26 normal-hearing children (NH children) at the age of 9 years. The objective assessment of nasalance values was performed with the Nasometer, perceptual evaluations of nasality by two experienced speech therapists on the basis of a nominal rating scale with consensus evaluation. Nasalance values were lower in CI and HA children for nasal stimuli and higher in oral stimuli than those of NH children. In addition, larger cul-de-sac resonance was found in CI and HA than in NH children. According to the perceptual evaluation, HA children were more hypernasal than NH children.

Naso-video-endoscopy may be used to exclude organic causes.

Voice Changes in Hearing Loss Lack of auditory feedback in hearing-impaired children has effects on voice function with incoordination of intrinsic and extrinsic laryngeal muscles, and

with disturbed contraction and relaxation of antagonistic muscles. Higher fundamental frequency, lack of loudness control and variable abnormal voice quality features have been reported in HL children, as well as incomplete mutational voice disorder or puberphonia. Voice has also been described as being monotonous because of the lack of prosodic information and acquisition of melodic patterns of language (Nickerson 1975). Nowadays, voice quality parameters found in children with profound hearing loss are more normalised than in former times, owing to the high technical standard of hearing aids and cochlear implants, and newborn hearing screening, early detection and intervention.

Garcia et al. (2010) found more altered voice quality in 62 children with profound HL supplied with cochlear implants than in such children wearing digital hearing aids, dependent on the degree of HL and the type of hearing prosthesis. The worst results were observed in children with analogue hearing aids. The children had to produce a sustained vowel /a:/ for 4–5 s. For evaluation of voice quality the authors focused on the analysis of F_0, jitter and shimmer. The control group comprised 54 NH children.

According to results in NH children, the authors defined a range of normal values for children 7–8 years old: F_0 253–270 Hz, jitter $\leq$ 1.250%, shimmer $\leq$ 0.400 dB.

The following quality values were achieved in children with profound hearing loss:

- Digital hearing aid users:
- F_0 265.50 Hz, jitter 1.009%, shimmer 0.486 dB.
- Cochlear implant users:
- F_0 287.93 Hz, jitter 1.344%, shimmer 0.526 dB.
- Analogue hearing aid users:
- F_0 323.80 Hz, jitter 1.999%, shimmer 0.687 dB.

Most important factors were degree of HL, type of prosthesis and hearing threshold reached with the prosthesis. The hearing age also has to be considered. Maturation of control mechanisms and adaptation of neuromuscular abilities to acquired hearing control by hearing devices have to be taken into account. The voice quality values were more normalised than found in the time before access to high technical standard hearing devices.

Campisi et al. (2006) described values of F_0, jitter and shimmer in 21 profoundly deaf children within the normal range and emphasised the importance of measuring Fundamental Frequency variation (vF0) and Peak Amplitude variation (vAM). According to their results, auditory deprivation causes reduced long-term control of frequency and amplitude during sustained phonation.

The phoniatrician/pedaudiologist has to be aware of possible functional effects by an insufficient hearing threshold reached with the prosthesis. In case of dysphonia, laryngoscopy with flexible optics may be necessary. Auditory perceptual analysis of the voice (throatiness, breathiness, hoarseness) and the average speaking pitch may be possible on the basis of spontaneous utterances. Depending on age, questionnaires, pitch range, standardised, phonetically balanced texts and acoustic analysis methods may be applied, the latter working with vocal expressions lasting a few seconds (Fuchs et al. 2007). For more details, see Sect. 5.16.

16.16.4 Evaluation of Non-verbal Communication

Preverbal Communication Skills To study preverbal communication skills in HA or CI children, the Tait video analysis is a suitable method for e.g. vocal turn-taking, non-looking vocal turns, gestural turn-taking, gestural autonomy and vocal autonomy (Tait et al. 2010). Vocal and early verbal developments may be monitored by video and audio recordings during parent–child interaction sessions, also observing developmental landmarks. Transcription should be performed by at least two experienced listeners as a consensus transcription procedure. Frequency of vocalisation, age at consistent babbling, consonantal inventory (place, manner), vowel inventory (height, place), mean syllable structure level and

patterns of syllable complexity in dependence on age are the parameters relating to vocal measures (Moeller et al. 2007a).

Sign Language Assessment An assessment tool of signed language skills is necessary to determine children's level of signed language proficiency, to monitor children's progress, to develop teaching goals and to give information to the parents.

The Assessing British Sign Language Development: Receptive Skills Test (BSL RST) (Herman et al. 1999) was developed for children aged 3–11 years. The BSL RST comprises a vocabulary check by a picture-naming task of 24 items and a video-based receptive test with 40 test items. The test items check grammatical structures, including negation, number and distribution, verb morphology and noun–verb distinction (Enns and Herman 2011).

Sign language raters should look at the candidate's performance in the following components:

- Sign production (its use and clarity of signs).
- Vocabulary knowledge.
- Use (or lack of use) of grammatical features.
- Fluency of the language to convey ideas, thoughts and opinions during the interview.
- Level of comprehension or receptive skills to judge the ease of understanding of what was signed.
- Use of culturally appropriate sign conversational strategies such as eye contact, appropriate turn-taking in dialogue and interruptions.

According to Johnston (2004), the BSL RST is the first worldwide standardised test of any signed language, normed on a population and tested for reliability.

An overview of existing sign language tests is given on the webpage http://www.signlang-assessment.info/index.php/home-en.html. These tests concern:

- Development of a sign language (L1).
- Learning a foreign sign language (L2).
- Linguistic research, e.g. concerning morphology, syntax.

16.16.5 Evaluation of Receptive Language/Comprehension With/Without Lip Reading, Narrative Skills, Supralinguistic Skills, Evaluation of Expressive Language with Phonetic, Phonological Levels, Semantic Levels, Working Memory and Word Finding, Morphological, Syntactic Levels, Prosody, Intelligibility and Pragmatics

The assessment of the developmental speech and language status of children is intensively explained in Sect. 11.3. The aim of this section is to present test instruments that are used for the assessment of children with hearing loss. In recent years, evaluation of speech communication in hearing-impaired children has focused on speech and language development of CI children in comparison with that of HA and NH children. A variety of test instruments is used for oral language assessment. Da Silva et al. (2011) performed a systematic literature survey on instruments assessing oral language in CI children and found 74 different tests, questionnaires and inventories used in different versions. We present the most-often used tests according to their results, and tests found in more current literature.

16.16.5.1 Evaluation of Receptive Language/Comprehension With/Without Lip Reading, Narrative Skills, Supralinguistic Measures

While evaluating receptive language skills, testing should be done in the auditory-only mode and in the audiovisual mode. If necessary, signing cues have to be used (Archer and Crosby-Quinatoa 2009). Before evaluation:

- The child's amplification should be checked.
- The testing environment should be quiet and free of visual distractions.

- The examiner should sit next to the child's best hearing ear (Archer and Crosby-Quinatoa 2009).
- Inadequate lighting of the examiner's face should be avoided and the child should watch him or her.

Non-formal assessment of language comprehension entails evaluating the child's understanding of speech aspects such as following a direction, answering a question, participating in a conversation and paraphrasing what has been said.

According to Kyle et al. (2013), prelingual children already use visual speech processing, which is important for phoneme discrimination/phoneme boundaries, and speech-reading ability improves similarly with age in deaf and in NH children. The authors emphasise the impact of speech-reading skills on word reading ability and vice versa.

Testing of lip reading should be performed at different psycholinguistic levels:

- Word level (lexicon and knowledge of using phonetic/semantic features are needed).
- Phrase/sentence level (higher-order linguistic skills and good working memory are needed).

It has to be taken into account that speech-reading accuracy decreases with complexity and length of the psycholinguistic requirement.

One example of formal testing is the Test of Child Speechreading (ToCS) developed by Kyle et al. (2013) which is a valid and reliable assessment of speech-reading ability in school-aged children:

- For testing of words/sentences the child watches a silent video clip of the male or female speaker saying the target word/sentence and then clicks on the correct picture out an array of four.
- For testing the comprehension of short stories the child sees a silent video clip of the male or female speaker telling a short story and is asked two questions by the tester, the child answers the question by selecting the correct picture from an array of four.

According to the systematic review of da Silva et al. (2011), the most-often used tests in CI children for receptive language are the Peabody Picture Vocabulary Test (PPVT) (see Dunn and Dunn 2007), the receptive parts of the Reynell Developmental Language Scales (RDLS) (see Edwards et al. 2011) and the Clinical Evaluation of Language Fundamentals (CELF) (for latest version, see Wiig et al. 2013). All these tests are available in different versions and translations.

A useful test to assess auditory comprehension is part of the fifth edition of the Preschool Language Scale (PLS-5) (Zimmerman et al. 2011) for children from birth to 7 years 11 months of age.

The Northwestern University Children's Perception of Speech Test (NU-CHIPS) (Elliott and Katz 1980), a closed-set picture-pointing task with four pictures per page, is designed for children with a vocabulary recognition age of at least two and a half years (Dobie and Van Hemel 2004).

The Common Phrases Test (six lists of ten sentences) measures the understanding of common phrases used in everyday situations. The material can be presented in the auditory-only (A), visual-only (V) and auditory + visual modality (AV) (Robbins et al. 1995). In 27 children with cochlear implants, the performance in the A condition was correlated with the ability to integrate visual speech information in the AV condition, which seems to be of predictive value in estimating the speech perception benefit with hearing devices (Kirk et al. 2012).

Kirk et al. (1995) found that CI children recognise acoustic-phonetic similarities among words and memorise words into similarity neighbourhoods in long-term memory. The Lexical Neighborhood Test (LNT) comprises two lists of 50 monosyllabic words, the Multisyllabic Lexical Neighborhood Test (MLNT) two lists of 24 two-to-three syllable words (audio-recorded in single-talker and multiple-talker conditions). In the MLNT, half of the words are easy because they are common in the language of young children and there are only few words that can be confused because of phonemic similarity. Half of the words are not easy and less common in early-acquired vocabulary and may be confused with more phonetically similar words.

On the basis of words used to develop the LNT and MLNT, five- to seven-word sentences were constructed including three key words. Twelve children with CIs, aged 5–14 years, showed better performance in the sentence than in the word task, and in sentences with lexically easy rather than lexically hard key words (20 test sentences, two lists, one with easy, one with hard key words) (Eisenberg et al. 2002).

For the Multimodal Lexical Sentence Test for Children (MLST-C), sentences by five male and five female talkers were audiovisually recorded to consider real-world listening. Twenty-one sentences were presented in the A, V and AV condition to 31 children in the age 4–12 years with HA or CI or both. Performance was poorer in the A than in the AV condition (perception of key words 81% and 91%, respectively), HA children correctly performed in 93%, CI children in 79% (Kirk et al. 2011).

Boons et al. (2013) studied *narrative skills* by the Bus Story subtest of the Renfrew Language Scales (Renfrew 1997) in 70 CI children (5–13.3 years) in comparison with NH children. CI children in general mentioned less-essential and subsidiary elements. The Comprehensive Assessment of Spoken Language (CASL) (Carrow-Woolfolk 1999) comprises amongst others *supralinguistic measures* to investigate if the child is able to comprehend complex language when meaning cannot directly be deduced from lexical or grammatical information.

16.16.5.2 Evaluation of Expressive Language with Phonetic, Phonological Levels, Semantic Levels, Working Memory and Word Finding, Morphological, Syntactic Levels, Prosody, Intelligibility and Pragmatics

According to da Silva et al. (2011), the most-often used instruments for expressive language in HL/CI children are the expressive parts of the Reynell Developmental Language Scales (RDLS) (see Edwards et al. 2011), The MacArthur

Communicative Development Inventories to assess lexical development (words, gestures, sentences) (MCDI) (Fenson et al. 2007), the Meaningful Use of Speech Scale (MUSS) (Robbins and Osberger 1990) and the expressive part of the Clinical Evaluation of Language Fundamentals (CELF) (for latest version, see Wiig et al. 2013). All these instruments are available in different versions and translations.

A useful test to assess expressive language in children from birth to 7 years 11 months is the corresponding part of the fifth edition of the Preschool Language Scale (PLS-5) (Zimmerman et al. 2011).

Evaluation of expressive language in hearing-impaired children should comprise phonetic, phonological, semantic, morphological, syntactic, prosodic and pragmatic levels:

Basic Phonetic Evaluation This method was introduced by Ling (1976). The tester produces a target sound and asks the child to imitate it. According to this author, the following skills were assessed:

- Vocalising on demand.
- Producing sound patterns: loud or soft, high or low pitched, sustained or brief.
- Producing all diphthongs and vowels with control.
- Producing consonant with /a/, /u/ and /i/.
- Producing initial and final consonant blends.

Phonetic Transcription Teoh and Chin (2007) performed phonetic transcriptions of 22 CI children to document the production of sounds with articulatory errors and distortions. The children labelled pictures, and the responses were recorded, digitised and edited. The transcription was performed with spectrographic support by two independent transcribers in phoneme-by-phoneme consensus.

Most common findings were:

- In place of articulation: inventories of coronal fricatives, nonstandard affricates, allophonic variants of /l/.

- In manner of articulation: substitution of dental stops for dental fricatives, spirantisation (i.e. the substitution of a fricative for a plosive), use of ejectives, glottalisation, flapping errors, partial nasality, gliding.
- In voicing: final obstruent devoicing, aspiration of voiced stops, unaspirated initial voiceless stops.
- In vowels: substitution of centralised vowels for /u/, errors of vowel length, use of nasal vowels for nasal consonants, lenition, monophthongisation, use of nonstandard diphthongs.

Archer and Crosby-Quinatoa (2009) use among others the Structured Photographic Articulation Test-Dudsberry II (by Dawson and Tattersall (2001), useful for ages 3–9 years) based on photographs of the golden retriever Dudsberry and the Arizona Articulation Proficiency Scale (Fudala 2001), a quick method for identifying misarticulations and most sensitive at preschool and early elementary school levels.

If a child knows how to articulate a sound correctly, this does not imply that the usage is correct in his spoken language.

Phonological Assessment This method investigates which phonetic elements (phonological contrasts) are used to achieve contrast of meaning in a specific language.

- Concerning vowels, any substitutions, neutralisation, diphthongisation and nasalisation of vowels are described.
- Concerning consonants, at least two presentations of all consonants of the language in initial, medial and final word positions are checked. Misarticulations of consonants are described in terms of voiced-voiceless errors, omission or distortion of initial and medial consonants, omission of consonants in blends, distortion of final consonants, substitution of one consonant for another, glottal replacement, final vowel additions and intrusive voicing between adjacent consonants. These non-developmental patterns should be differentiated from developmental processes such as final consonant deletion, reduplication, weak syllable deletion, cluster

reduction, context sensitive voicing, depalatalisation, fronting (fricatives and velars), alveolarisation (stops and fricatives), labialisation (stops), stopping (fricatives and affricates), gliding (fricatives and liquids), deaffrication, epenthesis, and metathesis (Flipsen and Parker 2008).

To study early phonological development in children with and without hearing loss, Moeller et al. (2007b) analysed recorded samples of mother–child interactions from 21 NH children and 12 HL children during the age span of 16–24 months. They defined vocal play, babble, jargon (babbled sequences with the intonation contours of spoken phrases), unintelligible communicative utterances, and words or word attempts.

The Mean Syllable Structure Level in Words, Percentage of Vowels Correct, Percentage of Consonants Correct, Phonological Mean Length of Utterance, Proportion of Whole Word Proximity, Word Shape Match and Words with Final Consonants were items of their analysis. In addition, the authors used parents' reports of vocabulary development from 10 to 30 months of age and at 36 months of age, based on spontaneous productions in a picture-naming task, the Goldman–Fristoe Test of Articulation-2 (Goldman and Fristoe 2000).

At 24 months of age, the HL toddlers produced fewer and less-complex words and were less accurate in consonant and word production. Delayed or limited use of syllables with consonants, vowel errors and limited production of recognisable words were found as indicators of atypical development.

Evaluation of Semantics, Working Memory and Word Finding Evaluating the meaning of words and utterances includes determining the number of single words uttered by the child, as well as evaluating complex use of vocabulary, including structures such as word categories, word relationships, synonyms, antonyms, figurative language, ambiguities and absurdities. In this respect, adjective, adverb, preposition, article and pronoun use is assessed. The response time in

selecting vocabulary words is also considered (word-finding problems such as circumlocutions, repetitions, frequent pauses). Over- or under-generalisation and frequent use of empty words such as 'thing', 'that', or the routinised expression 'you know' are all noted.

Archer and Crosby-Quinatoa (2009) use e.g. the Expressive Vocabulary Test-2nd Edition (EVT-2) (by Williams 2007) in children with cochlear implants. The child has to perform more complex tasks than only to label the pictured object or action. It seems that nowadays, owing to newborn-hearing screening and modern hearing devices, children with profound HL are also able to acquire a normal vocabulary with time. Ramos et al. (2015) could not find a significant difference from testing semantics in 18 CI children (9 and 10 years old) in comparison with the normal standard of NH children.

Marchman and Fernald (2008) found in NH children relations between word-recognition speed and vocabulary at 25 months with expressive language, IQ and especially working memory at age 8.

May-Mederake (2012) saw good results in an active vocabulary test in 28 CI children with early implantation in the first 2 years of life, but compared with their normative peers a poorer phonological working memory for nonsense words. Scientific work has still to be done to clarify the relationships between early perception, word learning and later language skills (Schwartz et al. 2013). Testing working memory seems to be a necessary step. Storing and processing of information were studied by Nittrouer et al. (2013) in 48 NH and 50 CI children, 8 years old. In CI children, less accurate recall of serial order was observed than in NH children but the rate of recall did not differ. The authors concluded that only storage is impaired in CI children.

An example of a word finding test is the Word Finding Vocabulary Test, a part of the Renfrew Language Scales (Renfrew and Mitchell 2015).

Evaluation of Morphology and Syntax Morphology assessment involves the evaluation of morphemes, the smallest units of language that have meaning.

A morpheme is a group of sounds that refers to a particular object, idea or action:

- Roots can stand alone (e.g. car, teach, tall).
- Affixes are bound, such as prefixes and suffixes, and when attached to root words change the meaning of the words (e.g. balls, baker, tallest, irresponsible).

Syntax assessment includes evaluating how the child uses the rules by which words are organised into phrases or sentences in their language. It refers to sentence structure.

This is typically assessed by referring to the mean length of utterance (MLU), the complexity of the sentence and word order in the sentence.

Boons et al. (2013) tested in 70 school-aged CI children (5–13.3 years) expressive morphological abilities by CELF Word Structure (CELF-WS) and expressive syntactic skills by CELF Formulating Sentences (CELF-FS), parts of the Dutch version CELF-4-NL (Kort et al. 2008). In comparison with the NH control group, the authors observed difficulties with morphological rules such as regular plurals, diminutives, irregular past participles, pronouns, comparative and superlative adjectives, demonstrative pronouns, articles and adjectives. Syntactical rules were more problematic for CI children with respect to nouns, verbs, adjectives, adverbs, conjunctions and prepositional expressions.

Testing of word ordering is part of the Test of Language Development: Intermediate (TOLD-I) (by Hammill and Newcomer 2001).

Evaluation of Prosody Prosody is defined by supra-segmental features of speech: stress, intonation, tone and duration (Kent and Kim 2008). To acquire prosody is important for the HL child because it concerns transmission of meaning and intelligibility of its utterances.

Evaluation of prosody comprises:

- Fundamental frequency patterns.
  - Average pitch: normal, too high or too low.
  - Pitch contour: appropriate or inappropriate.
  - Intonation: monotone, excessive variability or insufficient variability.
- Stress (emphasised or prominent units) normal, excessive or reduced.
- Temporal factors.
  - Rate appropriate, slow (<2 syllables per second) or fast (>4 syllables per second).
  - Duration of consonants and vowels: normal, increased or decreased.
  - Pause (juncture): normal or prolonged.
- Phrasing: syllable/word repetitions or syllable/word revisions.

Chin et al. (2012) studied prosody production in 15 CI (6.00–10.33 years) and 10 NH children (4.00–14.08 years) with the Prosodic Utterance Production (PUP) task (Bergeson and Chin 2008). Adults rated the performance of declarative, interrogative, happy and sad sentences. The percentage of correct scores was lower for CI children and the lowest ratings concerned interrogative intonation.

Evaluation of Intelligibility Speech intelligibility is either rated subjectively (poor, fair or good), quasi-objectively by rating scales, or by the ratio of intelligible words to the number of produced words (Ling 1976).

An example of a rating scale is the Speech Intelligibility Rating Test (SIR) (Cox and McDaniel 1989; Yoshinaga-Itano and Sedey 2000):

1. I always or almost always understand the child's speech with little or no effort.
2. I always or almost always understand the child's speech: however I need to listen carefully.
3. I typically understand about half of the child's speech.
4. I typically understand about 25% of the child's speech.
5. The child's speech is very hard to understand. I typically understand only occasional, isolated words or phrases.
6. I never or almost never understand the child's speech.

Chin et al. (2012) studied intelligibility in 15 CI (6.00–10.33 years) and 10 NH children (4.00–14.08 years) with the Beginner's Intelligibility Test (BIT; Osberger et al. 1994). This is a live-voice test of single sentences developed for CI children. The words are no longer than two syllables and are familiar to children. Adult listeners rated the performance in their study, the percentage of correct scores was higher for NH children than that of CI children, and better for children with longer hearing experience.

Evaluation of Pragmatics Pragmatic rules are needed to create interaction and transfer meaning, and comprise e.g. turn-taking, continuing a topic, adjoining information or questioning.

In order to assess pragmatic skills, the clinician has to observe the child in spontaneous, unstructured conversation with a partner.

The following communication skills should be commented on (Prutting 1982; DuCharme 1983):

- Following conversation rules for a topic: turn-taking, introducing and maintaining a topic, revising a message to fit a change in topic, modifying a message to repair breakdown in communication, and terminating conversation appropriately.
- Using language for different purposes: greeting, requesting, informing, demanding, promising.
- Changing language according to the needs of a listener or situation: talking differently to a baby and to an adult, giving background information to an unfamiliar listener, speaking differently in a classroom and on a playground.
- Abstraction: using sarcasm, understanding/responding to sarcasm, using idioms appropriately, understanding/responding appropriately to idioms.
- Visual/gestural cues: using appropriate eye contact, facial and body postures appropriately, using appropriate proximity/distance and physical contact and responding appropriately.

In HL children, acquiring pragmatic ability is delayed. Less-skilled pragmatic abilities may be turn-taking, repair strategies and maintaining a conversation topic; they use too many instructions instead of questions and have difficulty in multi-talker conversations (Rinaldi et al. 2013). Rinaldi et al. (2013) used Prutting and Kirchner's (1987) pragmatic protocol in 11 CI children and 13 HA children in comparison with 13 NH children (7 years old). They assessed verbal (e.g. response to the partner, cohesion, choosing conversation topic), paralinguistic (e.g. intelligibility, prosody, voice intensity, fluency) and non-verbal aspects (e.g. eye gaze, facial expression, physical contact). The videotaped child–adult conversations were analysed by two judges. CI and HA children showed more inappropriate use of the different pragmatic abilities than NH children. Most problematic were contingency (continuing the same topic, adding information), response and adjacency (continuing the same topic, immediately after the utterance of the conversational partner). Delayed or a different acquisition of pragmatic abilities in comparison with NH children may be explained by fewer opportunities for observing and practising an appropriate model of communication, *delayed language acquisition and a* failure to hear important cues (Rinaldi et al. 2013).

16.16.6 Evaluation of Auditory Perception Skills

To assess auditory perception skills, the hierarchy presented by Erber in 1982 is still a useful tool:

- Awareness/detection: The child responds by demonstrating absence or presence of sound.
- Discrimination: The child has to respond to whether two or more stimuli are similar or different.
  - Supra-segmentals with differences in duration–intensity–pitch–stress.
  - Segmentals: initial sound vocabulary–words varying in number of syllables–words with the same consonants but

varying vowels–words with the same vowel but varying consonants.

- Identification/recognition: The child responds by demonstrating recognition of what has been said by repeating or pointing to a picture or object as requested.
- Comprehension: The child demonstrates understanding of speech by:
  - Following a direction.
  - Answering a question.
  - Participating in a conversation.
  - Paraphrasing what has been said.
  - Answering questions about a story: open/closed set.

All these skills also to be tested in noisy environment.

Useful tools to measure auditory skills and progress over time may be the LittlEARS Auditory Questionnaire (May-Mederake et al. 2010) and the Evaluation of Auditory Responses to Speech (EARS) (Allum et al. 2000).

Among others the following tests are often used: the Early Speech Perception Test (Moog and Geers 1990), the Meaningful Use of Speech Scale (MUSS) (Robbins and Osberger 1990), the Meaningful Auditory Integration Scale (MAIS) (Robbins et al. 1991), the Test of Auditory Comprehension of Language (Carrow-Woolfolk 1985), the Ling 6 Sound Test (Ling 1989) and the Auditory Perception Test for the Hearing Impaired (Allen 2008).

For example, the BAS-II Digits Forward task (digit span) assesses auditory memory (GL Assessment 2011).

16.16.7 Evaluation of Visual Perception Skills

According to Berk (2000), the following parameters should be assessed for a basic visual perception evaluation: visual acuity, colour perception, focusing and tracking ability, depth perception, pattern recognition and object perception. For a full evaluation, the following should be assessed: visual coordination, visual discrimination, visual association, visual long-term memory, visual

Table 16.4 Examples of standardised tests to evaluate visual perception skills

Name of the test	Skills	Age range
Motor-Free Visual Perception Test, Fourth Edition (MVPT-4) by Colarusso and Hammill (2015)	– Spatial Relationship – Visual Closure – Visual Discrimination – Visual Memory – Figure Ground	4 through 80 years
Test of Visual Perceptual Skills, Fourth Edition (TVPS-4) by Martin (2017)	– Same as above plus: – Form Constancy – Visual Sequential Memory	5 through 21 years
Bender Visual-Motor Gestalt Test (Bender-Gestalt II) by Brannigan and Decker (2003)	– Visuospatial coordination – Visuomotor coordination	3 to 85+ years

short-term memory, visual sequential memory, visual vocal expression, visual motoric expression, visual figure ground discrimination, visual spatial relationships and visual form perception. Examples of standardised tests are shown in Table 16.4.

Testing of visual memory may also be useful. The Leiter-R Memory Screen is standardised on a deaf sample (Roid and Miller 1997).

16.16.8 Evaluation of Phonological Awareness, Reading, Writing (Details see Volume 2, Part III)

Phonological Awareness An important precursor of reading is the phonological awareness of syllables, rhymes and phonemes. In addition to the original test for phonological awareness by Bradley and Bryant (1983), a picture version has been developed by Harris and Beech (1998). The child is asked to point at two pictures out of three that share the same initial (e.g. boat, bow, rope), middle (hat, net, cat) or end sound (red, bed, pen).

To study phonological processing, Geers and Hayes (2011) used the following test instruments in 112 high school children with CI and found poorer phonological skills than in 46 NH peers:

- Woodcock Reading Mastery Test (WRMT) Revised (Woodcock 1987).
- Comprehensive Test of Phonological Processing (CTOPP) (Wagner et al. 1999).
- Children's Test of Nonword Repetition (CNRep) (Gathercole and Baddeley 1996).

Reading Assessment In Part III of Volume 2, reading assessment is intensively presented. Examples of formal reading assessment in HL children are:

- Test of Early Reading Ability: Deaf Hard of Hearing (TERA-D/HH) (Reid et al. 1991).
- Stanford Achievement Test for Hearing-Impaired Students (SAT-HI) (Gallaudet Research Institute 1983).

Geers and Hayes (2011) used the following tests in their study of 112 high school students with CI:

- Test of Reading Comprehension (TORC) (Brown et al. 1995).
- Peabody Individual Achievement Test (PIAT)-Revised (Dunn and Markwardt 1989).

Johnson and Goswani (2010) studied phonological awareness, vocabulary and reading in 21early and 22 late CI children, 16 HA children and 19 NH children (98–111 months old). They performed a rhyme test, an initial and final phoneme task, and for reading used the NARA-R test, the BAS-II single word reading subtest of the British Ability Scales and the Wordchains test (Miller Guron 1999), which measures visual word form familiarity. Phonological awareness, decoding, reading accuracy and reading comprehension were enhanced by early cochlear implantation.

Assessment of Writing In Part 3 of Volume II, assessment of writing is intensively presented. Evaluation of writing involves areas such as writing traits (examples include ideas, organisation, word choice, sentence structure and mechanics), writing process (the child's engagement in planning, composing and revision) and kinds of writing (the child's ability to utilise a variety of forms, such as essay, stories and reports).

To perform an informal assessment, a representative writing sample (or samples) is (are) collected. An example of an analysis scale is the following 'Written words rating scale' (syntactic complexity evaluation from written text) (Levitt et al. 1987) (Table 16.5).

In CI children shorter, less-complex sentences containing more errors were observed (Spencer et al. 2003). Although many CI children may achieve age-appropriate skills in literacy, in 112 high school students with CI Geers and Hayes (2011) found poorer skills in phonological processing tasks, spelling, and written expression in comparison with 46 NH peers. The authors used a picture spelling test and the Expository Writing with NTID Scoring (Schley and Albertini 2005). The four scoring categories comprised organisation and content of the assay, language use (e.g. spelling, grammatical structures) and vocabulary use. Although a wide variability in literacy outcomes was reported, better literacy skills are expected in general in CI children implanted at younger ages (Sarant 2012).

The Boehm Test of Basic Concepts (Boehm 1971) investigates basic concepts that are decisive for school performance. Children at risk for a learning difficulty can be identified from percentiles and performance ranges.

Table 16.5 Written words rating scale (Levitt et al. 1987)

Rating	Category description
1	No useful output (no words related to test material)
2	Single words related to the test material (labelling only, incorrect word order)
3	Some evidence of syntactic structure (words in correct word order, or use of verbs. Repetitive, fixed word order is not counted)
4	Essentially complete structure, although errors may be present
5	Substantial output, essentially complete structure

With kind permission from American Speech-Language-Hearing Association ASHA

16.17 Occupational Therapy Examinations

Jill Massey

16.17.1 Occupational Therapy: Definition and Special Needs in Hearing-Impaired Children

Occupational therapy employs a client-centred approach focusing on enabling an individual to participate in a variety of occupations to enhance health and wellbeing. The term 'occupations' refers to everything people do in the course of their daily life (College of Occupational Therapists (COT) 2015).

Occupation within the context of children and young people includes aspects of self-care such as developing their independence in dressing, eating a meal and using the toilet; work or being productive within school, college and university or caring for others; and leisure socialising and playing with friends and participating in hobbies or sports (COT 2015).

Promoting engagement, developing independence and preparing children and young people for independence in future life are core occupational therapy values. Occupational therapists work with those whose occupations are affected by injury, illness or disability, by family situations, and during changes of circumstances.

The impact of a hearing impairment for children and young people on development of language is widely documented, but it can be wide ranging with a profound effect that is often overlooked. Children who are hearing-impaired engage in fewer interactions with hearing peers (Simeonsson et al. 2001; Stinson and Liu 1999). Without this interaction, they do not experience the same levels of social or academic group participation as their hearing peers, nor do they receive the social and academic benefits that such participation provides. Young people with hearing impairment have been observed to develop limited life skills (Akamatsu et al. 2005). It is assumed these students experience limited opportunities and miss the incidental learning prospects to develop independence in life skills compared with typically developing peers.

Children with a hearing impairment or deafness must rely on other sensory systems. Therefore, they have been identified to be at greater risk of delays in sensory processing, motor skills, balance and the ability to carry out complex motor sequences (Gheysen et al. 2007; Schlumberger et al. 2004; Russel and Nagaishi 2010). These delays or deficits can inhibit occupational performance and development in the areas of self-care productivity and leisure.

Occupational therapists should be an integral member of a collaborative multidisciplinary team working with a child or young person who has a hearing impairment, and use their unique occupational lens to evaluate and ameliorate participation and development of daily occupations, by utilising adaptive and compensatory approaches, alongside planning and implementing education for the child, young person, their family and other professionals working with the child.

16.17.2 Evaluation

Gathering Information and Interview The occupational therapist's evaluation will include gathering information to form an occupational profile of the client. Initial referral information should include the student's type and degree of hearing loss, age of onset, cause of hearing loss, medical history comprising any additional disabilities and the student's level and preferred method of communication.

Through the use of a client-centred structured and semi-structured interview approach with the family, child and other key professionals such as the education team, the occupational therapist will then explore the child's daily life, routine occupations, needs and expectations, determine their strengths and how they are able to participate and identify any barriers or challenges that are influencing their successful participation.

In the case of interviewing a child with a hearing impairment, the occupational therapist will adapt their communication style to meet the needs of the student, depending on the student's preferred method of communication, age and literacy level. This may include use of simplified language, pictures and/or symbols; the most suitable method of communication should be discussed with the speech and language therapist and, where feasible, the specialist teacher of the deaf.

Observation A fundamental part of the occupational therapist's evaluation will involve contextual observation of the child's participating in his daily occupations. Where possible this is best undertaken within the natural environment. Analysis of the child's occupational performance along with the information gathered enables the therapist to determine what supports or limits the child's ability to participate in home, community and school settings. Activity demands, client factors and contexts in which the child performs occupations form part of the therapist's comprehensive assessment.

Assessment Tools Therapists also have a wide range of norm-referenced and criterion-referenced developmental assessment tools, which may typically be used in their practice, forming part of the comprehensive assessment. However, many rely on language for their standardised delivery; such tools need to be adapted or modified for their use with a child or young person with hearing impairment. Subsequently qualitative information can be taken and reported; standard scores should not be reported. Any reporting of information should include any amplification (if any) the children are using and details of how the assessment was modified taking into consideration their hearing impairment, e.g. their level of language and method of communication.

Goal Setting Having identified areas of important occupations, the occupational therapist will work with the child, family and other key people to evaluate what helps or hinders their involvement in daily life roles and to set client-centred meaningful goals for occupational therapy provision. As well as directing intervention, the goals can be reviewed after intervention and used as an outcome measure to determine the effectiveness of therapy with the child or young person.

16.17.3 Intervention

Working collaboratively with the child or young person, their family and key professionals, the occupational therapist will develop possible solutions, such as exploring alternative ways of doing things, developing skills through adapted or simplified approaches, using task analysis or making changes to the environment to support participation.

Deaf children have been identified as being at increased risk (anywhere between 30 and 50% more likely) of mental health difficulties compared with their hearing peers. Access to high-quality, effective mental health services is a key standard of the Children's National Service Framework in the UK. Within the UK occupational therapists who focus on the mental health difficulties of a young person with hearing impairment play a central role within the specialist of National Deaf Child and Adolescent Mental Health Service (CAMHS) team of professionals. Communication can be challenging for deaf families; it is also recognised that, for a variety of reasons, the developmental pathways for deaf children differ from those of their hearing counterparts. The social-emotional mental health needs of the child or young person who is hearing-impaired need to be properly considered for intervention to be effective. A developmental occupational therapist will often work together with the National Deaf CAMHS team to promote effective outcomes (Beresford et al. 2008).

16.17.4 Conclusion

The occupational therapists' holistic approach to understanding the strengths of and barriers to a hearing-impaired student's participation in routines and activities in all aspects of their daily life can help to improve participation in all aspects of occupation through modifications or adaptations to the environment. It is critical for occupational therapists to form part of the multi-disciplinary team supporting a child or young person with hearing impairment, in order to enable their maximum independence and engagement in meaningful occupation, social activities and opportunities for future life.

16.18 Evaluation of General Cognitive Developmental Stage

See Part III Sect. 11.7.

16.19 Child Psychological Examinations Including Tests to Rule Out Attention Deficit Disorders

See Part I, Chap. 3, Sect. 3.5 and Part III, Chap. 11, Sects. 11.7 and 11.8.

16.20 Aetiological Assessment After the Diagnosis of a Permanent Hearing Loss[2]

Thomas Wiesner

16.20.1 Introduction

In the case of a child diagnosed with a hearing loss, the literature provides diverse lists of examinations that are recommended for its aetiological assessment (Gürtler in press). Yet most of these lists are quite general and do not specify, for example:

- The details that should be requested when ordering a certain examination
- At what age the examination should be performed

---

[2]International Bureau for Audiophonology, Commission 12, adapted from the BIAP-Recommendation 12-7: Aetiological assessment after the diagnosis of a permanent hearing loss, April 2013, www.biap.org.

- Whether the examination must be repeated at certain intervals
- Which kind of hearing loss requires which examinations
- How the medical history and already existing test results affect the selection of additional examinations

To ensure that the necessary examinations are performed at the right time, and that unnecessary examinations can be prevented, the following text gives guidelines to the questions: *Which tests, what are the goals and at which age?*

16.20.2 Proposal for a Stepwise Aetiological Assessment Process

The examinations necessary for an aetiological assessment should be proposed to the parents of all children with a permanent hearing loss at the beginning of the rehabilitation process:

- Aetiological assessments should be carried out in parallel with, and without delaying, the further multidisciplinary assessment of the hearing loss itself.
- The choice of tests has to depend on the prior clinical examination and the case history.
- The goals for this completive assessment after the diagnosis of the hearing loss are:
  - To supplement and specify the auditory diagnosis
  - To initiate certain risk preventive actions (e.g. vaccination against *Haemophilus influenzae* and *Pneumococcus* in the case of a malformation of the internal ear, which increases the risk of meningitis as a complication of an ear infection)
  - To adjust and complete the information given to the parents in respect of the diagnosis, the therapeutic proposals and the follow-up
- Any aetiological assessment needs informed consent of the parents.

16.20.2.1 Elements of the Aetiological Assessment

These include searching for a clue that may lead to a possible cause of the deafness:

- Looking for risk factors according to the list of the JCIH (Joint Committee on Infant Hearing 2007).
- Reconsidering the family history, including parents and relatives of three generations (a questionnaire with specific questions is helpful).
- All hearing-impaired children need a careful paediatric examination including a paediatric neurology evaluation and an ENT clinical examination, especially searching for signs such as:
  - A white wick, unpigmented cutaneous spots, different eye colours or blue crystal eyes in combination with a bilateral sensorineural hearing loss would point to the diagnosis of a Waardenburg syndrome.
  - Cervical fistulas and pits with ear deformities suggesting branchio-oto-renal (BOR) syndrome.
  - Cleft lip/palate, down-slanting eyes, coloboma, low-set small external ears and mandible and maxillary hypoplasia in association with a conductive type of hearing loss, which would possibly indicate Treacher Collins syndrome.
  - Palatal and lip clefts in association with choanal atresia, external ear deformity and facial paralysis, which might raise the suspicion of CHARGE association or similar syndromes.
  - Cleft palate, velopharyngeal dysfunction and congenital heart defects (often already detected by prenatal sonography) may suggest a microdeletion 22q11.2 syndrome (DiGeorge syndrome, velocardiofacial syndrome).
  - Microcephaly that might be seen in association with perinatal CMV (cytomegalovirus) or rubella infection or other events such as birth asphyxia or brain underdevelopment.

- For reducing the strain on the families, the recommended examinations should be combined as far as possible to keep the number of appointments low.
- The timetable (Table 16.6) and the list of recommended examinations are not strict rules to be followed automatically but a proposal that must be adapted to the special situation of every child and its family.

The order of the recommended examinations refers to a very efficient proposal of De Leenheer et al. (2011). This proposal heavily relies on an early genetic evaluation. As this may not be accepted by all patients, the concept was not fully endorsed by the BIAP, but the proposed flowchart can be found in the publication of De Leenheer et al. (2011).

16.20.2.2 Specifications for the Diagnostic Procedures Named in the Timetable 16.6 (See Numbering in Table 16.6)

1. The examination algorithm to assess a congenital CMV infection is presented in Fig. 16.33.
2. The chances and limits of genetic testing must be discussed with the parents, such as which diagnoses the genetic tests are looking for and whether and how the knowledge of a certain diagnosis is helpful in the management and treatment of the child. The parents must be informed of the potential likelihoods of heredity transmission, but also that the results of the genetic assessment might concern not only the deaf child but also other members of his family. The testing is only allowed with the parent's permission. The counselling of the parents should be done by a geneticist specialised in hearing disorders (or a hearing specialist specially trained in genetic counselling).

   For the genetic testing, it is necessary to have as far as possible the complete medical history, a clinical paediatric examination and the results of the above recommended aetiological assessment including the audiometric results of the family members.

Table 16.6 Timetable for recommended examinations in the aetiological assessment

Timetable								
Type of hearing loss	Sensorineural (SNHL)						Conductive	
Degree of hearing loss	Profound		Other degrees progressive		Other degrees stable			
Examination	First test	Test repetition	First test	Test repetition	First test	Test repetition	First test	Test repetition
1. CMV screening	A.s.a.p.	–	A.s.a.p.	–	A.s.a.p.	–	–	–
2. Genetic	See remark in text							
3. MRI	<12 m	–	A.s.a.p.	–	When possible without sedation	–	–	–
4. CT scan	<12 m	–	–	–	–	–	When possible without sedation or before surgery	–
5. Ophthalmological examination	6 m	Every year	6 m	Every year	6 m	Every year	6 m	Every year
6. Searching for pre- and perinatal infections	<12 m A.s.a.p.	–	<12 m A.s.a.p.	–	<12 m A.s.a.p.	–	–	–
7. Haematuria/proteinuria screening + echo kidney	If malformation of external or middle ear	–	If malformation of external or middle ear	–	If malformation of external or middle ear	–	A.s.a.p.	–
8. ECG	<6 m	Once at ~18 m	–	–	–	–	If CHARGE syndrome in CT	–
9. ERG	>9 m	–	If clinical RP signs	–	–	–	–	–
10. Vestibular tests	<6 m	If first abnormal and pre and post CI	A.s.a.p.	If motor delay	<12 m A.s.a.p.	If motor delay	If hypotonia or if CHARGE syndrome	If hypotonia or if CHARGE syndrome

The numbering in the timetable corresponds to the numbering of the more detailed explanations of recommended examinations in the text

Comment: In case of a mixed hearing loss, the CT scan should be done <12 m. If this CT scan shows an inner ear malformation, follow the recommendation for the 'SNHL—other degrees stable'

MRI magnetic resonance imaging; *CT* computed tomography; *ECG* electrocardiography; *ERG* electroretinography; *RP* retinitis pigmentosa; *CI* cochlear implant; *a.s.a.p.* 'as soon as possible'; *m* month of age

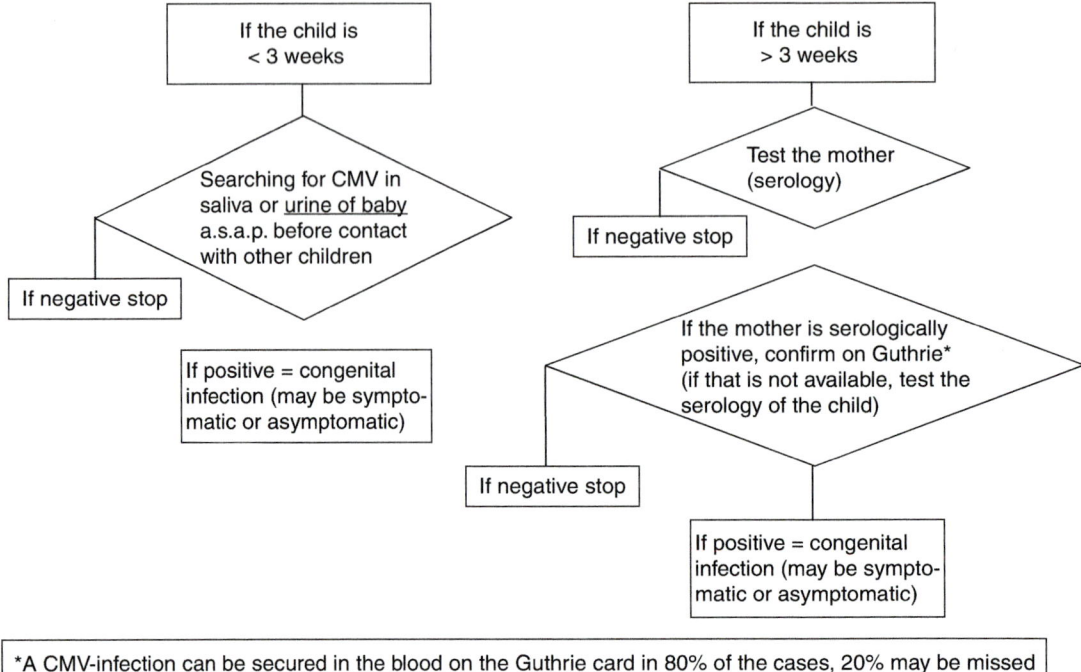

Fig. 16.33 Flowchart of an examination algorithm to assess a congenital CMV infection (Barbi et al. 2000; Boppana et al. 2011; Foulon et al. 2008, 2012; Soetens et al. 2008)

In case of an isolated cochlear SNHL, it is recommended first that a search for a mutation in connexin 26 and 30 genes be made, because it is the most frequent cause in this case.

In case of a motor developmental delay and vestibular problems, it is recommended that Usher syndrome is sought, provided that there are no additional clinical signs, e.g. pointing to CHARGE or other syndromic conditions with a developmental delay, and vestibular and hearing problems.

The decision on which kind of genetic test should be used will depend on whether a syndromic (Waardenburg, Pendred, Jervell, Alport, etc.) or an isolated non-syndromic cause of the hearing loss is being sought.

In the case of a non-syndromic hearing loss, the selection of genetic tests will be influenced by the preceding diagnostic findings of:

- Conductive or sensorineural
- Auditory neuropathy or auditory dyssynchrony spectrum (otoferlin)
- Inner ear malformation or not
- Outer ear or middle ear malformation
- Genetic transmission mode shown by the family history (mitochondrial type? X-linked? dominant? recessive?)

High-throughput next-generation sequencing (NGS) allows parallel screening of large panels of hearing-related genes with high accuracy, in a short time, at a cost lower than conventional Sanger sequencing (American College of Medical Genetics Expert Panel 2002). This can be achieved either by targeted capture of several dozens of genes or by direct sequencing of all exons present in the genome (so-called whole exome sequencing or WES). Targeted NGS screening would only detect genome variations in genes known to be involved in hearing loss. WES theoretically could uncover all DNA sequence variations, but laboratories that offer such WES may decide to filter the data and consider only pertinent genes (giving nevertheless the possibility of going back to the raw data to analyse further genes if necessary). Obviously, only targeted sequencing is convenient in a diagnostic setting. The strategy followed by the laboratory to which samples are sent must thus be clearly defined. At this point, the use of non-filtered WES data is limited to research. Parents must be informed before the examination whether the NGS screening will be in a diagnostic setting (i.e. focused on known hearing loss-causing genes) or whether the investigation is wider and may uncover unexpected negative findings, such as harmful mutations in genes predisposing to late-onset disorders. Genetic diagnosis and genetic counselling following the use of these new technologies require a close connection between clinicians and audiologists, clinical geneticists (or genetic counsellors) and molecular biologists, to avoid improper interpretation and for cross-validation between genotype and phenotype: even targeted NGS discloses a vast amount of DNA sequence variations whose significance may be unknown, or dubious. Genetic counselling based on NGS data may thus involve a number of ethical risks and questions that are not satisfactorily answered politically, juristically or by civil society.

3./4. Imaging should be performed by a specialist for paediatric radiology:

The decision whether to use a CT or MRI first will be influenced by whether one is searching for bony or soft tissue deficiencies (BAPA and BAAP 2008).

Temporal MRI scan and CT, general considerations:

- In case of a profound deafness.
- Before the end of the first year of life.
- For a CT a low radiation scanner should be used (e.g. cone beam scanner).
- A CT needs radiation but can be done so quickly that it can be performed during natural sleep (especially with very young children) or when under sedation.
- An MRI has no radiation but takes much longer and therefore normally needs general anaesthesia.

Aim of temporal MRI: searching for a malformation of the:

- Vestibular aqueduct (dilation)
- Cochlear or vestibular fibrosis
- Internal auditory canal

- The auditory, vestibular and facial nerve
- Central auditory pathways
- Brain (lesions)

Aim of CT: searching for a malformation of the:

- Ear (outer, middle and inner ear) and the vestibular organ
- Internal auditory canal
- Vestibular aqueduct (dilation)

5. **Aim** Searching for any impaired vision that might enhance the sensory deficit of the child and specifically for any signs of an 'oculo-auditory syndrome': coloboma, optic nerve abnormalities, oculomotor anomalies, refraction disorders, inflammation of the cornea or the retina, and cataract

   Exam Ophthalmological examination (incl. ocular motricity study and funduscopy) done by a specialist experienced in examining young children. (The early funduscopy does not rule out an 'Usher syndrome type I', because the specific signs of a retinitis pigmentosa occur later in childhood!)

   For the indication of an electroretinogram, see Point 8.

6. As with some infections such as CMV, toxoplasmosis and rubella, neither the mother nor the child might show obvious clinical signs of the infection, so one should also search for the following prenatal and perinatal infections in cases of an isolated, idiopathic hearing loss:

- CMV (see above)
- Toxoplasmosis
- Determination of antibodies (IgM and IgG) against *Toxoplasma gondii* in the hearing-impaired newborn should be performed, except in cases where the mother was known to be immune before pregnancy.
- Rubella
- If either maternal rubella immunisation by vaccination has not been performed or the maternal status is unknown, this diagnosis should be considered, and maternal and neonatal rubella-specific IgM and IgG should be determined.

As asymptomatic congenital infections of syphilis and herpes are very unlikely, routine serological screenings for these infections are not necessary in otherwise healthy hearing-impaired children.

16.20.2.3 Particular Situations Are an Indication for Complementary Testing

7. **Aim** Searching for a haematuria or proteinuria

    Exam Urine stick (a non-invasive procedure, but strong evidence to recommend this examination as a general screening is lacking; if any clinical signs of kidney malfunction occur, a thorough examination of the kidneys is necessary)

    Aim Searching for malformations of the kidney and urinary tract

    Exam Kidney sonography, if there are even minor malformations of the ear or a history of urinary and renal symptoms

8. **Aim** Searching for a prolongation of the QT interval in case of bilateral deafness (Jervell and Lange-Nielsen syndrome (BAPA and BAAP 2008)).

    Exam The ECG should be done by a paediatric cardiologist.

9. (see also Point 5)

    Aim Searching for 'Usher syndrome type I'. An abnormal ERG does not prove the Usher diagnosis in all cases; therefore a genetic assessment is additionally necessary. The diagnosis of an Usher syndrome should be communicated to the parents only by a clinician with specific experience in the management of patients with Usher syndrome.

    Exam An electroretinogram should be done in profoundly deaf children showing hypotonia or vestibular areflexia (not before the age of 9 months).

10. A vestibular examination should include otolithic functions and the semicircular canal functions.

16.21 Diagnostic Radiology

Sylva Bartel-Friedrich and Sabrina Kösling

16.21.1 Ear Malformations

16.21.1.1 Epidemiology

According to Weerda (2004), 50% of ENT malformations affect the ear. Congenital malformations (CMs) of the outer and middle ear occur mostly on the right side (58–61%), and the majority (ca. 70–90%) are unilateral. Inner ear CM may be found unilaterally or bilaterally. An incidence of 1:6000 to 1:6830 newborns has been reported for outer ear CM (Weerda 2004). Severe CM can be expected in 1:10000 to 1:20000 newborns (Ishimoto et al. 2005; Swartz and Harnsberger 1997; Weerda 2004). In terms of prevalence rates, the microtia is higher: ca. 2:10000 to 9:10000 births, depending on the data source (passive vs active surveillance systems) (EUROCAT 2013; Queißer-Luft and Spranger 2006; Schloss 1997).

CM can affect all three parts of the ear (outer ear (pinna and external auditory canal, EAC), middle ear, inner ear), not infrequently in combination. Inner ear CM frequencies of 11–47% in individuals with outer and middle ear CM have been reported (Kösling et al. 2009). CM of the middle ear can accompany CM of the outer ear at variable degrees and frequencies; according to Ishimoto, the ossicles are affected in 6–52% of cases, the round and oval window in 6–29%, the mastoid pneumatisation in 15–38%, the course of the facial nerve in 36–43% and the middle ear space in 0–15% (Ishimoto et al. 2005).

The most common form of CM is a combined deformity known as congenital aural atresia, involving severe CM of the pinna and the middle ear with the characteristic finding of an atretic EAC; there is accompanying CM of the inner ear in ca. 10% of cases, and the CMs are bilateral in 15–20% of patients. Nevertheless, the different embryogenesis of the outer/middle ear and inner ear results in CM of the outer or middle ear without inner ear CM and vice versa (Helms 1994). Overall, inner ear CM, middle ear CM and combined CM of all three parts of the ear are less frequent than congenital aural atresia.

Isolated middle ear CMs (often bilateral) without coexisting outer ear CM have been reported to occur in less than 10% of children with congenital conductive hearing loss (CHL) according to Lambert (2001).

The prevalence of inner ear CM in individuals with congenital deafness or sensorineural hearing loss (SNHL) varies from 2.3 to 28.4% depending on patient selection criteria. In groups of patients strictly selected for suspicion of CM, inner ear CMs were detected in 35% by means of CT and MRI, with MRI better at displaying the fine details (Kösling et al. 2003). In addition, as mentioned for CM of the outer and middle ear, the course of the facial nerve is found to be aberrant in ca. 15–32% of patients with cochleovestibular CM (Huang et al. 2012a).

CM can result from a developmental arrest, from irregular embryogenesis or from both, owing to spontaneous genetic mutations—this is the case for the majority of CM of the outer and middle ear—genetic transmission and exogenous factors (in about 10% of cases; e.g. teratogens such as retinoic acid, thalidomide and the immunosuppressant mycophenolate mofetil).

16.21.1.2 Congenital Malformations of the Outer and Middle Ear

Clinical Signs and Classification CM of the outer ear can involve the orientation, position, size and relief pattern of the pinna; anotia may also occur. Anterior to the pinna, ear tags, ear sinus and ear pits may be found. The EAC can be atretic (aplastic) or hypoplastic. Middle ear CM can affect the configuration and size of the middle ear spaces and the number, size and configuration of the ossicles. There may be anomalies of the oval window and, rarely, of the round window. On the whole, it can be stated that there is normally a correlation between the degree of CM of the pinna and that of the middle ear with the corresponding CHL. Nevertheless, normal auricles with atresia of the EAC and albeit rarely microtia combined with normal EAC and normal tympanic cavity have been reported (Klaiber and Weerda 2002). Tables 16.7 and 16.8 list the most commonly used classifications for CM of the outer ear (Fig. 16.34).

Table 16.7 Grades of dysplasia of the pinna with subgroups according to Weerda (2004)

Grade of dysplasia	Subgroups
I: First-degree CM	• Prominent ears • Macrotia • Cryptotia (pocket ear) • Coloboma (transverse cleft) • Scaphoid ear • Stahl ear • Satyr ear • Slight deformities (distinct Darwin tuberculum, absent crus of helix, deformities of tragus and antitragus) • Deformities of lobe (fixed lobe, hyperplasia or hypoplasia or aplasia or cleft of lobe) • Cup ear deformity type I • Cup ear deformity type IIa • Cup ear deformity type IIb Most structures of the normal pinna are recognisable. The reconstruction only occasionally requires the use of additional skin or cartilage

II: Microtia grade II, second-degree CM	• Cup ear deformity type III
	 • Mini-ear ('concha-type microtia')
	   – Hypoplasia of upper pinna
	   – Hypoplasia of middle pinna
	   – Hypoplasia (or aplasia) of lower pinna
	 Often combined with dystopia and EAC stenosis, rarely with EAC atresia, ear drum CM possible
	 Some structures of a normal auricle are recognisable. Partial reconstruction of the pinna requires the use of some additional skin and cartilage

III: Microtia grade III with anotia, third-degree CM	• Unilateral microtia grade III ('lobule-type microtia', Fig. 16.34) • Bilateral microtia grade III • Anotia often with dystopia and EAC atresia None of the normal structures of the pinna are recognisable. Total reconstruction requires the use of skin and large amounts of cartilage

Besides a wide range of findings within each grade of dysplasia, additional transitional forms have been noted, especially between grade II and grade III. Adapted from Weerda (2004) Thieme © 2004

Table 16.8 Classification of EAC malformations according to Weerda (2004)

Type of CM	Signs of CM
EAC stenosis type A	Marked narrowing of the EAC along with an intact skin layer[a]
EAC stenosis type B	Partial development of the EAC with an atresia plate at the medial part[b]
Type C	Complete bony EAC atresia[c]

Adapted from Weerda (2004) Thieme © 2004

[a]Type A, compared with atresia, carries a much greater risk of cholesteatoma, beginning at a canal opening of 4 mm or less. In ears with a bony canal opening of 2 mm or less, the risk of cholesteatoma formation increases to 91% by the age of 12 years (Declau et al. 2008). Thus, surgery is recommended for canals of 2 mm or less

[b]Depending on concomitant middle ear malformations or conductive hearing loss, it may be advisable to implement hearing aid treatment

[c]Often it is advisable to implement hearing aid treatment in view of the frequently concomitant middle ear malformations with conductive hearing loss

The classification of CM of the EAC according to Weerda (2004) includes three types, shown in Table 16.8.

The closely interrelated development of the EAC and the middle ear has led to the widely used classification of the combined CM termed congenital aural atresia according to Altmann (1955). Three degrees of severity are described, each based on its histopathological findings:

First-degree CM:	Stenosis of the EAC, normal or slightly hypoplastic tympanic cavity, deformed ossicles, well-aerated mastoid (Fig. 16.35)
Second-degree CM:	Blindly ending or absent EAC, narrow tympanic cavity, deformation and fixation of ossicles, decreased mastoid pneumatisation
Third-degree CM:	Absent EAC, absent mastoid pneumatisation (atresia plate), hypoplastic or rudimentary tympanic cavity, severely deformed ossicles (Fig. 16.36)

Ossicular CMs include fusion of the malleus and incus, fixation in the epitympanic recess, bony ankylosis of the neck of the malleus to the atresia plate, hypoplasia of the manubrium of the malleus and absent malleus and incus.

According to Müller (1991), three degrees of severity of isolated middle ear CM can be differentiated:

Mild CM:	Normal configuration of the tympanic cavity, ossicular dysplasia
Moderate CM:	Hypoplasia of the tympanic cavity, dysplastic or aplastic ossicles
Severe CM:	Aplastic or cleft-like tympanic cavity

Stapes CMs frequently occur in isolated 'minor' (mild) middle ear deformities. The most common type of isolated ossicular chain CM is a combined deformity of the stapes superstructure and of the incus, especially of its long process and lenticular process. There are frequently incudostapedial joint fusions and aplasia or hypoplasia of the stapes superstructures, such as snapped-off stapes head; thickening, thinning and fusion of the stapedial crura; and masses of bony or fibrotic tissue between the crura. Stapes fixation can result from bony plates or from apla-

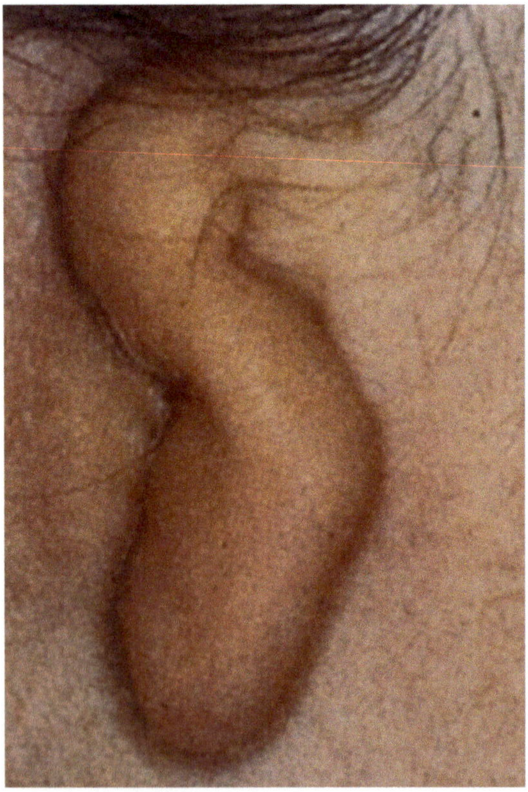

Fig. 16.34 Microtia grade III ('lobule-type microtia')

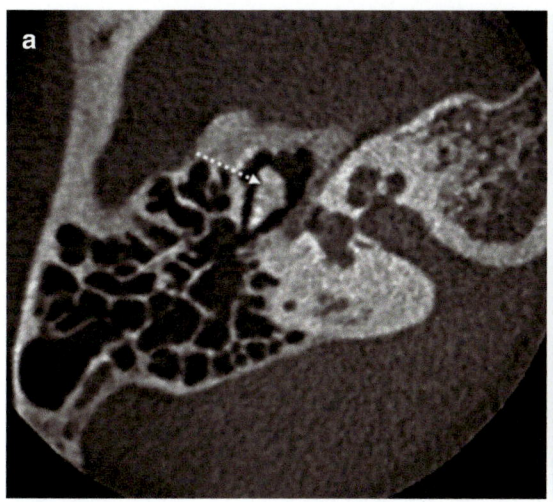

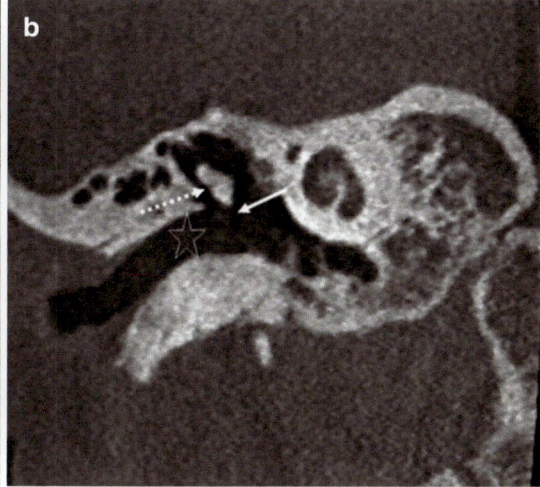

Fig. 16.35 CB-CT (A axial, B coronal) of a 13-year-old boy with unilateral auricular appendage, EAC stenosis and CHL of 45 dB. Narrowing of EAC (*star*), fused incudomalleolar joint (*dotted arrows*), absent malleolar manubrium (*arrow*), slightly smaller tympanic cavity than normal, normal pneumatisation and inner ear structures. Mild congenital aural atresia, grade I according to Altmann classification

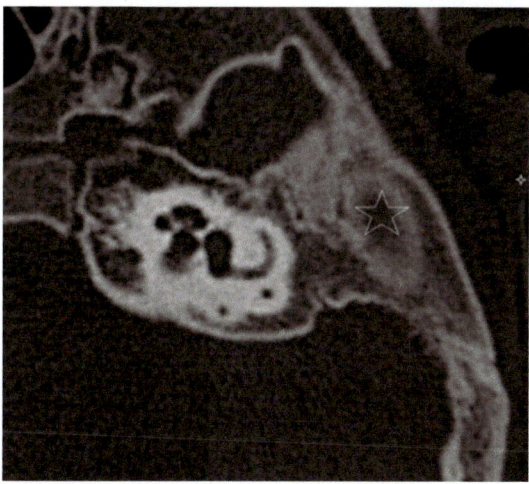

Fig. 16.36 Axial CT of a 6-year-old boy with unilateral microtia, atresia of EAC and severe CHL. Known Goldenhar syndrome. Absent tympanic cavity, broad atresia plate (*star*), normal inner ear. Severe congenital aural atresia, grade III according to Altmann classification

sia or dysplasia of the annular ligament. Moreover, stapes can be completely absent. On the basis of the frequent involvement of the stapes, Declau et al. (1999) proposed a modified classification.

Other changes viewed as malformations of the middle ear are cerebral spinal fluid (CSF)-middle ear fistulas (indirect translabyrinthine or direct paralabyrinthine CSF fistulas), congenital tumours (epidermoid) and dermoids (see Sect. 16.21.2 of this section).

CM of the outer and middle ear may be found in syndromes (Table 16.9), most commonly Franceschetti (Treacher Collins) syndrome, Goldenhar syndrome and Klippel Feil syndrome (Fig. 16.37).

Table 16.9 also lists syndromes in which hearing loss is a frequent or major component, but where malformations are not commonly detected by imaging.

The diagnosis of CM of the outer and middle ear is based on clinical examination and imaging.

Clinical Examination CMs of the outer and middle ear are diagnosed in early childhood in cases with deformities of the auricles or bilateral hearing impairment. If there is only unilateral hearing loss without external deformities, the diagnosis may be delayed. Thus, anamnesis plays an important role. The time of onset of the hearing problems should be established and other causes for hearing loss, e.g. infection, excluded. If CM is not suspected, CT is not frequently performed and the diagnosis is made during tympanotomy.

Table 16.9 Selected syndromes commonly associated with hearing loss and CM of the ear (Adapted from Beale and Madani 2008, Gorlin et al. 1990, Huang et al. 2012b)

Group of syndromes	Name of syndrome	Hearing loss			CM			
		CHL	SNHL	Mixed	Outer/middle ear	Inner ear	Facial nerve course	Not common on imaging
Otocraniofacial	Craniofacial microsomia, incl. Goldenhar	+	(+)	(+)	Pinna malformations, EAC atresia or stenosis, absent/abnormal ossicles, tegmen descent	IAC porus abnormally high	(+)	–
	Treacher Collins	+	(+)	(+)	Pinna malformations, EAC atresia, size-reduced attic/antrum, abnormal ossicles	Dysplastic lateral SCC	Altered	–
	BOR	+	+	+	EAC atresia or stenosis, abnormal ossicles	Hypoplasia of apical cochlear turn/Mondini deformity, vestibular dysplasia, SCC hypoplasia, LVA, short/bulbous/funnel-shaped IAC, CND	Obtuse angle of anterior genu	–
	CHARGE	+	+	+	Pinna malformations, EAC atresia or stenosis, abnormal ossicles, absent windows	Mondini deformity, absent SCC, vestibular dysplasia, CND	Abnormal	–
	X-linked deafness (with stapes gusher)	+	+	+	–	Enlarged/bulbous IAC, widened cochlear aperture, absence/deficiency of lamina cribrosa, cochlear hypoplasia, LVA	Widening of bony canal of labyrinthine segment	–
Cranio-synostoses	Crouzon	+	(+)	(+)	EAC atresia or stenosis, abnormal ossicles, petromastoid hypopneumatised, pyramid upward tilting	Large vestibule, dysplastic SCC	(+)	–
Otocervical	Klippel Feil and Wildervanck	+	+	+	Pinna malformations, EAC atresia or stenosis, abnormal ossicles	Mondini deformity, dysplastic SCC	(+)	–
	Pendred	–	+	–	–	Mondini deformity, modiolar deficiency, enlarged vestibule, LVA and sac	(+)	–
	Waardenburg	–	+	–	–	LVA, vestibule widening, decreased modiolus size, IAC hypoplasia, hypo-/aplasia of posterior SCC	(+)	–
Otoskeletal (bone dysplasias)	Osteogenesis imperfecta	+	+	+	Thin ossicles	Bone demineralisation within otic capsule	–	–
	Otodystrophies associated with sclerosis	–	–	+	(+)	Osteopetrosis with increased bone density	–	–
	Alport	–	+	–	–	–	–	+
	Jervell and Lange-Nielsen	–	+	–	–	–	–	+
	Norrie	–	+	–	–	–	–	+
	Stickler	–	+	–	–	–	–	+
	Usher	–	+	–	–	–	–	+

CM congenital malformation; *CHL* conductive hearing loss; *SNHL* sensorineural hearing loss; *BOR* branchio-oto-renal; *CHARGE* coloboma, *heart, atresia* of the choanae, retarded growth and development, genital hypoplasia and *ear* anomalies and/or deafness; *CND* cochlear nerve deficiency; *EAC* external auditory canal; *IAC* internal auditory canal; *LVA* large vestibular aqueduct; *SCC* semicircular canal

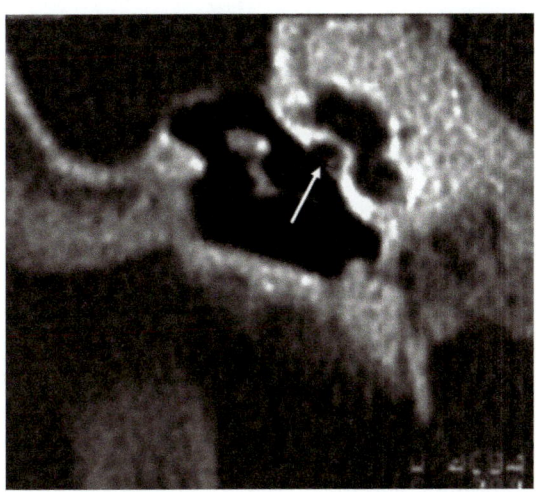

Fig. 16.37 Coronal CT of a 13-year-old boy with unilateral CHL of 40 dB. Known Klippel Feil syndrome. Moderate middle ear malformation and abnormal position of the facial nerve (arrow) in the oval window

Imaging Specific imaging of the temporal bone (not brain or skull imaging) has to be requested for patients with CM of the ear. CT or alternatively cone beam CT (CB-CT) is the method of choice in CM of the outer and middle ear. Conventional X-rays play no role in ear CM, and MRI delivers no diagnostic information. Diagnosis of CM requires optimal local resolution on CT. Primarily, this means low slice thickness (0.5–1 mm), use of a bone algorithm and a high zoom (small field of view). Radiation exposure can be lower than in tumour diagnostics, but cannot be as low as in low-dose CT of the paranasal sinuses because the increased image noise does not allow sufficient visualisation of small details, especially of the stapes. Nowadays a volume data set is acquired in only one plane from which images in any spatial orientation and of different character can be reconstructed.

Newborns with CM of the outer ear must undergo detailed physical investigation of craniofacial structures for possible underlying syndromes. Each major branch of the facial nerve has to be carefully examined. Additional malformations should be excluded by an interdisciplinary team.

Auditory assessment is the most important functional investigation in patients with ear CM. Patients with CM of the outer and middle ear suffer from CHL of variable extent. Severe congenital aural atresia is often accompanied by a complete conductive sound blocking of about 60 dB. In cases of unilateral congenital aural atresia, early testing of the apparently normal contralateral ear is important in order to detect or exclude bilateral hearing loss.

The assessment includes reflex and behavioural audiometry, tympanometry (impedance measurement) and otoacoustic emissions (OAE), as well as auditory brainstem response testing in bone and air conduction. In older children, puretone and speech audiometry are added. Repeated audiometry may be necessary in young infants or in children who are otherwise difficult to test, or in patients with multiple malformations.

CT and CB-CT have a high clarification rate in suspected CM of the outer and middle ear, including the detection of other causes of CHL. Only in a few cases can no cause be found. Even with modern techniques, it is difficult to diagnose isolated stapes fixation or visualise subtle detail of malformed ossicles. Nevertheless, CT or CB-CT is indicated in patients with suspected CM of the outer and middle ear and is absolutely necessary for presurgical planning.

The following structures and properties are analysed in detail:

Grade of temporal bone pneumatisation
Shape and width of EAC and tympanic cavity
Shape and localisation of ossicles, including inter-ossicular joints
Presence and morphology of windows
Course of facial nerve and bony canal of internal carotid artery (ICA)
Tensor tympani muscle and Eustachian tube
Inner ear/internal auditory canal (IAC) (see Sect. 16.21.1.3)

High-grade CMs affect nearly all of these structures, while in low- and medium-grade CM, normal and malformed structures are coexistent.

The imaging correlates of malformed structures include:

EAC	Bony or fibrous atresia
Pneumatised cells	Reduced, absent
Tympanic cavity	Hypoplastic, split (then often opacified and filled with non-resorbed embryonic or fibrotic tissue), absent, extra-cavitation
Ossicles	Aplasia/hypoplasia of an ossicle or parts of it, dysplasia, conglomerations or clots, displacement, fixation of malleus or incus on the tympanic wall
Joints	Separation, fusion, fragility (incudostapedial joint may exist only as fibrous connection—this is not identifiable on CT)
Window	Narrowed, closed, absent

Additionally, the following variants (without functional deficit) can be demonstrated:

Facial nerve	Lateralisation/anterior displacement of the tympanic or mastoid segment, dehiscence of tympanic segment, duplications/rarely bifurcation of labyrinthine or mastoid segment, displacement in the oval window or through stapes crura
ICA	Aberrant, lateralisation in the middle ear with or without bony canal dehiscence
Bulbus v. jugularis	Elevation with or without diverticulum
Sigmoid sinus	Lateralisation, anterior displacement with or without diverticulum

Only variants of the facial nerve occur more often in patients with CM than in healthy individuals or patients with other diagnoses. Imaging has limitations in the detection of some subtle forms of stapes CM.

At some institutions presurgical rating is performed. The decision to operate depends primarily on the degree of middle ear development as reflected by the size of the tympanum and the status of the ossicles and of the windows. A commonly used CT-BASED scale (Table 16.10) has been developed by Siegert et al. (1996) and Siegert (2010).

Depending on the score and whether the malformation is bilateral or unilateral, these authors recommend surgical or conservative therapy (for more details see Sects. 18.4 and 18.5):

In bilateral malformations: middle ear reconstruction of the better-hearing ear if the score is 15 or higher

In unilateral malformations: middle ear reconstruction if the score is at least 20, following a frank discussion with the patient/parents

In patients with lower scores: hearing aids only

Abnormal courses of arteries or of the facial nerve do not always preclude surgery, but they increase the risk of complications. Patients with a very atypical course of the facial nerve and those with severe middle ear malformations should not be considered for operative treatment. Thus, CT not only demonstrates suitability for surgery but also shows contraindications.

With regard to further treatment strategies, the bony thickness of the calvaria can be measured and 3D reconstructions of the temporal bone made in patients scheduled for insertion of the well-established bone-anchored hearing aid (BAHA) or implantable hearing aids.

16.21.1.3 Congenital Malformations of the Inner Ear

Clinical Signs and Classification Inner ear CMs cause hearing loss in ca. 20–30% of children with congenital SNHL. However, there is no clear correlation between severity of deformity seen on imaging and hearing loss. In some cases hearing loss develops after birth. This is particu-

Table 16.10 CT score according to Siegert, Mayer and Weerda (Siegert 2010; Siegert et al. 1996; Weerda 2004)

Structures	Configuration	Points
EAC	Normal/fibrotic atresia/bony atresia	2/1/0
Aeration of mastoid	Distinct/moderate/absent	2/1/0
Size of tympanic cavity	Large/moderate/eburnated	2/1/0
Aeration of tympanic cavity	Distinct/moderate/absent	2/1/0
Facial nerve	Normal/slightly aberrant/strongly aberrant	4/2/0
Course of arteries and veins	Normal/slightly aberrant/strongly aberrant	2/1/0
Malleus and incus	Normal/dysplastic/absent	2/1/0
Stapes	Normal/dysplastic/absent	4/2/0
Oval window	Open/closed	4/0
Round window	Open/closed	4/0
Maximum score		28

larly important in patients with large vestibular aqueduct syndrome (LVAS) or large endolymphatic duct and sac syndrome (LEDS). In these children, the onset of hearing loss may be delayed until adolescence or even longer (Bartel-Friedrich et al. 2008).

Aplasia, hypoplasia or dysplasia of the labyrinth and sensory patches in their entirety or in part has been described. Additionally, the vestibular aqueducts may be enlarged. The vestibuloacoustic ganglion cells are often reduced in number in inner ear CM. The IAC can also be affected by CM. Sennaroglu (2010) proposed a classification for cochleovestibular CM based on imaging and differentiated five main groups: malformations of the cochlea, of the vestibule, of the semicircular canals, of the IAC and of the vestibular or cochlear aqueduct. Cochlear CM (Table 16.11) has been divided into six categories

Table 16.11 Cochlear CM by time of developmental arrest according to Sennaroglu and Saatci (2002)

Cochlear malformations	Configuration
Michel deformity (arrest: 3rd week)	Complete absent of cochlear and vestibular structures, absent IAC, absent VA
Cochlear aplasia (arrest: late 3rd week)	Absent cochlea; normal, dilated or hypoplastic vestibule and SCC
Common cavity (arrest: 4th week)	Cochlea and vestibule build a common space without internal architecture, IAC more enlarged than narrow, normal VA
Incomplete partition type I (cystic cochleovestibular malformation) (arrest: 5th week)	Cystically enlarged cochlea without internal architecture, cystic dilated vestibule, enlarged IAC, normal VA
Cochlear hypoplasia (arrest: 6th week)	Distinctly recognisable separation of cochlear and vestibular structures, small cochlea bud, absent or hypoplastic vestibule, narrow or normal IAC, normal VA
Incomplete partition type II (Mondini deformity) (arrest: 7th week)	Cochlea with 1½ turns, cystically dilated middle and apical turn (cystic apex), nearly normal size of cochlea, slightly dilated vestibule, more enlarged IAC, enlarged VA

IAC internal auditory canal; *VA* vestibular aqueduct; *SCC* semicircular canal

of severity depending on the point of developmental arrest. In 2010, Sennaroglu (2010) updated their classification and provided more subgroups. For syndrome associations see Table 16.9.

The diagnosis of CM of the inner ear is based on clinical examination and imaging.

Clinical Examination As also mentioned in Sect. 16.1, a newborn with hearing loss or deafness must undergo detailed physical examination of craniofacial structures for possible underlying syndromes. Additional CM should be excluded by an interdisciplinary team.

Audiometry starts with the universal newborn hearing screening mostly by transient OAE (TOAE). Further investigations include tympanometry (impedance measurement), distortion product OAE (DPOAE) and early acoustically evoked potentials (auditory brainstem response, ABR). Older children are subjected to reflex and behavioural audiometric procedures, play techniques, pure-tone audiometry or speech reception threshold testing. The chosen test set depends on the age and development of the individual child. The objective measuring techniques (OAE and ABR in bone and air conduction) provide more reliable results. In the interests of accuracy, audiological testing should be repeated, particularly in young children and in patients with multiple malformations.

The testing of the labyrinthine vestibular organ has differential diagnostic value. The loss of the vestibular organ does not, however, exclude useful hearing.

Imaging Nowadays MRI of the temporal bone should be preferred in suspected CM of the inner ear. CT or CB-CT may detect such CM in nearly the same proportion of cases, but MRI delivers more detail.

For morphological analysis of the labyrinthine structures in the IAC and cerebellopontine angle (CPA), thin-slice (<0.7 mm) 3D T2-weighted sequences are used. Native T1-weighted sequences have to be performed for the differentiation of pathologies with high T1 contrast (blood, fat). The contrast-enhanced T1-weighted sequence is most sensitive in the detection of inflammation or tumours as differential diagnoses. With the addition of diffusion-weighted imaging (DWI), the diagnosis of cholesteatomas/epidermoids is often possible. Temporal bone MRI is performed with thin slices and a high matrix. The investigation takes much longer than CT or CB-CT. In young children sedation or anaesthesia is necessary, which represents a major disadvantage.

For inner ear CM, the following structures are analysed:

Labyrinth	Fluid signal
Cochlea	Shape, number of turns, relation of scala vestibuli to scala tympani, modiolus
Vestibule	Shape
Semicircular canals (SCC)	Shape
Endolymphatic	Presence and width duct and sac
Internal auditory canal (IAC)	Width, presence of facial, cochlear, superior and inferior vestibular nerve

Vascular loops with contact to cranial nerves can be observed in the cerebellopontine angle (CPA) and IAC. These are mostly normal variants.

On CT or CB-CT, the modiolus and scala vestibuli/scala tympani are harder to recognise. Cranial nerves in the IAC and CPA cannot be imaged. Rather than the endolymphatic duct itself, the canal through which it runs, the vestibular aqueduct, is visualised.

Compared with CM of the outer and middle ear, the clarification rate is lower in suspected inner ear CM. Only about 25% of cases have an imaging correlate. In other words, the imaging findings will be normal in the majority of patients.

The following changes are correlates of inner ear CM on MRI:

- Michel malformation: absent labyrinth and absent cochlear nerve
- Mondini malformation: cochlea with normal basal but fused middle and apical turn, dilated vestibule and enlarged endolymphatic duct/sac (Fig. 16.38)
- Common cavity: fusion of cochlea and vestibule
- LVAS = LEDS: large vestibular aqueduct (on CT: >1.5 mm)/large endolymphatic duct/sac (MRI) with or without other inner ear CM
- X-linked deafness (final diagnosis by verification of defect gene): bulbous enlargement of IAC with defect of the bony margin to the cochlea, small cochlea without modiolus, enlarged labyrinthine facial nerve canal and enlarged canal of inferior vestibular nerve
- Cochlear aplasia, hypoplasia of various grades (Giesemann et al. 2011) and incomplete partition (Sennaroglu 2010)
- Vestibule/SCC aplasia, hypoplasia, dilation, fusion of vestibule and SCC
- IAC stenosis, hypoplasia or absence of nerves (Fig. 16.39).

In many, though not all, cases of inner ear CM and hearing loss appropriate for scheduling CI, hearing restoration can be successful (for further details see Sect. 18.6).

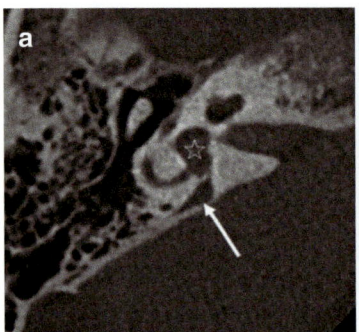 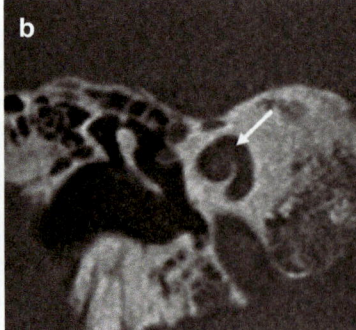 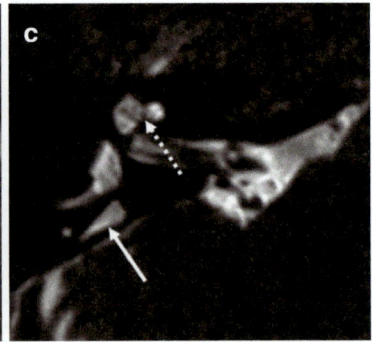

Fig. 16.38 CB-CT (**a** axial, **b** coronal) and axial T2-weighted MRI (**c**) of a 53-year-old woman, unilaterally nearly deaf. Mondini malformation: 1.5 cochlear turn (*arrow* in **b**), dilated vestibule (*star*), enlarged vestibular aqueduct (*arrow* in **a**) and endolymphatic duct (*arrow* in **c**). MRI additionally shows a hypoplastic modiolus (*dotted arrow* in **c**)

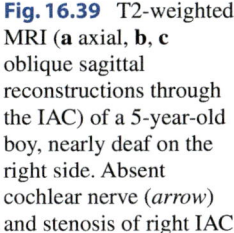

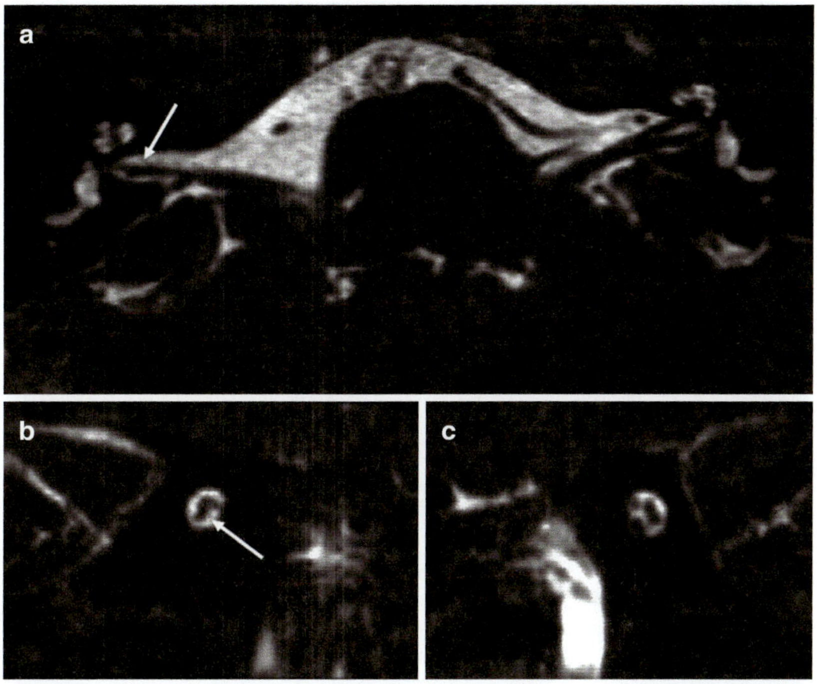

Fig. 16.39 T2-weighted MRI (**a** axial, **b**, **c** oblique sagittal reconstructions through the IAC) of a 5-year-old boy, nearly deaf on the right side. Absent cochlear nerve (*arrow*) and stenosis of right IAC

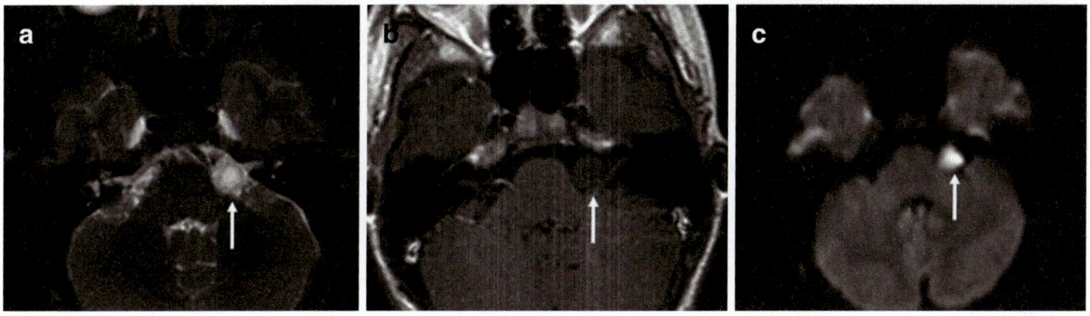

Fig. 16.40 Axial MRI (**a**) T2-weighted, (**b**) contrast-enhanced, (**c**) diffusion-weighted image showing an incidentally detected epidermoid in the left cerebellopontine angle (*arrows*) of right IAC

16.21.2   Paediatric Temporal Bone Tumours and Tumour-Like Lesions

Tumours of the temporal bone are rare in childhood. Congenital temporal bone lesions include epidermoids (Fig. 16.40; congenital cholesteatoma: 2–4% of all cholesteatomas, white mass medial to an intact tympanic membrane with normal pars tensa and flaccida, ranging from intratympanic pearls to destruction of the temporal bone), lipomas and arachnoid cysts (Fig. 16.41). Mostly these lesions are incidental findings, rarely the cause of hearing loss. They can be demon-strated and diagnosed by imaging. Furthermore, paediatric brain tumours can involve the temporal bone and adjacent regions (cerebellopontine angle, brainstem, cerebellum, posterior cerebral fossa) and may be accompanied by SNHL (including central hearing loss) or CHL or both, depending on the location and spread of the tumour. Some examples are listed in Table 16.12.

Examples of tumour-like lesions are cholesterol granuloma (rare in children, occurring anywhere from the middle ear to the petrous apex) and fibrous dysplasia.

Fibrous dysplasia is more frequent in the first two decades of life. It is a benign disease

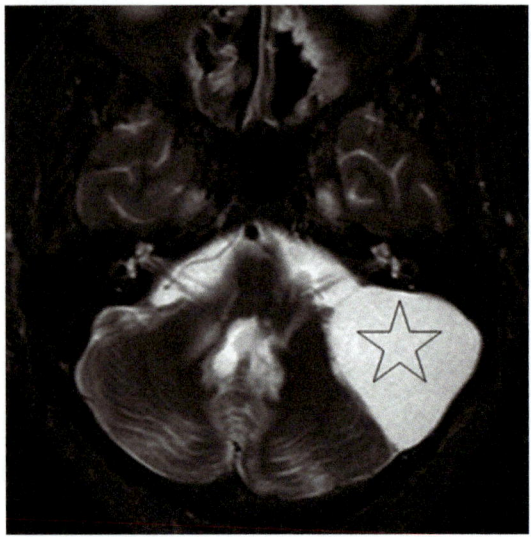

Fig. 16.41 Axial T2-weighted MRI showing an incidentally detected arachnoid cyst in the left cerebellopontine angle (*star*)

characterised by progressive replacement of normal bone elements with fibrous tissue, resulting in bone expansion. Temporal bone involvement, reported in ca. 20% of patients, can cause painless deformity and progressive CHL (occlusion of the Eustachian tube or of the EAC, or cholesteatoma formation secondary to obstruction) and sometimes SNHL (ca. 15% of patients, due to infection with ensuing cochlear destruction or to IAC stenosis and impingement of the eighth cranial nerve).

16.21.3 Imaging in Candidates for Cochlear Implantation

Before surgery can be planned, it has to be ascertained whether or not an electrode carrier can be implanted, whether complications are likely and

Table 16.12 Examples of paediatric central nervous system tumours assigned in part to the WHO histopathological categories

Tumours of neuroepithelial origin (56.4%[a])	Pilocytic astrocytoma (predominant in children 5–19 years of age) involving both the cerebellum and the brainstem; retrocochlear hearing loss can occur (Berg et al. 2005; Huang et al. 2012b; Mallur et al. 2008; Mirone et al. 2009)
Tumours of cranial and spinal nerves Tumours of the meninges	Meningiomas and nerve sheath tumours such as vestibular schwannoma within the temporal bone are rare in children. However, this entity diagnosed in a child, even if unilateral, should prompt confirmation or exclusion of a diagnosis of neurofibromatosis type 2 (NF-2). Hearing loss or tinnitus is described in ca. 20% of children, later diagnosed with this disease (Evans et al. 1999; Huang et al. 2012b; Neff and Welling 2005). In addition, NF-2 may be associated with multiple meningiomas and schwannomas of other cranial nerves
Lymphoma and haematopoietic neoplasms	Langerhans cell histiocytosis (also called histiocytosis X) can involve the temporal bone in ca. 20% of patients (De Foer et al. 2009; Fernández-Latorre et al. 2000; Robson et al. 1999). The disease results from clonal proliferation of Langerhans *cells*, abnormal cells deriving from *bone marrow*. Clinically, its manifestations range from isolated bone lesions to *multisystem disease*. In the multifocal unisystem subtype, fever, bone lesions and diffuse eruptions, usually on the scalp and in the ear canals, are characteristic. In cases with more extensive spread within the temporal bone, progressive otalgia, aural discharge, periauricular swellings and CHL can appear
Metastatic tumours	The most common metastatic neoplasms involving the temporal bone are leukaemia and neuroblastoma (Robson et al. 1999; Robson 2010). Depending on the site and size within the temporal bone, variable hearing loss can be present
Embryonal tumours (22.4%[a])	The 2006 Central Brain Tumor Registry of the United States (CBTRUS) reported that embryonal tumours, which encompass medulloblastomas, primitive neuroectodermal tumours and atypical teratoid/rhabdoid tumours (AT/RTs), are more prevalent among infants and children (0–4 years of age). Medulloblastoma is the second most frequent brain tumour in children after pilocytic astrocytoma and the most common malignant brain tumour in children (Gajjar et al. 2013). Originating from the cerebellar parenchyma and growing into the fourth ventricle and adjacent structures, medulloblastoma can lead to hearing loss combined with severe brain symptoms resulting from occlusion hydrocephalus
Mesenchymal tumours	Rhabdomyosarcoma (arising from immature mesenchymal cells that are committed to skeletal muscle lineage) is the most common primary malignancy of the temporal bone and is a highly aggressive lesion with a propensity for nervous system involvement and distant metastatic disease (De Foer et al. 2009; Robson et al. 1999). Clinical findings include a protruding tumour mass in the ear region, otorrhoea and bleeding from the outer ear canal, otalgia, hearing loss and facial weakness or palsy

[a]Frequencies according to Santi and Rushing (Santi and Rushing 2013)

whether electric signals will arrive at the central auditory cortex. To this end, imaging has to deliver the following information:

Configuration of the cochlea, detection/exclusion of fibrosis/ossification especially of the basal turn
Presence/absence of the cochlear nerve
Clarification of the individual anatomy including variants
Signs of gusher; inflammation

These points are best assessed by MRI and CT or CB-CT (Table 16.13).

According to Li et al. (2015), a stenosis of the internal auditory meatus or the cochlear nerve canal based on multi-slice spiral CT strongly hints at

Table 16.13 Strengths of CT/CB-CT and MRI (Adapted from Huang et al. 2012a)

CT/CB-CT	MRI
Better for bone details (pneumatic cell system, location of jugular vein bulb, sigmoid sinus, internal carotid artery, ossicular chain, course of facial nerve in tympanic and mastoidal segment)	Avoids radiation Superior soft tissue contrast High-resolution imaging of inner ear (fine details of cochlea) and brain
Width of IAC	Visualisation and fluid content of labyrinth
Patency of bony cochlear nerve canal (if IAC is narrow)	Nerve courses in IAC and CPA
Fibrous versus osseous obstruction of cochlea	
Lower cost	
Less time	
Sparing with sedation or anaesthesia	

hypo- or aplasia of the cochlear nerve demanding an additional MRI. Differentiation between hypo- and aplasia is of prognostic value, as the degree of malformation correlates with the audiological outcome after cochlear implantation (Wu et al. 2015). Morlet et al. (2017) found in about half of cases with cochlear nerve deficiency vestibular anomalies and in about one-third cochlear abnormalities. The technical aspects and systematic reviewing are the same as described in Sect. 16.21.1.

Functional MRI (fMRI) has the potential to ascertain the integrity of the central auditory pathways, but is not yet widely used.

Some centres employ intraoperative imaging requiring special technical equipment (Aschendorff 2011), whereby surgically problematic cases can be monitored.

Immediately after operation the position of the electrode carrier is documented by imaging (Fig. 16.42). Different centres use different methods: X-rays in special projection, CT, CB-CT and digital subtraction angiography with 3D capability. Owing to its low radiation exposure and its insensitivity to metal artefacts, as well as its superior spatial resolution, CB-CT is most suitable for demonstrating the intra-cochlear localisation of the electrode carrier.

After the initial postoperative phase, CT or CB-CT may detect opacifications of the mastoidectomy cavity or ossifications of the labyrinth as signs of inflammation.

In the event that MRI is needed to clarify disease, the manufacturer must be consulted as to whether or

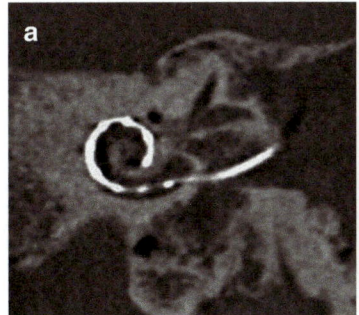 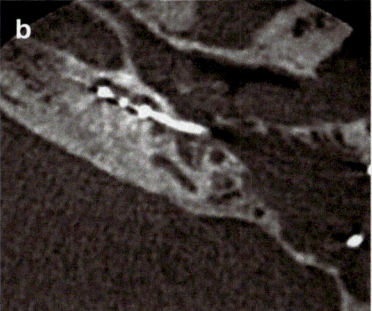 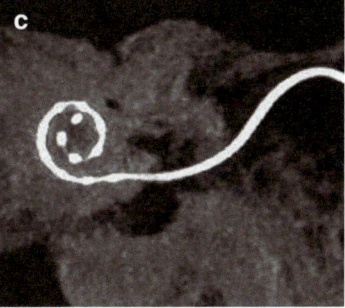

Fig. 16.42 CB-CT (an oblique coronal reconstruction, B axial, C maximum intensity projection) documenting correct position of an electrode carrier one day after implan- tation. At this time opacifications of the mastoidectomy cavity are normal postoperative changes

not the individual CI can be investigated with the on-site MRI device. Devices with field strength greater than 1.5 T are currently not allowed. Recently, rotatable magnets within the CI were developed, which reduce the risk of dislocation, but continue to shadow the MRI image. Owing to the strong artefacts caused by the electrode carrier, the evaluation of the posterior fossa, including the temporal bone, is not possible after cochlear implantation.

16.22 Genetic Testing

Pavel Seeman, Simona Poisson-Markova, Eva Seemanova, Antoinette am Zehnhoff-Dinnesen, and Hanno J. Bolz

DFNB1, which is caused by mutations in the *GJB2* gene, is by far the most common type of hereditary hearing impairment. Mutations in *GJB2* are responsible for up to 50% of cases of early non-syndromic genetic hearing impairment with autosomal recessive (AR) inheritance (Snoeckx et al. 2005). Diagnostic *GJB2* testing is therefore offered in many laboratories worldwide. It should be the first test in patients with prelingual non-syndromic deafness. Certain *GJB2* mutations have different prevalences in different populations. In Caucasian populations, initial diagnostic testing is therefore focused on the mutation c.35delG (Gasparini et al. 2000), in Asian populations on c.235delC (Yang et al. 2013), in Jewish populations on c.167delT (Morell et al. 1998; Sobe et al. 1999) and in Roma populations and in India on p.Trp24* (Minárik et al. 2003).

Attempts to correlate genotype and phenotype have shown a tendency of mutation c.35delG in *GJB2* to be more often related with severe to profound hearing loss (Beck et al. 2015).

Mutations in other known genes are less prevalent, and the probability of finding causal mutations in any other single gene in a patient previously excluded for DFNB1 is very low except of *STRC* gene (Marková et al. 2018). Testing mutations in the genes *STRC*, *SLC26A4*, *MYO15A* and *TMPRSS3* and in mitochondrial DNA is incidentally performed (Lechowicz et al. 2015), but recently developed genetic techniques, such as massively parallel sequencing (MPS), also called next-generation sequencing (NGS), allow testing of panels comprising all relevant genes (for non-syndromic deafness ~115) (Hereditary Hearing Loss 2019) in parallel for only a fraction of the cost of conventional sequencing. This new procedure improves the diagnostic yield for patients with already excluded mutations in the *GJB2* gene.

Even in cases with unilateral sensorineural hearing loss, genetic testing can be recommended according to the study of Gruber et al. (2016) showing *GJB2* mutations in 31.3% from affected children.

For further information, see Sect. 3.1 by Hanno J. Bolz.

Genetic testing has now begun to play a prominent role in diagnostics and genetic counselling, influencing the early management of disease and patients' subsequent quality of life. However, the importance of the physical examination when recommending genetic analyses should not be underestimated by clinicians.

16.23 Special Diagnostic Needs of Children with Multiple Handicaps: General Considerations

Mona Hegazi and Peter Matulat

16.23.1 Definition of Disability

The Convention on the Rights of Persons with Disabilities states to:

> provide those health services needed by persons with disabilities specifically because of their disabilities, including early identification and intervention as appropriate, and services designed to minimise and prevent further disabilities, including among children and older persons.
> UN General Assembly (2007)

The primary nosological framework for the classification of diagnoses, disorders and health conditions is the International Classification of Diseases (ICD) (World Health Organization 1992). The International Classification of Functioning, Disability and Health (ICF) (World

Health Organization 2001) focuses on functioning and disability associated with health conditions. The children and youth version (ICF-CY) of the ICF was developed to take into account that:

> the manifestations of disability and health conditions in children and adolescents are different in nature, intensity and impact from those of adults.
> World Health Organization (2007)

The ICF and ICF-CY provide a useful classification system with three levels: impairments, disabilities and handicaps. An impairment is primarily a problem of bodily function and structure (this part overlaps with the ICD). The term 'disabilities' includes impairments, activity limitations and participation restrictions. 'Handicap' refers to the result when an individual with an impairment or disability cannot fulfil a normal life role. 'Handicapped' is, however, not a medical term; it reflects the interaction between the individual's impairments and the social environment. The primary goal of these classifications is to allow the social participation of the handicapped child. Illum and Gradel (2015) found that a combination of the ICD and the ICF-CY could provide a helpful tool for the assessment of functioning in all children with different disabilities.

'Child with multi-handicaps' refers to a child who has more than one disabling health condition. The child typically has disabilities that are severe enough to require intensive support for handling the functions of daily living. In educational settings and according to the US Individuals with Disabilities Education Acts, the term 'multiple disabilities' refers to:

> concomitant (simultaneous) impairments (…), the combination of which causes such severe educational needs that they cannot be accommodated in special education programs solely for one of the impairments.
> USC (2004)

16.23.2 Prevalence of Disabilities

A European Union-funded study found that 1.9% of families contain a child with a disability (Di Giulio et al. 2014). The lowest level was found in Lithuania (0.58%) and the highest in Poland (4.0%).

The prevalence of disabilities concomitant with hearing impairment can be estimated by two approaches:

- Recording how many people with hearing disorders show characteristics of other disabilities
- Estimating the prevalence of hearing impairment among other disabilities

Estimates of deaf or hard-of-hearing children with additional disabilities vary according to the approach used. Various reports and reviews (Holden-Pitt and Diaz 1998; Picard 2004; Gallaudet Research Institute 2013; Cupples et al. 2014; Wakil et al. 2014) have estimated that from up to 20 to 40% of deaf or hard-of-hearing children have accompanying disabilities.

The following disorders, which sometimes coexist in children with hearing impairments, can cause a wide range of different disabilities and handicaps:

- Intellectual disability
- Disorders of psychological development:
  - Disorders of speech and language
  - Disorders of scholastic skills
  - Disorders of motor function
  - Pervasive developmental disorders (e.g. autism spectrum disorders)
- Behavioural or emotional disorders:
  - Hyperkinetic disorders
  - Conduct disorders
  - Emotional disorders
  - Disorders of social functioning
  - Nonorganic enuresis/encopresis
- Visual disturbances and blindness
- Various syndromes and many other medical, physical or motor problems (e.g. CHARGE syndrome, *cytomegalovirus (CMV)* infection, meningitis, cerebral palsy, Goldenhar syndrome, Waardenburg syndrome, various trisomy disorders)

The more common disorders that coexist with hearing impairment are learning and intellectual disabilities (16%), developmental delay (6%), attention deficit disorders (5.4%) and impaired vision or blindness (5%) (Gallaudet Research Institute 2013).

In practice, doctors and therapists are also confronted with models of impairments, from other professions, that are not shared by mainstream medical theory. The theoretical model of sensory integration dysfunction, developed by occupational therapists to describe hyper- or hyposensitivity to stimuli, and applied kinesiology, often used by chiropractors, are two such examples.

According to Wiley et al. (2011), the proportion of additional disabilities experienced by people with hearing impairment is approximately similar across all degrees of hearing loss (mild, moderate, severe, etc.).

16.23.3 The Diagnostic Challenge

Additional disabilities are strong predictors of poorer auditory and speech-language outcomes (Cupples et al. 2014). The assessment of children with additional disabilities and different needs is challenging for doctors and therapists involved in medical and developmental diagnosis. The examiner must be aware of the child's individual needs and strengths, and the choice of diagnostic methods depends upon the communicative possibilities of the child. A person-centred multidisciplinary approach is recommended.

In practice, the assessment of hearing in children with hearing loss and additional impairments is challenging because of:

- The wide variety of individual limitations, competence and potential in different children with multiple handicaps (Marschark and Spencer 2003).
- The lack of clinical staff familiar with all communication styles that may be used.
- The lack of psychometric tests for hearing impairment appropriate for children with additional disabilities (Illinois Service Resource Center 2011).
- The presence of certain characteristics that influence the assessment. These include (Snell 2002):
  - Limited communication
  - Difficulty in basic physical mobility
  - Tendency to forget skills through disuse
  - Trouble generalising skills from one situation to another
  - Limited alertness
- In general, the diagnostic procedure should answer the following questions:
  - What is the hearing condition and associated physical condition of the child?
  - Is the child able to perceive speech, vocalisations or environmental sounds?
  - Would the child benefit from hearing aids, amplification or noise reduction devices (such as an FM system) or cochlear implants?
  - What is the child's level of cognitive development?
  - In light of the above, what will the preferred mode of communication be?
  - Would this child benefit from talkers or other augmentative communication devices?

A full diagnostic profile for multi-handicapped children should include the assessment of the following areas (Center for Deaf and Hard of Hearing 2014):

- Audiological factors:
  - Age of onset and age of diagnosis
  - Age at starting to use full-time amplification
  - Auditory skills and use of residual hearing
  - Effectiveness of hearing technology
  - Aetiology of the hearing loss
  - Type and degree of hearing loss
- Behavioural factors:
  - Attitude and motivation level
  - Psychosocial behaviour
- Communication factors:
  - Augmentative communication devices; assistive technology
  - Primary language
  - Preferred mode of communication
- Educational, social, developmental and medical factors:
  - Attendance consistency and stability
  - Early education

- Family history including home language, cultural factors and hearing status of family members
- Genetic history
- Medical issues/concerns: risk factors
- Visual status

16.23.4   Evaluation of Cognitive, Social and Behavioural Functioning

In principle, an individual can be assessed with standard assessment batteries if he or she has normal auditory and visual modes of communication and can talk or respond adequately with at least one functional arm and hand (Johnson et al. 2001). If this is not possible, the use of developmental scales, which assess progress along a continuum rather than providing comparative performance data with peers, may be an appropriate alternative (Alvares and Sternberg 1994; Jones et al. 2007). With severe disabilities, it is important to conduct a functional skills assessment. This targets the skills needed in a given environment and activity and includes measures of social and adaptive functioning with a focus on basic life skills. It focuses on practical independent living skills. It also considers students' functioning in their environments and examines the process of learning and performance (Downing 2004).

Because speech and language therapists, clinical audiologists and teachers can provide important information regarding communication abilities, a multidisciplinary approach to psychological assessment is often best (Lutermann 2004).

In particular, visual or auditory disabilities combined with motor impairments or disabilities make accommodation and modification of the common testing conditions necessary. For these patients some hints for the adaptation of time/scheduling, test settings, administration/instructions, presentation format, response format and use of adaptive technology or computer-based testing can be found in the articles of Hill-Briggs et al. (2007) and Case (2005), which include:

- The adjustment of time limits and avoidance of speed tests
- The substitution of tests that do not require motor responses
- The management of test setting accommodation and accessibility
- The use of adapted administration and responding, rather than self-administration

Traxler (2000) points to the fact that deaf and hard-of-hearing children often have poor reading skills, which makes written instructions problematic and adaptations necessary. Children with a cochlear implant improve with respect to their readings skills (Vermeulen et al. 2007), but do not reach the level of normal-hearing children of the same age (Weisi et al. 2013).

However, one should always take into account that the adaptations above will often violate the assumptions of the test principle of 'standardisation' of the tests used.

Applied clinical and educational psychologists or neuropsychologists who work with children can use numerous psychological tests to evaluate intelligence (IQ), personality, adjustment, learning disabilities, memory difficulties, language skills, non-verbal skills, sensory and motor skills, executive functions and other neuropsychological skills.

Since not all tests are available in all languages, and country-specific norms are often lacking, recommendations of specific tests cannot be easily given.

To select a suitable test, the following questions should be answered:

- Can the test result produce information that helps answer one of the hypotheses concerning the child?
- Can the test items and the instructions be understood by the child in an appropriate style?
- Does the child have the communicative and motor skills required to respond to the test items?
- Are there national test norms for the age/sex/school grades of the child?

The starting point for a search could be special collections of psychological tests for deaf or hard-of-hearing children (Illinois Service Resource Center 2011) or test lists from members of the European Test Publisher Group (ETPG).

16.23.5 Visual Assessment

Visual impairment, as well as hearing impairment, has an impact on the child's cognitive, language, motor and social development.

The most common method of testing vision is to have the child verbally report what he or she sees. A satisfactory investigation is particularly challenging if the child has additional impairments. Visual function can be examined by functional and clinical vision assessments. Functional vision assessments focus on how children make use of their sight at school and play. In addition to careful observation of the child in their environment, electrophysiological techniques are used in order to assess the electrical activity of the visual pathway and occipital cortex of the brain. Children should also receive thorough eye examinations.

Two clinical visual acuity assessment techniques have gained wide acceptance for testing children with multiple handicaps (Mackie and McCulloch 1995), preferential looking (PL) and visual evoked potentials (VEPs):

- The preferential looking test (PL) is based on the fact that children prefer to fixate on patterned surfaces more than homogeneous ones and respond to visual stimuli by moving their eyes in the direction of the object of visual interest (Fantz 1965; Cohen and Cashon 2003).
- The visual evoked potential (VEP) is a bioelectrical signal generated in the visual cortex of the brain in response to visual stimulation.

16.23.6 Communicative Assessment

If a child with multiple disabilities communicates verbally, then standardised tests may be used for the evaluation of their communicative status (Guralnick 2000; Rowland 2005; Bagnato et al. 2007).

A functional communication assessment in preverbal children may consist of observing their behaviour in order to indicate different levels of particular communication skills that are suggested to be part of the language learning process (Johnson and Farroni 2007; Meltzoff and Brooks 2009; Van Hecke and Mundy 2007). The main steps are:

- Attending to and imitating faces and following a head turn:
  - Preferring to look at face-like stimuli
  - Imitating basic facial expressions
  - Following side-to-side head and eye movements
- Dyadic interaction with persons and objects:
  - Looking at a caregiver during social interactions or at objects
- Triadic interaction:
  - Sharing attention with an object with another person
- Responding to joint attention:
  - Responding to caregiver's attempts to coordinate attention during play
- Initiating joint attention:
  - Initiating interactions to coordinate attention with caregivers during play

Augmentative and alternative communication (AAC) is used in children with severe speech-language impairments to compensate for spoken or written language (ISAAC—International Society for Augmentative and Alternative Communication 2016).

This includes:

- Facial expression and vocalisations
- Gestures and sign languages
- Communication books
- Speech-generating devices (initiating or responding to communication by using hands, body parts, pointers, joysticks or switches and eye scanning devices)

The examination of the child's abilities and requirements for AAC should include their motor, visual, cognitive, language and communication strengths and weaknesses.

The evaluation should answer the following questions:

Receptive Language:
- What types of communicative behaviour does this child understand (spoken words, manual signs, gestures, facial expressions, vocal intonation, picture symbols, object symbols, etc.)?
- What messages or communicative functions does this child appear to understand (directives, greetings, requests, etc.)?
- Is prompting and support needed for the child to respond to a communication?

Expressive Language:
- How does the child make his or her needs and wishes known (body movements, gestures, facial expressions, vocalisations, words, sign language, picture symbols, object symbols, etc.)?
- Does the child's expressive behaviour appear to be intentional? Is it directed towards a goal? Does it appear that the child anticipates a response to the communication?
- How frequently does the child communicate?
- What specific messages or communicative functions does the child express (protests, requests, greetings, etc.)?
- Under what circumstances is the child most communicative (With whom? When? Where?)?
- Does the child need prompting or support to communicate clearly or consistently? What type of support?

16.24 Hearing Tests for Intellectually and Multiply Handicapped Children

Katrin Neumann

In paediatric audiology, the assessment of the hearing capacities of children with intellectual disabilities or multiple handicaps plays an important role and is particularly challenging.

Intellectual disability has a prevalence of about 3% in Western countries. Persons with intellectual disability are at increased risk of hearing impairment. Permanent hearing impairment in persons with intellectual disability occurs in about one quarter of the cases (Hild et al. 2008; Neumann et al. 2008). This high prevalence is mainly related to genetic reasons, syndromes or chronic otitis media, such as in Down syndrome where hearing impairment has been reported in 28% (Van Schrojenstein Lantman-de Valk et al. 1994) to 73% of cases (Squires et al. 1986). Auditory synaptopathy/auditory neuropathy (AS/AN) also occurs. Earwax is another major problem, because its production and self-cleaning, as well as ear canal anatomy, often differ from that in non-disabled persons (Evenhuis 1995; Neumann et al. 2008). These hearing impairments often remain undetected or underestimated because of information deficits among the parents, persons in care and medical professionals and because the intellectually disabled themselves are often unable to recognise and indicate such problems, in particular children. About three-quarters of the bilateral hearing loss identified in persons with intellectual disabilities who underwent a hearing screening during the German National Special Olympic games (sports games for people with intellectual disabilities) were unknown at the time (Hild et al. 2008). Similar findings have been made regularly during national and international Special Olympics games (Hild et al. 2008; Neumann et al. 2006). A high prevalence of hearing loss and many of the described conditions hold true for a large part of multiply handicapped children, too.

Ear and hearing disorders in children with intellectual disabilities or multiple handicaps can be well rehabilitated if treated early and continuously. For instance, multiply handicapped children have been shown to benefit from cochlear implantation, despite the rehabilitation of perceptual and verbal expressive abilities progressing slower than for profoundly deaf children with no additional disabilities (Waltzman et al. 2000). After medical or surgical treatment of chronic otitis media, Shott et al. (2001) found normal hearing levels in 98% of children with Down syndrome and stated that aggressive, meticulous and compulsory diagnosis and treatment of chronic ear disease in these children provide significantly improved hearing levels. In particular, it is necessary to 'carry' children with chronic otitis media with effusion through their childhood until tube ventilation and middle ear conditions have stabilised. Most children need regular cleaning of their external ear canals and fitting or check-ups of their hearing aids or implants, examination for necessary ear surgery as well as speech and hearing rehabilitation, which in most cases takes more time than for typically developed children. These specific tasks belong to the profile of a paediatric audiologist: to ensure such regular examinations of the children and always to act from an integrated view with interdisciplinary case conferences and professional parent counselling, taking care that all necessary constituents of rehabilitation are in place.

If left untreated, hearing impairments of intellectually disabled or multiply handicapped children aggravate their social and communicative problems, in particular in the period of language development which is often delayed anyhow (Neumann et al. 2006). Additionally, central auditory and language processing problems that occur regularly in persons with intellectual disabilities or multiple handicaps have to be faced. It has been shown that central auditory difficulties at the brainstem level have to be expected in about three-quarters, and at the cortical level in nearly two thirds, of intellectually disabled adults, depending on the specific processing category (Neumann et al. 2008). Auditory discrimination thresholds for non-speech (frequency, tone duration and level) and speech stimuli (voiced/unvoiced consonants, place of articulation) are reported to be at the level of <4- to 6-year-old children (Neumann et al. 2014). Grammatical abilities for plural forming scored on average in the range of those of 4-year-old children (Neumann et al. 2014). Therefore, it is necessary to use a specifically adapted, simplified speech in the communication with persons with intellectual disabilities.

To face all these problems, both a newborn hearing screening and regular otological and audiological check-ups are necessary for intellectually and multiply handicapped children. In the Netherlands, for example, systematic hearing screenings and examinations for people with intellectual disability have been implemented (Evenhuis 1996). The International Association of Scientific Studies on Intellectual Disability (IASSID) has published an international consensus on the early identification of hearing and visual impairment in children and adults with intellectual disability (Evenhuis and Nagtzaam 1998). For the audiological assessment of hearing loss in children with intellectual disabilities or multiple handicaps, objective methods such as the measurement of otoacoustic emissions, stapedius reflexes and in particular AEP (auditory evoked potentials) are the methods of choice (Hoth et al. 2015). The estimation of the hearing threshold needs to be done with both wide-frequency and frequency-specific ABR (auditory brainstem response). During recent years, the improvement in ASSR (auditory steady-state response) and chirp-based AEP technologies, by an optimisation of the stimuli and signal statistics, has made them well-suited methods, also for frequency regions below 1 kHz, for diagnosing precisely the kind and degree of hearing loss and for fitting hearing instruments properly (Hoth et al. 2015).

In most cases ABR and ASSR recordings in intellectually and multiply disabled children have to be performed under general anaesthesia, taking into consideration all medical, physical and psychic conditions of the child and his family. A careful analysis of level-latency functions and level-amplitude functions of ABR enables the specification of the type of hearing loss, the extent of a sound conduction component and the presence of a recruitment in case of a sensorineural hearing loss. For the latter, the level-latency curve is steeper for lower sound levels and flows into the normative range for higher levels. For children with Down syndrome or craniofacial anomalies, a conductive or combined hearing loss is frequent, and it is often challenging to separate the single components of a hearing loss. A conductive component can be confirmed either by a bone-conduction ABR recording or by estimating the extent of a horizontal deviation of the wave JI latency from its normal range in an air-conduction ABR recording. It has to be considered that in case of paracentesis, which is performed frequently before an AEP measurement, remains of blood or secretion or inflammatory processes in the middle ear may lead to a non-permanent conductive component of a hearing loss.

A flatter than normal curve of the wave JV latency in the level-latency diagram may indicate a neural hearing disorder. Figure 16.43 demonstrates an ABR finding of the right ear of a 2-year-old boy with a mitochondriopathy and a right-sided hearing loss with both a peripheral and a central component. In such cases the recording of middle and late-latency auditory evoked responses may indicate the central component and compensation of the hearing loss.

The safest method for the objective examination of the inner ear function is electrocochleography (ECochG), which demonstrates the sensorineural activity of pre- and postsynaptic processes during the transformation of acoustic stimuli in neural excitation. In intellectually disabled or multiply handicapped children, an ECochG is performed under general anaesthesia and mainly if there is a suspicion of a profound hearing loss or deafness or of an auditory synaptopathy/auditory neuropathy (AS/AN). The acoustic stimulation is performed via insertion phones and the recording by a needle electrode fixed on the promontory. The cochlear microphonics (CMs) and the summation potentials (SP) reflect the functioning of the outer and the inner hair cells and the compound action potentials (CAP) the functioning of the auditory nerve. For details see Hoth et al. (2015).

Pure-tone audiometry (PTA) has been shown to reveal reliable results for persons with intellectual disabilities, if performed properly. This includes suprathreshold training, short performance time and direct verbal or hand raising responses of the examined children if play audiometry is not understood satisfactorily. For younger or severely handicapped children, visual reinforcement audiometry or behavioural observational audiometry may reveal reliable results,

too. Recently it has been shown that an adaptive self-assessment procedure such as the multiple-choice auditory graphic interactive check (MAGIC®) even assesses hearing thresholds with more sensitivity than a classical PTA (Neumann et al. in press). Results of speech audiometry are less reliable in most cases than those from PTA because it requires higher cognitive functions. Nevertheless, because it is needed for hearing aid or implant fitting and because a discrepancy between speech in quiet and in noise measurements indicates the neural or central component of the hearing difficulties, speech audiometry in quiet and noise shall be performed with tests adjusted to the cognitive capacities of a handicapped child.

Electrophysiological methods to assess central aspects of hearing difficulties of intellectually and multiply disabled children measure middle latency and late cortical evoked potentials. For example, the combination of normal PTA results, normal or near to normal ABR but disturbed perception of speech or music or environmental or animal sounds, a pathological reflex decay as well as degraded or lacking middle latency and late cortical evoked potentials indicates a central hearing loss (Hoth et al. 2015).

Procedures using speech or music or other complex stimuli have mainly been used for research purposes so far and may gain greater importance for the clinical routine assessment of auditory functions of children in the near future. Such methods include the measurement of cortical evoked responses in 32–64 up to 128 channels, event-related responses (ERP), ABR with complex sounds (cABR; Russo et al. 2010) and frequency-modulated auditory evoked responses (FMAER; Duffy et al. 2013), also called frequency following responses (FFR). These stimulation settings, which decode the quickly changing stream of segmented sounds such as speech or music, enable the hemisphere-specific analysis of the morphology and distribution of evoked potentials (brain mapping) on the cortical, subcortical and even brainstem level, or a dipole source analysis. They are particularly useful for neurologically motivated questions aimed at a precise localisation of a functional cerebral

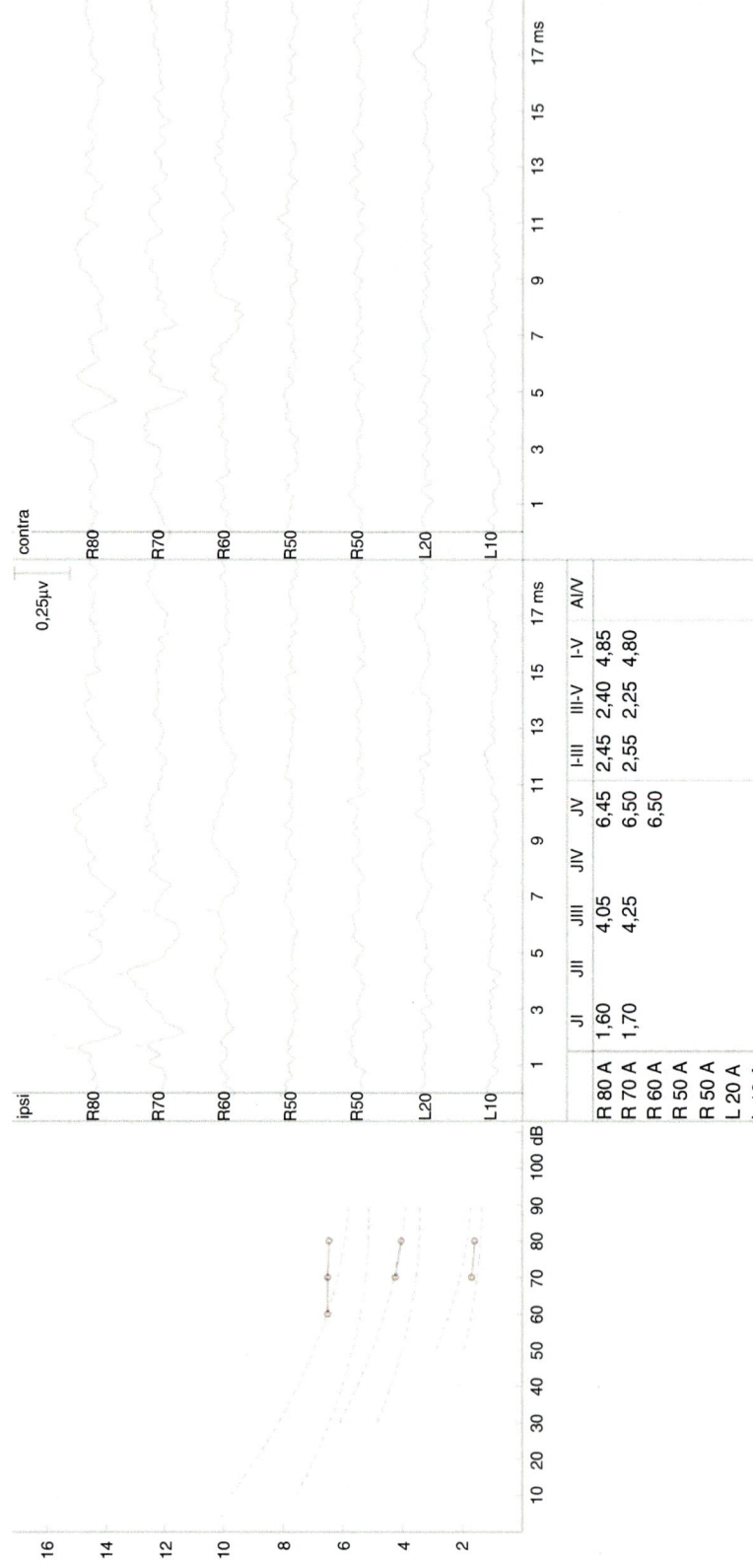

Fig. 16.43 ABR with click stimuli of the right ear indicating the peripheral and the central component of a right-sided hearing loss of a 2-year-old boy with a mitochondriopathy: stimulus-response threshold at 60 dB nHL with abnormal potential morphology, reduced amplitude of wave IV, immaturity-related elongated interpeak and absolute latencies and flat level-latency curves (Modified from Hoth et al. (2015)). Reprinted with permission from Springer Nature

lesion or on the assessment of specific auditory processing capacities (Hall et al. 2011).

16.25 Management of Psychological Sequelae for Parents After Diagnosis

Peter Matulat and Mona Hegazi

> ...and its [sic] not just a sentence, every word is important because you are hanging on to everything they say and you will remember every word that they say, it sticks in your mind. They need to really plan their sentences and their words because this is going to stay with you for the rest of your life.
> Parent, Informing Families Focus Groups
> Harnett (2007)

16.25.1 Parental Reactions and Coping

Parents of children who have been newly diagnosed with a hearing impairment usually have little or no experience with hard-of-hearing or deaf people. An appropriate emotional evaluation of an event depends greatly on previous experience, and most parents do not have a framework for making an appropriate evaluation. Perceived stress depends upon self-efficacy and the ability to master a situation by the individual's own competent action (Scholz et al. 2002). The initial emotions experienced after receiving a diagnosis of chronic illness—such as a hearing impairment—often include fear, shock, confusion, anger, frustration, depression, sadness, loneliness and blame (Kurtzer-White and Luterman 2003). In parents of newly diagnosed infants, these feelings may impede their natural interaction with the child (Horsch 2008; Spencer and Meadow-Orlans 1996; Koester and Lahti-Harper 2010).

The cognitive, emotional and behavioural strategies of parents' adaptation to the child's illness are called coping. Coping is process-orientated and has numerous interindividual variations. There are gender differences. Phase models are often used to describe the grieving process (Kricos 1993). Other authors focus more on the adaptation process (Ulrich and Bauer 2003).

Hintermair (2004) emphasised the importance of a sense of coherence (SOC)—in addition to experienced social support, the effects of the severity of the hearing loss and additional handicaps of the child—as a crucial personal resource in the coping process and as having a strong influence on the perceived quality of life. The Salutogenese model (Antonovsky and Sourani 1988) conceptualises the SOC as a combination of the subjective feelings of understandability, manageability and meaningfulness of the new situation.

16.25.2 Counselling and Intervention

Counselling and intervention are seen as the primary approach in helping to strengthen the resources of parents by promoting the ability for independent and self-determined action (empowerment). National principles and guidelines (Joint Committee on Infant Hearing 2013) and an international consensus statement (Moeller et al. 2013) on best practices for family-centred early intervention for children with hearing impairments have been created. Intervention programmes for parents and children have been developed (Holzinger et al. 2011; Reichmuth et al. 2013; Stredler-Brown and Abraham 2002). Early paedaudiologic care combined with family-centred educational intervention is predictive for a successful speech development of hearing-impaired children (Moeller 2000; Yanbay et al. 2014; Yoshinaga-Itano 2003; Meinzen-Derr et al. 2011; Fulcher et al. 2012).

Since a child with chronic illness will face new challenges in its childhood and adolescence (Compas et al. 2012; Laugen et al. 2016), the child's coping process must also be considered by doctors.

16.25.3 Informing Parents of the Diagnosis

The expectations of parents on the content and conditions of a medical diagnostic interview vary greatly between individuals. An evaluation of retrospective studies (Römer 2007) revealed that the following factors positively affect the experience for parents:

- The presence of a familiar person (e.g. a partner or close friend)
- Openness and directness of information sharing
- Clarity of the information (including written information)
- Familiarity with the doctor
- Awareness of support services
- Opportunity to ask questions

Very detailed descriptions of the necessary conditions for an appropriate setting can be found in the Irish national best practice guidelines for informing families of their child's disability (Harnett 2007). These hints are presented on the basis of the basic principles:

- Family-centred disclosure
- Respect for child and family
- Sensitive and empathetic communication
- Appropriate and accurate information
- Positive and realistic messages and hope
- Team approach and planning

These principles can certainly be applied to various diseases.

References

Akamatsu CT, Mayer C, Farrelly S (2005) An investigation of two-way text messaging use with deaf students at the secondary level. J Deaf Stud Deaf Educ 11(1):120–131

Alexiades G, Hoffmann RA (2008) Medical evaluation and medical management of hearing loss in children. In: Madell JR, Flexer C (eds) Pediatric audiology: diagnosis, technology, and management. Thieme, New York

Alfelasi M, Piron JP, Mathiolon C et al (2013) The transtympanic promontory stimulation test in patients with auditory deprivation: correlations with electrical dynamics of cochlear implant and speech perception. Eur Arch Otorhinolaryngol 270(6):1809–1815

Allen SG (2008) Auditory Perception Test for the Hearing Impaired-Revised (APT/HI-R). Plural Publishing, San Diego, CA

Allen JB, Hall JL, Jeng PS (1990) Loudness growth in 1/2-octave bands (LGOB)—a procedure for the assessment of loudness. J Acoust Soc Am 88(2):745–753

Allum JHJ, Greisiger R, Straubhaar S et al (2000) Auditory perception and speech identification in children with cochlear implants tested with the EARS protocol. Br J Audiol 34(5):293–303

Altmann F (1955) Congenital aural atresia of the ear in men and animals. Ann Otol Rhinol Laryngol 64(3):824–858

Alvares R, Sternberg L (1994) Communication and language development. In: Sternberg L (ed) Individuals with profound disabilities. Pro-Ed, Austin, TX

American Academy of Audiology (2010) Guidelines for the diagnosis, treatment, and management of children and adults with central auditory processing disorder. http://audiology-web.s3.amazonaws. com/migrated/CAPD%20Guidelines%208-2010. pdf_539952af956c79.73897613.pdf. Accessed 29 Dec 2015

American College of Medical Genetics Expert Panel (2002) Genetic evaluation of congenital hearing loss. Genet Med 4(3):162–171

American Speech-Language-Hearing Association (1978) Guidelines for manual pure-tone threshold audiometry. ASHA 20(4):297–301

American Speech-Language-Hearing Association (1996) Central auditory processing: current status of research and implications for clinical practice. Am J Audiol 5(2):41–54

American Speech-Language-Hearing Association (2005a) (Central) Auditory processing disorders: the role of the audiologist. http://www.asha.org/policy/ PS2005-00114.htm. Accessed 23 Sept 2013

American Speech-Language-Hearing Association (2005b) (Central) Auditory processing disorders (Technical Report). www.asha.org/policy. Accessed 12 July 2018

Amitay S, Ahissar M, Nelken I (2002) Auditory processing deficits in reading disabled adults. J Assoc Res Otolaryngol 3(3):302–320. https://doi.org/10.1007/ s101620010093

Antonovsky A, Sourani T (1988) Family sense of coherence and family adaptation. J Marriage Fam 50(1):79–92

Archer JC, Crosby-Quinatoa G (2009) Strategies for treating children with hearing impairment in the schools. http://www.asha.org/Events/convention/ handouts/2009/1431_Archer_Jamy_Claire. Accessed 18 Mar 2017

Aschendorff A (2011) Imaging in cochlear implant patients. GMS Curr Top Otorhinolaryngol Head Neck Surg 10:Doc07

Aslin RN, Smith LB (1988) Perceptual development. Annu Rev Psychol 39:435–473

Australian Hearing (2013) CAPD service offered by Australian Hearing. http://www.hearing.com.au/capd-service-offered-australian-hearing/. Accessed 12 Mar 2015

Bagnato SJ, Wolfe PS, Rubina R (2007) How can we effectively assess for severe disabilities? In: Bagnato SJ (ed) Authentic assessment for early childhood intervention. Best practices. Guilford Press, New York, pp 178–204

Baguley D, McFerran D, Hall D (2013) Tinnitus. Lancet 9904:1600–1607

Barbi M, Binda S, Primache V et al (2000) Cytomegalovirus DNA detection in Guthrie cards: a powerful tool for diagnosing congenital infection. J Clin Virol 17(3):159–165

Barry JG, Moore DR (2014) Evaluation of Children's Listening and Processing Skills (ECLiPS). MRC-T, London

Barry JG, Tomlin D, Moore DR et al (2015) Use of questionnaire-based measures in the assessment of listening difficulties in school-aged children. Ear Hear 36(6):e300–e313

Bartel-Friedrich S, Fuchs M, Amaya B et al (2008) Der erweiterte Ductus und Saccus endolymphaticus, Teil 2: Klinische Manifestationen. HNO 56(2):225–230

Baudonck N, Van Lierde K, D'haeseleer E et al (2015) Nasalance and nasality in children with cochlear implants and children with hearing aids. Int J Pediatr Otorhinolaryngol 79(4):541–545

Beale TJ, Madani G (2008) Imaging of the Deaf Child. In: Graham JM, Scadding GK (eds) Bull PD Pediatric ENT. Springer, Berlin, Heidelberg

Beck DL, Speidel DP, Petrak M (2007) Auditory steady-state response: a Beginner's guide. Hear Rev 14(12):34–37

Beck C, Pérez-Álvarez JC, Sigruener A et al (2015) Identification and genotype/phenotype correlation of mutations in a large German cohort with hearing loss. Eur Arch Otorhinolaryngol 272(10):2765–2776

Benton C, Brough JE, Dodd MC (2004) Analysis of the middle ear. In: McCormick B (ed) Paediatric audiology 0–5 years, 3rd edn. Whurr Publishers, London

Beresford B, Greco V, Clarke S et al (2008) An evaluation of specialist mental health services for deaf children and young people. Social Policy Research Unit University of York, York

Berg AL, Olson TJ, Feldstein NA (2005) Cerebellar pilocytic astrocytoma with auditory presentation: case study. J Child Neurol 20(11):914–915

Bergeson TR, Chin SB (2008) Prosodic utterance production. Indiana University School of Medicine, Manuscript

Berk LE (2000) Child development, 5th edn. Allyn and Bacon, Boston

Bischoff C, Klingelhöfer J, Conrad B (1989) Decay and recovery of the stapedial reflex by prolonged stimulation in the diagnosis of myasthenia gravis. J Neurol 236(6):343–348

Boehm AE (1971) Boehm test of basic concepts manual. Psychological Corporation, New York

Boons T, De Raeve L, Langereis M et al (2013) Expressive vocabulary, morphology, syntax and narrative skills in profoundly deaf children after early cochlear implantation. Res Dev Disabil 34(6):2008–2022

Boothroyd A, Cawkwell S (1970) Vibrotactile thresholds in pure tone audiometry. Acta Otolaryngol 69(6):381–387

Boppana SB, Ross SA, Shimamura M et al (2011) For the National Institute on Deafness and Other Communication Disorders CHIMES Study. Saliva Polymerase-Chain-Reaction. Assay for Cytomegalovirus Screening in Newborns. N Engl J Med 364(22):2111–2118

Bradley L, Bryant PE (1983) Categorizing sounds and learning to read: a causal connection. Nature 301(5899):419–421

Brand T, Hohmann V (2002) An adaptive procedure for categorical loudness scaling. J Acoust Soc Am 112(4):1597–1604

Brannigan G, Decker S (2003) Bender visual-motor gestalt test, 2nd edn. (Bender-Gestalt II). http://www.wpspublish.com/store/p/2678/bender-visual-motor-gestalt-test-second-edition-bender-gestalt-ii. Accessed 27 Feb 2017

British Association of Paediatricians in Audiology (BAPA), British Association of Audiological Physicians (BAAP) (2008) Guidelines for the aetiological investigation of infants with congenital hearing loss identified through newborn hearing screening. http://www.baap.org.uk/Resources/Documents,GuidelinesClinicalStandards.aspx. Accessed Jan 2012

British Society of Audiology (2011a) Recommended procedure: pure-tone air-conduction and bone-conduction threshold audiometry with and without masking. British Society of Audiology, Berkshire, UK

British Society of Audiology (2011b) Recommended Procedure. Determination of uncomfortable loudness levels. British Society of Audiology, Berkshire, UK

British Society of Audiology (2013) Recommended procedure: tympanometry. http://www.thebsa.org.uk/wp-content/uploads/2014/04/BSA_RP_Tymp_Final_21Aug13_Final.pdf. Accessed 5 Jan 2017

British Society of Audiology (2014) Tinnitus in children and teenagers. http://www.thebsa.org.uk/wp-content/uploads/2014/06/Paed-Tin-Guide-Pub-Consul-Compressed.pdf. Accessed 23 Feb 2017

British Society of Audiology APD SIG (2011a) Position statement: Auditory Processing Disorder (APD). www.thebsa.org.uk/images/stories/docs/BSA_APD_PositionPaper_31March11_FINAL.pdf. Accessed 28 June 2018

British Society of Audiology APD SIG (2011b) Practical guidance: an overview of current management of auditory processing disorder. www.thebsa.org.uk/images/stories/docs/BSA_APD_Management_1Aug11_FINAL_a_mended17Oct11.pdf. Accessed 28 June 2018

British Society of Audiology APD SIG (2018) Position Statement and Practice Guidance Auditory Processing Disorder (APD). http://www.thebsa.org.uk/wp-content/uploads/2018/02/Position-Statement-and-Practice-Guidance-APD-2018-1.pdf. Accessed 28 June 2018

Brown CJ (2003) Clinical uses of electrically evoked auditory nerve and brainstem responses. Curr Opin Otolaryngol Head Neck Surg 11(5):383–387

Brown VL, Hammill DD, Wiederholt JL (1995) Test of Reading Comprehension (TORC-3). ProEd Publishing, Austin, TX

Brunner M, Seibert A, Dierks A et al (1998) Heidelberger Lautdifferenzierungstest (HLAD). Westra Elektroakustik, Wertingen

Burns E, Arehart K, Campbell S (1992) Prevalence of spontaneous otoacoustic emissions in neonates. J Acoust Soc Am 91(3):1571–1575

Cacace AT, McFarland DJ (2013) Factors influencing tests of auditory processing: a perspective on current issues and relevant concerns. J Am Acad Audiol 24(7):572–589. https://doi.org/10.3766/jaaa.24.7.6

Campbell NG, Bamiou DE, Sirimanna T (2012) Current progress in auditory processing disorder. ENT Audiol News 21(2):86–90

Campbell NG, Grant P, Rosen S, Moore DR (2019) Auditory processing disorder in children. BATOD Foundation. http://www.meshguides.org/guides/node/1432

Campisi P, Low AJ, Papsin BC (2006) Multidimensional voice program analysis in profoundly deaf children: quantifying frequency and amplitude control. Percept Mot Skills 103(1):40–50

Canadian Interorganizational Steering Group for Speech-Language Pathology and Audiology (2012) Canadian guidelines on auditory processing disorder in children and adults: assessment and intervention. www.sac.oac.ca/sites/default/files/resources/Canadian-Guidelines-on-Auditory-Processing-Disorder-in-Children-and-Adults-English-2012.pdf. Accessed 28 June 2018

Carhart R, Jerger JJ (1959) Preferred method for clinical determination of pure-tone thresholds. J Speech Hear Disord 24:330–345

Carney AE (1996) Audition and the development of oral communication competency. In: Bess FH et al (eds) Amplification for children with auditory deficits. Bill Wilkerson Center, Nashville, pp 29–54

Carrow-Woolfolk E (1985) TACL-R: test for auditory comprehension of language, Part 1. DLM Teaching Resources, Allen, TX

Carrow-Woolfolk E (1999) Comprehensive assessment of spoken language. American Guidance Service, Circle Pines, MN

Case JC (2005) Accommodations to improve instruction and assessment of students who are deaf or hard of hearing. Policy Report. Pearson Education, London, UK

Casselbrant M, Mandel E, Sparto P et al (2010) Longitudinal posturography and rotational testing in children three to nine years of age: normative data. Otolaryngol Head Neck Surg 142(5):708–714

Center for Deaf and Hard of Hearing (2014) Guidelines for the assessment and educational evaluation of deaf and hard of hearing children in Indiana. http://www.state.in.us/isdh/files/Assessment_Guideline__finalized_January_2015.pdf. Accessed 13 Sept 2016

Chermak GD, Hall JW III, Musiek FE (1999) Differential diagnosis and management of central auditory processing disorder and attention deficit hyperactivity disorder. J Am Acad Audiol 10(6):289–303

Chermak GD, Tucker E, Seikel JA (2002) Behavioral characteristics of auditory processing disorder and attention-deficit hyperactivity disorder: predominantly inattentive type. J Am Acad Audiol 13(6):332–338

Chin SB, Bergeson TR, Phan J (2012) Speech intelligibility and prosody production in children with cochlear implants. J Commun Disord 45(5):355–366

Chou YF, Chen PR, Yu SH et al (2012) Using multistimulus auditory steady state response to predict hearing thresholds in high-risk infants. Eur Arch Otorhinolaryngol 269(1):73–79

Cohen LB, Cashon CH (2003) Infant perception and cognition. Handbook of psychology. Dev Psychol 2:6389

Colarusso RP, Hammill DD (2015) Motor-Free Visual Perception Test-4 (MVPT-4). https://www.wpspublish.com/store/p/3303/motor-free-visual-perception-test-4-mvpt-4. Accessed 27 Feb 2017

Cole EB, Flexer C (2011) Children with hearing loss: developing listening and talking, birth to six. Plural Publishing, San Diego

College of Occupational Therapists (2015) Occupational therapy evidence fact sheet: occupational therapy with children and young people. https://www.cot.co.uk/sites/default/files/commissioning_ot/public/OT-with-children-and-young-people-updated-April2015.pdf. Accessed 20 May 2015

Compas BE, Jaser SS, Dunn MJ et al (2012) Coping with chronic illness in childhood and adolescence. Annu Rev Clin Psychol 8:455–480

Coninx F (2005) Konstruktion und Normierung des Adaptiven Auditiven Sprach-Test (AAST). 100 Jahre Phoniatrie in Deutschland. 22. Jahrestagung der Deutschen Gesellschaft für Phoniatrie und Pädaudiologie, 24. Kongress der Union der Europäischen Phoniater. September 16th–18th, 2005, Berlin. http://www.egms.de/en/meetings/dgpp2005/05dgpp045.shtml#. Accessed 12 May 2018

Coninx F, Moore JM (1997) The multiply handicapped deaf child. In: McCracken W, Kemp L (eds) Audiology in education. Whurr Publishers, London, pp 107–135

Cox RM, McDaniel DM (1989) Development of the Speech Intelligibility Rating [SIR] Test for hearing aid comparisons. J Speech Hear Res 32(2):347–352

Cupples L, Ching TYC, Crowe K et al (2014) Outcomes of 3-year-old children with hearing loss and different types of additional disabilities. J Deaf Stud Deaf Educ 19(1):20–39

da Silva MP, Comerlatto AAJ, Bevilacqua MC et al (2011) Instruments to assess the oral language of children fitted with a cochlear implant: a systematic review. J Appl Oral Sci 19(6):549–553. https://doi.org/10.1590/S1678-77572011000600002

Dau T, Wegner O, Mellert V et al (2000) Auditory brainstem responses with optimized chirp signals compensating basilar-membrane dispersion. J Acoust Soc Am 107(3):1530–1540

Dawson JI, Tattersall PJ (2001) Structured Photographic Articulation Test—DII. Janelle Publications, DeKalb, IL

De Foer B, Kenis C, Vercruysse JP et al (2009) Imaging of temporal bone tumors. Neuroimaging Clin N Am 19(3):339–366

De Leenheer EMR, Janssens S, Padalko E et al (2011) Etiological diagnosis in the hearing impaired newborn: proposal of a flow chart. Int J Pediatr Otorhinolaryngol 75(1):27–32. https://doi.org/10.1016/j.ijporl.21010.05.040

De Wit E, Neijenhuis K, Luinge MR (2017) Dutch position statement children with listening difficulties (Translated version of The Dutch Position Statement Kinderen met Luisterproblemen). Federation of Dutch Audiological Centres, Utrecht

Declau F, Cremers C, Van de Heyning P (1999) Diagnosis and management strategies in congenital atresia of the external auditory canal. Br J Audiol 33(5):313–327. Review

Declau F, Van de Heyning P, Cremers C (2008) Diagnosis and management strategies in congenital middle and external ear anomalies. In: Graham JM et al (eds) Pediatric ENT. Springer, Berlin, Heidelberg

Delaroche M (2001) Audiométrie comportementale du très jeune enfant. De Boeck Université, Bruxelles

Delaroche M, Thiebaut R, Dauman R (2004) Behavioural audiometry: protocols for measuring hearing thresholds in babies aged 4-18 months. Int J Pediatr Otorhinolaryngol 68(10):1233–1243

Delaroche M, Thiebaut R, Dauman R (2005) Behavioural audiometric measurements obtained using the 'Delaroche protocol in babies aged 4-18 months suffering from bilateral sensorineural hearing loss. Int J Pediatr Otorhinolaryngol 70(6):993–1002

Delaroche M, Gavilan-Cellié I, Maurice-Tison S et al (2011) Is behavioral audiometry achievable in infants younger than 6 months of age? Int J Pediatr Otorhinolaryngol 75(12):1502–1509

Di Giulio P, Philipov D, Jaschinski I (2014) Families with disabled children in different European countries. Families and Societies Working Paper Series (23). http://www.familiesandsocieties.eu/wp-content/uploads/2014/12/WP23GiulioEtAl.pdf. Accessed 13 Sept 2016

Dillon H, Cameron S, Glyde H et al (2012) An opinion on the assessment of people who may have an auditory processing disorder. J Am Acad Audiol 23(2):97–105. https://doi.org/10.3766/jaaa.23.2.4

Dobie RA, Van Hemel S (2004) Chapter 7: Hearing loss in children. In: Hearing loss: determining eligibility for social security benefits. National Academies Press, Washington, DC, pp 18–223. https://www.ncbi.nlm.nih.gov/books/NBK207837/. Accessed 12 Feb 2017

Dobie RA, Wilson MJ (1996) A comparison of t test, F test, and coherence methods of detecting steady-state auditory-evoked potentials, distortion-product otoacoustic emissions, or other sinusoids. J Acoust Soc Am 100(4 Pt 1):2236–2246

Downing JE (2004) Communication skills. In: Orelove FP et al (eds) Educating students with multiple disabilities: a collaborative approach. Paul H. Brooks, Baltimore

Dršata J, Havlík R et al (2015) Foniatrie—Sluch. Tobiáš, Havlíčkův Brod, p 136

DuCharme R (1983) The test of pragmatic skill. Pragmatic skills checklist from Communication Skill Builders, The Learning Clinic

Duffy FH, Eksioglu YZ, Rotenberg A et al (2013) The frequency modulated auditory evoked response (FMAER), a technical advance for study of childhood language disorders: cortical source localization and selected case studies. BMC Neurol 13:12

Dunn LM, Dunn DM (2007) Peabody picture vocabulary test, 4th edn. American Guidance Service, Circle Pines, MN

Dunn L, Markwardt FC (1989) Peabody individual achievement test-revised. American Guidance, Circle Pines, MN

Edwards S, Letts C, Sinka I (2011) The new reynell developmental language scales. GL Assessment, London

Eisenberg LS (2016) Clinical management of children with cochlear implants, 2nd edn. Plural Publishing, San Diego. http://pluralpublishing.com/publication_cmcci2e.htm. Accessed 28 Feb 2017

Eisenberg LS, Martinez AS, Holowecky SR et al (2002) Recognition of lexically controlled words and sentences by children with normal hearing and children with cochlear implants. Ear Hear 23(5):450–462

Eisenberg LS, Martinez AS, Boothroyd A (2007) Assessing auditory capabilities in young children. Int J Pediatr Otorhinolaryngol 71(9):1339–1350

Elberling C (1999) Loudness scaling revisited. J Am Acad Audiol 10(5):248–260

Elberling C, Don M, Cebulla M et al (2007) Auditory steady-state responses to chirp stimuli based on cochlear travelling wave. J Acoust Soc Am 122(5):2772–2785

Elliott LL, Katz DR (1980) Northwestern University children's perception of speech: (NU-CHIPS). Auditec of St Louis, St. Louis

Ellison J, Keefe D (2008) Audiometric predictions using SFOAE and middle-ear measurements. Ear Hear 26(5):487–503

Emanuel DC (2009) Acoustic Reflex Threshold (ART) patterns: an interpretation guide for students and supervisors. AudiologyOnline. http://www.audiologyonline.com/articles/acoustic-reflex-threshold-art-patterns-875. Accessed 5 Jan 2017

Emanuel DC, Ficca KN, Korczak P (2011) Survey of the diagnosis and management of auditory processing disorder. Am J Audiol 20(1):48–60. https://doi.org/10.1044/1059-0889(2011/10-0019)

Enns C, Herman R (2011) Adapting the assessing British Sign Language development: receptive skills test into American Sign Language. J Deaf Stud Deaf Educ 16(3):362–374

Erber N (1982) Auditory training. Alexander Graham Bell Association, Washington DC, pp 92–94

Erber NP, Alencewicz CM (1976) Audiologic evaluation of deaf children. J Speech Hear Disord 41(2):256–267

Esser G, Anderski CH, Birken A et al (1987) Auditive Wahrnehmungsstörungen und Fehlhörigkeit bei Kindern im Schulalter. Sprache-Stimme-Gehör 11:10–16

European Surveillance of Congenital Anomalies (EUROCAT) (2013) Prevalence Tables. http://www.eurocat-network.eu/ACCESSPREVALENCEDATA/PrevalenceTables. Accessed 16 Apr 2013

Evans DG, Birch JM, Ramsden RT (1999) Paediatric presentation of type 2 neurofibromatosis. Arch Dis Child 81(6):496–499

Evenhuis HM (1995) Medical aspects of ageing in a population with intellectual disability: II. Hearing impairment. J Intellect Disabil Res 39(Pt 1):27–33

Evenhuis HM (1996) Dutch consensus in diagnosis and treatment of hearing impairment in children and adults with intellectual disability. J Intellect Disabil Res 40(Pt 5):451–456

Evenhuis HM, Nagtzaam LMD (1998) Early identification of hearing and visual impairment in children and adults with an intellectual disability. International Consensus Statement, IASSID. http://iassid.org/pdf/sensory-imp-consensus. Accessed 16 Nov 2014

Eviatar L, Eviatar A (1979) The normal nystagmic response of infants to caloric and perrotatory stimulation. Laryngoscope 89(7 pt 1):1036–1045

Fabijańska A, Smurzyński J, Hatzopoulos S et al (2012) The relationship between distortion product otoacoustic emissions and extended high-frequency audiometry in tinnitus patients. Part 1: normally hearing patients with unilateral tinnitus. Med Sci Monit 18(12):CR765–CRC770

Fantz RL (1965) Visual perception from birth as shown by pattern selectivity. Ann N Y Acad Sci 118(21):793–814

Fenson L, Marchman VA, Thal DJ et al (2007) The MacArthur communicative development inventories: user's guide and technical manual, 2nd edn. Brookes, Baltimore

Ferguson MA, Hall RL, Riley A et al (2011) Communication, listening, cognitive and speech perception skills in children with auditory processing disorder (APD) or specific language impairment (SLI). J Speech Lang Hear Res 54(1):211–227. https://doi.org/10.1044/1092-4388(2010/09-0167

Ferm I, Lightfoot G, Stevens J (2013) Comparison of ABR response amplitude, test time, and estimation of hearing threshold using frequency specific chirp and tone pip stimuli in newborns. Int J Audiol 52(6):419–423

Fernández-Latorre F, Menor-Serrano F, Alonso-Charterina S et al (2000) Langerhans' cell histiocytosis of the temporal bone in pediatric patients: imaging and follow-up. AJR 174(1):217–321

Fife T, Tusa R, Furman J et al (2000) Assessment: vestibular testing techniques in adults and children. Neurology 55(10):1431–1441

Flipsen PJ, Parker RG (2008) Phonological patterns in the conversational speech of children with cochlear implants. J Commun Disord 41(4):337–357

Foudriat BA, DiFabio RP, Anderson JH (1993) Sensory organisation of balance responses in children 3-6 years of age: a normative study with diagnostic implications. Int J Pediatr Otorhinolaryngol 27(3):255–271

Foulon I, Naessens A, Foulon W et al (2008) A 10-year prospective study of sensorineural hearing loss in children with congenital cytomegalovirus infection. J Pediatr 153(1):84–88

Foulon I, Naessens A, Faron G et al (2012) Hearing thresholds in children with a congenital CMV infection: a prospective study. Int J Pediatr Otorhinolaryngol 76(5):712–717. https://doi.org/10.1016/j.ijporl.2012.02.026

Franks JR (2001) Hearing measurement. In: Goelzer B et al (eds) Occupational exposure to noise: evaluation, prevention and control. World Health Organization, Geneva, Switzerland, pp 183–232. http://www.who.int/occupational_health/publications/noise8.pdf. Accessed 9 Sept 2016

Fuchs M, Fröhlich M, Hentschel B et al (2007) Predicting mutational change in the speaking voice of boys. J Voice 21(2):169–178

Fudala JB (2001) Arizona articulation proficiency scale, 3rd Revision (Arizona-3). Western Psychological Services, Torrance, CA. http://li129-107.members.linode.com/downloads/compendium_instruments_publishers.pdf. Accessed 17 Mar 2017

Fulcher A, Purcell AA, Baker E et al (2012) Listen up: children with early identified hearing loss achieve age-appropriate speech/language outcomes by 3 years-of-age. Int J Pediatr Otorhinolaryngol 76(12):1785–1794

Gajjar A, Packer RJ, Foreman NK et al (2013) Children's Oncology Group's 2013 blueprint for research: central nervous system tumors. Pediatr Blood Cancer 60(6):1022–1026. Review

Gallaudet Research Institute (1983) Norm tables: 1982 Stanford Achievement Test, 7th Edition, Form E for use with hearingimpaired students. Gallaudet University, Washington, DC

Gallaudet Research Institute (2013) Regional and National Summary Report of Data from the 2011–12 Annual Survey of Deaf and Hard of Hearing Children and Youth. Gallaudet University, GRI

Garcia JV, Rovira JM, González Sanvicens L (2010) The influence of the auditory prosthesis type on deaf children's voice quality. Int J Pediatr Otorhinolaryngol 74(8):843–848

Gasparini P, Rabionet R, Barbujani G et al (2000) High carrier frequency of the 35delG deafness mutation in European populations. Genetic Analysis Consortium of GJB2 35delG. Eur J Hum Genet 8(1):19–23

Gathercole SE, Baddeley A (1996) The children's test of non-word repetition. Psychological Corporation Europe, London

Geers A, Hayes H (2011) Reading, writing, and phonological processing skills of adolescents with 10 or more years of cochlear implant experience. Ear Hear 32(1):49S–59S

German Society of Phoniatrics and Pedaudiology (GSPP) (2014) Auditory processing and perception disorders: definition. Professional guidelines. German Society for Phoniatry and Pediatric Audiology

Germiller JA (2007) Hearing loss in children. In: Wetmore RF (ed) Pediatric otolaryngology: the requisites in pediatrics. Mosby Elsevier, Philadelphia

Gheysen F, Loots G, Van Waelvelde H (2007) Motor development of deaf children with and without cochlear implants. J Deaf Stud Deaf Educ 13(2):215–224

Gibbin KT (2007) Management of the deaf child. In: Graham JM et al (eds) Pediatric ENT. Springer, Berlin, Heidelberg

Giesemann AM, Goetz F, Neuburger J et al (2011) Appearance of hypoplastic cochlea in CT and MRI: a new subclassification. Neuroradiology 53(1):49–61

GL Assessment (2011) British ability scales, 3rd edn, The leading standardised battery for assessing children's current intellectual functioning. http://www.gl-assessment.co.uk/products/bas3. Accessed 10 Aug 2016

Goldman R, Fristoe M (2000) Goldman-Fristoe-2 Test of articulation. Pearson Assessments, Minneapolis MN

Goodman S (2011) Comparison of high-frequency TEOAEs and DPOAEs for monitoring ototoxicity in pediatric cancer patients. Lecture presented at Illinois Speech-Language-Hearing Association. https://clas.uiowa.edu/sites/clas.uiowa.edu.comsci/files/groups/arl/pubs/goodman_isha_2011.pdf. Accessed 21 Jan 2017

Gorga MP, Johnson TA, Kaminski JR et al (2006) Using a combination of click- and tone burst-evoked auditory brain stem response measurements to estimate pure-tone thresholds. Ear Hear 27(1):60–74

Gorlin RJ, Cohen MM, Levin LS (1990) Syndromes of the head and neck, 3rd edn. Oxford University Press, New York, Oxford

Govaerts PJ, Daemers K, Yperman M et al (2006) Auditory Speech Sounds Evaluation (A(section)E): a new test to assess detection, discrimination and identification in hearing impairment. Cochlear Implants Int 7(2):92–106

Gruber M, Brown C, Mahadevan M et al (2016) The yield of multigene testing in the management of pediatric unilateral sensorineural hearing loss. Otol Neurotol 37(8):1066–1070

Guralnick MJ (ed) (2000) Interdisciplinary clinical assessment of young children with developmental disabilities. Paul H. Brookes Publishing, Baltimore

Gürtler N (in press) Studie: Prospektive multizentrische Studie zur Abklärung der Ätiologie der bilateralen kongenitalen Schwerhörigkeit. Nicolas Gürtler HNO-Klinik, Kantonsspital Aarau AG, Aarau

Hall JW (1999) Handbook of Otoacoustic Emissions. Singular Publishing Group, San Diego, p 643. ISBN: 1-56593-873-9

Hall JW, Bantwal AR, Ramkumar V et al (2011) Electrophysiological assessment of hearing with auditory middle latency and auditory late responses. In: Seewald R, Tharpe AM (eds) Comprehensive handbook of pediatric audiology. Plural Publishing, San Diego, CA, pp 449–482

Hammill DD, Newcomer PL (2001) Test of language development-intermediate, 3rd edn. http://cirrie.buffalo.edu/database/20818/. Accessed 4 June 2017

Harnett A (2007) Informing families of their child's disability. National best practice guidelines. Consultation and Research Report. The National Federation of Voluntary Bodies Providing Services to People with Intellectual Disability, Oranmore, Galway. ISBN: 978-0-9557833-0-2

Harris M, Beech JR (1998) Implicit phonological awareness and early reading development in prelingually deaf children. J Deaf Stud Deaf Educ 3(3):205–216

Haskins HL (1949) A phonetically balanced test of speech discrimination for children. Doctoral Thesis, Northwestern University

Health and Safety Authority (2007) Guidelines on hearing checks and audiometry under the safety, health and welfare at work (general application) regulations 2007, Control of Noise at Work. Health and Safety Authority. http://www.hsa.ie/eng/Publications_and_Forms/Publications/Occupational_Health/audiometry.pdf. Accessed 9 Sept 2016

Heinz MG, Colburn HS, Carney LH (2001) Rate and timing cues associated with the cochlear amplifier: level discrimination based on monaural cross-frequency coincidence detection. J Acoust Soc Am 110(4):2065–2084

Helms J (1994) Mittelohrmissbildungen. In: Helms J (ed) Oto-Rhino-Laryngologie in Klinik und Praxis, vol 1. Thieme, Stuttgart, pp 545–563

Henningsson G, Kuehn DP, Sell D et al (2008) Universal parameters for reporting speech outcomes in individuals with cleft palate. Cleft Palate Craniofac J 45(1):1–17

Henry JA (2016) "Measurement" of tinnitus. Otol Neurotol 37(8):e276–e285

Henry JA, Meikle MB (2000) Psychoacoustic measures of tinnitus. J Am Acad Audiol 11(3):138–155

Henry JA, Stewart BJ, Abrams HB et al (2014) Tinnitus functional index—development and clinical application. Audiol Today 26(6):40–48

Henry JA, Griest S, Zaugg TL et al (2015) Tinnitus and hearing survey: a screening tool to differentiate bothersome tinnitus from hearing difficulties. Am J Audiol 24(1):66–77

Hereditary Hearing Loss (2019). http://hereditaryhearingloss.org. Accessed 20 June 2019

Herman R, Holmes S, Woll B (1999) Assessing British Sign Language development: receptive skills test. Forest Bookshop, Gloucestershire

Hild U, Hey C, Baumann U et al (2008) High prevalence of hearing disorders at the Special Olympics indicate need to screen persons with intellectual disability. J Intellect Disabil Res 52(Pt 6):520–528

Hill-Briggs F, Dial JG, Morere DA et al (2007) Neuropsychological assessment of persons with physical disability, visual impairment or blindness, and hearing impairment or deafness. Arch Clin Neuropsychol 22(3):389–404

Hind SE, Haines-Bazrafshan R, Benton CL et al (2011) Prevalence of clinical referrals having hearing thresholds within normal limits. Int J Audiol 50(10):708–716. https://doi.org/10.3109/14992027.2011.582049

Hintermair M (2004) Sense of coherence: a relevant resource in the coping process of mothers of hearing-impaired children? J Deaf Stud Deaf Educ 9(1):15–26

Holden-Pitt L, Diaz J (1998) Thirty five years of the annual survey of the deaf and hard of hearing children and youth: a glance over the decades. Am Ann Deaf 143(2):72–76

Holube I, Böld T, Gerdes T et al (2011) Internationales Sprachtestsignal (ISTS) als fluktuierender Maskierer im Satztest. 14. Jahrestagung der Deutschen Gesellschaft für Audiologie, March 9th–12th, 2011, Jena

Holzinger D, Fellinger J, Beitel C (2011) Early onset of family centred intervention predicts language outcomes in children with hearing loss. Int J Pediatr Otorhinolaryngol 75(2):256–260

Horsch U (2008) Dialog und Bildung in der Vorsprachlichkeit—Zur Situation hörgeschädigter Kinder in der Frühpädagogik. Sprache Stimme Gehör 32(1):18–25

Hoth S, Mühler R, Neumann K et al (2015) Objektive Audiometrie im Kindesalter. (Objective audiometry in children), 1st edn. Springer, Heidelberg

Huang BY, Zdanski C, Castillo M (2012a) Pediatric sensorineural hearing loss, part 1: practical aspects for neuroradiologists. AJNR Am J Neuroradiol 33(2):211–217. Review

Huang BY, Zdanski C, Castillo M (2012b) Pediatric sensorineural hearing loss, part 2: syndromic and acquired causes. AJNR Am J Neuroradiol 33(3):399–406. Review

Hugdahl K, Westerhausen R, Alho K et al (2009) Attention and cognitive control: unfolding the dichotic listening story. Scand J Psychol 50(1):11–22. https://doi.org/10.1111/j.1467-9450.2008.00676.x

Iliadou V, Ptok M, Grech H et al (2017) A European perspective on auditory processing disorder-current knowledge and future research focus. Front Neurol 8:622. https://doi.org/10.3389/fneur.2017.00622

Illinois Service Resource Center (2011) Guidelines for psychological testing of deaf and hard of hearing students. http://www.isrc.us/sites/default/files/pdf/psych-guidelines2011.pdf. Accessed 13 Sept 2016

Illum ON, Gradel KO (2015) Assessing children with disabilities using WHO International Classification of Functioning, Disability and Health Child and Youth Version Activities and Participation D Codes. Child Neurol Op 1-9

ISAAC—International Society for Augmentative and Alternative Communication (2016). https://www.isaac-online.org/. Accessed 17 Mar 2016

Ishimoto S, Ito K, Yamasoba T et al (2005) Correlation between microtia and temporal bone malformation evaluated using grading system. Arch Otolaryngol Head Neck Surg 131(4):326–329

ISO 16832 (2006) Acoustics—Loudness scaling by means of categories

ISO 60645-5 (2005) Electroacoustics—Audiometric equipment—Part 5: Instruments for the measurement of aural acoustic impedance/admittance

ISO 8253-1 (2010) Acoustics—Audiometric Test Methods—Part 1: Pure tone air and bone conduction audiometry

Janse E, Newman RS (2013) Identifying nonwords: effects of lexical neighborhoods, phonotactic probability, and listener characteristics. Lang Speech 56(Pt 4):421–441

Jedrzejczak WW, Blinowska KJ, Kochanek K et al (2008) Synchronized spontaneous otoacoustic emissions analyzed in a time-frequency domain. J Acoust Soc Am 124:3720. https://doi.org/10.1121/1.2999556

Jerger J (1970) Clinical experience with impedance audiometry. Arch Otolaryngol 92(4):311–324

Jerger JF, Hayes D (1976) The cross-check principle in pediatric audiometry. Arch Otolaryngol 102(10):614–620

Jewett DL (1970) Volume conducted potentials in response to auditory stimuli as detected by averaging in the cat. Electroencephalogr Clin Neurophysiol 28(6):609–618

Jewett DL, Romano MN, Williston JS (1970) Human auditory evoked potentials: possible brain stem components detected on the scalp. Science 167(3924):1517–1518

John MS, Lins OG, Boucher BL et al (1998) Multiple auditory steady-state responses (MASTER): stimulus and recording parameters. Audiology 37(2):59–82

Johnson TA, Brown CJ (2005) Threshold prediction using the auditory steady-state response and the tone burst auditory brain stem response: a within-subject comparison. Ear Hear 26(6):559–576

Johnson MH, Farroni T (2007) The neurodevelopmental origins of eye gaze perception. In: Flom R et al (eds) Gaze-following: its development and significance. Lawrence Erlbaum Associates, Mahwah, NJ, pp 1–16

Johnson C, Goswani U (2010) Phonological awareness, vocabulary, and reading in deaf children with cochlear implants. J Speech Lang Hear Res 53(2):237–261

Johnson MR, Wilhelm C, Eisert D et al (2001) Assessment of students with motor impairments. In: Simeonsson RJ, Rosenthal SL (eds) Psychological and developmental assessment. Guilford Press, New York, pp 205–224

Johnston T (2004) The assessment and achievement of proficiency in a native sign language within a sign bilingual program: the pilot Auslan receptive skills test. Deafness Educ Int 6(2):57–81

Joint Committee on Infant Hearing (2007) Year 2007 position statement: principles and guidelines for early hearing detection and intervention. Appendix 1: Risk Indicators Associated with Permanent Congenital, Delayed-Onset, or Progressive Hearing Loss in Childhood. www.asha.org/policy. Accessed 11 June 2017. Reproduced with permission from Pediatrics, 120:898–921

Joint Committee on Infant Hearing (2013) Supplement to the JCIH 2007 position statement: principles and guidelines for early intervention after confirmation that a child is deaf or hard of hearing. Pediatrics 131(4):1324–1349

Jones MW, Morgan E, Shelton JE (2007) Primary care of the student with cerebral palsy. J Pediatr Health Care 21(4):226–237

Jozefowicz-Korczynska M, Ciechomska EA, Pajor AM (2005) Electronystagmography outcome and neuropsychological findings in tinnitus patients. Int Tinnitus J 11(1):54–57

Keith RW (2009) SCAN–3:C tests for auditory processing disorders for children. Pearson, London

Kemp D (1978) Stimulated acoustic emissions from within the human auditory system. J Acoust Soc Am 64(5):1386–1391

Kemp D (2002) Otoacoustic emissions, their origin in cochlear function, and use. Br Med Bull 63:223–241

Kent RD, Kim Y (2008) Acoustic analysis of speech. In: Ball MJ et al (eds) The handbook of clinical linguistics. Blackwell, Malden, MA, pp 360–380

Kentish RC, Crocker SR, McKenna L (2000) Children's experience of tinnitus: a preliminary survey of children presenting to Psychology department. Br J Audiol 34(6):335–340

Khater AM, Afifi PO (2016) Video head-impulse test (vHIT) in dizzy children with normal caloric responses. Int J Pediatr Otorhinolaryngol 87:172–177

Kim EY, Yoon MS, Kim NH et al (2012) Characteristics of nasal resonance and perceptual rating in prelingual hearing impaired adults. Clin Exp Otorhinolaryngol 5(1):1–9

Kirk KI, Pisoni DB, Osberger MJ (1995) Lexical effects on spoken word recognition by pediatric cochlear implant users. Ear Hear 16(5):470–481

Kirk KI, Eisenberg LS, French BF et al (2011) The multimodal lexical sentence test for children: performance of children with hearing loss. Paper presented at the 13th symposium on cochlear implants in children, Chicago, IL, 14–16 June 2011

Kirk KI, Prusick L, French B et al (2012) Assessing spoken word recognition in children who are deaf or hard of hearing: a translational approach. J Am Acad Audiol 23(6):464–475. https://doi.org/10.3766/jaaa.23.6.8

Klaiber S, Weerda H (2002) BAHA bei beidseitiger Ohrmuscheldysplasie und Atresia auris congenita. HNO 50(10):949–959

Koester LS, Lahti-Harper E (2010) Mother-infant hearing status and intuitive parenting behaviors during the first 18 months. Am Ann Deaf 155(1):5–18

Korczak P, Smart J, Delgado R et al (2012) Tutorial Auditory steady-state responses. J Am Acad Audiol 23(3):146–170

Kort W, Schittekatte M, Compaan EL (2008) CELF-4-NL: clinical evaluation of language fundamentals-vierde-editie. Pearson Assessment and Information BV, Amsterdam

Kösling S, Jüttemann S, Amaya B et al (2003) Stellenwert der MRT bei Verdacht auf Innenohrmissbildung. Fortschr Röntgenstr 175(12):1639–1646

Kösling S, Omenzetter M, Bartel-Friedrich S (2009) Congenital malformations of the external and middle ear. Eur J Radiol 69(2):269–279. Review

Kricos P (1993) The counseling process: children and parents. In: McCarthy P, Alpiner J (eds) Rehabilitative audiology: children and adults, 2nd edn. Williams and Wilkins, Baltimore, MD, pp 211–237

Kuk FK, Tyler RS, Russell D et al (1990) The psychometric properties of a tinnitus handicap questionnaire. Ear Hear 11(6):434–445

Kummer AW (2008) Cleft palate and craniofacial anomalies: effects on speech and resonance, 2nd edn. Thomson Delmar Learning, New York, Chapter 14

Kunze S, Nickisch A, von Voss H et al (2016) Stapediusreflexe von Kindern mit und ohne auditive Verarbeitungs- und Wahrnehmungsstörungen. HNO 65(4):328–336. https://doi.org/10.1007/s00106-016-0271-2

Kurtzer-White E, Luterman D (2003) Families and children with hearing loss: grief and coping. Ment Retard Dev Disabil Res Rev 9(4):232–235

Kuwada S, Batra R, Maher VL (1986) Scalp potentials of normal and hearing-impaired subjects in response to sinusoidally amplitude-modulated tones. Hear Res 21(2):179–192

Kyle FE, Campbell R, Mohammed T et al (2013) Speechreading development in deaf and hearing children: introducing the test of child speechreading. J Speech Lang Hear Res 56(2):416–426

Lambert PR (2001) Congenital aural atresia. In: Bailey BJ (ed) Head and neck surgery—otolaryngology. Lippincott Williams & Wilkins, Philadelphia, pp 1745–1757

Laugen NJ, Jacobsen KH, Rieffe C et al (2016) Predictors of psychosocial outcomes in hard of hearing preschool children. J Deaf Stud Deaf Educ 21(3):259–267

Lechowicz U, Pollak A, Oldak M (2015) Novel trends in the molecular genetics of hearing loss. J Hear Sci 5(3):9–13

Lehnhardt E, Laszig R (eds) (2009) Praxis der Audiometrie. Thieme, Stuttgart, New York, p 140

Lesinski A, Littmann X, Battmer RD et al (1997) Comparison of preoperative electrostimulation data using an ear-canal electrode and a promontory needle electrode. Am J Otol 18(6 suppl):88–89

Levitt H, McGarr N, Geffner D (1987) Development of language and communication skills in hearing-impaired children: introduction. ASHA Monogr 26:1–8

Li Y, Yang J, Liu J et al (2015) Restudy of malformations of the internal auditory meatus, cochlear nerve canal and cochlear nerve. Eur Arch Otorhinolaryngol 272(7):1587–1596

Lightfoot GR (1979) Air-borne radiation from bone conduction transducers. Br J Audiol 13(2):53–56

Lightfoot GR (2000) Audiometer calibration: interpreting and applying the standards. Br J Audiol 34(5):311–316

Lightfoot GR, Hughes JB (1993) Bone conduction errors at high frequencies: implications for clinical and medico-legal practice. J Laryngol Otol 107(4):305–308

Lightfoot G, Kennedy V (2006) Cortical electric response audiometry hearing threshold estimation: accuracy, speed, and the effects of stimulus presentation features. Ear Hear 27(5):443–456

Limberger A, Bohnert A, Lippert, KL et al (2007) Verschiedene Sondentöne in der Tympanometrie. Paper presented at 78th annual meeting of the German Society of Oto-Rhino-Laryngology, Head and Neck Surgery, Munich, 16–20 May 2007. German Medical Science GMS Publishing House, Düsseldorf. http://www.egms.de/static/en/meetings/hnod2007/07hnod042.shtml. Accessed 30 Dec 2016

Lin K, Hsu Y, Young Y (2010) Brainstem lesion in benign paroxysmal vertigo children: evaluated by a combined ocular and cervical vestibular-evoked myogenic potential test. Int J Pediatr Otorhinolaryngol 74(5):523–527

Ling D (1976) Speech and the hearing-impaired child: theory and practice. Alexander Graham Bell Association for the Deaf, Washington, DC

Ling D (1989) Foundations of spoken language for the hearing-impaired child. Alexander Graham Bell Association for the Deaf, Washington, DC

Lins OG, Picton TW (1995) Auditory steady-state responses to multiple simultaneous stimuli. Electroencephalogr Clin Neurophysiol 96(5):420–432

Lutermann D (2004) Children with hearing loss and special needs. The Volta Review, Washington, DC

Luts H, Desloovere C, Wouters J (2006) Clinical application of dichotic multiple-stimulus auditory steady state responses in high-risk newborns and young children. Audiol Neurootol 11(1):24–37

MacDougall HG, Weber KP, McGarvie LA et al (2009) The video head impulse test: diagnostic accuracy in peripheral vestibulopathy. Neurology 73(14):1134–1141

Mackie RT, McCulloch DL (1995) Assessment of visual acuity in multiply handicapped children. Br J Ophthalmol 79(3):290–296

Madell JR, Flexer C (2008) Pediatric audiology: diagnosis, technology and management. Thieme, New York

Mallur PS, Wisoff JH, Lalwani AK (2008) Steroid responsive fluctuating sensorineural hearing loss due to juvenile pilocytic astrocytoma involving the cerebellopontine angle. Int J Pediatr Otorhinolaryngol 72(4):529–534

Marchman VA, Fernald A (2008) Speed of word recognition and vocabulary knowledge in infancy predict cognitive and language outcomes in later childhood. Dev Sci 11(3):1–9

Marková SP, Brožková DŠ, Laššuthová P, Mészárosová A, Krůtová M, Neupauerová J, Rašková D, Trková M, Staněk D, Seeman P (2018) STRC gene mutations, mainly large deletions, are a very important cause of early-onset hereditary hearing loss in the czech population. Genet Test Mol Biomarkers 22(2):127–134. https://doi.org/10.1089/gtmb.2017.0155

Margolis RH (1993) Detection of hearing impairment with the acoustic stapedius reflex. Ear Hear 14(1):3–10

Margolis RH (2015) The Vanishing Air-Bone Gap—Audiology's Dirty Little Secret. http://www.audiologyonline.com/articles/vanishing-air-bone-gap-audiology-901. Accessed 21 Oct 2016

Margolis RH, Wilson RH, Popelka GR et al (2015) Distribution characteristics of normal pure-tone thresholds. Int J Audiol 54(11):796–805

Marschark M, Spencer PE (2003) Oxford handbook of deaf studies, language and education. Oxford University Press, New York

Martin N (2017) Test of Visual Perceptual Skills–Fourth Edition (TVPS-4). Pro Ed, Austin

May-Mederake B (2012) Early intervention and assessment of speech and language development in young children with cochlear implants. Int J Ped Otorhinolaryngol 76(7):939–946

May-Mederake B, Kuehn H, Vogel A et al (2010) Evaluation of auditory development in infants and toddlers who received cochlear implants under the age of 24 months with the LittlEARS Auditory Questionnaire. Int J Ped Otorhinolaryngol 74(10):1149–1155

Meikle MB, Vernon J, Johnson RM (1984) The perceived severity of tinnitus. Some observations concerning a large population of tinnitus clinic patients. Otolaryngol Head Neck Surg 92(6):689–696

Meinzen-Derr J, Wiley S, Choll ID (2011) Impact of early intervention on expressive and receptive language development among young children with permanent hearing loss. Am Ann Deaf 155(5):580–591

Meltzoff AN, Brooks R (2009) Social cognition and language: the role of gaze following in early word learning. In: Colombo J et al (eds) Infant pathways to language: methods, models, and research directions. Erlbaum, Mahwah, NJ, pp 169–194

Miller Guron L (1999) Wordchains: word reading test. NFER Nelson, Windsor, UK

Miller CA, Wagstaff DA (2011) Behavioral profiles associated with auditory processing disorder and specific language impairment. J Commun Disord 44(6):745–763. https://doi.org/10.1016/j.jcomdis.2011.04.001

Minárik G, Ferák V, Feráková E et al (2003) High frequency of GJB2 mutation W24X among Slovak Romany (Gypsy) patients with non-syndromic hearing loss (NSHL). Gen Physiol Biophys 22(4):549–556

Mirone G, Schiabello L, Chibbaro S et al (2009) Pediatric primary pilocytic astrocytoma of the cerebellopontine angle: a case report. Childs Nerv Syst 25(2):247–251

Moeller MP (2000) Early intervention and language development in children who are deaf and hard of hearing. Pediatrics 106(3):e43

Moeller MP, Hoover B, Putman C et al (2007a) Vocalizations of infants with hearing loss compared with infants with normal hearing: Part I—phonetic development. Ear Hear 28(5):605–627

Moeller MP, Hoover B, Putman C et al (2007b) Vocalizations of infants with hearing loss compared with infants with normal hearing: Part II—transition to words. Ear Hear 28(5):628–642

Moeller MP, Carr G, Seaver L et al (2013) Best practices in family-centered early intervention for children who are deaf or hard of hearing: an international consensus statement. J Deaf Stud Deaf Educ 18(4):429–445

Moog JS, Geers AE (1990) Early Speech Perception Test of profoundly hearing-impaired children. Central Institute for the Deaf, St. Louis, MO

Moore BCJ (2001) Dead regions in the cochlea: diagnosis, perceptual consequences, and implications for the fitting of hearing aids. Trends Amplif 5(1):1–34

Moore DR (2012) Listening difficulties in children: bottom-up and top-down contributions. J Commun Disord 45(6):411–418. https://doi.org/10.1016/j.jcomdis.2012.06.006

Moore DR, Hunter LL (2013) Auditory processing disorder (APD) in children: a marker of neurodevelopmental syndrome. Hear Balance Commun 11(3):160–167

Moore JM, Thompson G, Thompson M (1975) Auditory localization of infants as a function of reinforcement conditions. J Speech Hear Disord 40(1):29–34

Moore BCJ, Huss M, Vickers DA et al (2000) A test for the diagnosis of dead regions in the cochlea. Br J Audiol 34(4):205–224

Moore DR, Ferguson MA, Edmondson-Jones AM et al (2010) Nature of auditory processing disorder in children. Pediatrics 126(2):e382–e390. https://doi.org/10.1542/peds.2009-2826

Moore DR, Rosen S, Bamiou D-E et al (2013) Evolving concepts of developmental auditory processing disorder (APD): a British Society of Audiology APD Special Interest Group 'white paper'. Int J Audiol 52(1):1499–2027

Morell RJ, Kim HJ, Hood LJ et al (1998) Mutations in the connexin 26 gene (GJB2) among Ashkenazi Jews with nonsyndromic recessive deafness. N Engl J Med 339(21):1500–1505

Morlet T, Pazuniak M, O'Reilly R et al (2017) Cochlear nerve deficiency and brain abnormalities in pediatric patients. Otol Neurotol 38(3):429–440

Mühlenberg L, Schade G (2012) Frühe akustisch evozierte Potentiale: Low-Chirp-BERA versus Notched-Noise-BERA. (A comparison of low-chirp- and notched-noise-evoked auditory brainstem response). Laryngo-Rhino-Otologie 91(8):500–504

Müller KHG (1991) Missbildungen des Schläfenbeins. In: Mödder U, Lenz M (eds) Klinische Radiologie, Gesichtschädel, Felsenbein, Speicheldrüsen, Pharynx, Larynx, Halsweichteile. Springer, Berlin, p 170

Munro KJ, Agnew N (1999) A comparison of inter-aural attenuation with the Etymotic ER-3A insert earphone and the Telephonics TDH-39 supra-aural earphone. Br J Audiol 33(4):259–262

National Acoustics Laboratory (2015) NAL position statement on auditory processing disorder. www.capd.nal.gov.au/capd-position-statement.shtml. Accessed 28 June 2018

National Centre for Health Statistics (2003) National health and nutrition examination survey: audiometry procedures manual. http://www.cdc.gov/nchs/data/nhanes/nhanes_03_04/au.pdf. Accessed 1 Sept 2016

Neff BA, Welling DB (2005) Current concepts in the evaluation and treatment of neurofibromatosis type II. Otolaryngol Clin N Am 38(4):671–684. Review

Neumann K, Dettmer G, Euler HA et al (2006) Auditory status of persons with intellectual disability at the German Special Olympic games. Int J Audiol 45(2):83–90

Neumann K, Ludwig A, Montgomery J et al (2008) Special Olympics as research platform of hearing disorders in people with intellectual disabilities. In: Wegner M, Schulke HJ (eds) Kieler Schriften zur Sportwissenschaft—Behinderung, Bewegung, Befreiung: Gewinn von Lebensqualität und Selbständigkeit durch Wettbewerb und sportliches Training bei Menschen mit geistiger Behinderung. Christian-Albrechts-Universität zu Kiel, Kiel, pp 25–28

Neumann K, Waschkies L, Thomas JP et al (2014) Hearing and communication situation of persons with intellectual disability (ID). Paper presented at the Coalition for Global Hearing Health conference, Oxford, July 25–26, 2014, Book of Abstracts

Neumann K, Rosenberger D, Euler HA et al (in press) The adaptive MAGIC® test measures fast and reliably the pure tone hearing threshold of persons with intellectual disabilities. Manuscript in preparation

Newman CW, Jacobson GP, Spitzer JB (1996) Development of the tinnitus handicap inventory. Arch Otolaryngol Head Neck Surg 122(2):143–148

Nguyen LH, Allegro J, Low A et al (2008) Effect of cochlear implantation on nasality in children. Ear Nose Throat J 87(3):138–143

Nickerson RB (1975) Characteristics of the speech of deaf persons. Volta Rev 77(6):342–362

Nickisch A, Gross M, Schönweiler R et al (2015) Auditive Verarbeitungs- und Wahrnehmungsstörungen (AVWS): Zusammenfassung und aktualisierter Überblick. HNO 63:434–438

Nittrouer S, Caldwell-Tarr A, Lowenstein JH (2013) Working memory in children with cochlear implants: problems are in storage, not processing. Int J Pediatr Otorhinolaryngol 77(11):1886–1898

Northern JL, Downs MP (2001) Hearing in children. Lippincott Williams & Wilkins, Philadelphia

O'Reilly R, Grindle C, Zwicky E et al (2011) Development of the vestibular system and balance function: differential diagnosis in the pediatric population. Otolaryngol Clin N Am 44(2):251–271

Osberger MJ, Robbins AM, Todd SL et al (1994) Speech intelligibility of children with cochlear implants. Volta Rev 96(5):169–180

Petrak MR, Bahner C, Beck DL (2013) Video Head Impulse Testing (vHIT): VOR Analysis of High Frequency Vestibular Activity. The Hearing Review. http://www.hearingreview.com/2013/08/video-head-impulse-testing-vhit-vor-analysis-of-high-frequency-vestibular-activity/. Accessed 20 Apr 2017

Piaget J, Inhelder B (1969) The psychology of the child. Basic Books, New York

Picard M (2004) Children with permanent hearing loss and associated disabilities: revisiting current epidemiological data and causes of deafness. Volta Rev 104(4):221236

Picton TW (2011) Human auditory evoked potentials. Plural Publishing, San Diego

Picton TW, Ouellette J, Hamel G et al (1979) Brainstem evoked potentials to tonepips in notched noise. J Otolaryngol 8(4):289–314

Picton TW, John MS, Dimitrijevic A et al (2003) Human auditory steady-state responses. Int J Audiol 42(4):177–219

Potsic WP, Lando T (2012) Introduction to pediatric otology. In: Wetmore RF et al (eds) Pediatric otolaryngology: principles and practice pathways. Thieme, New York

Pruszewicz A, Obrębowski A (2010) Clinical audiology edd.IV. Med Univ Poznań, Poznań

Prutting C (1982) Observational protocol for pragmatic behaviors' (Clinic manual). Developed for the University of California Speech and Hearing Clinic, Santa Barbara

Prutting C, Kirchner D (1987) A clinical appraisal of the pragmatic aspects of language. J Speech Hear Disord 52(2):105–119

Queißer-Luft A, Spranger J (2006) Fehlbildungen bei Neugeborenen. Dtsch Arztebl 103(38):A 2464–A 2471

Ramos JA, Kristensen SGB, Beck DL (2013) An overview of OAEs and normative data for DPOAEs. Hearing Review. http://www.hearingreview.com/2013/10/an-overview-of-oaes-and-normative-data-for-dpoaes/. Accessed 2 Nov 2016

Ramos D, Jorge JX, Teixeira A et al (2015) The impact of cochlear implant in the oral language of children with congenital deafness. Acta Medica Port 28(4):442–447. Epub 2015 Aug 31

Rance G, Roper R, Symons L et al (2005) Hearing threshold estimation in infants using auditory steady-state responses. J Am Acad Audiol 16(5):291–300

Reichmuth K, Embacher AJ, Matulat P et al (2013) Responsive parenting intervention after identification of hearing loss by universal newborn hearing screening: the concept of the Muenster Parental Programme. Int J Pediatr Otorhinolaryngol 77(12):2030–2039

Reid DK, Hammill D, Wiltshire S, Hresko W (1991) Test of Early Reading Ability Deaf or Hard of Hearing (TERA-D/HH) Hresko. Pro Ed, Austin

Renfrew C (1997) Bus story test (Renfrew language scales), 4th edn. Winslow Press, Bicester

Renfrew C, Mitchell P (2015) Word finding vocabulary test (the Renfrew language scales). Routledge, London

Rinaldi P, Baruffaldi F, Burdo S et al (2013) Linguistic and pragmatic skills in toddlers with cochlear implant. Int J Lang Commun Disord 48(6):715–725. https://doi.org/10.1111/1460-6984.12046. Epub 2013 Jul 29

Rizzi MD, Dunham BP (2014) Congenital malformations of the nose and nasopharynx. In: Elden LM, Zur KB (eds) Congenital malformations of the head and neck. Springer, New York

Robbins AM, Osberger MJ (1990) Meaningful Use of Speech Scale (MUSS). Indiana University School of Medicine, Indianapolis

Robbins AM, Renshaw JJ, Berry SW (1991) Evaluating meaningful auditory integration in profoundly hearing-impaired children. Am J Otol 12(Suppl):144–150

Robbins AM, Renshaw JJ, Osberger MJ (1995) Common phrases test. Indiana University School of Medicine, Indianapolis

Robinette M, Glattke T (2007) Otoacoustic emissions: clinical applications. Thieme, New York

Robinette MS, Cevette MJ, Probst R (2007) Otoacoustic emissions and audiometric outcomes across cochlear and retrocochlear pathology. In: Robinette MS, Glattke TJ (eds) Otoacoustic emissions: clinical applications, 3rd edn. Thieme Publishing, New York, pp 236–237

Robson CD (2010) Imaging of head and neck neoplasms in children. Pediatr Radiol 40(4):499–509

Robson CD, Robertson RL, Barnes PD (1999) Imaging of pediatric temporal bone abnormalities. Neuroimaging Clin N Am 9(1):133–155. Review

Roid GH, Miller LJ (1997) Leiter international performance scale-revised. Stoelting, Wood Dale, IL

Römer TA (2007) Retrospektives Erleben von Eltern zur Diagnosestellung einer chronischen Stoffwechselerkrankung bei ihrem Kind. Dissertation, Universität Hamburg

Ross HW (1979) Wepman Test of Auditory Discrimination (WADT): what does it discriminate. J Sch Psychol 17(1):47–54

Rowland C (2005) But what CAN they do? Assessment of communication skills in children with severe and multiple disabilities. Perspect Augment altern commun 14(1):1–5

Ruben JR (2001) The pediatric otolaryngic assessment of the child with a suspected hearing loss. In: Gerber SE (ed) The handbook of pediatric audiology. Gallaudet University Press, Washington

Russel E, Nagaishi P (2010) Service for children with visual or hearing impairments. In: Case-Smith J (ed) Occupational therapy for children, 6th edn. Maryland Heights, Mosby/Elsevier, MO, pp 744–784

Russo NM, Hornickel J, Nicol T et al (2010) Biological changes in auditory function following training in children with autism spectrum disorders. Behav Brain Funct 6:60

Santi S, Rushing EJ (2013) Tumors of the pediatric central nervous system. In: Keating RF et al (eds) Neurosurgery, 2nd edn. Thieme Medical Publisher, New York

Sarant J (2012) Cochlear implants in children: a review. The University of Melbourne Australia. http://cdn.intechopen.com/pdfs-wm/33875.pdf. Accessed 11 Aug 2016

Scherg M (1991) Akustisch evozierte Potentiale. In: Baumgartner A et al (eds) Psychiatrie, Neurologie, Klinische Psychologie. Kohlhammer, Stuttgart

Schley S, Albertini J (2005) Assessing the writing of deaf college students: reevaluating a direct assessment of writing. J Deaf Stud Deaf Educ 10(1):96–104

Schloss MD (1997) Congenital anomalies of the external auditory canal and the middle ear. Surgical management. In: Tewfik TL, Der Kaloustian VM (eds) Congenital anomalies of the ear, nose, and throat. Oxford University Press, New York, pp 119–124

Schlumberger E, Narbona J, Manrique M (2004) Nonverbal development of children with deafness with and without cochlear implants. Dev Med Child Neurol 46(9):599–606

Schmidt CM, Knief A, Deuster D et al (2007) Melatonin is a useful alternative to sedation in children undergoing brainstem audiometry with an age dependent success rate—a field report of 250 investigation. Neuropediatrics 38(1):2–4

Schmidt CM, Huebner JR, Deuster D et al (2012) A positive wave at 8 ms (P8) and modified auditory brainstem responses measurement in auditory neuropathy spectrum disorder. Int J Pediatr Otorhinolaryngol 76(5):636–641

Schmuziger N, Probst R, Smurzynski J (2004) Test-retest reliability of pure-tone thresholds from 0.5 to 16 kHz using Sennheiser HDA 200 and Etymotic Research ER-2 earphones. Ear Hear 25(2):127–132

Scholz U, Gutiérrez-Doña B, Sud S et al (2002) Is general self-efficacy a universal construct? Psychometric findings from 25 countries. Eur J Psychol Assess 18(3):242–251

Schwartz RG, Steinman S, Ying E et al (2013) Language processing in children with cochlear implants: a preliminary report on lexical access for production and comprehension. Clin Linguist Phon 27(4):264–277

Sennaroglu L (2010) Cochlear Implantation in inner ear malformations—a review article. Cochlear Implants Int 11(1):34–41

Sennaroglu L, Saatci I (2002) A new classification for cochleovestibular malformations. Laryngoscope 112(12):2230–2241

Shahnaz N, Bork K, Polka L et al (2009) Energy reflectance and tympanometry in normal and otosclerotic ears. Ear Hear 30(2):219–233

Sharma M, Purdy SC, Kelly AS (2009) Comorbidity of auditory processing, language, and reading disorders. J Speech Lang Hear Res 52(3):706–722. https://doi.org/10.1044/1092-4388(2008/07-0226)

Sherlock LP, Formby C (2005) Estimates of loudness, loudness discomfort, and the auditory dynamic range: normative estimates, comparison of procedures, and test-retest reliability. J Am Acad Audiol 16(2):85–100

Shetye A, Kennedy V (2010) Tinnitus in children: an uncommon symptom? Arch Dis Child 95(8):645–648

Shinjo Y, Jin Y, Kaga K (2007) Assessment of vestibular function of infants and children with congenital and acquired deafness using ice-water caloric test, rotational chair test and vestibular-evoked myogenic potential recording. Acta Otolaryngol 127(7):736–747

Shoman NM, Samy RN, Choo DI (2014) Congenital malformations of the ear. In: Elden LM, Zur KB (eds) Congenital malformations of the head and neck. Springer, New York

Shott SR, Joseph A, Heithaus D (2001) Hearing loss in children with Down syndrome. Int J Pediatr Otorhinolaryngol 61(3):199–205

Siegert R (2010) Combined reconstruction of congenital auricular atresia and severe microtia. Adv Otorhinolaryngol 68:95–107

Siegert R, Weerda H, Mayer T et al (1996) Hochauflösende Computertomographie fehlgebildeter Mittelohren. Laryngo-Rhino-Otologie 75(4):187–194

Simeonsson RJ, Carlson D, Huntington GS et al (2001) Students with disabilities: a national survey of participation in school activities. Disabil Rehabil 23(2):49–63

Sismanis A (2011) Pulsatile tinnitus: contemporary assessment and management. Curr Opin Otolaryngol Head Neck Surg 19(5):348–357

Smits C, Goverts ST, Festen JM (2013) The digits-in-noise test: assessing auditory speech recognition abilities in noise. J Acoust Soc Am 133(3):1693–1706

Smoorenburg GF, Willeboer C, van Dijk JE (2002) Speech perception in Nucleus CI24M cochlear implant users with processor settings based on electrically evoked compound action potential thresholds. Audiol Neurootol 7(6):335–347

Snell ME (2002) Severe and multiple disabilities, education of individuals with multiple disabilities—definition and types of severe and multiple disabilities. http://www.encyclopedia.com/doc/1G2-3403200553.html. Accessed 13 Sept 2016

Snoeckx RL, Huygen PL, Feldmann D et al (2005) GJB2 mutations and degree of hearing loss: a multicenter study. Am J Hum Genet 77(6):945–957

Sobe T, Erlich P, Berry A et al (1999) Letter to the editor. High frequency of the deafness-associated 167delT mutation in the connexin 26 (GJB2) gene in Israeli Ashkenazim. Am J Med Genet 86(5):499–500

Soetens O, Vauloup-Fellous C, Foulon I et al (2008) Evaluation of different cytomegalovirus (CMV) DNA PCR protocols for analysis of dried blood spots from consecutive cases of neonates with congenital CMV infections. J Clin Microbiol 46(3):943–946

Spearman C (1904) "General intelligence," objectively determined and measured. Am J Psychol 15(2):201–209

Spencer PE, Meadow-Orlans KP (1996) Play, language, and maternal responsiveness: a longitudinal study of deaf and hearing infants. Child Dev 67(6):3176–3191

Spencer LJ, Barker BA, Tomblin JB (2003) Exploring the language and literacy. Outcomes of pediatric cochlear implant users. Ear Hear 24(3):236–247

Squires N, Ollo C, Jordan R (1986) Auditory brain stem responses in the mentally retarded: audiometric correlates. Ear Hear 7(2):83–92

Stapells D (2002) Cortical event-related potentials to auditory stimuli. In: Katz J (ed) Handbook of clinical audiology. Lippincott Williams & Wilkins, Philadelphia

Stapells DR (2011) Frequency-specific threshold assessment in young infants using the transient ABR and the brainstem ASSR. In: Seewald RC, Trahpe AM (eds) Comprehensive handbook of pediatric audiology. Plural Publishing, San Diego, pp 409–448

Stapells D, Oates P (1997) Estimation of the pure-tone audiogram by the auditory brainstem response: a review. Audiol Neurootol 2(5):257–280

Stavroulaki P, Apostolopoulos N, Segas J et al (2001) Evoked otoacoustic emissions—an approach for monitoring cisplatin induced ototoxicity in children. Int J Pediatr Otorhinolaryngol 59(1):47–57

Steindl R, Kunz K, Schrott-Fischer A et al (2006) Effect of age and sex on maturation of sensory systems and balance control. Dev Med Child Neurol 48(6):477–482

Stinson MS, Liu Y (1999) Participation of deaf and hard-of-hearing students in classes with hearing students. J Deaf Stud Deaf Educ 4(3):191–202

Stredler-Brown A, Abraham H (2002) Colorado Home Intervention Program (CHIP) Manual. The Keystone Project. Colorado School for the Deaf and Blind, Colorado

Stuart A, Stenstromb R, Tompkins C et al (1991) Test-retest variability in audiometric threshold with supraaural and insert earphones among children and adults. Audiology 30(2):82–90

Studebaker GA (1967) Intertest variability and the air-bone gap. J Speech Hear Disord 32(1):82–86

Stürzebecher E, Cebulla M, Elberling C et al (2006) New efficient stimuli for evoking frequency-specific auditory steady-state responses. J Am Acad Audiol 17(6):448–461

Swartz JD, Harnsberger HR (1997) Imaging of the temporal bone, 3rd edn. Thieme, New York

Tait M, Nikolopoulos TP, De Raeve L et al (2010) Bilateral versus unilateral cochlear implantation in young children. Int J Pediatr Otorhinolaryngol 74(2):206–211

Teoh AP, Chin SB (2007) Phonetic transcriptions of children with cochlear implants. Poster presented at the 11th International Conference on Cochlear Implants in Children. Charlotte, North Carolina, 11–14 June 2007

Thomsen KA (1955) The Metz recruitment test and a comparison with the Fowler method. Acta Otolaryngol 45(6):544–552

Tlumak AI, Rubinstein E, Durrant JD (2007) Meta-analysis of variables that affect accuracy of threshold estimation via measurement of the auditory steady-state response (ASSR). Int J Audiol 46(11):692–710

Tlumak AI, Durrant JD, Delgado RE et al (2012) Steady-state analysis of auditory evoked potentials over a wide range of stimulus repetition rates: profile in children vs. adults. Int J Audiol 51(6):480–490

Traxler CB (2000) The Stanford Achievement Test, 9th Edition: national norming and performance standards for deaf and hard-of-hearing students. J Deaf Stud Deaf Educ 5(43):337–348

Ulrich ME, Bauer AM (2003) Levels of awareness: a closer look at communication between parents and professionals. Teach Except Child 35(6):20–24

UN General Assembly (2007) Convention on the rights of persons with disabilities. http://www.refworld.org/docid/45f973632.html. Accessed 13 Sept 2016

United States Congress (USC) (2004) Individuals with Disabilities Education Act, 20

Valente LM (2007) Maturational effects of the vestibular system: a study of rotary chair, computerized dynamic posturography, and vestibular evoked potentials with children. J Am Acad Audiol 18(6):461–481

Valente L (2011) Assessment techniques for vestibular evaluation in pediatric patients. Otolaryngol Clin N Am 44(2):273–290

Van Hecke V, Mundy P (2007) Neural systems and the development of gaze following and related joint attention skills. In: Flom R et al (eds) Gaze-following: its development and significance. Lawrence Erlbaum Associates, Mahwah, NJ, pp 17–51

Van Lierde KM, Vinck BM, Baudonck N et al (2005) Comparison of the overall intelligibility, articulation, resonance, and voice characteristics between children using cochlear implants and those using bilateral hearing aids: a pilot study. Int J Audiol 44(8):452–465

Van Maanen A, Stapells DR (2010) Multiple-ASSR thresholds in infants and young children with hearing loss. J Am Acad Audiol 21(8):535–545

Van Schrojenstein Lantman-de Valk HJM, Havemann MJ, Maaskant MA et al (1994) The need for assessment of sensory functioning in ageing people with mental handicap. J Intellect Disabil Res 38(Pt 3):289–298

Vermeulen AM, van Bon W, Schreuder R et al (2007) Reading comprehension of deaf children with cochlear implants. J Deaf Stud Deaf Educ 12(3):283302

Wagner R, Torgesen J, Rashotte C et al (1999) Comprehensive test of phonological processing. ProEd Publishing Co, Austin, TX

Wakil N, Fitzpatrick EM, Olds J et al (2014) Long-term outcome after cochlear implantation in children with additional developmental disabilities. Int J Audiol 53(9):587–594

Walger M, Mühler R, Hoth S (2014) In: Hoth S et al (eds) Objektive Audiometrie im Kindesalter. Springer, Berlin, pp 140–157

Waltzman SB, Scalchunes V, Cohen NL (2000) Performance of multiply handicapped children using cochlear implants. Am J Otol 21(3):329–335

Wang S, Yeh T, Chang C et al (2008) Consistent latencies of vestibular evoked myogenic potentials. Ear Hear 29(6):923–929

Watson CS, Kidd GR (2009) Associations between auditory abilities, reading, and other language skills in children and adults. In: Cacace AT, McFarland DJ (eds) Controversies in central auditory processing disorders. Plural Publishing, San Diego, pp 217–242

Weerda H (2004) Chirurgie der Ohrmuschel. Verletzungen, Defekte und Anomalien. Thieme, Stuttgart, pp 105–226

Wegner O, Dau T (2002) Frequency specificity of chirp-evoked auditory brainstem responses. J Acoust Soc Am 111(3):1318–1329

Weisi F, Rezaei M, Rashedi V et al (2013) Comparison of reading skills between children with cochlear implants and children with typical hearing in Iran. Int J Pediatr Otorhinolaryngol 77(8):1317–1321

Wiig EH, Semel E, Secord WA (2013) Clinical evaluation of language fundamentals–Fifth Edition (CELF-5). Pearson, Ontario

Wilber LA (2002) Calibration: puretone, speech, and noise signals. In: Katz J (ed) Handbook of clinical audiology, 5th edn. Lippincott Williams & Wilkins, Philadelphia, pp 50–68

Wiley S, Arjmand E, Meinzen-Derr J et al (2011) Findings from multidisciplinary evaluation of children with permanent hearing loss. Int J Pediatr Otorhinolaryngol 75(8):1040–1044

Williams KT (2007) Expressive vocabulary test, 2nd edn. http://images.pearsonclinical.com/images/Products/EVT-II/evt2.pdf. Accessed 4 June 2017

Wilson WJ, Arnott W (2013) Using different criteria to diagnose (central) auditory processing disorder: how big a difference does it make? J Speech Lang Hear Res 56(1):63–70

Wilson PH, Henry J, Bowen M et al (1991) Tinnitus reaction questionnaire: psychometric properties of a measure of distress associated with tinnitus. J Speech Hear Res 34(1):197–201

Woodcock RW (1987) Woodcock reading mastery test. Teaching Resources. Revised edition. American Guidance Services, Circle Pines, Allen, TX

World Health Organization (1992) International statistical classification of diseases and related health problems, 10th Revision (ICD-10). WHO, Geneva

World Health Organization (2001) International classification of functioning, disability and health (ICF). WHO, Geneva

World Health Organization (2007) International classification of functioning, disability and health—children and youth. WHO, Geneva

World Health Organization (2013) WHO methods and data sources for global burden of disease estimates 2000–2011. WHO, Geneva. http://www.who.int/healthinfo/statistics/GlobalDALYmethods_2000_2011.pdf. Accessed 4 Jan 2017

Wu CM, Lee LA, Chen CK et al (2015) Impact of cochlear nerve deficiency determined using 3-dimensional magnetic resonance imaging on hearing outcome in children with cochlear implants. Otol Neurotol 36(1):14–21

Yanbay E, Hickson L, Scarinci N et al (2014) Language outcomes for children with cochlear implants enrolled in different communication programs. Cochlear Implants Int 15(3):121–135

Yang T, Wei X, Chai Y et al (2013) Genetic etiology study of the non-syndromic deafness in Chinese Hans by targeted next-generation sequencing. Orphanet J Rare Dis 8:85

Yoshinaga-Itano C (2003) From screening to early identification and intervention: discovering predictors to successful outcomes for children with significant hearing loss. J Deaf Stud Deaf Educ 8(1):11–30

Yoshinaga-Itano C, Sedey A (2000) Early speech development in children who are deaf or hard of hearing: interrelationships with language and hearing. Volta Rev 100(5):181–211

Ziegler JC, Pech-Georgel C, George F et al (2005) Deficits in speech perception predict language learning impairment. Proc Natl Acad Sci U S A 102(39):14110–14115. https://doi.org/10.1073/pnas.0504446102

Ziegler JC, Pech-Georgel C, George F et al (2009) Speech-perception-in-noise deficits in dyslexia. Dev Sci 12(5):732–745. https://doi.org/10.1111/j.1467-7687.2009.00817.x

Zigmond AS, Snaith RP (1983) The hospital anxiety and depression scale. Acta Psychiatr Scand 67(6):361–370

Zimmerman IL, Steiner VG, Pond E (2011) Preschool Language Scales–Fifth Edition (PLS-5). Pearson Assessments, San Antonio

Prevention of Disorders of Hearing Development

17

Antoinette am Zehnhoff-Dinnesen, Hanno J. Bolz, Gwen Carr, Manfred Gross[†], Ross Parfitt, Simona Poisson-Markova, Debbie Rix, Pavel Seeman, Eva Seemanova, and Monika Tigges

17.1 Universal Newborn Hearing Screening

Manfred Gross

17.1.1 Risk Screening and Universal Newborn Hearing Screening (UNHS)

Although there is no experimental proof from a randomised prospective study that hearing loss leads to major developmental problems, there is enough empirical evidence that language abilities and intellectual, social and emotional development largely depend on normal hearing in early childhood. Owing to a prevalence of 1–3 children in 1000 newborns in developed countries and up to a rate of 1% in low- and middle-income countries, permanent hearing loss has been a major issue in all health systems worldwide. It also has become clear that there is only a small time window in the first months of life where synaptic connections of the hearing system, as the basis of a well-organised hearing system, may grow. This synaptic sprouting is dependent on a sensory stimulation. Downs and Yoshinaga-Itano (1999) found

[†] Deceased

A. am Zehnhoff-Dinnesen · R. Parfitt
Clinic of Phoniatrics and Pedaudiology, University Hospital Münster, Münster, Germany
e-mail: am.zehnhoff@uni-muenster.de;
ross.parfitt@ukmuenster.de

H. J. Bolz
Senckenberg Centre for Human Genetics, Frankfurt am Main, Germany
e-mail: h.bolz@senckenberg-humangenetik.de

G. Carr
UCL Ear Institute, University College London, London, UK
e-mail: gwencarr@ehdiprofessional.com

M. Gross
Department of Audiology and Phoniatrics, Campus Virchow-Klinikum, Berlin, Germany
e-mail: Manfred.gross@charite.de

S. Poisson-Markova · P. Seeman · E. Seemanova
Department of Child Neurology, 2nd Medical School of Charles University Prague, Prague, Czech Republic
e-mail: s.markova@lfmotol.cuni.cz;
Pavel.seeman@lfmotol.cuni.cz;
Eva.seemanova@lfmotol.cuni.cz

D. Rix
Wandsworth Hearing Support Service, Linden Lodge School, London, UK
e-mail: rix@wandsworthhis.org.uk

M. Tigges
Städt. Klinikum Karlsruhe GmbH, ENT Clinic, Phoniatrics and Pedaudiology, Karlsruhe, Germany
e-mail: monika.tigges@klinikum-karlsruhe.de

© Springer-Verlag GmbH Germany, part of Springer Nature 2020
A. am Zehnhoff-Dinnesen et al. (eds.), *Phoniatrics I*, European Manual of Medicine,
https://doi.org/10.1007/978-3-662-46780-0_17

that normal cognitive development may be realised only if hearing loss, irrespective of its grade, is diagnosed in the first 6 months of life.

As with other diseases, there are three categories of prevention. Primary prevention of hearing loss can be realised by, e.g. immunisation against rubella, in low-income countries by vitamin- and mineral-enriched food (Schmitz et al. 2010), by ototoxic drug administration under serum level control, by counselling for family planning in families with inherited hearing loss, etc. (Smith and Bale Jr 2005).

Secondary prevention is intended to stop or slow down the progress of hearing loss in its earliest stage, with the aim of limiting its consecutive disabilities. In order to identify children with hearing loss, risk screening was performed in many countries until the 1990s. This meant clinicians checking whether there were anamnestic hints for potentially pathogenic constellations resulting in childhood hearing loss, e.g. genetic hearing loss in the family, rubella infection during pregnancy, asphyxia during delivery, etc. If so, these children underwent a complete clinical examination of the hearing abilities. This methodology of risk screening was very expensive and insufficient because a rather high percentage (more than 30%) of the newborns with hearing loss was not identified. Simultaneously a new method for hearing examination was developed, otoacoustic emissions. This was an objective, easy-to-realise examination with high sensitivity and specificity that could be applied in sleeping newborns and that usually did not last more than 5–10 min. Since then the measurement of transitory-evoked otoacoustic emissions (TEOAE) became a preferred procedure for hearing screening, which allowed checking hearing, including the outer, middle and inner ear. As soon as the algorithms for the measurement of auditory brainstem responses became more sophisticated, it was possible to automate this procedure (AABR) and reduce the needed time. In contrast to the risk screening, screening with otoacoustic emissions and AABR must be performed universally, in all newborns without any exception.

17.1.2 Effectiveness

Granell et al. (2008) found a statistically significant difference in the percentage passing in the first step, favouring ABR over OAE (99.7% vs 91.8%; $p < 0.0005$). Cost evaluation indicates a decreasing difference between both methods. Wolff et al. (2010) found in a systematic review widely varying results from 0.5 to 1.0 for sensitivity and from 0.49 to 0.97 for specificity of OAE compared with AABR; owing to improved technology, the sensitivity and specificity have grown continuously to values of more than 96–98% (Morton and Nance 2006), but compared with biochemical screening, these results are still of less sensitivity and specificity. The personnel who perform the neonatal screening do not need to be audiologists or physicians (Yee-Arellano et al. 2006). Tranebaerg (2008) reported that after the implementation of UNHS, the average age of identification of moderate-profound hearing loss decreased to 1–3 months of age.

Colgan et al. (2012) reviewed the literature for distinct observational or modelled evaluations of effectiveness. They found only two publications that clearly compared universal newborn hearing screening with risk factor screening for bilateral permanent congenital hearing impairment. Of these one examined the long-term costs and outcomes and concluded that universal newborn hearing screening could be "cost-saving if early intervention led to a substantial reduction in future treatment costs and productivity losses" (Grosse and Ross 2006).

Universal newborn hearing screening seemed to be the solution because in many countries delivery is mostly hospital-based, and therefore under these circumstances, a high capture rate is possible. In other countries without hospital-based delivery, the first contact with healthcare providers, e.g. for immunisation, is used to perform a hearing screening.

In a cohort of children with very low birth weight, Cristobal and Oghalai (2008) found a substantially higher rate of permanent hearing loss, including progressive and late-onset hearing loss. They recommend performing not only otoacoustic emissions but also AABR.

17.1.3 Screening Principles and Methods

Wilkinson and Jiang (2006) pointed out that ABR is the objective method that enables detection of early brain damage, delayed neural conduction in the central nervous system, neurological abnormalities and hearing loss. ABR may be recorded as early as week 26 of gestational age and can be used thereafter rapidly. Seven waves can usually be identified, representing different anatomical structures (I and II represent the extra- and intracranial portion of N VIII, wave III is generated in the cochlear nucleus, wave IV is generated in the superior olivary complex, wave V is derived from the lateral lemniscus and the inferior colliculus). Waves VI and VII are also thought to originate from the inferior colliculus. In normal-hearing children, ABRs demonstrate rapid maturational changes in the first 2 years of age, and thereafter results become similar to those of adults. The most prominent waves are waves I, III and V (Wilkinson and Jiang 2006). The Joint Committee on Infant Hearing (1995) recommended ABR for several risk factors such as "family history of hearing loss, in utero infections, craniofacial anomalies, birth weight <1500 g, severe hyperbilirubinaemia, ototoxic medications, bacterial meningitis, perinatal asphyxia, mechanical ventilation for more than five days and stigmata suggestive of a syndrome associated with hearing loss". The Joint Committee on Infant Hearing (2000) defined in its position statement craniofacial anomalies, including abnormalities of the pinna and ear canal, family history of hereditary childhood sensorineural hearing loss, neonatal intensive care unit admission for more than 2 days, rubella or other foetal infection (e.g. herpes, *Cytomegalovirus*) and syndromes associated with hearing loss (e.g. Usher's syndrome, Waardenburg's syndrome) as risk factors for childhood hearing loss. According to that recommendation, ABR is still the preferred method in these patients. The prevalence of hearing loss in newborns with specific risk factors is up to 20 times higher than in the general newborn population. The US Preventive Services Task Force (2008) identified the following risk factors to be associated with permanent bilateral congenital hearing loss: NICU admission for ≥2 days, family history of hereditary childhood sensorineural hearing loss, craniofacial abnormalities, certain congenital syndromes and infections.

In many countries a two-step procedure is recommended. The first step usually is performed in the maternity hospital. In case the newborn does not pass this test or an immediate repetition of the screening test, a second test is recommended within the following 4 weeks by means of AABR (De Barros Boishardy et al. 2005; Gross 2005; Martini et al. 2013; Neumann et al. 2009; Olusanya et al. 2008; Prpić et al. 2007; Vos et al. 2013; Weichbold et al. 2006 and many others). If the newborn does not pass the second test again, a confirmation test will be performed in order to find out the exact hearing threshold. Depending on the result, hearing loss can be excluded or confirmed. A therapy of any hearing loss should be started immediately after a positive confirmation test.

According to Morton and Nance, a second prerequisite had been met when Yoshinaga-Itano et al. (1998) demonstrated that the early identification of children with hearing loss improves cognitive development dramatically.

Choo and Meinzen-Derr (2010) assumed that the most birthing facilities worldwide implemented otoacoustic emissions and automated auditory brainstem response (AABR). The advantages and disadvantages of these methods are described in Table 17.1.

In order to reduce the false-positive rate because of middle ear fluid or vernix, the combination of OAE and AABR with the measurement of wideband reflectance had been recommended.

17.1.4 Limitations of the UNHS and Dealing with Screening Failures

As long as there is no governmental regulation of UNHS, it is hard to cover a large percentage of newborns (Kaye 2006).

The test failure rate ranges from 2 to 4% and is dependent on the training of the personnel

Table 17.1 Comparison of OAE and ABR newborn hearing screening technologies (Choo and Meinzen-Derr 2010)

	(Automated) transitory-evoked otoacoustic emissions testing	Automated auditory brainstem response testing
Advantages	Simple testing technique (relatively minimal training needed to perform OAE testing)	Superior evaluation of the auditory system (vs assessment of outer hair cell function alone as in OAE)
	Cheaper than AABR screening	Likely provides better detection of infants with auditory neuropathy
	Fast	
Disadvantages	Limited assessment of the auditory system	Requires more operator knowledge than OAE testing
	Impacted by middle ear fluid issues	Potential for electrical and noise artefact yielding poor screening
	Potentially impacted by vernix or wax in the ear canal	Requires sleeping or quiet infant
	Optimal to perform in a quiet environment	Optimally performed in a quiet environment
		Requires longer times than OAE screening
		Typically more costly than OAE screening

With kind permission from Wolters Kluwer Health, Inc.

conducting the UNHS (Morton and Nance 2006). Thus the extraordinarily low failure rates of metabolic screening procedures cannot be met.

Permanent hearing loss is defined as hearing loss of more than 40 dB in the UK and of more than 35 dB in the USA (Morton and Nance 2006). Consequently, in many countries, UNHS is limited to hearing loss of more than 35 or 40 dB. For this reason mild hearing loss is not taken into consideration although its negative implications are well known. Although more than 90% of the newborns are screened in the USA, mild bilateral hearing loss and unilateral hearing loss (UHL) are still a problem because they seem to be under-identified (Ross et al. 2008). The authors concluded that the newborn prevalence of UHL was 0.35/1000 newborns and 0.16/1000 for mild bilateral hearing loss. In contrast Choo and Meinzen-Derr (2010) advanced the opinion that the sensitivity and specificity of OAE and AABR are effective enough.

Some cases of early-onset hearing loss are not apparent at birth. There is no alternative to UNHS performed with otoacoustic emissions and AABR, but improvement is necessary in order to identify prelingual hearing loss, which is not apparent shortly after birth because many of the parents trust in the results of UNHS and do not react adequately when language acquisition is delayed. Morton and Nance (2006) recommend

combining the UNHS with tests on blood samples which had been collected on Guthrie cards. GJB2 deafness, the mitochondrial A1555G mutation (showing aminoglycoside-induced hearing loss) and SLC26A4 (associated with Pendred syndrome), as well as a test for the presence of *Cytomegalovirus* infection, should additionally be performed, in order to identify delayed-onset prelingual hearing loss (Morton and Nance 2006). Choo and Meinzen-Derr (2010) also argue that almost 1% of the newborns are infected with *Cytomegalovirus*. Tranebaerg (2008) recommends an early aetiological examination for persons without known aetiology, including the examination of the parents, a three-generation pedigree, a temporal bone imaging, a physical examination from top to toe and a genetic screening for a GJB2 mutation.

In case a newborn does not pass the OAE screening, there are several technical possibilities why the examination failed:

- Ear probe blocked
- Outer ear canal blocked by debris, amniotic fluid or cerumen
- Ear probe positioned against the outer ear canal
- Ear probe too small
- Child is not quiet
- Too loud an environment

An ideal precondition for AABR is that the child:

- Is full and sleeping (very tired)
- Has no cream applied to its face
- Does not sweat

In case a newborn fails AABR, there are also several procedural reasons:

- Environment or the child is too loud
- Myogenic artefacts (child is fretful)
- Impedance at the electrodes is too high
- External electronic emission
- Position of the headphone (out of place)

Another problem of the newborn hearing screening protocols is the under-identification of auditory neuropathy/dyssynchrony disorders (ANDD). Usually newborns with ANDD pass the OAE screening because the OAE signals are robust. In order to diagnose ANDD reliably, a newborn hearing screening protocol that includes both OAE and AABR is needed. However, most of the protocols implement a two-step protocol starting with the cheaper and faster OAE, followed by AABR when the newborn does not pass the OAE examination (Choo and Meinzen-Derr 2010).

From the high frequency of viral and genetic aetiologies, it may be foreseen that future hearing screening protocols will develop in this direction.

17.1.5 Setting Up a Screening Programme

Setting up a screening programme in a district means:

- To motivate the birthing centres to perform UNHS.
- To build up a tracking centre. The aim of a tracking centre is to follow every newborn until normal hearing is proved or until the hearing-impaired baby has started a specific phoniatric-(ped)audiologic therapy.

- To motivate ENT specialists to perform a second screening test in those babies who failed the first one or who did not participate in a screening test in the birthing centre.
- To motivate specialists in phoniatrics and pedaudiology to perform confirmatory diagnostics.
- To monitor and audit the screening programme.

17.1.6 Early Hearing Detection and Intervention Programmes

It is reasonable to combine early hearing detection with an intervention programme (e.g. ASHA: Early Hearing Detection and Intervention (EHDI) 2016) and early aetiological investigations because there are some aetiologies that are characterised by progressive hearing loss or crucial associated anomalies.

17.1.7 Management of Control Intervals/Screenings for Late-Onset Hearing Loss

Control intervals should be kept as short as possible. In general diagnostics of hearing loss and hearing aid fitting should be completed within the first 3–6 months of age. It is the main activity of the tracking centres to motivate the parents to attend the screening tests even when the parents are convinced that their child is able to hear correctly.

Barreira-Nielsen et al. (2016) found in 47.9% of 330 hearing-impaired children (251 exposed to NHS) progression of hearing loss and recommend close audiological monitoring after early hearing loss detection.

Holzinger et al. (2016) collected data from a complete sample of hearing-impaired school-aged children born in 1997–2001 in the Austrian federal state Carinthia. 85.2% of them had undergone NHS and 50% of those had passed this early screening. The observed rate of hearing impairment was twice the rate detected in newborns.

Skarżyński and Piotrowska (2012) presented the European Consensus Statement on Hearing Screening of Pre-School and School-Age Children to develop hearing screening programmes for these age groups.

Louw et al. (2017) successfully tested smartphone-based hearing screening at primary healthcare clinics in South Africa even in 3-year-old children.

17.1.8 Early Aetiological Investigations

To know the aetiology of permanent childhood hearing loss will disburden many mothers who are threatened by self-doubt because they fear to have caused the hearing loss by some misconduct during pregnancy. It is also important to know the aetiology in the context of family planning, the prognosis of the hearing loss as well as the prognosis of associated anomalies in syndromic hearing loss. Principally the aetiology of hearing loss is divided into pre-, peri- and post-natally acquired and into syndromic and non-syndromic genetic hearing loss. The most important pre- and peri-natal aetiologies are listed according to their frequency in the "year 2000 position statement: principles and guidelines for early hearing detection and intervention programs" (Joint Committee on Infant Hearing 2000). CMV infections have gained importance during recent years, and new therapy programmes promise to reduce CMV-related hearing loss (Gandhi et al. 2010; de Vries et al. 2011). Because we find ourselves in a phase of extremely fast developments in genetic diagnostics, it is foreseeable that in the coming years we can expect an increasingly complete genetic diagnosis and, derived from that, new therapy options. Until then it is recommended to repeat aetiological investigations at the age of 3–6 years, at the age of 9–12 years and in early adulthood because, especially in syndromic hearing loss, many signs and symptoms that had not been present before become obvious with increasing age (e.g. retinitis pigmentosa in Usher's syndrome).

17.1.9 Role of Immunisation

Vaccination is an important way to prevent hearing loss. The aim of national and international vaccination programmes is to reduce the rate of foetal infections such as rubella. The most important infections are summarised under the acronym TORCH which stands for:

- T = Toxoplasmosis
- O = Others
- R = Rubella
- C = *Cytomegalovirus*
- H = Herpes

For some authors the acronym is extended to STORCH where S stands for syphilis. The prevalence of this sexually transmissible disease is growing again mainly in eastern European countries after many years of reduced morbidity. In most of the European nations, comprehensive vaccination programmes have been introduced, and prenatal care is an essential healthcare issue as well. However, in some countries without compulsory vaccination, it has become fashionable to forgo vaccinations. There are also significant differences in the prevalence of these diseases. For example, toxoplasmosis, which appears much more frequently in Belgium, is a matter of prenatal care. Reviewing five studies about toxoplasmosis and hearing loss, Brown et al. (2009) pointed out a prevalence of toxoplasmosis-associated hearing loss from 0 to 26%. In utero toxoplasmosis infection may lead to delayed-onset or progressive hearing loss and therefore can be overlooked in UNHS. When an antiparasitic therapy was started before 2.5 months of age and continued for 12 months, no children (0%) developed hearing loss. The authors stressed that it seemed to be important that the compliance with the treatment needs to be monitored.

Without any doubt *Cytomegalovirus* infections are underdiagnosed dramatically in childhood hearing loss. *Cytomegalovirus* infections are the most common infections in newborns (Gandhi et al. 2010). According to de Vries et al. (2011), 7 out of 1000 newborns are infected, and 85–90% of these are without any symptoms.

17.1.10 How to Communicate the Results of UNHS

It is important to communicate the test results to the parents in adequate terms. It is not helpful to use terms such as fail, suspicious, etc. These terms may induce adverse reactions because in such a situation many of the parents are highly irritated, depressed and agitated. Often they do not accept having to wait a few days for a further examination. Parental anxiety is natural and can be expected when their children fail hearing screening, but may be reduced if counselling is done by skilled and empathetic professionals (Low et al. 2005) using terms indicating that the results are insecure as long as there are no distinct results that exclude a hearing loss or that confirm it in detail. In the Anglo-Saxon language area, the euphemism "refer" has been adopted to indicate a failed screening test.

17.2 Programmes for Enhancing Parental Communication Skills

Debbie Rix and Gwen Carr

17.2.1 Introduction

Newborn hearing screening is now the accepted standard of care in many countries and is being increasingly adopted in others. The advantages of early identification and advances in technology enable children with hearing loss to develop language and communication at a similar rate to that of hearing peers. The meaningful and effective involvement of parents and family, however, has been shown to be the single most effective predictor of a newly identified child's success (Yoshinaga-Itano 2000), and late engagement and limited family involvement have been shown to be associated with significant developmental delay in children's language skills (Moeller 2000; DesJardin 2006).

For this reason, much attention has been directed towards the development of family-centred service delivery in early intervention for children with hearing loss. An international consensus statement on Best Practices in Family-Centred Early Intervention with Deaf and Hard of Hearing Children (Moeller et al. 2013) detailed ten research and evidence-based key principles supporting positive outcomes for children with hearing loss. In addition to principles relating to the broader context of early support, specific early intervention provider behaviours are highlighted in relation to parent-infant interaction and progress monitoring that underpin all approaches to promoting language and communication development.

The emotional impact of diagnosis leaves many parents of deaf children feeling underskilled. This has a significant impact on the parents' capacity to interact with their child naturally and to partner confidently with professionals (Beazley and Moore 1995). In recent times, family-centred services have sought to develop parents' communication skills in order to:

- Promote their child's language and communication.
- Partner effectively with professionals and develop self-advocacy skills.

17.2.2 Examples of Enabling Parents to Promote Their Child's Language

Following diagnosis, the teacher of the deaf or speech and language pathologist will support the parents in understanding their child's communication and language needs and how these may be met. Ongoing assessment and monitoring of the child's developing communication skills is undertaken in partnership with parents/caregivers. The practitioner and parent then agree on short-term goals for the deaf child, and the professional coaches the parent on how to build maximum opportunities for language growth within typical daily routines.

The specialist input also includes regular training on features of communication that most enhance deaf children's understanding and expression (Janjua et al. 2002) (see Fig. 17.1). Such features include:

- Establishing eye contact and eye gaze
- Promoting turn taking
- Following the child's lead in conversation
- Enabling language rather than correcting
- Being emotionally attuned in terms of facial expression (see Fig. 17.2)
- Providing pauses to enable the child to process

Two of the most widely used formal approaches to supporting parents to develop spoken language in their deaf and hard-of-hearing children are:

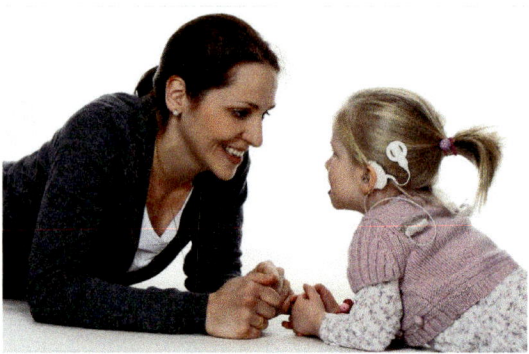

Fig. 17.1 Positive interaction between parent and child demonstrating the essential eye contact. The child is wearing a cochlear implant. Photo with kind permission of the parents

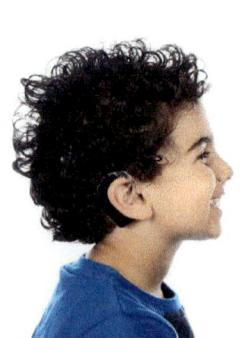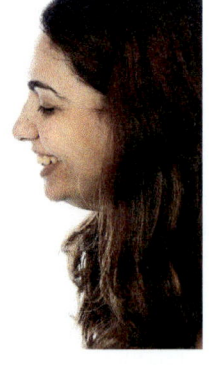

Fig. 17.2 Emotionally attuned facial expressions in parent and child. The child is wearing a cochlear implant. Photo provided with kind permission of the parents

- The Hanen Parent Education Programme, in which:

  the parent is encouraged to enhance the quality of interaction in spontaneously occurring events using a number of techniques (Baxendale and Hesketh 2003)

  and which focuses on empowering parents to foster both early language and social communication development.

- Auditory-verbal therapy, an approach to early habilitation, in which:

  caregivers and therapists provide the children with maximal acoustic stimulation to develop listening, speech, and language skills. (Easterbrooks et al. 2000)

17.2.3 Example of Enabling Parents to Partner Effectively with Professionals

A five-session training course has been developed at the authors' centre (Wandsworth Hearing Support Service) to train parents in communicating effectively with professionals. Parents develop skills in assertiveness, understanding models of disability, effective listening and preparing for meetings. One hundred per cent of parents who attend report a significant shift in their ability to advocate for their child. Information on the parent training course can be obtained from info@wandsworthhis.org.uk.

17.3 Stimulation of Language Development

See Part III Sect. 12.2.

17.4 Family Audiometry

Monika Tigges

Family audiometry may be helpful in some cases of a hearing disorder in a child.

If a child has been diagnosed with a hearing disorder, family members (at the minimum siblings and parents) should undergo audiometric examination. As the risk for a sibling to have a hearing disorder is high, i.e. 25% in an autosomal recessive disorder, younger siblings especially may benefit from an early diagnosis to prevent or minimise speech development impairment (White 2004). The aim is to demonstrate any hearing loss that may be present. Additionally, patients with bilateral hearing loss of unknown aetiology more frequently have relatives with undiagnosed mild or unilateral hearing loss, hinting at a genetic background (Tharpe and Sladen 2008).

If the type of hearing impairment is uncertain (e.g. sensorineural or conductive hearing loss, low frequency hearing loss), the audiogram readings of family members can give pointers regarding the nature of the hearing impairment (e.g. time point of manifestation, affected frequency range, progression, degree; see Table 17.2) and thus indicate appropriate methods for the further evaluation (e.g. frequency-specific electrical response audiometry), advice and counselling.

Examples of audiograms showing non-syndromic hearing losses are presented in Fig. 17.3a–f.

Furthermore, the results of audiometric evaluation of several family members may provide useful hints of a genetic disorder (non-syndromic/syndromic hearing disorder) and permit establishment of a family pedigree that will improve the quality of genetic counselling (Kochhar et al. 2007) (see Sect. 17.5). In family members with a hearing disorder, special attention should be paid to morphological changes, i.e. craniofacial abnormalities that might be related to syndromic hearing disorders. On the other hand, if an individual is diagnosed with syndromic hearing loss, family members should be examined for symptoms related to the respective syndrome. Syndromic hearing disorders are described in Sect. 14.11.

17.5 Genetic Counselling

Pavel Seeman, Simona Poisson-Markova, Eva Seemanova and Hanno J. Bolz

The aims of genetic counselling usually include determining the recurrence risk for the offspring of the patient, his parents and other relatives and the estimation of the clinical prognosis. However, defining the patient's needs is a prerequisite for genetic counselling.

The most important requirement for estimating the genetic prognosis of a defect is the identification of its aetiology (Fig. 17.4). Genetic counselling must be non-directive. The genetic counsellor/clinical geneticist should inform the patient and family about the genetic risk, the clinical prognosis and the feasibility of therapy for the defect in question (European Board of Medical Genetics 2010); for further details, see Sects. 3.1, 3.2, 14.10, 14.11 and 18.26.

Because technical possibilities rapidly advance in diagnostics (NGS, preimplantation diagnosis), assisted reproduction- and gene editing-related questions may be addressed by patients who plan to have children. Because hearing loss is treatable by hearing aids and cochlea implantation, prenatal testing is the exception in case of this condition and confined to severe syndromes. The clinical geneticist/genetic counsellor faces the challenge of balancing technical feasibility with ethical concerns.

Table 17.2 Phenotypes of non-syndromic sensorineural hearing loss distinguished by several parameters (Konigsmark and Gorlin 1976; Toriello et al. 2004)

Audiogram shape	Rate of progression	Age of onset	Severity
Downsloping (high-frequency)	Stable	Congenital	Mild
U-shaped (mid-frequency)	Progressive	Early	Moderate
Upsloping (low-frequency)		Late onset	Severe
Residual hearing (measurable frequencies only in low frequencies)			Profound

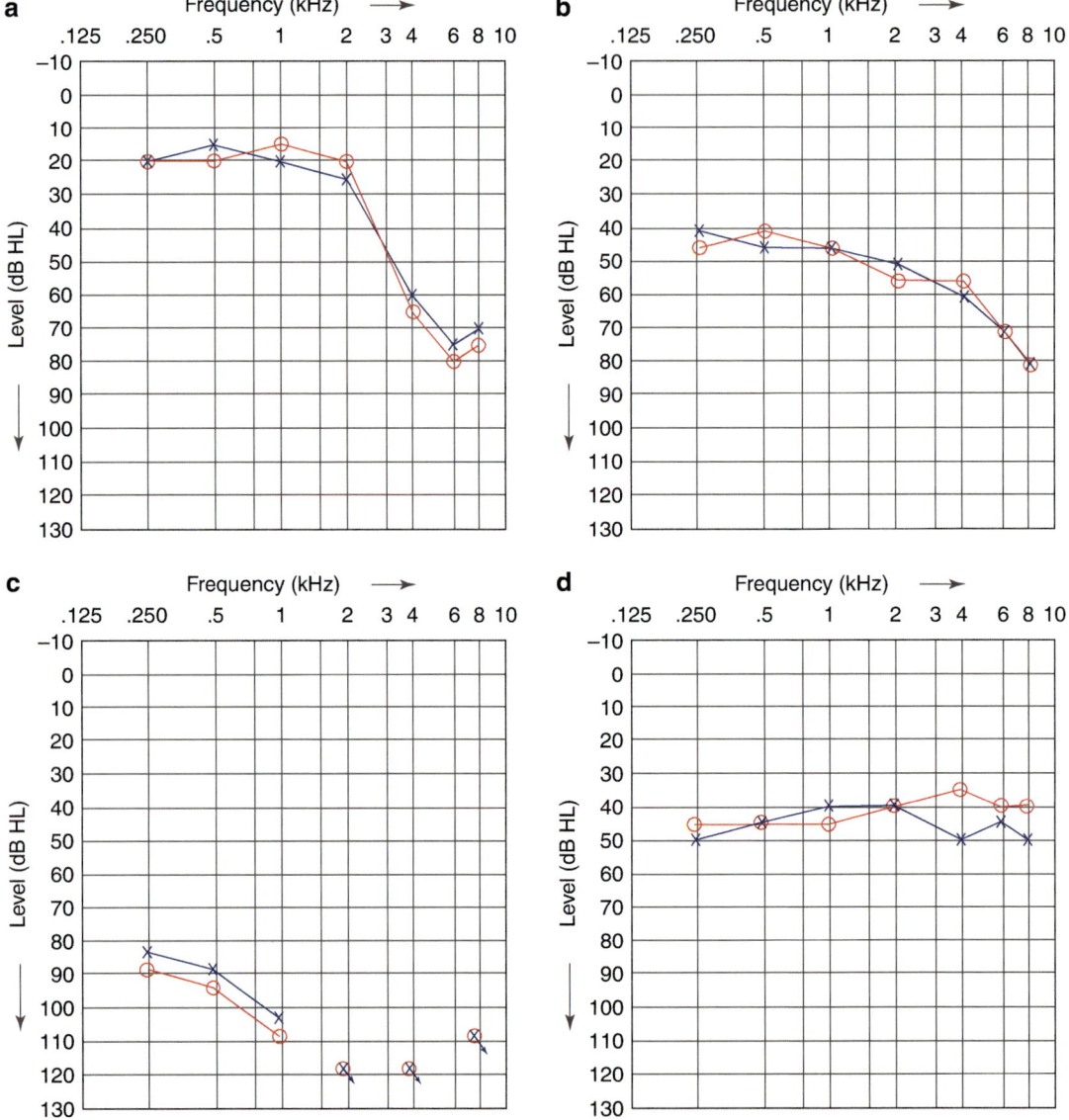

Fig. 17.3 (**a–f**) Examples of audiograms showing non-syndromic hearing losses. (**a**) Sharply downsloping, (**b**) gently downsloping, (**c**) residual, (**d**) flat, (**e**) U-shaped and (**f**) upsloping. All hearing losses shown are sensori-neural, but bone-conduction thresholds have been omitted for clarity of presentation. Audiograms adapted from Liu and Xu (1994), copyright © 1994 by SAGE Publications, Inc. Reprinted by Permission of SAGE Publications, Inc.

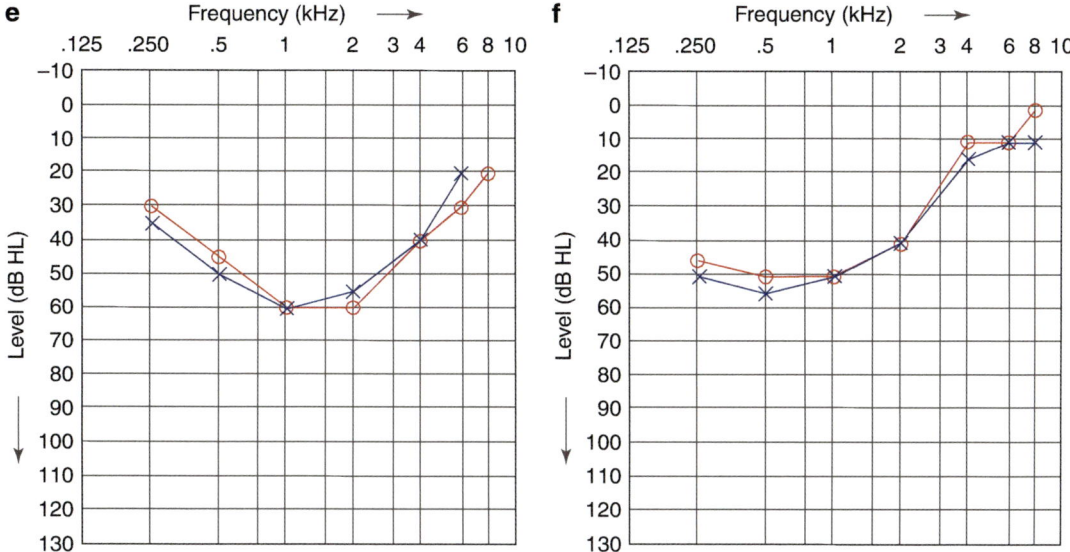

Fig. 17.3 (continued)

17.6 Parental Guidance in Respect of Hearing Conservation

Antoinette am Zehnhoff-Dinnesen and Ross Parfitt

17.6.1 Preventing Head Trauma in Large Endolymphatic Duct and Sac Syndrome

Large endolymphatic duct and sac syndrome (LEDS) is the most common inner ear malformation, with a prevalence of 1.7% in the normal population and 7.2–13.8% in the population of children who are suspected of having an inner ear malformation or are being prepared for cochlea implantation (Bartel-Friedrich et al. 2008a). LEDS may be combined with further inner ear malformations and may occur uni- or bilaterally. Clinically, children show a progressive or fluctuating progressive hearing loss of pre- or peri-lingual onset predominantly affecting the high frequencies or total deafness (Bartel-Friedrich et al. 2008b). Vertigo, dizziness and tinnitus are also possible. Bartel-Friedrich et al.

(2008b) found in progressive cases that episodes of acute hearing loss were not rare and, as with hearing loss progression, happened predominantly in later childhood and adolescence. The authors observed that triggers, such as minimal head trauma or physical exertion when giving birth, could provoke the acute hearing loss.

Important advice for parents and children/adolescents with LEDS is to avoid head trauma, even slight trauma. Variations in intracranial pressure should be prevented. In case of pregnancy, Caesarean section is to be preferred to avoid hearing damage of the mother. Early diagnosis is necessary, including radiological investigations. Parents and children/adolescents should have information about the possible course of the disease (Bartel-Friedrich et al. 2008b).

The National Institute on Deafness and Other Communication Disorders (NIDCD) (2017) recommends:

- Avoiding sports that involve a risk of head injury
- Wearing head protection, e.g. when riding a bicycle or skiing
- Avoiding barotrauma, e.g. from scuba diving
- Not using hyperbaric oxygen treatment

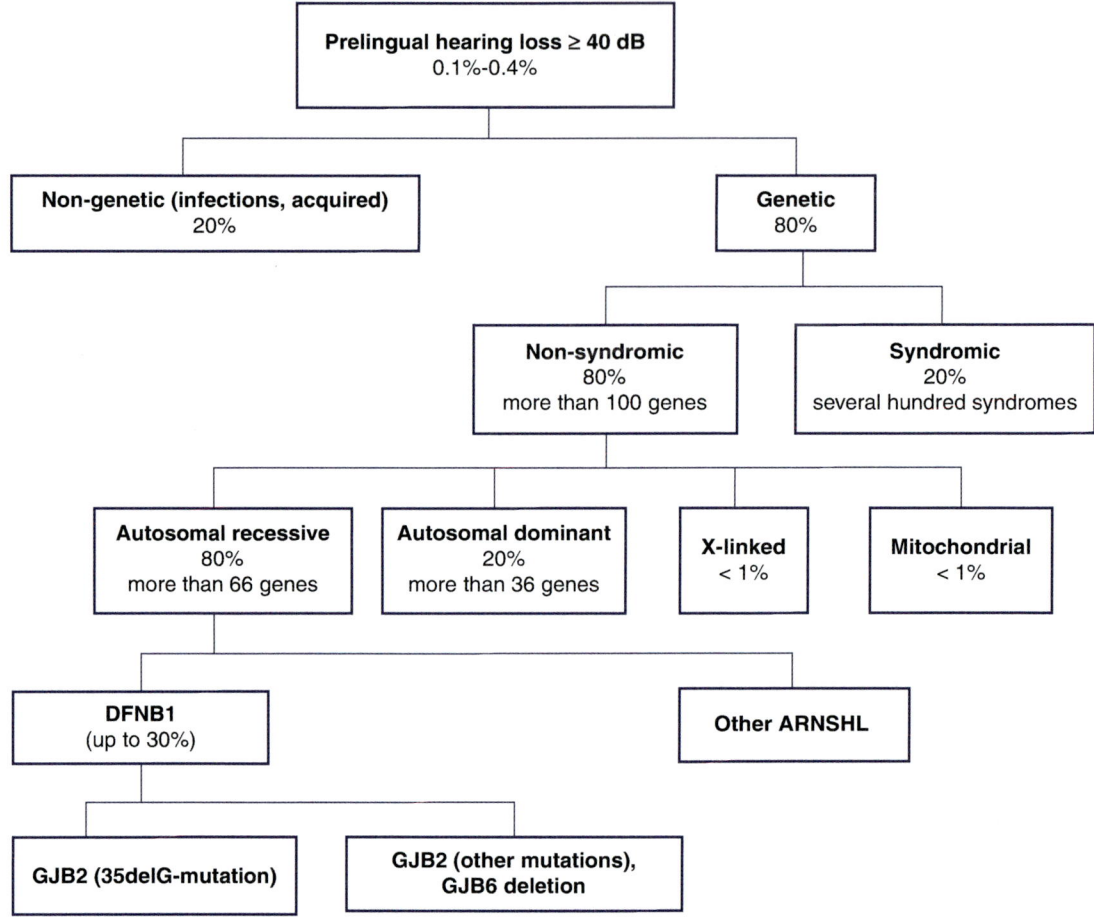

Fig. 17.4 Causes and distribution of prelingual hearing loss modified after Shearer et al. (2017) Gene Reviews https://www.ncbi.nlm.nih.gov/books/NBK1434/. With kind permission from © University of Washington 1993–2017. *DFNB1* deafness type B1, non-syndromic hearing loss and deafness, autosomal recessive, *ARNSHL* autosomal recessive non-syndromic hearing loss, *GJB2* gap junction beta-2 protein, encoding connexin 26, *GJB6* gap junction beta-6 protein, encoding connexin 30

- Using nasal decongestants in case of cold or flu when travelling by air (air travel in commercial aircraft seems to be of low risk)

According to the American Speech-Language-Hearing Association (ASHA), frequent monitoring of hearing is necessary, especially in infants and toddlers, who are not able to offer information about their own perceived change in hearing. Given the unstable constitution of the inner ear in cases of fluctuating and progressive hearing loss,

careful fitting and close monitoring of amplification are recommended (Oyler 2007).

Noordman et al. (2015) found reduced hearing sensitivity in 34% of patients with enlarged vestibular aqueduct (EVA) in a meta-analysis of 179 patients with 351 EVA, documenting a significant association between acute hearing loss after minor head trauma and pre-existing fluctuation of hearing. The authors discuss whether the above-mentioned stringent lifestyle advice should be confined to patients with fluctuating hearing loss or hearing loss after minor head trauma.

17.6.2 Preventing Noise-/Music-Induced Hearing Loss

Noise-induced hearing loss (NIHL) used to be a topic just for professionals in workplaces with high intensities of background sound. The risk of hearing impairment in this group has been reduced through legislation, guidelines and safety factors. These days, however, NIHL is increasingly becoming a serious concern for children and adolescents (Harrison 2012). The prevalence of noise-induced hearing loss is estimated to be 12–15% in school-aged children/adolescents (Harrison 2008), and many researchers attribute this largely to the use of portable music devices, such as MP3 players, and attending music events, such as nightclubs and live amplified concerts.

Manufacturers and distributors of portable listening devices (such as MP3 players) and electronic gaming systems include warnings in their packaging. Despite this, Vogel et al. (2009), who studied music-listening behaviour in 1687 12-to-19-year-olds, revealed that 90% listened to music through earphones on MP3 players, 48% used high-volume settings and only 6.8% used a noise limiter to restrict the maximum sound output levels of the device. They found a correlation between frequent use of MP3 players and risky listening to music at high levels, especially in adolescents in practical prevocational schools. Portnuff et al. (2011), however, found that only 16% of adolescents who used portable listening devices listened at potentially unsafe levels.

Early symptoms of NIHL include tinnitus (ringing in the ears), often associated with music exposure (le Clercq et al. 2016), temporary threshold shifts (often reflected by a sensation of dulled hearing) and decreased sound tolerance/hypersensitivity to sound (Women's and Children's Health Network 2017). The effects of noise exposure are cumulative, with clinical manifestation occurring later. There is a serious risk of permanent hearing impairment from frequent exposure to loud sound (Harrison 2012). Noise can also affect the cardiovascular system and may cause psychological stress and impair cognitive function (Münzel et al. 2014).

In a study by Sekhar et al. (2011), 11th graders had to answer a questionnaire concerning exposure to MP3 players, cell phones, lawn mowers, musical instruments and woodwork/metalwork classes in school. Pure-tone audiometry was performed. Correlations with the presence of a notch around 4 kHz in the audiogram indicated that the use of an MP3 player with headphones presented a greater risk than the use of earbuds (in-ear earphones) and stereo connection/docking systems. Tinnitus was significantly associated with the noise notch in the audiogram. The authors recommended a school hearing screening that includes the high frequencies. Gilles et al. (2012) provided a questionnaire to 145 university students and found that approximately 89.5% experienced transient tinnitus after loud music exposure, with a higher prevalence in female students. Permanent noise-induced tinnitus was observed in 14.8%.

European legislation (European Union 2003) for industry sets a level of 85 dB A (dB A is a weighted scale for sound-pressure level measurements that has a similar frequency response to human loudness sensitivity) over 8 h per day as the point at which workers must wear hearing protection. This is approximately equivalent to the level of a shouting voice at a distance of 1 m. This level is not specific to industrial noise, and such risk assessment can also apply to sound exposure in other settings, such as listening to music, using power tools or riding a motorbike.

The level of the noise and duration of exposure are critical parameters—the higher the level and the longer the duration, the greater the risk. This may explain why exposure to loud music in nightclubs seems to be one of the more damaging activities (Women's and Children's Health Network 2017)—because of the high sound levels and length of time that people spend in clubs. Every 3 dB increase in average sound intensity requires that the duration be reduced by half in order to stay at the same level of risk.

The maximum output levels of various portable music devices have been measured at 101–107 dB A (Keith et al. 2008). The equivalent risk of sound at these levels to the necessary action level mentioned in the European legislation (85 dB A over 8 h) would be reached after 3–12 min. Peak sound levels at rock concerts can reach 122 dB A and above (e.g. Cabot et al. 1979; Sataloff 1998), for which the equivalent risk would be reached after 9 s.

Wearing hearing protection lowers the sound level for the listener. Ear protectors that reduce sound levels by just 15 dB would allow the extremely high-level 122 dB A rock concert to be heard for 3 min with the same level of risk (rather than just 9 s without hearing protection). A more moderate (though still loud) rock group playing at an average 105 dB A could be listened to for 2.5 h with the same risk.

What kind of hearing protection is available? Industrial hearing protection typically involves large supra-aural headphones (see Fig. 17.5), but in-ear hearing protectors (usually known as ear-

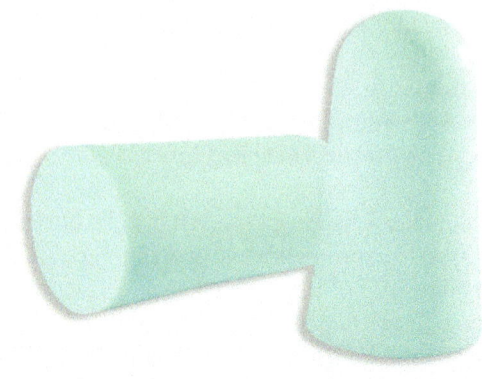

Fig. 17.6 Earplugs from foam. Image copyright and kind permission from UVEX SAFETY GROUP

plugs) are most common outside industry. Earplugs range from very cheap pieces of foam (see Fig. 17.6) to much more expensive "musicians' earplugs" (see Fig. 17.7a, b). The main difference between these earplugs is not the level of protection offered but the effect on how music sounds when wearing them. Basic foam earplugs reduce general sound levels very well but give much more reduction at high frequencies than low frequencies, with the effect that music often sounds muffled (e.g. Fligor 2012). Musicians' earplugs are tailor-made to the shape of the individual's ears and have essentially equal attenuation across the frequency spectrum. This gives a much more realistic percept to the music being heard.

Simply having hearing protection available is not the only way to reduce the risks of noise exposure for young people, not least because earplugs generally cannot be used at the same time as a portable listening device. Education would seem to be essential. Gilles et al. (2012), for example, reported that the level of knowledge of the risks presented by noise exposure was low amongst university students and that the use of hearing protection was uncommon. Sekhar et al. (2011) found that many adolescent MP3 users were unaware of the potential harm caused by loud noise but that most were willing to turn down the volume of the electronic device, to reduce the time spent using it and to use a volume-

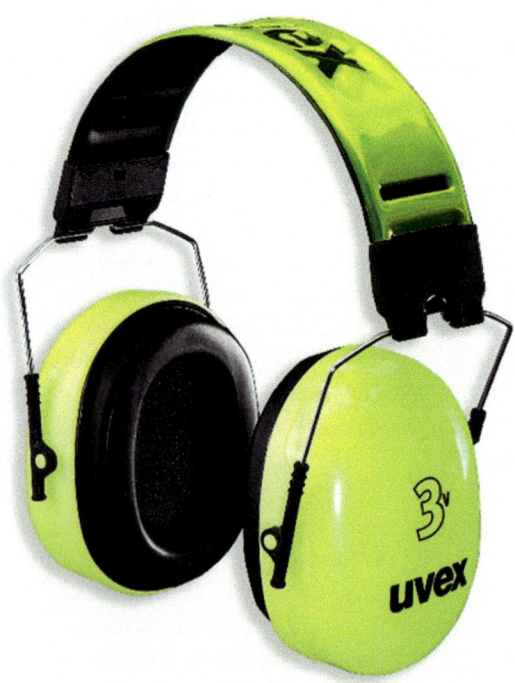

Fig. 17.5 Supra-aural headphones. Image copyright and kind permission from UVEX SAFETY GROUP

Fig. 17.7 (**a**) Musicians' earplugs. Custom-fit filtered earplugs with special filters that produce balanced frequency response. Photo courtesy and used by kind permission of Sensaphonics, Inc. (**b**) Musicians' earplug Musicians Ultraflex. Image copyright and kind permission from Starkey

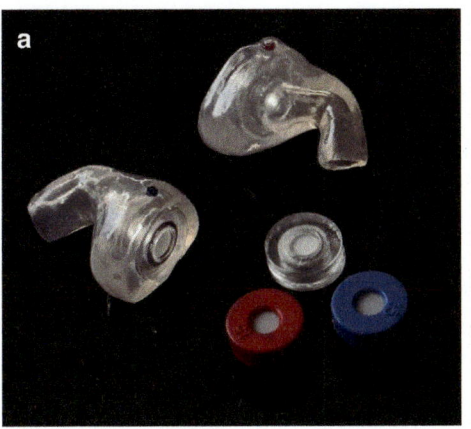
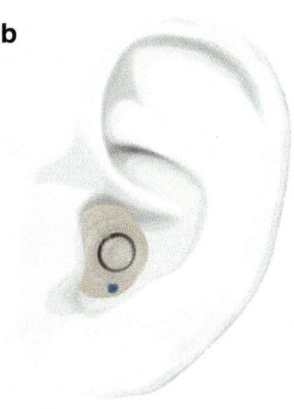

limiting device when informed about the risk. Gilles and Van de Heyning (2014) found significant changes in attitudes towards noise and use of hearing protection in high-school students after a governmental campaign on the dangers posed by noise. Some other studies support the benefit of governmental/educational programmes, but there is very little recent quality literature on the long-term impact.

Campaigns such as the British Tinnitus Association's "Plug'em" campaign have taken a different approach to formal education programmes, by recruiting well-known musicians and DJs to report their experience of tinnitus and hearing impairment and to encourage and normalise the use of hearing protection. Anecdotally, the use of hearing protection at concerts and in nightclubs seems to be much more common and more acceptable socially than 10 years ago.

Further research to understand patterns of risky listening behaviour and to provide information about possible risk-reduction strategies would be highly beneficial. Portnuff (2016) gives an excellent overview of research that considers demographic factors within adolescence, adolescents' broader attitudes towards noise and music (such as their experience-mediated behaviour, self-perception of invulnerability, the impact of socially normative behaviour, sensation seeking and risk judgement) as well as other psychological aspects of music listening. He follows this research to propose strategies for engendering change in listening behaviour, including the following:

- Following the 80/90 rule, by which the listener monitors their own behaviour, following an upper limit of 80% of the maximum output level of the device for a maximum of 90 min per day.
- Use of headphones/earbuds that reduce background noise as well as playing music. This proposal reflects the finding that the music levels most people choose for listening are usually related to having a positive signal-noise level (i.e. the music is noticeably louder than background noise, such as environmental sounds or public transport) rather than absolute level.
- Development of educational programmes based on established health-behaviour models that take account of social and psychological aspects of the listening behaviour of young people and that do not demonise the act of listening to music. Challenging beliefs around invulnerability, possibly with the use of hearing-loss simulations, is important.
- Individual advice from healthcare professionals, including assessing the risk presented by an individual's listening behaviour and giving tailored advice on suitable levels, duration, suitable headphones and environment.

According to a study by scientists from the Boston Children's Hospital, listening for 1 h a day to a portable music player with headphones may be relatively safe if the volume is 60% of the potential maximum loudness (Harrison 2008): the 60/60 rule in contrast to Portnuff's (2016) 80/90 rule.

The following recommendations may also be helpful:

Regarding portable listening devices:

- Earbuds that fit tightly into the ear canal can reduce noise from outside; the transmission of high levels of sound into the closed space of the ear canal has to be avoided.
- Parents and children should try to find a comfortable listening level together.
- Using a noise limiter built in to the device can be beneficial, though consciously monitoring the level and duration of use may be better.
- Periodic 15–20-min breaks whilst listening to music give the inner ear the opportunity to recover (Harrison 2012).

Regarding other listening environments:

- Try to avoid particularly loud environmental sound, such as being close to exploding fireworks, gunfire and power tools. Many high-level sound sources, such as power tools, are especially loud indoors or on a resonating surface (Women's and Children's Health Network 2017).
- Use hearing protection, such as earplugs, in environments where sound is loud, for example, concerts and nightclubs (American Academy of Otolaryngology, Head and Neck Surgery 2017).
- If parents wear earplugs at a concert, their children/teenagers may be more motivated to use them as well.
- Going to nightclubs often has a higher risk. It may be worth setting a limit, such as maximum once a week. The highest sound levels in nightclubs are on the dancefloor, so do not spend all of the time there. Try to spend more time in areas where it is possible to have a conversation. Visiting different loud venues on the same night does not reduce the risk (Women's and Children's Health Network 2017).
- If noise is unavoidable, e.g. in working in a noisy environment, hearing protection must be worn. Organisations such as the European Agency for Safety and Health at Work provide legislation and guidelines. A compendium was created by the Centers for Disease Control

and Prevention (2016). Noise measurements and audiometric monitoring must be performed, employees need to have appropriate training and hearing protection devices must be regularly checked.
- Educational sessions at school should be performed about the risk of noise exposure; see, e.g. The Hearing Foundation of Canada (2013), Dangerous Decibels (2017) and Harrison (2008). Public awareness should be increased (World Health Organization 2009).

April 27 each year is International Noise Awareness Day. It was founded by the Center for Hearing and Communication, New York City, in 1996 (Center for Hearing and Communication 2017).

17.6.3 Avoidance of Noise in Combination with Ototoxic Drugs

Cochlear cells may retain aminoglycosides for 6 months or longer. After application of aminoglycosides, patients should be monitored for cochleotoxic and vestibulotoxic damage for as long as 6 months after cessation of the treatment, and these patients should avoid noise for at least this time span (Li and Steyger 2009). These authors describe the synergistic toxicity of simultaneous noise and aminoglycosides (e.g. for newborns in the neonatal intensive care unit) or a sub-damaging dose of aminoglycosides that intensifies the effect of noise. Sub-damaging noise exposure may also intensify the toxic effect of aminoglycosides.

Similarly, the synergistic effect of noise has to be considered where another ototoxic drug is applied, e.g. during and after chemotherapy with a platinum compound.

17.6.4 General Advice Concerning Hearing Conservation

In order to avoid complications, treatment should start immediately in cases of middle ear infection and be guided by an otorhinolaryngologist. Head trauma, even slight head trauma such as a slap in the face, may cause a commotio labyrinthi and should be avoided. More severe head trauma can cause damage to the tympanic membrane or the ossicular chain. Ototoxic drugs should be applied carefully, and it is important to avoid combinations of ototoxic drugs with simultaneous noise exposure. Children and adolescents should be informed about the risks of listening to loud music and using electronic gaming devices with headphones. Sound-hazardous environments should be avoided. In case of hearing loss, any amplification has to be fitted carefully, hearing thresholds should be monitored closely and any effects of hearing aid supply should be monitored. Stress, especially due to noise, should be avoided.

References

American Academy of Otolaryngology, Head and Neck Surgery (2017) Noise-induced hearing loss in children. Available via http://www.entnet.org/content/noise-induced-hearing-loss-children. Accessed 17 June 2017

ASHA (2016). http://www.asha.org/advocacy/federal/ehdi/. Accessed 27 June 2016

Barreira-Nielsen C, Fitzpatrick E, Hashem S et al (2016) Progressive hearing loss in early childhood. Ear Hear 37(5):e311–e321

Bartel-Friedrich S, Amaya B, Rasinski C et al (2008a) Der erweiterte Ductus und Saccus endolymphaticus. Teil 1: Analyse bildgebender Befunde. (Large endolymphatic duct and sac syndrome (LEDS): part I: analysis of imaging findings). HNO 56(2):219–224

Bartel-Friedrich S, Fuchs M, Amaya B et al (2008b) Der erweiterte Ductus und Saccus endolymphaticus. Teil 2: Klinische Manifestationen. (Large endolymphatic duct and sac syndrome: part 2: clinical manifestations). HNO 56(2):225–230

Baxendale J, Hesketh A (2003) Comparison of the effectiveness of the Hanen Parent Programme and traditional clinic therapy. Int J Lang Commun Dis 38(4):397–415

Beazley S, Moore M (1995) Deaf children, their families and professionals. David Fulton Publishers, London

Brown ED, Chau JK, Atashband S et al (2009) A systematic review of neonatal toxoplasmosis exposure and sensorineural hearing loss. Int J Pediatr Otorhinolaryngol 73(5):707–711. https://doi.org/10.1016/j.ijporl.2009.01.012. Epub 2009 Feb 11

Cabot RC, Genter CR, Lucke T (1979) Sound levels and spectra of rock music. J Audio Eng Soc 27:267–283

Center for Hearing and Communication (2017) International Noise Awareness Day 23rd anniversary. Available via http://chchearing.org/noise/day/. Accessed 17 June 2017

Centers for Disease Control and Prevention (2016) Hearing protector device compendium. Available via www.cdc.gov/topics/noise/hpdcomp. Accessed 17 June 2017

Choo D, Meinzen-Derr J (2010) Universal newborn hearing screening in 2010. Curr Opin Otolaryngol Head Neck Surg 18(5):399–404. https://doi.org/10.1097/MOO.0b013e32833d475d

Colgan S, Gold L, Wirth K et al (2012) The cost-effectiveness of universal newborn screening for bilateral permanent congenital hearing impairment: systematic review. Acad Pediatr 12(3):171–180. https://doi.org/10.1016/j.acap.2012.02.002

Cristobal R, Oghalai JS (2008) Hearing loss in children with very low birth weight: current review of epidemiology and pathophysiology. Arch Dis Child Fetal Neonatal Ed 93(6):F462–F468. https://doi.org/10.1136/adc.2007.124214

Dangerous Decibels (2017) Noise-induced hearing loss can be prevented. Available via www.dangerousdecibels.org. Accessed 17 June 2017

De Barros Boishardy A, Lenoir FM, Kapella M et al (2005) Universal hearing screening: 10,835 newborns tested in maternity wards of the geographical Department of Eure, France. Ann Otolaryngol Chir Cervicofac 122(5):223–230

de Vries JJ, Vossen AC, Kroes AC et al (2011) Implementing neonatal screening for congenital cytomegalovirus: addressing the deafness of policy makers. Rev Med Virol 21(1):54–61. https://doi.org/10.1002/rmv.679. Epub 2011 Jan 18

DesJardin JL (2006) Family empowerment: Supporting language development in young children who are deaf or hard of hearing. Volta Rev 106(3):275–298

Downs MP, Yoshinaga-Itano C (1999) The efficacy of early identification and intervention for children with hearing impairment. Pediatr Clin N Am 46(1):79–87

Easterbrooks SR, O'Rourke CM, Todd NW (2000) Child and family factors associated with deaf children's success in auditory-verbal therapy. Am J Otol 21(3):341–344

European Board of Medical Genetics (2010) Core competences for genetic counsellors. Available via https://www.eshg.org/fileadmin/eshg/committees/EBMG/EBMGCoreCompetencesForGeneticCounsellors.pdf. Accessed 8 Dec 2016

European Union (2003) Directive 2003/19/EC. Available via http://eur-lex.europa.eu/LexUriServ/LexUriServ.do?uri=OJ:L:2003:042:0038:0044:EN:PDF. Accessed 17 June 2017

Fligor B (2012) Clinical verification of custom-fitted musicians' earplugs. Available via Audiology Online. http://www.audiologyonline.com/articles/clinical-verification-custom-fitted-musicians-11373. Accessed 12 Apr 2017

Gandhi RS, Fernandez-Alvarez JR, Rabe H (2010) Management of congenital cytomegalovirus infection: an evidence-based approach. Acta Paediatr 99(4):509–515. https://doi.org/10.1111/j.1651-2227.2009.01655.x. Epub 2009 Dec 24

Gilles A, Van de Heyning P (2014) Effectiveness of a preventive campaign for noise-induced hearing damage in adolescents. Int J Pediatr Otorhinolaryngol 278(4):604–609

Gilles A, De Ridder D, Van Hal G et al (2012) Prevalence of leisure noise-induced tinnitus and the attitude toward noise in university students. Otol Neurotol 33(6):899–906

Granell J, Gavilanes J, Herrero J et al (2008) Is universal newborn hearing screening more efficient with auditory evoked potentials compared to otoacoustic emissions? Acta Otorrinolaringol Esp 59(4):170–175

Gross M (2005) Universelles Hörscreening bei Neugeborenen—Empfehlungen zu Organisation und Durchführung des universellen Neugeborenen-Screenings auf angeborene Hörstörungen in Deutschland. (Universal hearing screening in newborns—recommendations for organizing and conducting universal hearing screening for congenital hearing loss in Germany). Laryngorhinootologie 84(11):801–808

Grosse SD, Ross DS (2006) Cost savings from universal newborn hearing screening. Pediatrics 117(4):1101–1112

Harrison RV (2008) Noise-induced hearing loss in children: a 'less than silent' environmental danger. Paediatr Child Health 13(5):377–382

Harrison RV (2012) The prevention of noise induced hearing loss in children. Int J Pediatr 2012:473541. Published online 2012 Dec 13. https://doi.org/10.1155/2012/473541

Holzinger D, Wieshaupt A, Fellinger P et al (2016) Prevalence of 2.2 per mille of significant hearing loss at school age suggests rescreening after NHS. Int J Pediatr Otorhinolaryngol 87:121–125

Janjua F, Woll B, Kyle J (2002) Effects of parental style of interaction on language development in very young severe and profound deaf children. Int J Pediatr Otorhinoalaryngol 64(3):193–205

Joint Committee on Infant Hearing (1995) 1994 position statement. Pediatrics 95(1):152–156

Joint Committee on Infant Hearing (2000) Year 2000 position statement: principles and guidelines for early hearing detection and intervention programs. Pediatrics 106(4):798–817

Kaye CI (2006) Introduction to the newborn screening fact sheets. Pediatrics 118(3):1304–1312

Keith SE, Michaud DS, Chiu V (2008) Evaluating the maximum playback sound levels from portable digital audio players. J Acoust Soc Am 123(6):4227–4237

Kochhar A, Hildebrand MS, Smith RJ (2007) Clinical aspects of hereditary hearing loss. Genet Med 9(7):393–408

Konigsmark BW, Gorlin RJ (eds) (1976) Genetic and metabolic deafness. WB Saunders, Philadelphia

le Clercq CM, van Ingen G, Ruytjens L et al (2016) Music-induced hearing loss in children, adolescents, and young adults: a systematic review and meta-analysis. Otol Neurotol 37(9):1208–1216

Li H, Steyger PS (2009) Synergistic ototoxicity due to noise exposure and aminoglycoside antibiotics. Noise Health 11(42):26–32

Liu X, Xu L (1994) Nonsyndromic hearing loss: an analysis of audiograms. Ann Otol Rhinol Laryngol 103(6):428–433

Louw C, Swanepoel W, Eikelboom RH et al (2017) Smartphone-based hearing screening at primary health care clinics. Ear Hear 38(2):e93–e100

Low WK, Pang KY, Ho LY et al (2005) Universal newborn hearing screening in Singapore: the need, implementation and challenges. Ann Acad Med Singap 34(4):301–306

Martini A, Marchisio P, Bubbico L et al (2013) Permanent childhood hearing impairment: universal newborn hearing screening, PCHI management. Minerva Pediatr 65(2):231–250

Moeller MP (2000) Early intervention and language development in children who are deaf and hard of hearing. Pediatrics 106(3):E43

Moeller MP, Carr G, Seaver L et al (2013) Best practices in family-centered early intervention for children who are deaf or hard of hearing: an international consensus statement. J Deaf Stud Deaf Educ 18(4):429–445. https://doi.org/10.1093/deafed/ent034

Morton CC, Nance WE (2006) Newborn hearing screening—a silent revolution. N Engl J Med 354(20):2151–2164

Münzel T, Gori T, Babisch W et al (2014) Cardiovascular effects of environmental noise exposure. Eur Heart J 35(13):829–836

National Institute on Deafness and Other Communication Disorders (2017) Enlarged vestibular aqueducts and childhood hearing loss. Available via https://www.nidcd.nih.gov/health/enlarged-vestibular-aqueducts-and-childhood-hearing-loss. Accessed 17 June 2017

Neumann K, Nawka T, Wiesner T et al (2009) Autorengruppe im Auftrag der DGPP: Qualitätssicherung eines universellen Neugeborenen-Hörscreenings. Empfehlungen der Deutschen Gesellschaft für Phoniatrie und Pädaudiologie. (Quality assurance of a universal newborn hearing screening. Recommendations of the German Society of Phoniatrics and Pediatric Audiology). HNO 57(1):17–20

Noordman BJ, van Beeck Calkoen E, Witte B et al (2015) Prognostic factors for sudden drops in hearing level after minor head injury in patients with an enlarged vestibular aqueduct: a meta-analysis. Otol Neurotol 36(1):4–11

Olusanya BO, Wirz SL, Luxon LM (2008) Hospital-based universal newborn hearing screening for early detection of permanent congenital hearing loss in Lagos, Nigeria. Int J Pediatr Otorhinolaryngol 72(7):991–1001

Oyler AL (2007) Large vestibular aqueduct (LVA) disorders. ASHA. Available via http://www.asha.org/Articles/Large-Vestibular-Aqueduct-Disorders. Accessed 17 June 2017

Portnuff CDF (2016) Reducing the risk of music-induced hearing loss from overuse of portable listening devices: understanding the problems and establishing strategies for improving awareness in adolescents. Adolesc Health Med Ther 7:27–35

Portnuff CDF, Fligor BJ, Arehart KH (2011) Teenage use of portable listening devices: a hazard to hearing? J Am Acad Audiol 22(10):663–677

Prpić I, Mahulja-Stamenković V, Bilić I et al (2007) Hearing loss assessed by universal newborn hearing screening-the new approach. Int J Pediatr Otorhinolaryngol 71(11):1757–1761

Ross DS, Holstrum WJ, Gaffney M et al (2008) Hearing screening and diagnostic evaluation of children with unilateral and mild bilateral hearing loss. Trends Amplif 12(1):27–34. https://doi.org/10.1177/1084713807306241

Sataloff RT (1998) Rock concert audience noise exposure: a preliminary study. J Occup Hear Loss 1:97–99

Schmitz J, Pillion JP, LeClerq SC et al (2010) Prevalence of hearing loss and ear morbidity among adolescents and young adults in rural southern Nepal. Int J Audiol 49(5):388–394

Sekhar DL, Rhoades JA, Longenecker AL et al (2011) Improving detection of adolescent hearing loss. Arch Pediatr Adolesc Med 165(12):1094–1100

Shearer AE, Hildebrand MS, Smith RJH (2017) Hereditary hearing loss and deafness overview. Gene Reviews [Internet]. Available via https://www.ncbi.nlm.nih.gov/books/NBK1434/. Accessed 28 Nov 2017

Skarżyński H, Piotrowska A (2012) Screening for preschool and school-age hearing problems: European Consensus Statement. Int J Pediatr Otorhinolaryngol 76(1):120–121

Smith RJ, Bale JF Jr (2005) Sensorineural hearing loss in children. Lancet 365(9462):879–890

Tharpe AM, Sladen DP (2008) Causation of permanent unilateral and mild bilateral hearing loss in children. Trends Amplif 12(1):17–25

The Hearing Foundation of Canada (2013) Sound sense. Available via www.soundsense.ca. Accessed 17 June 2017

Toriello HV, Reardon W, Gorlin RJ (2004) Hereditary hearing loss and its syndromes. Oxford Monographs on Medical Genetes no. 50. Oxford University Press, Oxford

Tranebaerg L (2008) Genetics of congenital hearing impairment: a clinical approach. Int J Audiol 47(9):535–545. https://doi.org/10.1080/14992020802249259

US Preventive Services Task Force (2008) Universal screening for hearing loss in newborns: US Preventive Services Task Force recommendation statement. Pediatrics 122(1):143–148

Vogel I, Verschuure H, van der Ploeg CP et al (2009) Adolescents and MP3 players: too many risks, too few precautions. Pediatrics 123(6):e953–e958. https://doi.org/10.1542/peds.2008-3179

Vos B, Lagasse R, Levêque A (2013) The organisation of universal newborn hearing screening in the Wallonia-Brussels Federation. B-ENT Suppl 21:9–15

Weichbold V, Nekahm-Heis D, Welzl-Mueller K (2006) Universal newborn hearing screening and postnatal hearing loss. Pediatrics 117(4):e631–e636

White KR (2004) Early hearing detection and intervention programs: opportunities for genetic services. Am J Med Genet A 130A(1):29–36

Wilkinson AR, Jiang ZD (2006) Brainstem auditory evoked response in neonatal neurology. Semin Fetal Neonatal Med 11(6):444–451. Epub 2006 Oct 2

Wolff R, Hommerich J, Riemsma R et al (2010) Hearing screening in newborns: systematic review of accuracy, effectiveness, and effects of interventions after screening. Arch Dis Child 95(2):130–135

Women's and Children's Health Network (2017) Parenting and child health. Child and youth health. Noise and hearing. Available via http://www.cyh.com/HealthTopics/HealthTopicDetails.aspx?p=114&np=304&id=1584. Accessed 17 June 2017

World Health Organization (2009) Children and noise. Children's health and the environment. Available via www.who.intr/ceh/capacity/noise. Accessed 17 June 2017

Yee-Arellano HM, Leal-Garza F, Pauli-Muller K (2006) Universal newborn hearing screening in Mexico: results of the first 2 years. Int J Pediatr Otorhinolaryngol 70(11):1863–1870. (PubMed: 16914209)

Yoshinaga-Itano C (2000) Successful outcomes for deaf and hard of hearing children. Semin Hear 21:4

Yoshinaga-Itano C, Sedey AL, Coulter DK et al (1998) Language of early- and later-identified children with hearing loss. Pediatrics 102(5):1161–1171

Rehabilitation and Prognosis of Disorders of Hearing Development

18

Songul Aksoy, Antoinette am Zehnhoff-Dinnesen,
Ahmet Atas, Doris-Eva Bamiou,
Sylva Bartel-Friedrich, Claire Benton,
Steffi Johanna Brockmeier, Nicole G. Campbell,
Gwen Carr, Marco Caversaccio, Hatice Celik,
Jakub Dršata, Kate Hanvey, Mona Hegazi,
Reinhild Hofmann (born Glanemann), Malte Kob,
Martin Kompis, Peter Matulat, Wendy McCracken,
David R. Moore, Dirk Mürbe, Haldun Oguz,
Levent N. Ozluoglu, Kayhan Öztürk, Ross Parfitt,
Stefan Plontke, Ute Pröschel, Karen Reichmuth,
Debbie Rix, Charlotte Rogers, Mustafa Asim Safak,
Tony Sirimanna, Konstance Tzifa, Christoph von
Ilberg, Thomas Wiesner, and Katherine Wilson

Electronic Supplementary Material The online version
of this chapter (https://doi.org/10.1007/978-3-662-46780-
0_18) contains supplementary material, which is available
to authorized users.

S. Aksoy
Department of Audiology, Hacettepe University,
Sıhhiye-Ankara, Turkey

A. am Zehnhoff-Dinnesen · P. Matulat · R. Parfitt ·
K. Reichmuth
Clinic of Phoniatrics and Pedaudiology, University
Hospital Münster, Münster, Germany
e-mail: am.zehnhoff@uni-muenster.de;
matulat@uni-muenster.de;
ross.parfitt@ukmuenster.de;
karen.reichmuth@ukmuenster.de

R. Hofmann (born Glanemann)
ICBF Germany International Talent Centre, Westphalian
Wilhelms-University Munster, Münster, Germany
e-mail: r.hofmann@uni-muenster.de

A. Atas
Department of Audiology, Faculty of Health Science,
Istanbul University Cerrahpasa, İstanbul, Turkey

Department of ENT—Audiology and Speech
Pathology, Faculty of Medicine, İstanbul University
Cerrahpasa, İstanbul, Turkey

D.-E. Bamiou
National Hospital for Neurology and Neurosurgery,
London, UK
e-mail: d.bamiou@ucl.ac.uk

S. Bartel-Friedrich · S. Plontke
Department of Otorhinolaryngology—Head and
Neck Surgery, University Hospital
Martin Luther University Halle-Wittenberg,
Halle (Saale), Germany
e-mail: sylva.bartel-friedrich@uk-halle.de;
stefan.plontke@uk-halle.de

C. Benton
Nottingham Audiology Services, Ropewalk House,
Nottingham, UK
e-mail: claire.benton@nuh.nhs.uk

C. Rogers
Leicester School of Allied Health Sciences,
De Montfort University, Hawthorn Building,
Leicester, UK
e-mail: charlotte.rogers@dmu.ac.uk

© Springer-Verlag GmbH Germany, part of Springer Nature 2020
A. am Zehnhoff-Dinnesen et al. (eds.), *Phoniatrics I*, European Manual of Medicine,
https://doi.org/10.1007/978-3-662-46780-0_18

S. J. Brockmeier
ENT Clinic, Audiology, Phoniatrics, Neuro-Otology,
Kantonsspital Aarau AG,
Aarau, Switzerland
e-mail: hanna.brockmeier@ksa.ch

N. G. Campbell
Auditory Implant Service, University of
Southampton, Southampton, UK
e-mail: N.G.Campbell@soton.ac.uk

G. Carr
UCL Ear Institute, University College London,
London, UK
e-mail: gwencarr@ehdiprofessional.com

M. Caversaccio
Universitätsklinik für Hals-, Nasen- und
Ohrenkrankheiten (HNO), Kopf- und Halschirurgie,
Inselspital, Bern, Switzerland
e-mail: marco.caversaccio@insel.ch

H. Celik
Department of Otorhinolaryngology, Ankara Training
and Research Hospital, Ankara, Turkey

J. Dršata
Department of Otorhinolaryngology and Head and
Neck Surgery, University Hospital Hradec Kralove,
Hradec Kralove, Czech Republic
e-mail: drsata@fnhk.cz

K. Hanvey
Aston University Day Hospital, Birmingham
Children's Hospital, The Midlands Hearing Implant
Programme, Birmingham, UK
e-mail: kate.hanvey@bch.nhs.uk

M. Hegazi
ENT Department, Ain Shams University,
Cairo, Egypt

M. Kob
Detmold University of Music, Erich Thienhaus
Institute, Music Acoustics and Theory of Music
Transmission, Detmold, Germany
e-mail: kob@hfm-detmold.de

M. Kompis
Universitätsklinik für Hals-, Nasen- und
Ohrenkrankheiten, Inselspital, Bern, Switzerland
e-mail: martin.kompis@insel.ch

W. McCracken
School of Psychological Sciences, University of
Manchester, Manchester, UK
e-mail: Wendy.mccracken@manchester.ac.uk

D. R. Moore
Communication Sciences Research Center,
Cincinnati Children's Hospital, Cincinnati, OH, USA
e-mail: david.r.moore@cchmc.org

D. Mürbe
Department of Audiology and Phoniatrics,
Charité— University Medicine Berlin, Berlin,
Germany
e-mail: dirk.muerbe@charite.de

H. Oguz
Fonomer, Ankara, Turkey

L. N. Ozluoglu
Department of Otolaryngology, Baskent University,
Etimesgut/Ankara, Turkey
e-mail: leventozluoglu@baskent-ank.edu.tr

K. Öztürk
Department of Otolaryngology, Selcuk University,
School of Medicine, Yeni Istanbul, Caddesi,
Konya, Turkey

U. Pröschel
Institut für Phoniatrie und Pädaudiologie, Vestische
Kinder- und Jugendklinik Datteln, Datteln, Germany
e-mail: U.Proeschel@kinderklinik-datteln.de

D. Rix
Wandsworth Hearing Support Service, Linden Lodge
School, London, UK
e-mail: rix@wandsworthhis.org.uk

M. A. Safak
Department of Otolaryngology, Near East University,
Lefkosa, Turkey

T. Sirimanna
Audiological Medicine and Cochlear Implant
Department, Great Ormond Street Hospital,
London, UK
e-mail: Tony.Sirimanna@gosh.nhs.uk

K. Tzifa
Birmingham Children's Hospital, Birmingham, UK
e-mail: info@tzifa.eu

C. von Ilberg
Meniere-Center-Frankfurt,
Frankfurt am Main, Germany

T. Wiesner
Department of Phoniatrics and Pediatric Audiology,
Werner Otto Institut gGmbH, Hamburg, Germany
e-mail: twiesner@werner-otto-institut.de

K. Wilson
St Thomas' Hearing Implant Centre, St Thomas'
Hospital, London, UK
e-mail: katherine.wilson@gstt.nhs.uk

18.1 Team Building in the Care for Hearing-Impaired Children

Steffi Johanna Brockmeier

18.1.1 Multidisciplinary Team

Concepts of team working are complex, and the terminology is often used inconsistently or incorrectly (McCallin 2001). A "multidisciplinary team" is generally accepted as being:

> a team or collaborative process where members of different disciplines assess or treat patients independently and then share the information with each other.
>
> Sorrels-Jones (1997)

Interdisciplinary teams work closely, with care plans for individual patients being discussed and developed together. Crucial to the effectiveness of any team structure is having shared goals and values, good communication, clearly defined roles and respect for and understanding of the different areas of expertise (Pearson and Spencer 1995).

Specifically regarding paediatric hearing services, Baguley et al. (2000) state that

> it is the parental role that is central: the role of the team is to facilitate that role.

Structuring a multidisciplinary team with the parental role as the centre recognises the parents' own expertise regarding their child and enables the realisation of the legal and moral right of the parent to drive the process. In order to work together truly for the benefit of the parent and child, individual team members may therefore need to:

> reassess exclusive claims to specialist knowledge and authority.
>
> Mental Health Commission (2006)

Hearing-impaired children are usually cared for by a multidisciplinary team (American Speech-Language-Hearing Association 2015; National Center for Hearing Assessment and Management, Utah State University 2011). The participants of this team, however, vary widely between countries and within countries and institutions; therefore, this article represents the experience of the author and may differ, to varying degrees, from those of the reader.

The paedaudiologist, either in the form of a paedaudiologically specialised physician or an audiologist specialised in children, will be notified through the neonatal hearing screening programme that a child needs follow-up. All technical and physical examinations to assess hearing loss will be performed or initiated by this person. The need for a hearing aid or other measures will be discussed with the parents, and the actions needed will be set into motion.

Before neonatal hearing screening was established, the paediatrician or the general practitioner who knew the family and the child well might suspect hearing loss usually when milestones of speech development had not been met. Bonding between parents and child as well as the doctor would have been a sound foundation for the management of diagnostic and therapeutic procedures involved with hearing loss, as well as the psychological impact caused. However, today when a hearing loss is detected, the paedaudiologist must be aware of the consequences for the family and needs to have the expertise to manage the situation when the parent-child relationship is vulnerable during the neonatal period.

After the diagnostic period, regular follow-up visits and later visits to monitor development of hearing and speech are also provided by these services. Initially, intervals of 3–6 months are recommended between the consultations. If the child develops well and hearing is stable, one visit a year might be considered sufficient.

A hearing aid specialist, who may be part of the audiological team, will provide hearing aids for children diagnosed with hearing loss, as needed. Especially in the case of very young children, this person should have an additional paediatric qualification.

Teachers of the deaf are employed to provide audiological education to the family, as well as to support the speech development of the child and to facilitate the child's inclusion in local schools. Their feedback is of utmost importance when decisions have to be made on the necessity to move from a conventional hearing aid to an implantable solution, as they can best judge the performance of the individual in everyday life.

As around 30% of all children with hearing loss also have additional physical impairments, paediatricians need to consider, e.g. cardiac and nephrological anomalies as well developmental delays. An ophthalmologist should also be involved to assess visual impairment. The policy concerning the stage at which radiological diagnostics are performed varies widely; this is also true for genetic counselling. For children with conductive hearing loss and for those who are provided with an implantable hearing solution, an ENT surgeon is needed. Additionally, the following professions are often involved in the diagnosis and treatment of children with hearing loss: speech and language pathologists and therapists, psychologists and an anaesthesiologist. Occasionally an occupational therapist, physiotherapist or those from similar professions are involved (see Sects. 13.3 and 16.17).

Ideally, all these specialists should have gained special knowledge in the context of hearing loss in children and will continue to keep in touch with the progress in their respective fields. Exchange of information, not only on a case-by-case basis, is essential to link the professional groups.

18.1.2 Sharing Information

Optimising the care of an individual subject is highly dependent on the information available. Therefore, the exchange of information is the core of fruitful cooperation.

Consent needs to be obtained from the primary caregiver of the child in order to share information. It might allow details to be passed on to all professional groups involved, or the consent might limit the exchange by excluding individual persons or professional groups. The decisions taken in this area are legally binding and serve as the basis for a trusting relationship between the caregiver and professionals. The duty of disclosure of information to health insurance or other financing authorities is subject to national requirements.

As the amount of information that needs to be handled by service providers can be over-whelming when considering the number of reports and of potential patients, the selection of relevant details needs to be checked carefully. Clear statements and conclusions in reports are helpful, as is information about the actions taken and the arrangements needed. In most cases, exchange of information is managed via a letter sent either by standard mail or electronically, if security allows. All service providers for the respective child should be notified. Sometimes it is helpful to have a meeting that includes all the professional groups involved. Especially when services or cooperation is initiated, it is suggested that regular meetings and discussions take place in order to enhance understanding and communication between the individual groups and persons of the team involved in the care of a hearing-impaired child. If services share many patients, regular meetings are suggested as personal contact enhances paving the way for efficient handling of critical situations (National Deaf Children's Society UK 2015).

18.2 Therapeutic Parental Guidance Programmes

Debbie Rix and Gwen Carr

The Global Coalition of Parents of Children who are Deaf or Hard of Hearing (2010) strongly express the view that:

> A well-adjusted successful child who is deaf or hard of hearing is the product of a well-adjusted successfully supported family.

The Coalition emphasises the fact that such support should be culturally competent, taking into account:

> the distinctive nature of families - their configuration, cultural considerations, beliefs, values, emotional reactions, coping styles, family dynamics and other issues.

Family-centred services for deaf children acknowledge that each family is unique and that the role of the professional is to enable, not control (Moeller et al. 2013). Through this approach, parents move from a position of loss of control at diagnosis to self-efficacy and competence. The importance of direct parent-to-parent support has also been identified as playing a key role in programmes, both in promoting the social and emotional well-being of families and in enabling the development of self-advocacy. The conceptual framework developed by Henderson et al. (2014) deepens understanding of how parent-to-parent support can operate to enhance the effectiveness of overall parent and family support and guidance programmes.

Any parent guidance or parent support programme is "therapeutic" only to the extent that it promotes positive outcomes and meets the developmental needs of the child within the context of supporting the social and emotional well-being of the parents and family. Skilled and qualified professionals need to ensure that their guidance:

- Recognises and builds on families' strengths
- Supports parents and caregivers to provide an environment that optimises the child's development
- Gives confidence in order to enhance skills and competence, enabling families to use language stimulation strategies that are known to promote early development within their typical daily lives
- Fosters natural interactions between parents/caregivers and the child that maintain a joyful relationship
- Is underpinned by regular monitoring and assessment of the child's progress and child and family outcomes

In response to the recognition of the centrality of the family in promoting best outcomes for children with hearing loss, many services have now adopted the Family Partnership Model to create a service delivery approach at all levels, which both creates an increased sense of well-being (see Fig. 18.1) and autonomy among parents and increases engagement with services (Davis and Day 2010).

The model includes the following features:

- An emphasis on including all family members
- Listening actively to understand in depth a family's priorities and concerns

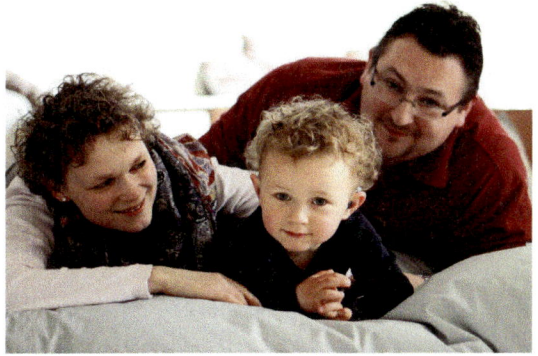

Fig. 18.1 Family with a sense of well-being. The child is wearing hearing aids. Photo with kind permission of the parents ©privat

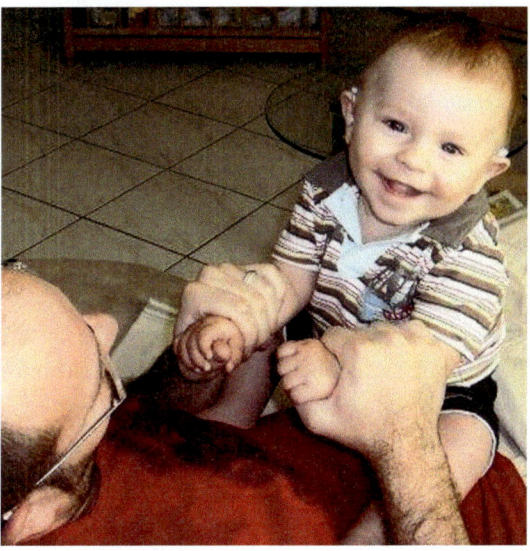

Fig. 18.2 Playful interaction between parent and child. The child is wearing hearing aids. Photo with kind permission of the parents

- Building a trusting relationship between professionals and parents
- Understanding that each family is unique

Implementation of the model follows a training programme in which practitioners develop the communication skills to support parents. It has been successfully applied across education and health networks in the UK and overseas. Ultimately, whilst the programme is of benefit to parents (and professionals), research indicates the positive impact on child developmental outcomes (see Fig. 18.2).

18.3 The Concept of the Muenster Parental Programme

Reinhild Hofmann (born Glanemann) and
Karen Reichmuth

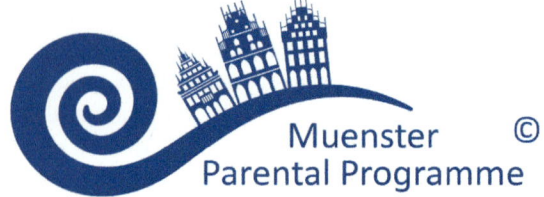

Fig. 18.3 Logo of the Muenster Parental Programme

18.3.1 Need for Family-Centred Early Intervention After Diagnosis of Hearing Loss (HL)

Newborn hearing screening (NHS) programmes and the early provision of hearing aids have improved the perspective of children with HL to develop the best possible speech-language and auditory skills. However, the early detection and the early provision of technical aids are not considered to be sufficient for successful speech-language development. Another significant factor is the early start of a family-centred early intervention that highlights the parents' central role in their child's communicative development (Moeller 2000; Holzinger and Fellinger 2013; Sarimski et al. 2013). Following the modern paradigms in early intervention and the guidelines for best practice of hearing-impaired infants, the focus should be on family-child interaction, rather than on child-directed therapy (Moeller et al. 2013).

Normally, for hearing parents, the diagnosis HL is unexpected. It may irritate parents in their communicative interaction with the infant and can impede their intuitive parental skills (Koester and Lahti-Harper 2010). However, a language-rich stimulation during natural interaction is most influential for successful communication development of children with HL (Szagun and Stumper 2012). Parents themselves wish for early and close-meshed support after the diagnosis (Young and Tattersall 2007).

18.3.2 The Muenster Parental Programme (MPP)

The *MPP* (see Fig. 18.3) is an evidence-based responsive parenting intervention specific to the needs of parents of infants with HL identified by newborn hearing screening (NHS) (Reichmuth et al. 2013; Glanemann et al. 2013). The concept of the *MPP* draws upon current research findings concerning early speech and language development of normally hearing children and of children with HL. It follows the principle of communication-orientated and natural auditory-oral approaches for children with HL. These concepts emphasise the importance of natural parent-child communication in everyday life (e.g. Batliner 2012; Clark 2007). The *MPP* incorporates essential elements of existing responsive parenting programmes for normally hearing children that focus on parents' communication towards their child (international overview by Brady et al. 2009). These elements have been extended and modified to satisfy the needs of families who have a child with HL. Moreover, the *MPP* matches the demands of national (German) and international guidelines (Moeller et al. 2013; DGPP 2013).

Fundamentally, the *MPP* follows two main goals in optimising the conditions for the child to develop the best possible speech-language competence. First, parents get reinforcement concerning their intuitive parental skills and competences – especially in being responsive – and they are supported in communicating and interacting with their child (see Fig. 18.4). In working with the parents, the programme is respectful of individual differences and recognises each family's strengths and natural skills. Second, the group sessions allow early contact and exchange with other families and offer mutual social and emotional support.

The *MPP* is a short intervention of 3 months and combines six multifamily parent-group sessions with four single-family parent sessions. It is designed for parents of hearing-impaired children who are at the preverbal level and who do not yet use words (age 3–18 months). The children may

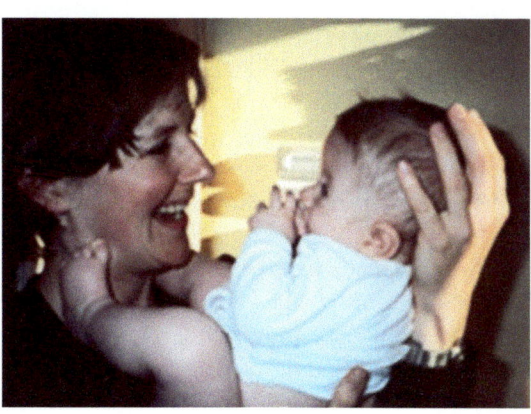

Fig. 18.4 Example of interaction between parent and child. Image with kind permission of the parent

Case Study 18.1

The video shows the interaction between a 5-month-old baby with bilateral moderate sensory hearing loss, who has worn hearing aids for 2 months, and its mother, who participated in the *Muenster Parental Programme*. She shows a well-made responsive parenting style by following the child's lead through the interaction. For this she has learned to first observe the non-verbal and vocal signals of her child and then to mirror and imitate these signals in a naturally exaggerated manner and to observe and wait again. By this, turn-taking can emerge. The child itself seems to become more and more aware of this turn-taking and starts to join in.

have a risk of an additional developmental delay. If the child is a candidate for cochlea implantation, the *MPP* serves as a valuable activity to bridge the time until implantation. Parents can already establish a sound basis for successful parent-child communication. Following the implantation parents can build on what they have experienced and learnt during the preoperative period.

In small groups without children, parents learn about communicative strategies, such as responsiveness, which nurture their child's speech-language and auditory development (see Reichmuth et al. 2013 for more details on further contents). In two of the single sessions, parents learn to recognise their child's communicative attempts and to be responsive to them. Here, they are guided by means of individual video feedback to employ and intensify responsive strategies in the interaction with their child. By this, parents often realise that they already use a great part of these strategies and (re)start to appreciate their own parenting skills.

In addition to the 3-month programme in early infanthood, there is an individual refresher session with video feedback when the child is at the early verbal stage, around 24–30 months of age. Embedded in dialogic picture book reading, as a typical and joyful interactive situation at that age, parents learn to transfer the *MPP* strategies to the now raised verbal level of their child (see Reichmuth et al. 2013 for more details on this concept).

18.3.3 Study Results

The accompanying study (prospective group design) showed by video analysis that parents who participated in the *MPP* could intensify their communication-enhancing behaviour towards their child more than parents of a control group (see Figs. 18.5 and 18.6). Moreover, at the end of

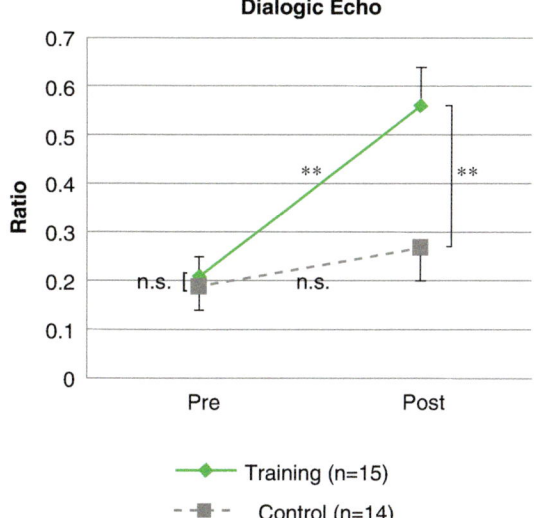

Fig. 18.5 Parental dialogic echo (ratios) (error bars = SEM standard error of the mean) before (pre) and after (post) the *MPP*: ** significant at the <0.01 level. Courtesy of Int J Pediatr Otorhinolaryngol, reprinted from Glanemann et al. (2013), with permission from Elsevier

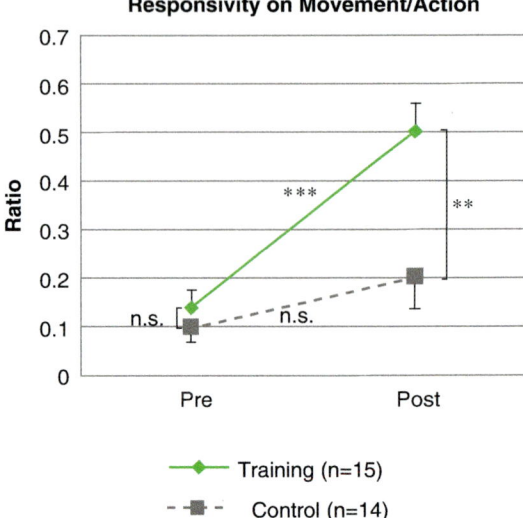

Fig. 18.6 Parental responsiveness on movement/action of the child (ratios) (error bars = SEM) before (pre) and after (post) the *MPP*: ** significant at the <0.01 level. *** significant at the <0.001 level. Courtesy of Int J Pediatr Otorhinolaryngol, reprinted from Glanemann et al. (2013), with permission from Elsevier

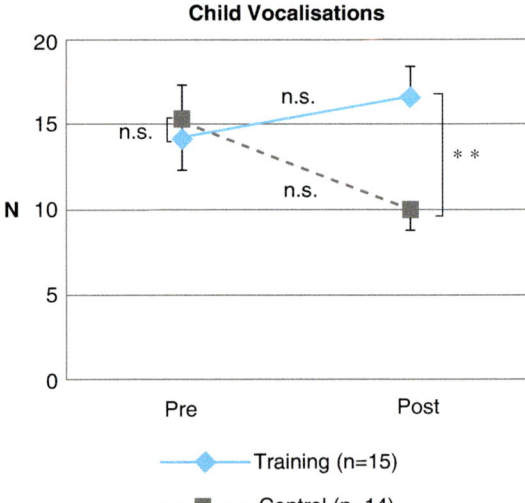

Fig. 18.7 Total number of child vocalisations (error bars = SEM) before (pre) and after (post) the *MPP*: ** significant at the <0.01 level. Courtesy of Int J Pediatr Otorhinolaryngol, reprinted from Glanemann et al. (2013), with permission from Elsevier

the 3-month programme, children of participating parents vocalised more than children of the control group (see Fig. 18.7).

The feedback from participating parents was very affirmative. Specifically, they valued the exchange with other parents of affected children and the individual single sessions with video feedback. Altogether, they would recommend the *MPP* to other parents in a comparable situation (Glanemann et al. 2016).

The evidence-based *Muenster Parental Programme* fulfils the demands of modern family-centred early intervention (Moeller et al. 2013) and is a module of comprehensive early intervention. As such it can be recommended after early identification of HL.

18.4 Fitting and Evaluation of Hearing Devices Including Audiometric Validation and Technical Verification

Thomas Wiesner

18.4.1 Introduction

The aim of a hearing aid fitting is to make sounds and especially speech audible for the hearing-impaired person. As most people with a sensorineural hearing loss have a limited hearing range between their hearing threshold and their uncomfortable loudness threshold, the amplified sound has to be compressed into the remaining dynamic field so that soft sounds can be heard again and loud sounds do not get uncomfortably loud. To make a hearing aid wearable, it is also necessary to miniaturise the electronic components (see Fig. 18.8), including the microphone and receiver, as much as possible, but that still implies a number of restrictions especially concerning the sound quality and the bandwidth of the receiver. Therefore a certain amount of hearing loss is necessary for the unavoidable degradation of the sound passing through the miniature components of the hearing aid to be outperformed by the benefit that can be achieved through the amplification of the sound.

The individual hearing and communication needs, the degree and the configuration of the

Fig. 18.8 Key components of a hearing aid. Image copyright and with kind permission of Oticon

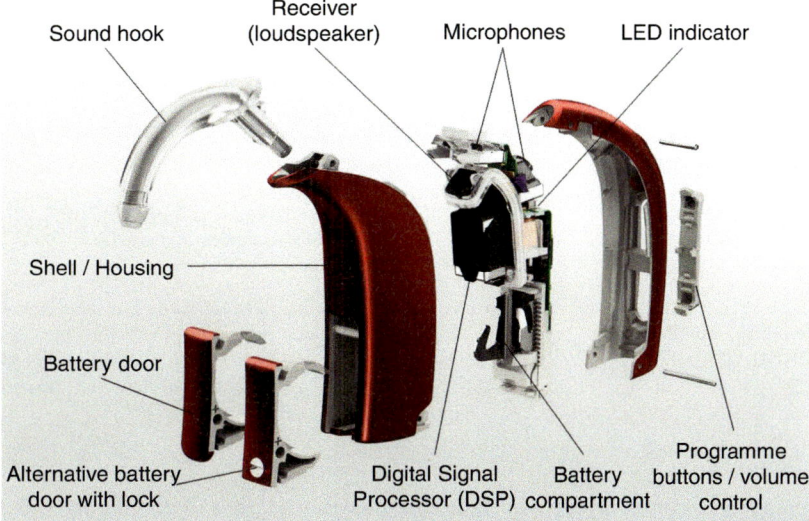

Sound hook   Receiver (loudspeaker)   Microphones   LED indicator

Shell / Housing

Battery door

Alternative battery door with lock   Digital Signal Processor (DSP)   Battery compartment   Programme buttons / volume control

hearing loss and a careful review of the achieved benefit have to be considered in combination with a rigorous fitting and verification protocol for a hearing aid to be successful.

18.4.2 Audiological Candidacy and Audiometric Preconditions

The basis for any hearing aid fitting is an as precise as possible audiometric evaluation, including a frequency-specific threshold. Whenever possible these data should be completed by an estimate of the residual dynamic range, speech audiometric data and a measurement of acoustic characteristics of the outer ear and ear canal. The extent of individual audiometric data that can be collected will depend on the hearing-impaired person's ability to cooperate.

For children the audiometric assessment will depend on their developmental age (DGPP 2012):

- From 0 to 6 months, the estimate of the threshold will be based on the frequency-specific ABR (auditory brainstem response) in combination with the results of a BOA (behavioural observation audiometry).
- Above 6 months, hearing reactions near the threshold can be achieved through VRA

(visual reinforcement audiometry), additionally used to estimate a frequency-specific hearing threshold.
- For children older than 2–3 years, it will be possible to teach them play audiometry.

Depending on the size of the ear canal and the air volume under the headphone, or between the tip of the ear mould and the eardrum, the sound pressure level at the eardrum differs from the reading at the dial of the audiometer. The sound pressure level will be higher at the eardrum for the smaller ear canals of children than at the bigger ear canals of adults. These differences can be calculated by taking into account the transfer characteristics of the transducer together with a measured correction factor for the individual ear canal. This calculated sound pressure level at the eardrum should then be the starting point for the programming algorithm of the hearing aid. For the verification process, it is additionally necessary to convert threshold data and measured hearing aid performance into the same scale unit (Fig. 18.9). For this purpose the data are mostly converted to dBSPL.

For children the programming algorithm also has to incorporate additional gain that is needed to give children enhanced audibility of speech sounds for their language acquisition, as they still do not have the capacity to "fill in the blanks" for

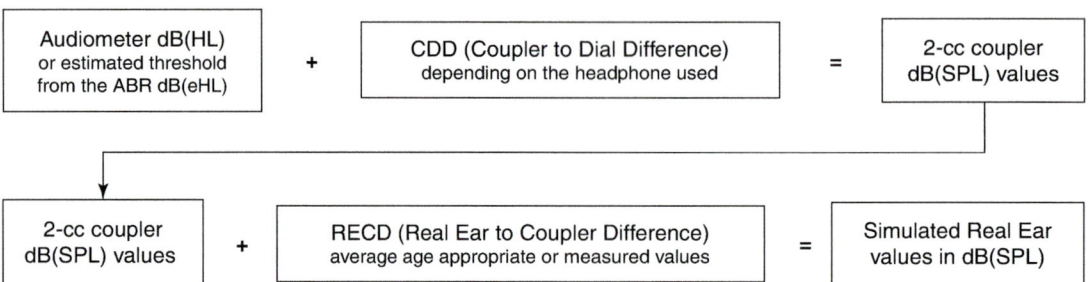

Fig. 18.9 Correcting for the increased sound pressure level in small volume ear canals, from "audiometer dB(HL) threshold values" to "simulated real ear values in dB (SPL)": flowchart describing the transformation of audiometer or ABR threshold values calibrated for the ear canal volume of adults in dB(HL) or dB (eHL estimated hearing level) into the corresponding dB(SPL) levels at the eardrum of the child by taking into account the smaller volume of the child's ear canal

inaudible sounds in the way that adult listeners do (American Academy of Audiology 2013).

As they still have to acquire their language skills, a hearing aid fitting should also be considered for children with very mild hearing losses of less than 30 dB and for children with unilateral hearing loss. After a trial period, the long-term provision of the hearing aid can only be justified if it can be proved that usable gain is provided and that a benefit in audibility can be expected.

For deaf children with additional needs, the assessment and the fitting should be provided by an experienced multi-professional team. For some of these children, the effect of their hearing loss on their development will be intensified by their additional handicaps, but for others hearing may be not their most urgent priority, or they may be very sensitive and easily overwhelmed by too much sound that they cannot differentiate.

18.4.3 Preparation of the Audiometric Data for Hearing Aid Fitting to Young Children

For the necessary conversions, some pre-existing correction factor tables can be used, such as dBHL to dBSPL, or the CDD values (coupler-to-dial difference), which are for a given transducer the difference between the audiometer dial reading and the corresponding sound pressure level in a 2 cc-coupler (which is used for measuring hearing aids). Other correction factors have to be measured individually, such as the RECD (real ear-to-coupler difference), which is the individual difference between the sound pressure level in the patient's ear canal and that of the same sound delivered to a 2 cc-coupler (Fig. 18.9). The RECD can even be measured in babies, but average RECD values for monthly age intervals are available (DGPP 2012; Western University of Ontario National Centre for Audiology 2014). To keep the necessary corrections as small as possible, it is highly recommended to use insert earphones for measuring tone audiometry as well as ABR thresholds with children.

By combining these correction factors, threshold values in dBHL from the audiometer (or ABR) can be converted to the corresponding dBSPL at the eardrum. When using ABR threshold data, one additionally has to bear in mind that, depending on the kind of stimulus (e.g. click, toneburst, notch-noise, chirp), the kind of method (classic ABR or ASSR) and the type of machine, the results will vary in regard to how close they get to the "real" threshold in different frequency areas. So for tonebursts or for most ASSR measurements at low frequencies such as 500 Hz, threshold levels that are 30 dB (±20 dB) louder than the "real" threshold are common. Therefore the use of frequency-specific corrections to get from the dial reading of the ABR machine (dBnHL decibel above normal adult hearing) to an estimate of the "real" threshold is necessary (Fig. 18.10).

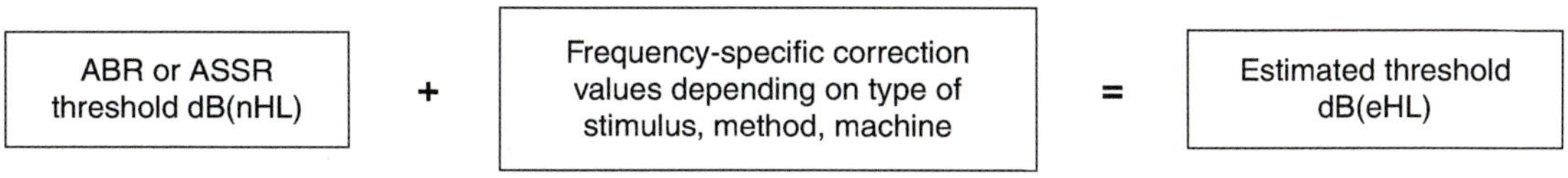

| ABR or ASSR threshold dB(nHL) | **+** | Frequency-specific correction values depending on type of stimulus, method, machine | **=** | Estimated threshold dB(eHL) |

Fig. 18.10 Correction factors and calculations for ABR results: flowchart describing the calculation of the "estimated threshold" by adding frequency-specific correction factors to the ABR/ASSR results

These corrections will differ from clinic to clinic (depending on their equipment) and can therefore only be performed by the professional who did the ABR measurement. But the final threshold estimate that will be used for the hearing aid fitting should not only include the data from the ABR but also a summary of all the audiometric data available at the end of the diagnostic process. The threshold estimate should be as close as possible to the threshold in dBHL that would be expected from the hearing-impaired person if he were able to cooperate fully in a tone audiometry procedure. These values can then be used in the hearing aid fitting software without further "ABR corrections" provided by the fitting software itself (this function must then be disabled in the software!).

18.4.4 Types of Hearing Aid

Hearing aids can be classified in very different ways, by the:
- Style of wearing: behind the ear (BTE), in the ear (ITE), in the ear canal (ITC), attached to glasses, body-worn, bone-anchored, partially or fully implanted (see Fig. 18.11)
- Amount of gain and maximum output
- Type of amplification: analogue, digital programmable, digital
- Type of sound processing: linear, compression, wideband compression, the number of frequency and compression channels, the number and kind of sound-processing programmes for different hearing situations, the way of switching between these programmes
- Type of receiver and the way of coupling the receiver to the ear: air conduction with standard tube and ear mould, with slim-tube, open fitting, external receiver in the ear canal, bone conduction

- Routing of signals: monaural, bilateral, contralateral routing of signal (CROS) with a microphone on the worse hearing side and the receiver in an open fitting on the better (normal)-hearing side or BiCROS with a microphone on both sides connected to one receiver on the better-hearing side
- Additional features that are available in a hearing aid: directional microphones, noise reduction, feedback cancellation
- Special features for children: a switch and volume control that can be deactivated, a tamper-proof battery compartment, moisture-resistant, an LED indicating the functioning of the hearing aid

In regard to the complexity of many digital hearing aids with a high number of additional features and the option of attaching further hearing devices directly to the hearing aid (streamer, FM systems, telephones, etc.), many professionals today prefer the term "hearing system" instead of "hearing aid".

The most widely used hearing aids in Europe are fully digital hearing aids with multi-frequency and multi-compression channels. For children up to primary school age, it is reasonable to use BTE hearing aids (American Academy of Audiology 2013), as they are the most robust devices and the ear moulds can be easily exchanged whenever the child grows and the ear mould starts leaking sound and produces feedback problems.

18.4.5 Types of Ear Mould

Ear moulds are necessary to channel the sound into the ear canal and to retain the hearing aid at the ear. The higher the gain of the hearing aid, the tighter the seal of the ear mould must be, to

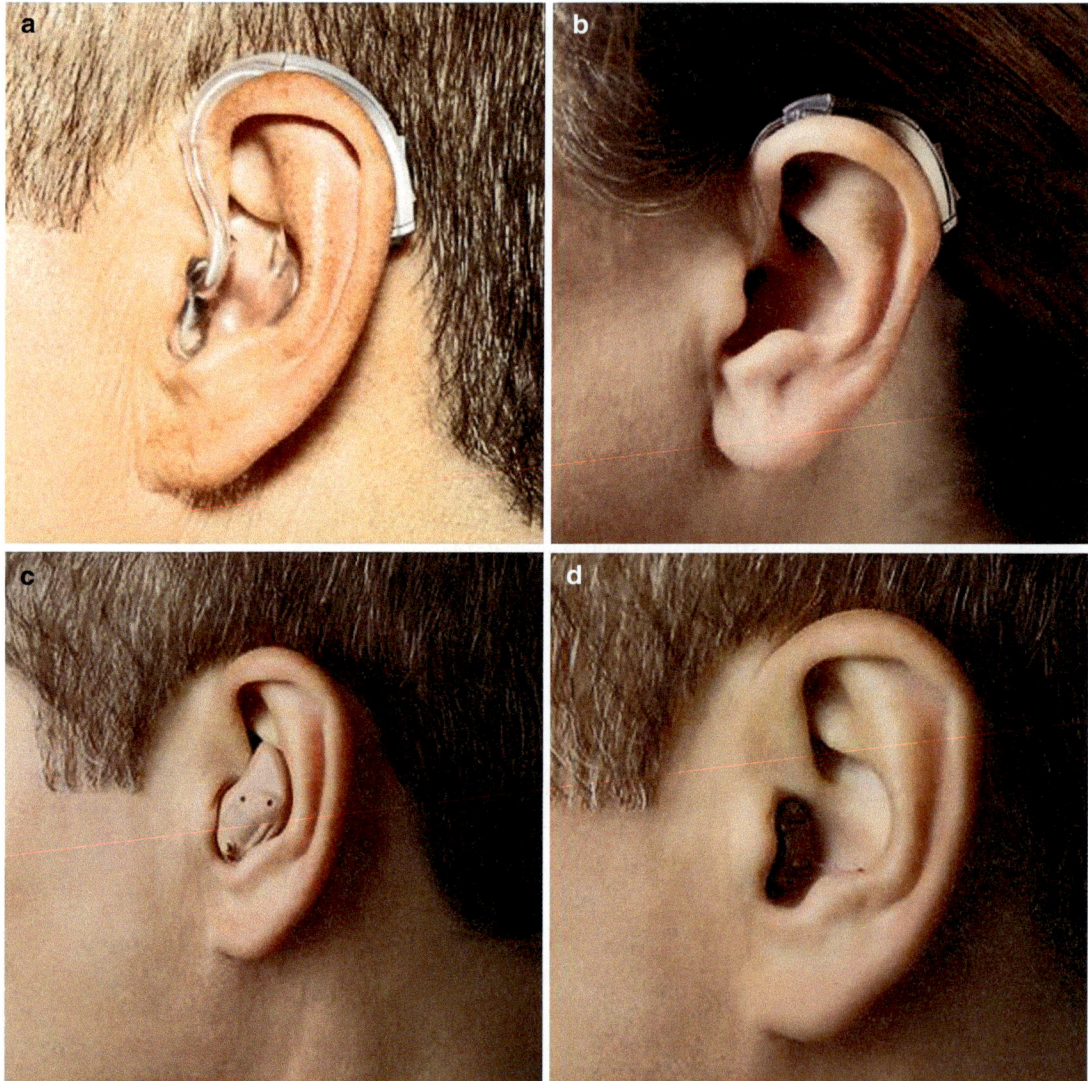

Fig. 18.11 Common hearing aid styles: (**a**) behind the ear (BTE) with ear mould, (**b**) BTE open fit, (**c**) in the ear (ITE), (**d**) in the canal (ITC). Images provided by Starkey

prevent feedback (whistling) (Fig. 18.12a). The length of the ear canal part of the ear mould determines the air volume that is left in front of the eardrum, and the smaller this volume is, the higher the sound pressure level at the eardrum becomes. The length, the diameter and the shape of the tubing in the ear mould influence significantly the frequency transmission into the ear canal. Therefore the ear mould is a part of the overall sound transmission of the hearing system, and it can enhance or degrade the performance

of a hearing aid. So the effect of the ear mould has to be taken into account with any verification process.

Ear moulds can be classified for their shape and function (Fig. 18.12a–g). Ear moulds may be "vented" by a second borehole in the ear mould that reduces the occlusion effect (complaints of fullness in the ear) and warms and ventilates the otherwise quite humid space between the ear mould and the eardrum. Especially in any case of otitis externa, a humid chamber may further

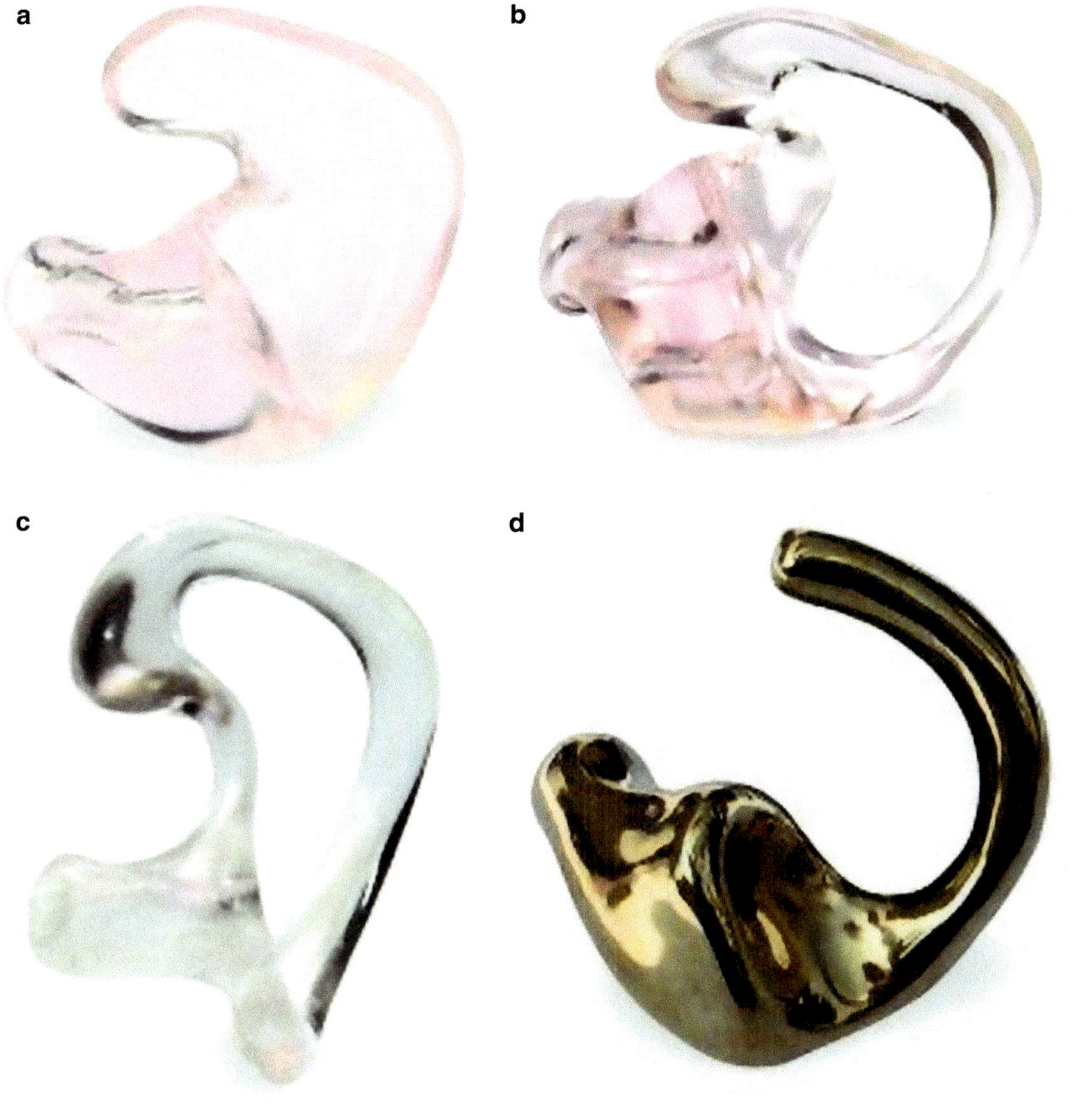

a

b

c

d

Fig. 18.12 (**a**) Shell ear mould. (**b**) Open ear mould fitting and venting. (**c**) Open ear mould fitting. (**d**) Gilded ear mould. (**e**) Titan ear mould. (**f**) THERMOtec® ear mould. (**g**) Ear mould with petal application. (**a–g**) Common varieties of ear mould. Images and copyright with kind permission by HEBA Otoplastik

e

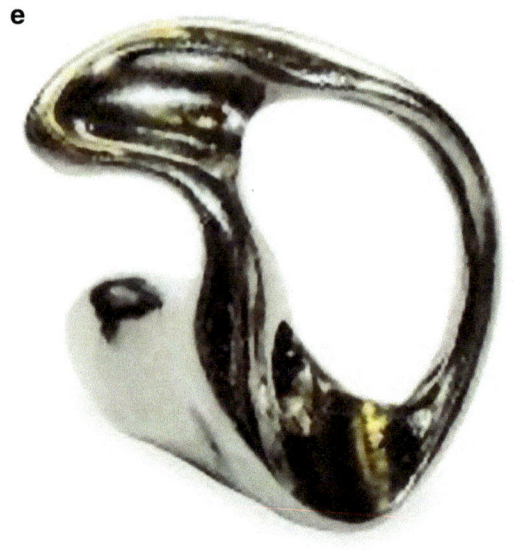

f

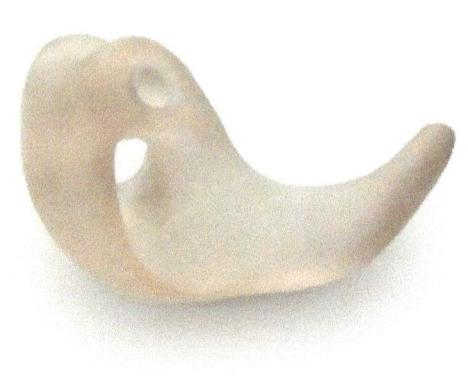

g

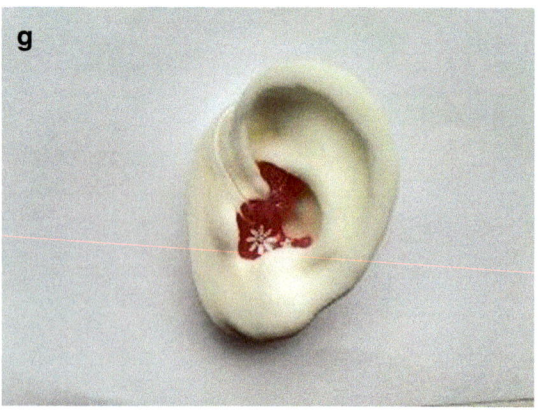

Fig. 18.12 (continued)

enhance the growth of bacteria and fungi in the ear canal.

Hearing loss of a lesser degree allows open ear mould fitting, which reduces the amount of occlusion and the contact to the skin of the ear canal and the pinna (Fig. 18.12b, c). Feedback cancellation systems or an increased distance between microphone and receiver may be necessary to avoid whistling artefacts.

For children the ear mould should be made from soft (normally silicone) material. In case of an allergy against one of the ear mould materials, there are alternative hypoallergenic materials available as well as special coatings (such as gilding of the ear mould or titanium ear moulds,

Fig. 18.12d, e). For more than moderate hearing losses, the length of the ear canal part should reach the second bend of the ear canal (American Academy of Audiology 2013; BIAP 2012), and the outlet of the ear mould must point in the direction of the eardrum. As children grow and the softer tissue of a child's ear will widen initially by the use of the ear mould, it may be necessary to renew ear moulds in babies every few weeks (BIAP 2012; DGPP 2012; Western University of Ontario National Center for Audiology 2014). Well-fitted and well-sealed ear moulds for babies with high-power hearing aids can prove to be a piece of art that needs a lot of experience and dedication.

A better sealing may be reached by a thermoplastic material (e.g. THERMOtec, Fig. 18.12f), which softens at body temperature, but it is more expensive, and because of the surface condition, more intensive cleaning (disinfection, ultrasonic cleaning) is necessary.

Ear moulds are available in many colours and with applications (e.g. comic motives or strass stones) suitable for children (Fig. 18.12g).

Please keep in mind that the making of any good ear mould starts with a perfect impression. During impression taking, penetration of the impression material in the middle ear through an unintended or pre-existent perforation of the eardrum is rarely reported but should strictly be avoided by careful handling and use of protective means in the ear canal, especially in patients with eardrum perforation or a tympanostomy tube (Silva et al. 2015).

As babies and young children cannot themselves complain specifically about hearing aid or ear mould problems that bother them, a tight quality control by the professionals is necessary. If there is any question of whether the sealing effect of an ear mould is sufficient, the seal of an ear mould should be measured. The necessary devices are available from the quality control measurements for noise protectors.

18.4.6 Selection and Fitting of the Hearing Aid

The degree and type of hearing loss will determine the amount of gain and maximum output level that is needed to make speech audible again. The age, the living conditions and the personal requirements of the hearing-impaired person will affect the choice of hearing aid type and hearing aid features. For children a robust hearing aid with a reliable repair service, a tamper-proof battery compartment, a volume control and switch that can be deactivated, a water-resistant shell and a direct audio input port to attach an FM receiver would be a suitable choice. It should be a digital, multichannel compression device (>4 channels) with a feedback-cancelling algorithm that does not affect the overall gain of the hearing aid.

In the programming software, select a fitting algorithm (prescription method) that is developed and validated for paediatric use and takes into account the unique developmental and auditory needs of children.

> Validation studies indicate high levels of speech recognition in controlled and real world environments when hearing aids are fitted using prescriptive targets generated by independently developed formulae such as the Desired Sensation Level (DSL) or National Acoustics Laboratories (NAL) prescriptions.
>
> (Quotation from American Academy of Audiology Clinical Practice Guidelines: Pediatric Amplification, June 2013) (American Academy of Audiology 2013; DGPP 2012; Western University of Ontario National Center for Audiology 2014).

Any person with bilateral hearing loss should be fitted bilaterally with hearing aids. There may be exemptions to this rule if it can be shown in the validation process that the second hearing aid compromises the hearing and understanding through the leading ear. In cases of asymmetrical losses, one should try to use the same hearing aid model on both sides. In the case of very asymmetrical losses, it may be necessary to use a more powerful hearing aid on the poorer hearing side, but it has to be shown that this hearing aid provides at least some benefit. With very young children, that proof of a benefit may not be achievable; therefore one may try to fit a hearing aid on the worse side as long as it is tolerated and does not provide feedback problems. In case of a profound hearing loss on the worse side, one may also consider a bimodal intervention with a cochlear implant on the profound side and a hearing aid on the better-hearing side.

(See also the paragraph "special issues".)

18.4.7 Selection of Hearing Aid Features

In addition to a number of frequency channels with wide range dynamic compression and an effective feedback suppression system, modern hearing aids may provide such features as an extended high-frequency bandwidth, techniques for frequency lowering (making high frequencies audible in the mid-frequency range), adaptable directional microphones, digital noise reduction and an automatic switching between different hearing programmes depending on the hearing situation of the child. The aims of the advanced features are an improvement in the perception of speech or music as well as in hearing comfort in adverse hearing situations. For children the use of these advanced features and especially the age at which these features should be activated have been discussed controversially for many years:

- One group of professionals argues that children in their first few years of life need the challenge of difficult hearing situations (without the help of advanced signal-processing features of the hearing aid) to develop their directional hearing skills and their skills to detect, differentiate and understand speech sounds in noisy situations.
- A second group of professionals argues that for the speech development of hearing-impaired children, it is necessary to provide them with the best quality of auditory input by using all technical means that are available. Therefore they advocate, for example, an early use of directional microphones and noise reduction systems. They also argue that until now (2016) the effectiveness of even the most advanced features is still limited and that under real-life circumstances, the systems may even lose up to 50% of their effectiveness compared with laboratory situations (such as those in the audiometry booth). So any side effects of these advanced features may also be much less than expected.

Very beneficial and in most cases not controversial are the following features:

- Binaural signal processing to provide the correct interaural time and loudness differences.
- Water resistance or even waterproof housings of the hearing aid, so that the hearing aid better survives moisture (when sweating) or the bathtub or swimming pool.
- Visual control for the caregivers (parents, teachers) of the functioning of a hearing aid

such as a control LED on the hearing aid or a bidirectional remote control, which informs them about the actual status of the hearing aid (on/off, battery status, programme). All acoustic control signals of the hearing aid, which can only be heard by the child and which are meaningless to the young child, should be switched off.
- Automated detection of a telephone next to the hearing aid and the channelling of the telephone sound into both hearing aids (not only the hearing aid on the side with the telephone receiver), when the child starts to use a telephone on its own. It should be deactivated for babies to avoid interference when the baby is on the mother's arm and the mother is using her phone.
- Reduction of wind noise to improve the comfort of hearing, as long as it does not decrease speech perception. Therefore the better options are algorithms that actively enhance speech recognition under wind noise conditions, which may be a relevant safety feature when cycling with a child.
- Wireless connection features that exceed the FM compatibility, by providing direct connections of the hearing aid to devices such as a smart phone. Such a feature can even be used by an app on the smart phone to locate and find a lost hearing aid (one of the nightmares for parents with hearing-impaired children).

It seems to be that in the recent past, more professionals are tending to follow the argument of the second group, for a more active use of the advanced features of hearing aids even with very young children, and especially utilising directional microphones and noise reduction systems. For the fitting of frequency-lowering techniques, see also the paragraph "verification". The use of directional microphones should not be started until the baby is more upright and no longer lying most of the time in its bed; otherwise the contact of the directional microphones with the pillows may add a lot of rubbing noises to the hearing signal.

As children and especially very young children are not able to switch between different hearing aid programmes according to their actual needs in different hearing situations (such as quiet, noisy, multi-talker background, music, external wireless microphones, etc.), they need a precise-as-possible automated classification of the hearing situation and an automatic adaptation of the hearing aid mode/programme to the hearing situation. Studies seem to indicate that children need different classification boundaries for switching the hearing aid mode than do adults and that these special needs for children may even be age-dependent. Manufacturers are just starting to implement these findings into their fitting algorithms.

As most children in Europe get good-quality hearing aids, but not the high-end hearing aids, the features that are available in the mid-range hearing aids are less sophisticated, or some of them even unavailable, compared with the hearing aid models that were used for the scientific studies. But with fewer frequency channels and reduced classification capabilities, even the features still available may be less useful or produce more side effects than the more sophisticated algorithms in the hearing aids used in the studies. So for directional microphones, only adaptive systems are acceptable that ensure in quiet situations that directionality is switched off and in noisy situations that dominant speakers located to the side of or behind the child can also be understood. To minimise any negative effect on the speech perception of the child, noise reduction systems need as many frequency channels as possible that can be separately regulated and a very good child- and age-related hearing situation classification algorithm that can make use of a variety of specialised hearing programmes. These necessary requirements tend to be only available in the most advanced (and therefore most expensive) high-end hearing aids. Until now it is an open question in most countries how this technology can be made available to all or at least most children. If only limited automated algorithms are available in a hearing aid, the risk increases for a number of hearing situations that inappropriate features may be activated by the hearing aid. For these hearing aids, it may be more advisable to restrict the activation of features

such as directional microphones or noise reduction systems to an often difficult case-by-case decision.

Some help for making the decision on whether and how to fit advanced data-logging algorithms may come from the data logging system of the hearing aids. Data-logging can provide an overview about the distribution of hearing situations that the child is confronted with in daily life (percentage of time in a quiet environment, in a noisy environment, in a multi-talker environment). An even better overview of the listening environment of children can be achieved by using sound recordings and communication analysis by the LENA system (LENA Research Foundation 2016).

18.4.8 Verification

Any hearing aid fitting requires a verification that the prescribed target gain, frequency range and prescribed maximum output levels are achieved for the individual conditions in the ear canal of the client. It has to be proved that the long-term average speech spectrum is made audible again. Such a technical control of the hearing aid performance is indispensable, especially when fitting hearing aids to children, as validation measurements are much more difficult and less reliable than with adults. Audibility and how well the hearing aid output data match the prescribed targets can be best evaluated when targets, output data and the hearing threshold of the patient are displayed in one graph. Such a display can be achieved with an SPLogram or with a percentile measurement (Fig. 18.13).

As most advanced hearing aids use speech-sensitive processing algorithms, it is necessary to use speech itself as a stimulus for the verification measurements, such as the International Speech Test Signal ISTS (American Academy of Audiology 2013; BIAP 2012; DGPP 2012). With this signal the performance of the hearing aid for soft, moderate and loud speech can be tested. For testing the maximum output tonebursts, warble and sinus tones at 90 dB are used. With these the maximum output level of digital

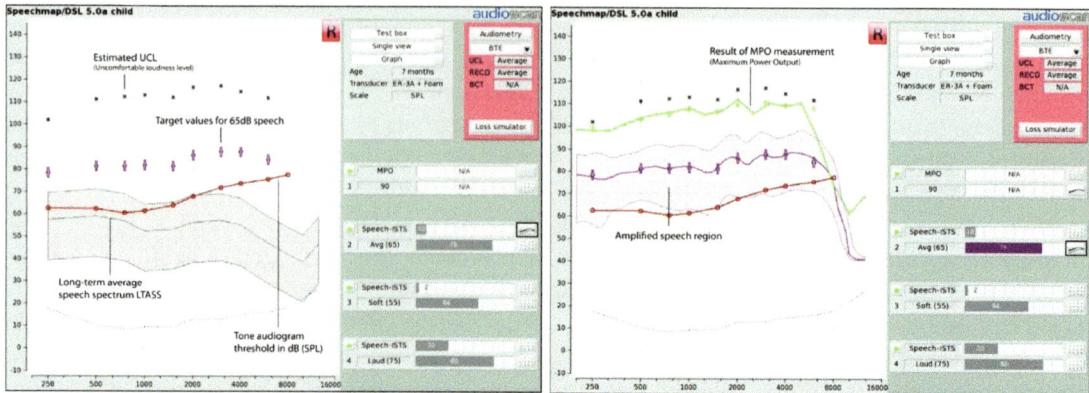

Fig. 18.13 The SPLogram (or a percentile measurement) gives a comprehensive overview of the audibility of the long-term average speech spectrum (LTASS) that can be achieved through the hearing aid amplification, by dis-playing the patient's hearing threshold, the targets of the fitting algorithm and the verification measurements of the hearing aid all in the same diagram (example from a measurement with the Audioscan Verifit®)

multi-compression hearing aids may be underestimated; therefore more suitable broadband test signals are in preparation.

The SPLogram or the percentile measurement provides an easy-to-read overview for the audiologist but also for other professionals (early interventionist, teachers, speech therapists) and for the parents, comprising:

- Whether the full frequency range of speech sounds is audible.
- In which frequency area a need for optimisation still exists or even a change of the hearing aid model or technology is necessary to meet the prescribed targets.
- Whether the dynamic field is well used.
- Whether even after maximum effort of optimisation, including an optimisation of the ear mould characteristics, a significant lack of speech audibility still remains, so that different means of amplification such as cochlear implants have to be considered.

The SPLogram or the percentile measurement also provides a unique opportunity for a well-controlled and well-targeted approach for finding the cause of complaints by the client or a rejection of a hearing aid by a child. These measurements will also provide the necessary data to enhance certain frequency areas when the speech audiometry, speech testing or the speech development shows deficits for some speech sounds.

For the verification of some hearing aid features, specific tests are necessary:

- As the effectiveness of directional microphone systems in hearing aids can be very different and can be over- or under-estimated from the technical data provided by the manufacturers, a visualisation of the directional microphone effect can be obtained from some of the hearing aid test box systems.
- Frequency-lowering techniques may provide an alternative for achieving audibility for high-frequency speech sounds if all other means of amplification fail, especially with moderate-to-profound high-frequency hearing loss. The benefit of such systems must be controlled through an SPLogram with special high-frequency test signals or through behavioural validation (e.g. phoneme tests).

> Frequency lowering should be treated as a form of distortion purposefully introduced to the amplified pathway. Fine tuning and the accompanying verification and outcome assessment should have the goal of providing the least possible effect (distortion) that allows access to high frequency sound.
>
> (Quotation from American Academy of Audiology Clinical Practice Guidelines: Pediatric Amplification, June 2013)

18.4.9 Validation

The hearing test options to validate the benefit of hearing aids are often the same procedures that are used in the diagnostic process before the hearing aid fitting, so that the test results without amplification can be compared with the results from the hearing device. The choice of testing options again depends on the developmental age, the ability to cooperate and, for speech audiometry, the speech and language skills of the hearing aid wearer:

- Hearing reactions with hearing aids: BOA for children who are too young for VRA
- Aided thresholds (American Academy of Audiology 2013; BIAP 2012; DGPP 2012):
  - VRA-aided threshold
  - Play audiometry-aided threshold
- Speech sound detection, discrimination and identification (e.g. LING Test, A§E)
- Speech audiometry (close set, open set, adaptive)
- Speech in noise
- Testing of directional hearing
- Loudness scaling in different frequency areas
- Testing the tolerance for loud sounds and noise
- Anamnesis including parents, therapist, early interventionist, kindergarten teacher, etc.
- Age-appropriate questionnaires (BIAP 2012; DGPP 2012)

All these tests may provide valuable information about the performance and benefit, or the still remaining deficiencies, of a hearing aid fitting. But each of these tests has its strengths and pitfalls.

For aided thresholds (American Academy of Audiology 2013):
- They prove the audibility of soft sounds in the tested frequency range.
- The results may be corrupted by poor cooperation of the child.
- They do not provide information from moderate and loud input levels.

- The test stimulus (warble tone, narrow band noise) may be processed differently by the hearing aid than speech.
- They cannot substitute verification measurements (as can the SPLogram)!

Speech sound detection, discrimination and identification:
- It is possible to get reliable results even through VRA and VRA with an oddball paradigm.
- With young children, experienced staff and frequent testing sessions are needed to have sufficient access to time slots when the child is in a good to optimal testing condition and to replicate results.

Speech audiometry:
- Speech audiometry tackles one of the major goals of most hearing aid fitting, how much improvement in word and sentence understanding can be achieved by the hearing aids.
- The test results strongly depend on the ability to concentrate and cooperate; the vocabulary, speech, language and cognitive skills; and the ability to fill in missing parts of speech information.
- For children, testing material that is adequate for their developmental age is necessary, and for children with limited expressive vocabulary, a picture-pointing task is necessary to assess their understanding of the test items.
- To assess small speech discrimination differences between different hearing aids or hearing aid settings, a speech audiometry test with a steep discrimination function is necessary.

Speech in noise:
- Speech-in-noise testing tries to simulate degradation of speech understandability in everyday life. The results are an important indicator of how well the hearing-impaired person will cope in difficult listening situations.
- The type of noise, the loudspeaker setting (e.g. direction of the speech and the noise) and the room acoustics significantly affect the test results. The type of noise and the loudspeaker

setting should always be documented together with the test results.

- Computer-controlled adaptive measurements of the signal-to-noise ratio (SNR) can be a reliable and time-efficient way to test speech in noise with children. As part of an adaptive procedure, children even tolerate and cooperate with the difficult testing for an SNR aimed at the understanding of just 50% of the test items, because the adaptive paradigm ensures that the children cannot fail a test totally, but always experience a partial success of 50%.

As any audiometry testing with the hearing aids can only provide data that are limited by the special and sometimes quite "artificial" test circumstances, the validation procedure must include a good anamnesis of the hearing performance and difficulties in daily life, as well as any concerns about the use of the hearing aids. The anamnesis can be supported by a questionnaire in the form of a structured interview. Questionnaires are also an efficient way of obtaining information about the progress of the child with the hearing aids from other team members, and they permit a good opportunity to monitor the progress of a hearing aid fitting process.

Memory box: A hearing aid fitting of children should only be finalised if audibility of speech sounds is secured as far as possible. This has to be documented by a measurement of the hearing aid output in relation to the child's hearing threshold and the child's uncomfortable loudness threshold (e.g. through an SPLogram or percentile measurement). The hearing aid benefit must be additionally validated by audiometric tests (speech audiometry and aided thresholds) as well as reports by the child's caregivers.

18.4.10 Interdisciplinary Cooperation

Audiological assessment, hearing aid fitting and early intervention have to be a part of a holistic family-centred approach to meet the needs of a hearing-impaired child and its family. All stakeholders in this approach have to cooperate closely and transparently. Everyone has to ensure that the other professionals receive information and data that they need to fulfil their task timely and in a way that the data can be used with a minimised risk of misinterpretation. Any doubts and criticism should be exchanged directly and respectfully among the professionals. The different supplementary points of view can provide the opportunity of self-control and self-reflection. Such interdisciplinary cooperation also provides valuable self-protection in the difficult assessment and intervention process, so that needs of improvement and change can be identified as early as possible. Important steps in the intervention process, such as finalising the hearing aid fitting, suggesting a cochlear implantation or changing the mode of communication, should be taken in consent with the other professionals involved.

18.4.11 Special Issues

Mild Hearing Loss Because of newborn hearing screening, mild hearing losses are increasingly often detected very early. As children still have to develop language, even a mild hearing loss may affect their development or their performance at school. Therefore one may advocate that children try out hearing aids even at the limit between the upper range of "normal" hearing and the lower end of the mild hearing loss range (BIAP classification). In any case the pros and cons have to be well discussed with the parents. Until now insufficient data are available about the age when a hearing aid fitting has to be started. Depending on the amount of hearing loss in Germany, we recommend trying out hearing aids within the first year of life (BIAP 2012). Before starting a hearing aid fitting, the hearing threshold of the child has to be confirmed. On this basis one has to verify through an SPLogram or percentile measurement that an increase in audibility can be achieved and that the hearing aids have to be well accepted by the child. Internal noise of the hearing aid should be as small as possible.

Unilateral Hearing Loss Unilateral hearing losses affect especially directional hearing and speech understanding in noise. These two areas of concern become more relevant for children when they enter kindergarten and later on school. But directional hearing and understanding in noise must be learned by the child; animal experiments suggest that this learning has to take place in the first few years of life. Therefore binaural hearing should be established through hearing devices (BIAP 2012):

- 0–30 dB unilateral hearing loss: a hearing aid will not provide significant benefit, and the asymmetry of hearing will be at least partly compensated for by central processing.
- 30–60 dB unilateral hearing loss: a hearing aid may lead to a bilateral hearing with some directional hearing and better understanding in noisy situations.
- >60 dB unilateral hearing loss: it is increasingly difficult to achieve a quality and loudness level on the hearing-impaired ear that reaches the range of the normal-hearing ear, and therefore it will no longer be possible to achieve an effective binaural hearing. In these cases a cochlear implant may provide a solution.
- Remember: a CROS system cannot provide binaural hearing, as the sound from the hearing-impaired ear is channelled to the normal-hearing ear, and one still hears only with one ear. Such a system should only be prescribed for patients who can selectively switch the CROS microphone on and off, depending on whether there is just noise or useful information on the hearing-impaired side (American Academy of Audiology 2013; BIAP 2012). This may be feasible for adolescents.

For children who are already 4–5 years old and who may be already too old for learning directional hearing, a BiCROS system with fully automatic adaptive directional microphones may provide some help in noisy situations, such as at school. To enhance the SNR at school, the use of a FM system can be an option.

Auditory Synaptopathy BR thresholds do not provide a reliable basis for a hearing aid fitting; therefore subjective thresholds are necessary. With babies it may be necessary to wait for a hearing aid fitting until these subjective thresholds can be established (e.g. through VRA). The hearing aids will then be programmed according to the subjective threshold results. Hearing and understanding that can be achieved by hearing aids may be worse than with other types of hearing loss. Therefore the hearing performance and speech development have to be closely monitored. If hearing aids cannot provide sufficient benefit, a cochlear implant may bring better results (BIAP 2012).

Atresia A bilateral hearing loss should be treated with a bone conduction hearing aid before the age of 6 months, as for any moderate or severe sensorineural hearing loss. For babies the bone conduction hearing aid will mostly be fixed with a headband. Later a bone-anchored hearing aid or an implanted bone conduction or middle ear implant may provide further options. With a unilateral atresia, the fitting of a single-sided bone conductor should be tried within the first year of life.

Chronic Otitis Media with Effusion The usual remedy will be the provision of grommets. If repeated grommets prove unsuccessful, or if a child cannot get general anaesthesia for the insertion of grommets, the fitting of hearing aids may be an effective way to compensate a long-lasting conductive hearing loss.

Dead Regions Providing amplification in a dead region area may lead to off-frequency hearing and uncomfortable and distorted sounds. Therefore maximum amplification in dead region areas should be avoided. One should try to transpose the information from the frequency area of the dead regions into an area where hair cells and hearing are still preserved.

Steep-Sloping High-Frequency Hearing Loss High-frequency speech sound information is essential for speech understanding, articulation and perceiving and learning grammatical cues of language. It is therefore necessary to provide, verify and validate sufficient audibility of high-frequency speech sounds. A better transmission of these speech sounds may be supported by hearing aids with an extended high-frequency bandwidth, by the use of external receivers and by special trumpet-like tubes in the ear mould. If all these efforts cannot provide enough audibility of high-frequency speech sound, "frequency-lowering techniques" (such as transposition or frequency compression) may make high-frequency speech information usable again.

Low-Frequency Hearing Loss Especially if there is still nearly normal hearing in the higher-frequency areas, amplification just in the lower frequencies needs to be carefully considered, as many environmental noises have their maximum impact in the lower-frequency areas, and an amplification of environmental noises can lead to a masking of speech sounds and consecutively to less speech understanding.

Bimodal: Hearing Aid and CI In case of an asymmetrical hearing loss, a cochlear implant on the side with the profound hearing loss and a conventional hearing aid on the better-hearing side can be the most adequate way of amplification, as the better transmission of the lower frequencies by the hearing aid and the better transmission of the higher frequencies by the cochlear implant can supplement each other (American Academy of Audiology 2013). After fitting the cochlear implant and the hearing aid individually to the target values (especially optimising speech understanding), it is necessary to balance the loudness perception through both devices to equal levels. "Loudness scaling" can help to achieve this goal.

Multiple Disabilities Hearing-impaired children with additional handicaps often have complex needs and provide a number of challenges for their parents and the professionals that may result in:

- Fewer diagnostic data
- Less reliable thresholds
- Less reliable ABR
- More middle ear problems
- Less cooperation

Therefore it is necessary always to crosscheck all test results, e.g. ABR versus VRA or BOA data, and the audiometric data versus reports about hearing reactions by the parents! Only a conclusive summary of all these data sources can be an acceptable basis for a diagnosis and basis for a hearing aid fitting.

The developmental delays and a different ability of perception may also lead to different goals for a fitting of hearing aids and eventually to different fitting strategies:

- To ensure a short distance to the auditory input, these children often need a very close and direct contact with the speaker.
- The hearing aid should make sounds and speech audible to these children, but as speaking on their own may be a secondary and more long-term goal, the speech development mostly cannot be used as a scale for the success of a hearing aid fitting.
- Being able to hear sounds can already be very valuable to these children, as it makes the environment for the child more predictable, and the voices and noises by the family are reassuring for the child.

Concerning the amount of amplification, one may have to consider that multiple disabilities may magnify the effect of hearing loss and therefore emphasise the need of compensation, but some of these children can also get more easily overwhelmed by sound and noise as they are less able to pick and listen selectively to the relevant sound source in a noisy environment. A well-documented verification of the applied gain and output characteristics provides the necessary data for a targeted fine-tuning of the hearing aid according to the needs, reactions and acceptance by the child.

These children can be highly selective in the sounds they are reacting to. Therefore listen to the family and ask about sounds that are familiar and of interest to the child. Try to integrate these sounds into your hearing evaluation (with and without hearing aids).

Please also keep in mind that for some multi-handicapped children, their hearing problem may be an important but not the most urgent problem the families have to deal with first, so that diagnostic procedures and hearing rehabilitation efforts have to be postponed. But even then keep in touch with family, and try to find the most appropriate way of assessment and support for this family.

18.5   Special Knowledge of Bone-Anchored Hearing Aids and Implantable Hearing Aids

Martin Kompis

18.5.1 Implantable Hearing Aids

Today, the majority of all implanted hearing aids are semi-implantable, i.e. they consist of an implanted part, always containing at least the interface, which delivers acoustic energy to some part of the ear or the skull of the user, and an externally worn part, which contains at least the energy source of the device, the microphone and an interface, which allow communication with the implanted part. From the considerable number of devices that have been developed and presented so far, the majority has been abandoned, and only a few systems have been implanted in more than 1000 users. However, implantable hearing aids are a very active area of research, so new designs and devices can be expected to become available in the future.

Implantable hearing aids can be classified according to different features. From the audiological point of view, it is useful to differentiate between:

(a) Devices that inject their acoustic output signal along the normal air conduction path or close to it, i.e. at the tympanic membrane, or

one of the ossicles, including the stapes footplate or the round window
(b) Devices that use the bone conduction (BC) path to transfer acoustic energy to the skull at some point at least some distance away from the physiological air conduction path
(c) Cochlear implants, which stimulate the inner ear directly electrically

Today, implantable or semi-implantable hearing aids of the type described by (a) that drive the ossicular chain are used only relatively rarely in children. At some centres, they are used to treat aural atresia in children. Currently, however, at most centres even for this indication, one of the solutions of type (b) discussed further below is preferred. Indications for cochlear implants (c), finally, will be covered in Sect. 18.6.

18.5.2 Bone-Conduction (BC) Hearing Aids

BC hearing aids can be subdivided into implantable and non-implantable systems, both of which are used regularly in children (McDermott and Sheehan 2011). Some special features are shared by both kinds of system; some are specific to either implantable or non-implantable systems.

18.5.2.1 General Audiological Features of All Bone-Conduction Hearing Systems

There are a number of important audiological differences between conventional (i.e. air conduction) hearing aids and BC hearing systems, either implantable or non-implantable (Stenfelt 2011). Here is a short list:

Stimulation at the Inner Ear Is Largely Independent of a Conductive Component As the normal conductive pathway through the external auditory canal and the middle ear is bypassed, the effective stimulation of the inner ear is (almost) independent of the amount of conductive hearing loss. This can be a desirable feature, e.g. in children with a fluctuating conductive hearing loss, as the subjective impression will be almost independent of the current state of the middle ear without the need of any adjustments to the aid.

Limited Maximum Power Output (MPO) and Amplification Bone conduction is an inefficient way to transfer acoustic energy to the inner ear. As a consequence, the MPO is much lower in BC aids than in conventional hearing aids, often as low as an equivalent stimulation with 56–85 dB HL (Snik 2017). This includes very recent high-power devices such as the Baha 5 superpower in which a cable connects the power transducer to a behind-the-ear (BTE) sound processor. Likewise, amplification is limited by the MPO, as too high amplification would compress everyday sound levels to values close to the MPO and feedback problems may arise in certain situations.

Binaural Stimulation As the transcranial attenuation is much lower (order of magnitude 5–15 dB with a large variability both individually and across frequencies) than that for air conduction (at least 50 dB, depending on the acoustic transducer used), usually both inner ears are stimulated, even if only one BC hearing aid is used. This feature is exploited for so-called BC-CROS stimulation in unilateral profound sensorineural deafness. It is interesting to note, and of practical importance, that true binaural hearing is nevertheless possible and useful for patients, who use two BC hearing aids bilaterally.

Correction Is Limited Almost Completely to the Conductive Component of a Hearing Loss As a consequence of the above-listed features, bone conduction hearing aids are excellent for the correction of conductive hearing losses, even if they are very large, but rather poor when used to correct sensorineural hearing losses or sensorineural components of hearing losses. The only noteworthy exception is BC-CROS for unilateral sensorineural deafness, where the deafness is not truly corrected, but rather the signal is transmitted to the better-hearing ear. As inner ear function is often perfect in children, results with BC hearing aids are often better in children than in adults.

Unusual Feedback Paths In BC hearing aids, acoustic feedback paths, which are different from those of air conduction hearing aids, can occur. One important additional path is the vibration of the entire skull by the BC hearing aid, which then emits low-level acoustic signal from the head surface to the microphones of the hearing aids both at the ipsilateral and the contralateral side of the head.

18.5.2.2 Non-Implantable Bone-Conduction Hearing Aids

Non-implantable BC hearing aids are easy to use and can be fitted quickly in children. No surgery is needed, and several different systems from different manufacturers, as well as a number of methods to attach the transducer to the head of the child, are available (Verstraeten et al. 2009). Figure 18.14 shows a girl wearing a BC aid on a softband, and Fig. 18.15 a shows the same aid attached to a headband. At some centres, BC hearing aids are not fitted much before the age of approximately 6 months, as indentations in the softer skull of very young children are more frequent. A number of current systems are shown in

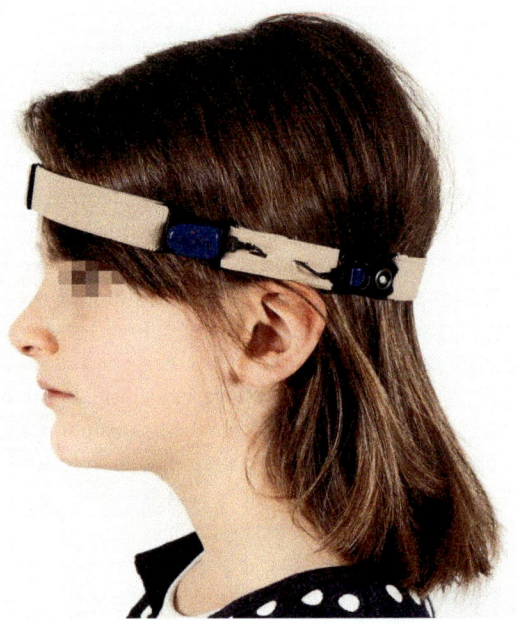

Fig. 18.14 Example of a non-implantable bone conduction hearing aid in use (contact mini, with kind permission from BHM Inc.). For better visibility, the transducer is worn over the hair for this photo only. In practice, it is worn under the hair, in contact with the skin. Photo with kind permission from the parents

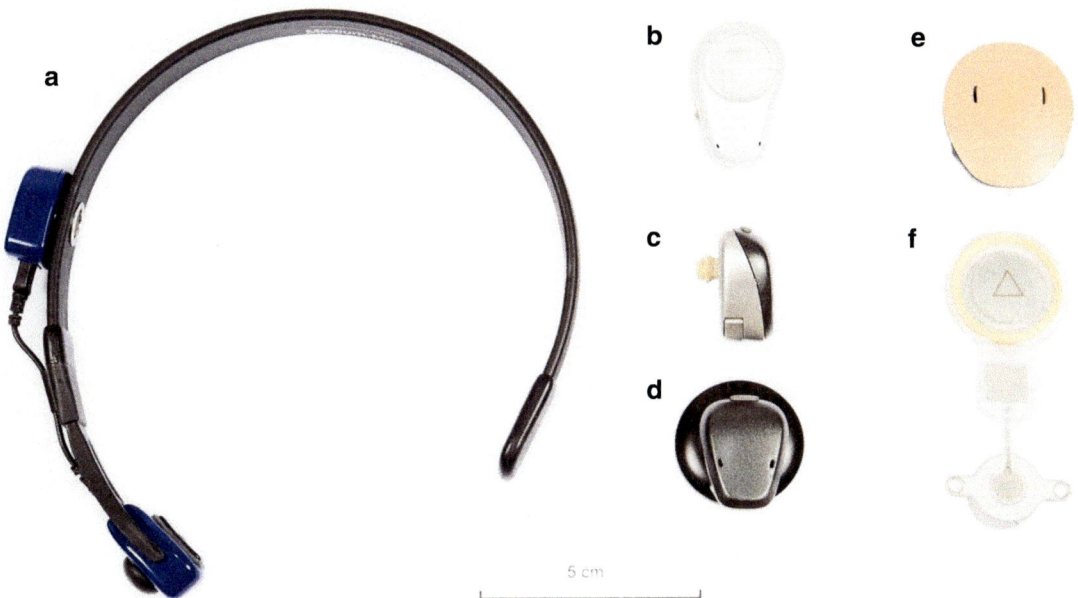

Fig. 18.15 Selection of several current implantable and non-implantable bone-conduction (BC) hearing aids. (**a**) BC aid worn on a headband (contact mini, with kind permission from BHM). (**b**) and (**c**) BC sound processors: (**b**) Ponto plus (with kind permission from Oticon Medical) and (**c**) Baha 5 (with kind permission from Cochlear Inc.). (**d**) Transcutaneous device with external magnetic plate attached, Baha Attract (with kind permission from Cochlear Inc.). (**e**) and (**f**) Active transcutaneous BC devices (Vibrant Bonebridge, with kind permission from MED-EL Inc.) with the (**e**) sound processor and the (**f**) implant with the transducer

Figs. 18.14 and 18.15. They include strictly non-implantable devices, such as the contact mini (BHM Inc., Figs. 18.14 and 18.15a), the Ponto series devices (Oticon Medical, Fig. 18.15b) and the Baha series devices (Cochlear Inc., Fig. 18.15c), which can be used either with headbands, softbands or implants.

Currently, new systems are introduced frequently. Figure 18.16 shows two recent additions. In the ADHEAR system (MED-EL Inc., Fig. 18.16a), an adhesive adapter is placed behind the ear and can stay there for several days, before it is replaced by a new adhesive adapter. An audio processor is then snapped on the protruding adapter pin of the adhesive part. In the SoundArc System (Cochlear Inc., Fig. 18.16b), a sound processor is attached to a flexible arc, which is worn just above the ears and passes behind the head of the user, thus improving the cosmetic aspect considerably, when compared to the softband or the headband. One or two processors can be worn on the same arc.

Acoustic overstimulation of the inner ear is not possible with any of the current devices.

18.5.2.3 Implantable Bone-Conduction Hearing Aids

Currently, three basic types of implantable BC hearing aid are available. The oldest principle, the bone-anchored aid, has now been used for over 35 years. It consists of a percutaneous titanium implant to which an external sound processor is attached (Kurz et al. 2013). Figure 18.15b, c shows current sound processors, and Fig. 18.16b shows a model of such a system.

For the second type of implantable BC hearing aid, the same sound processors can be used, but the coupling to the skull is transcutaneous (Kurz et al. 2014). An implanted magnetic plate is connected to the skull and attracts an external magnetic plate, to which a sound processor is attached. The skin between the two magnetic plates remains intact and results in a small attenuation predominantly at

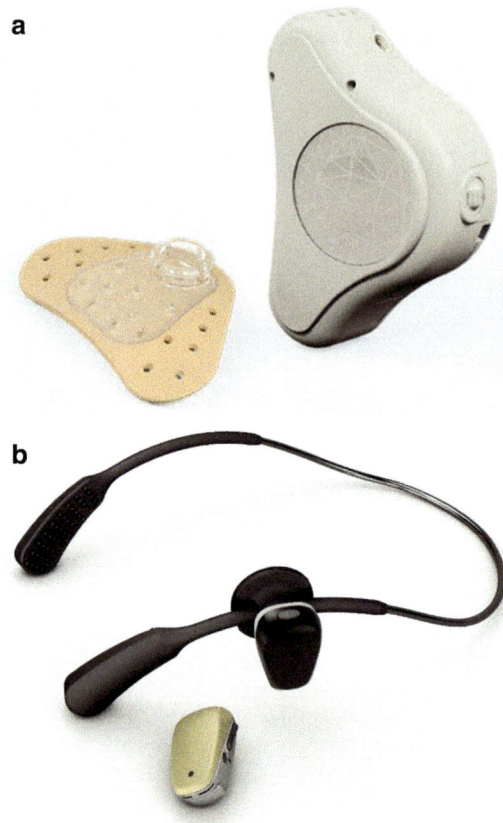

a

b

Fig. 18.16 Two recent additions to the selection of methods to wear a non-implantable BC hearing aid: (**a**) ADHEAR system (MED-EL Inc.) with an adhesive adapter to be placed behind the ear and a matching sound processor and (**b**) the SoundArc (Cochlear Inc.) to which one or two sound processors can be attached in an unobtrusive way. Images copyright and with kind permission of MED-EL Inc. and Cochlear Inc., respectively

frequencies above 2 kHz. Figures 18.15d and 18.17 a show the external components of such a transcutaneous system.

Similarly, the skin remains intact in the third type of implantable BC-device, shown in Fig. 18.15e, f (Zernotti and Sarasty 2015). Here, the transducer is implanted and is therefore attached directly to the skull, ensuring good acoustic coupling.

For children with a perfect inner ear function, the performance of these three types of implantable BC hearing aid can be expected to be comparable.

18.6 Cochlear Implant: Technology, Candidacy and Rehabilitation

Dirk Mürbe

18.6.1 Cochlear Implantation: Basic Principles

Cochlear implantation is an accepted method of treatment for children and adults with severe-to-profound hearing loss who derive insufficient benefit from conventional hearing devices (Wilson and Dorman 2008; Holden et al. 2013). A cochlear implant (CI) evokes auditory sensation via direct electrical stimulation of the auditory pathways by converting acoustic signals into coded electrical pulses. These electrical pulses stimulate nerve fibres in the cochlea. The auditory nerve transmits the signals to the brain where they are interpreted as sounds (Clark 2003; Peterson et al. 2010).

A CI consists of internal components, which are surgically implanted under the skin, and external components, which are worn behind the ear (Fig. 18.18).

CI provision is not limited to the surgical issue of implantation which is presented in Sect. 18.24.

CI provision includes careful preoperative (ped)audiologic assessment and counselling and post-operative (re)habilitation. The latter starts with the initial fitting of the implant and covers a period of 2–3 years, depending on the CI user's age and communication status.

18.6.2 Cochlear Implant Technology

Components The internal components of a CI, which are surgically placed under the skin behind the ear, consist of (1) the implant, including the receiver and the magnet, and (2) the electrode array, including the electrode contacts. The implant contains the electronic device for signal processing. The electrode array is surgically placed within the cochlea and contains 12–22 electrodes for

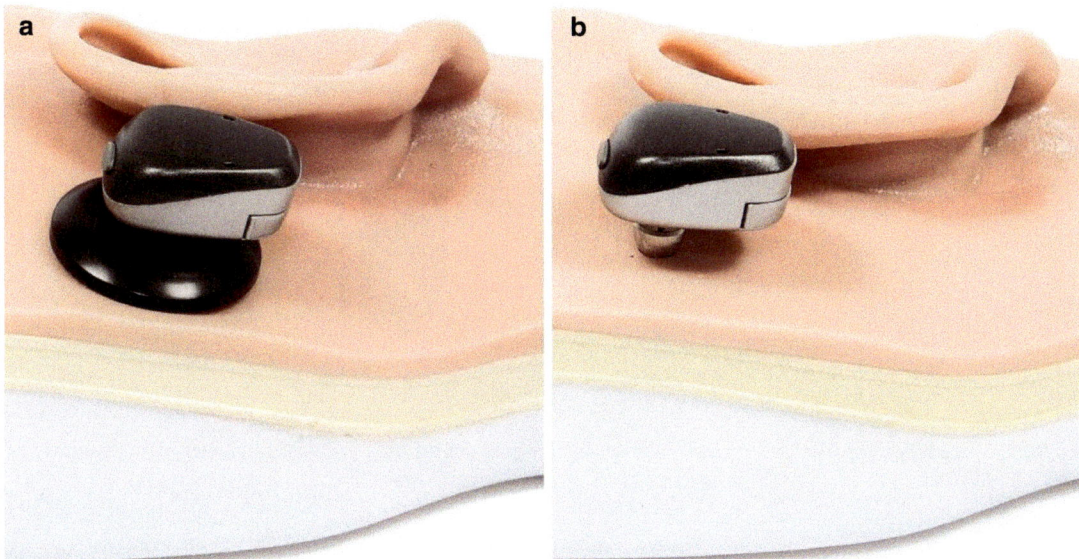

Fig. 18.17 Models of (**a**) a transcutaneous BC system showing the external magnetic plate and (**b**) a percutaneous BC system with the titanium implant visible, both using the same sound processor (Baha 5, with kind permission from Cochlear Inc.)

Fig. 18.18 Cochlear implant system with implanted internal components and the external behind-the-ear processor (courtesy of MED-EL, Austria)

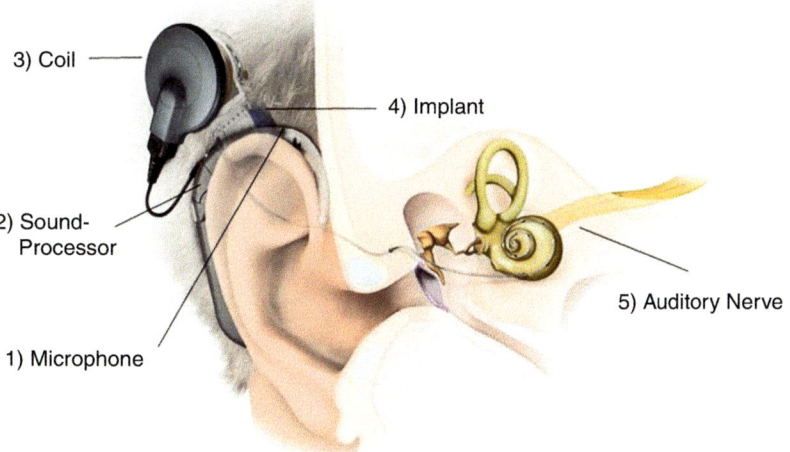

stimulating the nerve fibres within the cochlea. The external components are worn behind the ear and consist of the sound processor with microphone, the battery pack, the coil, the magnet and a cable connecting the sound processor and the coil. The sound processor contains the electronic device for signal processing (Zeng et al. 2008). The external coil is held in place behind the ear via external and internal magnets (Fig. 18.19).

Signal Processing The starting point of signal processing is the microphone of the external sound processor, which converts acoustic sound into an electrical signal. The electronic device of the sound processor analyses and codes this signal into a special pattern of digital information by using a coding strategy. The coil transcutaneously transmits the coded electrical signal to the receiver. The internal electronic device decodes

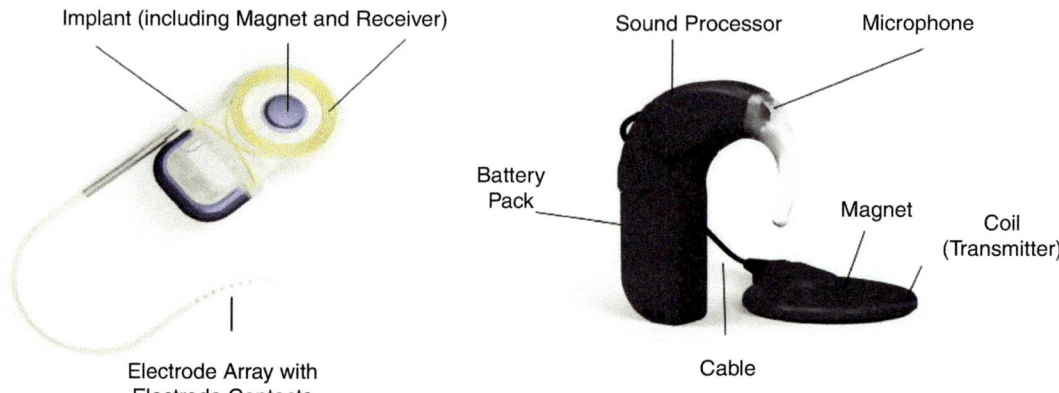

Fig. 18.19 Internal components (left) and external components (right) of a cochlear implant system (courtesy of MED-EL, Austria)

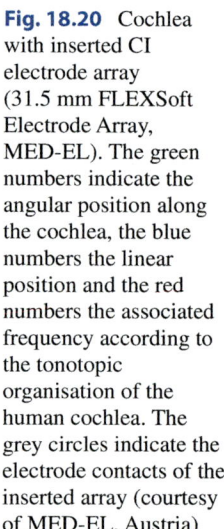

Fig. 18.20 Cochlea with inserted CI electrode array (31.5 mm FLEXSoft Electrode Array, MED-EL). The green numbers indicate the angular position along the cochlea, the blue numbers the linear position and the red numbers the associated frequency according to the tonotopic organisation of the human cochlea. The grey circles indicate the electrode contacts of the inserted array (courtesy of MED-EL, Austria)

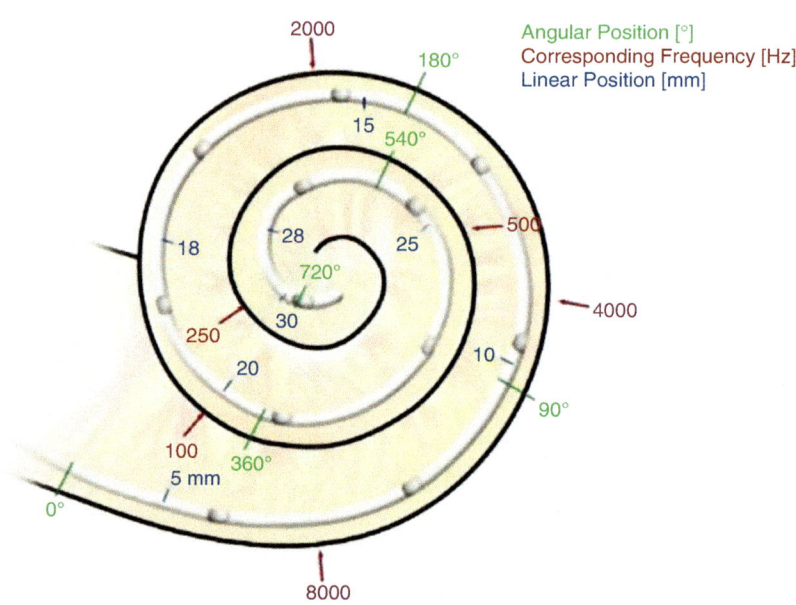

the transmitted signal and forwards it to the electrode array by means of specific electrical pulses of individual electrodes. These electrical pulses stimulate the nerve fibres within the cochlea (Rubinstein 2004). The aim of the signal processing of the cochlear implant is to produce electrical stimuli which closely resemble the stimuli that intact hair cells would produce with the same acoustic input. Hearing perception depends on the characteristics of the electrical stimulus and on the place of the stimulation. Accordingly, CI technology uses certain characteristics of signal processing/stimulating and the tonotopic organisation of the cochlea.

The tonotopy of the human cochlea describes the relationship between frequency and place of stimulation, meaning that an acoustic signal with a specific frequency results in the stimulation of auditory nerve fibres in a specific region of the cochlea (Greenwood 1990). The basal part of the cochlea is associated with high frequencies, and the apical part of the cochlea is associated with low frequencies (see Fig. 18.20). Accordingly, cochlear implants map high frequencies to basal electrodes and low frequencies to apical electrodes (Oxenham et al. 2004).

Cochlear implants can cover a frequency range of approximately 100–8500 Hz, in which each electrode is assigned to a certain frequency band. For example, for spectral fractionising, a frequency range (188–7938 Hz) is assigned to 22 frequency bands. The final amplitude of the electric current pulse of a specific electrode is proportional to the energy of the amplitude of the acoustic input of the associated frequency band. Here mainly the signal amplitude changes over time, the so-called envelope information is taken into account, whereas the spectral information is largely reduced. In most cases, the shape of the electrical stimulus is a charge balanced biphasic pulse. The duration of the electrical pulses is very small (usually <50 μs). The characteristic of

the signal processing for converting the acoustic input to the final electrical stimulus is defined by the coding strategy. Various coding strategies are available, for example, ACE (advanced combination encoder), CIS (continuous interleaved sampling), SPEAK (spectral peak coding), HiRes120 (high-resolution fidelity—120 virtual channels), FSP (fine structure processing) and FS4 (fine structure processing on 4 channels).

Figure 18.21 shows the colour-mapped intensity of the electrical pulses for the acoustic signal corresponding to the spoken German word "Zeit" (tsait). Here the signal coding strategy ACE (advanced combination encoder) was used, segmenting the acoustic signal into 22 frequency bands. For each time instant, the frequency bands that feature the highest acoustical energy were chosen in order to stimulate the associated electrodes simultaneously. The colour mapping

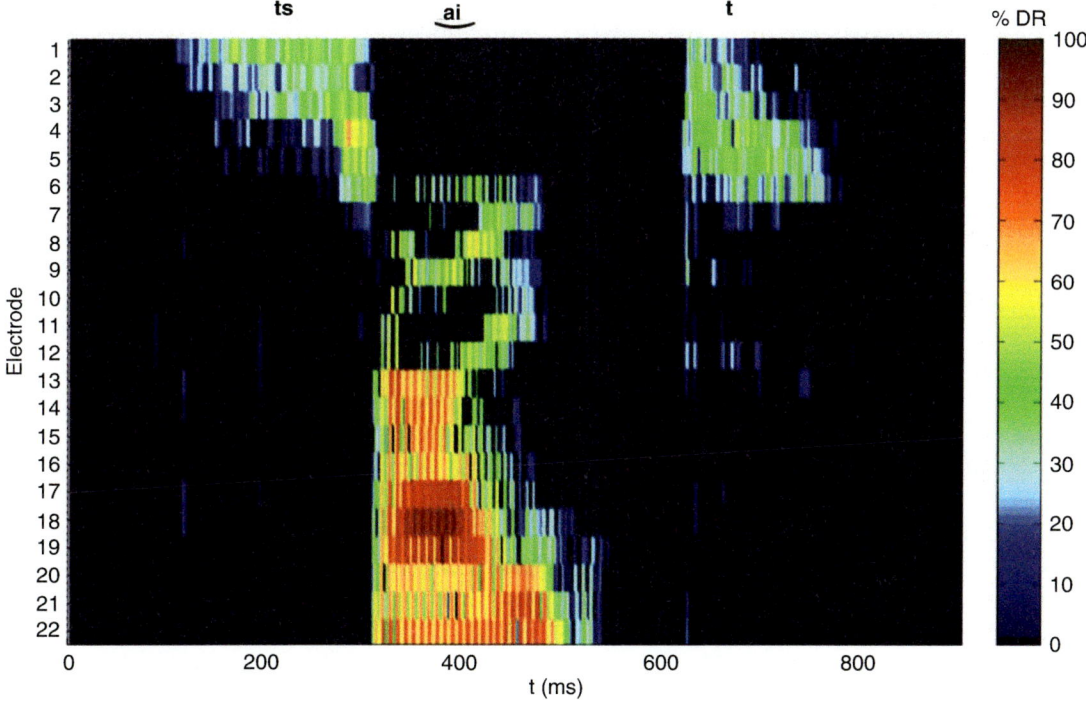

Fig. 18.21 Illustration of the electrical stimulation of the converted spoken German word "Zeit" (tsait). Electrode number 1 is associated with the basal end and electrode 22 with the apical end of the array. The high-frequency parts of the word ("ts", "t") result in stimulating the basal part of the cochlea. The low-frequency part ("i") of the word results in stimulating the apical part of the cochlea. The colour mapping illustrates the intensity of the electrical stimulus, according to the intensity of the acoustic signal, specified as a percentage of the dynamic range (DR) of each electrode. The absolute intensity and the absolute size of the DR are defined by the Threshold Level (THR) and the Maximum Comfortable Level (MCL) of each electrode (courtesy of Cochlear Limited)

---

illustrates the intensity of the electrical stimulus according to the intensity of the acoustic signal, specified as a percentage of the dynamic range (DR) of each electrode. The colour-mapped intensity is a relative (%) not an absolute value. The absolute intensity of this current flow is an individual quantity which has to be determined for each CI user and for each electrode individually. This process is called cochlear implant fitting (see next section).

18.6.3 Cochlear Implant Fitting

Hearing through a CI differs greatly from normal hearing, and the (re)habilitation process and the ultimate performance show great variability across CI users (Peterson et al. 2010). Adequate fitting of the CI is the centrepiece of this gradual process. It is important to emphasise that these fitting processes require parallel aural rehabilitation approaches that include speech and language therapy, psychosocial support, etc. Thus, postoperative therapy entails more than just regular fitting sessions. This is particularly true for children, who should participate in multidisciplinary (re)habilitation programmes for the entire period of their speech and language development. However, adults also need support by therapists of different professional backgrounds to become accustomed to the changing hearing impressions over time.

Basically, cochlear implant fitting means determining a CI user's Threshold (THR or T-Level) and Maximum Comfortable Level (MCL or C-Level) for each electrode referring to the electrical current flow and the duration of this current flow for each individual electrode (Shapiro and Bradham 2012). Figure 18.22 shows a screenshot of the fitting software "Custom Sound". To determine the MCL and THR of individual channels, single electrode stimulation is performed within the fitting section. MCL is defined as the current flow which produces a loud but still comfortable perception when stimulating a certain electrode (or the maximum loudness of the comfortable region). The corresponding THR is defined as the current flow at the hearing threshold (a current flow less than the THR is not perceptible for the CI user). An objective measurement of neural responses to electrical stimulations—neural response telemetry (NRT)—can support the fitting procedure. Normally, the first fitting procedure is executed about 3 weeks after implantation. Since the perception of these pulses is not consistent over time, it is necessary to repeat the fitting procedure regularly. This reflects the learning process that occurs as the CI user becomes increasingly accustomed to stimulation through the implant. Thus, after the initial fitting of the CI, CI users will need to return to the CI rehabilitation centre regularly for subsequent refitting within the (re)habilitation paradigm. Frequent refitting is required, especially during the first year of implant use. After the first year, less frequent sessions will be required. Later on, most CI users continue to require occasional adjustments (yearly or twice a year) for as long as they use their implant.

18.6.4 Candidacy and Indication in Children

The implementation of universal newborn hearing screening has been enhancing the prospects of early clinical diagnostics and therapy of hearing-impaired infants. As early intervention facilitates speech and language acquisition, physicians specialised in communication disorders, notably paedaudiologists, are challenged to provide reliable diagnosis within the first months of life. With respect to early cochlear implantation, an essential concern is the issue of diagnostic specificity and reliability in young infants: the risk of implanting a child without severe-to-profound hearing loss (Sampaio et al. 2011).

High standards and multidisciplinarity are therefore crucial for the assessment of candidacy for v implantation, and the final recommendation should be given by an experienced council of specialists. The diagnostic procedure needs to be appropriate to the developmental status and to the age of the child. Thus, audiometric

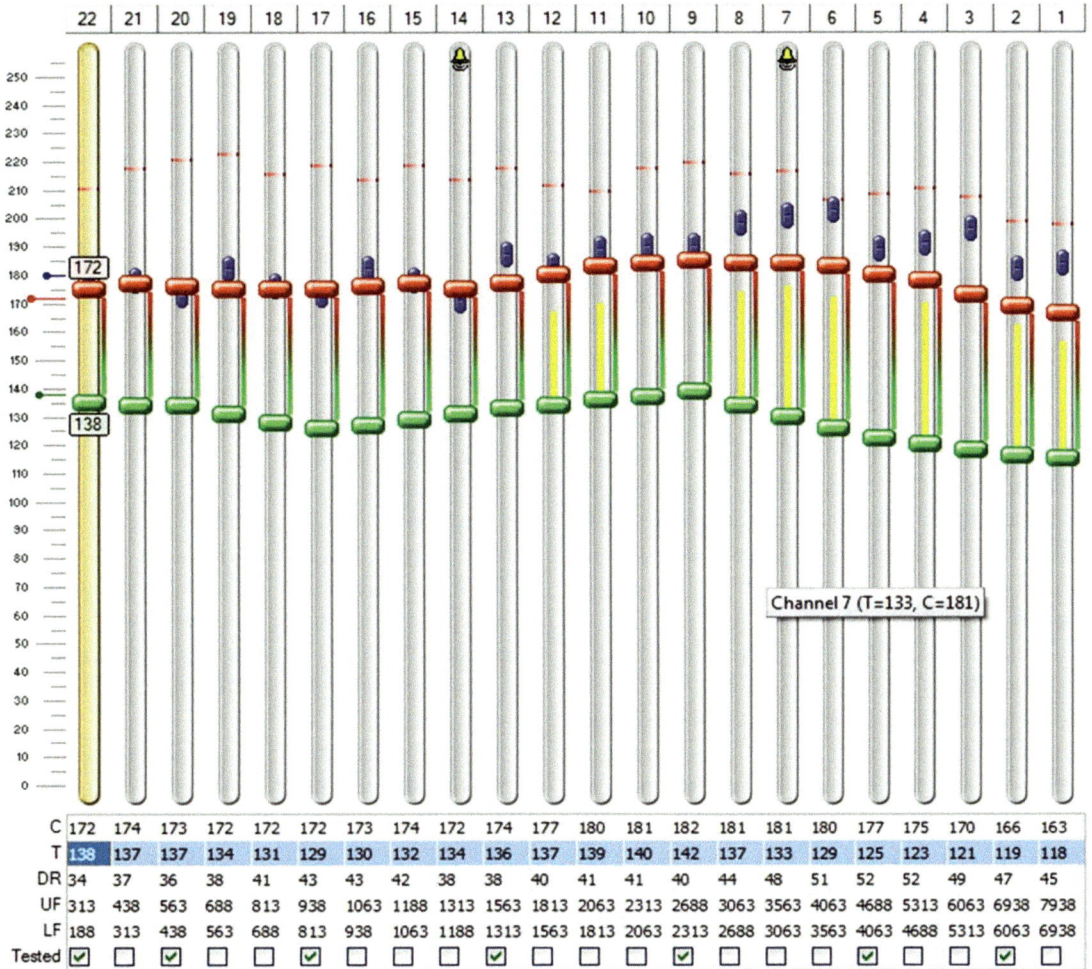

Fig. 18.22 Screenshot of the fitting software Custom Sound, visualising the MCL (here C-Level, red symbols) and the THR (here T-Level, green symbols) of 22 electrodes (current units), resulting in a certain dynamic range (DR) of the electrical output [current units]. The duration of the stimulus is named pulse-width (PW) (µs). Upper and lower frequencies (UF and LF) indicate the frequency band (Hz). The blue symbols indicate the NRT thresholds, obtained with an objective measurement of neural responses to electrical stimuli (current units). The yellow bars visualise the stimulation of a spoken sibilant sound stimulating the high-frequency region mainly. The lowest row: "tested" can be used to indicate which electrode the THR was tested for. The slim red lines indicate the maximum current level the power supply is able to deliver (compliance) (courtesy of Cochlear Limited)

assessment should include behavioural observation audiometry, visual reinforcement audiometry, play audiometry or pure-tone audiometry. Electrophysiological testing incorporates tympanometry, stapedial reflex measurements, otoacoustic emissions, frequency-specific ABR or auditory steady-state responses (ASSR).

As ABR thresholds can change, at least two ABR measurements should be performed before initiating a cochlea implantation (Louza et al. 2016). Special attention is mandatory for infants treated in the neonatal intensive care unit, who often show a significant improvement of ABR thresholds in their development in comparison to the initial ABR measures (Morimoto et al. 2010).

For a detailed description of audiometric and electrophysiological testing, see Chap. 16. Since most of the infants with hearing loss initially receive hearing aids, verification measurements are essential to compare the performance with and without hearing aids (see Sect. 18.4). Further assessment includes diagnostic interviews of parents, age-related detailed evaluation of verbal and non-verbal communication skills (see Sect. 16.16) and the estimation of the general cognitive developmental stage (see Sect. 16.18). Another major aspect of candidacy assessment is the radiological examination of the cochlea and auditory pathway with particular consequences in cases of cochlear malformation (see Sect. 16.21). An extended individual diagnostic procedure needs to be provided for children with multiple disabilities (see Sects. 16.23 and 16.24). Generally, the interdisciplinary diagnostic approach described allows a confident assessment of a child's hearing loss within the first 12 months of life, including a hearing aid trial.

In principle, there is an indication for cochlear implantation for individuals with severe-to-profound hearing loss who obtain little or no benefit from acoustic amplification in the best-aided condition and show no progress in spite of auditory training and speech and language therapy. In contrast to the former requirement of bilateral deafness, most devices now are approved for use in patients with severe-to-profound hearing loss, even including asymmetric and unilateral losses. The above-mentioned interdisciplinary diagnostic approach clarifies that candidacy not only depends on audiometric findings. Age and developmental status also determine the relevance of the different measures for decision-making. For example, electrophysiological measures, in particular frequency-specific ABR and prelinguistic evaluation of communication skills, are of special importance in candidacy assessment in infants after 9–12 months of life with congenitally profound hearing loss. In contrast, in a toddler with progressive hearing loss, a detailed evaluation of the different levels of speech communication might be of particular importance to assess the handicaps' severity. With regard to the developmental status, it is important to understand that ABR may fail in preterm children in the first months of life and in other children with disturbance of brain function or retarded maturation. Since reversible ABR abnormalities are common among neonates and infants at high risk of hearing loss, a control ABR some months later or repetitive measurements are necessary for precise threshold assessment (Psarommatis et al. 2017).

Recent publications have suggested guidance values with respect to mean pure-tone thresholds in unaided conditions. These authors recommend that children presenting with pure-tone thresholds worse than 75–85 dB HL should be considered as candidates for cochlear implantation (Leigh et al. 2011; Lovett et al. 2015). In cases of bilateral severe-to-profound hearing loss, bilateral cochlear implantation is recommended. Apart from general limitations of unilateral CI supply in binaural CI candidates, it has been shown that left ear placement resulted in restricted long-term language outcomes in comparison to initial right ear cochlear implantation (Geers et al. 2016).

In patients suffering from asymmetrical hearing loss, a bimodal provision can be advised with a cochlear implant on the side with profound hearing loss and a conventional hearing aid on the opposite ear (see Sect. 18.4). Recently it has been further shown that children with unilateral hearing loss benefit from cochlear implantation owing to successful binaural processing and integration of electrical and acoustic stimulation (Hassepass et al. 2013). For patients with stable low-frequency residual hearing, specific devices for electro-acoustic stimulation should be considered (see Sect. 18.7). Apart from severe-to-profound sensorineural hearing loss, cochlear implants might also be suitable in special sorts of hearing disorders such as auditory neuropathy. In the case of deafness resulting from meningitis, immediate implantation is necessary owing to the risk of cochlear fibrosis and rapid ossification, which can be assessed by MRI (see Sect. 16.21).

For many years, the lower age limit for implantation was 1–2 years. There is increasing evidence that early implantation in children before 12 months of age provides a significant advantage for spoken language achievement (see, e.g. Nicholas and Geers 2013). However, such a treatment modality should be decided cautiously and only after obtaining valid and stable objective and subjective hearing thresholds especially in children with high potential of recovery of an abnormal ABR (Psarommatis et al. 2011).

Apart from the challenges in diagnosis and anaesthetic and surgical management, a cochlear implantation in these very young children requires an adequate provision of post-operative rehabilitative resources.

For deaf children who are not cochlear implant candidates owing to cochlear nerve aplasia, the auditory brainstem implant (ABI) might be a reasonable option although providing inferior speech and language outcome perspectives in comparison with CI provision (Noij et al. 2015).

18.6.5 Post-Operative (re) Habilitation and Follow-Up

Beside preoperative audiologic assessment and surgery, the post-operative (re)habilitation is a centrepiece of the three-part way of CI provision. In principle, adults with a post-lingual acquired hearing loss need a specified rehabilitation programme for restoration of hearing and speech understanding. In contrast, prelingual deafened children enter a habilitation process for the acquisition of speech and communication skills. Commonalities and differences of habilitation and rehabilitation approaches have to be considered in the therapeutic content, the structure and the duration of the different programmes.

Speech and language therapy and cochlear implant fitting represent central aspects of habilitation programmes in children. Special focus is on early intervention and therapeutic parental guidance programmes with respect to intra-familial communication skills. Further therapeutic issues include principles of linguistic enrichment, augmentative communication and literacy training in the hearing-disabled children. It encourages training in respect of specific deficits, i.e. training of compensatory strategies, and might include alternative modes of communication. However, rehabilitation programmes are not limited to speech therapy and fitting but require a holistic approach to coordinate a multidisciplinary collaboration. Among others, this includes the management of psychological and socio-emotional sequelae for the child and its family and the consideration of educational needs. Further, because of the incidence of vestibular loss in children with cochlear implants and missing spontaneous recovery after implantation, a specific vestibular rehabilitation might be considered (Janky and Givens 2015). For a detailed description of aural rehabilitation approaches as applied after cochlear implantation, see Sect. 18.13.

The structures of (re)habilitation programmes after cochlear implantation show regional differences depending on health insurance funds, national legal regulations of special support and local developments. To provide focused clinical experience in the requested multidisciplinary programmes, they are commonly offered by specialised institutions (cochlear implant rehabilitation centres). These centres integrate the work of different professions: in particular physicians specialised in communication disorders, speech and language therapists, physicists or engineers, psychologists, occupational or music therapists and administration staff.

Generally, (re)habilitation starts with the initial fitting about 3–4 weeks after implantation. Often, speech and language therapists have already been introduced to the family owing to their counselling and diagnostic work before surgery. In prelingual deaf children, the multidisciplinary rehabilitation programme should run at least 3 years. Depending on the individual communication status and the local preconditions, the children and their families get regular appointments in the centre. However, cochlear-implanted patients require a lifelong follow-up care. Thus, also after completion of the rehabilitation programme, the patients have routine access to the specialists to check the device and to address problems associated with their handicap. In children this commonly includes educational and inclusion issues. In case of multiply handicapped children, the rehabilitative approach is particularly challenging and requires a specific individualisation and extension of the programme contents.

18.6.6 Bilateral Cochlear Implantation

Binaural hearing describes the integration of information that the brain receives from the two ears. By means of the head shadow effect and the central processing of listening cues based on timing, frequency and level between both ears, binaural hearing clearly enhances sound localisation and speech understanding in noise.

In many patients with profound hearing loss in both ears, unilateral cochlear implantation provides sufficient speech understanding in quiet. However, these unilaterally implanted patients frequently complain about difficulties in everyday listening conditions, such as impossible sound localisation, often creating a safety issue, and hearing restrictions in noise. Consequently, these patients should be considered for bilateral implantation because of the expectancy of improved speech intelligibility and sound localisation with two devices. This is supported by the psychoacoustic findings of the importance of bilateral hearing for normal-hearing people and hearing aid recipients.

Bilateral implantation can be undertaken either simultaneously or sequentially. Simultaneous surgery of both implants during one operation is commonly performed in children with bilateral deafness. Sequential surgery means a patient initially receives one implant and then later on decides to have the other ear implanted as often experienced in patients with progressive hearing loss.

Recently, a European Bilateral Pediatric Cochlear Implant Forum consensus statement was published: "Currently we feel that the infant or child with unambiguous cochlear implant candidacy should receive bilateral cochlear implants simultaneously as soon as possible after definitive diagnosis of deafness to permit optimal auditory development; an atraumatic surgical technique designed to preserve cochlear function, minimise cochlear damage, and allow easy, possibly repeated re-implantation is recommended" (Ramsden et al. 2012).

In patients with asymmetrical hearing loss and adequate residual hearing on the better side, a bimodal supply should be advised with a CI on the side with profound hearing loss and a conventional hearing aid on the opposite ear (see Sect. 18.4).

18.7 Knowledge of Electric-Acoustic Stimulation: Basic Principles, Application and Results

Katherine Wilson, Kate Hanvey,
Christoph von Ilberg, and Konstance Tzifa

18.7.1 Electric-Acoustic Stimulation (EAS): Basic Principles

Traditionally, cochlear implants (CI) have been provided to children who have severe-to-profound sensorineural hearing loss. More recently, owing to better sound processing techniques, advances in technology and improved hearing preservation (HP) surgery, children with functional low-frequency hearing and severe-to-profound or even complete high-frequency hearing loss can also be considered as candidates for CI (see Fig. 18.23). Individuals with this type of hearing loss are often referred to as having "partial hearing" because they are able to hear well at low frequencies.

Partial deafness can be congenital or acquired. Kuthubutheen et al. (2012) have identified the more frequent causes of partial deafness in children as genetic variation, very low birth weight in premature babies or drug-induced hearing loss due to ototoxic antibiotic or cisplatin.

The strategy from which these children can benefit is "electric-acoustic stimulation (EAS)", first described by von Ilberg et al. (1999). Children who are fitted with EAS are able to exploit the advantages of using both electric and acoustic stimulation in the same ear. Electric stimulation of the auditory system is transmitted via the CI

Fig. 18.23 Audiometric candidacy for electric-acoustic stimulation (EAS)

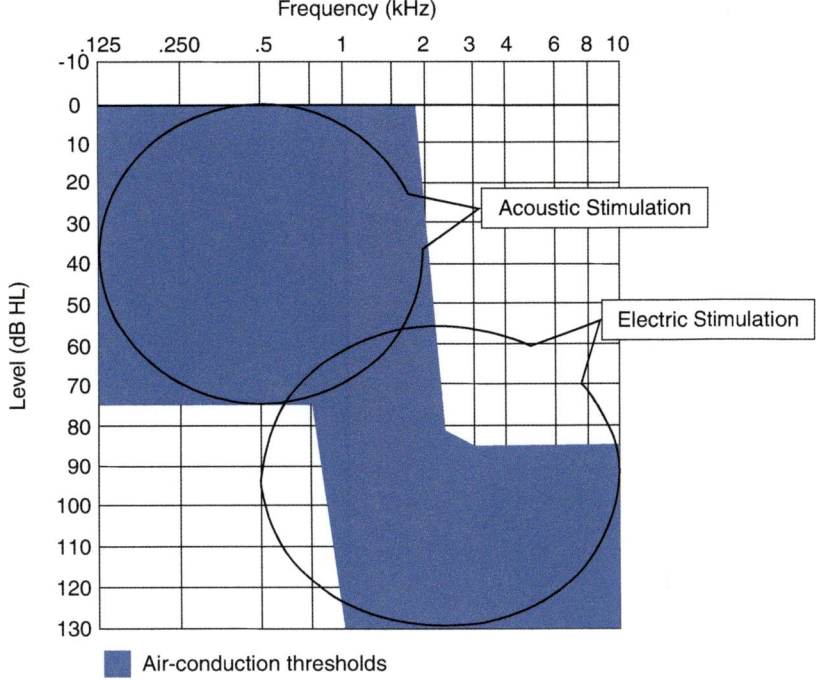

Air-conduction thresholds

(to provide audibility to the very poor high-frequency hearing at the base of the cochlea), and the acoustic stimulation is via the hearing aid in the same ear (to maintain frequency resolution and waveform fine structure to residual low-frequency hearing at the apical part of the cochlea). As depicted in Fig. 18.24a, both the CI and the hearing aid are integrated in a single behind-the-ear (BTE) sound processor. In cases where the child has *normal* low-frequency hearing, unamplified acoustic stimulation can occur in combination with a CI in the same ear.

In addition to a conventional cochlear implant, an acoustic stimulator is integrated in the BTE housing (see Fig. 18.24a) in order to transmit the low frequencies into the outer ear canal. The characteristic of the acoustic stimulator is depicted in Fig. 18.24b. Its maximal gain of 40–50 dB SPL is restricted to the frequency range 125–1500 Hz.

EAS is typically realised in the same ear (see Fig. 18.24a), but the combination of acoustic and electric stimulation can be clinically implemented in different modalities (see Fig. 18.25).

Ipsilateral EAS	Combined EAS speech processor in one ear
Bimodal	CI in one ear; hearing aid in the opposite ear
Bilateral EAS	Combined EAS speech processor in both ears
Binaural EAS	Combined EAS speech processor in one ear; hearing aid in the opposite ear
Electric complement	CI for high frequencies only; no amplification at low frequencies needed

The EAS combination helps to compensate for some of the deficits of CIs, such as small electrical dynamic ranges and poor temporal information. It is well documented that the amount of speech information available to children via a CI alone is quite limited (Wilson and Dorman 2008), especially in challenging and noisy environments. EAS offers a new possibility for regaining satisfactory hearing and speech perception, above and beyond what hearing aids alone can achieve, or what CIs alone can provide, in children who suffer from *severe or total high-frequency hearing loss*. EAS is particularly effective in situations

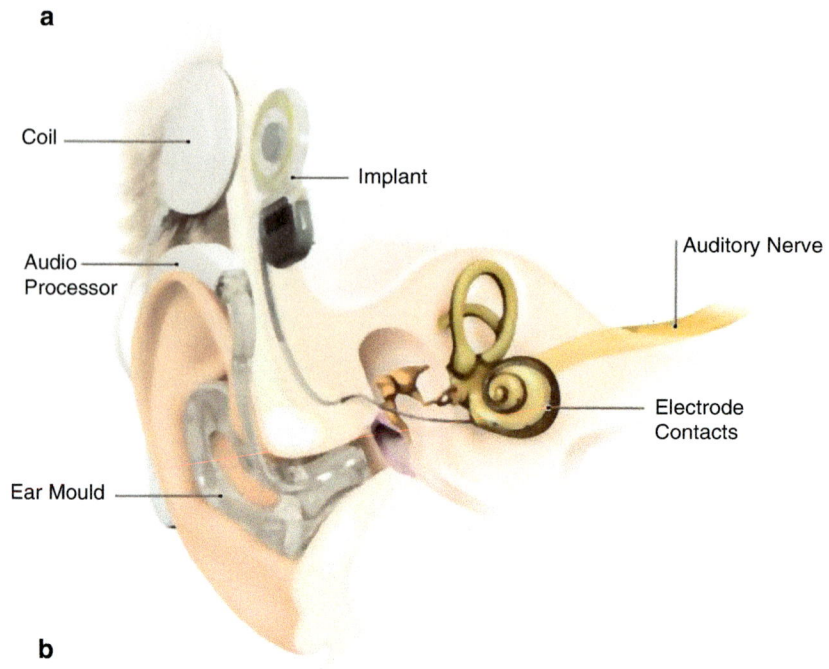

Fig. 18.24 (**a**) The combination of cochlear implant and EAS processor (Picture: with kind permission from MED-EL). (**b**) Characteristic of the acoustic stimulator

a

Coil

Implant

Auditory Nerve

Audio Processor

Electrode Contacts

Ear Mould

b

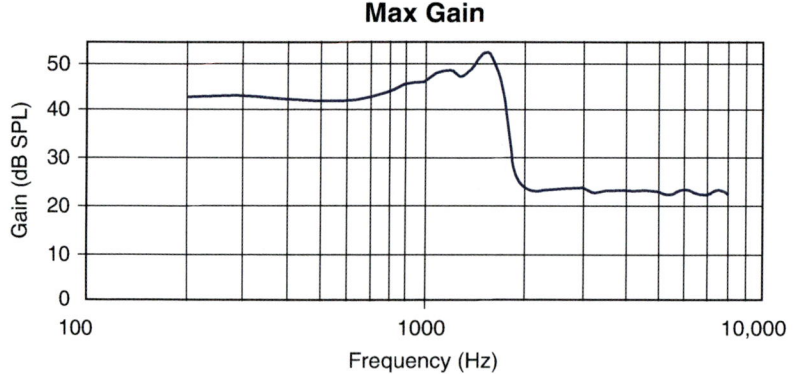

Max Gain

with competing sound, especially where there are multiple talkers. It has not only an additive but in many cases a synergistic effect (Wilson and Dorman 2008).

18.7.2 Hearing Preservation

As the performance of EAS largely depends on the amount of residual acoustic low-frequency hearing, a meticulous surgical technique is necessary to minimise trauma to the delicate intracochlear structures. It is particularly important not to interfere with the still functioning auditory system of the apical region during the insertion of the electrode carrier.

Consequently, the insertion depth of the electrode should correspond to the amount of residual hearing: the more low-frequency hearing to be preserved, the shorter the electrode should be. However, in order to guarantee a fully functioning CI system in the rare cases of subsequent partial or complete hearing loss, the insertion depth should not fall below 22 mm. Furthermore, the individual length of the cochlear duct, which can vary considerably (Erixon et al. 2009), has to

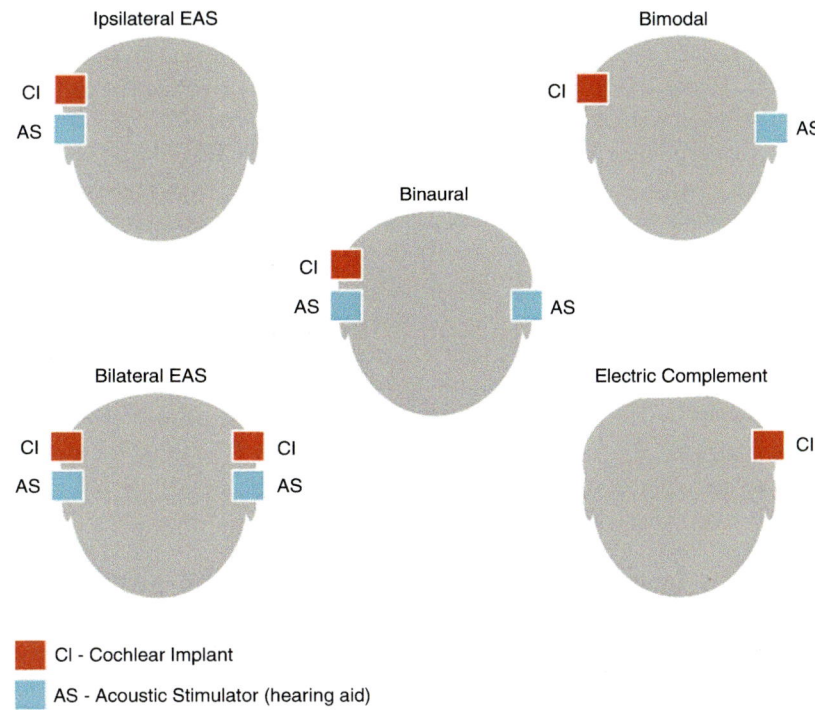

Fig. 18.25 Different EAS configurations for children with partial hearing

be determined preoperatively by high precision imaging. Owing to the development of softer electrodes of smaller diameter, there is now a tendency to use longer electrodes, and successfully, in hearing and structure preservation surgery. This is particularly reasonable in cases with a progressive hearing loss.

In addition to the hearing and structure preservation surgery, other factors such as pre-, intra- and post-operative steroid application (Sweeny et al. 2015) and gene therapy—as a future option (Staecker et al. 2007)—are applied to support the amount of early and long-term preservation of acoustic hearing.

Under these conditions, with the use of a 20 mm electrode array, the risk of losing residual hearing in children was assessed by Skarżyński and Lorens (2010) to be less than 15%. Comparable HP results in children have also been found with longer electrode arrays of 24 mm. Thus Rajan et al. (2012) reported an average loss of hearing in children of 3 dB (±1.2 dB standard deviation). Considering that even small amounts of acoustic hearing can be important for speech recognition, *any attempt* should be made to preserve it, even

though a subsequent successful implementation of EAS cannot be precisely predicted.

18.7.3 Limitation of Hearing Aids with a Significant High-Frequency Hearing Loss

Children with partial hearing, i.e. severe-to-complete high-frequency hearing loss, usually wear bilateral high-power hearing aids and are often reported to be "doing well" because they are compared with other severe-to-profound hearing-impaired children. This results in a misunderstanding of the child's hearing difficulties and an underestimation of the child's true potential.

These children will have great difficulty perceiving speech cues associated with the manner and place of articulation, even with the best hearing aids available. The substantial loss of inner hair cells in the high-frequency region of the cochlea prevents the transmission of temporal and spectral cues to the brain (Turner et al. 2004). This will inhibit the neural coding of these speech cues that define various phonemes. The use of frequency-lowering and frequency-compression aids may result in good detection of high-frequency sounds, but the child will not be able to discriminate between them with accuracy (Gifford et al. 2007). Therefore, inadequate high-frequency amplification results in perception of sounds that lacks the quality and clarity important for word discrimination and speech understanding in noise.

Children need to be able to hear and discriminate high-frequency speech sounds in order to develop them in their own speech. Inaccurate speech patterns developed through compromised hearing may be irreversible, even with remedial intervention. Persistent inadequate access to sound can result in impaired speech intelligibility and quality, subtle language delays and vocabulary gaps that can worsen as the child gets older. Delage and Tuller (2007) observed language delays in over 50% of adolescents with prelingual mild-to-moderate hearing loss. Additionally, Yoshinaga-Itano et al. (2010) observed that a higher proportion of children with severe-to-profound hearing loss who use hearing aids are "gap openers" (i.e. the gap between their age-equivalent language scores and chronological age increases over time), compared with their matched peers with profound hearing loss and CI, who are more likely to be "gap closers" (i.e. the gap between their age-equivalent language scores and chronological age closes over time).

18.7.4 EAS Indication in Children

Apart from the given audiological limits (Fig. 18.23), specific guidelines regarding CI for children with partial hearing have yet to be established (Gratacap et al. 2015). It is therefore imperative that any EAS candidate has individual evaluation. As a consequence, professionals must understand the limitations of hearing aid technology and the potential impact these limitations have on a child's speech and language development. Increasing awareness about the consequences of partial deafness, together with early detection and intervention, can prevent permanent speech and language impairment in these children (Jayawardena et al. 2012).

Early intervention with CI is an established principle for *congenitally severe-to-profound* deaf children (see Sect. 18.6). In the same way, unless there is early intervention of children with *congenital partial hearing*, functional outcomes will be compromised. Therefore, families should be counselled on the possibility of CI and EAS, preferably within the first year of their child's life or diagnosis of hearing loss. They need to understand the long-term implications of high-frequency hearing loss and be reassured about HP. Waiting for their child to fail linguistically or academically is leaving the referral too late.

18.7.5 EAS Assessment Test Battery

Ascertaining the amount of benefit that a child receives from hearing aids versus the potential benefit of CI can be challenging in this client group (see Fig. 18.26 and Table 18.1). Not only does it require detailed assessment but also ongoing extensive counselling with the family. Owing to the progress in speech understanding and speech performance in the early years, parents might be of the opinion that their child is hearing adequately enough with their hearing aids. Furthermore, parents may worry that any low-frequency hearing will be irreversibly damaged during CI surgery, thereby focusing more on what the child has to lose, rather than on what the child could gain from EAS.

A complete pre-implant assessment test battery of hearing thresholds, developmentally appropriate speech perception in quiet *and in noise*, speech and language development, cognitive abilities, educational attainment and quality of life is required (see Fig. 18.26). It may also be necessary to repeat certain tests at specified intervals, in order to ascertain if the predicted rate of progress is being achieved with hearing aids alone.

In addition to determining hearing thresholds, functional hearing ability must be assessed, in each ear separately in quiet, to determine if there is an interaural difference. This will help in

Fig. 18.26 The multidisciplinary EAS assessment

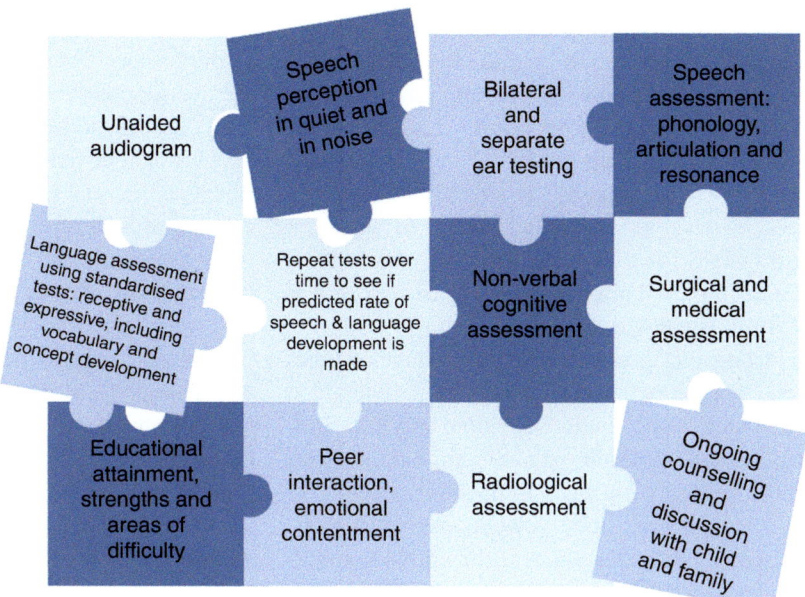

Table 18.1 Comparison between hearing aids and EAS showing the potential advantages (in green) versus disadvantages (in orange) of hearing aids and EAS

	Hearing aids	EAS
Invasiveness	No surgery required	Surgery required
Cosmetics	Often smaller than an EAS sound processor	Often larger than a hearing aid; requires both earmould in ear and coil on head
Acoustic feedback	Whistling can occur, owing to high gain required at high frequencies	No acoustic feedback as high frequencies are stimulated electrically, not acoustically
Sound clarity	Frequency compression provides good detection of speech sounds, but poor discrimination and clarity of speech	Temporal resolution provided acoustically and audible frequency resolution provided electrically = good detection, discrimination, and identification of speech sounds
Hearing in noise	Poor understanding in noise because of poor clarity of high frequency sounds	Better understanding in noise due to clear, audible sound across the speech frequency range
Opportunities for age-appropriate language and clear speech, leading to higher academic potential and successful peer relationships	Age-appropriate language with clear speech very hard to achieve in many cases of congenital partial hearing	Age-appropriate language with clear speech easier to achieve in many cases of congenital partial hearing, *if CI is performed early enough in childhood*

determining whether unilateral implantation (i.e. the child uses bimodal stimulation) or bilateral implantation is more appropriate. If implanted unilaterally, generally the *poorer* functioning ear is implanted, leaving the *better* ear for the hearing aid. This is contrary to traditional thinking. *Speech perception tests carried out in noise are particularly important* because the detrimental effects of partial hearing may only be apparent in adverse listening conditions.

Alongside pre-recorded assessments, functional speech perception tests may include aided live voice Ling sound detection and discrimination and minimal pair discrimination with particular focus on high frequencies and VCV/CVC (vowel-consonant-vowel/consonant-vowel-consonant) discrimination. If the child is preverbal, then tests of discrimination may include the auditory speech sounds evaluation (A(section)E) (Govaerts et al. 2006), which does not require the child to understand words.

Receptive and expressive language must be carefully evaluated by using standardised language assessments, and if more evidence is still required to determine whether EAS is appropriate, then the tests should be re-administered over a specified period of time to see whether the predicted amount of progress has been made. Children learn spoken language through incidental listening. Whilst it is possible for children with partial hearing to learn reasonable functional communication, they are likely to have some delays. Detailed assessment, including vocabulary and concepts if appropriate, will highlight any difficulties the child may be experiencing.

The EAS pre-implant assessment can also involve standardised cognitive tests to determine if the child is accessing enough sound to develop their speech and language properly. Comparisons between non-verbal cognitive test results with verbal cognitive test scores and language assessment scores can be made in order to see if there is a mismatch. A child not reaching his verbal potential may be indicative of compromised hearing.

Formal and informal quality of life measures, either through questionnaires or simple discussions with the family, can provide insight into peer interaction, the ability to cope in different communication situations and the child's overall emotional contentment. Information gleaned through these discussions can also contribute to the overall picture of how the child's hearing loss is impinging on their development.

Throughout the assessment described above, it is essential that there is ongoing feedback, discussion and counselling with parents, the child (if old enough) and the child's team of support professionals. Some parents may need help to shift their focus to what the child has to *gain* from EAS, instead of being solely concerned about what they might *lose*. Parents therefore need to understand what each assessment is for, the results of each and the overall prognosis for their child's speech, language and educational attainment. They are then in a position to make an informed choice on behalf of their child.

18.7.6 Results with EAS

EAS studies to date have mainly been carried out on adults. Those studies have shown that EAS can significantly improve speech perception in quiet but particularly in challenging noisy conditions. A European multicentre clinical trial was conducted by Gstoettner et al. (2008). In the best-aided condition with bilateral hearing aids, preoperative open-set sentence scores were 24% in quiet and 14% in noise. Twelve months after EAS, the speech recognition scores had significantly increased to 76% in quiet and 60% in noise. Studies in adults have also shown an improvement in music enjoyment and natural sound quality with EAS when compared with CI alone (Brockmeier et al. 2010).

In those rare cases where partial hearing cannot be primarily preserved, or when the preserved hearing deteriorates over time, it is possible to increase electrical input into the lower frequencies gradually until the EAS user has switched over to full electrical stimulation. Outcomes of partially hearing adults who lost their residual hearing post-EAS still show better results with a CI than the hearing aid that they had worn before surgery (Lorens et al. 2008). Furthermore, if reimplantation is required owing to device failure, preservation of residual hearing is possible, as described by Jayawardena et al. (2012).

There is no reason to believe that children should not benefit from EAS in the same way as adults; indeed, Skarżyński et al. (2002) published the first cases of HP surgery with EAS and "electrical component" strategies in children and found that the children performed equally well as, or even better than, comparable adult recipients.

For congenital partial hearing loss in children, early implantation for EAS yields better results in the same way as for "traditional" CI candidates (Gratacap et al. 2015). Wilson et al. (2016) found that the speech intelligibility of younger children with congenital partial hearing consistently improved after CI, but not for children who were implanted when older.

Whilst children with partial hearing may already function "well" with their hearing aids in a quiet environment, the greatest benefit is often in noise. Skarżyński and Lorens (2010) showed children's open-set word scores in noise improved from 7% (best aided before EAS) to 47% (after EAS).

18.7.7 Summary

Children with partial hearing can gain significant benefit from EAS, particularly if they are implanted before language gaps or irreversible speech patterns become established. A growing body of research and clinical evidence is now able to show surgical success with hearing preservation techniques in children; moreover, the evidence demonstrates the significant gains that EAS has over hearing aids in challenging listening situations. Professionals working with families of children with partial hearing have a crucial role in providing information and reassurance in order to facilitate timely referrals to CI teams.

18.8　Training in Handling Hearing Devices/Cochlear Implants

Thomas Wiesner and Dirk Mürbe

Studies show that the hours of hearing aid/cochlear implant (CI) use can vary significantly depending on the confidence and the acceptance of the device by the caregivers. Parents who are less confident with the handling and troubleshooting of their child's hearing aid/CI will be more frustrated, less willing and simply less able to keep the devices on their child's ears. A child who senses the uncertainty of its parents will be more likely to feel less at ease with the device, and this may cause more trouble wearing the aids. Therefore a considerate training (and ongoing coaching) of all relevant caregivers is necessary.

It is essential that the parents are taught until they feel comfortable in:

- How to place the ear mould easily and securely in the child's ear, preferably by including written and video instruction material
- How to keep the hearing aid/CI behind the ear, if necessary by including the use of a retention device such as a thin baby cap and a "hooky system" or the use of special tape or, in the case of CI, the use of an appropriate magnet
- Making sure that the hearing aid/CI cannot get lost, even when the child removes the device from the ear, by the use of a hearing aid/CI retainer cord.
- Being equipped with a stethoclip, a battery tester and a cleaning and a drying kit (DGPP 2012) and learning how to:
  - Check the hearing aid and ensure that it is functioning properly, by using a stethoclip and a battery tester (ASHA 2017)
  - Clean and dry the hearing aid/CI, including the use of an electrical hearing aid dryer (which may include ultraviolet light for disinfecting the hearing aid and the ear mould at the same time)
  - Clean and if necessary sanitise the ear mould and prevent the spread of an infection from one ear canal to the other
- Checking daily the hearing aid/CI and the child's hearing, by teaching the child to respond to the speech sounds of the Ling test
- Learning to find and troubleshoot minor problems, such as a blocked or torn tube or, in the case of CI, a cable break
- Having the ears checked and cleaned regularly, to prevent a buildup of earwax in the ear canal at the end of the ear mould

- Teaching their child as early as possible to learn to participate in the handling and maintenance of the hearing aid/CI

Additionally, the hearing aid/CI, the ear mould and the child's hearing threshold should be checked regularly by a professional: every professional should check the child's hearing devices before any rehabilitation session. With babies, ear moulds may have to be replaced, even after a few weeks. For older children, ear moulds must be replaced whenever they are leaking and cause feedback, and soft ear moulds should be replaced at least once a year for hygiene reasons. A professional full technical checkup of the child's hearing aids should be made at least three to four times a year. In CI patients the position and fit of the transmission coil must be checked for pressure, skin irritation, atrophy or turgor. Such checks must be conducted, even if the patient reports no problems with the device (Knief et al. 2015).

To help parents to understand, accept and cooperate in the rehabilitation and early intervention process, parents need the opportunity to:

- Understand the test results (e.g. to read a diagram of the hearing threshold) so that they get a realistic understanding of the child's hearing capacity with and without devices. Such knowledge will make it easier for the parents to adjust their communicative behaviour to the needs of the child.
- Obtain basic knowledge about the components and functioning of a hearing aid/CI, which will additionally help them to understand the causes and impact (such as severe distortion) of feedback and what can be done to prevent it.
- Learn how to support and enhance the hearing and communication development of their child.
- Experience how a language-rich environment can provide the child with the necessary stimuli to learn to process and understand sounds and language.
- Acquire communication tactics in the relationship with their child that make it easier, or for some children just possible, to pick up meaningful language.

- Meet other parents of hearing-impaired children as well as hearing-impaired adults and profit from their knowledge and experience.
- Get an overview of accessory devices that can provide solutions for special hearing tasks and difficult listening environments such as FM systems, wireless audio streamer (TV, mp3, telephone, etc.) and vibration and flashing alarm systems (doorbell, telephone, alarm clock, etc.).
- Feel invited to ask and come back for further training whenever needed.
- Get most of the information in an adequate, written form, so that it can be reread and shared at home (DGPP 2012). Additionally, all manual tasks should be demonstrated and practically trained.

The counselling and training is part of a multi-professional approach involving at least the phoniatrician, the paediatric audiologist, the paediatric acoustician and the early interventionist. All professional team members should be able to participate in the counselling process of the parents and to provide coherent information founded on an open-minded but evidence-based and concerted team concept. In cases of CI patients, this counselling and training is usually included in the structured rehabilitation that is entered after implantation. Well-informed parents will feel less helpless and be empowered to take responsibility and to make the informed choices that suit the needs of their family.

Whereas most of the above-mentioned aspects are valid both for the external components of a CI system and for hearing aids, there is a need for additional information concerning the internal components of a CI system. For these components it is essential to provide information about relevant warnings and precautions. These details should also be provided in an adequate, written form, since they are essential for CI patients/parents. Warnings include:

- Medical treatments generating induced currents: for example, electrosurgery, diathermy, neuro-stimulation, electroconvulsive therapy, ionising radiation therapy and ultrasound close to the implant.

- Magnetic resonance imaging (MRI): not all implants are permitted for MRI. CI companies have defined instructions for MRI investigations in CI patients depending on the CI type. In more modern CI devices, the magnet is surgically removable and replaceable, but the use of 1.5 T MRI seems to be possible without magnet removal, which requires informed consent of the parents/patients. A compression headwrap should be used to avoid magnet torsion/displacement. This procedure is allowed in Europe and countries with similar guidelines but is not in accordance with the Food and Drug Administration guidelines, which still require magnet removal before MRI for most CI devices (Young et al. 2016).
- Head trauma: risk of damaging the implant.

Relevant precautions to be addressed in counselling include:

- Theft- and metal-detection systems might be activated by the implant. Further, these systems may induce distorted sound sensation for CI patients when passing through or near one of these devices.
- Mobile telephones may interfere with the operation of a CI creating distorted sound sensation.
- Regarding air travelling, CI manufacturers recommend switching off the external CI components during take-off and landing.
- Scuba diving may require limited diving depths owing to variable robustness of the implant against pressure changes.

18.9 Tinnitus Management: A Medical Perspective

Ahmet Atas, Songul Aksoy, Levent N. Ozluoglu, Haldun Oguz, Mustafa Asim Safak, and Ross Parfitt

Introduction A careful medical and audiological evaluation is necessary in order to guide the management of the tinnitus patient. Selection of an appropriate rehabilitation method and its application should be agreed between the individual patient and an experienced professional. Use of an unsuitable treatment method or inappropriate application could cause the severity of a patient's tinnitus to heighten and possibly increase his resistance to further treatment. General aims of treatment include eliminating the source of tinnitus or modifying the tinnitus signal itself (pharmacology, surgery, sound therapy), reducing tinnitus-related distress (psychological approaches and psychotropic agents) and minimising the involvement of the limbic and autonomic systems (e.g. tinnitus retraining therapy). Section 18.10 discusses the management of tinnitus in children and teenagers.

Drug Treatment Various medical treatment modalities for subjective tinnitus have been proposed, including vascular circulation regulators, antidepressants, anxiolytics, local anaesthetics and glutamate antagonists, among others (see Baguley et al. 2013 and Allman et al. 2016, from which sources the following brief overview has been taken). These approaches have, however, found very little success.

Vascular circulation regulators, such as diuretics, anticoagulants and vasodilators, have not been found to be successful in the treatment of tinnitus. Betahistine dihydrochloride can be beneficial in the treatment of Ménière's disease (of which tinnitus is a key symptom), but not for other tinnitus aetiologies. Glutamate antagonists, such as memantine, flurtipine and neramexane, have not been found to be effective, despite their logical appeal given the importance of glutamate as an auditory neurotransmitter.

Intravenous injection of the local anaesthetics lidocaine, bupivacaine or procaine can have an inhibitory effect on the central auditory pathway, thereby temporarily relieving tinnitus. But there are considerable risks in this method of application. Evidence on the effectiveness of tricyclic antidepressants and anxiolytics does not support their use for the elimination of tinnitus. They may, however, be beneficial in reducing tinnitus-related distress.

No evidence has been found in support of paramedical treatment for tinnitus such as ginkgo biloba homoeopathy or acupuncture (Savage and Waddell 2014).

Sound Therapy Neurological theories of tinnitus suggest that a reduced level of stimulation from the peripheral organ leads to central changes causing the perception of tinnitus (e.g. Brozoski et al. 2012). The converse of this would imply that an enhanced sound environment, for example, through the use of a hearing aid or sound generator, would improve the symptoms of tinnitus. A 2012 Cochrane Review suggests that the evidence available in the literature is not sufficiently strong (Hobson et al. 2012) to support the use of sound therapy for tinnitus, but audiologists and hearing aid acousticians will recognise a wealth of anecdotal evidence in its support.

Hearing aids are commonly used as a rehabilitative strategy for individuals with hearing impairment. Given the great overlap between tinnitus and hearing impairment (see Davis and El Rafaie 2000), hearing aids often form a part of tinnitus treatment. Sixty percent of hearing aid wearers receive some level of improvement in their symptoms through wearing hearing aids, with 22% experiencing major relief and only 2% reporting that their tinnitus worsens, according to a survey of 230 hearing care professionals (Kochkin and Tyler 2008).

The use of specific devices, such as wearable white noise generators or bedside sound generators, is often referred to as tinnitus masking (Vernon 1988). The aim, however, should not be to render the tinnitus percept inaudible by playing sounds that are immediately louder than it (as would be implied by the meaning of the term "masking" in other audiological contexts), but to provide relief by enhancing the sound environment through constant low-level auditory stimulation (see Henry et al. (2002) for an overview of misconceptions of tinnitus masking). The main objective of masking tinnitus is to reduce the perception of tinnitus and to eliminate its conscious perception completely. Newer technology combining the functionality of a hearing aid with masking/sound therapy capability is available.

Residual Inhibition Residual inhibition, another effect of auditory stimulation on tinnitus, was observed by Feldmann (1971). He noted that specific auditory stimuli led to inhibition of the tinnitus percept for approximately 1 min. Henry (2016) has proposed that further research to develop optimal stimuli could be beneficial for the development of a new therapeutic approach. Stein et al. (2015) showed in patients with chronic tonal tinnitus a reduction of subjective tinnitus loudness after listening to music passing through a notch filter gauged to the individual tinnitus frequency. Magnetoencephalographic measurements showed a correlative reduction of temporal and frontal activation aroused by the tinnitus tone. The inhibition-induced effect persisted and accumulated over 3 days.

Tinnitus Retraining Therapy A specific form of sound therapy and counselling called tinnitus retraining therapy (TRT), derived from the neurophysiological model of tinnitus (Jastreboff and Hazell 1993), is a good and effective therapeutic tool (Graham and Butler 1984). TRT facilitates habituation to tinnitus by suppressing negative reactions and associations caused by tinnitus, with the result that the perception and its associations are suppressed. TRT is typically combined with the use of sound therapy devices.

Other Rehabilitative Tools Research into the neurological underpinnings of tinnitus and potential therapeutic strategies, including auditory and even electrical stimulation designed to modulate neural processing, is ongoing at various centres. Concerning acoustic coordinated reset neuromodulation based on a desynchronisation technique, see Tass et al. (2012). Positive results were seen in a clinical trial by Folmer et al. (2015) with application of repetitive transcranial magnetic stimulation (rTMS). Noh et al. (2017) found significant effects in tinnitus suppression by dual-site rTMS in the auditory cortex and the dorsolateral prefrontal cortex.

Interpersonal, interactive educational interventions for noise-induced hearing loss (NIHL) and tinnitus prevention are aimed at improving knowledge, attitudes and intentional behaviour regarding sound exposure and appropriate use of hearing protection in children. The Dangerous Decibels classroom programme run by the University of Northern Colorado, for example, is reported to be more effective and longer-lasting than self-directed learning experiences (Martin et al. 2013).

Questionnaires, such as the Tinnitus Handicap Inventory (Newman et al. 1996), that measure the severity and impact of tinnitus can be invaluable in measuring the benefit of rehabilitative interventions and progress during follow-up.

18.10 Management of Tinnitus in Children and Teenagers: A Specialist Paediatric Audiology and Hearing Therapy Perspective

Claire Benton and Charlotte Rogers

Tinnitus Management A good explanation of tinnitus forms a solid foundation for all management strategies. It is important to be led by the child and its family and offer reassurance. Many families are concerned that tinnitus can damage hearing or is a sign of hearing loss. Thus normalising tinnitus and offering reassurance that other children hear noises in their ears help to develop a sense of control, and suggestions can be given for simple practical strategies for the family to adopt. Helping the children develop their own strategies and solutions to the difficulties they experience is also often effective in promoting control over their experience and ability to manage their tinnitus.

Effective management needs to address the impact of tinnitus upon the child, its psychological well-being, educational progress and life stressors, both at home and at school, which exacerbate tinnitus distress.

In forming your dialogue with the patients, consider their age and cognitive ability. Younger children appreciate explanations that are within their realm of experience. For example, tinnitus can be explained as the sound that our ears sometimes make when they are working, in the same way as the sound we make when breathing. Older children have developed the linguistic and cognitive skills to understand the relationship between tinnitus symptoms and thoughts, emotions, physiological reactions and life events. Tinnitus models can be adapted by replacing words with images or thoughts, worries or feelings; if children can produce their own images, this increases their feelings of ownership (Emond and Kentish 2013).

Tinnitus management strategies focus on sound enrichment, coping strategies and psychological management. Sound devices are often used as a filter for tinnitus sounds for that child. Where a hearing loss is present, hearing aid amplification is usually provided, and open ear mould fitting is recommended where appropriate for these children (Gabriels 1996). There is little evidence for the effectiveness of the use of wearable sound generators in children. Environmental sounds such as music, white noise and nature sounds can provide the same effects. It is equally important to explore useful coping strategies with the child. These can sometimes be a change in current behaviour, adopting a method of relaxation or altering a routine.

Healthcare professionals need to ensure that they identify children in need of psychological support and refer them onwards to appropriate services where necessary. Tinnitus can be associated with anxiety overlay, and it is also important to address issues that may perpetuate this anxiety. The use of cognitive behavioural therapy techniques is widely recognised in the literature for adult tinnitus patients, and narrative therapy may prove a useful tool for younger children to explore and help manage their tinnitus.

18.11 Knowledge of Hearing Assistive Technology

Thomas Wiesner

18.11.1 Introduction

Hearing aids (HA) and cochlear implants (CI) can compensate for the loudness deficit of a sensorineural hearing loss. But any such loss is not only characterised by its loudness deficit but also by a degradation of the quality of hearing with respect to the discrimination of small frequency and time differences and distortion. Furthermore, the passage of the sound through the tiny microphone and especially the tiny receiver of a hearing aid, or the limited number of channels of a CI, already provides a signal of restricted sound quality and bandwidth to the ear. In summary, even after an optimal fitting of a HA or CI, "normal hearing" cannot be restored by these devices; therefore hearing and understanding can still be very difficult and sometimes impossible, especially in noisy environments.

Further improvement is possible (and necessary) through the use of additional listening devices such as loop systems or wireless sound transmitter systems, e.g. the former FM systems (frequency modulation systems) and now digital wireless transmitter systems or Bluetooth streamers, which feed the sound signal from a remote microphone, TV set or telephone directly into the hearing aid. A classic example of using a wireless transmitter system for hearing-impaired children would be in school, where the teacher would wear a wireless microphone (Fig. 18.27), which picks up the voice of the teacher near his mouth and sends it wirelessly to a receiver that is attached to the pupil's hearing aids (Fig. 18.28) providing the pupil with a clear speech signal of the teacher.

More and more competing and technically sophisticated systems are coming on the market, but a number of the systems work only within the range of products of one specific

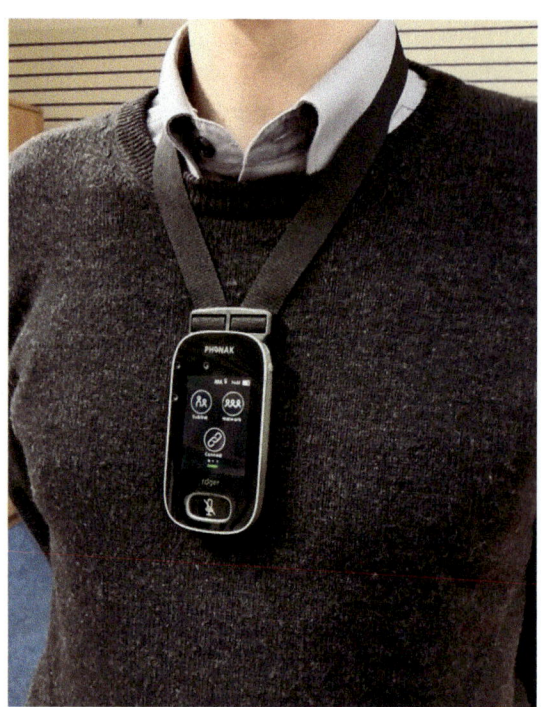

Fig. 18.27 Wireless microphone worn around the neck (model featured is the Phonak Roger). Photo courtesy of and copyright Connevans Limited

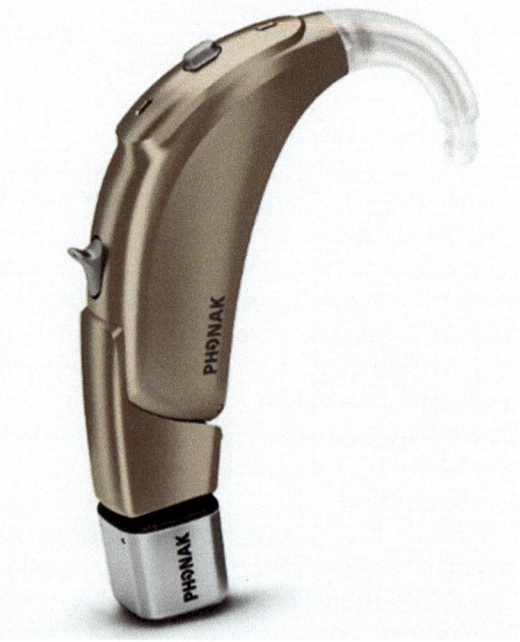

Fig. 18.28 FM receiver attached to a hearing aid (model featured is the Phonak Roger X attached to a Phonak Naida V SP). Photo courtesy of and copyright Phonak

manufacturer and cannot be used with a hearing aid from a different manufacturer. Therefore for some of these systems, one has to see them as a combined package of the two hearing aids together with a wireless transmitter system tailored to the individual needs of the hearing-impaired (adult or adolescent) person.

Infants and children who are still learning to decode and understand speech need a higher signal-to-noise ratio for speech comprehension than that of adults with well-developed auditory systems and communication skills. Without a good positive signal-to-noise ratio, children cannot detect grammatical markers such as unvoiced word endings. Only a reliable and consistent input of these grammatical markers and all soft speech sounds allows the children to develop their grammatical knowledge and later on their phonological awareness. Depending on their degree of hearing loss and the challenges of their acoustic environment, a wireless microphone system can be necessary even for infants starting around 1 year of age.

For children the guideline for wireless microphone systems ("FM systems") should be:

- In most of the cases, the wireless transmitter system will have to last more than the "lifetime" of one pair of hearing aids before any new reimbursement is possible. Therefore the receiver of the wireless system should be attached to the hearing aid by an adapter shoe, so that it can also be used with different hearing aids just by changing the adapter.
- Any wireless transmitter system should be tried out under the daily life conditions where it will be used later on. Only a system that will be regularly used is a worthwhile prescription, as unused systems will be overtaken by new technical developments quite easily and may be already outdated when they may finally come into use years later. Any trial of a wireless transmitter system should be under the supervision and guidance of a professional trained to fit and use these systems.

- The transmitter has to be rugged and tamper-proof. It should provide different microphone options such as a lapel microphone or a boom microphone. It needs different frequency channels so that one can always find an unobstructed frequency. The system may automatically change frequencies when the child changes classrooms.
- Systems with a fully digital transmission are preferred, as they provide less stray pick-up and advanced noise reduction algorithms.
- For most children the best solution will be to attach the receiver to the direct audio input of the hearing aid. Therefore children should only be fitted with hearing aids that provide such a direct audio input option. In some cases the receiver can also be worn with a telecoil loop around the neck. Some children may also attach the wireless microphone receiver to their individual streaming device, which will transmit the audio signal directly into their hearing aids.
- In higher school classes especially, the dialogue in the class may be less and less dominated by the teacher and more by contributions of other pupils. Then one transmitter microphone that stays with the teacher may not be sufficient, and a system with more than one microphone is needed. Most fully digital systems provide such a multi-microphone option.

18.11.2 Fitting, Verification and Validation of Wireless Microphone Systems

When fitting a wireless transmission system, these goals should be achieved with the system:

- Providing full audibility and intelligibility of speech that is equal to their best speech recognition performance in ideal listening conditions
- Maintaining full audibility of oneself and others
- Reducing the deleterious effects of distance, noise and reverberation

For technical verification of the output response curve of the hearing aid with the attached wireless microphone (for details see the recommendation of the American Academy of Audiology (2011) or the EUHA Leitlinie (2016)):

- Moderate input levels of 65 dB(SPL) at the microphone of the wireless transmitter system (set to HA+FM) should achieve the same output levels as feeding the same input signal into the microphones of the hearing aid itself.
- For the measurement, the hearing aid with the attached FM receiver is coupled to the test microphone and placed outside the test chamber (in a quiet room). The wireless microphone is placed inside the test chamber next to the speaker providing the test signal.

For audiometric validation of the benefit of a wireless microphone system attached to the hearing aids (for details see the recommendation of the American Academy of Audiology (2011) or the EUHA Leitlinie (2016)):

- It is recommended to place the wireless microphone next to the loudspeaker with the speech test signal in front of the child and the loudspeaker with the noise behind the child (180°).
- Speech recognition performance with the HA+FM in noise should be significantly improved over performance in noise with the HA alone. Speech recognition results from the HA+FM in noise should be equal to speech recognition performance in ideal listening conditions.
- Speech recognition results should be unchanged between the HA alone and with the HA+FM active in ideal listening conditions.
- Speech recognition results should be unchanged between the CI alone and with the FM active in ideal listening conditions. Speech recognition performance with the FM in noise should be significantly improved over the per-formance in noise with the CI alone. Speech recognition results from the FM in noise should match speech recognition performance in ideal listening conditions.

As wireless microphone systems (FM) or other assistive listening devices are often coupled to hearing aids or cochlear implants that do not come from the same manufacturer, and as these combined systems are used in a wide range of environments such as TV sound transmitters or telephone amplifiers at home; loop systems in churches, cinemas or theatres; and FM systems in schools, universities or conferences, it is not possible to take into account in the clinical test situation all the sources of interference that might influence the performance in real life. Therefore any complaint by the child should be taken seriously, and the complete system of hearing aid and assistive listening device has to be checked not only in the laboratory but also with simultaneous inputs to FM and HA to judge the overall signal quality. The relationship of the FM level to the hearing aid microphone has to be performed under the conditions of actual use of the system.

18.11.3 Special Issues

If important sounds such as alarm bells, telephones, doorbells or alarm clocks, and even the sound of a crying baby, cannot be made audible enough for the hearing-impaired person, electronic systems can transform these sound signals into a visible signal (e.g. a flashing light) or a tactile signal (e.g. a vibration). For this purpose wired and wireless alarm systems are available. Before purchasing one of these systems, testing the system is always recommended.

If speech can no longer be made audible, or to relieve the strains of difficult listening situations, it is necessary to use text or signing. SMS and Internet with email, video telephone or speech-to-text services provide a number of easily accessible communication options.

18.12 Improvement of Classroom Acoustics

Malte Kob

18.12.1 Room Acoustics of Classrooms

Most classrooms are designed to provide space for a maximum number of pupils whilst offering free line of sight to the lecture desk of the teacher. These conditions might be optimal for the visual aspects of "talk and chalk" teaching style but are often problematic because of the sound field distribution in classrooms.

Sound Insulation and Interior Noise Sources The predominant condition for optimal teaching in classrooms is the absence of disturbing visual and auditive cues. Such unwanted acoustic fields can either originate from neighbouring rooms, corridors or the outside, or they can be produced inside the classroom.

Sound from outside the classroom reaches the listeners inside through bounding areas of the classroom: walls, doors, floor and ceiling. Another source of incident sound can be ventilation ducts that can transfer sound from other parts of the building or the outside into the classroom.

Sound inside the classroom can be as disturbing: sources can be electrical devices, heating, ventilation or sounds and speech produced by the pupils.

Balance of Direct and Diffuse Field Speech intelligibility depends on the ability of listeners to identify speech segments without errors. A large level difference between unwanted sounds and the teacher's voice signal is an important condition for high speech intelligibility. This can be achieved by either raising the teacher's voice level or reducing the unwanted sound level.

Every sound source in the classroom—whether wanted or not—will increase the background noise level (BNL). The BNL also depends on the reverberation of the classroom: the BNL increases in rooms with few absorbent and many hard reflecting surfaces. A measure of reverberation is the reverberation time, which should not exceed 1 s in classrooms (Schick et al. 2003; Kob et al. 2006, 2008; ANSI/ASA 2010; ISO/TR 1974).

The perceived teacher's voice level (TVL) depends on the distance between listener and speaker: the smaller the distance, the larger is the TVL and the level difference between BNL and TVL. This difference is called the signal-to-noise ratio (SNR).

In classrooms the SNR depends on the location of the listener: pupils in the first row experience a larger SNR and pupils in the back row a smaller or even negative SNR.

Recommended Limit Values of Acoustic Parameters Guidelines exist about the BNL, reverberation times and other acoustic measures in classrooms (ANSI/ASA 2010). The A-weighted BNL should not exceed 35 dB(A), and the C-weighted BNL should be below 55 dB(C). The reverberation time in octave bands at midband frequencies (500–2000 Hz) should not be longer than 0.7 s, preferably smaller. In addition to these recommendations, noise criteria (NC) curves can be measured to identify too noisy rooms. The intelligibility of speech from the teacher's location to the listener's position can be assessed by measurement of the speech transmission index for public address systems (STIPA; see Sect. 1.6 and ISO/TR 1974).

18.12.2 Improvement of Classroom Acoustics

A number of methods can be applied to improve the acoustics in classrooms. Some of them require major changes of the room boundaries and might require costly structural modifications of walls and floors. Some are easy to implement if no such modifications are necessary. The decision on the extent and potential impact on acoustic measures can be made once the nature and intensity of the present unfavourable sound field and the envisaged improvement are defined.

Reduction of Diffuse Field A first approach would aim at the minimisation of the background sound field in the classroom. The damping of external sources by sound insulation of all boundaries of the classroom to the outside should be improved, and potential noise sources inside the room should be avoided. Secondly, to reduce the growth of the diffuse field by the teacher's and pupils' voices, the attenuation of sound waves at the walls, ceiling and floor of the classroom should be improved by adding sound-absorbing material. The amount of absorption should not be too high: a loss of speech intelligibility results when early reflections are completely cancelled (see Sect. 1.6).

Increase of Perceived Speech Level Voice intelligibility can be improved by the increase of the speakers' voice level at the source or at the receiver. The first would result in a more loaded voice that could potentially be at risk of voice disorders (see Sects. 5.1 and 5.2).

The other, acoustic, method would be the design of early reflections that support the direct sound of the speaker without increasing the BNL. These early reflections would enhance the power of the direct sound and therefore support the projection of the speaker's voice. These reflections can be realised by adding lateral or suspended reflective building elements such as plates or walls. Such installations should be designed and dimensioned by an acoustic consultant.

If none of these methods are applicable, the electro-acoustic amplification of the teacher's voice can be a way to raise the TVL. Whereas this concept reduces the loading of the teacher's voice, it does not necessarily improve the SNR for all listeners.

18.13 Knowledge of Aural Rehabilitation Programmes

Debbie Rix and Gwen Carr

18.13.1 Aural Habilitation Programmes

Deaf children today have wonderful opportunities to develop language and listening through advanced hearing aid technology. However, providing the equipment is only the start of the journey, not an end in itself. Clinicians must work closely with educators and parents to optimise the opportunities available.

It is also important that professionals provide families with unbiased information on the full range of approaches available and be skilled in supporting families to consider and make properly informed choices (Doherty-Sneddon 2003; Young et al. 2006). Each family is unique and influenced by its own complex tapestry of personal history and cultural experience. A communication approach that suits one child and family may not be right for another, and it is important for families to have access to unbiased and independent information to support them in deepening their own understanding of their potential choices (Carr 2015).

At diagnosis most families have had no prior experience of deafness. For many their main concern is whether they will be able to communicate with their child. One approach that practitioners can successfully use is to reassure parents that communication approaches can be changed as their child's needs change. It is important to use a flexible approach that acknowledges the child's personal strengths and preferences and that is based on high expectations. State-of-the-art amplification has meant that the majority of deaf children without significant other needs achieve intelligible and meaningful spoken language. It is now recognised that for some young children, whose auditory access through conventional hearing aids is inadequate to support the development of spoken language, signed approaches can support the growth of language and communication as they await cochlear implantation. It is also interesting to note that some older implanted children who develop full fluency in spoken language later choose to learn sign as a second language, enabling them total flexibility in their communication modes.

Features of Effective Language Enrichment Programmes

- Programmes are personalised so that each child's strengths and areas for improvement are carefully assessed and understood.
- Adults use a consistent approach based on shared goals.
- The programme has high expectations of developmental progress but is delivered at an appropriate pace in achievable steps.
- The programme develops communication in its widest sense as a means to enabling the child to enjoy and achieve relationships and learning.
- Communication and language is linked to the development of higher-order thinking skills (Doherty-Sneddon 2003).
- The programme is based on the child's unique interests and personal experiences.
- Parents actively contribute to the planning and delivery of targets and take a leading role.
- Adults are prepared to change the activity and goals according to the child's interests and developing needs.

Principles of Effective Auditory Training

- The deaf child/young person must have audiological equipment that is appropriately selected, well-fitted and managed at an optimum level.
- Every session must be preceded by careful checking of the equipment.
- Sessions should take place in favourable acoustic conditions, ideally in a room free from environmental noise.
- Sessions should be planned according to the child's developmental rather than chronological age although high expectations for the rate of progress must be maintained.

- Detailed assessment of children's listening skills should dictate the planning and review of the programme.
- Opportunities should be created for the deaf child to generalise the skills acquired in everyday life.
- Activities are based on a listening hierarchy so that children progress from an understanding of sound/no sound to understanding conversation through incremental stages.

Features of Effective Language and Auditory Programmes for Children up to 3 Years

- Parents are the child's main educator, so any communication programme needs to both empower and prioritise the parent's role.
- There needs to be a holistic approach to the child's development so that communication is developed alongside play, social and emotional needs and other milestones.
- Communication needs to be developed through child-centred play activities, particularly those that develop the child's thinking and imaginative skills.
- Amplification needs to be optimum and worn consistently.
- The language and listening environment needs to be quiet, stimulating and safe.
- Adults need to be emotionally attuned to the child and follow the child's lead.

The main types of aural habilitation programmes are categorised below:

Auditory Verbal Therapy (AVT) Widely used following cochlear implantation as well as with children who are conventionally aided, it is delivered by a trained practitioner who may be a teacher of the deaf, speech and language therapist or audiologist. The AV practitioner teaches the child to learn to listen in carefully structured developing stages. A key aspect of the approach is the practitioner's coaching of others, for example, the parent or child's teacher, to teach in this way. The approach is underpinned by optimum audiological management and a detailed understanding of the child's listening skills (Easterbrooks et al. 2000).

Oral-Aural/Natural Auralism In this approach deaf children are exposed to spoken language alone (i.e. no sign language and very limited gestures). Practitioners and educational provisions will vary greatly in the way they use this approach. Some will prioritise direct teaching of new vocabulary and language; others will use a more conversational approach. The approach is underpinned by excellent audiological management, development of good listening skills and the use of spoken language only for receptive (understanding) and expressive (use of) communication.

Total Communication Whilst this method is not strictly an aural approach, as it embraces a wide range of communication support features, it does include maximising auditory potential and supports the development and use of spoken language. It may be used alongside cochlear implant habilitation (Robbins 2002) but also in a wide variety of other settings and situations.

It can be likened to a tool box from which the practitioner can take any means of communication to develop both the child's understanding and expressive language. These tools include speech, sign, facial expression, audition and gesture.

The above are communication approaches/ methods of teaching rather than languages in their own right.

18.13.2 Alternative and Supplementary Modes of Communication

For some children, aural approaches alone are not sufficient to support the development of language and communication competence. This might be due to one or more of the following factors:

- Lack of sufficient access to audition to access the sounds of speech effectively
- Late diagnosis of deafness
- Difficulty extracting meaning from sound/ auditory processing disorder
- Other developmental needs, e.g. deaf-blindness
- Learning disability

For these children there are a number of options available to accelerate their ability to communicate and learn effectively:

Cued Speech This method can also be incorporated into signed approaches but is most frequently used in conjunction with oral/aural approaches. The parent or teacher uses hand shapes close to the mouth to give deaf children additional information (or cues) regarding the sounds being made. It therefore provides a visual reinforcement of the auditory message. Exponents of the method link its use to higher levels of language and literacy development.

Sign-Supported English The adult/teacher and child use speech but add simultaneously signs taken from British Sign Language. This forms both a visual and auditory delivery. The user either signs most words spoken or simply the key ones.

Signed English In addition to the sign system described above, some grammatical markers are also signed. This might include, for example, apostrophes and past tenses.

Makaton Makaton (du Feu and Fergusson 2003) incorporates signs and symbols to support children's communication. It can be introduced from an early age. Down syndrome children with additional hearing difficulties often benefit from the system. Most deaf children in the UK would not be introduced to Makaton unless they have an additional learning disability.

Picture Exchange Communication System (PECS) This is one of the more widely used forms of augmentative and assistive communication approaches originally devised for autistic children. Given the increasing number of deaf children with complex additional needs, practitioners in the field may use it. It involves the child's selecting a picture and giving it to the parent or teacher who then responds in turn.

British Sign Language Some families may choose sign language as their child's primary mode of communication. British Sign Language is a complete language in its own right, rather than just a communication method of instruction (Densham 1995). It is wholly visual with its own grammatical structure and no auditory component. Whilst its use is rare following the introduction of cochlear implantation, it does occur. Children and families choosing British Sign Language need access to a number of resources. These include:

- Access to deaf role models
- Access to other children using sign language
- Sign language instruction classes
- Interpreters including ones in an educational provision

18.13.3 Speech and Language Therapy for Deaf Children and Young People

In the UK some therapists have additional training and become specialist therapists working with deaf children. These therapists work in a variety of settings, including cochlear implant programmes, within education services for deaf children, within the National Health Services and in voluntary sector organisations that specialise in working with deaf children and families. They work jointly with teachers of the deaf, general speech and language therapists and parents to plan, deliver and review programmes of listening and language.

In addition to the delivery of individual and small group therapy, speech and language therapists make specialist assessments of language. These might include tests for differential diagnosis whereby the practitioner assesses whether the child has a language disorder over and above their deafness, for example, dyspraxia. Where deaf children have an additional language disorder, they receive specialist intervention programmes such as the Nuffield Dyspraxia Programme (Williams and Stephens 2010).

Additionally, because of, inter alia, problems with nasality/resonance, lack of intensity/frequency control and altered intonation, voice quality should be improved applying different techniques and exercises (Coelho et al. 2015).

18.13.4 Use of Computer/ Technological Devices to Develop Communication

Teachers of the deaf are increasingly harnessing the power of technology to motivate and develop deaf children's interest in communication. This is particularly true of iPad devices. Pre-schoolers can access iPads and delight in some of the more imaginative and creative apps. Further information can be obtained via the following sources:

- www.pathstoliteracy.org/technology/ipad-ipod-iphone
- www.wonderbaby.org

18.14 Rehabilitation and Prognosis for Children with Auditory Processing Disorder

David R. Moore, Nicole G. Campbell, Doris-Eva Bamiou, and Tony Sirimanna

Introduction Current intervention strategies can be divided into four main categories: (1) listening strategies, (2) modifying the listening environment, (3) auditory training and (4) compensatory strategies (BSA 2011, 2018; Chermak and Musiek 2013). The strategies listed under "Modifying the Listening Environment" are more evidence-based than the other strategies. Several "auditory training" approaches have been tested rigorously, with mixed results. "Compensatory strategies" are widely advocated but have not been well validated (BSA 2018). The lack of an agreed diagnostic procedure makes it more challenging to conduct traditional case-control studies in which those with the disorder are compared with carefully matched controls who lack the disorder. Also, there is no agreement on what the "gold standard" should be against which the sensitivity or specificity of a candidate intervention should be compared. Finally, the high co-occurrence of APD with other disorders can make the use of interventions for specific difficulties of limited general effectiveness. Nevertheless, there is no shortage of suggestions as to what may work (BSA 2011; Chermak and Musiek 2013), and there is increasing evidence that some approaches may improve listening in general.

New technologies, such as remote microphone devices (also referred to as assistive listening devices or wireless listening devices), personal sound amplification products ("PSAPs") and "apps", are promising (Smart et al. 2018) but require further investigation. Remote microphone devices are also proving to be beneficial to those with language and attention difficulties, as the technology allows better access to the primary signal, reducing background noise and reverberation (Schafer et al. 2014).

Listening Strategies There is no doubt that fixating a speaking face improves speech perception (Everdell et al. 2007; Vo et al. 2012), but observation of normal-hearing listeners suggests that this is not something we all do routinely unless we are having difficulty hearing, in which case an individual will intuitively look directly at the speaker. For a person with a listening difficulty (APD), it is the simplest way to improve listening. For a child, it may be something they have never been taught to do (Truesdale 1990). Asking a speaker to direct speech towards a listener and to ensure their face is uncovered is also a good idea.

Modifying the Listening Environment Increasing the signal (speech) level relative to that of the background noise (signal/noise ratio; S/N) will usually result in enhanced perception. This may be achieved in a low-tech way, for example, by sitting or standing closer to a speaker. Reducing the noise level of a listening environment may also be feasible and has been shown to be helpful, for example, in schools

(Shield et al. 2015). In addition to reducing the level of a bothersome sound, reducing reverberation within an environment commonly used for communication is advised (Klatte et al. 2013). This may be achieved through passive acoustic methods such as carpets, curtains, doors, seals and rubber tips on furniture legs and the installation of noise-absorbent partitions or screens. Other aspects that can be considered are architectural design of buildings (e.g. double-glazed windows) and interventions to improve the S/N, including preferential seating (BSA 2018).

Wireless listening devices, also known as "FM systems", have been used for many years to improve the S/N. The principle of wireless listening devices is simple. A target sound source is amplified relative to prevailing noise. This can be achieved without creating an overloud signal by using a closed-loop system in which the listener wears headphones or other receiver (e.g. insert earphones), usually connected wirelessly to a microphone and transmitter, which may be worn by or placed close to the speaker. FM and "Bluetooth" (2.4 GHz) wireless listening devices are becoming simpler to use, more affordable and smaller. Recent evidence suggests that such systems can improve learning outcomes, auditory perception and the fidelity with which the auditory brainstem encodes speech signals (Hornickel et al. 2012; Smart et al. 2018). Although one of these studies targeted children with reading disorders (Hornickel et al. 2012), about half of those children were likely to have APD (Sharma et al. 2009). It may therefore be assumed that the improved outcomes observed would also be seen in children with APD.

Auditory Training There is overwhelming evidence that auditory training results in "near" learning, hearing of stimuli that are the same as, or closely related to, those used during training (e.g. Ferguson et al. 2014). A systematic review (Loo et al. 2010) suggested that current software provides robust "on-task" learning of the exact skill trained, but little or no transfer of learning to untrained tasks or skills. However, a crucial issue in evaluating the rehabilitation benefits of training is whether the observed learning transfers to untrained tasks (Wright and Zhang 2009), especially those that cause difficulty in hearing and listening in everyday life. For example, does music training, or playing computer games involving simple acoustic stimuli (e.g. tones, phonemes), transfer to improved speech perception in noisy environments or reduced inattention of a child to the parent or teacher they need to communicate with? On this issue, the evidence is more equivocal (BSA 2018). There seems reasonable agreement that some short-term, computer-based sensorimotor training can transfer to untrained stimuli (Anguera et al. 2013), but there are also several examples of well-controlled studies where short-term training (i.e. less than about 3 months of daily or near-daily exercises) has been ineffective (Halliday et al. 2012; Murphy et al. 2015). Musical training has been found beneficial for learning important auditory skills and tuning underlying brain processes (Strait et al. 2013; Alain et al. 2014). However, the extent of benefit and transfer to real-world tasks and settings is controversial. In further research it is essential to control carefully for therapist-contact, and to use active control groups, and robust outcome measures to prevent false-positive results (Halliday 2014). It is important that intervention addresses core difficulties and results in improvement in daily functioning, rather than improvement in only a discrete skill that is trained and then remeasured.

Compensatory Strategies Training in metacognitive and metalinguistic strategies can also be considered. These strategies include self-regulation and problem-solving, by identifying individual listening strengths and weaknesses and listening situations that are more challenging. Possible solutions include use of visual material, visual imagery or "chunking" to remember and recall verbal information or writing information down to stay focused and for remembering. Verbal rehearsal may be used to commit verbal information to memory. These strategies, though widely advocated, have not been scientifically tested (BSA 2018).

Long-Term Benefit To the extent that good listening strategies and acoustic enhancement may be lifelong changes in behaviour, we can assume that the benefits of those interventions will persist. Persistence of benefit is likely to be enhanced by making tasks easier, more attractive or more accessible, but these requirements should be balanced against the need for close attention to and engagement with the speaker. Performance may even improve over time owing to long-term learning effects. Similarly, as with other forms of training, continuing engagement with relevant, demanding listening tasks, either during training or in the course of everyday life, may lead to benefits of the sort reported following prolonged musical or language training. There is evidence that various forms of perceptual learning are persistent (Molloy et al. 2012) and that skill acquisition or recovery, especially earlier in life, may be retained without further specific intervention. Finally, the activity for which there is the best evidence for the retention and enhancement of cognitive function, underpinning all aspects of hearing and listening, is aerobic exercise (Hillman 2014; Hillman et al. 2008), and higher physical activity is associated with reduced age-related hearing loss (Curhan et al. 2013). Research of the effect of exercise on children's listening skills could be fruitful. The APD MESHGuide, a new evidence-based resource, offers practical guidance (Campbell et al. 2019).

18.15 Placement, Support and Inclusion of Deaf and Hard-of-Hearing Children

Wendy McCracken and Debbie Rix

Every country has specific statutory requirements regarding the education of all children. These are guided by wider international recommendations such as the Salamanca agreement (UNESCO 1994), the European Convention on the Exercise of Children's Rights, Strasbourg (Council of Europe 1996), the UN (2006) and the Council of Europe (2003, 2006). Whilst the importance of meeting an individual child's needs is recognised, the overriding move has been towards including children's special educational needs within mainstream education. This has led to a diminishing role of special schools for the deaf and a growth of mainstream placements. In England 76% of deaf children are within mainstream education; 79% communicate by using spoken English only; 12% use another spoken language, either on its own or in combination with another language; and only 9% of such children use sign language (Consortium for Research in Deaf Education (CRIDE) 2013).

An appropriate placement for any child rests on the use of appropriate assessment tools. Where there is a newborn hearing screening programme in place that allows very early identification of permanent childhood deafness, access to an appropriate multidisciplinary team can support families and help to ensure optimum outcomes. There is no simple relationship between the degree of hearing loss and the type of placement; thus a child with profound degree of hearing loss may be appropriately placed in a mainstream setting, whereas a child with a moderate loss may need more support and be better placed in a resourced school where such support is available daily. The heterogeneity that typifies any group of deaf children means that making any decisions about the type of placement that is suitable has to be informed by detailed individualised assessment of needs. To meet such diversity, it is important that a continuum of provision is available nationally.

A mainstream setting offers the opportunity for attending school locally the potential to build friendships and fully join in the life of the school and home. In such a setting, reliance on radio amplification and the support of a qualified teacher of the deaf (ToD) are essential. A ToD provides training for mainstream staff who are unlikely to have any experience of deafness; this includes appropriate use of the child's amplification package (hearing aids, radio aids, cochlear implants, sound field amplification) and support to the individual child to facilitate access to the curriculum. Such support is tailored to help meet individual needs (Hyde and Power 2004; Foster and Cue 2009). For children who require more focused time and support, placement would be within a mainstream school that has a resource base within it: in such settings children can

potentially receive significantly more support. These settings also provide access to other children with permanent childhood deafness (PCD); such a peer group offers the opportunity for meeting, playing and working with other deaf children. Such resource bases have the disadvantage of being at a distance from most children's homes. This means daily travel, sometimes over long distances, and makes it harder for a child to establish friendship patterns at home. Currently in England 8.4% of all children with PCD are in resourced provision (CRIDE 2013).

The highest level of needs is met in special schools for deaf children. The reduction in the number of such schools in the UK means they are now highly specialised, seeking to meet the needs of children who, for a variety of reasons, cannot attend mainstream or resources provision. This currently accounts for 3.3% of all children with PCD in England (CRIDE 2013). This may be because of late identification of hearing loss, preference for a specific mode of communication or the presence of additional learning needs, for example, a specific language impairment. A number of schools for the deaf in the UK have a significant proportion of children with complex additional needs, including intellectual disability, physical impairment, autistic spectrum disorder or other social emotional problems. There are a significant number of children who have additional special educational needs attending institutions with provisions to meet them and who are also deaf; in England 11.9% of all children with PCD are in such settings (CRIDE 2013).

18.16 Educational Provision Planning/Management

Wendy McCracken and Debbie Rix

18.16.1 Planning Support Services

Each country and local area is likely to have its own governance and legal framework to underpin the planning of support services for deaf children.

In the UK there is a law, the Children and Families Act 2014 (UK Legislation 2014), which outlines the responsibilities of education, health and social care providers in terms of the planning and delivery of services to deaf children, from diagnosis to the age of 25 years.

There are several principles enshrined in this Act that other countries may wish to consider in the planning of their own services and provisions:

- Multi-professional collaboration and communication between services is fundamental to achieving the best outcomes for children with hearing impairment (Abbot et al. 2005; Atkinson et al. 2007; Office for Standards in Education, Children's Services and Skills 2012).
- Children and families need to be at the centre of planning services through involvement at every level in strategic thinking and delivery.
- Parents and deaf young people need choices and control over the services they select.

A further consideration is that the services that might be appropriate in one area or locality may be very different from those most needed in another. When planning services, commissioners/managers need to understand fully the population they are aiming to serve through detailed data collection and analysis. In addition, this needs to be reviewed periodically so that services remain current and appropriate.

Data on the population to be served might include:
- The age profile of deaf children and young people in the locality
- The level of need and consideration of trends in the population, for example, the number of deaf-blind children or those with a particular aetiology
- The distances involved between the patients and services, for example, how accessible the services provided are
- The cultural and linguistic needs of families
  - Once the population of deaf children and their families is fully understood and mapped out, services can then be allocated and developed.

It is likely that services in whichever country they are located will need to demonstrate efficiency and value for money. One key aspect will be the service's readiness for change and ability to plan in a proactive way for what might be needed in the future. Those services that do not demonstrate the ability to take on new practices and approaches are likely to be less effective. Change management needs to involve professionals, parents and children. A SWOT analysis (an analysis of the Strengths and Weaknesses of a service, the Opportunities open to it and the Threats it faces) is an effective means of gathering viewpoints and ensuring that all aspects are considered.

When planning support services, the monitoring of services needs to be carefully considered. The views of stakeholders, including children, young people and their parents, need to be obtained, and performance indicators need to be both introduced and publicised so that a continual drive towards excellence is achieved. The use of performance indicators based on quantifiable data, such as the time delay between diagnosis and referral to habilitation, is invaluable but needs to be shared alongside the qualitative feedback from deaf children and families. This can be achieved through questionnaires and semi-structured interviews.

It is recommended that services report annually on both their activity and their outcomes. Qualitative and quantitative data can be used to inform the next year's introduction of or improvements to existing services.

Some services may commission an external body or agency to carry out quality assurance on the services provided (UK National Screening Committee 2012–2013). Where a service has been commissioned, for example, by education or health, it is important that there be a shared understanding between commissioners and providers on what service is expected and how its impacts and outcomes are measured. Increasingly commissioners will have a choice of services, and this competition means that providers will need to ensure as a priority that the service meets the needs and expectations of deaf children and families.

18.16.2 Integration Between Health and Education Services

The UK has benefited enormously from the historical partnership between the departments of health and education in determining provision for deaf children and their families. There is a strong tradition of the two agencies working in partnership, underpinned by the values of:

- Mutual respect for each other's roles
- Strong communication
- Co-location where possible
- Clarity and transparency regarding roles and responsibilities
- Joint commitment to achieving the best outcomes

When newborn hearing screening was introduced into the UK, collaboration between the departments of health and education was further strengthened. Areas were assessed on their ability to combine services and jointly plan and deliver services. Some areas developed single-care pathways to achieve seamless delivery of services.

A fundamental concern of any screening programme is that by identifying a need, there is an ability to respond and achieve better outcomes. In the case of deafness, the diagnosis by health professionals requires the timely and effective response of educational habilitationists, usually the teacher of the deaf. One cannot function without the other. There are certain approaches that facilitate team working; these include:

- Joint training
- Joint clinics and assessments
- Joint strategic planning and oversight of service delivery
- Using similar terminology, i.e. avoiding jargon
- Joint IT systems to ease the secure electronic transfer of information

A starting point for services wishing to review their joint practice might be to survey patients and their parents/carers to find out whether their experience of the services provided are in fact seamless. All too often the professionals may consider that they work closely with other agencies, but this takes place "behind the scenes" and does not filter down to the patient experience.

In the UK there is a national network of strategic bodies known as the CHSWG or Children's Hearing Services Working Group. These committees include representatives from education, health, social care and the voluntary sector and, crucially, parents of deaf children. The aim of the CHSWG is to reflect regularly on the joint strategic planning within the area and continually improve it (CHSWG 2017).

Where services demonstrate the highest levels of seamless service delivery, there appear to be common features that are not always dependent on joint funding:

- Commitment from managers and leaders to release staff for joint strategic planning and training
- A joint understanding and commitment to clinical governance
- A common IT system and rigorous data protection systems
- Mutual respect and trust
- The ability jointly to solve problems and develop solutions
- Clear systems for the sharing of information that are process- not personality-driven
- Services that centre on the child and family experience

An example of a successful initiative in Wandsworth, South West London, has been for the head of the educational audiology service, together with the consultant audiological physician in a joint meeting, to meet families of deaf children within days of the diagnosis. At the meeting the care pathway is agreed with families, including discussion of how both education and health will work together to achieve the best outcomes for both parents and deaf children. The meeting is carefully planned so that the professionals work together to explain their different but complementary roles. Through this approach, partnership working is demonstrated from the start.

In *summary*, features of well-planned services include:

- Robust data collection and analysis on the needs of the population to be served
- A skills matrix on the professional team to inform workforce planning
- A shared vision and values framework
- Annual service improvement planning
- A range of performance indicators and outcome measures
- A change management process via a systemic understanding of the whole organisation both internally and externally
- Openness to best practice elsewhere and collaborative working
- Regular involvement of both internal and external stakeholders
- Development of health and education joint care pathways
- Adoption of a health and education joint service improvement approach to patient care

18.17 Teaching and Assessing Literacy Skills in Deaf Children

Wendy McCracken and Debbie Rix

18.17.1 Key Components Underpinning Achievement in Literacy

Being literate is a key skill in life that opens up opportunities to academic achievement at school and helps to secure employment. It was widely considered, historically, that deaf children would inevitably achieve lower reading ages than their hearing peers and would reach a ceiling of attainment beyond which they were unlikely to progress (Conrad 1977). Fortunately, this is no longer inevitable, although deaf children remain at risk of underachievement in literacy (Luckner et al. 2005/2006; Mayer 2007; Easterbrooks et al. 2008). It has been shown that deaf children

who do not have a learning difficulty in addition to their deafness are not only able to reach comparable reading ages to their hearing peers but also exceed them.

The reasons for this are multi-faceted and include the following:
- Modern expectations of educational achievement and attainment being higher
- Earlier diagnosis of deafness
- Cochlear implantation of profoundly deaf children
- Advancements in hearing aid technology
- Research into the reading attainment of deaf children feeding into practice

Four key components underpin the ability to read: the language base, world experience, code knowledge and phonological awareness.

Language Proficiency Hearing children typically bring language competence to the task of reading; they have implicit knowledge of plural, possessive and tense forms. For a child with permanent childhood deafness (PCD), language competence relies on having exposure to both quality and quantity of an accessible language used by a competent native language user (Mayer 2007). The introduction of newborn hearing screening programmes makes it possible to identify hearing loss and fit hearing aids earlier than at any other point in history.

Where amplification provides access to the speech frequencies, there is growing evidence that children are able to develop age-appropriate language (Archbold et al. 2008; Desjardins et al. 2008). However, where parents are unable to ensure that infants wear hearing aids (Moeller 2000) or young children have repeated bouts of otitis media with effusion (OME), the development of age-appropriate language skills is unlikely to be achieved. For children with profound deafness, access to spoken language may be delayed depending on the approach taken, whether a parent chooses to opt for cochlear implantation or the use of sign language. Hearing aids and cochlear implants need to provide access to the spoken word, but children live in acoustically challenging situations, and such devices alone will not ensure access to the speech signal in the car, supermarket and park or at playgroups. In fact any situation that is acoustically hostile will mean that children using amplification are at risk of not hearing. Even in quiet situations, children with PCD are unlikely to benefit from incidental learning (overhearing words in conversations) (Maasaro and Light 2004; Pittmann 2008). The early use of radio aid amplification could help to meet this challenge (Mullah 2011).

In order to access written text, children need access to spoken language, as this is literally what is on the page. Native sign language users therefore need to have spoken language skills in order to access written text. Many deaf children are benefiting from methods of literacy teaching based on the work of Pie Corbett (e.g. Corbett and Strong 2011), which emphasises the link between spoken language and the written word. This is not a new development in deaf education, but it is being optimised with the greater participation of deaf children into inclusive education settings where conversation and everyday conversational speech can be accessed.

World Experience The wider a child's experience, the wider its understanding of the world around it. This is termed world knowledge. If a child has been to a farm, it will be easier to understand any discussion of a farm. Any experiences of making a drink or sandwich, going to a party, shopping or visiting a park all provide opportunities not only to develop language but also to develop an underlying conceptual understanding of that activity.

A mechanistic approach to the teaching of literacy to deaf children will potentially limit the child's ability to achieve fluency and enjoyment. It is important that deaf children read for enjoyment and for information and parents are engaged in this process from diagnosis. Too often deaf children are limited by the interventions of adults who may create a sense of reading being a task-driven exercise with a pass or fail outcome. An approach that links literacy to real-life experiences and creative narratives is more likely to bear fruit.

Code Knowledge The majority of spoken languages have a written format. Code knowledge incorporates the form of the print, the direction of print, the alphabetic principles of a sound being represented by a letter and groups of letters making words and the function of print (that combinations of letters carry meaning). Very young children are typically exposed to print both through the medium of books and through print in the environment. It has been demonstrated that simple exposure to books is not adequate for gaining code knowledge. Shared reading, where attention is drawn to pictures and pauses are introduced to help reflection and consideration, has been shown to be effective in aiding children's understanding (National Early Literacy Panel NELP 2008), as has print referencing, where a child's attention is directly drawn to the text through comments or questions or by tracking the text with a finger. Both techniques are important in helping children gain code knowledge. A rich spoken language environment, where parent and child are relaxed, is the most conducive to supporting a child's development. Optimum listening environments will directly support this, but, in many instances, homes are acoustically hostile, and amplification may be inadequate to meet these challenges unless directly addressed.

Phonological Awareness Understanding the underlying sound structure of language is an area that a child with PCD will of course find difficult as a direct result of his or her hearing loss. The language base itself is more complex for some children. For example, in a phonetically based language, where there is a one-to-one correspondence between the spoken sound and the written letter, the task is considerably easier than, for example, English, where 44 sounds are represented by 26 letters. Phonological awareness refers to the ability to recognise sounds and words of spoken language but also to identify similarities and differences between phonemes that make up a word, as well as being able to manipulate these (Gillion 2000; Beal-Alvarez et al. 2011). Whilst children with PCD have been shown to develop phonological awareness in the same sequence as their hearing peers

(Desjardins and Ambrose 2010), it is developed at a slower rate (Spencer and Tomblin 2009). This is an area that requires direct teaching. It actively depends on optimal individual fitting, verification and continuous validation of personal amplification. Those working with the child, both parents and professionals, should initially use words that are accessible acoustically, short in duration and meaningful. Words should be used in a way that engages and interests the child. Phonological skills should be built up through the use of natural language. The hierarchy of skills should be built up logically, with increasing complexity. Children will need to be supported by the use of a range of activities to build their skills in this area (Yopp and Yopp 2000). The National Deaf Children's Society (2013) in the UK has published guidance on the teaching to deaf children of phonics (a method of teaching literacy skills that focuses initially on the phonemes used within a language before linking them to the letters of the language). This includes daily practice on phonics in quiet listening conditions.

In learning a new word, hearing children will typically have heard it used in a variety of settings before they develop an understanding of its meaning and usage. Children with PCD need more experience than hearing peers but typically get less, as a result of reduced ability to discriminate sounds and lack of opportunity to overhear (Pittman 2008). It is thus important for new words to be directly taught to help increase vocabulary knowledge in these children. It is not only the size of a child's vocabulary that is important but the depth of meaning attached to a word. Work focusing on synonyms can be very helpful (Luckner et al. 2005/2006), and shared reading can be used to support a child in this area. Using both auditory and listening goals is a very useful approach (Zuplan and Dempsey 2013).

The more a child understands and is able to use spoken language, the more knowledge he or she will have of the structure of that language. This helps to ensure that a child is not simply decoding print but is unlocking the meaning of the text (Mayer 2007). The smallest unit of oral language is a morpheme, which provides important information about the meaning of words

(house/houses) and about the syntactic relationship to other words (Neilsen et al. 2011). Hearing children starting school bring with them implicit knowledge of morphological markers, for example, child/children, happy/unhappy and shoe/shoes. There is a paucity of research in this area related to children with PCD, but morphological markers in English tend to be high frequency, short duration and unstressed, which makes them hard to access (Stelmachowicz et al. 2004).

18.17.2 Assessing Literacy Skills in Deaf Children

The assessment of literacy among deaf children needs to involve a number of approaches. First, whilst practitioners may be keen to compare reading ages with hearing peers, it is important that an overall judgement is made regarding the deaf child's interest in text and motivation to read. Deaf children may have difficulties with the pragmatics of language, and it can be important to note whether the child has access to both non-fiction and fiction texts and has an exposure to the rich repertoire of fairy tales and folk tales that characterise early children's understanding of narrative.

A range of assessments is available. However, assessments are typically not standardised on deaf children, given the low incidence. This means that when reporting the reading ages of deaf children, reference needs to be made to a score standardised for hearing children and needs to be interpreted with some caution.

It is important that workers identify assessments that reflect the phonological system of the child's first language. Reading assessments that focus simply on word recognition are of limited value to deaf children. It is important that reading assessments are diagnostic and can identify multiple aspects of the reading process, such as knowledge of syntax and comprehension.

A potential drawback in the teaching of literacy to deaf children is the overemphasis of the teaching of vocabulary. This results in children with good sight vocabulary but poor comprehension skills. Assessment of deaf children's reading through a diagnostic profile can reveal strengths and weaknesses that can inform teaching programmes. This is a far more useful approach than simply a reading age by itself.

In *summary*, effective teaching of literacy to deaf children is underpinned by:

- Detailed assessment of children's phonological, comprehension and word recognition skills, for example, the Phonological Abilities Test (Easterbrooks et al. 2000) and Edinburgh Reading Test (Robbins 2002)
- Careful tracking of deaf children's progress over time so that strengths and areas for improvement are continually reviewed
- Opportunities for deaf children to see adults enjoy and use text
- Reading stories based on their personal interests and everyday experience
- Developing deaf children's use of phonics in quiet listening environments
- Being encouraged to relax whilst reading and find a quiet uninterrupted space
- Frequent praise and encouragement—never overcorrection or chastisement
- Professionals need to seize on the current potential for deaf children to develop as motivated and proficient readers, understanding the significant link between literacy and self-esteem (du Feu and Fergusson 2003)

18.18 Management of Psychological and Socio-Emotional Sequelae and Cultural Influences

Peter Matulat and Mona Hegazi

18.18.1 Psychological and Socio-Emotional Sequelae

Communication with others is regarded as an essential element of human functioning. For a long time, the concept of hearing impairment as a disability has been the premise behind the assessment and rehabilitation of the children affected. Intervention has often focused on improving their hearing and speech and language performance (Butler et al. 2001), but the ICF-CY reframed this by establishing a conceptual framework describing impairment in terms of activity limitations and participation restriction, in combination with environmental and personal factors, rather than just bodily function.

In general, severe-to-profound hearing impairment makes interaction with the outside world difficult. Research has long demonstrated the considerable negative social and psychological effects (Carlsson et al. 2015; Hogan et al. 2015; Hallberg et al. 2008). Communication barriers surrounding hearing-impaired individuals have an impact on their social lives, leading to a spectrum of problems ranging from isolation, loneliness and withdrawal, through anger, stress and irritability, to learning disabilities and maladaptive behaviour. These problems have strongly negative effects upon the individual's quality of life. Consequences of hearing loss cannot be predicted from audiometric data alone (Hallberg et al. 2008). Carlsson et al. (2015) propose "extended audiological rehabilitation" focused on the psychosocial consequences in addition to technical audiological rehabilitation.

Hearing impairment has serious consequences for the individual's physical, cognitive and social functioning. However, it is also a family disease. It has long been considered a social stigma that adversely affects not only the child born with hearing loss but also its family. In 2001 the World Health Organization (WHO 2007) defined the term "third-party disability" to describe negative effects on family members due to the health condition of their close relatives (Scarinci et al. 2009).

On the surface, childhood hearing disability appears only to affect the communication between the child and its parents adversely. But parents (and other family members) also experience other problems secondary to hearing impairment. These include:

- Negative emotions (e.g. frustration and anxiety)
- Reduced social activities
- Relationship problems

- Mental health problems (e.g. depression and anxiety)

The professional development of family members and the financial opportunities facing the family can also be affected.

In clinical practice, professionals have tended to focus on bodily functions when assessing hearing-impaired children. In recent years, however, checklists and questionnaires based on the ICF-CY have been developed for various disabilities to address all relevant factors influencing bodily function, activity and participation and environmental and personal factors. Ibragimova et al. (2009) showed that ICF-CY-based instruments are beneficial in assessment before intervention. McLeod and Threats (2008) focused on a set of ICF codes for children with communication disabilities, whilst Morettin et al. (2013) and Zhang et al. (2016) examined patients using cochlear implants.

Intervention programmes for parents and children have been developed, e.g. the:
- Colorado Home Intervention Program (CHIP) (Colorado School for the Deaf and the Blind CSDB 2017)
- Familienzentriertes Linzer Interventionsprogramm (FLIP) (Barmherzige Brüder Konventhospital Linz 2016)
- Muenster Parental Programme (MPP) (Reichmuth et al. 2013)

The aim of such programmes is to strengthen the resources of the family for independent and self-determined action (empowerment) (Ciciriello et al. 2016). The provision of early pedaudiological care combined with family-centred educational intervention is predictive of successful outcomes for hearing-impaired children, such as improved speech development (e.g. Moeller 2000; Yanbay et al. 2014).

Family-centred care involves family members in rehabilitation services not only as supporters of the hearing-impaired child but also as people with their own needs and difficulties and with individual characteristics, strengths and preferences. Parents' socio-economic circumstances,

their work schedules, their willingness to participate in rehabilitation and the availability of nearby training centres are among factors that govern parents' choices and have an impact on the outcome of management options (Gravel and O'Gara 2003). Findings from Ekberg et al. (2015) show that family members would also like a family-orientated approach to be taken within practical audiology.

Appropriate (external) psychotherapeutic measures should be initiated in cases of mental health problems (in the child or family members) according to the International Classification of Diseases (e.g. for depression or anxiety disorder).

18.18.2 Cultural Influences on Rehabilitation

> Disability is defined by culture. The tendency to categorise all people with different impairments as 'disabled' is a fairly recent phenomenon emanating from Western societies.
>
> Coleridge (1993)

Individuals' health beliefs and behaviour are influenced by their social and cultural background. They play an important role in influencing attitudes towards disability and rehabilitation (Thomas and Thomas 1998). Changing demographics within Europe, where doctors are seeing a growing number of patients from different backgrounds (including the Deaf culture) in clinical practice, require doctors to be more multiculturally (and linguistically) competent.

Culture-sensitive communication and cultural competence allow organisational barriers (e.g. diversity in the leadership and workforce of healthcare organisations), structural barriers (e.g. lack of interpreter services in doctor-patient communication) and clinical barriers (e.g. sociocultural factors and health beliefs and behaviour) to be taken into account as influencing factors in the effective care of patients (Betancourt et al. 2003).

Even such subtle details as the way questions are posed, body language and intensity of eye contact can be interpreted as rude or invasive behaviour.

In addition to the question of how adequate communication can be ensured, cultural competence combines patient-/family-centred care with an understanding of social and cultural influences that affect the quality of medical services and treatment. The awareness and understanding of the key roles played by these factors in the patient-doctor relationship is important.

The Association for Multicultural Counseling and Development (AMCD) provides an overview of the areas of competence relevant to multicultural counselling, including awareness of one's own cultural values and biases, the client's worldview and appropriate intervention strategies (Arredondo et al. 1996). From this perspective, cultural competence is seen a set of congruent behaviour, attitudes and skills, based on self-awareness and cross-cultural knowledge.

The project Culturally Competent in Medical Education (Suurmond 2016) aims to help medical educators and students "provide high quality care to patients from diverse backgrounds" (Diversity in Medicine and Health DIMAH Group 2016). It was funded with the support of the Education, Audiovisual and Culture Executive Agency (EACEA) ERASMUS Lifelong Learning Programme (2013–2015). The main aims of this project (which has partners in 12 countries) are to identify the sorts of competence required by medical educators, to develop a core curriculum, to identify teacher training needs and to develop online modules. First online modules can be found on the website of the Diversity in Medicine and Health Group (DIMAH Group 2016).

18.19 Rehabilitation of Children with Multiple Handicaps

Mona Hegazi and Peter Matulat

Risk of Additional Handicaps 20–40% of all children with hearing loss (HL) have one or more additional handicaps (Cupples et al. 2014). In a literature review, the National Deaf Children's Society (2012) found speech-language disorders (61–88%), visual impairments (4–57%) and neurodevelopmental disorders (2–14%) to be most frequently associated with hearing loss. Children with a HL have a 14 times greater relative risk of a coexisting autistic spectrum disorder (ASD) than the general population (Do et al. 2017). Hearing disorders occur particularly frequently in children with ASD (2–4.2%), cerebral palsy (2–13%) and pervasive developmental disorders (2%).

Team Approach Rehabilitative services provided to individuals who have multiple disabilities generally depend upon the aetiology and specific combination of disabling conditions. They require a team in which a broad range of skills is covered, including medical, therapeutic and educational personnel (Ewing and Jones 2003). Family members play a key role in the process of rehabilitation, and they should be supported in gaining access to the right services. For this reason, empowerment and resource orientation are the current focus in family-centred care (Hintermair 2000, 2006).

The skills taught to children with severe and multiple disabilities should meet their needs and resources and improve their social participation (World Health Organization 2001, 2007). Typically, this includes offers to improve functional, language and self-care skills, visual and auditory training and mobility training. Orientation and mobility specialists help the visually impaired child to develop knowledge of the environment and to enhance the ability of spatial orientation. Physical and occupational therapists work on gross motor development, muscle relaxation and fine motor control. Speech and language therapists/logopaedics assist with speech and language development and feeding problems.

Goals of Intervention Early intervention can have positive outcomes in terms of reducing the level and intensity of support needed as an adult and increasing levels of independence, community presence and quality of life.

Role of Amplification Children with all types of hearing loss and other disabilities are entitled to be provided with amplification devices once hearing loss is confirmed. Some autistic children, though, may be hypersensitive to sound. In these cases, amplification devices should be introduced gradually, using plenty of reinforcement and behavioural management techniques.

As cochlear implants (CI) have become more widely used, the question of whether children with hearing loss and additional disabilities should be provided with them has become a more common subject for debate (Stacey et al. 2006). Schlumberger et al. (2004) argued that early implantation enhances the improvement of non-verbal capacities and that auditory stimulation plays a role in what they called "building the brain". More recent research confirms that children with additional disabilities do benefit from CI (Youm et al. 2013; Lee et al. 2010; Waltzman et al. 2000; Wiley et al. 2005; Hamzavi et al. 2000; Berrettini et al. 2008), although at a slower rate and to a lesser degree than if hearing loss were the only disability. In one study (Cupples et al. 2014), the degree of benefit in language acquisition obtained from CI in children with additional disabilities was found to be significantly related to the level of maternal education.

Communicative Rehabilitation Approaches It is important to consider the development of verbal language after providing appropriate amplification in children with less severe disabilities. Children with more severe disabilities may fail to develop language, so an appropriate mode of communication should be chosen according to each case. Some children may only be taught a few signals to indicate their needs, whilst others may use wider augmentative and alternative communication (AAC) systems. For more information, visit the homepage of the International Society for Augmentative and Alternative Communication (ISAAC) (https://www.isaac-online.org/), or see Communication Matters (2017) which is the working name of ISAAC (UK). An overview of technical aids can be found in Scherer (2017).

Anything that augments speech or accomplishes communicative function is known as augmentative communication. Augmentative communication may be aided or unaided.

- Unaided approaches use signals, codes, gestures and signs (including standard sign language).
- Aided approaches may be low-tech or high-tech.
  - Low-tech approaches include communication boards and communication books.
  - High-tech approaches include speech synthesisers such as voice output communication aids (VOCA), also known as speech-generating devices (SGD).

Choosing the most suitable augmentative and alternative communication method should also depend on the presence and severity of a visual or motor handicap. Ongoing assessments of progress achieved by children in rehabilitation are important components of the therapy programme.

For children with ASD, the TEACCH (Treatment and Education of Autistic and Related Communication Handicapped Children) programme (Mesibov et al. 2004) may be appropriate because it adopts a highly visual teaching method, utilises a clearly defined structured environment and actively involves the parents in all activities. Other approaches that use speech-generating devices also exist (Lorah et al. 2013; Achmadi et al. 2012).

Deaf-blind children have special needs that require adaptations to communication strategies. According to Dammeyer and Larsen (2016), 23% of deaf-blind children use tactile language, 32% oral language and 39% visual sign language. Principles for evidence-based best practice in early identification and intervention can be found in Wiley et al. (2016). The most useful communication method for an individual child varies according to the degree of visual impairment. The most frequently used communication methods are (Welch and Huebner 1995):

- Touch cues: communication prompts that are made on a child's body, such as a light touch on the lips for eating. Touch cues encourage the child to anticipate the next activity and to begin to respond appropriately.

- Object cues: communication prompts that are made with objects that touch the child's body or are presented visibly to the child. For example, a washcloth touched to the face can indicate the activity of washing the face. An object cue encourages the child to anticipate an activity and can be the precursor for using objects as symbols.
- Gestures: mutually understood natural movements or signals, such as pointing or waving goodbye, that are used to communicate specific ideas consistently. Gestures can be used to prepare a child for the use of signs as symbols.
- Vocalisations: sounds made with the voice that can be used to get attention, make wants and needs known and communicate specific things to others. Vocalisations may precede speech.
- Print-on-palm: "writing" on a person's palm with the index finger.
- Tangible symbols: items, such as objects (either partial or whole), pictures or textured materials, that can be used to represent a concept or activity. Their use does not require the level of cognitive ability that formal language does, and they can be readily manipulated to convey an idea (Rowland and Schweigert 2000).
- Sign language: a formal language that uses hand and arm movements, natural gestures, body and facial movements and expressions symbolically.
- Tactile sign language: sign language that is based on touch. It is very similar to sign language but differs linguistically. In a dialogue the two participants sit opposite each other and sign in the other's hand.
- Spoken language: the use of speech to articulate concepts.
- Braille: written language that is embossed, so it can be read by touch.
- Large print: writing that is made large for people who are visually impaired, so they can read it more easily.

In recent years, a growing number of technical devices have been developed for communication between deaf-blind people and people without disabilities (Sharma et al. 2017; Choudhary et al. 2015).

Although technical approaches are very helpful as tools, the multidisciplinary team and the family are still the main decisive pillars of the rehabilitation process.

18.20 General Therapeutic Principles for Childhood Ear Disorders

Hatice Celik and Haldun Oguz

18.20.1 Introduction: Treatment of Childhood Sensorineural Hearing Loss (SNHL)

A multidisciplinary team consisting of an otorhinolaryngologist/phoniatrician, audiologist/paedaudiologist, speech therapist, genetic specialist and educational specialist must evaluate the patient for the proper treatment plan. Hearing aids, special educational programmes supporting hearing development, speech therapy, lip-reading, sign language, fingerspelling, cued speech and hearing tactics strategies and cochlear implant are the modalities used, taking the degree of the hearing loss into account (Lalwani 2002; Joint Committee on Infant Hearing Position Statement 2007).

Although cochlear implants have made great progress in introducing or reintroducing people with hearing impairment to society, SNHL does not still have a definitive therapy. Progress in cell transplantation and regenerative medicine is hoped to lead to pioneering new treatment modalities (Okano and Kelley 2012).

In the following, general therapeutic approaches to treat childhood ear disorders that cause different types of hearing loss are presented.

18.20.2 Medical Treatment of Middle Ear Infections

Acute Otitis Media Clinical observation and antibiotics are the treatment options in acute otitis media (OM) according to the otitis media diagnosis and treatment guide revised by the American Academy of Pediatrics in 2013 (Lieberthal 2013). Clinical observation without antibiotics is recommended in 6–23-month-old children with unilateral and mild OM. High-dose amoxicillin is the first-line antibiotic for those whose clinical findings get worse in the first 48–72 h of the observation, those younger than 6 months of age and those with severe disease. Amoxicillin-clavulanate is regarded as the second-line antibiotic for the above-mentioned cases or may be used as the first line for beta-lactam-resistant infections.

Recurrent Otitis Media Preventive measures including control of the risk factors, immunisation and surgical methods have been used for the treatment of recurrent OM. Basic preventive measures are informing the parents about taking care of the child at home, the harmful effects of smoking at home, breastfeeding the child for at least 6 months and the incorrect use of antibiotics. Antibiotic prophylaxis has been replaced by active immunisation and surgical methods such as ventilation tube insertion and adenoidectomy, owing to the development of resistant pneumococcus species (Lieberthal 2013).

Otitis Media with Effusion In otitis media with effusion (OME), the duration of effusion, accompanying predisposing factors, alterations in the eardrum and middle ear, the status of hearing and language development are all taken into consideration in the treatment plan. A guideline published in 2004 reported that 80% of the cases with OME improved spontaneously. The first stage of treatment is observation for 3 months in cases without an indication for emergency treatment or accompanying risk factors (Rosenfeld et al. 2004). Antibiotics are not recommended in the routine treatment. In case of refusal of surgical therapy by the family, antibiotic treatment can be used. Antihistamines, decongestants, non-steroidal anti-inflammatory drugs and corticosteroids are not recommended for the treatment of OME. Antihistamines can only be administered when OME is together with allergy. The efficacy of mucolytics is debated in OME treatment.

Chronic Otitis Media In chronic suppurative otitis media, topical antibiotics, topical corticosteroids, topical antiseptics, systemic antibiotics and cleansing and acidification of the ear (aspiration) can be used alone or in combination for the resolution of otorrhoea in adults. There is a consensus for a combination of topical cleansing of the ear, under appropriate magnification, with non-ototoxic topical antibiotics (Acuin 2007).

18.20.3 Medical Treatment of Ear Traumata

Acoustic Trauma Avoiding acoustic trauma and administering systemic and transtympanic steroids, hyperbaric oxygen treatment (HOT) and antioxidants are the treatment choices that have been recommended in studies based on clinical experience and author opinions and in expert committee reports (Katz et al. 2009; Arslan et al. 2012).

Barotrauma In order to avoid middle and inner ear barotrauma during flight, pressure equalisation manoeuvres (yawning, swallowing, chewing gum and the Valsalva manoeuvre) can be beneficial in uncomplicated cases. However, if the tubal orifice is blocked by oedema due to an upper respiratory tract infection, antibiotics, oral and nasal decongestants, anti-inflammatory agents and topical steroids must be used before flying. HOT can be used for inner ear decompression sickness (Klingmann 2004).

Temporal Bone Fractures Temporal bone fractures occur very rarely as isolated injuries and are associated with brain and other organ trauma in most patients. Neurosurgeons and otorhinolaryngologists must cooperate to prevent or treat properly complications such as intracranial haemorrhage, cerebral contusion, cerebrospinal fluid leak, meningitis, hearing loss, vertigo and facial paralysis, including both medical and surgical treatment. Intravenous corticosteroids are used for treating sensorineural hearing loss (SNHL) and facial paralysis. Vestibular suppressants can be used for a short time in benign paroxysmal positional vertigo (Patel and Groppo 2010).

18.20.4 Medical Treatment of Inner Ear Diseases

Autoimmune Inner Ear Disease First-line treatment is with corticosteroids in primary autoimmune inner ear disease or involvement of the inner ear in systemic autoimmune disorders. Cytotoxic chemotherapeutics such as long-term methotrexate and cyclophosphamide can be used in cases unresponsive to steroids. Enoxaparin and rituximab can be used, and cochlear implants can be applied in cases with bilateral deafness (Cohen et al. 2011). Plasmapheresis is suitable only for immune-mediated disorders (Bianchin et al. 2010). There are current investigations on cell and gene therapies.

Idiopathic Sudden Sensorineural Hearing Loss Spontaneous recovery is seen in 32–65% of cases with sudden SNHL. Recovery is associated with a number of factors including the age of the patient, presence of vertigo at the beginning of the disease, the degree of hearing loss, audiometric configuration and the duration between disease onset and beginning of treatment. In a clinical practice guideline published in 2002, corticosteroids were suggested as the initial treatment in idiopathic sudden SNHL (Stachler et al. 2012). Recovery

is usually seen in the first 2 weeks. Intratympanic steroid perfusion is usually reserved as a salvage therapy, in case of incomplete recovery or treatment failure; however, it may be used as a first-line treatment together with systemic steroids as well (Kilic et al. 2007; Arslan et al. 2011). HOT is beneficial in profound and severe hearing loss when used within the first 3 months. Other pharmacological agents (antivirals, thrombolytics, vasodilators, vasoactive substances, antioxidants) are not used in routine treatment. They can be used on an individual basis, with patient-specific indications.

Menière's Disease None of the treatment modalities preserve hearing in the long-term. The disease can be controlled with current medical treatment in 80% of patients. Proposed treatment regimens are, in acute crisis, intravenous injection of hypertonic serum + corticosteroids + symptomatic treatment of nausea + benzodiazepine and, between crises, betahistine, regulation of life style (avoidance of triggering factors, salt restriction) and relaxation therapy. In the event of instability, it is necessary to propose vestibular rehabilitation (VR) if the compensation is not completely realised. Chemical intratympanic treatment involves chemical destruction of the reached vestibule + VR (Coelho and Lalwani 2008; Garduno-Anaya et al. 2005; Junicho et al. 2008).

In Menière's disease (MD), which is thought to be an inflammatory or immune-mediated disease, steroids are used on the basis of their success in autoimmune HL and tinnitus. Intratympanic steroids (ITS) may be efficient for the recovery of hearing loss in sudden SHL; however they have no effect on hearing in MD. Despite improvement in vertigo, there may not be significant changes in hearing and tinnitus.

ITS injections may be beneficial in patients refractive to medical treatment, before any aggressive surgical approaches are planned (Coelho and Lalwani 2008; Garduno-Anaya et al. 2005; Junicho et al. 2008). The efficacy of vasodilators is debated in MD treatment.

There are no evidence-based data on gingko biloba, niacin, bioflavonoids, lipoflavonoids, ginger root and other herbal supplements or devices that aim to increase the fluid exchange in the inner ear (Meniette device).

18.20.5 Medical Treatment of Other Ear Disorders

Hearing Loss Secondary to Cerebellopontine Masses Three treatment modalities of the cerebellopontine masses are follow-up, microsurgical dissection and radiation (stereotactic radiosurgery/radiotherapy) after considering the site, nature and size of the tumour. The aim is prevention of the poor outcome by diagnosing them at an early stage. Agents such as anti-VEGF (bevacizumab) and anti-EGFR (erlotinib) have been tried in the medical treatment of neurofibromatosis II progressive vestibular schwannoma (Plotkin et al. 2009, 2010).

Hearing Loss Secondary to Neurological Disorders The treatment of hearing loss due to nervous system diseases is through treatment of the causative specific disease.

Hearing Loss Secondary to Pharmaceutical Agents (Ototoxicity) Currently, there is no curative therapy. Current treatment is directed towards prevention of ototoxicity. Many protective agents including KR-22332, thymoquinone, intratympanic dexamethasone, free oxygen radical scavengers, phosphomycin, sodium thiosulphate and lipoid acid have given promising results for prevention of cisplatin ototoxicity (Shin et al. 2012; Sagit et al. 2012; Shafik et al. 2013).

Glutathione, thyroxine, poly-L-aspartic acid, neurotrophin-3, salicylates, Q-ter (a soluble formulation of coenzyme Q) (Patel and Groppo 2010) and siRNA-mediated knock-down of NOX3, NecroX and many other agents have been suggested to be effective for preventing aminoglycoside ototoxicity (Fetoni et al. 2012; Park

et al. 2012; Lautermann et al. 1995; Hulka et al. 1993; Rybak et al. 2012).

Labyrinthitis Treatment depends on the cause of labyrinthitis. Antibiotics and antiviral agents are directed to the cause, whilst antiemetics, sedatives and hypnotics are used for symptom control in the case of a vertigo attack. For patients with sudden sensorineural hearing loss, a short course of oral corticosteroids is considered the standard of care.

Perilymphatic Fistula Most of the patients may improve spontaneously. Restriction of activity and strict bed rest are recommended. In the presence of Eustachian tube obstruction due to an upper respiratory tract infection or allergy, decongestants, allergy medication and ventilating tubes are recommended. Agents such as diazepam, meclizine and promethazine can be used for symptomatic treatment (Weber et al. 2003; Gacek 1998).

Tinnitus Today, there is no standard and ideal therapy for tinnitus. A disease-specific treatment must be given if there is a known disease causing tinnitus. General aims of the treatment are:

- Eliminating or modifying the tinnitus signal or its source (pharmacological and surgical methods, acoustic treatments)
- Eliminating the stress caused by the tinnitus signal (psychological approaches and psychotropic agents)
- Eliminating the limbic and autonomic system links of the tinnitus signal (tinnitus retraining therapy and neuromonics)

There is no evidence supporting the efficacy of paramedical approaches (herbal preparations such as ginkgo biloba homoeopathy, acupuncture) (Savage and Waddell 2012).

Juvenile Otosclerosis At the onset of otosclerosis, different pharmacological agents can be used to prevent progressive hearing loss or to delay its progression. Sodium fluoride and bisphosphonates have not been found to be successful in otosclerosis. Bioflavonoids may ameliorate otosclerosis-related tinnitus; however, there are no data for their long-term use or their effects on SNHL. Corticosteroids or non-steroidal anti-inflammatory agents may be effective at the initial phase of the disease, but they may cause significant adverse effects with long-term systemic use. There are insufficient data on immunosuppressive treatment. Investigations on pharmacological treatment directed at inflammation and bone metabolism (vitamin D administration, etc.) are current (Liktor et al. 2013). In the future, treatments with osteoprotegerin, receptor activator of nuclear factor kappa ligand, cathepsins and Wnt-β-catenin pathway components may also become current issues.

Hearing Loss Secondary to Vascular Disorders Hearing loss may be seen in a number of vascular disorders (congenital or idiopathic vascular disorders, vascular tumours, thrombosis of the anterior inferior cerebellar artery, vertebrobasilar ischaemia, systemic cardiovascular diseases, etc.). A common treatment modality does not exist for use in all disorders. Disease-specific medical or surgical treatments are performed (Moller et al. 1993; Guevara et al. 2008).

18.21 Conservative Management of Auditory Tube Dysfunction

Kayhan Öztürk and Haldun Oguz

18.21.1 Anatomy, Physiology and Dysfunction of the Eustachian Tube

Anatomy of the Eustachian Tube The Eustachian tube (ET) is a unique connection between the middle ear cavity and the nasopharynx. The ET consists of three parts including a cartilage portion, a bony portion and a junctional portion, which is between the bony and cartilaginous portions. It is almost 3–4 cm in adults and is

directed downwards, forwards and medially (Ishijima et al. 2002).

Physiology of the Eustachian Tube Protection, clearance and ventilation of the middle ear are the main functions of the ET. The cartilaginous part of the ET is closed at rest and protects the middle ear from contamination. Secretions of the middle ear and mastoid cavity are transported to the nasopharynx. The ventilation function of ET ensures that air pressures in the middle ear and the atmosphere are equalised. The tensor veli palatini muscle (TVPM) and levator veli palatini muscle (LVPM) open the ET when they contract during swallowing, yawning or chewing. These muscles are innervated by the trigeminal nerve. The ET is shorter in children and is located nearly horizontally (Ishijima et al. 2002; Bluestone 2005; Ozturk et al. 2011).

Eustachian Tube Dysfunction ET dysfunction is defined as a disturbance of its clearance and ventilation functions. Generally, ET dysfunction is caused by congestion or blockage, secondary to upper respiratory tract infections (URTI) (Casselbrant and Mandel 2004). The tympanic membrane does not vibrate properly because of the air pressure difference between the middle ear and the atmosphere. Hearing loss, autophonia and feeling of fullness in the middle ear are the main symptoms (Catalano et al. 2012). The ET should be closed during rest. If it remains open, the entity is called patulous (patent) ET. The symptoms of patulous ET are autophonia and objective tinnitus (O'Connor and Shea 1981).

18.21.2 Aetiology of Eustachian Tube Dysfunction

Congenital Anomalies Cleft palate, craniofacial abnormalities and Down syndrome can increase the risk of ET dysfunction and related diseases (Catalano et al. 2012).

Infections Clinical and experimental studies demonstrate that viral URTI (common cold, sinusitis or adenoiditis) is a major risk factor for ET dysfunction and ET-related diseases (Casselbrant and Mandel 2004).

Allergy Respiratory allergens may lead to inflammation of ET, hypersecretion and nasal obstruction and cause ET dysfunction (Casselbrant and Mandel 2004; Gentile and Skoner 2004).

Reflux Reflux of gastric contents from the nasopharynx to the middle ear is possible because of immaturity of the ET in children. Gastrooesophageal reflux may play a role in the aetiology of middle ear and ET inflammations (Keles et al. 2004).

Environmental Factors It has been shown that passive smokers have an increased risk of ET dysfunction and otitis media (Murphy 2006).

Otitis Media Otitis media (OM) is the inflammation of mucosal lining of the middle ear. In the following subtypes are listed:

- *Acute Otitis Media*
  - Acute OM is very common among children. Acute OM is usually a bacterial infection. *Streptococcus pneumoniae*, *Haemophilus influenzae* and *Moraxella catarrhalis* are the most common bacterial agents. Group A streptococcus, *Staphylococcus aureus* and viral agents are less common causes. There are four stages of the disease including inflammation, exudation, suppuration and complication or resolution. The main symptoms are otalgia, fullness, hearing loss, autophonia and fever. The tympanic membrane is red, bulging and thick. If perforation occurs, suppurative ear discharge may be seen (Pichichero 2004).
- *Recurrent Otitis Media*
  - Four or more acute OM attacks in 1 year, or three or more attacks in 6 months, are called recurrent acute OM (Leach and Morris 2006).
- *Otitis Media with Effusion*
  - When the ET dysfunction and obstruction continue, fluid is collected in the middle ear secondary to negative pres-

sure and called OM with effusion. The symptoms of acute OM are not present in OM with effusion. The patients complain about hearing loss and sometimes balance problems (Smith and Greinwald 2011). The chronic inflammation can cause structural tympanic membrane abnormalities, tympanosclerosis, ossicular erosion or cholesteatoma.
- *Chronic Otitis Media*
  - Prolonged ET dysfunction and obstruction may cause chronic adhesive OM, chronic suppurative OM or chronic suppurative otitis media with cholesteatoma.

> ET dysfunction, OM with effusion and chronic OM are strongly associated with hearing loss. This may cause important speech and language development delays in children.
>
> Ruben (2004)

18.21.3 Conservative Management of Eustachian Tube Dysfunction

There is no consensus on the management of uncomplicated ET dysfunction, acute otitis media and otitis media with effusion. Watchful waiting and treatment of symptoms are alternative approaches for these diseases (Pichichero 2004). ET dysfunction usually resolves in 1 week.

Antibiotics There is some controversy over the use of the antibiotics for acute otitis media and otitis media with effusion. Evidence-based analysis shows that antibiotics are helpful in the rapid resolution of symptoms of uncomplicated AOM and middle ear effusion. Antibiotics reduce complications. Amoxicillin is generally offered as the first-line selection. Macrolides or trimethoprim-sulfamethoxazole should be offered for children with penicillin allergy. Amoxicillin-clavulanate or new-generation cephalosporins may be selected for resistance or recurrence cases (Pichichero 2004).

Decongestants The aim is to treat inflammation by vasoconstriction around and in the ET and in the middle ear. They are generally effective on nasal obstruction and may also reduce nasopharyngeal mucous, but a prospective study by Ovari et al. (2015) showed no improvement in Eustachian tube opening by nasal decongestants when tube manometry and the pressure equalisation test were used (see Sect. 18.22).

Topical and systemic decongestants may be selected to improve nasal ventilation:

- *Topical Decongestants*
  - Topical intranasal decongestants can only be used for 3 to 5 days. It is really helpful to manage nasal obstruction but patients suffer from rebound obstruction. Doctors should be alert to the possibility of rhinitis medicamentosa.
- *Systemic Decongestants*
  - The most commonly used systemic decongestant is pseudoephedrine. Systemic side effects such as nervousness, insomnia, irritability, headache and palpitations, tachycardia, high blood pressure, raised intraocular pressure and urinary obstruction should be considered when this is selected.

Antihistamines Antihistamines are recommended for patients with allergic rhinitis or food allergy.

Topical Steroids Intranasal steroids have been used for treatment of allergic rhinitis and chronic rhinosinusitis. They have an advantage in preventing systemic complications of steroids. Although some authors (Gluth et al. 2011) have not found a difference between children who used intranasal steroids or placebo, intranasal steroids are generally recommended for the treatment of ET dysfunction.

Others Autoinsufflation is offered by some authors to treat ET dysfunction. Banigo et al. (2016) could show in their randomised single-blind controlled trial that application of the Ear Popper® improves hearing in children with OM with effusion and reduces the necessity of ventilation tube insertion (see Fig. 18.29). The system should be used in the absence of nasal infection

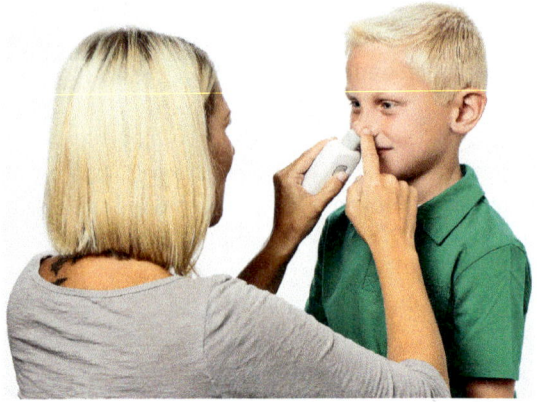

Fig. 18.29 Application of Ear Popper® Image Courtesy of Summit Medical, Inc. Photo with kind permission from the parents

because otherwise there is an increased risk of bacterial and viral inoculation of the middle ear (Perera et al. 2006).

Laryngopharyngeal reflux should be considered in chronic ET dysfunction (Keles et al. 2004; Grimmer and Poe 2005). Balloon dilation of the ET may be useful for chronic ET dysfunction (Catalano et al. 2012). Paracentesis is an option in cases of high pressure in acute otitis media to prevent inner ear damage.

18.22 Indications and Surgical Procedures for Eustachian Tube Dysfunction

Haldun Oguz, Mustafa Asim Safak, and Antoinette am Zehnhoff-Dinnesen

18.22.1 Anatomy, Physiology and Pathologies of the Eustachian Tube

Anatomy of the Eustachian Tube (ET) The ET connects the tympanic cavity to the nasopharynx. The medial two-thirds of the ET is fibrocartilaginous and is in close relation with the tensor veli palatini, levator veli palatini, tensor tympani and salpingopharyngeus muscles. The narrowest part of the ET is at the bone-cartilage junction, and the internal carotid artery is just anterior to this point. The course of the ET is nearly horizontal to the sagittal plane in early childhood, but it develops a superior inclination of 30–40 degrees from medial to lateral by growth of the child to adult ages. The nasopharyngeal orifice of the ET is called the torus tubarius, which is built from a hook-shaped cartilaginous tube, muscle endings and Ostmann's fat pad (Cunsolo et al. 2010).

Physiology of the ET The ET remains closed unless it is opened by contraction of its muscles during swallowing or yawning. The functions of the ET are pressure regulation of the tympanic cavity, protection and clearance of the middle ear.

ET Pathologies ET pathologies may arise from obstruction, improper functioning (dysfunction) or patency of the tube. Obstruction of the ET may arise from oedema secondary to an inflammation in the nasopharynx, such as adenoiditis, adenoid vegetation, sinusitis, passive smoking, etc. (Gryczynska et al. 1999). Neoplastic masses such as angiofibroma or nasopharyngeal carcinoma may also lead to ET obstruction. Diseases that affect the mucosa, such as infections, allergic reactions and ciliary dyskinesis, may also obstruct the lumen of the ET (Takasaka and Kawamoto 1985). Finally, any kind of nasal obstruction may change the nasopharyngeal airflow dynamics and result in obstruction of the ET. Craniofacial malformations such as cleft palate, Down syndrome, craniosynostosis syndromes, Pierre Robin sequence, hemifacial microsomia and Treacher Collins syndrome can change the position and proper functioning of the ET and result in ET dysfunction without an exact obstruction (Kemaloglu et al. 1999). Diseases and disorders of the muscular system such as myopathies or muscular dystrophy may spoil the muscle functions of ET and cause ET dysfunction. Normally

the ET is closed at rest, but rarely it can be open throughout its full length. This condition is called *patulous ET*. There is no ventilation problem in this condition, but the prevention function of the ET is especially disturbed (Grimmer and Poe 2005).

18.22.2 Diagnostic Evaluation of the Eustachian Tube

ET disorders cause middle ear problems. Obstruction or dysfunction of the tube will always result in ventilation difficulties of the middle ear. At the early stage of the disease, when negative pressure increases in the tympanic cavity, some complaints such as slight hearing difficulty, sensation of blockage in the ear and sometimes tinnitus arise. When the problem becomes chronic, fluid accumulates behind the tympanic membrane (TM), and the complaints become more marked. At this stage, some TM findings are visible by otoscopy or otomicroscopy: enlargement of vessels of the TM, prominently visible processus brevis of the malleus, air-fluid level or air bubbles behind the TM and colour changes (yellow to brownish) of the TM are the most significant. The movements of the TM are diminished during pneumatic otoscopy (Rosenkranz et al. 2012). Type B or C tympanograms may be detected by tympanometry.

Tube opening quality can, e.g. be examined by tube manometry according to the Estève method (application into the nose of an air pressure bolus, which by swallowing reaches the nasopharyngeal ostium of the ET and measuring the effect by a pressure probe in the external ear canal) and by the pressure equalisation test (test for ears with a perforated tympanic membrane, swallowing at negative and positive external ear canal pressures) (Ovari et al. 2015). Scintigraphic evaluations may also be used to assess ET dysfunctions (Celen et al. 1999). Further tests, e.g. Bluestone's nine-step test (inflation-deflation test with a tympanometer) and sonotubometry (sound is conveyed from the nose to the Eustachian tube after swallowing or similar manoeuvres; an increased sound level can be recorded by a microphone placed in the external auditory canal depending on tube function), are presented in updates by Borangiu et al. (2014) and Smith et al. (2017).

The diagnosis may be clarified with a direct or endoscopic upper respiratory tract inspection. This would reveal mostly a mass in the nasopharynx such as adenoid vegetation or a focal infection. If there is a craniofacial malformation, a computed tomographic (CT) evaluation may be needed.

In the case of patulous ET, the patients suffer from hearing their own respiration sounds and describe autophonia. This may have a negative impact on quality of life (Bayar Muluk and Carpar 2011; Oguz and Felek 2012). The synchronised movement of the TM with respiration may easily be seen during otoscopy. Owing to failure of the protection function of the ET, the nasopharyngeal content may easily reach the tympanic cavity and cause frequent attacks of acute otitis media.

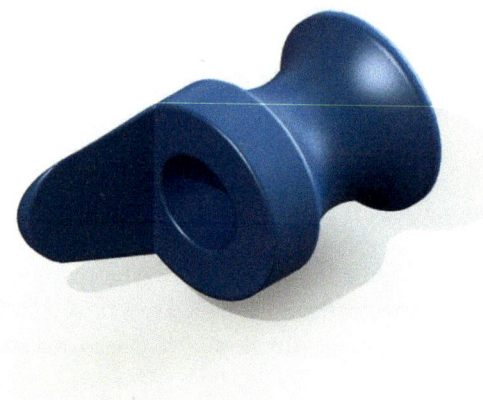

Fig. 18.30 Shepard type ventilation tube. Image copyright and with permission from Summit Medical, Inc

18.22.3 Surgery for Eustachian Tube Dysfunctions

Surgery to Improve Tube Opening Quality/ Ventilation of the Tympanic Cavity The treatment modalities focus on relieving the middle ear physiology. The first important objective is to interfere with the ventilation of the tympanic cavity. To insert a ventilation tube into the TM is a very easy and effective treatment (American Academy of Family Physicians, American Academy of Otolaryngology-Head and Neck Surgery, American Academy of Pediatrics Subcommittee on Otitis Media with Effusion 2004). For primary surgical treatment, the ventilation tube we usually prefer is a Shepard type (Fig. 18.30). For recurrent ventilation tube application needs, or when there is a need for a longer period of the tube in the tympanic membrane, we usually prefer a T-type tube (Fig. 18.31). Söderman et al. (2016) saw significantly more extrusion from short-shaft than long-shaft ventilation tubes and a higher incidence of otorrhoea by fluoroplastic than by silicone tubes in a prospective randomised controlled trial in children with bilateral recurrent acute otitis media or otitis media with effusion

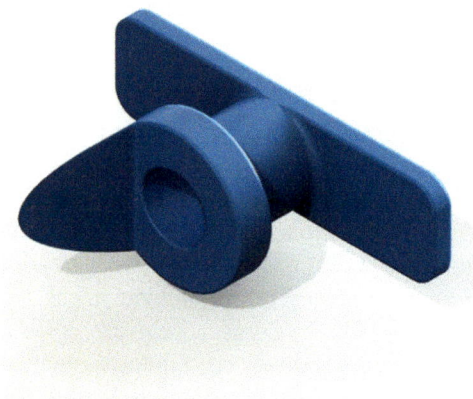

Fig. 18.31 T-shaped (T-type) ventilation tube SuperSoft. Image copyright and with permission from Summit Medical, Inc

after 12 months post tube insertion. In tubed ears the risk of tympanosclerosis was found by the Multicentre Otitis Media Study Group, UK (2012), to be 27%, of otorrhoea <2% and of permanent perforation <1%. The risk of persistent tympanic membrane perforations after tympanostomy tube surgery increases with longer follow-up, repeated insertion, older age at insertion and female sex (Alrwisan et al. 2016).

The second important objective is to treat the obstructive pathologies. If adenoid vegetation is detected, adenoidectomy is advised. The

Multicentre Otitis Media Study Group, UK 2012), found haemorrhage in 1 of 165 children (0.6%) with adenoidectomy. Adenoidectomy in combination with ventilation tube insertion extended better hearing through the second postoperative year and reduced eligibility for repeat tube surgery.

According to the study by Yegin et al. (2015), ventilation tube insertion was more effective than myringotomy alone, in association with adenoidectomy, in improving hearing of children with otitis media with effusion. This result was valid for the whole audiological follow-up period until 1 year after surgery.

For the other (non-adenoid) masses, except in suspicion of an angiofibroma, a biopsy is required for exact pathological diagnosis. Septoplasty or conchoplasty may be performed in suitable indications. The techniques for enlargement of the ET are not yet in routine practice (Catalano et al. 2012). In cases of craniofacial abnormalities, many specific operative techniques are described according to the type of the pathology.

Surgery for Patulous ET The closure techniques, such as injecting different materials into the torus tubarius or suturing the limbs of it, are not useful. Ventilation tube insertion may reveal the symptom of hearing one's own respiration sounds, but it is not so effective for other complaints (Chen and Luxford 1990).

18.23 Indications and Surgical Procedures Concerning Congenital Malformations of the Ear

Sylva Bartel-Friedrich and Stefan Plontke

18.23.1 Indications for Surgical Treatment of Congenital Malformations (CM) of the Ear

The indications for surgical treatment of minor CM of the pinna (found in up to ca. 5% of the population) are psycho-emotional stress from teasing, decline in health-related quality of life associated with reduced school or work performance, social avoidance and loss of self-confidence (see Fig. 18.32a, b).

In patients who have higher-grade CM of the outer ear (auricle and external auditory canal, EAC; see Figs. 18.33 and 18.34) with severe aesthetic, and in bilateral cases functional, consequences, the primary indications for surgical treatment are psychosocial pressure and the suffering of the patient (Berghaus et al. 2010).

The functional surgical repair of atresia should follow the recommendations of Siegert (2010) or Jahrsdoerfer et al. (1992) (criteria listed below). As functionally excellent alternatives for hearing rehabilitation, partially implantable hearing devices can be offered, either bone-anchored (e.g. Baha® by Cochlear Corp., Melbourne, Australia, and Bonebridge® by Vibrant MED-EL, Innsbruck, Austria) or with direct stimulation of the ossicular chain or the round window membrane (e.g. Vibrant Soundbridge (VSB) by Vibrant MED-EL, Innsbruck, Austria).

For inner ear CM with profound hearing loss or deafness, surgery for hearing rehabilitation is focused on cochlear implantation. The indication for operative treatment is hearing loss that cannot be sufficiently ameliorated by hearing aids (open speech understanding of approximately ≤50% of monosyllables at 65 dB SPL with an optimal hearing aid or a hearing threshold of 80–90 dB HL or worse at 1000 Hz and higher (Mlynski and Plontke 2013)). The appropriate electrodes or insertion techniques should be chosen with respect to the underlying cause of hearing loss, the shape of the pure-tone audiogram and the (radiological) anatomy.

18.23.2 Surgical Procedures in CM of the Outer and Middle Ear

Plastic and aesthetic surgery of low-grade auricular dysplasia—most frequently protruding ear—is suggested to be medically and surgically optimal at the age of 5–6 years, just before school age. However, current developments in the legal

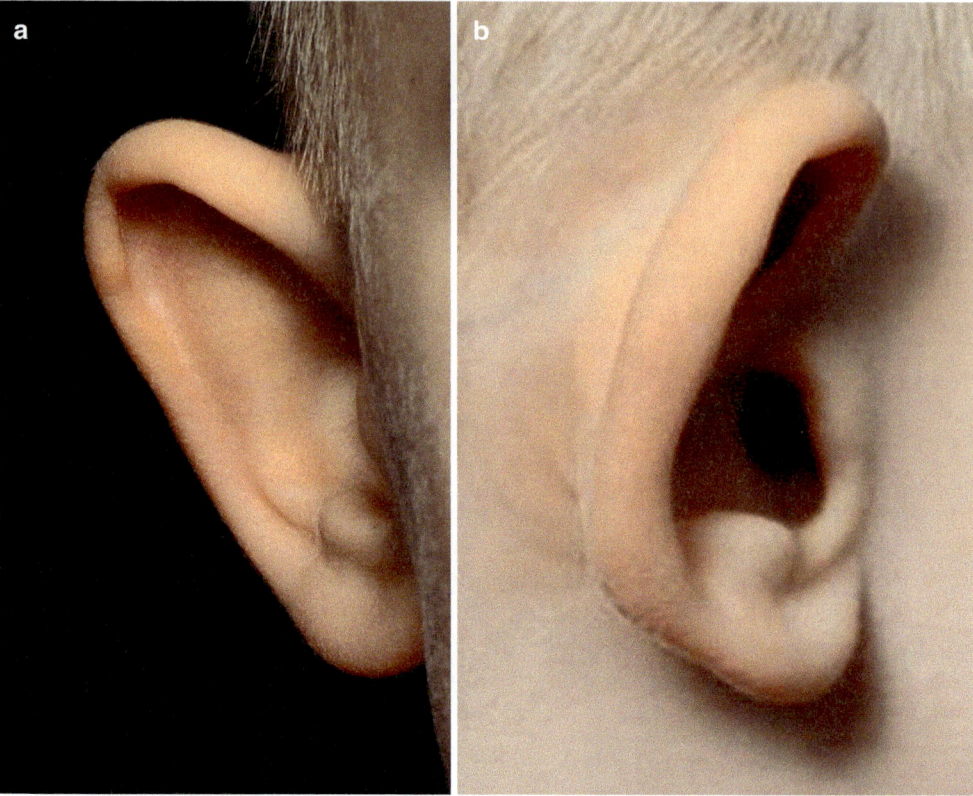

Fig. 18.32 (**a** and **b**) Grade I microtia with protruding auricle, flattening of antihelix and poorly developed crura anthelicis (prominent ear). Patent external auditory canal and normal hearing were present

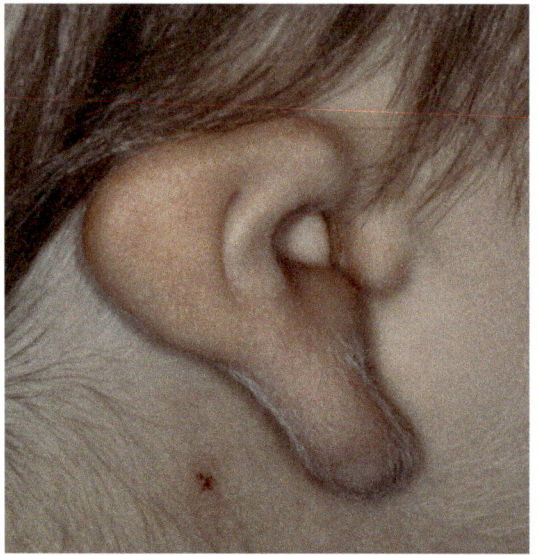

Fig. 18.33 Grade II microtia with the absence of the upper auricle and thickened helix of the middle third of the auricle, whilst tragus, antitragus and lobule are present. Additional right-sided findings were cartilaginous external auditory canal stenosis, mild-to-moderate middle ear malformation and severe conductive hearing loss

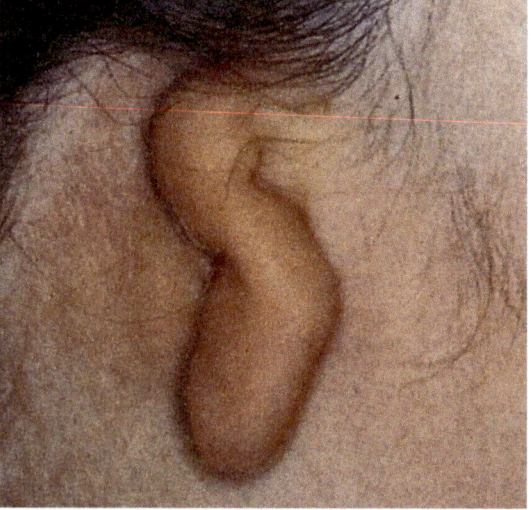

Fig. 18.34 Grade III microtia with rudimentary remnant of the lower auricle (peanut ear, lobule-type microtia) and external auditory canal atresia. Additional findings showed severe middle ear malformations and a severe conductive hearing loss

aspects of plastic and aesthetic surgery in children need to be considered. Various techniques are used, which can be grouped into three categories: sculpting, suturing and combinations of the two (Park et al. 2010). *Sculpting* comprises the superficial scoring/rasping/scratching/incision technique, mostly in the region of the anterior surface of the antihelical cartilage (the Stenstrom method), cartilage or skin excisions, and thinning of the posterior surface of the cartilage by means of a diamond burr (burring). *Suturing* comprises antihelical tubing (Mustardé method), conchal setback and cavum conchae rotation with concha-mastoid sutures (Goldstein and Furnas method) and lobule correction with a concha-lobule suture (Weerda method). The converse method combines suturing and posterior incisions of the cartilage for remodelling of the auricular vaults without involvement of the anterior perichondrium. Suturing techniques are commonly used in patients with soft and pliable cartilage and yield good to excellent results (Braun et al. 2010b; Heppt 2008). Other techniques such as incisions, scoring, burring and combined methods may be used in the case of thick, stiff and unyielding cartilages and for revision surgery and can achieve pleasing results depending on careful selection of surgical technique and the surgeon's experience.

Complications following otoplasty can be subdivided into early and late (Table 18.2). According to Park et al. (2010), the cumulative incidence of early complications varies from 0 to 8.4% and that of late complications from 0 to 47.3%. Only in a low proportion of patients (1.6–4.8% according to Braun et al. (2010b)) are suturing techniques followed by major complications (othaematoma, relapse, asymmetry, keloid, thread granuloma) necessitating revision.

Patients with second-degree malformations can also undergo surgery at the age of 5–6 years, provided sufficient cartilage exists to form the new ear. Reconstruction of higher-grade auricular dysmorphia is complex and usually requires multiple interventions with autologous costal cartilage. Various one- to six-stage procedures have been described (Brent 1999; Nagata 1995; Weerda 2007). In most cases two- to three-stage techniques are used, following the Nagata approach

Table 18.2 Early and late complications following otoplasty (modified from Braun et al. 2010b, Heppt 2008 and Park et al. 2010)

Early complications (up to 14 days after surgery)	Late complications
Haematoma	Suture extrusion
Bleeding	Scarring
Infection	Hypersensitivity
Skin necrosis	Asymmetry
Wound dehiscence	Pain
Allergic reaction to local materials	Keloid
Paraesthesia	Thread granuloma
Pain	Excess of skin/annoying shape of ear
Hypersensitivity	Unaesthetic results
	Overcorrection, undercorrection, reprotrusion (relapse, 2–13% (Heppt 2008)), telephone deformities, reverse telephone deformities, cartilage irregularities
	Rigidification of upper helix

or variations of it. Each operation for auricular reconstruction contains three basic elements:

- Construction and placement of the costal cartilage framework
- Rotation of the lobule, conchal excavation and tragal construction
- Elevation of the helical rim

An axial temporal fascia flap or galeal fascia muscle flap can be raised to cover the elevated framework. To close the retroauricular skin defect, either local skin flaps or full-thickness or split-thickness skin grafts (e.g. obtained from the groin, the opposite postauricular region or another hair-bearing part of the head) are placed over the fascia flap. In the case of unfavourable local conditions (injuries, scars), one-step procedures involving an axial fascia flap can be used (Katzbach et al. 2006). As a rule, plastic reconstruction of microtia is recommended from the age of 8–10 years. The rate of success, assessed by comparing the appearance (shape, curve, size) of the reconstructed ear with the normal ear and by the emotional benefit to the patient, varies between 60 and 100% (Declau et al. 2008). Complications following microtia repair can be

Table 18.3 Complications at the donor and graft sites following microtia repair using autologous costal cartilage

Complications at donor site	Complications at graft site
Pneumothorax	Seroma and haematoma
Chest wall deformity	Flap necrosis
Scarring	Extrusion of framework
Discomfort and anaesthesia	Resorption of framework
–	Pressure necrosis due to sleeping position
–	Incorrect positioning of ear
–	Poorly designed cartilage framework
–	Disruption of helix-baseplate attachment
–	Hypertrophic scars and keloid

Table 18.4 Complications following auricular reconstruction with porous polyethylene frameworks (adapted from Braun et al. 2010a and Naumann 2011)

Region of reconstructed ear	Region of donor site of skin transplants	Region of temporoparietal fascia flap
Scars	Scars	Scar without hair growth
Discomfort	Hair loss	Numbness
Unpleasing shape/position	Numbness	Lesion of temporal branch of facial nerve
Numbness	–	–
Unpleasing skin colour	–	–
Extrusion of implant	–	–
Flap necrosis	–	–
Hair growth within auricle (rare)	–	–
Increased skin dryness and odour (rare)		

subdivided into those at the donor site and those at the graft site (Table 18.3). The latter may arise in 2–10% of cases (Declau et al. 2008).

As an alternative to autologous costal cartilage, alloplastic materials can be used in reconstruction. The material currently most often used is porous polyethylene (MEDPOR®, Porex Surgical, Newnan, GA, USA). With porous polyethylene, reconstruction can already be successfully carried out at preschool age in a single operation, with a second step only rarely required (Berghaus et al. 2010; Naumann 2011; Reinisch and Lewin 2009). The one-step procedure involves insertion of the implant, completely enveloped in a highly vascularised flap, e.g. from the temporal parietal fascia; skin covering of the ventral aspect of the ear with local flaps and full-thickness skin obtained from the contralateral ear; and covering of the post-auricular skin defects with full-thickness grafts obtained from the groin or abdomen. Braun et al. (2010a) reported a high rate of patient satisfaction (adults 72.7%, children/parents 85%/73.7%) and patient benefit (adults 75.6%, children 100%) for this intervention. Complications following auricular reconstruction with porous polyethylene frameworks can be divided into those affecting the reconstructed ear, the donor site of skin transplants and the region of the temporoparietal fascia flap (Table 18.4). Naumann (2011) reported an overall complication rate of less than 4% in the hands of experienced surgeons.

Individual children may experience problems attaching the clip of a bone conduction hearing aid or wearing an earring or psychological rejection of the new ear.

The production of autologous cartilage by means of tissue engineering is the subject of intensive research. Furthermore, an episthesis can be used for aesthetic rehabilitation, especially in patients with failed autogenous reconstruction and in cases of severe soft tissue or skeletal hypoplasia (Park et al. 2010).

Higher-grade dysplasia of the auricle is often accompanied by CM of the EAC or the middle ear, and by no means all EAC and middle ear reconstructions (atresia repair) yield the desired hearing improvement. According to Jahrsdoerfer et al. (1992), only 50% of patients with aural atresia are candidates for repair. The decision to operate depends primarily on the degree of middle ear development as reflected by the size of the tympanum and the status of the ossicles. Lambert (2001) states that the chances of a successful hearing result are increased if the middle ear and mastoid are at least two-thirds of the normal size and if all three ossicles, although deformed, can be identi-

Table 18.5 CT score according to Siegert, Mayer and Weerda (Siegert 2010 and Siegert et al. 1996)

Structures	Configuration	Points
EAC	Normal/fibrotic atresia/bony atresia	2/1/0
Aeration of mastoid	Distinct/moderate/absent	2/1/0
Size of tympanic cavity	Large/moderate/eburnated	2/1/0
Aeration of tympanic cavity	Distinct/moderate/absent	2/1/0
Facial nerve	Normal/slightly aberrant/strongly aberrant	4/2/0
Course of arteries and veins	Normal/slightly aberrant/strongly aberrant	2/1/0
Malleus and incus	Normal/dysplastic/absent	2/1/0
Stapes	Normal/dysplastic/absent	4/2/0
Oval window	Open/closed	4/0
Round window	Open/closed	4/0
Maximum score		28

Table 18.6 CT score according to Jahrsdoerfer et al. (1992)

Temporal bone parameter	Points
Stapes present	2
Oval window open	1
Middle ear space	1
Course of facial nerve	1
Malleus-incus complex	1
Mastoid pneumatisation	1
Incus-stapes connection	1
Round window (open)	1
Appearance of outer ear	1
Maximum score	10

© 1992, The American Journal of Otology, Inc. With kind permission from Wolters Kluwer Health, Inc

fied. On the basis of clinical findings (EAC present, tympanic membrane of any size) and CT scans, Frenzel et al. (2012) integrated canaloplasty/tympanoplasty into the auricular reconstruction procedure. To avoid failures, the indication for atresia repair surgery should be assessed from the Siegert or Jahrsdoerfer scales (Tables 18.5 and 18.6).

Depending on the score and whether the malformation is bilateral or unilateral, Siegert and co-workers recommend surgical or conservative therapy:

- In bilateral malformations, middle ear reconstruction of the better-hearing ear if the score is 15 or more

- In unilateral malformations, middle ear reconstruction if the score is at least 20, following a frank discussion with the patient/parents
- In patients with lower scores, hearing aids only

Patients with a preoperative score of 8 or more were considered suitable candidates. A score of 5 or less disqualifies the patient for surgery. According to Jahrsdoerfer et al. (1992), whether the ear malformation is unilateral or bilateral plays no part in the decision.

The prospect of hearing improvement after surgery is good only in the presence of favourable anatomical conditions or a sufficiently high score (Jahrsdoerfer et al. 1992; Siegert 2010; Siegert et al. 1996). For example, 82% of patients with scores of 8/10 achieve a post-operative speech reception threshold of 15–25 dB, and 89% of those with a score above 8 achieve 0–10 dB, thus attaining normal or near-normal hearing (Jahrsdoerfer et al. 1992). Repair should take place after the age of 6 years and in experienced hands (Declau et al. 2008).

Bilateral microtia and congenital aural atresia are usually accompanied by normal inner ear function. Therefore, children should be provided with bone conduction hearing aids from the first weeks of life in order to ensure normal language development. Initially a headband with a bone conduction device is used. This can be replaced by surgically implanted bone-anchored hearing aids (Baha®; Cochlear Corp., Melbourne, Australia) or a Ponto R bone-anchored hearing aid (Oticon Medical, Göteborg, Sweden) from approximately the age of 4 years (depending on the thickness of the skull). A newer alternative is the Bonebridge® bone conduction hearing device (Vibrant MED-EL, Innsbruck, Austria), which is approved for children from age 5 (Rahne et al. 2016). Sufficient volume of the mastoid needs to be present for placement of the Bonebridge's Floating Mass Transducer, which can be assessed by preoperative planning (Plontke et al. 2014).

The recommended timing of microtia-atresia surgery depends on the chosen reconstruction technique (age 8–10 years if using autologous costal cartilage, or preschool age if using porous polyethylene frameworks) and the atresia score.

If the latter is poor/marginal or worse ($\leq$5 of 10 points on the Jahrsdoerfer scale), EAC/middle ear surgery should not be performed; in these cases, hearing devices should be continued or offered. If the Jahrsdoerfer score indicates a CM suitable for surgery, atresia repair can be started from the age of approximately 6 years, with one-, two- or three-stage procedures. Jahrsdoerfer and Kim (2004) favour performing the auricular reconstruction first, to avoid any scar formation. Weerda (2004) recommends starting primary auricular surgery at the age of 8–10 years; the middle ear reconstruction is then carried out simultaneously with the second step of auricular reconstruction, following CT evaluation. Siegert (2010) described a special operative procedure for the reconstruction of the entire sound conduction system combined with auricular surgery with a three-stage procedure starting at the age of 9 years. In his series of integrated tympanoplasty, 59% and 76% of patients achieved post-operative air-bone gaps of 25 dB or less and 30 dB or less, respectively.

The primary goal of atresia surgery is to establish sound and speech reception without hearing aids. According to Wollenberg et al. (2007), however, an acceptable residual air-bone gap of $\leq$20 dB HL can only be achieved for approximately 20–25% of patients even at highly experienced surgical centres. Higher reported success rates are most likely due to very restrictive selection criteria, a higher residual air-bone gap, or partially unavailable long-term follow-up data. At least, surgery should enable hearing rehabilitation by the use of conventional hearing aids. However, this can be challenging in patients who have undergone auricular reconstruction and canaloplasty. In addition, the air-bone gap may increase owing to restenosis of the EAC and lateralisation of the tympanic membrane reconstruction. In this context, new treatment options for hearing restoration have been developed with the aim of avoiding complications associated with the Baha bone anchor (e.g. skin infection or loss of osseous integration) or atresia repair. Alternative approaches include other partially implantable bone conduction hearing devices (e.g. Bonebridge®, Vibrant MED-EL, Innsbruck, Austria; Alpha 2®, Sophono, Inc., Boulder,

CO, USA) and the active middle ear implants (e.g. Vibrant Soundbridge®) for direct stimulation of the ossicular chain or the round window membrane.

Nevertheless, surgeons considering the use of these implants must take into account various aspects, such as the individual anatomical conditions, the kind and degree of hearing loss, the psychological impact and the limitations for future MR imaging after surgical hearing rehabilitation with implantable hearing aids. Ongoing studies have developed a score, based on CT scans, for more precise risk stratification and decision-making for active middle ear implant (aMEI) candidates (Frenzel et al. 2013). The VSB can achieve good hearing results (Clarós and Pujol-Mdel 2013; Cremers et al. 2010; Frenzel et al. 2012). Further studies must determine the prognostic/predictive value of the aMEI score for hearing outcomes.

Frenzel et al. (2012) developed the "Lübeck Flowchart" for functional and aesthetic rehabilitation of ear atresia and microtia (Fig. 18.35). This can serve as a basis for decision-making and intervention planning for malformed ears. Moreover, beyond the flowchart, the aMEI and other implants can be used later in life, in combination with auricle reconstruction or in cases where a Baha has to be removed owing to complications such as recurrent infection.

It has long been assumed that unilateral hearing loss (UHL) can be considered a minimal hearing loss and will not influence a child's development. However, UHL is accompanied by significant functional impairment (Welsh et al. 2004), and there is increasing evidence that school-age children with UHL appear to have increased rates of grade failures, need for additional educational assistance and perceived behavioural problems in the classroom (Lieu 2004). A relevant number of children with lack of binaural hearing show significant difficulties in their language, academic and socio-emotional development (Yoshinaga-Itano et al. 2008). Binaural hearing in normal-hearing listeners results in better speech understanding in the quiet and in noise, and it is necessary for spatial hearing and sound localisation. Additional

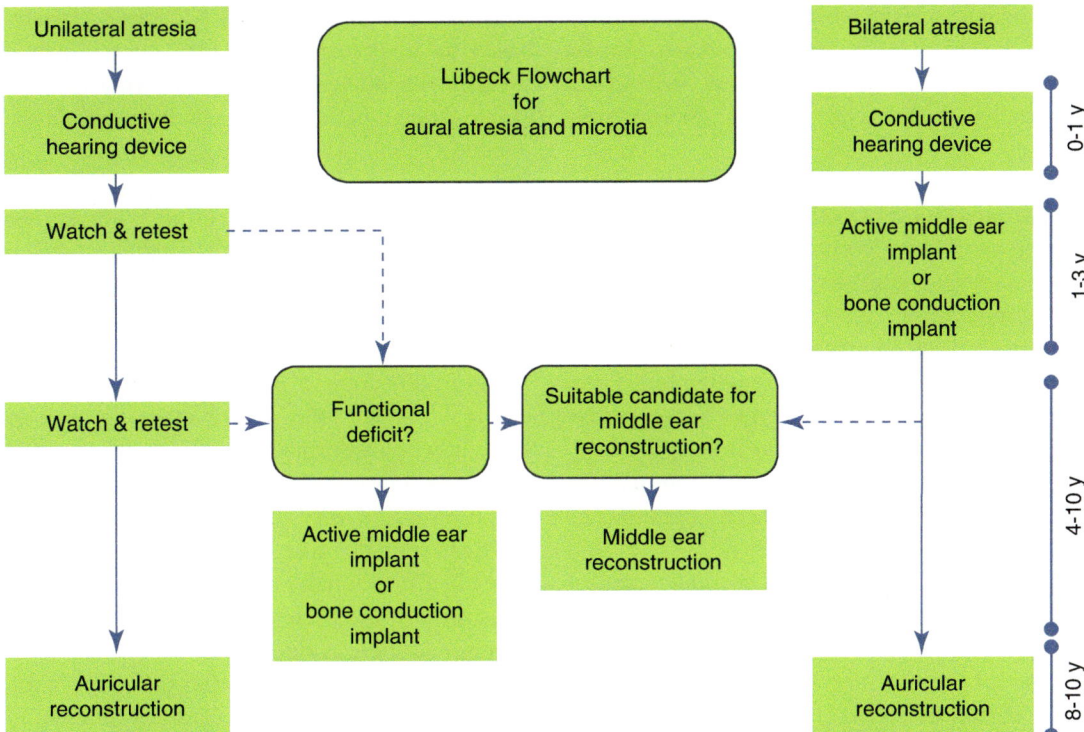

Fig. 18.35 The "Lübeck Flowchart" for aural atresia and microtia adapted from Frenzel et al. (2012). Patients with bilateral atresia are provided with a bilateral conductive hearing device (headband) as soon as possible. Before the age of 2, the conductive hearing device is replaced by a permanent solution. The auricular reconstruction with autologous rib cartilage is performed at ages 8–10 years. Patients with unilateral atresia are provided with a unilat- eral conductive hearing device (headband). With a given indication, the conductive hearing device is changed into a permanent solution. The auricular reconstruction is per- formed at ages 8–10 years. Patients with suitable anatomy are considered for canaloplasty/tympanoplasty. The pro- cedure is integrated into the auricular reconstruction. With kind permission from Wolters Kluwer Health, Inc.

benefits of binaural hearing are a more natu- ral hearing, a reduced listening effort and an improved quality of life. Therefore, it is advis- able to supply a hearing aid in the first year of life, before complete maturation of the central auditory pathway, to avoid impairments particu- larly in directional hearing and noise-disturbed hearing (Sommer and Schönweiler 2004). This prevents unfavourable consequences for com- munication, behaviour, intellectual development and school and career performance, which seem to occur in approximately one-third of unilateral atresia patients lacking fully functional compen- sation (Bess and Tharpe 1984; Kiese-Himmel and Kruse 2001; Lieu 2004, Weerda 2004). Furthermore, early amplification of the affected side allows for symmetrical maturation of the auditory pathways improving the physiologi- cal basis for hearing benefit following definitive solutions planned at a later time point.

18.23.3 Surgical Procedures in CM of the Inner Ear

Malformations of the inner ear are observed in approximately 20% of patients with congeni- tal sensorineural hearing loss. Mainly because of the risk of insertion failures and meningitis, CI was considered a contraindication in com- plex inner ear malformations. Nowadays CI is no longer contraindicated in inner ear congeni- tal malformations with profound hearing loss or deafness. Exceptions are the Michel deformity and cochlear aplasia, where the cochlea is absent and no neural structures can be expected. In most other cases, CI can be accomplished successfully by detailed preoperative imaging, appropriately selected electrodes and insertion techniques. Close attention must be paid, however, to a possible aberrant course of the facial nerve, or a gusher phenomenon. An algorithm that—depending on the pathology—considers intraoperative facial nerve monitoring, electrophysiological testing (electrically evoked stapedial reflex and electrically evoked compound action potential), intraoperative navigation and imaging (intraoperative X-ray, CT or cone beam CT) with possible cerebrospinal fluid drainage or total obliteration of the middle ear cavity has been suggested by Arndt et al. (2010).

Absence (aplasia) of the vestibulocochlear nerve is a contraindication to cochlear implantation. Nevertheless, some positive results of CI in cases of cochlear nerve deficiency (Marangos 2002; Zhang et al. 2012) have reopened critical discussion on this topic. Cochlear nerve deficiency (CND) is defined as a diameter of the midportion of the IAC less than that of the adjacent facial nerve (FN) or the absence of the IAC, either congenital or acquired, in the reconstructed parasagittal oblique plane (Zhang et al. 2012). CND can be associated with other inner ear CM and is classified according to Govaerts' system (Govaerts et al. 2003), on the basis of the affected branch of the nerve and the related labyrinthine CM on MRI findings (Table 18.7).

In a small number of CND cases, mostly based on mild response to loud environmental sounds with bilateral powerful hearing aids, or very restricted but demonstrable language development (babbling, few monosyllabic words) as well as the parents' aspirations, and following detailed audiological and neuroimaging assessments together with in-depth parental counselling, CI may achieve an improvement in hearing thresholds resulting in possible improvements in sound or word perception (Zhang et al. 2012). These results support data showing that even a minimal number of CN branches can deliver some acoustic information to the higher central auditory pathways (Zanetti et al. 2006). It can be supposed that a very thin CN, undetectable on MRI, intermingles with facial or vestibular nerve fibres in a functionally combined trunk and then turns towards the cochlea, permitting signal processing via these auditory nerve fibres. In addition, these undetectable branches may explain the unexpected improvement in auditory function in those cases where MRI, with insufficient spatial resolution for identification of a very thin CN, and subtle motion artefacts point to CND.

Even if hearing results after cochlear implants in congenital inner ear malformations show a large variability, they can generally be considered as good (Birman et al. 2012), and, with the exception of (definite) cochlear nerve aplasia and cochlear aplasia, profound hearing loss or deafness due to CM of the inner ear can be successfully surgically treated with a CI.

Table 18.7 Govaerts' system for classification of cochlear nerve deficiency (CND) (Govaerts et al. 2003)

	MRI				
Classification	CN	VN	FN	CT	Comment
Type I	Absent	Absent	Present	CM possible	Reported cochleovestibular labyrinth CM: IAC stenosis, absence of BCNC, VSCM, IP I, IP II
Type IIa	Absent or hypoplastic	Present	Present	CM of cochleovestibular labyrinth	
Type IIb	Absent or hypoplastic	Present	Present	Normal morphology of cochleovestibular labyrinth	IAC stenosis possible

CN cochlear nerve, *VN* vestibular nerve, *FN* facial nerve, *IAC* internal auditory canal, *VSCM* vestibular and semicircular canal CM, *BCNC* bony cochlear nerve canal, *IP I* incomplete partition type I, *IP II* incomplete partition type II

18.24 Indications and Surgical Procedures Concerning Bone-Anchored Hearing Aids, Implantable Hearing Aids and Cochlear Implants

Martin Kompis and Marco Caversaccio

18.24.1 Indications

Indications for implantable hearing system do not depend solely on the device in question, its known benefits and limitations but also on the success rate, performance, cost and ease of use of all competing solutions. As a consequence, indications can and do change over time and may also depend on external factors, such as insurance coverage. Therefore, indications may or will vary over time and, to a certain extent, between countries.

18.24.1.1 Implantable Bone Conduction (BC) Hearing Aids Including Bone-Anchored Systems

Today, implantable BC hearing aids encompass percutaneous bone-anchored hearing aids (Arnold et al. 2011), such as the Baha® (Cochlear) or Pontois™ (Oticon Medical) systems, as well as transcutaneous systems (Riss et al. 2014) such as the Bonebridge™ (MED-EL) and the Baha Attract (Cochlear). These systems are shown and described in more detail in Sect. 18.5.

In most cases implantable BC hearing aids can be viewed as a therapeutic modality, which is either alternative or superior to either conventional hearing aids or, more frequently, non-implantable BC hearing aids. They can be indicated in any kind of purely conductive hearing loss including conductive hearing loss due to congenital malformations such as ear canal atresia, draining ears, syndromic hearing losses, e.g. due to Goldenhar or Down syndrome, or after previous ear surgeries. Indications include unilateral or bilateral hearing losses. In bilateral hearing losses, monaural fittings are possible, but bilateral implan-

tation does clearly improve bilateral hearing. In unilateral hearing losses, the hearing threshold of the other ear can lie anywhere between normal values and complete deafness. Small additional sensorineural components of the hearing loss are much less frequent in children than in adults and can be compensated, but the indication needs to be carefully examined if BC thresholds are above approximately 30 dB. An additional indication is single-sided deafness, where a BC hearing aid is placed on the side of the deaf ear to allow a bone conduction-CROS (contralateral routing of signals) fitting. Today, this last indication is usually reserved for adults and older children.

In contrast to conventional hearing aids, BC implants can be used even in draining ears, and in ears without ear canals, and provide a constant acoustic stimulation even in fluctuating conductive hearing losses. Compared with non-implantable BC hearing aids, aesthetics and mechanical robustness are often better, and skin attenuation is lower for most systems (exception: Baha Attract). On the other hand, MRI, especially on the ipsilateral side of the head, is limited or complicated if the implant contains a magnetic component.

Usually, implantations do not take place before the age of 2, and parents often opt for even later implantations. The prerequisites for surgery, as listed below, must be met.

18.24.1.2 Implantable Hearing Aids Not Using the Bone-Conduction (BC) Pathway

Today, some implantable hearing aids not using the BC pathway, such as the DACS, are not used in children at all; others, such as the Vibrant Soundbridge® system (MED-EL), are used predominantly in congenital aural atresia.

18.24.1.3 Cochlear Implants

Cochlea implants (CI) are currently by far the most frequently used active auditory implants. Their usefulness especially for small children is clearly proven. Historically, the first and still most important indication is a bilateral profound cochlear deafness (Tajudeen et al. 2010). No threshold limit is given here, as this limit has moved in the last decades from formerly over 90 dB towards lower values and seems to continue to do so. As a general rule, a CI is indicated when the expected outcome is better than with the best conventional hearing aid fitting. Note that hearing may be lost during CI surgery. Today, many children with a congenital hearing loss receive their first CI before or around the age of 1 year. Late implantations, i.e. after age 2 or 3, show systematically poorer results. In acquired deafness, implantation should be performed as soon as possible. This is especially important after bacterial meningitis, where ossification of the cochlea may impede later implantation.

Apart from bilateral profound deafness, two newer indications are accepted today: profound high-frequency hearing loss and unilateral deafness. In the former, only moderately increased or even perfect hearing thresholds up to 1000 Hz are accepted. Preservation of this low-frequency hearing is sought through careful, atraumatic surgery. The aim is to combine electrical (high-frequency region) and acoustical (lower frequency) stimulation in the same ear. In single-sided deafness, the experience with children is so far too limited to define generally valid indication criteria (Friedmann et al. 2016).

18.24.2 Prerequisites and Surgical Procedures

Before surgery, not only the audiological indications but also the surgical prerequisites must be considered.

18.24.2.1 Prerequisites to Surgery

For bone-anchored hearing aids (Baha, Ponto), a sufficient bone thickness and bone quality are necessary. Usually, children should be more than 2 years old and have a skull bone thickness of at least 2.5 mm. When fitting a child with a transcutaneous Baha Attract System (c.f. Fig. 18.15 in Sect. 18.5), a skin thickness of at least 3 mm is required. If a child does not meet these conditions, BC hearing devices mounted on headbands can be used for the time until surgery. A

preoperative CT scan is recommended to assess bone quality and bone thickness, which is important for the decision of the implant length (3 or 4 mm).

The Bonebridge device (c.f. Fig. 18.15e, f in Sect. 18.5) has been certified for children of age 5 years and older. Surgically, the key limiting factor is usually the size of the cylindrical transducer (approximately 16 mm across and 9 mm deep), which must fit safely and reasonably well behind the ear of the child. The so-called lifts, i.e. small spacers attached to the transducer, can help the surgeon in implantations, where only a part of the transducer is placed beneath the surface level of the skull.

For cochlear implants, the presence and sufficient patency of the cochlea are the most important anatomical prerequisites. Imaging, usually including CT and MRI, is used to detect malformations of the cochlea and the vestibular system, to assess the path of cranial nerve VII and the existence and appearance of cranial nerve VIII. From the configuration and the liquid-filled length of the cochlea, first inferences about the ideal length of the electrode array can be derived.

18.24.2.2 Surgical Procedures

Various surgical procedures have been proposed and are used at different centres. This diversity is particularly pronounced for bone-anchored hearing aids (Arnold et al. 2011). Owing to the limited scope of this section, the following subsections describe only one possible method for each implant type.

Bone-Anchored Devices (Baha, Ponto)
Although bone-anchored implants can be placed under local anaesthesia in adults, in young children surgeries are performed regularly under general anaesthesia.

The implant is placed retro-auricularly, starting with a small linear incision. A hole of 3 mm diameter is drilled at the place of the future implant. It is important to keep the direction of the drill strictly perpendicular to the skin surface, as sound processors, which are placed on skewed implants, may touch the surrounding tissue and cause acoustic feedback later. The next and most central step is shown in Fig. 18.36. The implant (in children usually 3 mm long), which is also a self-tapping screw, is driven into the opening by a dedicated power instrument developed by the manufacturer. The abutment, the upper part of which will later hold the sound processor, is already connected to the implant at this stage. After closure, a so-called healing cap, i.e. a circular disc, clicking onto the abutment is placed above the dressing around the implant. With some of the current implants, a speech processor can be used as soon as 2 weeks after surgery.

In Baha Attract surgery, only the implant itself, without, i.e. the abutment, is implanted. After it

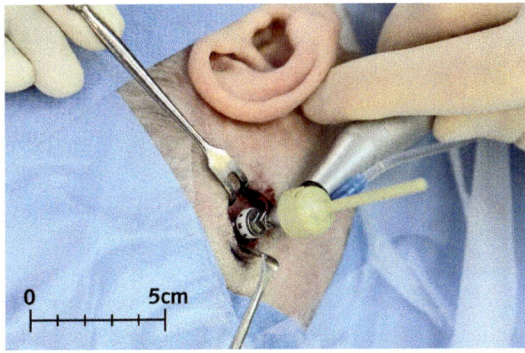

Fig. 18.36 Implantation of a bone-anchored device (here: Baha, with kind permission from Cochlear): placement of the implant. The abutment is already attached to the implant at this stage

is ensured that the implanted magnetic disc does not touch the skull anywhere, it is screwed to the implant. Skin thickness above the implant should be between 3 and 6 mm.

Besides general complications such as bleeding, infection, scarring and paraesthesia of the skin, further risks may be failure of osseointegration of the screw and damage to the dura mater.

BC Devices with Implanted Transducers (Bonebridge) Implantation of BC devices with implanted transducers such as the Bonebridge (MED-EL) is usually performed under general anaesthesia in children. The particular challenge of Bonebridge implantations in children is to find a safe placement for the transducer (Wimmer et al. 2015) (approximately 9 mm thick and 16 mm in diameter, right-hand part of Fig. 18.37). CT and preoperative planning (left-hand part of Fig. 18.37) are strongly recommended. If the transducer does not fit fully into the mastoid cavity, which is frequent in children, the above-mentioned lifts (spacers) can be used. In this case, a substantial portion of the transducer will remain above the former bone surface level. The transducer is screwed to the bone. The two screws are the most important acoustic path, at least during the first time after surgery. The coil/magnet/stimulator unit is placed and fixed further to the rear and the wound is closed. Possible risks are similar to those of surgical complications mentioned above.

Fig. 18.37 Implantation of a bone conduction hearing aid with an implanted transducer (here: Bonebridge, with kind permission from MED-EL). Left panel: preoperative planning showing sufficient bone thickness in white and green (courtesy of Dr. W. Wimmer). Right-hand side: cavity after burring and with and without the transducer in place (sigmoid sinus, ss; dura mater, dm)

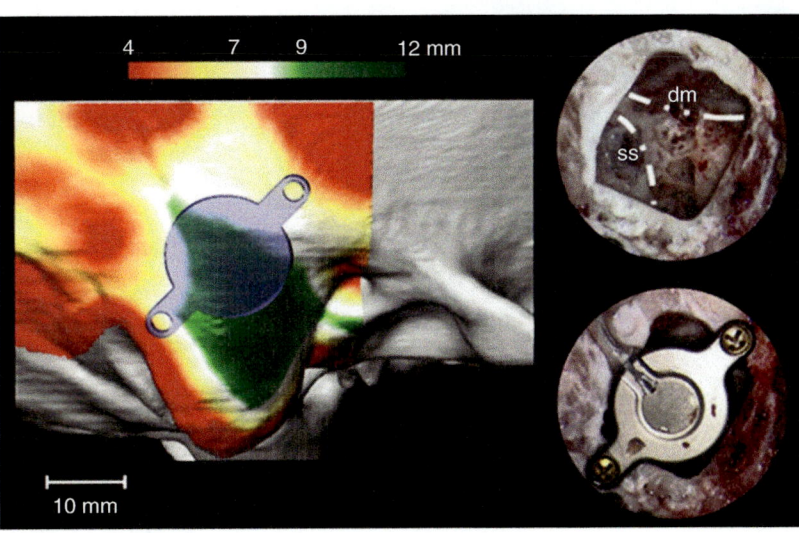

Cochlear Implants Cochlear implantation can be performed unilaterally or bilaterally during the same surgery under general anaesthesia. Figure 18.38 shows the retroauricular access to the middle ear cavity. After conservative mastoidectomy and posterior tympanotomy, in the round window approach, the bony overhang is reduced by drilling. Today, measures are usually taken to preserve any residual hearing, and corticosteroids are applied along with antibiotics. The electrode array is placed carefully into the scala tympani, aiming to avoid damage to the basilar membrane. The length of the inserted electrode array should ideally match the frequency region intended to be stimulated electrically. This is especially important for electrical and acoustical stimulation in the same ear.

The implant body is fixed and the wound is closed. Usually, telemetry of the implant and the measurement of the neural response through the implant are performed towards the end of the

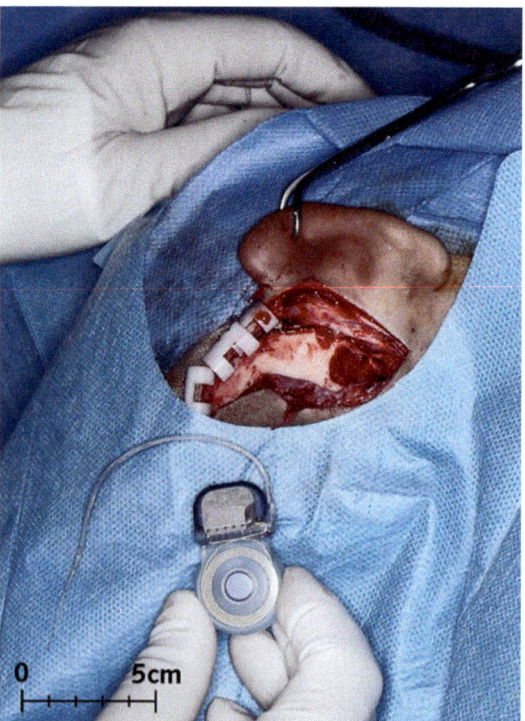

Fig. 18.38 Cochlear implantation in a child: view of the retroauricular access. Synchrony, with kind permission from MED-EL

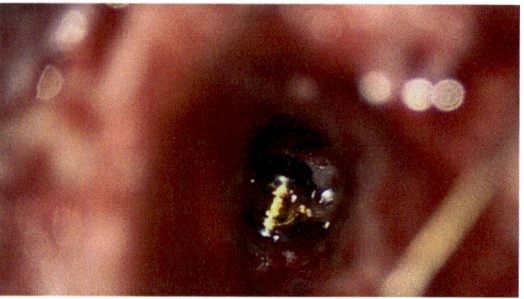

Fig. 18.39 The transducer of a Vibrant Soundbridge system (with kind permission from MED-EL), in situ during surgery. The transducer is approximately 2 mm long and 1 mm in diameter

surgery. Possible risks are general complications as mentioned above and dizziness, leakage, meningitis, facial nerve paralysis and dysgeusia.

Implantable Hearing Aids Not Using the BC Pathway (Vibrant Soundbridge) Implantation of a Vibrant Soundbridge system is, up to a certain point, similar to a cochlear implantation. However, instead of directly accessing the cochlea, the acoustic transducer, which is roughly 2 mm long and 1 mm in diameter, is attached to a structure in the middle ear. This structure is most frequently the incus but, using different couplers available from the manufacturer, can also be the round window or the head of the stapes. Figure 18.39 shows a transducer in situ during surgery. The complication rate is lower than the one in percutaneous systems.

18.25 Cooperation in Surgical Management in Children with Different Stages of Cleft Palate

Ute Pröschel

Children with cleft palate or additional cleft lip may suffer from several restrictions: hypernasality, reduced speech intelligibility, hearing disorders, dysphagia and reduced facial appearance. This might have a significant impact on the child's quality of life. The outcome of the treatment can be improved if therapy is offered by an experienced multidisciplinary team in a cleft centre. The core team of the cleft centre should include an oral surgeon, an orthodontist, a phoniatrician, a speech and language therapist and an audiological physician. Members of other disciplines such as psychology, genetics, paediatric dentistry, restorative dentistry, paediatrics and obstetrics are desirable but optional.

One task of the phoniatrician and the audiological physician is the continuous monitoring of the child's middle ear function and hearing. Children with cleft palate suffer more often from middle ear affections resulting in conductive hearing loss than do children without a cleft palate. This is due to the impaired function of the cleft musculature opening the Eustachian tube and achieving ear clearing, i.e. musculus levator palatini and musculus tensor veli palatini.

The middle ear function and the child's hearing should be checked before every (oral) surgical intervention. The incidence of serous otitis media is close to 100% before the primary closure of the cleft palate. If serous otitis media persists, the insertion of grommets is necessary to restore accurate hearing and prevent impaired speech development due to impaired hearing. Anaesthesia can then be used for the closure of the cleft as well as for insertion of the grommets.

Short-term grommets might not be sufficient if otitis media with effusion appears recurrently (Fig. 18.40). The use of permanent T-tubes however bears the highest long-term risk of perforations. Thus in cases of recurrent or chronic otitis media with effusion, the insertion of intermediate-type tubes is recommended (Baik

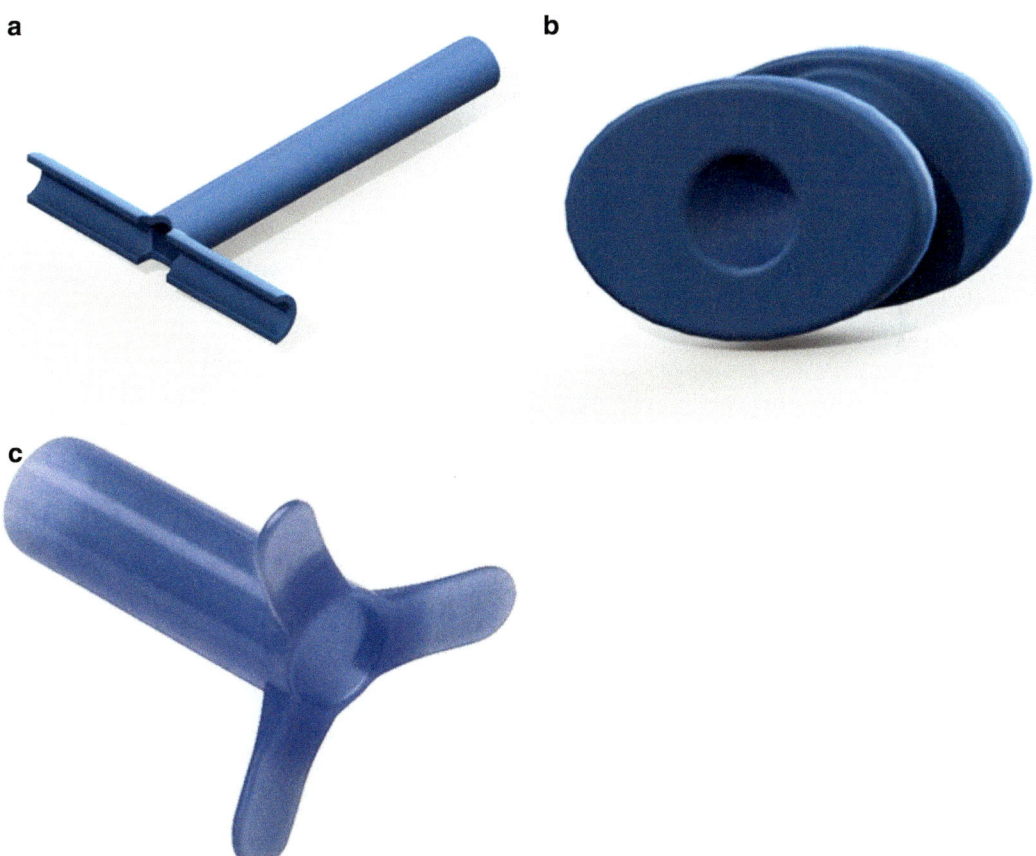

Fig. 18.40 Various types of grommets/tympanostomy tubes. (**a**) A permanent T-tube. (**b**) A short-term grommet (type shown is a Pope grommet). (**c**) An intermediate T-tube (type shown is a Triune tube). Images **a** and **b** copyright and with kind permission of Summit Medical, USA. Image **c** copyright and with kind permission from Grace Medical

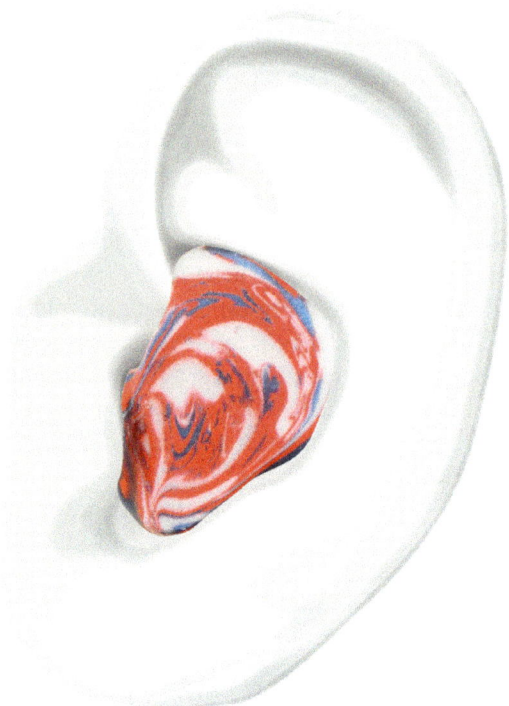

Fig. 18.41 Floatable swim plug. Image copyright and with kind permission from Starkey

and Brietzke 2015). Contemporary guidelines concerning tympanostomy tubes may be found in the review of Jefferson and Hunter (2016). In case of allergy gold-plated grommets may be used, swim plugs protect the middle ear when bathing or swimming (Fig. 18.41).

After functional closure of the cleft palate, the middle ear problems are more often reduced in children with combined cleft lip and palate than in children with cleft palate only. The intra-individual differences of ongoing middle ear problems range from complete recovery to recurrent middle ear affections resulting in chronic otitis media such as cholesteatoma. If no other surgery is necessary, the treatment of the middle ear affection then has to take place independently.

Adenoidectomy is a risk to velopharyngeal function as the nasal airway is enlarged, but adenoidectomy does not necessarily lead to velopharyngeal incompetence. To minimise the risk of velopharyngeal insufficiency and hyper-

nasality, endoscopic partial adenoidectomy is recommended (Stern et al. 2006; Tweedie et al. 2009; Askar and Quriba 2014; Abdel-Aziz et al. 2015).

In some cases of hearing loss due to middle ear problems such as extensive myringosclerosis, it might not be possible to insert grommets to restore good hearing. Depending on the amount of hearing loss, it then is necessary to fit hearing aids.

The second important task of the phoniatrician is to monitor the speech development of the children with cleft palate. This includes the possible occurrence of hypernasality and its treatment. If surgical treatment of hypernasality is considered, a thorough investigation by the phoniatrician of the amount and kind of velopharyngeal insufficiency is important. This aspect is covered in detail elsewhere (see Vol. 2, Part I).

If the cleft team decides on a velopharyngoplasty, it is important to perform an adenoidectomy before this; otherwise the ventilation of the middle ears as well as the nasal breathing might be severely impaired.

18.26 Genetic Treatment Options

Antoinette am Zehnhoff-Dinnesen

New Therapeutic Strategies In addition to conservative and surgical therapeutic practices, gene therapy is discussed as a future option (Sun et al. 2011) to preserve and to restore hearing ability. Recent insights into the genetics of the cochlea and in molecular mechanisms involved in cell repair and apoptosis open up opportunities to:

- Correct mutations.
- Support the body's own protective pathways.
- Induce proliferation/regeneration of hair cells.
- Use optogenetic stimulation of auditory pathway structures.

An overview is given, e.g. in the reviews of Sun et al. (2011) and Kohrman and Raphael (2013). For genetic studies on mammalian audition, mouse mutants are the model organisms of choice, shedding light on the function of the key genes and the key complexes underlying the development, functioning and deterioration of the auditory system. Understanding the molecular background of hearing and hearing loss is the basis of new therapeutic strategies (Brown et al. 2008). In the following, recent exemplary studies paving the way for genetic treatment options are presented.

Correction of Mutations Mianné et al. (2016) could correct the auditory phenotype in mice with the $Cdh23^{ahl}$ allele, predisposing to age-related progressive hearing loss. In C57BL/6NTac zygotes, the specific DNA sequences of the mutation could be removed and the correct gene built in by targeted CRISPR/Cas9-mediated homology-directed repair (HDR). From 456 injected embryos and 104 live pups, 15 mice were transgenic of which 4 carried the correct $Cdh23^{753A>G}$ repair. The subsequent whole-genome sequencing showed only sequence changes near the defective gene to have been corrected, but no unintentional lesions at any of the predicted off-target sites. Scanning electron microscopy of dissected cochleae from 36-week-old mice verified the correction of progressive loss of sensory hair cell stereocilia bundles, and audiological measurements in mice at 24 and 36 weeks of age demonstrated the correction of the phenotype progressive hearing loss. Because of mosaicism in founder animals, the genotype and phenotype data should be acquired from subsequent generations.

In Usher syndrome 1C, the $Ush1c$ gene, which encodes harmonin, an important protein for the framework of hair cells, is altered. Without harmonin hair cells degenerate, and affected individuals develop hearing loss and vestibular problems. The team from Gwenaelle Géléoc (Pan et al. 2017) delivered wild-type $Ush1c$ into the inner ear of knock-in mice with the $Ush1c$ c.216G>A mutation by using the synthetic adeno-associated viral vector Anc80L65. Hearing and balance behaviour recovered in the treated mice with Usher syndrome type 1C.

Support of the Body's Own Protective Pathway The LIM-homeodomain transcription factor Is/1 is expressed in prenatally developing auditory hair cells. Huang et al. (2013) created a transgenic mouse model with overexpression of Is/1 in postnatal hair cells, which showed normal function. In comparison with wild-type controls, in Is/1 transgenic mice, age-related hearing loss was significantly reduced with survival of hair cells. Furthermore, Is/1 transgenic mice were protected from noise-induced hearing loss.

Induced Proliferation/Regeneration of Hair Cells Kelly et al. (2012) could show proliferation of extra sensory hair cells in a transgenic mouse line in the postnatal stage induced by a gene called $Atoh1$. According to Robas (2015), $Atoh1$ functions as a switch to turn on hair cell growth, but in mammals it is usually turned off after birth. Virus-delivered $Atoh1$ (CGF166) could restore hearing in animal models. Researchers have started a clinical trial in patients with acquired hearing loss (ClinicalTrials.gov 2017).

Optogenetic Stimulation of Auditory Pathway Structures To overcome the limited frequency resolution of cochlear implants and to improve the perception of speech, prosody and music, scientific work was performed on optical stimulation of spiral ganglion neurons genetically altered to express the light-gated ion channel channelrhodopsin-2 (ChR2). Such optogenetic stimulation with µLEDs showed innervation in response to light and could restore auditory activity in deaf mice (Hernandez et al. 2014).

Conclusion Nowadays, in diagnostic terms genetic knowledge and techniques provide opportunities to screen children with hereditary hearing loss by high-tech genetic sequencing, a time- and cost-saving simultaneous analysis of known deafness genes. Possibly in the future, gene-based therapy options could be transferred from animal studies and clinical trials to clinical application.

18.27 Prognosis of Developmental Hearing Disorders

Jakub Dršata and Ross Parfitt

18.27.1 Introduction

The consequences of childhood hearing impairment can be wide-reaching, affecting not only the sensitivity of a child's hearing but also the ability to perceive speech, music and environmental sound clearly, to express itself through spoken language and to access and progress in formal education; a range of other abilities and characteristics are affected (e.g. Powers 1996; Moeller 2007; Moeller et al. 2007). In short, permanent childhood hearing impairment can have significant consequences for the individual's quality of life as a whole. With this in mind, it is clear that when considering the prognosis of childhood hearing disorders, audiological outcome is not the only relevant issue.

The prognosis of childhood hearing impairment depends upon a host of factors, including the type of hearing disorder diagnosed; its severity, laterality and time of onset; the time points at which the hearing impairment was detected and treatment begun; the nature and quality of the treatment; the nature and quality of professional and family support; and the presence of associated disorders or health issues. Essentially, better prognoses are found for hearing losses that are identified earlier and treated effectively, but the later the onset of hearing loss, the better the typical outcome. Hearing loss in isolation has a better prognosis than that in combination with other disorders, such as visual impairment or learning difficulty.

18.27.2 Factors Influencing the Prognosis of Childhood Hearing Impairment

Type of Diagnosis, Severity and Laterality of Hearing Loss Conductive hearing losses (CHL) have favourable prognosis in general because many are temporary and hearing can recover without intervention in many cases. Other reasons for this more favourable prognosis include the possibility of essentially normal hearing being restored following surgery in some cases, the theoretical worst-case conductive hearing loss being no worse than 60 dB HL (i.e. moderate hearing loss) and positive outcomes resulting from the use of conventional or bone-anchored hearing aids where long-term CHL is evident.

The prognosis of sensorineural hearing losses (SNHL) is generally worse than for CHL. SNHL is permanent in almost all cases, and auditory thresholds can range up to levels in excess of 120 dB HL (i.e. profound/total hearing loss).

Hearing disorders with a greater central auditory system component have less clear prognoses. In the case of auditory processing disorder (see Sects. 15.2, 16.8 and 18.14), for example, there is no generally accepted diagnostic procedure or rehabilitation strategy, so the prognosis must be dependent upon the degree to which the individual is handicapped by their symptoms and the level of benefit gained from highly individualised therapy. Subjective tinnitus (see Sects. 15.4, 16.5, 16.6, 18.9 and 18.10) has a similarly unclear prognosis, depending very much upon the management strategies employed and psychological characteristics of the individual.

The severity of the hearing loss has a significant effect on the prognosis. The impact of mild and unilateral hearing losses on developmental outcomes has been disputed (see Walker et al. 2015), but there is no dispute about the impact of severe-to-profound hearing losses. However, this lack of clarity means that children with mild or unilateral hearing losses face an uncertain future: if their handicap is not judged to be severe enough, they often do not receive the support needed (Holstrum et al. 2008).

In the case of mild bilateral hearing losses, some beneficial effects of hearing devices (hearing aids and FM systems) on speech perception and general language development have been reported (e.g. Anderson and Goldstein 2004; Walker et al. 2015). A growing body of evidence suggests that unilateral hearing loss is associated with various educational and communication difficulties (see Fitzpatrick et al. 2010). Audiological and educational outcomes for children with unilateral hearing loss may be improved by wearing a hearing aid in the affected ear (e.g. McKay 2002; see also Sect. 18.4).

In cases of more severe hearing loss, patients benefit nowadays from modern digital hearing aid technology, and cochlear implants render speech comprehension possible in profound hearing loss.

Time of Onset, Detection and Treatment of Hearing Impairment More severe bilateral hearing losses obviously present more significant problems for speech reception, and, although considerable progress has been made in technological and rehabilitative strategies around hearing aids and cochlear implants, outcomes are still dependent on a variety of factors, such as times of onset, detection and treatment of the hearing impairment.

One of the more important factors influencing the prognosis of more severe bilateral SNHL is the time of its onset. Congenital or prelingual hearing losses risk greatly impeding language development. The prognosis regarding language development, communication and social skills, educational attainment and quality of life is far worse in this group than in those for whom the hearing loss occurs later (e.g. Yoshinaga-Itano et al. 1998).

It is therefore crucial that hearing impairment is identified as early as possible. Parental suspicion of hearing loss in their own child has been reported to be as low as 44% in infants with severe-profound bilateral hearing loss (Watkin et al. 1990). Newborn hearing screening programmes, which aim to identify hearing loss early without having to rely on the suspicion of parents and others, have significantly lowered the age of initial diagnosis to a matter of months, rather than years (e.g. Harrison et al. 2003; see also Sect. 17.1). Many screening programmes have driven audiological service development to the extent that they are fully integrated into subsequent management pathways (such as the

UK's Neonatal Hearing Screening Programme (NHSP)). Such integrated services enable treatment to begin rapidly after identification, and the benefits can be seen in the better developmental outcomes of children diagnosed via this process than via traditional approaches (Korver et al. 2010). The linguistic, social and emotional outcomes for children in whom treatment begins before 6 months of age are significantly better than for those who start later (Yoshinaga-Itano 2003), so the positive impact of early identification and treatment enabled by neonatal screening on the prognosis of childhood hearing loss is clear.

Appropriate Management of Hearing Loss Management of hearing loss must not only be timely but appropriate and high-quality. These needs should be met by evidence-based treatment (see Sect. 2.3) that is tailored to the individual patient and their family, discussed and agreed with them and provided by well-resourced, experienced, competent agencies working closely together (e.g. Baguley et al. 2000) (and see Sects. 18.1–18.3, 18.15, and 18.16).

Details regarding best practice and outcomes of specific interventions, such as surgery and the use of hearing devices, can be found in Sects. 18.4–18.8 and 18.11 (hearing aids, cochlear implants and others) and Sects. 18.22–18.25 (surgery). Management of the auditory aspects of hearing impairment does not occur in isolation, and other sections in this chapter detail other essential elements of rehabilitation, such as parental support, principles of social and educational support and other specific rehabilitation strategies. All of these aspects are important for the prognosis of hearing loss. Of course, the prognosis of specific interventions depends upon the quality of the work at each stage, from assessment and diagnosis, counselling and communication, selection and planning of the intervention, performance, verification and validation of the intervention and regular follow-up.

Given the importance of access to information, diagnostic and support services to the prognosis for people with hearing disorders, it is clear that socio-economic factors themselves (such as poverty, lower educational level, greater additional health concerns and reduced access to support networks) must have an impact upon the well-being of children with hearing loss. Shargorodsky et al. (2010), for example, found a significantly higher odds of hearing loss in US adolescents living below the federal poverty line than above it. Campaigns to promote awareness within specific communities and to provide key information regarding the causes of hearing loss and strategies for prevention and management (such as that run by the World Health Organization (2016)) play a vital role internationally in improving the prognosis for those with hearing loss.

Morton and Nance (2006) point out that the benefits of early identification and intervention are the same regardless of the mode of communication which the child and their family select, be it oral, manual (sign language) or both; linguistic, social and emotional development can progress at an appropriate rate (Yoshinaga-Itano 2003). Where manual communication has been chosen, adequate support within the family and the deaf community, as well as from professionals, is essential.

Associated Disorders 20–40% of children with hearing losses have associated disorders (various authors; see Sect. 16.23), and 50% of them have more than one (Fortnum and Davis 1997). The presence of associated disorders or health issues in addition to hearing loss can have a significant effect on auditory and speech-language outcomes (Cupples et al. 2014) (see Sects. 14.11, 16.23, 16.24 and 18.19 for details of associated conditions). The management strategy must therefore take associated disorders into account.

Hearing losses associated with visual impairment or blindness occur in 5% of cases of permanent childhood hearing loss (Gallaudet Research Institute 2013) and represent the most severe combination of sensory handicap. Usher syndrome is a typical example. It is usually progressive and offers an unfavourable prognosis for both sight and hearing. The combination

of hearing loss and intellectual disability, such as in cases of cerebral palsy, occurs in 16% of cases (Gallaudet Research Institute 2013). For such individuals, the prognosis is very variable; increasing comorbidity (including the level of neuropsychological development) is a strongly associated factor indicating quality of life (Tessier et al. 2014). Syndromes associated with serious somatic impairment (including intellectual disability) present great challenges for the rehabilitation of hearing. Ensuring the functioning of vital bodily systems (cardiovascular, respiratory and central nervous systems) is always the priority. Communication, however, is extremely important in such situations, so the provision of adequate hearing support within the limits of available medical care should be sought in order to ensure the best possible quality of life.

References

Abbott D, Watson D, Townsley R (2005) The proof of the pudding: what difference does multi agency working make to families with disabled children with complex health care needs? Child Fam Soc Work 10(3):229–230

Abdel-Aziz M, Khalifa B, Shawky A et al (2015) Transoral endoscopic partial adenoidectomy does not worsen the speech after cleft palate repair. Braz J Otorhinolaryngol 82(4):422–466. (Epub ahead of print). https://doi.org/10.1016/j.bjorl.2015.08.025

Achmadi D, Kagohara DM, van der Meer L et al (2012) Teaching advanced operation of an iPod-based speech-generating device to two students with autism spectrum disorders. Res Autism Spec Disord 6(4):1258–1264

Acuin J (2007) Chronic suppurative otitis media. BMJ Clin Evid 02:507

Alain C, Zendel BR, Hutka S et al (2014) Turning down the noise: the benefit of musical training on the aging auditory brain. Hear Res 308:162–173

Allman BL, Schormans AL, Typlt M et al (2016) Past, present, and future pharmacological therapies for Tinnitus. In: CG LP et al (eds) Translational research in audiology, neurotology, and the hearing sciences, vol 58, pp 165–195

Alrwisan A, Winterstein AG, Antonelli PJ (2016) Epidemiology of persistent tympanic membrane perforations subsequent to tympanostomy tubes assessed with real world data. Otol Neurotol 37(9):1376–1380

American Academy of Audiology (2011) Clinical practice guidelines: remote microphone hearing assistance technologies for children and youth from birth to 21 years, Supplement A.4

American Academy of Audiology (2013) Clinical practice guidelines: pediatric amplification. http://audiology-web.s3.amazonaws.com/migrated/PediatricAmplificationGuidelines.pdf_539975b3e7e9f1.74471798.pdf. Accessed Jun 2013

American Academy of Family Physicians, American Academy of Otolaryngology-Head and Neck Surgery, American Academy of Pediatrics Subcommittee on Otitis Media With Effusion (2004) Otitis media with effusion. Pediatrics 113(5):1412–1429

American Speech-Language-Hearing Association (2015) Permanent childhood hearing loss: section treatment. http://www.asha.org/PRPSpecificTopic.aspx?folderid=8589934680&section=Treatment. Accessed 13 Nov 2016

Anderson KL, Goldstein H (2004) Speech perception benefits of FM and infrared devices to children with hearing aids in a typical classroom. Lang Speech Hear Serv Sch 35(2):169–184

Anguera JA, Boccanfuso J, Rintoul JL et al (2013) Video game training enhances cognitive control in older adults. Nature 501(7465):97–101. https://doi.org/10.1038/nature12486

ANSI/ASA S12.60-2010/Part 1 (2010) American National Standard: Acoustical Performance Criteria, Design Requirements, and Guidelines for Schools, Part 1: Permanent Schools

Archbold SM, Harris M, O'Donoghue G et al (2008) Reading abilities after cochlear implantation: the effect of age of implantation on outcomes at 5 and 7 years after implantation. I J Pediatr Otorhinolaryngol 72(1):471–478

Arndt S, Beck R, Schild C et al (2010) Management of cochlear implantation in patients with malformations. Clin Otolaryngol 35(3):220–227

Arnold A, Caversaccio MD, Mudry A (2011) Surgery for the bone-anchored hearing aid. Adv Otorhinolaryngol 71:47–55

Arredondo P, Toporek R, Pack Brown S et al (1996) Operationalization of the multicultural counseling competencies. J Multicult Counsel Dev 24:42–78. Association for Multicultural Counseling and Development AMCD: Multicultural Counseling Competencies, Alexandria, VA. http://www.healthalt.org/uploads/2/3/7/5/23750643/amcd_multicultural_counseling_competencies.pdf. Accessed 12 Dec 2016

Arslan N, Oğuz H, Demirci M et al (2011) Combined intratympanic and systemic use of steroids for idiopathic sudden sensorineural hearing loss. Otol Neurotol 32(3):393–397

Arslan HH, Satar B, Serdar MA et al (2012) Effects of hyperbaric oxygen and dexamethasone on proinflammatory cytokines of rat cochlea in noise-induced hearing loss. Otol Neurotol 33(9):1672–1678

ASHA (2017) Daily care for the hearing aid. http://www.asha.org/uploadedFiles/AIS-Hearing-Aids-Troubleshooting.pdf. Accessed Apr 2017

Askar SM, Quriba AS (2014) Powered instrumentation for transnasal endoscopic partial adenoidectomy in children with submucosal cleft palate. Int J Pediatr Otorhinolaryngol 78(2):317–322

Atkinson M, Jones M, Lamont E (2007) Multi Agency Working and its implications for practice. A review of the literature NFER. CfBT Education Trust, Hyderabad Children and Families Act (2014). http://www.legislation.gov.uk/ukpga/2014/6/contents/enacted. Accessed 9 Mar 2017

Baguley D, Davis A, Bamford J (2000) Principles of family-friendly hearing services for children. Brit Soc Audiol New 29:35–39

Baguley D, McFerran D, Hall D (2013) Tinnitus. Lancet 382(9904):1600–1607

Baik G, Brietzke S (2015) How much does the type of tympanostomy tube matter? A utility-based Markov decision analysis. Otolaryngol Head Neck Surg 152(6):1000–1006

Banigo A, Hunt A, Rourke T et al (2016) Does the EarPopper® device improve hearing outcomes in children with persistent otitis media with effusion? A randomised single-blinded controlled trial. Clin Otolaryngol 41(1):59–65

Barmherzige Brüder Konventhospital Linz (2016) FLIP—Familienzentriertes Linzer InterventionsProgramm. https://www.barmherzige-brueder.at/pages/issn/kommunikationsprache/paedoaudiologberattherapi/flip. Accessed 16 Mar 2017

Batliner G (2012) Frühförderung nach dem natürlichen hörgerichteten Ansatz. In: Leonhardt A (ed) Frühes Hören—Hörschädigungen ab dem Ersten Lebenstag erkennen und therapieren. Ernst Reinhardt Verlag, München, pp 194–205

Bayar Muluk N, Carpar O (2011) Tinnitus and quality of life. Near East Med J 1(2):95–100

Beal-Alvarez JS, Lederberg AR, Easterbrookes SR (2011) Grapheme-phoneme acquisition of deaf pre-schoolers. J Deaf Stud Deaf Educ 17(1):39–60

Berghaus A, Stelter K, Naumann A et al (2010) Ear reconstruction with porous polyethylene implants. Adv Otorhinolaryngol 68:53–64

Berrettini S, Forli F, Genovese E et al (2008) Cochlear implantation in deaf children with associated disabilities: challenges and outcomes. Int J Audiol 47(4):199–208

Bess FH, Tharpe AM (1984) Unilateral hearing impairment in children. Pediatrics 74(2):206–216

Betancourt JR, Green AR, Carrillo JE et al (2003) Defining cultural competence: a practical framework for addressing racial/ethnic disparities in health and health care. Public Health Rep 118(4):393–302

Bianchin G, Russi G, Romano N et al (2010) Treatment with HELP-apheresis in patients suffering from sudden sensorineural hearing loss: a prospective, randomized, controlled study. Laryngoscope 120(4):800–807

Birman CS, Elliott EJ, Gibson WP (2012) Pediatric cochlear implants: additional disabilities prevalence, risk factors, and effect on language outcomes. Otol Neurotol 33(8):1347–1352

Bluestone CD (2005) Anatomy and physiology of the Eustachian tube system. In: Bailey BJ et al (eds) Head & neck surgery–otolaryngology, 4th edn. Lippincott Williams & Wilkins, Philadelphia, pp 1253–1263

Borangiu A, Popescu CR, Purcarea VL (2014) Sonotubometry, a useful tool for the evaluation of the Eustachian tube ventilatory function. J Med Life 7(4):604–610

Brady N, Warren SF, Sterling A (2009) Interventions aimed at improving child language by improving maternal responsivity. Int Rev Res Ment Retard 37:333–357

Braun T, Gratza S, Becker S et al (2010a) Auricular reconstruction with porous polyethylene frameworks: outcome and patient benefit in 65 children and adults. Plast Reconstr Surg 126(4):1201–1212

Braun T, Hainzinger T, Stelter K et al (2010b) Health-related quality of life, patient benefit, and clinical outcome after otoplasty using suture techniques in 62 children and adults. Plast Reconstr Surg 126(6):2115–2124

Brent B (1999) Technical advances in ear reconstruction with autogenous rib cartilage grafts: personal experience with 1200 cases. Plast Reconstr Surg 104(2):319–334. discussion 335-338

British Society of Audiology (2011) An overview of current management of auditory processing disorder. http://www.thebsa.org.uk/wp-content/uploads/2014/04/BSA_APD_Management_1Aug11_FINAL_amended17Oct11.pdf. Accessed 29 Dec 2015

British Society of Audiology APD SIG (2018) Practical Guidance: An overview of current management of auditory processing disorder. www.thebsa.org.uk/wp-content/uploads/2018/02/Position-Statement-and-Practice-Guidance-APD-2018-1.pdf. Accessed 12 Jul 2018

Brockmeier SJ, Peterreins M, Lorens A et al (2010) Music perception in electric acoustic stimulation users as assessed by the Mu.S.I.C. test. Adv Otorhinolaryngol 67:70–80

Brown SD, Hardisty-Hughes RE et al (2008) Quiet as a mouse: dissecting the molecular and genetic basis of hearing. Nat Rev Genet 9(4):277–290. https://doi.org/10.1038/nrg2309

Brozoski T, Odintsov B, Bauer C (2012) Gamma-aminobutyric acid and glutamic acid levels in the auditory pathway of rats with chronic tinnitus: a direct determination using high resolution point-resolved proton magnetic resonance spectroscopy (1H-MRS). Front Syst Neurosci 6:9. https://doi.org/10.3389/fnsys.2012.00009

Bureau International d'Audiophonologie (2012) Recommendation 06/12: Earmoulds for newborn infants and young children. http://www.biap.org/en/recommandations/recommendations/tc-06-hearing-aids/225-rec-06-12-en-earmoulds-for-newborn-infants-and-young-children/file. Accessed Jun 2013

Butler R, Skelton T, Valentine G (2001) Language barriers: exploring the world of the deaf. Disabil Stud Q 21(4):42–52

Campbell NG, Grant P, Rosen S, Moore DR (2019) Auditory processing disorder in children, BATOD Foundation. Available at: http://www.meshguides.org/guides/node/1432

Carlsson P-I, Hjaldahl J, Magnuson A et al (2015) Severe to profound hearing impairment: quality of life, psychosocial consequences and audiological rehabilitation. Disabil Rehab 37(20):1849–1856

Carr G (on behalf of the National Deaf Children's Society) (2015) Communicating with your deaf child. http://www.ndcs.org.uk/document.rm?id=10296. Accessed 20 April 2017

Casselbrant ML, Mandel EM (2004) Risk factors for otitis media. In: Alper C, Bluestone CD (eds) Advanced therapy of otitis media. BC Decker, London, pp 26–31

Catalano PJ, Jonnalagadda S, Yu VM (2012) Balloon catheter dilatation of Eustachian tube: a preliminary study. Otol Neurotol 33(9):1549–1552

Celen Z, Kanlikama M, Bayazit AY et al (1999) Scintigraphic evaluation of the Eustachian tube functions. Rev Laryngol Otol Rhinol (Bord) 120(2):123–125

Chen DA, Luxford WM (1990) Myringotomy and tube for relief of patulous Eustachian tube symptoms. Am J Otol 11(4):272–273

Chermak GD, Musiek FE (2013) Handbook of central auditory processing disorder, comprehensive intervention, vol 2, 2nd edn. San Diego, CA, Plural

Children's Hearing Services Working Group (2017). www.ndcs.org.uk. Accessed 14 Mar 2017

Choudhary T, Kulkarni S, Reddy P (2015) A Braille-based mobile communication and translation glove for deaf-blind people. In: International Conference on Pervasive Computing (ICPC) 14. IEEE, January 8–10, 2015, Pune, India, pp 1–4

Ciciriello E, Bolzonello P, Machi R et al (2016) Empowering the family during the first months after identification of permanent hearing impairment in children. Acta Otorhinolaryngol Ital 36(1):64–70

Clark G (ed) (2003) Cochlear implants: fundamentals and applications. Springer, New York

Clark M (2007) A practical guide to quality interaction with children who have a hearing loss. Plural, Abingdon

Clarós P, Pujol-Mdel C (2013) Active middle ear implants: Vibroplasty™ in children and adolescents with acquired or congenital middle ear disorders. Acta Otolaryngol 133(6):612–619

ClinicalTrials.gov (2017) Safety, tolerability and efficacy for CGF166 in patients with bilateral severe-to-profound hearing loss. https://clinicaltrials.gov/ct2/show/NCT02132130. Accessed 18 Jun 2017

Coelho DH, Lalwani AK (2008) Medical management of Ménière's disease. Laryngoscope 118(6):1099–1108

Coelho AC, Malta Medved D, Ghedini Brasolotto A (2015) Hearing loss and the voice. In: Bahmad F Jr (ed) Update on hearing loss medicine. IntechOpen, Rijeka

Cohen S, Roland P, Shoup A et al (2011) A pilot study of rituximab in immune-mediated inner ear disease. Audiol Neurootol 16(4):214–221

Coleridge P (1993) Disability and culture. disability, liberation and development. Oxfam and ADD. http://english.aifo.it/disability/apdrj/selread100/disability_culture_coleridge.pdf. Accessed 12 Dec 2016

Colorado School for the Deaf and the Blind (CSDB) (2017) Colorado Home Intervention Program (CHIP). http://www.csdb.org/programs-services/outreach-programs-3/early-education-services/colorado-home-intervention-programchip/. Accessed 12 Dec 2016

Communication Matters (2017) National Standards for AAC services. http://www.communicationmatters.org.uk/page/national-standards-aac-services. Accessed 4 Apr 2017

Conrad R (1977) The deaf schoolchild: language and cognitive function. Harper and Row, New York

Consortium for Research in Deaf Education (CRIDE) (2013) 2013 survey on provision for deaf children in England. www.ndcs.org.uk/data. Accessed 10 Mar 2014

Corbett P, Strong J (2011) Talk for writing across the curriculum: how to teach non-fiction writing 5-12 years. Open University Press, Milton Keynes

Council of Europe (1996) European convention on the exercise of children's rights Strasbourg. https://rm.coe.int/CoERMPublicCommonSearchServices/DisplayDCTMContent?documentId=090000168007c daf. Accessed 29 Jan 2015

Council of Europe (2006) Action plan to promote the rights and full participation of people with disabilities: improving the quality of life of people with disabilities in Europe for and through full participation 2006–2015. https://rm.coe.int/CoERMPublicCommonSearchServices/DisplayDCTMContent?documentId=0900001680595206. Accessed 29 Jan 2015

Council of Europe Political Declaration (2003) Improving the quality of life of people with disabilities: enhancing a coherent policy for and through full participation. http://sid.usal.es/idocs/F8/FDO7134/improving_the_quality_of_life_of_people_with_disabilities.pdf. Accessed 10 Jan 2015

Cremers CW, O'Connor AF, Helms J et al (2010) International consensus on Vibrant Soundbridge® implantation in children and adolescents. Int J Pediatr Otorhinolaryngol 74(11):1267–1269

Cunsolo E, Marchioni D, Leo G et al (2010) Functional anatomy of the Eustachian tube. Int J Immunopathol Pharmacol 23(1 Suppl):4–7

Cupples L, Ching TY, Crowe K et al (2014) Outcomes of 3-year-old children with hearing loss and different types of additional disabilities. J Deaf Stud Deaf Educ 19(1):20–39

Curhan SG, Eavey R, Wang M et al (2013) Body mass index, waist circumference, physical activity, and risk of hearing loss in women. Am J Med 126(12):1142. e1141–1142.e1148. https://doi.org/10.1016/j.amjmed.2013.04.026

Dammeyer J, Ask Larsen F (2016) Communication and language profiles of children with congenital deafblindness. Br J Vis Impair 34(3):214–224

Davis H, Day C (2010) Working in partnership: the family partnership model. Pearson Education, London

Davis A, Rafaie EA (2000) Epidemiology of tinnitus. In: Tyler RS (ed) Tinnitus Handbook. Singulair, San Diego, CA

Declau F, Van de Heyning P, Cremers C (2008) Diagnosis and management strategies in congenital middle and external ear anomalies. In: Graham JM et al (eds) Pediatric ENT. Springer, Berlin

Delage H, Tuller L (2007) Language development and mild to moderate hearing loss: does language normalize with age? J Speech Lang Hear Res 50(5):1300–1313

Densham J (1995) Deafness, children, and the family: a guide to professional practice. Arena, Suffolk

Desjardins JL, Ambrose SE (2010) The importance of the home literacy environment for developing literacy skills in young children who are deaf or hard of hearing. Young Except Child 13(5):28–44

Desjardins JL, Ambrose SE, Eisenberg LS (2008) Literacy skills in children with cochlear implants: the importance of early oral language and joint storybook reading. J Deaf Stud Deaf Educ 14(1):22–43

Deutsche Gesellschaft für Phoniatrie und Pädaudiologie (DGPP) (2012) Konsenspapier der DGPP zur Hörgeräte-Versorgung bei Kindern, Vers. 3.5. http://www.dgpp.de/cms/modules/download_gallery/dlc.php?file=42&id=1353870245. Accessed Nov 2012

Deutsche Gesellschaft für Phoniatrie und Pädaudiologie (DGPP) (2013) S2k-Leitlinie: Periphere Hörstörungen im Kindesalter-Langform. AWMF-Register Nr. 049/010. http://www.dgpp.de/cms/media/download_gallery/Hoerstoerungen%20Kinder%20lang.pdf. Accessed 5 May 2015

Diversity in Medicine and Health DIMAH Group (2016) Training support—DIMAH. http://www.dimah.co.uk. Accessed 12 Dec 2016

Do B, Lynch P, Macris EM et al (2017) Systematic review and meta-analysis of the association of Autism Spectrum disorder in visually or hearing impaired children. Ophthalmic Physiol Opt 37(2):212–224

Doherty-Sneddon G (2003) Children's unspoken language. Jessica Kingsley, London

du Feu M, Fergusson K (2003) Sensory impairment and mental health advances in psychiatric treatment. Adv Psychiatr Treat 9(2):95–103

Easterbrooks SR, O'Rourke CM, Todd NW (2000) Child and family factors associated with deaf children's success in auditory-verbal therapy. Am J Otolarynol 21(3):341–344

Easterbrooks SR, Lederberg AR, Miller EM et al (2008) Emergent literacy skills during early childhood in children with hearing loss: strengths and weaknesses. Volta Rev 108(2):91–114

Education, Audiovisual and Culture Executive Agency EACEA ERASMUS LifeLong Learning Programme (2013-2015). http://eacea.ec.europa.eu/llp/index_en.php. Accessed 11 Jul 2017

Ekberg K, Meyer C, Scarinci N et al (2015) Family member involvement in audiology appointments with older people with hearing impairment. Int J Audiol 54(2):70–76

Emond A, Kentish R (2013) Tinnitus counselling with children. Audacity 2013(2):26–29

Erixon E, Högstorp H, Wadin K et al (2009) Variational anatomy of the human cochlea: implications for cochlear implantation. Otol Neurotol 30(1): 14–22

EUHA (2016) EUHA Leitlinie. Drahtlose Übertragungsanlagen—Messtechnischer Nachweis des individuellen Nutzens und Überprüfung der Anlage, Version 0.9 (Entwurf), Stand 06.09.2016. http://www.euha.org/assets/Uploads/Arbeitskreis-Perzentile/EUHA-Leitlinie-Drahtlose-Uebertragungsanlagen.pdf. Accessed Nov 2016

Everdell IT, Marsh HO, Yurick MD et al (2007) Gaze behaviour in audiovisual speech perception: asymmetrical distribution of face-directed fixations. Perception 36(10):1535–1545

Ewing KM, Jones TW (2003) An educational rationale for deaf students with multiple disabilities. Am Ann Deaf 148(3):267–271

Feldmann H (1971) Homolateral and contralateral masking of tinnitus by noise-bands and by pure tones. Audiology 10(3):138–144

Ferguson MA, Henshaw H, Clark DP et al (2014) Benefits of phoneme discrimination training in a randomized controlled trial of 50- to 74-year-olds with mild hearing loss. Ear Hear 35(4):e110–e121. https://doi.org/10.1097/aud.0000000000000020

Fetoni AR, Eramo SL, Rolesi R et al (2012) Antioxidant treatment with coenzyme Q-ter in prevention of gentamycin ototoxicity in an animal model. Acta Otorhinolaryngol Ital 32(2):103–110

Fitzpatrick EM, Durieux-Smith A, Whittingham J (2010) Clinical practice for children with mild bilateral and unilateral hearing loss. Ear Hear 31(3):392–400

Folmer RL, Theodoroff SM, Casiana L et al (2015) Repetitive transcranial magnetic stimulation treatment for chronic tinnitus: a randomized clinical trial. JAMA Otolaryngol Head Neck Surg 141(8):716–722

Fortnum H, Davis A (1997) Epidemiology of permanent childhood hearing impairment in trent region, 1985–1993. Br J Audiol 31(6):409–446

Foster S, Cue K (2009) Roles and responsibilities of itinerant specialist teacher of deaf and hard of hearing students. Am Ann Deaf 153(5):435–449

Frenzel H, Schönweiler R, Hanke F et al (2012) The Lübeck flowchart for functional and aesthetic rehabilitation of aural atresia and microtia. Otol Neurotol 33(8):1363–1367

Frenzel H, Sprinzl G, Widmann G et al (2013) Grading system for the selection of patients with congeni-

tal aural atresia for active middle ear implants. Neuroradiology 55(7):895–911

Friedmann DR, Ahmed OH, McMenomey SO et al (2016) Single-sided deafness Cochlear implantation: candidacy, evaluation, and outcomes in children and adults. Otol Neurotol 37(2):e154–e160

Gabriels P (1996) Children with Tinnitus. In: Reich G, Vernon J (eds) Proceedings of the Fifth International Seminar. The American Tinnitus Association, Portland, OR, pp 270–274

Gacek RR (1998) Perilymphatic fistula: pathophysiology, diagnosis and management. Otorhinolaryngol Nova 8(4):177–181

Gallaudet Research Institute (2013) Regional and National summary report of data from the 2011-12 annual survey of deaf and hard of hearing children and youth. GRI, Geallaudet University, Washington, DC

Garduno-Anaya MA, Couthino De Toledo H, Hinojosa-González R et al (2005) Dexamethasone inner ear perfusion by intratympanic injection in unilateral Ménière's disease: a two-year prospective, placebo-controlled, double-blind, randomized trial. Otolaryngol Head Neck Surg 133(2):285–294

Gentile DA, Skoner DP (2004) Allergy testing/treatment for otitis media. In: Alper C, Bluestone CD (eds) Advanced therapy of otitis media. BC Decker, London, pp 146–151

Gifford RH, Dorman MF, Spahr AJ et al (2007) Effect of digital frequency compression (DFC) on speech recognition in candidates for combined electric and acoustic stimulation (EAS). J Speech Lang Hear Res 50(5):1194–1202

Gillion GT (2000) The efficacy of phonological awareness intervention for children with spoken language impairment. Lang Speech Hear Serv Sch 31(2):126–141

Glanemann R, Reichmuth K, Matulat P et al (2013) Muenster Parental Programme empowers parents in communicating with their infant with hearing loss. Int J Pediatr Otorhinolaryngol 77(12):2023–2029

Glanemann R, Reichmuth K, am Zehnhoff-Dinnesen A (2016) Muenster parental programme – feedback from parents: How do parents evaluate an early intervention programme for improving the communication with their baby or toddler with hearing impairment? [Münsteraner Elternprogramm – Elternfeedback: Wie beurteilen Eltern die Frühintervention zur Kommunikationsförderung von Säuglingen und Kleinkindern mit Hörschädigung?] HNO 64(2):101–110

Global Coalition of Parents of Children who are Deaf and Hard of Hearing (2010) Position statement and recommendations for family support in the development of newborn hearing screening systems and early hearing and detection systems worldwide. https://sites.google.com/site/gpodhh/Home/position_statement. Accessed 17 Jun 2017

Gluth MB, McDonald DR, Weaver AL et al (2011) Management of eustachian tube dysfunction with nasal steroid spray: a prospective, randomized, placebo-controlled trial. Arch Otolaryngol Head Neck Surg 137(5):449–455

Govaerts PJ, Casselman J, Daemers K et al (2003) Cochlear implants in aplasia and hypoplasia of the cochleovestibular nerve. Otol Neurotol 24(6):887–891

Govaerts PJ, Daemers K, Yperman M et al (2006) Auditory speech sounds evaluation (ASSE): a new test to assess detection, discrimination and identification in hearing impairment. Cochlear Implants Int 7(2):92–106

Graham J, Butler J (1984) Tinnitus in children. J Laryngol Otol 9:236–241

Gratacap M, Thierry B, Rouillon I et al (2015) Pediatric cochlear implantation in hearing candidates. Ann Otol Rhinol Laryngol 124(6):443–451

Gravel JS, O'Gara J (2003) Communication options for children with hearing loss. Ment Retard Dev Disabil Res Rev 9(4):243–251

Greenwood DD (1990) A cochlear frequency position function for several species-29 years later. J Acoust Soc Am 87(6):2592–2605

Grimmer JF, Poe DS (2005) Update on eustachian tube dysfunction and the patulous eustachian tube. Curr Opin Otolaryngol Head Neck Surg 13(5):277–282

Gryczynska D, Kobos J, Zakrzewska A (1999) Relationship between passive smoking, recurrent respiratory tract infections and otitis media in children. Int J Pediatr Otorhinolaryngol 49(Suppl 1):S275–S278

Gstoettner WK, Van de Heyning P, Fitzgerald O'Connor A et al (2008) Electric acoustic stimulation of the auditory system: results of a multi-centre investigation. Acta Otolaryngol 128(9):968–975

Guevara N, Deveze A, Buza V et al (2008) Microvascular decompression of cochlear nerve for tinnitus in capacity: pre-surgical data, surgical analyses and long-term follow-up of 15 patients. Eur Arch Otorhinolaryngol 265(4):397–401

Hallberg LRM, Hallberg U, Kramer SE et al (2008) Self-reported hearing difficulties, communication strategies and psychological general well-being (quality of life) in patients with acquired hearing impairment. Disabil Rehabil 30(3):203–212

Halliday LF (2014) A tale of two studies on auditory training in children: a response to the claim that 'discrimination training of phonemic contrasts enhances phonological processing in mainstream school children' by Moore, Rosenberg and Coleman (2005). Dyslexia 20(2):101–118. https://doi.org/10.1002/dys.1470

Halliday LF, Taylor JL, Millward KE et al (2012) Lack of generalization of auditory learning in typically developing children. J Speech Lang Hear Res 55(1):168–181. https://doi.org/10.1044/1092-4388(2011/09-0213)

Hamzavi J, Baumgartner WD, Egelierler B et al (2000) Follow up of cochlear implanted handicapped children. Int J Pediatr Otorhinolaryngol 56(3):169–174

Harrison M, Roush J, Wallace J (2003) Trends in age of identification and intervention in infants with hearing loss. Ear Hear 24(1):89–95

Hassepass F, Aschendorff A, Wesarg T et al (2013) Unilateral deafness in children: audiologic and sub-jective assessment of hearing ability after cochlear implantation. Otol Neurotol 34(1):53–60

Henderson RJ, Johnson A, Moodie S (2014) Parent-to parent support for parents with children who are deaf or hard of hearing: a conceptual framework. Am J Audiol 23(4):437–448

Henry JA (2016) "Measurement" of Tinnitus. Otol Neurotol 37(8):e276–e285

Henry JA, Schechter MA, Nagler SM et al (2002) Comparison of tinnitus masking and tinnitus retrain-ing therapy. J Am Acad Audiol 13(10):559–581

Heppt WJ (2008) Otoplasty and common auricular deformities. In: Graham JM et al (eds) Pediatric ENT. Springer, Berlin

Hernandez VH, Gehrt A, Reuter K et al (2014) Optogenetic stimulation of the auditory pathway. J Clin Invest 124(3):1114–1129

Hillman CH (2014) I. An introduction to the relation of physical activity to cognitive and brain health, and scholastic achievement. Monogr Soc Res Child Dev 79(4):1–6. https://doi.org/10.1111/mono.12127

Hillman CH, Erickson KI, Kramer AF (2008) Be smart, exercise your heart: exercise effects on brain and cognition. Nat Rev Neurosci 9(1):58–65. https://doi.org/10.1038/nrn2298

Hintermair M (2000) Children who are hearing impaired with additional disabilities and related aspects of parental stress. Except Child 66(3):327–332

Hintermair M (2006) Parental resources, parental stress, and socioemotional development of deaf and hard of hearing children. J Deaf Stud Deaf Educ 11(4):493–513

Hobson J, Chisholm E, El Refaie A (2012) Sound therapy (masking) in the management of tinnitus in adults. Cochrane Database Syst Rev (12):CD006371. https://doi.org/10.1002/14651858

Hogan A, Phillips RL, Brumby SA et al (2015) Higher social distress and lower psycho-social wellbe-ing: examining the coping capacity and health of people with hearing impairment. Disabil Rehabil 37(22):2070–2075

Holden LK, Finley CC, Firszt JB et al (2013) Factors affecting open-set word recognition in adults with cochlear implants. Ear Hear 34(3):342–360

Holstrum WJ, Gaffney M, Gravel JS (2008) Early inter-vention for children with unilateral and mild bilateral degrees of hearing loss. Trends Amplif 12(1):35–41

Holzinger D, Fellinger J (2013) Moderne Ansätze evi-denzbasierter familienzentrierter Frühintervention bei Kindern mit Schwerhörigkeit oder Gehörlosigkeit. Sprache·Stimme·Gehör 37(01):e1–e6

Hornickel J, Zecker SG, Bradlow AR et al (2012) Assistive listening devices drive neuroplasticity in children with dyslexia. Proc Natl Acad Sci USA 109(41):16731–16736. https://doi.org/10.1073/pnas.1206628109

Huang M, Kantardzhieva A, Scheffer D et al (2013) Hair cell overexpression of Islet 1 reduces age-related and noise-induced hearing loss. J Neurosci 33(38):15086–1509.4. https://doi.org/10.1523/JNEUROSCI.1489-13.2013

Hulka GF, Prazma J, Brownlee RE et al (1993) Use of poly-l-aspartic acid to inhibit aminoglycoside cochlear ototoxicity. Am J Otol 14(4):352–356

Hyde M, Power D (2004) The personal and professional characteristics and work of itinerant teachers of the deaf and hard of hearing in Australia. Volta Rev 104(2):51–68

Ibragimova N, Granlund M, Björck-Åkesson E (2009) Field trial of ICF version for children and youth (ICF-CY) in Sweden: Logical coherence, developmental issues and clinical use. Dev Neurorehabil 12(1):3–11

Ishijima K, Sando I, Balaban CD et al (2002) Functional anatomy of levator veli palatini muscle and tensor veli palatini muscle in association with Eustachian tube cartilage. Ann Otol Rhinol Laryngol 111(6):530–536

ISO/TR 3352:1974 (1974) Acoustics—assessment of noise with respect to its effect on the intelligibility of speech

Jahrsdoerfer R, Kim JHN (2004) Chirurgie des missgebildeten Mittelohres. Technik und Ergebnisse. In: Weerda H (ed) Chirurgie der Ohrmuschel. Thieme, Stuttgart, pp 240–249

Jahrsdoerfer RA, Yeakley JW, Aguilar EA et al (1992) A grading system for the selection of patients with congenital aural atresia. Am J Otol 13(1):6–12

Janky K, Givens D (2015) Vestibular, visual acuity and balance outcomes in children with cochlear implants: a preliminary report. Ear Hear 36(6):e364–e372

Jastreboff PJ, Hazell JW (1993) A neurophysiological approach to tinnitus: clinical implications. Br J Audiol 27(1):7–17

Jayawardena J, Kuthubutheen J, Rajan G (2012) Hearing preservation and hearing improvement after reimplantation of pediatric and adult patients with partial deafness: a retrospective case series review. Otol Neurotol 33(5):740–744

Jefferson ND, Hunter LL (2016) Contemporary guidelines for tympanostomy tube placement. Curr Treat Options Peds 2:224–235

Joint Committee on Infant Hearing Position Statement (2007) Principles and guidelines for early hearing detection and intervention. Pediatrics 120(4):898–921

Junicho M, Aso F, Fujisaka M et al (2008) Prognosis of low-tone sudden deafness—does it inevitably progress to Meniere's disease? Acta Otolaryngol 128(3):304–308

Katz J, Medwetsky L, Burkard R et al (eds) (2009) Handbook of clinical audiology. Chap 31. Lippincott W & W, Philadelphia

Katzbach R, Klaiber S, Nitsch S et al (2006) Ohrmuschelrekonstruktion bei hochgradiger Mikrotie. HNO 54(6):493–514

Keles B, Oztürk K, Günel E et al (2004) Pharyngeal reflux in children with chronic otitis media with effusion. Acta Otolaryngol 124(10):1178–1181

Kelly MC, Chang Q, Pan A et al (2012) Atoh1 directs the formation of sensory mosaics and induces cell proliferation in the postnatal mammalian cochlea in vivo. J Neurosci 32(19):6699–6710. https://doi.org/10.1523/JNEUROSCI.5420-11.2012

Kemaloglu YK, Kobayashi T, Nakajima T (1999) Analysis of the craniofacial skeleton in cleft children with otitis media with effusion. Int J Pediatr Otorhinolaryngol 47(1):57–69

Kiese-Himmel C, Kruse E (2001) Unilateral hearing loss in childhood. An empirical analysis comparing bilateral hearing loss. Laryngo-Rhinootol 80(1):18–22

Kilic R, Şafak MA, Oğuz H et al (2007) Intratympanic methylprednisolone for sudden sensorineural hearing loss. Otol Neurotol 28(3):312–316

Klatte M, Bergstrom K, Lachmann T (2013) Does noise affect learning? A short review on noise effects on cognitive performance in children. Front Psychol 4:578. https://doi.org/10.3389/fpsyg.2013.00578

Klingmann C (2004) Behandlung akuter kochleovestibulärer Schädigungen nach dem Tauchen. HNO 52(10):891–896

Knief A, am Zehnhoff-Dinnesen A, Deuster D (2015) Überträgerspulen von Cochlea-Implantaten: Sitzt die Spule gut? In: Proceedings of the Deutsche Gesellschaft für Phoniatrie und Pädaudiologie. 32. Wissenschaftliche Jahrestagung der Deutschen Gesellschaft für Phoniatrie und Pädaudiologie (DGPP). Oldenburg 24.-27.09.2015. German Medical Science GMS Publishing House, Düsseldorf. https://doi.org/10.3205/15dgpp32

Kob M, Behler G, Kamprolf A et al (2006) In: Kruse E (ed) Untersuchung des Raumeinflusses auf die Stimmgebung von Lehrern einer Aachener Hauptschule. 23. Wissenschaftliche Jahrestagung der Deutschen Gesellschaft für Phoniatrie und Pädaudiologie (DGPP), Heidelberg. Programmheft, DGPP, Nürnberg, pp 1–6

Kob M, Behler G, Kamprolf A et al (2008) Experimental investigations of the influence of room acoustics on the teacher's voice. Acoust Sci Technol 29(1):86–94

Kochkin S, Tyler R (2008) Tinnitus treatment and the effectiveness of hearing aids: hearing care professional perceptions. Hear Rev 15(13):14–18

Koester LS, Lahti-Harper E (2010) Mother–infant hearing status and intuitive parenting behaviors during the first 18 months. Am Ann Deaf 155(1):5–18

Kohrman DC, Raphael Y (2013) Gene therapy for deafness. Gene Ther 20(12):1119–1123

Korver AM, Konings S, Dekker FW et al (2010) Newborn hearing screening vs later hearing screening and developmental outcomes in children with permanent childhood hearing impairment. JAMA 304(15):1701–1708

Kurz A, Caversaccio M, Kompis M (2013) Hearing performance with two different high-power sound processors for osseointegrated auditory implants. Otol Neurotol 34(4):604–610

Kurz A, Flynn M, Caversaccio M et al (2014) Speech understanding with a new implant technology: a comparative study with a new non-skin penetrating Baha® system. BioMed Research International 2014:416205. https://doi.org/10.1155/2014/416205

Kuthubutheen J, Hedne CN, Krishnaswamy J et al (2012) A case series of paediatric hearing preservation cochlear implantation: a new treatment modality for children with drug-induced or congenital partial deafness. Audiol Neurotol 17(5):321–330

Lalwani A (2002) Evaluation of childhood sensorineural hearing loss in the post-genome world. Arch Otolaryngol Head Neck Surg 128(1):88–89

Lambert PR (2001) Congenital aural atresia. In: Bailey BJ (ed) Head and neck surgery—otolaryngology. Lippincott Williams & Wilkins, Philadelphia, pp 1745–1757

Lautermann J, McLaren J, Schacht J (1995) Glutathione protection against gentamicin ototoxicity depends on nutritional status. Hear Res 86(1-2):15–24

Leach AJ, Morris PS (2006) Antibiotics for the prevention of acute and chronic suppurative otitis media in children. Cochrane Database Syst Rev (4):CD004401

Lee YM, Kim LS, Jeong SW et al (2010) Performance of children with mental retardation after cochlear implantation: speech perception, speech intelligibility, and language development. Acta Oto-Laryngol 130(8):924–934

Leigh J, Dettman S, Dowell R et al (2011) Evidence-based approach for making cochlear implant recommendations for infants with residual hearing. Ear Hear 32(3):313–322

LENA Research Foundation (2016) Early talk shapes a child's life. http://www.lenafoundation.org. Accessed 18 Jun 2017

Lieberthal AS (2013) Revised AOM guideline emphasizes accurate diagnosis. AAP News 34(3):4

Lieu JE (2004) Speech-language and educational consequences of unilateral hearing loss in children. Arch Otolaryngol Head Neck Surg 130(5):524–530

Liktor B, Szekanecz Z, Batta TJ et al (2013) Perspectives of pharmacological treatment in otosclerosis. Eur Arch Otorhinolaryngol 270(3):793–804

Loo JHY, Bamiou DE, Campbell N et al (2010) Computer-based auditory training (CBAT): benefits for children with language- and reading-related learning difficulties. Dev Med Child Neurol 52(8):708–717

Lorah ER, Tincani M, Dodge J et al (2013) Evaluating picture exchange and the iPad™ as a speech generating device to teach communication to young children with autism. J Dev Phys Disabil 25(6):637–649

Lorens A, Polak M, Piotrowska A et al (2008) Outcomes of treatment of partial deafness with cochlear implantation: a DUET study. Laryngoscope 118(2):288–294

Louza J, Polterauer D, Wittlinger N (2016) Threshold changes of ABR results in toddlers and children. Int J Pediatr Otorhinolaryngol 85:120–127

Lovett RE, Vickers DA, Summerfield AQ (2015) Bilateral cochlear implantation for hearing-impaired children: criterion of candidacy derived from an observational study. Ear Hear 36(1):14–23

Luckner JL, Sebald AM, Cooney J et al (2005/2006) An examination of the evidence based literacy research in deaf education. Am Ann Deaf 150(5):443–456

Maasaro DW, Light J (2004) Improving the vocabulary of children with hearing loss. Volta Rev 104(3):141–174

Marangos N (2002) Dysplasien des Innenohres und inneren Gehörganges. HNO 50(9):866–881

Martin WH, Griest SE, Sobel JL et al (2013) Randomized trial of four noise-induced hearing loss and tinnitus prevention interventions for children. Int J Audiol 52(Suppl 1):41–49

Mayer C (2007) What really matters in the early literacy of deaf children. J Deaf Studies Deaf Educ 12(4):411–413

McCallin A (2001) Interdisciplinary practice—a matter of teamwork: an integrated literature review. J Clin Nurs 10(4):419–428. https://doi.org/10.1046/j.1365-2702.2001.00495.x

McDermott AL, Sheehan P (2011) Paediatric Baha. Adv Otorhinolaryngol 71:56–62

McKay S (2002) To aid or not to aid: children with unilateral hearing loss. http://www.audiologyonline.com/articles/to-aid-or-not-children-1167. Accessed 23 Mar 2017

McLeod S, Threats TT (2008) The ICF-CY and children with communication disabilities. Int J Speech Lang Pathol 10(1-2):92–109

Mental Health Commission (2006) Multidisciplinary team working: from theory to practice: discussion paper. Available via Lenus: The Irish Health Repository. http://hdl.handle.net/10147/43830. Accessed 15 Nov 2016

Mesibov GB, Shea V, Schopler E (2004) The TEACCH approach to Autism spectrum disorders. Springer, New York

Mianné J, Chessum L, Kumar S et al (2016) Correction of the auditory phenotype in C57BL/6N mice via CRISPR/Cas9-mediated homology directed repair. Genome Med 8(1):16. https://doi.org/10.1186/s13073-016-0273-4

Mlynski R, Plontke S (2013) Cochleaimplantatversorgung bei Kindern und Jugendlichen. HNO 61(5):388–398

Moeller MP (2000) Early intervention and language development in children who are deaf and hard of hearing. Pediatrics 106(3):43–52

Moeller MP (2007) Current state of knowledge: psychosocial development in children with hearing impairment. Ear Hear 28(6):729–739

Moeller MP, Tomblin JB, Yoshinaga-Itano C et al (2007) Current state of knowledge: language and literacy of children with hearing impairment. Ear Hear 28(6):740–753

Moeller MP, Carr G, Seavers L et al (2013) Best practices in family-centered early intervention for children who are deaf or hard of hearing: an international consensus statement. J Deaf Stud Deaf Educ 18(4):429–445

Moller MB, Moller AR, Jannetta PJ et al (1993) Vascular decompression surgery for severe tinnitus: selection criteria and results. Laryngoscope 103(4 Pt 1):421–427

Molloy K, Moore DR, Sohoglu E et al (2012) Less is more: latent learning is maximized by shorter training sessions in auditory perceptual learning. PLoS One 7(5):e36929. https://doi.org/10.1371/journal.pone.0036929

Morettin M, Cardoso MR, Delamura AM et al (2013) Use of the International classification of functioning, disability and health for monitoring patients using cochlear implants. CoDAS 25(3):216–223

Morimoto N, Taiji H, Tsukamoto K et al (2010) Risk factors for elevation of ABR threshold in NICU-treated infants. Int J Pediatr Otorhinolaryngol 74(7):786–790

Morton CC, Nance WE (2006) Newborn hearing screening—a silent revolution. N Engl J Med 354:2151–2164

Multicentre Otitis Media Study Group (2012) Adjuvant adenoidectomy in persistent bilateral otitis media with effusion: hearing and revision surgery outcomes through 2 years in the TARGET randomised trial. Clin Otolaryngol 37(2):107–116

Mullah I (2011) Early use of FM amplification. Thesis, University of Manchester. https://www.escholar.manchester.ac.uk/uk-ac-man-scw:138160. Accessed 9 Mar 2017

Murphy T (2006) Otitis media, bacterial colonization and the smoking parent. Clin Infect Dis 42(7):904–906

Murphy CF, Moore DR, Schochat E (2015) Generalization of auditory sensory and cognitive learning in typically developing children. PLoS One 10(8):e0135422

Nagata S (1995) Total auricular reconstruction with a three-dimensional costal cartilage framework. Ann Chir Plast Esthet 40(4):371–399. discussion 400-403

National Center for Hearing Assessment and Management, Utah State University (NCHAM) (2011) The role of a Multi-disciplinary Team Clinic. http://www.infanthearing.org/meeting/ehdi2011/ehdi_2011_presentations/topical1/Sandra_Gabbard.pdf. Accessed 13 Nov 2016

National Deaf Children's Society (2012) Prevalence of additional disabilities with deafness: A review of the literature. National Deaf Children's Society, London

National Deaf Children's Society (2013) Phonics Guidance. National Deaf Children's Society, London

National Deaf Children's Society (2015) Supporting the achievement of hearing impaired children in early years settings. www.ndcs.org.uk/document.rm?id=9422. Accessed 17 Jun 2017

National Early Literacy Panel (NELP) (2008) Developing early literacy: report of the National Early Literacy Panel. Literacy Information and Communication System. https://lincs.ed.gov/publications/pdf/NELPReport09.pdf. Accessed 9 Mar 2017

Naumann A (2011) Rekonstruktion mittel- bis hochgradiger Ohrdefekte mit Hilfe poröser Polyethylenimplantate. HNO 59(2):197–212. quiz 213-214

Neilsen DC, Leutke B, Stryker DS (2011) The importance of morpheme awareness in reading achievement and the potential of signing morphemes to support reading development. J Deaf Stud Deaf Educ 16(3):275–288

Newman CW, Jacobson GP, Spitzer JB (1996) Development of the Tinnitus Handicap Inventory. Arch Otolaryngol Head Neck Surg 122(2):143–148

Nicholas JG, Geers AE (2013) Spoken language benefits of extending cochlear implant candidacy below 12 months of age. Otol Neurotol 34(3):532–538

Noh TS, Kyong JS, Chang M et al (2017) Comparison of Treatment Outcomes Following Either Prefrontal Cortical-only or Dual-site Repetitive Transcranial Magnetic Stimulation in Chronic Tinnitus Patients: A Double-blind Randomized Study. Otol Neurotol 38(2):296–303

O'Connor AF, Shea JJ (1981) Autophony and the patulous eustachian tube. Laryngoscope 91(9 Pt 1):1427–1435

Office for Standards in Education, Children's Services and Skills (2012) Communication is the key. https://www.gov.uk/government/uploads/system/uploads/attachment_data/file/419049/Communication_is_the_key.pdf. Accessed 9 Mar 2017

Oguz H, Felek S (2012) Tinnitus ve Yasam Kalitesi. Kulak Burun Bogaz'da Guncel Yaklasim Dergisi 8:70–72

Okano T, Kelley MV (2012) Stem cell therapy for the inner ear: recent advances and future directions. Trends Amplif 16(1):4–18

Ovari A, Buhr A, Warkentin M et al (2015) Can nasal decongestants improve the Eustachian tube function? Otol Neurotol 36(1):65–69

Oxenham AJ, Bernstein JG, Penagos H (2004) Correct tonotopic representation is necessary for complex pitch perception. Proc Natl Acad Sci USA 101(5):1421–1425

Ozturk K, Snyderman CH, Sando I (2011) Do mucosal folds in the eustachian tube function as microturbinates? Laryngoscope 121(4):801–804

Pan B, Askew C, Galvin A et al (2017) Gene therapy restores auditory and vestibular function in a mouse model of Usher syndrome type 1c. Nat Biotechnol 35(3):264–272

Park C, Yoo YS, Hong ST (2010) An update on auricular reconstruction: three major auricular malformations of microtia, prominent ear and cryptotia. Curr Opin Otolaryngol Head Neck Surg 18(6):544–549. Review

Park MK, Lee BD, Chae SW et al (2012) Protective effect of NecroX, a novel necroptosis inhibitor, on gentamicin-induced ototoxicity. Int J Pediatr Otorhinolaryngol 76(9):1265–1269

Patel A, Groppo E (2010) Management of temporal bone trauma. Craniomaxillofac Trauma Reconstr 3(2):105–113

Pearson P, Spencer J (1995) Pointers to effective teamwork: exploring primary care. J Interprof Care 9(2):131–138

Perera R, Haynes J, Glasziou P et al (2006) Autoinflation for hearing loss associated with otitis media with effusion. Cochrane Database Syst Rev (4):CD006285. Accessed 18 Oct 2006

Peterson NR, Pisoni DB, Miyamoto RT (2010) Cochlear implants and spoken language processing abilities: review and assessment of the literature. Restor Neurol Neurosci 28(2):237–250

Pichichero ME (2004) First-line treatment of acute otitis media. In: Alper C, Bluestone CD (eds) Advanced therapy of otitis media. BC Decker, London, pp 32–38

Pittman AL (2008) Short term word-learning rate in children with normal hearing and children with hearing loss with a limited and extended high frequency bandwidths. J Speech Lang Hear Res 51(3):1785–1797

Plontke SK, Radetzki F, Seiwerth I et al (2014) Individual computer-assisted 3D planning for surgical placement of a new bone conduction hearing device. Otol Neurotol 35(7):1251–1257

Plotkin SR, Stemmer-Rachamimov AO, Barker FG II et al (2009) Hearing improvement after bevacizumab in patients with neurofibromatosis type 2. N Engl J Med 361(4):358–367

Plotkin SR, Halpin C, McKenna MJ et al (2010) Erlotinib for progressive vestibular schwannoma in neurofibromatosis 2 patients. Otol Neurotol 31(7):1135–1143

Powers S (1996) Deaf pupils' achievements in ordinary subjects. J Br Assoc Teachers Deaf 20:111–123

Psarommatis I, Florou V, Fragkos M et al (2011) Reversible auditory brainstem responses screening failures in high risk neonates. Eur Arch Otorhinolaryngol 268(2):189–196

Psarommatis I, Voudouris C, Kapetanakis I et al (2017) Recovery of abnormal ABR in neonates and infants at risk of hearing loss. Int J Otolaryngol Article 5:1–8. https://doi.org/10.1155/2017/7912127

Rahne T, Schilde S, Seiwerth I et al (2016) Mastoid dimensions in children and young adults: consequences for the geometry of transcutaneous bone-conduction implants. Otol Neurotol 37(1):57–61

Rajan GP, Kuthubutheen J, Hedne N et al (2012) The role of preoperative, intratympanic glucocorticoids for hearing preservation in cochlear implantation: a prospective clinical study. Laryngoscope 122(1): 190–195

Ramsden JD, Gordon K, Aschendorff A et al (2012) European bilateral pediatric cochlear implant forum consensus statement. Otol Neurotol 33(4):561–565

Reichmuth K, Embacher AJ, Matulat P et al (2013) Responsive parenting intervention after identification of hearing loss by universal newborn hearing screening: the concept of the Muenster Parental Programme. Int J Pediatr Otorhinolaryngol 77(12):2030–2039

Reinisch JF, Lewin S (2009) Ear reconstruction using a porous polyethylene framework and temporoparietal fascia flap. Facial Plast Surg 25(3):181–189

Riss D, Arnoldner C, Baumgartner WD et al (2014) Indication criteria and outcomes with the Bonebridge transcutaneous   bone-conduction   implant. Laryngoscope 124(12):2802–2806

Robas N (2015) Testing the world's first gene therapy for hearing loss. https://www.actiononhearingloss.org.uk/live-well/our-community/our-blog/first-gene-therapy-for-hearing-loss/. Accessed 28 Aug 2016

Robbins A (2002) How does total communication affect cochlear implant performance in children? Paper presented at the 4th ACFOS International Conference the

impact of scientific advances on the education of deaf children. Paris, Nov 8-10:2002

Rosenfeld RM, Culpepper L, Doyle KJ et al (2004) American Academy of Pediatrics Subcommittee on Otitis Media with Effusion; American Academy of Family Physicians; American Academy of Otolaryngology - Head and Neck Surgery. Clinical practice guideline: Otitis media with effusion. Otolaryngol Head Neck Surg 130(5 Suppl):S95–S118

Rosenkranz S, Abbott P, Reath J et al (2012) Promoting diagnostic accuracy in general practitioner management of otitis media in children: findings from a multimodal, interactive workshop on tympanometry and pneumatic otoscopy. Qual Prim Care 20(4):275–285

Rowland C, Schweigert P (2000) Tangible symbols, tangible outcomes. Augment Altern Commun 16(2):61–78

Ruben RJ (2004) Management of otitis media and otitis media with effusion in the speech-delayed child. In: Alper CM, Bluestone CD, Casselbrandt ML et al (eds) Advanced therapy of otitis media. BC Decker, London, pp 203–206

Rubinstein JT (2004) How cochlear implants encode speech. Curr Opin Otolaryngol Head Neck Surg 12(5):444–448

Rybak LP, Mukherjea D, Jajoo S et al (2012) siRNA-mediated knock-down of NOX3: therapy for hearing loss? Cell Mol Life Sci 69(14):2429–2434

Sagit M, Korkmaz F, Akcadag A et al (2012) Protective effect of thymoquinone against cisplatin-induced ototoxicity. Eur Arch Otorhinolaryngol 270(8):2231–2237

Sampaio AL, Araújo MF, Oliveira CA (2011) New criteria of indication and selection of patients to cochlear implant. Int J Otolaryngol 2011:573968

Sarimski K, Hintermair M, Lang M (2013) Familienorientierte Frühförderung von Kindern mit Behinderung. Ernst Reinhardt Verlag, Munich

Savage J, Waddell A (2012) Tinnitus. BMJ Clin Evid (Online) 2012. pii: 0506

Savage J, Waddell A (2014) Tinnitus. Systematic review 506. BMJ Clinical Evidence. http://clinicalevidence.bmj.com/x/systematic-review/0506/overview.html. Accessed 11 Nov 2016

Scarinci N, Worrall L, Hickson L (2009) The ICF and third-party disability: its application to spouses of older people with hearing impairment. Disabil Rehabil 31(25):2088–2100

Schafer EC, Florence S, Anderson C et al (2014) A critical review of remote-microphone technology for children with normal hearing and auditory differences. J Educ Audiol 20:1–11

Scherer MJ (2017) Enhancing appropriate use of adaptive/assistive technology. In: Budd MA et al (eds) Practical psychology in medical rehabilitation. Springer International, Berlin, pp 353–360

Schick A, Klatte M, Meis M et al (2003) Hören in Schulen. Beiträge zur Psychologischen Akustik. Isensee, Oldenburg, pp 359–377

Schlumberger E, Narbona J, Manrique M (2004) Nonverbal development of children with deafness with and without cochlear implants. Dev Med Child Neurol 46(9):599–606

Shafik AG, Elkabarity RH, Thabet MT et al (2013) Effect of intratympanic dexamethasone administration on cisplatin-induced ototoxicity in adult guinea pigs. Auris Nasus Larynx 40(1):51–60

Shapiro WH, Bradham TS (2012) Cochlear implant programming. Otolaryngol Clin North Am 45(1):111–127

Shargorodsky J, Curhan SG, Curhan GC et al (2010) Change in prevalence of hearing loss in US adolescents. JAMA 304(7):772–778. https://doi.org/10.1001/jama.2010.1124

Sharma M, Purdy SC, Kelly AS (2009) Comorbidity of auditory processing, language, and reading disorders. J Speech Lang Hear Res 52(3):706–722. https://doi.org/10.1044/1092-4388(2008/07-0226)

Sharma R, Bhateja V, Satapathy SC et al (2017) Communication device for differently abled people: a prototype model. In: Satapathy S et al (eds) Proceedings of the International Conference on Data Engineering and Communication Technology. Advances in Intelligent Systems and Computing. Vol 469. Springer, Singapore

Shield B, Conetta R, Dockrell J et al (2015) A survey of acoustic conditions and noise levels in secondary school classrooms in England. J Acoust Soc Am 137(1):177–188. https://doi.org/10.1121/1.4904528

Shin YS, Song SJ, Kang S et al (2012) A novel synthetic compound, 3-amino-3-(4-fluoro-phenyl)-1H-quinoline-2,4-dione, inhibits cisplatin-induced hearing loss by the suppression of reactive oxygen species: in vitro and in vivo study. Neuroscience 232:1–12

Siegert R (2010) Combined reconstruction of congenital auricular atresia and severe microtia. Adv Otorhinolaryngol 68:95–107

Siegert R, Weerda H, Mayer T et al (1996) Hochauflösende computer tomographie fehlgebildeter Mittelohren. Laryngo Rhino Otol 75(4):187–194

Silva C, Amorim AM, Gapo C et al (2015) Complications of ear mold impressions: two case reports. Eur Arch Otorhinolaryngol 272(1):253–255

Skarżyński H, Lorens A (2010) Electric acoustic stimulation in children. In: Van de Heyning P, Kleine Punte A (eds) Cochlear implants and hearing preservation. Adv Otorhinolaryngol 67:135–143

Skarżyński H, Lorens A, D'Haese P et al (2002) Preservation of residual hearing in children and post-lingually deafened adults after cochlear implantation: an initial study. ORL 64(4):247–253

Smart JL, Purdy SC, Kelly AS (2018) Impact of personal frequency modulation systems on behavioral and cortical auditory evoked potential measures of auditory processing and classroom listening in school-aged children with auditory processing disorder. J Am Acad Audiol 29(7):568–586

Smith N, Greinwald J Jr (2011) To tube or not to tube: indications for myringotomy with tube placement. Curr Opin Otolaryngol Head Neck Surg 19(5):363–366

Smith ME, Zou CC, Baker C et al (2017) The repeatability of tests of eustachian tube function in healthy ears. Laryngoscope 127(11):2619–2626. https://doi.org/10.1002/lary.26534

Snik ADF (2017) Auditory implants. Amplification options for conductive and mixed hearing loss; an introduction. (Chapter 2). Blog. http://www.snikimplants.nl/. Accessed 29 Jun 2017

Söderman AC, Knutsson J, Priwin C et al (2016) A randomized study of four different types of tympanostomy ventilation tubes—one-year follow-up. Int J Pediatr Otorhinolaryngol 89:159–163

Sommer H, Schönweiler R (2004) Hörgeräteversorgung bei Atresia auris congenita. In: Weerda H (ed) Chirurgie der Ohrmuschel. Thieme, Stuttgart, pp 253–256

Sorrells-Jones J (1997) The challenge of making it real: interdisciplinary practice in a 'seamless' organisation. Nur Adm Q 21(2):20–30

Spencer LJ, Tomblin JB (2009) Evaluating phonological skills in children with prelingual deafness who use a cochlear Implant. J Deaf Stud Deaf Educ 14(1):1–21

Stacey PC, Fortnum HM, Barton GR et al (2006) Hearing-impaired children in the United Kingdom, I: Auditory performance, communication skills, educational achievements, quality of life, and cochlear implantation. Ear Hear 27(2):161–186

Stachler RJ, Chandrasekhar SS, Archer SM et al (2012) Clinical practice guideline: sudden hearing loss. Otolaryngol Head Neck Surg 146(3):1–35

Staecker H, Praetorius M, Baker K et al (2007) Vestibular hair cell regeneration and restoration of balance function induced by math1 gene transfer. Otol Neurotol 28(2):223–231

Stein A, Engell A, Junghoefer M et al (2015) Inhibition-induced plasticity in tinnitus patients after repetitive exposure to tailor-made notched music. Clin Neurophysiol 126(5):1007–1015

Stelmachowicz PG, Pittman AL, Hoover BM et al (2004) The importance of high frequency audibility in the speech and language development of children with hearing loss. Arch Otolaryngol Head Neck Surg 130(5):556–562

Stenfelt S (2011) Acoustic and physiologic aspects of bone conduction hearing. Adv Otorhinolaryngol 71:10–21

Stern Y, Segal K, Yaniv E (2006) Endoscopic adenoidectomy in children with submucosal cleft palate. Int J Pediatr Otorhinolaryngol 70(11):1871–1874

Strait DL, Parbery-Clark A, O'Connell S et al (2013) Biological impact of preschool music classes on processing speech in noise. Dev Cog Neurosci 6:51–56

Sun H, Huang A, Cao S (2011) Current status and prospects of gene therapy for the inner ear. Hum Gene Ther 22(11):1311–1322. https://doi.org/10.1089/hum.2010.246

Suurmond J (2016) Culturally Competent in Medical Education (C2ME) (2013-2015). Academic Medical

Centre/University of Amsterdam. http://ec.europa.eu/chafea/documents/health/migrants-health-actions/Suurmond%20Janny_C2ME.pdf. Accessed 12 Dec 2016

Sweeny A, Carlson ML, Zuniga MG et al (2015) Impact of perioperative oral steroid use on low-frequency hearing preservation after cochlear implantation. Otol Neurotol 36(9):1480–1485

Szagun G, Stumper B (2012) Age or experience? The influence of age at implantation and social and linguistic environment on language development in children with cochlear implants. J Speech Lang Hear Res 55(6):1640–1654

Tajudeen BA, Waltzman SB, Jethanamest D et al (2010) Speech perception in congenitally deaf children receiving cochlear implants in the first year of life. Otol Neurotol 31(8):1254–1260

Takasaka T, Kawamoto K (1985) Mucociliary dysfunction in experimental otitis media with effusion. Am J Otolaryngol 6(3):232–236

Tass PA, Adamchic I, Freund H-J et al (2012) Counteracting tinnitus by acoustic coordinated reset neuromodulation. Restor Neurol Neurosci 30(2):137–159

Tessier DW, Hefner JL, Newmeyer A (2014) Factors related to psychosocial quality of life for children with cerebral palsy. Int J Pediatr 2014:204386. https://doi.org/10.1155/2014/204386

Thomas M, Thomas MJ (1998) Influence of cultural factors on disability and rehabilitation in developing countries. Paper presented at the 7th European Regional Rehabilitation Conference of Rehabilitation International, Jerusalem, Israel, November 29–December 3, 1998. http://www.dinf.ne.jp/doc/english/asia/resource/apdrj/z13jo0400/z13jo0403.html. Accessed 12 Dec 2016

Truesdale SP (1990) Whole body listening: developing active auditory skills. Lang Speech Hear Serv Sch 21(3):183–184

Turner CW, Gantz BJ, Vidal C et al (2004) Speech recognition in noise for cochlear implant listeners: benefits of residual acoustic hearing. J Acoust Soc Am 115(4):1729–1735

Tweedie DJ, Skilbeck CJ, Wyatt ME et al (2009) Partial adenoidectomy by suction diathermy in children with cleft palate, to avoid velopharyngeal insufficiency. Int J Pediatr Otorhinolaryngol 73(11):1594–1597

UK Legislation (2014) Children and Families Act 2014. http://www.legislation.gov.uk/ukpga/2014/6/contents/enacted/data.htm. Accessed 8 Jul 2017

UK National Screening Committee (2012-13) Report of the 4th cycle of the Newborn Hearing Screening Quality assurance Programme (NHSP QA). http://webarchive.nationalarchives.gov.uk/20150408181648/http://hearing.screening.nhs.uk/siteqareports. Accessed 8 Jul 2017

UNESCO (1994) The Salamanca Statement and Framework for Action on Special Education Needs, Paris: UNESCO. http://www.unesco.org/education/pdf/SALAMA_E.PDF. Accessed 29 Jan 2015

United Nations (2006) United Nations Convention on the rights of persons with disabilities and its optional protocol. UN. http://www.ohchr.org/EN/HRBodies/CRPD/Pages/ConventionRightsPersonsWithDisabilities.aspx. Accessed 29 Jan 2015

Vernon JA (1988) Current use of masking for the relief of tinnitus. In: Kitahara M (ed) Tinnitus: pathophysiology and management. Igaku-Shoin, Tokyo, pp 96–106

Verstraeten N, Zarowski AJ, Somers T et al (2009) Comparison of the audiologic results obtained with the bone-anchored hearing aid attached to the headband, the testband, and to the "snap" abutment. Otol Neurotol 30(1):70–75

Vo ML, Smith TJ, Mital PK et al (2012) Do the eyes really have it? Dynamic allocation of attention when viewing moving faces. J Vis 12(13). https://doi.org/10.1167/12.13.3

von Ilberg CA, Kiefer J, Tillein J et al (1999) Electric-acoustic stimulation of the auditory system: new technology for severe hearing loss. ORL J Otorhinolaryngol Relat Spec 61(6):334–340

Walker EA, Holte L, McCreery RW et al (2015) The influence of hearing aid use on outcomes of children with mild hearing loss. J Speech Lang Hear Res 58(5):1611–1625

Waltzman SB, Scalchunes V, Cohen NL (2000) Performance of multiply handicapped children using cochlear implants. Am J Otol 21(3):329–335

Watkin PM, Baldwin M, Laoide S (1990) Parental suspicion and identification of hearing impairment. Arch Dis Child 65:846–850

Weber PC, Bluestone CD, Perez B (2003) Outcome of hearing and vertigo after surgery for congenital perilymphatic fistula in children. Am J Otolaryngol 24(3):138–142

Weerda H (2004) Chirurgie der Ohrmuschel. Verletzungen, Defekte und Anomalien. Thieme, Stuttgart, pp 105–226

Weerda H (2007) Surgery of the auricle, 2nd edn. Thieme, New York

Welch TR, Huebner KM (1995) The deaf-blind child and you (Module 1). In: Huebner KM et al (eds) Hand in hand. Essentials of communication and orientation and mobility for your students who are deaf-blind, vol 1. AFB Press, New York

Welsh LW, Welsh JJ, Rosen LF et al (2004) Functional impairments due to unilateral deafness. Ann Otol Rhinol Laryngol 113(12):987–993

Western University of Ontario National Centre for Audiology (2014) University of Western Ontario Pediatric Audiological Monitoring Protocol Version 1.0 (UWO PedAMP v1.0). http://www.dslio.com/wp-content/uploads/2014/03/2_UWO_PedAMP_v1.0_for_printing_Revision_2_Dec_11.pdf. Accessed Nov 2016

Wiley S, Jahnke M, Meinzen-Derr J et al (2005) Perceived qualitative benefits of cochlear implants in children with multi-handicaps. Int J Ped Otorhinolaryngol 69(6):791–798

Wiley S, Parnell L, Belhorn T (2016) Promoting early identification and intervention for children who are deaf/hard of hearing, children with vision impairment, and children with deaf-blind conditions. J Early Hear Detect Interv 1(1):26–33

Williams P, Stephens H (2010) The Nuffield Centre dyspraxia programme. In: Williams AL et al (eds) Interventions for speech sound disorders in children. Brookes, Baltimore, MD, pp 159–177

Wilson BS, Dorman MF (2008) Cochlear implants: a remarkable past and a brilliant future. Hear Res 242(1-2):3–21

Wilson K, Ambler M, Hanvey K et al (2016) Cochlear implant assessment and candidacy for children with partial hearing. Cochlear Implants Int 17(Suppl 1):66–69. https://doi.org/10.1080/14670100.2016.1152014

Wimmer W, Gerber N, Guignard J et al (2015) Topographic bone thickness maps for Bonebridge implantations. Eur Arch Otorhinolaryngol 272(7):1651–1658

Wollenberg B, Beltrame M, Schönweiler R et al (2007) Integration des aktiven Mittelohrimplantates in die plastische Ohrmuschelrekonstruktion. HNO 55(5):349–356

World Health Organization (2001) International classification of functioning, disability and health (ICF). WHO, Geneva

World Health Organization (2007) International classification of functioning, disability, and health-children and youth. WHO, Geneva

World Health Organization (2016) Childhood hearing loss: act now, here's how. http://www.who.int/pbd/deafness/world-hearing-day/WHD2016_Brochure_EN_2.pdf. Accessed 23 Mar 2017

Wright BA, Zhang Y (2009) A review of the generalization of auditory learning. Philos Trans R Soc Lond B Biol Sci 364(1515):301–311. https://doi.org/10.1098/rstb.2008.026

Yanbay E, Hickson L, Scarinci N et al (2014) Language outcomes for children with cochlear implants enrolled in different communication programs. Cochlear Implants Int 15(3):121–135. https://doi.org/10.1179/1754762813Y.0000000062

Yegin Y, Celik M, Olgun B et al (2015) Is ventilation tube insertion necessary in children with otitis media with effusion? Otolaryngol Pol 69(6):39–44

Yopp HK, Yopp RH (2000) Supporting phonemic awareness in the classroom. Read Teach 54(2):130–143

Yoshinaga-Itano C (2003) Early intervention after universal neonatal hearing screening: impact on outcomes. Ment Retard Dev Disabil Res Rev 9(4):252–266

Yoshinaga-Itano C, Sedey AL, Coutler DK et al (1998) Language of early and later identified children with hearing loss. Pediatrics 102(5):1161–1171

Yoshinaga-Itano C, DeConde JC, Carpenter K et al (2008) Outcomes of children with mild bilateral hearing loss and unilateral hearing loss. Sem Hear 29(2):196–211

Yoshinaga-Itano C, Baca RL, Sedey AL (2010) Describing the trajectory of language development in the presence of severe to profound hearing loss: a closer look at children with cochlear implants versus hearing aids. Otol Neurotol 31(8):1268–1274

Youm HY, Moon IJ, Kim EY et al (2013) The auditory and speech performance of children with intellectual disability after cochlear implantation. Acta Oto-Layngol 133(1):59–69

Young A, Tattersall H (2007) Universal newborn hearing screening and early identification of deafness: parents' responses to knowing early and their expectations of child communication development. J Deaf Stud Deaf Educ 12(2):209–220

Young AM, Carr G, Hunt R et al (2006) Informed choice and deaf children: underpinning concepts and enduring challenges. J Deaf Stud Deaf Educ 11(3):322–336

Young NM, Rojas C, Deng J et al (2016) Magnetic resonance imaging of cochlear implant recipients. Otol Neurotol 37(6):665–671

Zanetti D, Guida M, Barezzani MG et al (2006) Favorable outcome of cochlear implant in VIIIth nerve deficiency. Otol Neurotol 27(6):815–823

Zeng FG, Rebscher S, Harrison W et al (2008) Cochlear implants: system design, integration, and evaluation. IEEE Rev Biomed Eng 1:115–142

Zernotti ME, Sarasty AB (2015) Active bone conduction prosthesis: Bonebridge. Int Arch Otorhinolaryngol 19(4):343–348

Zhang Z, Li Y, Hu L et al (2012) Cochlear implantation in children with cochlear nerve deficiency: a report of nine cases. Int J Pediatr Otorhinolaryngol 76(8):1188–1195

Zhang M, Malysa C, Huettmeyer F et al (2016) Using the International Classification of functioning model to gain new insight into the impact of cochlear implants on prelingually deafened recipients. J Speech Pathol Ther 1:117. https://doi.org/10.4172/2472-5005.1000117

Zuplan B, Dempsey L (2013) Facilitating emergent literacy skills in children with hearing loss. Deaf Educ Int 15(3):130–148

List of Video Examples, Audio Samples and Related Images

Video = isolated video example

Audio = isolated audio sample

Case Study-Video, Case Study-Audio, Case Study-Image (voice range profile (VRP)) = belong to a case study (isolated case studies without electronical material are not mentioned here but included in the numbering)

Relation for Audio 1.1-1.8: Part 1, Chapter 1, Section 1.6

Audio Sample 1.1 Singing voice is demonstrated by a passage from Pamina's Aria in 'Die Zauberflöte' sung without accompaniment in a studio. Singing voice, original recording

Audio Sample 1.2 Singing voice is demonstrated by a passage from Pamina's Aria in 'Die Zauberflöte' sung without accompaniment in a studio. Singing voice, in a dry room

Audio Sample 1.3 Singing voice is demonstrated by a passage from Pamina's Aria in 'Die Zauberflöte' sung without accompaniment in a studio. Singing voice, in a room with medium reverberation time

Audio Sample 1.4 Singing voice is demonstrated by a passage from Pamina's Aria in 'Die Zauberflöte' sung without accompaniment in a studio. Singing voice, in a wet room with long reverberation time

Audio Sample 1.5 Running speech is demonstrated by the standard text 'Der Nordwind Und Die Sonne' (The North Wind and the Sun) recorded in a studio under the same conditions as the aria passage. Running speech, original recording

Audio Sample 1.6 Running speech is demonstrated by the standard text 'Der Nordwind Und Die Sonne' (The North Wind and the Sun) recorded in a studio under the same conditions as the aria passage. Running speech, in a dry room

Audio Sample 1.7 Running speech is demonstrated by the standard text 'Der Nordwind Und Die Sonne' (The North Wind and the Sun) recorded in a studio under the same conditions as the aria passage. Running speech, in a room with medium reverberation time

Audio Sample 1.8 Running speech is demonstrated by the standard text 'Der Nordwind Und Die Sonne' (The North Wind and the Sun) recorded in a studio under the same conditions as the aria passage. Running speech, in a wet room with long reverberation time

Relation for Video 1.1 and 1.2 and Audio 1.9 and 1.10: Part 1, Chapter 1, Section 1.12

Audio Sample 1.9 Synthesised speech (German), "Hallo, wie geht es dir?"

Audio Sample 1.10 Synthesised speech (German), "Lea und Doreen mögen Bananen"

Video 1.1 Two examples demonstrating articulatory movements of the vocal tract when singing. Synthesised vocal tract articulation. Round "Dona nobis pacem", sung by bass and tenor

Video 1.2 Two examples demonstrating articulatory movements of the vocal tract when singing. Synthesised vocal tract articulation. "Salvete", voice and orchestral accompaniment

A. am Zehnhoff-Dinnesen et al. (eds.), *Phoniatrics I*, European Manual of Medicine, https://doi.org/10.1007/978-3-662-46780-0

Relation for Case Study Video etc 4.1-4.6: Part 2, Chapter 4, Section 4.4

Case Study Video 4.1 Breathy voice

Case Study Audio Sample 4.1 Breathy voice

Case Study Image 4.1 Voice range profile breathy voice

Case Study Video 4.2 Normal male voice

Case Study Audio Sample 4.2 Normal male voice

Case Study Image 4.2 Voice range profile normal male voice

Case Study Video 4.3 Normal female voice

Case Study Audio Sample 4.3 Normal female voice

Case Study Image 4.3 Voice range profile normal female voice

Case Study Video 4.4 Rough male voice

Case Study Audio Sample 4.4 Rough male voice

Case Study Image 4.4 Voice range profile rough male voice

Case Study Video 4.5 Ventricular fold voice woman

Case Study Audio Sample 4.5 Ventricular fold voice woman

Case Study Image 4.5 Voice range profile ventricular fold voice woman

Case Study Video 4.6 Distortion of vocal fold vibration by adducting the ventricular folds

Case Study Audio Sample 4.6 Vocal sound Louis Armstrong

Relation for Case Study Video etc 5.1 and 5.2: Part 2, Chapter 5, Section 5.1

Case Study Video 5.1 Hypofunction

Case Study Audio Sample 5.1 Hypofunction

Case Study Image 5.1 Voice range profile hypofunction

Case Study Video 5.2 Hyperfunction

Case Study Audio Sample 5.2 Hyperfunction

Case Study Image 5.2 Voice range profile hyperfunction

Relation for Case Study Video etc 5.3 and 5.4: Part 2, Chapter 5, Section 5.2

Case Study Video 5.3 Marginal oedema due to occupational vocal load

Case Study Audio Sample 5.3 Marginal oedema due to occupational vocal load

Case Study Image 5.3 Marginal oedema due to occupational vocal load

Case Study Video 5.4 Vocal fold nodules due to occupational vocal load

Case Study Audio Sample 5.4 Vocal fold nodules due to occupational vocal load

Case Study Image 5.4 Vocal fold nodules due to occupational vocal load

Relation for Case Study Video etc 5.5-5.8: Part 2, Chapter 5, Section 5.3

Case Study Video 5.5 Female pop singer nodules

Case Study Audio Sample 5.5 Female pop singer nodules (**a**) spoken language

Case Study Audio Sample 5.5 Female pop singer nodules (**b**) singing voice

Case Study Image 5.5 Voice range profile female pop singer nodules

Case Study Video 5.6 Male pop singer oedema

Case Study Audio Sample 5.6 Male pop singer oedema (**a**) spoken language

Case Study Audio Sample 5.6 Male pop singer oedema (**b**) singing voice

Case Study Image 5.6 Voice range profile male pop singer oedema

Case Study Video 5.7 Female singer soprano oedema

Case Study Audio Sample 5.7 Female singer soprano oedema (**a**) spoken language

Case Study Audio Sample 5.7 Female singer soprano oedema (**b**) singing voice

Case Study Image 5.7 Voice range profile female singer soprano oedema

Case Study Video 5.8 Male singer baritone inflammation

Case Study Audio Sample 5.8 Male singer baritone inflammation (**a**) spoken language

Case Study Audio Sample 5.8 Male singer baritone inflammation (**b**) singing voice

Case Study Image 5.8 Voice range profile male singer baritone inflammation

Relation for Case Study Video etc 5.9-5.16: Part 2, Chapter 5, Section 5.4

Case Study Video 5.9 Polyp

Case Study Audio Sample 5.9 Polyp

Index

© Springer-Verlag GmbH Germany, part of Springer Nature 2020
A. am Zehnhoff-Dinnesen et al. (eds.), *Phoniatrics I*, European Manual of Medicine,
https://doi.org/10.1007/978-3-662-46780-0